Case-Based Textbook of Echocardiography

Anita Sadeghpour • Azin Alizadehasl
Editors

Case-Based Textbook of Echocardiography

Springer

Editors
Anita Sadeghpour, MD, FACC, FASE
Rajaie Cardiovascular, Medical and Research Center, Echocardiography Research Center
Iran University of Medical Sciences
Tehran
Iran

Azin Alizadehasl, MD, FACC, FASE
Rajaie Cardiovascular, Medical and Research Center, Echocardiography Research Center
Iran University of Medical Sciences
Tehran
Iran

ISBN 978-3-030-09808-7 ISBN 978-3-319-67691-3 (eBook)
https://doi.org/10.1007/978-3-319-67691-3

This Springer imprint is published by Springer Nature, under the registered company Springer International Publishing AG
The registered company address is: Gewerbestrasse 11, 6330 Cham, Switzerland

Preface

Echocardiography is the most frequently used imaging modality for the evaluation of all cardiovascular diseases in that it can provide precise information regarding the heart's structure, function, and hemodynamic abnormalities. However, it requires a high level of knowledge, capability, and expertise in ultrasound physics, anatomy, physiology, and also clinical cardiology, and it also requires one to carry out a substantial number of echocardiography studies in order to attain and maintain the practice skills.

For all the excellent textbooks and reviews on echocardiography, we felt the need for a step-by-step educational textbook covering basic to advanced echocardiography besides focusing on practical points in real cases and latest published guidelines.

It is noteworthy to mention that each chapter can serve as an overview for introduction to the subject and subsequently as a concise review of echocardiography, and questions at the end of each chapter will provide a useful method of self-assessment.

We hope that this book will be an ideal companion to all cardiovascular imagers and cardiologists by covering all that is required in echocardiography training. The compilation of this book would not have become possible without the contributions of our indefatigable expert editors, who wrote their respective chapters. Needless to say, our work comes with its shortcomings and we look forward to addressing them with the aid of your valuable comments.

Tehran, Iran — Anita Sadeghpour
Tehran, Iran — Azin Alizadehasl

Acknowledgments

We dedicate this book to our mentors, patients, and dear families. Numerous individuals have made invaluable contributions to the compilation of *Case-Based Textbook of Echocardiography*, particularly our expert contributors, who wrote their respective chapters and shared their experiences and cases from around the world.

Many other individuals have also contributed directly and indirectly to the conclusion of this volume with their extensive experience in various fields, and we hereby especially appreciate the efforts of our colleagues in Rajaie Cardiovascular Medical and Research Center including Marzieh Pakbaz, Farshad Amouzadeh, Mahdieh Azimi, Shahnaz Sheikh, and Solmaz Jafari.

Finally, we give special recognition to the publisher, Springer, for its unwavering moral and technical support and inspiration throughout the project. Our friends at Springer, not least Grant Weston, Evanjalin Hephsibah, and Ramamoorthy Jeyashree, deserve considerable appreciation for their kindness and helpfulness in accommodating our numerous requests.

Contents

Abbreviations

2D	Two-dimensional
2DE	Two-dimensional echocardiography
3D	Three-dimensional
3DE	Three-dimensional echocardiography
4C	Four chamber
A	Peak velocity of the mitral (or tricuspid) valve atrial wave inflow (cm/s)
A.Ao	Ascending aorta
A′	TDI of the mitral annulus
a′	Peak velocity of the mitral (or tricuspid) annulus atrial phase motion (cm/s)
AA	Ascending aorta
ACC	American College of Cardiology
ACCF	Appropriateness criteria of the American College Of Cardiology Foundation
AF	Atrial fibrillation
AHA	American Heart Association
AIDS	Acquired immune deficiency syndrome
AL PM	Anterolateral papillary muscle
ALC	Anterolateral commissure
AMI	Acute myocardial infarction
AML	Anterior mitral leaflet
AO	Aorta
AoV	Aortic valve
AP2	Apical 2-chamber
AP3	Apical 3-chamber
AP4	Apical 4-chamber
APS	Antiphospholipid syndrome
AR	Pulmonary valve atrial reversal
ARVD/C	Arrhythmogenic right ventricular dysplasia/cardiomyopathy
AS	Aortic stenosis
ASA	American Society of Anesthesiologists
ASC	Ascending
ASD	Atrial septal defect
ASE	American Society of Echocardiography
ASH	Asymmetric septal hypertrophy
AT	Acceleration time
ATMV	Accessory tissue mitral valve
ATRAMI	Autonomic tone and reflexes after myocardial infarction
AUC	Appropriate use criteria
AV	Aortic valve
AVA	Aortic valve area
AVF	Arteriovenous fistula
AVR	Aortic valve replacement
AVSD	AV septal defect

AZ	Azygos
BAAT	Biatrial anastomosis technique
BBB	Bundle branch block
BCAT	Bicaval anastomosis technique
BIS	Bispectral index
BMI	Body mass index
BMPR2	Bone morphogenetic protein receptor type 2
BP	Blood pressure
BSA	Body surface area
CABG	Coronary artery bypass graft surgery
CAD	Coronary artery disease
CATs	Calcified amorphous tumors
CAV	Cardiac allograft vasculopathy
CCTGA	Congenitally corrected transposition of the great arteries
CE	Cardiac echinococcosis
CFI	Color flow imaging
CFR	Coronary flow reserve
CFVR	Coronary flow velocity reserve
CHD	Congenital heart disease
CHFpEF	CHF with preserved EF
CHFrEF	CHF with reduced EF
CMR	Cardiac magnetic resonance
CO	Cardiac output
COA	Coarctation
CP	Constrictive pericarditis
CPR	Cardiopulmonary resuscitation
CRP	C-reactive protein
CRT	Cardiac resynchronization therapy
CS	Coronary sinus
CSA	Cross-sectional area
CT	Computed tomography
CTED	Chronic thromboembolic disease
CTEPH	Chronic thromboembolic pulmonary hypertension
CV	Cardiovascular
CW	Continuous wave
CX	Circumflex branch of the left coronary artery
D	Diameter
DA	Ductus arteriosus
DC	Direct cardioversion
DCM	Dilated cardiomyopathy
DD	Diastolic dysfunction
DF	Diastolic function
DILV	Double inlet left ventricle
DORV	Double outlet right ventricle
DPG	Diastolic pressure gradient
DSE	Dobutamine stress echocardiography
DT	Doppler tissue
DT	Deceleration time
d-TGA	Complete transposition of the great arteries
DTI	Doppler tissue imaging
DVI	Doppler velocity index
DVT	Deep venous thrombosis
E	Peak E-wave velocity of the mitral valve (cm/s)

E′	Tissue Doppler index of the mitral valve annulus
E/A	Ratio of early to atrial inflow velocity (respectively mitral or tricuspid)
E/e′	Ratio of early inflow velocity to early annulus velocity (respectively mitral or tricuspid)
E′	TDI of the mitral annulus
e′	Peak velocity of the mitral (or tricuspid) annulus early phase motion (cm/s)
e′/a′	Ratio of early to atrial phase of annulus velocity (respectively mitral or tricuspid)
EACVI	European Association of Cardiovascular Imaging
EAT	Epicardial adipose tissue
EBD	Endocardial border delineation
ECG	Electrocardiogram
EDV	End-diastolic volume
EF	Ejection fraction
EI	Eccentricity index
EKG	Electrocardiogram
EOA	Effective orifice area
ERO	Effective regurgitant orifice
EROA	Effective regurgitant orifice area
ESRD	End-stage renal disease
ESV	End-systolic volume
ET	Ejection time
FA	Femoral artery
FAC	Fractional area change
FC	Functional class
FDA	Food and Drug Administration
FED	Fibroelastic deficiency
FMR	Functional mitral regurgitation
FPS	Frame per second
FV	Femoral vein
GCS	Global circumferential strain
GLS	Global longitudinal strain
HAPE	High altitude pulmonary edema
HbA1C	Glycosylated hemoglobin
HCM	Hypertrophic cardiomyopathy
HF	Heart failure
HHD	Hypertensive heart disease
HIV	Human immunodeficiency virus
HOCM	Hypertrophic obstructive cardiomyopathy
HPRF	High pulse repetition frequency
HR	Heart rate
HT	Heart transplantation
HTN	Hypertension
HU	Hunsfiel unit
HV	Hepatic vein
HVR	High volume rate
I	Inversus
IAS	Inter-atrial septum
ICA	Internal carotid artery
ICD	Implantable cardioverter defibrillators
ICU	Intensive care unit
Idiopathic RCM	Idiopathic restrictive cardiomyopathy
IE	Infective endocarditis

I-I	Inner edge–to–inner edge
IL1; 6;16	Interleukin 1, 6;16
IMH	Intramural hematoma
IMT	Intima-media thickness
INR	International normalized ratio
IV	Intravenous
IVA	Isovolumic acceleration
IVC	Inferior vena cava
IVCT	Isovolumic contraction time
IVG	Intraventricular gradients
IVRT	Isovolumic relaxation time
IVS	Interventricular septum
IVUS	Intravascular ultrasound
JNC	Joint national committee
LA	Left atrium
LAA	Left atrial appendage
LAP	Left atrial pressure
LAPV	Left upper pulmonary vein
LAV	Left atrial volume
LAVI	Left atrial volume index
LAX	Long axis
LCA	Left coronary artery
LCC	Left coronary cusp
LDL	Low density lipoprotein
LE	Lower esophageal
LGE	Late gadolinium enhancement
LGE/CMR	Late gadolinium enhancement/cardiovascular magnetic resonance
LHC	Left-sided heart catheterization
LHD	Left heart disease
L-L	Leading edge–to–leading edge
LLPV	Left lower pulmonary vein
LMCA	Left main coronary artery
LPA	Left pulmonary artery
LSCA	Left subclavian artery
LUPV	Left upper pulmonary vein
LV	Left ventricular
LV/LA	Left ventricular/left atrial
LVAD	Left ventricular assist device
LVED	Left ventricular end-diastolic
LVEDD	Left ventricular end-diastolic dimension
LVEDP	Left ventricular end-diastolic pressure
LVEF	Left ventricular ejection fraction
LVES	Left ventricular end-systolic
LVESD	Left ventricular end-systolic dimension
LVH	Left ventricular hypertrophy
LVIDd	Left ventricular internal diameter
LVM	Left ventricular mass
LVNC	Left ventricular non-compaction
LVO	Left ventricular opacification
LVOT	Left ventricular outflow tract
LVOT VTI	LVOT subvalvular velocity time integral
MAC	Mitral annulus calcification
MADIT-II	Multicenter automatic defibrillator implantation trial II

MB	Moderator band
MBF	Myocardial blood flow
MCE	Myocardial contrast echocardiography
MCSs	Mechanical circulatory supports
MDCT	Multidetector computed tomography
ME	Mid-esophageal
MHz	Megahertz
MI	Myocardial infarction
M-mode	Motion mode
MPA	Main pulmonary artery
MPAP	Mean pulmonary artery pressure
MPG	Mean pressure gradient
MPI	Myocardial performance index
MPR	Multiplanar reconstruction
MR	Mitral regurgitation
MRI	Magnetic resonance imaging
MS	Mitral stenosis
MTHFR	Methylene tetrahydrofolate reductase
MV	Mitral valve
MVA	Mitral valve area
MVLs	Mitral valve leaflets
MVP	Mitral valve prolapse
MVR	Mitral valve replacement
MVs	Myxomatous valves
NAFLD	Nonalcoholic fatty liver disease
NCC	Noncoronary cusp
NSAID	Nonsteroidal anti-inflammatory drug
NSVT	Nonsustained ventricular tachycardia
NYHA	New York Heart Association
OHT	Orthotopic heart transplantation
P	Posterior
PA	Pulmonary artery
PADP	Pulmonary artery diastolic pressure
PAEDP	Pulmonary artery end-diastolic pressure
PAH	Pulmonary artery hypertension
PAP	Pulmonary arterial pressure
PAPVC	Partial anomalous pulmonary venous connection
PASP	Pulmonary artery systolic pressure
PAT	Pericardial adipose tissue
PCWP	Pulmonary capillary wedge pressure
PDA	Patent ductus arteriosus
PE	Pulmonary embolus
PET	Positron emission tomography
PFO	Patent foramen ovale
PFT	Pulmonary function test
PH	Pulmonary hypertension
PISA	Proximal isovelocity surface area
PLAX	Parasternal long axis
PM	Papillary muscle
PM PM	Posteromedial papillary muscle
PMC	Posteromedial commissure
POCUS	Point of care ultrasound
PO-TEE	Perioperative transesophageal echocardiography

PPM	Prosthesis–Patient mismatch
PR	Pulmonary regurgitation
PREDV	Pulmonary regurgitation end-diastolic velocity
PRF	Pulse repetition frequency
PSAX	Parasternal short axis
PSID	Pocket size imaging device
PSLAX	Parasternal long axis
PTE	Pulmonary thromboembolism
PTMC	Percutaneous transvenous mitral commissurotomy
PV	Pulmonic valve
PV AR	Pulmonary valve atrial reversal
PVd(D)	Diastolic component of the pulmonary vein
PVR	Pulmonary vascular resistance
PVs	Pulmonary veins
PVs1	First systolic component of the pulmonary vein
PVs2	Second systolic component of the pulmonary vein
PVT	Prosthetic valve thrombosis
PW	Pulsed wave
PW	Posterior wall
QT	QT interval in ECG
RA	Rheumatoid arteritis
RA	Right atrium/right atrial
RAA	Right atrial appendage
RAP	Right atrial pressure
RCA	Right coronary artery
RCC	Right coronary cusp
RCM	Cardiomyopathies, restrictive cardiomyopathy
RF	Regurgitant fraction
RH	Right heart
RHC	Right heart catheterization
RIMP	Right ventricular index of myocardial performance
RLPV	Right lower pulmonary vein
ROI	Region of interest
RPA	Right pulmonary artery
RUPV	Right upper pulmonary vein
RV	Right ventricle
RV	Regurgitant volume
RV S’	Tissue Doppler index of the tricuspid valve annulus
RVFAC	Right ventricular fractional area change
Rvol	Regurgitant volume
RVOT	Right ventricular outflow tract
RVOT VTI	RVOT subvalvular velocity time integral
RVSP	Right ventricular systolic pressure
RWM	Regional wall motion
RWMA	Regional wall motion abnormalities
RWT	Relative wall thickness
S	Solitus
SAM	Systolic anterior motion
SAX	Short axis
SCD	Sudden cardiac death
SCD-HeFT	Sudden cardiac death in heart failure trial
SE	Stress echocardiography
SLE	Systemic lupus erythematosus
SPAP	Systolic pulmonary artery pressure

SR	Strain rate
STE	Speckle-tracking echocardiography
STEMI	ST-segment myocardial infarction
STJ	Sinotubular junction
SV	Stroke volume
SVC	Superior vena cava
TA	Tricuspid atresia
TAPSE	Tricuspid annular plane systolic excursion
TAPVC	Total anomalous pulmonary venous connection
TAR	Traumatic aortic rupture
TAVI	Transcatheter aortic valve implantation
TAVR	Transcatheter aortic valve replacement
TB	Tuberous sclerosis
TCO	Tricuspid valve opening time
TCO	Tricuspid closure-opening time
TDI	Tissue Doppler imaging
TEE	Transesophageal echocardiography
TFC	Task force criteria
TGA	Transposition of the great arteries
TNF α	Tumor necrosis factor A
TR	Tricuspid regurgitation
TRV	Tricuspid regurgitation velocity
TS	Tricuspid stenosis
TTE	Transthoracic echocardiography
TTR	Transthyretin
TV	Tricuspid valve
TVI	Time velocity integral
TVLs	Tricuspid valve leaflets
UCA	Ultrasound contrast agent
V	Vertebra
V/Q	Ventilation–perfusion
VA	Ventriculo-arterial
VADs	Ventricular assist devices
VC	Vena contracta
VHD	Valvular heart disease
Vp	Velocity propagation
VSD	Ventricular septal defect
VTI	Velocity time integral
WMSI	Wall motion score index

1 Basic Principles of Echocardiography

Anita Sadeghpour and Azin Alizadehasl

Abstract

Echocardiography which is the most commonly used noninvasive cardiac imaging modality is called ultrasonography of the heart. It provides real-time images from the heart and gives comprehensive information regarding the cardiac structure, function and the hemodynamic at a relatively inexpensive cost. Echocardiography uses harmless ultrasound waves (1–10 MHz) to visualize the heart.

This book is a practical echocardiography book; nonetheless, sonographers and clinicians should be familiar with the basic physics of ultrasound to obtain better images and avoid artifacts. In this chapter we tried to point out some useful data regarding ultrasound Physics, transducer Types, Echocardiography Modes, Tissue Harmonic Imaging, Principles of Doppler Echocardiography and Doppler-Based Hemodynamic Assessment.

Keywords

Echocardiography · Ultrasonography · Transducer Doppler · Tissue harmonic imaging · Artifact

Abbreviations

CFI	Color flow imaging
CSA	Cross-sectional area
CW	Continuous wave
D	Diameter
HPRF	High pulse repetition frequency
LV	Left ventricular
LVOT	Left ventricular outflow tract
PRF	Pulse repetition frequency
PW	Pulsed wave
SV	Stroke volume
TEE	Transesophageal echocardiography
TTE	Transthoracic echocardiography
Vp	Velocity propagation
VTI	Velocity time integral

A. Sadeghpour, MD, FACC, FASE
Professor of Cardiology, Echocardiography Research Center, Rajaie Cardiovascular Medical and Research Center, Iran University of Medical Science, Tehran, Iran

A. Alizadehasl, MD, FACC, FASE (✉)
Associate Professor of Cardiology, Echocardiologist, Echocardiography and Cardiogenetic Research Centers, Cardio-Oncology Department, Rajaie Cardiovascular Medical and Research Center, Tehran, Iran

Definition and General Principles in Echocardiography

- Echocardiography is ultrasonography of the heart. It is the most commonly used noninvasive cardiac imaging modality (Fig. 1.1).
- Echocardiography is unique for the following reasons:

1. It provides real-time images from the heart.
2. Images can be obtained quickly with the least patient discomfort.
3. It is designed to be portable and used as a bedside imaging modality.
4. It gives comprehensive information regarding the cardiac structure and function and the hemodynamic flow at a relatively inexpensive cost.

History

- First record of heart movement captured by using ultrasound was reported by Edler and Hertz in 1954 [1, 2].
- 2D echocardiography was developed in the mid 1970s. It quickly established itself as a very useful tool for imaging the morphology and function of the heart.

A. Sadeghpour, A. Alizadehasl (eds.), *Case-Based Textbook of Echocardiography*, https://doi.org/10.1007/978-3-319-67691-3_1

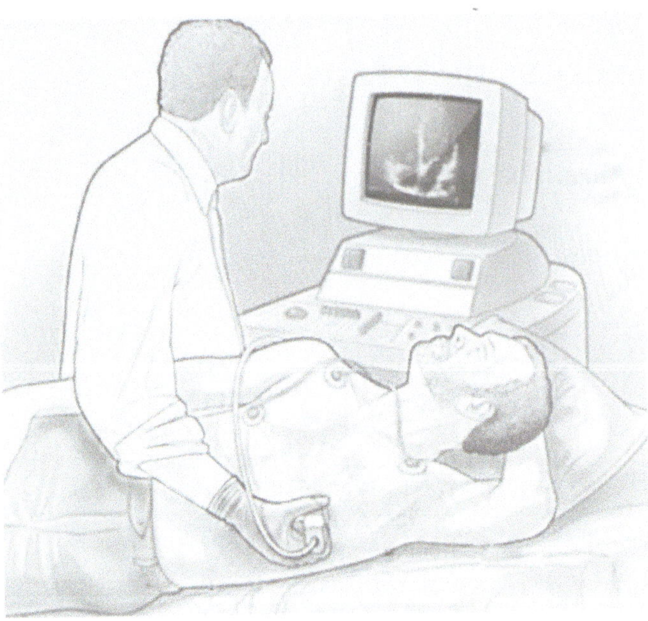

Fig. 1.1 Bedside transthoracic echocardiography on a patient in the left lateral decubitus position

- 2D echocardiography was followed by the development of Doppler and color Doppler in 1980.
- Although the concept of transesophageal echocardiography (TEE) dates backs to 1970s, the common practice of TEE began in 1987 [3, 4].

Ultrasound Physics

- 2D echocardiography images are produced by the reflection of ultrasound waves from the cardiac structure.
- Standard transthoracic echocardiography (TTE) comprises M-Mode, 2D, and all spectral Doppler study, which encompasses continuous wave (CW), pulsed wave (PW), color Doppler, and tissue Doppler imaging (Fig. 1.2).
- TTE can be complemented by 3D echocardiography, TEE, and stress echocardiography.
- In all types of echocardiography, image acquisition and interpretation is operator-dependent and needs considerable training and skill.

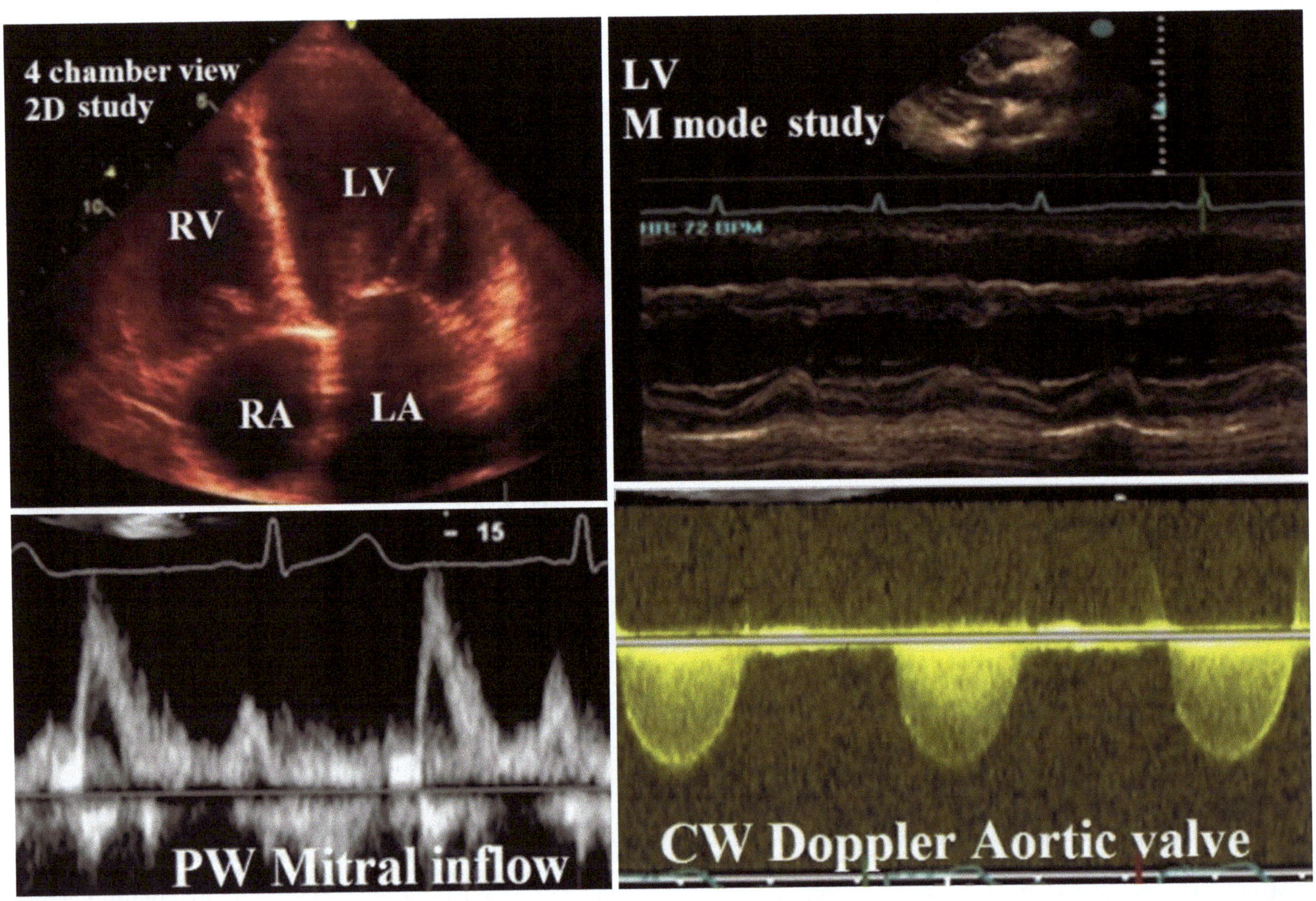

Fig. 1.2 Transthoracic echocardiography (TTE), showing 2D study (left upper), M-mode study (right upper), PW Doppler study (left lower), and CW Doppler study (right lower). *PW*, pulsed wave; *CW* continuous wave

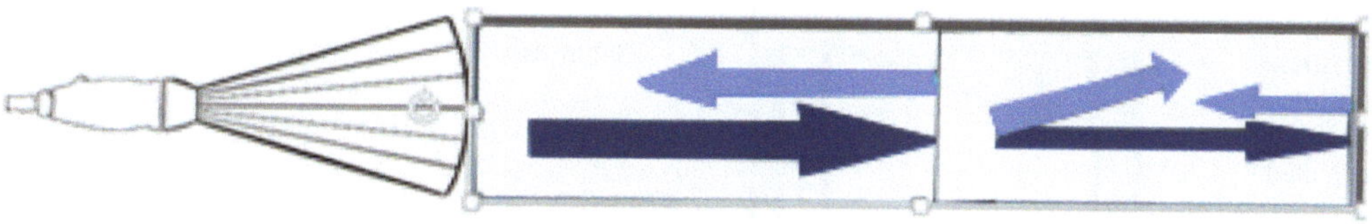

Fig. 1.3 Left: Ultrasound waves can be directed and focused in a beam. Right: The beam has the characteristics of refraction and reflection, which constitute the basics of image production

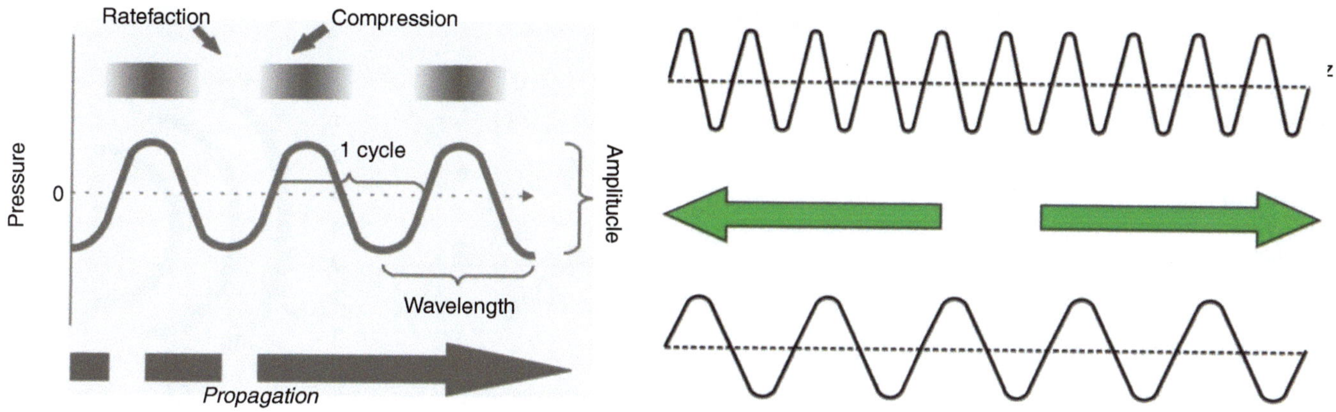

Fig. 1.4 Ultrasound waves are series of sine waves with compression and rarefaction or peaks and troughs

Ultrasound Physics

- Ultrasound uses sound waves with much higher frequencies than the human hearing range. (Humans can hear sounds at 20–20,000 Hz.)
- Cardiac ultrasound uses harmless ultrasound waves (1–10 MHz) to visualize the heart.
- Advantage of ultrasound waves in terms of imaging modality is that these waves can be directed and focused in a beam and when this beam passes through a medium and encounters structures with different acoustic properties, it manifests the characteristics of refraction and reflection (Fig. 1.3).
- However, there is a major disadvantage to the ultrasound beam: It is poorly transmitted through air.
- As ultrasound waves propagate, they attenuate. The greater the acoustic mismatch, the more the energy reflected rather than transmitted.
- Sound waves are produced by mechanical vibration and are graphically depicted as a sine wave with peaks and troughs or compression and rarefaction (Fig. 1.4).

This book is a practical echocardiography book; nonetheless, sonographers and clinicians should be familiar with the basic physics of ultrasound to obtain better images and avoid artifacts. Some basic parameters and definitions are provided below.

Ultrasound waves: Series of sine waves with peaks and troughs, denoting compression and rarefaction areas.

Cycle: Sum of 1 compression and 1 rarefaction.

Wavelength (λ): Distance between 2 similar points or 1 complete cycle.

Frequency: Number of wavelengths per unit of time, measured in hertz (number of cycles per second).

Velocity: Speed of the sound wave in a medium. The ultrasound velocity in soft tissue is 1540 m/s.

- Frequency has an inverse relation with wavelength based on the following equation:

$$\text{velocity of the sound wave}(\mathrm{V}) = \text{frequency}(f) \times \text{wavelength}(\lambda)$$

$$\mathrm{V} = f \times \lambda$$

- Ultrasound travels in the soft tissue at a relatively constant velocity (at about 1540 m/s [1.54 m/ms]); consequently, the wavelength of a 3.0-MHz (3,000,000 cycles/s) transducer would be $\lambda = V/f$. (1.54 divided by 3 is about 0.51 mm.)
- This equation is important since a transducer with a higher frequency provides a shorter wavelength and consequently better resolution, but shallower penetration.
- Transducer frequency can be changed by a thin or thick chest wall. The common frequency of the transducer for adults is 2 to 3 MHz to 5 MHz in a thin chest wall and 5 to 7.5 MHz for pediatrics and 3.5 to 7 MHz for TEE probes.

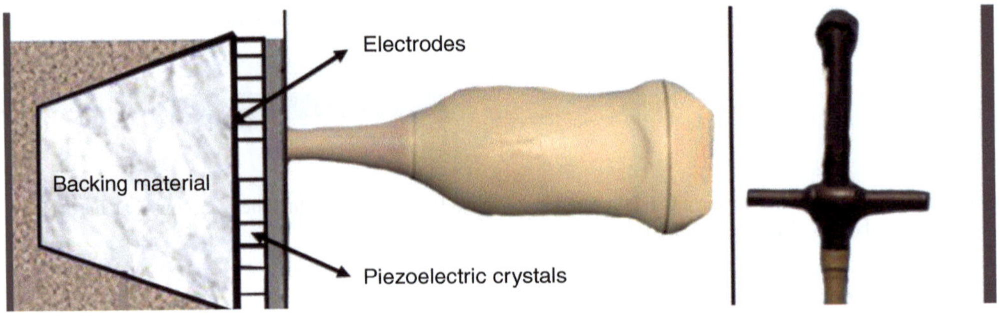

Fig. 1.5 Left: Internal component of an ultrasound transducer. Middle: Adult transducer, Right: Non imaging Doppler dedicated probe

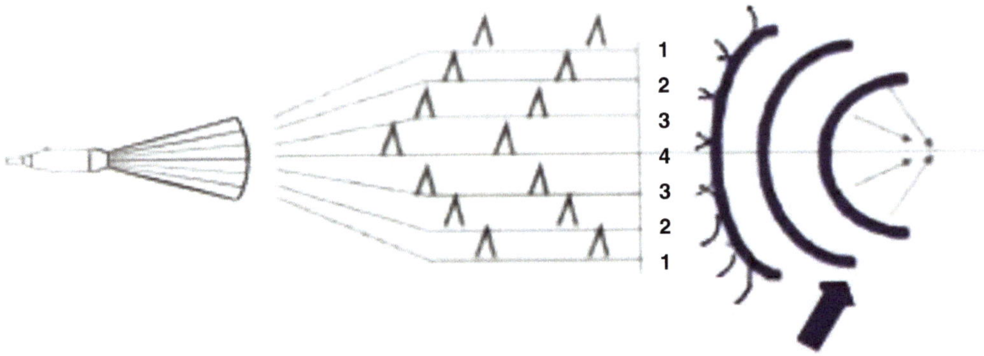

Fig. 1.6 Phased-array transducers, consisting of a series of piezoelectric crystals. Electrical steering and focusing is done by adjusting the timing of excitation

Transducers

- Transducers are devices that can convert 1 form of energy to another form.
- Curvilinear probes with their small footprints are the most suitable probes for echocardiography.
- Fundamental components of transducers are piezoelectric crystals, which are carefully arranged and interconnected. Indeed, had it not been for the development of piezoelectric crystals, imaging by ultrasound would not have become possible (Fig. 1.5).
- Piezoelectric crystals have the capability of vibrating during alternating electrical currents, which means that electrical signals are transformed to ultrasound waves.
- This transformation occurs oppositely. In other words, as piezoelectric crystals receive reflected sound energy, they transform the sound wave (as mechanical energy) to electric impulses and finally generate images [3–5].
- For clinical implications, the ultrasound beam should be focused and steered either mechanically or electronically.
- In the modern era, almost all transducers are phased-array transducers, consisting of a series of piezoelectric crystals. Electrical steering is done by adjusting the timing of excitation (Fig. 1.6).
- Gel is used on the transducer to facilitate the transmission of ultrasound from the transducer to the skin and the heart as ultrasound cannot pass the bone and air.
- Ability to distinguish small objects separately and in close proximity is called "resolution". Resolution is categorized as spatial, temporal, and contrast.
- Spatial resolution denotes the smallest distance between 2 objects that can be separately differentiated. It is dependent on the wavelength. (Resolution is about half of the wavelength.) In a transducer with a 2.5-MHz frequency, the spatial resolution is about 0.3 mm.
- Contrast resolution refers to the ability to distinguish different shades of the gray scale in an image.
- Temporal resolution or the frame rate means the ability to track a moving object over time.
- Transducer design has an important role in optimal image acquisition. The transducer should be small to be placed between the ribs.

Echocardiography Modes

Ultrasound creates an image by sending pulses and then receiving them. Since the velocity of sound is known, the time and consequently the distance between the transducer and the image are calculated and the received data are traditionally displayed as A mode (amplitude mode), B mode (brightness), and M mode (motion). Indeed, 2D echocardiographic shows the structure and function of the heart and Doppler echocardiography is the mainstay of cardiovascular hemodynamic assessment.

2D Echocardiography

By placing the transducer on the chest, between the ribs, the phased array transducer sends the ultrasound beam. The beam is constructed from multiple scan lines and can be focused and steered electronically. It creates a fan-shaped sector (Fig. 1.7).

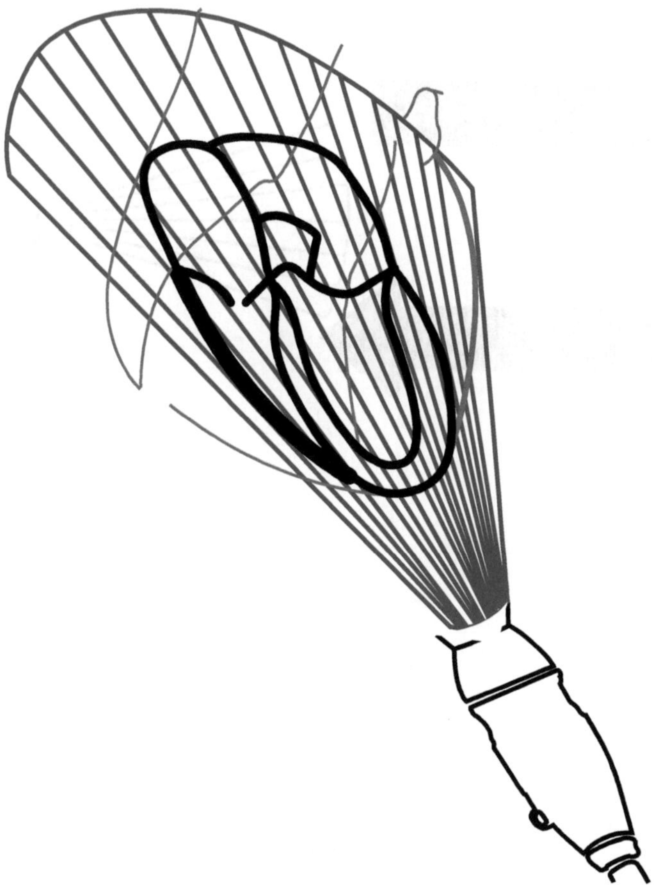

Fig. 1.7 A fan-shaped beam, constructed from multiple scan lines

Given the heart's motion, 25 images per second is the minimum number of images needed to obtain a good image quality.

Limitation of 2D Study

- Obtaining good image quality in TTE needs optimal patient window. Sometimes image quality is suboptimal because of small acoustic windows, obesity, and hyperinflated lungs in chronic lung disease and in early postoperative cardiothoracic surgery.
- Image quality decreases in 2D imaging due to attenuation. Attenuation denotes a decrease in the intensity of the ultrasound wave as the beam travels in the tissue. It is caused by absorption, refraction, and reflection.
- However, there are a few buttons in the setting which help to optimize 2D images. The buttons enable the operator to alter the gain, time gain compensation depth, sector width, and focus.
- 2D echocardiography can provide not only real-time high-resolution images of the heart but also a framework for M-mode, Doppler, and color flow imaging (CFI).

Tissue Harmonic Imaging

- Tissue harmonic imaging is an echocardiography mode that can significantly augment image quality.
- Most recent transducers have the capability of tissue harmonic imaging by using the resonance feature of the tissue.
- It means that the tissue vibrates in harmonic frequencies when it receives a specific frequency. Therefore, by sending the ultrasound waves in a wide bandwidth, the tissue vibrates at multiple frequencies ($2F$, $3F$, $4F$, etc.) of the transmitted frequency. The received frequency is higher than the fundamental frequency, which enhances the signal-to-noise ratio and decreases artifacts (Fig. 1.8) [4, 8].

M-Mode Echocardiography

- M-mode echocardiography is a relatively old echocardiography mode and is still a part of standard echocardiography.
- In M-mode echocardiography, a single scan line is sent from the transducer to the moving heart and yields a repetitive 1D image on the y-axis and time on the x-axis (Fig. 1.9).
- High temporal resolution (at least 1000 lines per second in comparison to 25 images per second in 2D study) is a unique feature of the M-mode study and records detailed motions heart movements.
- 2D–guided M-mode study is derived by placing a cursor through the heart structure.
- M-mode is used for the measurement of the left ventricular (LV) size, LV hypertrophy, and LV mass. Also, it can display subtle heart structure motions in specific cardiac diseases (Fig. 1.10) [3, 4, 6].

Principles of Doppler Echocardiography

- In 1842, Christian Doppler discovered "the Doppler effect", which constitutes the cornerstone of Doppler echocardiography and the backbone of cardiovascular hemodynamic study.
- Principle of the Doppler effect is based on the decrease or increase in the frequency of the sound wave frequency as it strikes the moving red blood cells. The ultrasound wave, graphically illustrated as a sine wave, has several parameters and definitions.

Doppler effect: This effect is defined as the increment in sound frequency as the target moves toward the transducer and the decrease in sound frequency as the target moves away from the transducer. In a stationary target, both transmitted and received frequencies will be identical. In the cardiovascular system, the red blood cells are the moving target.

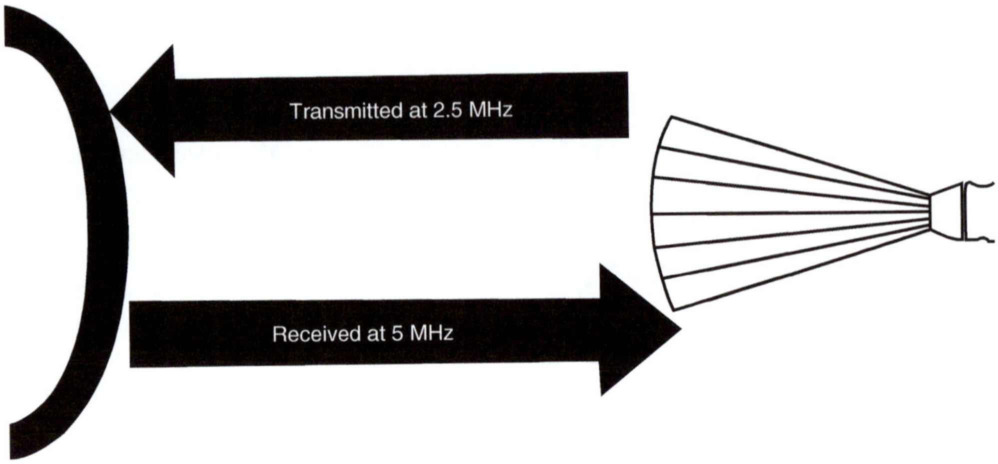

Fig. 1.8 Tissue harmonic imaging mode, sending ultrasound waves at a 2.5-MHz frequency *(F)* and receiving ultrasound waves at a 5-MHz frequency

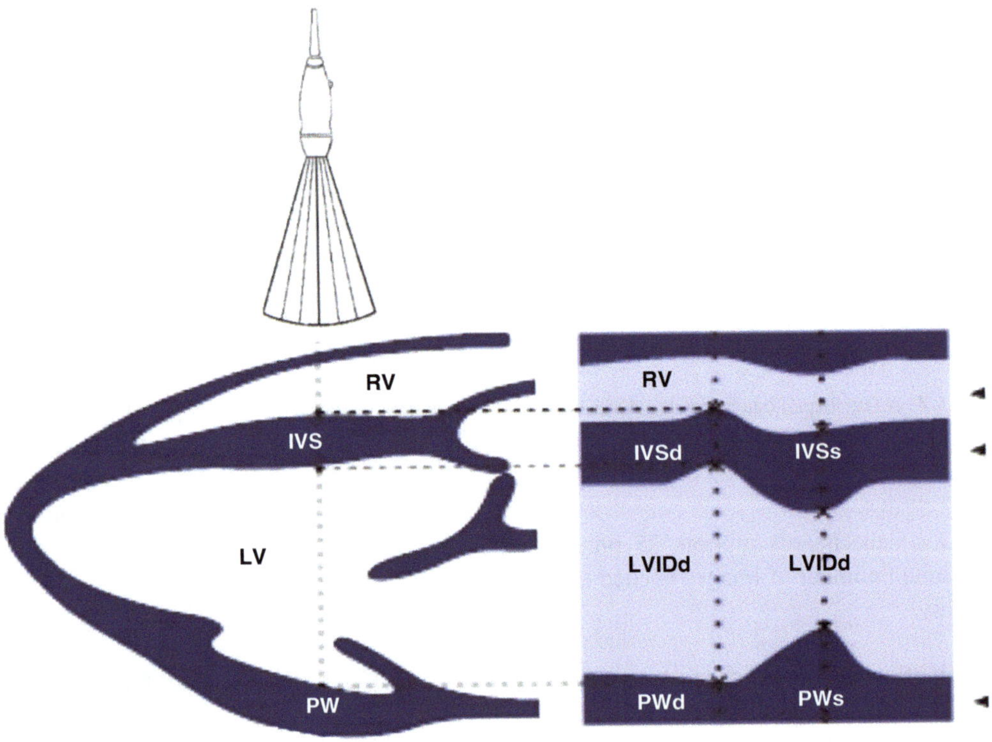

Fig. 1.9 Systolic and diastolic movements of a 1D slice of the moving heart. *RV*, right ventricle; *IVS*, interventricular septum; *PW*, posterior wall

Doppler shift ($\Delta f = f0 - fr$): This shift is defined as the difference between the transmitted (*f0*) and received (*fr*) ultrasound frequencies.

Doppler equation: The frequency shift is associated with the velocity of the moving target (v), transmitted frequency (*f0*), speed of sound (c), and angle between the interrogated beam and the blood flow (cos ø) (Fig. 1.11). As the speed of ultrasound in blood (c) and *f0* is known, the Doppler shift depends on v and cos ø:

$$\Delta f = 2f0 \times v \times \cos\phi \,/\, c$$

Doppler equation correlates with the transmitted frequency (*f0*), received frequency (*fr*), angle of incidence (cos ø), and speed of sound (c).

- When the ultrasound beam is parallel to the blood flow, ø is 0°, the cosine value is 1, and the maximum velocity is recorded. As ø increases, maximum velocity is progressively underestimated; and beyond 20°, the underestimation becomes significant.
- Blood flow velocity is calculated based on the following equation:

$$v = \Delta f \times c \,/\, 2f0 \times \cos\phi$$

Spectral analysis, which is a complex process, determines the Doppler shift and yields information regarding the flow velocity, direction of the flow (Doppler trace above the baseline means that the blood flow moves toward the transducer

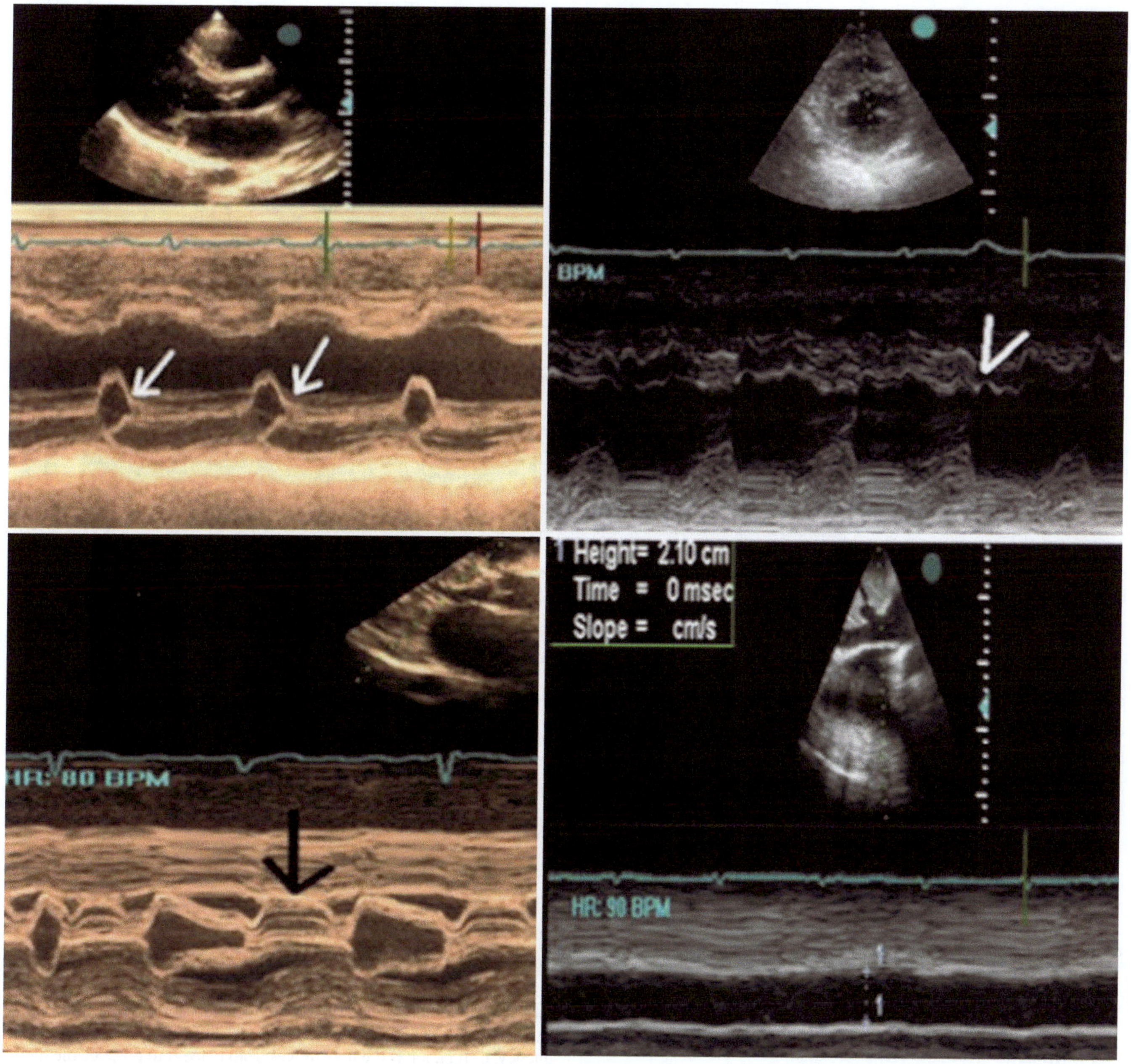

Fig. 1.10 M-mode study in different heart diseases. Left upper: White arrow shows the early closure of the mitral valve in the setting of acute aortic regurgitation. Right upper: M-mode study shows thickened pericardium and septal bounce (arrow head) in constrictive pericarditis. Left lower: Systolic anterior motion of the anterior mitral leaflet. Right lower: Plethora of the inferior vena cava and a dilated hepatic vein in restrictive cardiomyopathy

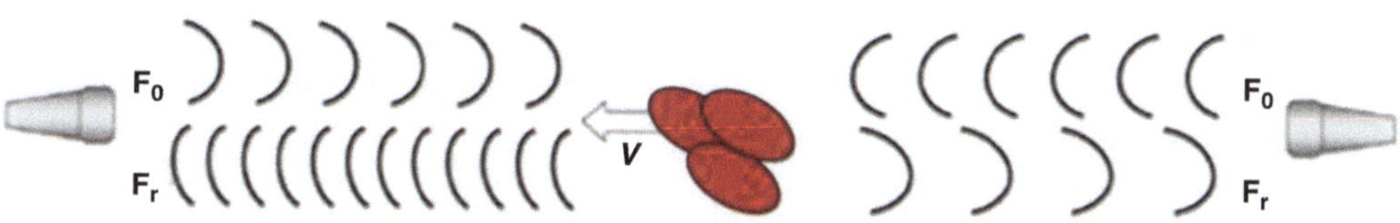

Fig. 1.11 Basic principle of the Doppler effect as the increase in sound frequency as the target moves toward the transducer and the decrease in sound frequency as the target moves away from the transducer

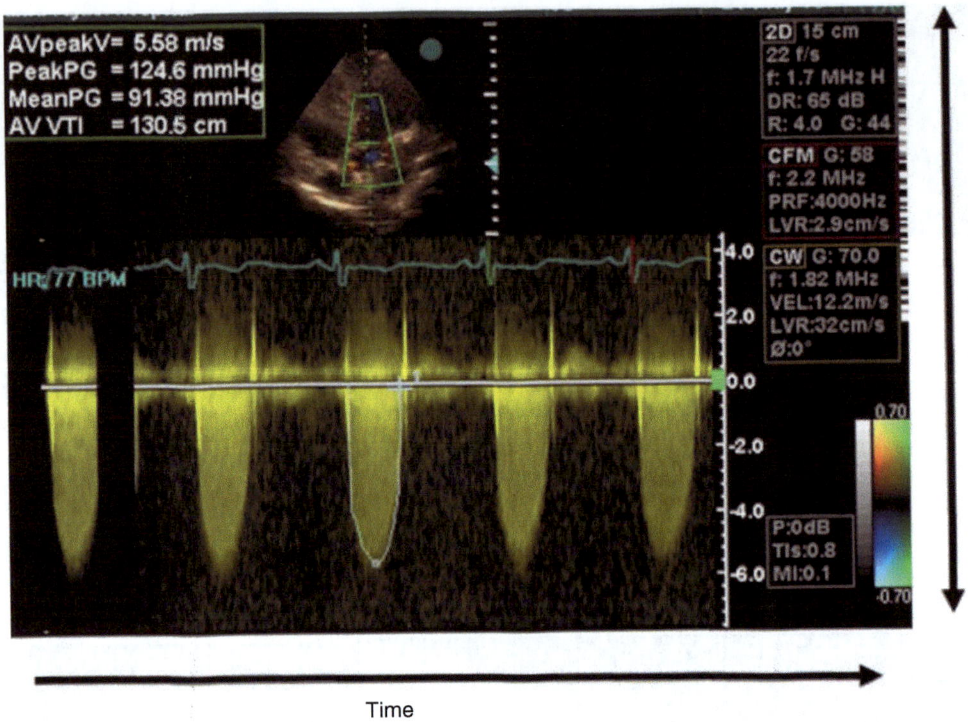

Fig. 1.12 By tracing pulsed-wave or continuous-wave Doppler study, peak velocity, peak and mean pressure gradients, and VTI are automatically calculated. *VTI*, velocity time integral

and under the baseline means that the blood flow moves away from the transducer), timing of the flow, and power of the flow signal.

There are different forms of Doppler imaging [7–9]:

1. CW
2. PW
3. High pulse repetition frequency (HPRF) or multigated PW Doppler, containing multiple sample volumes
4. Color flow imaging (CFI)
5. Color Doppler M-mode (using M-mode on CFI)

Most common basic types of Doppler imaging are PW and CW.

Spectral Doppler gives a graph demonstrating velocities over time (flow velocity in the y-axis and time in the x-axis).

Peak velocities can be measured and by tracing the PW or CW envelope.

Velocity time integral (VTI) is automatically calculated, which corresponds to the stroke distance (Fig. 1.12).

Pulsed-Wave Doppler

- In the PW mode, a single crystal sends intermittent bursts of ultrasound waves and the same crystal waits to receive the returning signals.
- PW can measure the blood flow velocities from a specific location in the heart by using the sample volume.

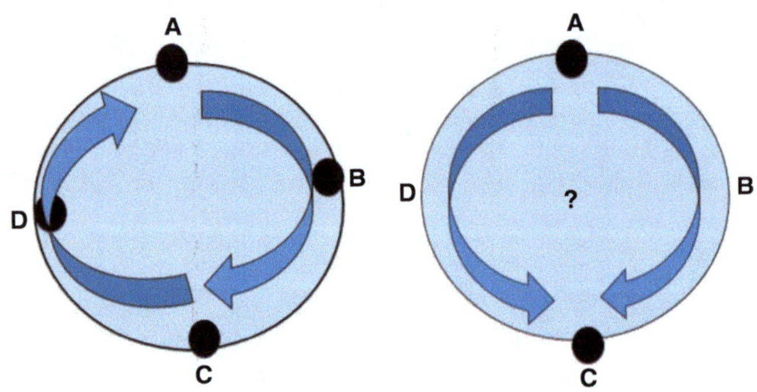

Fig. 1.13 Measurement of a blood flow velocity based on the Doppler frequency. It needs sampling the wave for at least twice the wave frequency. Left panel: If the flow moves from place A to place C, the blood should be sampled at point B; otherwise, the direction of the blood is not clear (right panel)

- Main weakness of PW is aliasing, which means PW cannot measure high blood flow velocities. The accurate measurement of a Doppler frequency needs sampling the wave for at least twice the wave frequency (Fig. 1.13). The maximum velocity, which can be measured by PW without the occurrence of aliasing, is called the Nyquist frequency limit, which is one-half of the pulse repetition frequency (PRF = the number of pulses transmitted in each second).

$$\text{Nyquist frequency limit} = \text{PRF} / 2$$

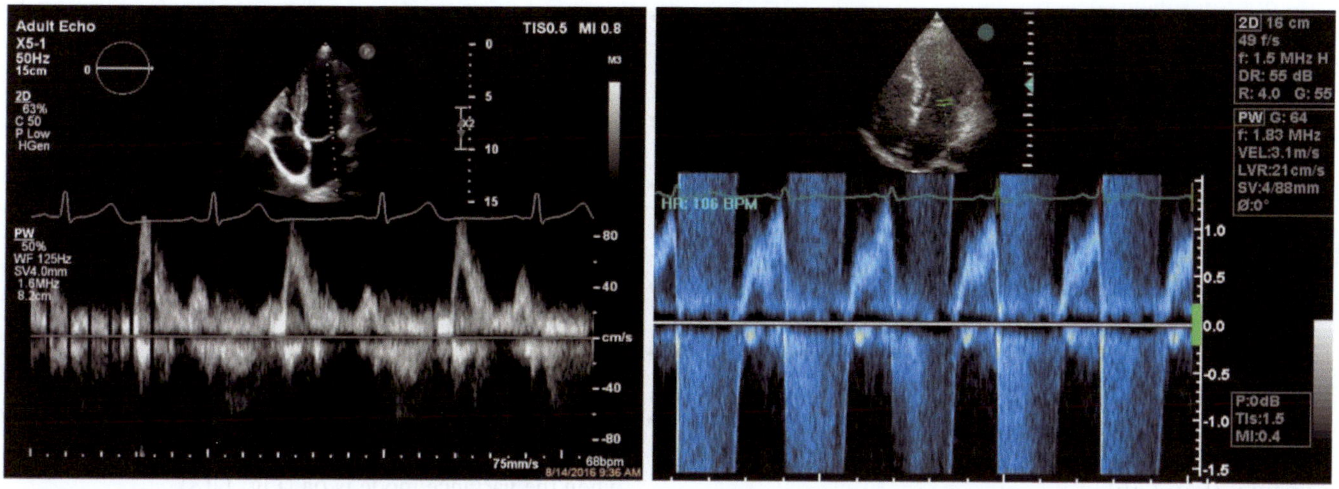

Fig. 1.14 Left panel: Normal PW study of the mitral inflow. Right panel: PW study of the mitral valve in the presence of mitral regurgitation with a high MR jet velocity. Aliasing is seen as a cutoff of velocity and Doppler signal wrap around the baseline: It results in confusion for accurate peak velocity measurement and flow direction. *PW*, pulsed wave; *MR*, mitral regurgitation

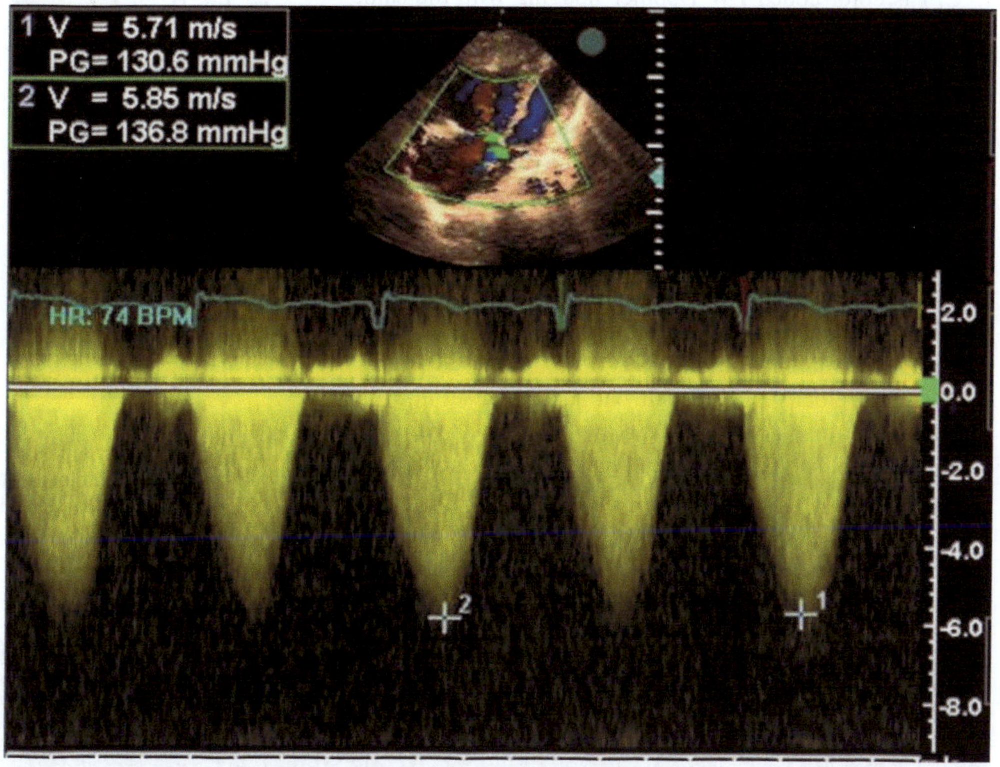

Fig. 1.15 CW Doppler study measures high velocity tricuspid regurgitation without aliasing

- When the frequency shift or velocity is higher than the Nyquist frequency, aliasing occurs. It results in the inability of PW Doppler to correctly record velocities more than 1.5 to 2 m/s (Fig. 1.14).
- Overcoming aliasing and measuring the peak velocity of high speed flows accurately require the utilization of CW. Additionally, decreasing the depth can be useful.

Continuous Wave Doppler

CW Doppler study utilizes a transducer that contains 2 crystals: One of them continuously transmits and the other one continuously receives the signals.

CW can accurately measure the maximum velocity without the occurrence of aliasing (Fig. 1.15). However, it has the disadvantage of not recognizing the location of the sampling since all the velocities along the Doppler beam have been recorded. In the normal heart, most velocities are less than 1.5 m/s and can be measured via PW Doppler.

In pathological conditions with abnormal, high-velocity blood flows, CW Doppler should be used to obtain the highest flow velocity [4, 7].

High Pulse Repetition Frequency (HPRF)

HPRF mode is a combination of PW and CW Doppler modes that uses multiple sample volumes (additional sample volumes are not in high-velocity areas) along the beam which increases the Nyquist limit and allowing measuring higher velocities (Fig. 1.16).

Color Flow Imaging (CFI)

1. CFI is color-coded PW Doppler imaging with the same strengths and weaknesses as PW Doppler imaging.
2. By convention:

- Flow toward the transducer is displayed in red and away from the transducer is displayed in blue (blood flow direction [BART]: blue away and red toward).
- CFI provides a colorized box on real-time 2D imaging which displays BART and blood flow velocity.
- Color bar at the right side of the image contains 2 basic colors: red and blue with multiple shades from dark red to light and dark blue to light blue.
- Aliasing velocity of the color bar should be set at 50 to 70 cm/s.
- Gain of CFI should be adjusted just below the noise.
- Normal blood flow patterns in the heart and great vessels are laminar flows.
- High velocity and turbulent flow create multiple directions, and velocities of the blood flow that exceed the Nyquist limit appear in a mosaic pattern.
- Aliasing velocity of the color bar should be set at 50 to 70 cm/s.
- Lighter shades of each color means higher velocities, and when the blood velocity exceeds the Nyquist limit, aliasing occurs.
- Variance means that the mosaic pattern of the turbulent flow turns green (Fig. 1.17).
- Aliasing in CFI means that the color is repeatedly inverted to the opposite color, creating a mosaic pattern.
- When using CFI, the operator can easily recognize an abnormal flow pattern as a mosaic pattern or green color when the variance mode is on (Fig. 1.18).

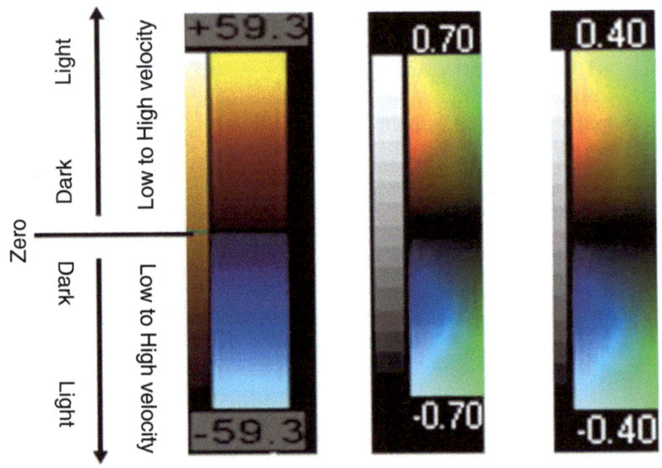

Fig. 1.17 Color bar in the color flow imaging mode. Left: Different shades of blue and red colors as lighter shades are assigned to higher velocities. Middle: Superimposition of variance on the color map. Right: Low Nyquist limit

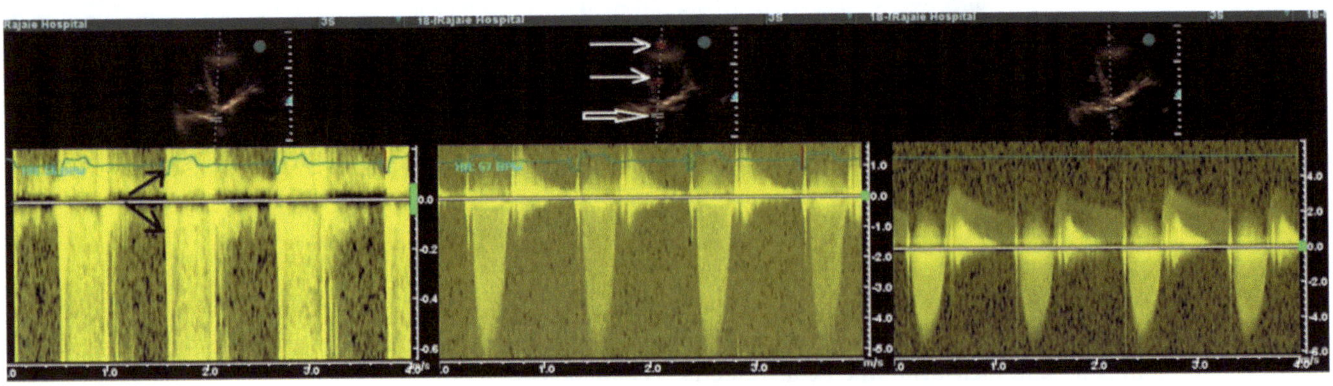

Fig. 1.16 Doppler study in a patient with Aortic stenosis. Left: Aliasing in PW study (black arrow) Middle: High pulse repetition frequency mode increase the Nyquist limit the main sample volumes is placed in high-velocity area. Right: CW Doppler study measures high velocity without aliasing

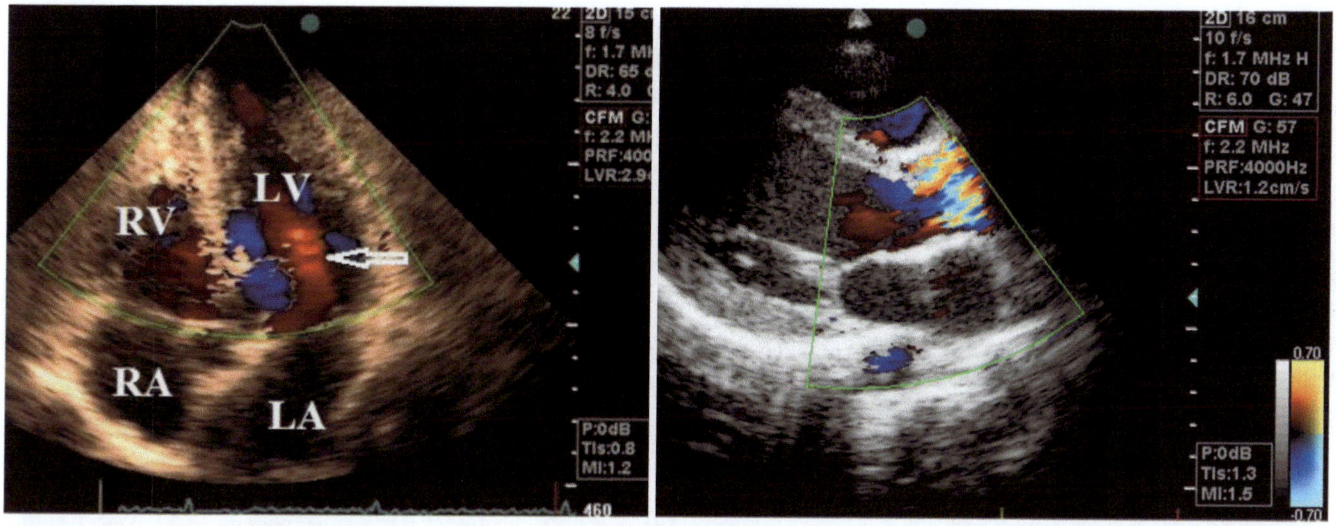

Fig. 1.18 Left panel: Normal flow pattern of the mitral inflow shown as dark red color by color flow imaging (arrow). Right panel: Aliasing and turbulent flow at the aortic valve level, suggestive of aortic valve stenosis

- CFI is very useful for the diagnosis of an abnormal turbulent flow, which occurs in discrete stenosis, high velocity regurgitation, or shunt lesions [10, 11].

Color Doppler M-Mode Imaging

- Color Doppler M-mode is achieved by superimposing CFI on traditional M-mode images.
- It has the advantages of high spatial and temporal resolution along the interrogated line.
- It helps to determine the duration and precise timing of the regurgitation flow (Fig. 1.19).

Doppler-Based Hemodynamic Assessment

- Doppler echocardiography is the basis of noninvasive hemodynamic assessment and measurement of the blood flow velocity.
- It is noteworthy that Doppler echocardiography measures blood *velocity*, not absolute pressure in the chambers, pressure gradient, or the flow directly.
- Intracardiac pressures, pressure gradients, and stroke volume (SV) can be estimated based on 2 important equations: the Bernoulli equation and the continuity equation.

Bernoulli Equation

The blood velocity in the heart is dependent on the pressure gradient between the chambers; accordingly, based on the Bernoulli equation and the measurement of the blood velocity by Doppler shift, the pressure gradient between the 2 chambers (**P1-P2 = ΔP**) can be estimated (Fig. 1.20).

- Indeed the Bernoulli equation converts the velocity to the pressure gradient.
- Original Bernoulli equation is a complex formula that encompasses convective acceleration, flow acceleration, and viscous friction. That is why the following simplified form has been suggested:

$$P1 - P2(\Delta P) = 4\left(V_2^{\,2} - V_1^{\,2}\right)$$

- Bernoulli equation-based calculated pressure gradient has been validated by invasive hemodynamic study.
- In most patients with aortic stenosis, Doppler echocardiography provides trans-aortic jet velocity and mean and peak pressure gradients by using the modified Bernoulli equation, which obviates the need for cardiac catheterization (Fig. 1.21).
- It is important to know that Doppler echocardiography measures the maximum instantaneous peak velocity; consequently, the Bernoulli equation estimates the maximum instantaneous pressure gradient, which is higher than the catheter-based measured peak-to-peak gradient [4, 6, 8].

Continuity Equation

- Based on the concept of the conservation of mass, whatever comes into the heart and passes through the valves should go out from the other heart valve.
- Consequently, in the absence of regurgitation or intracardiac shunting, the flow across all the cardiac valves should be equal.
- Flow across a valve is equal to the product of the flow velocity and the cross-sectional area (CSA) of the valve: flow = CSA × velocity

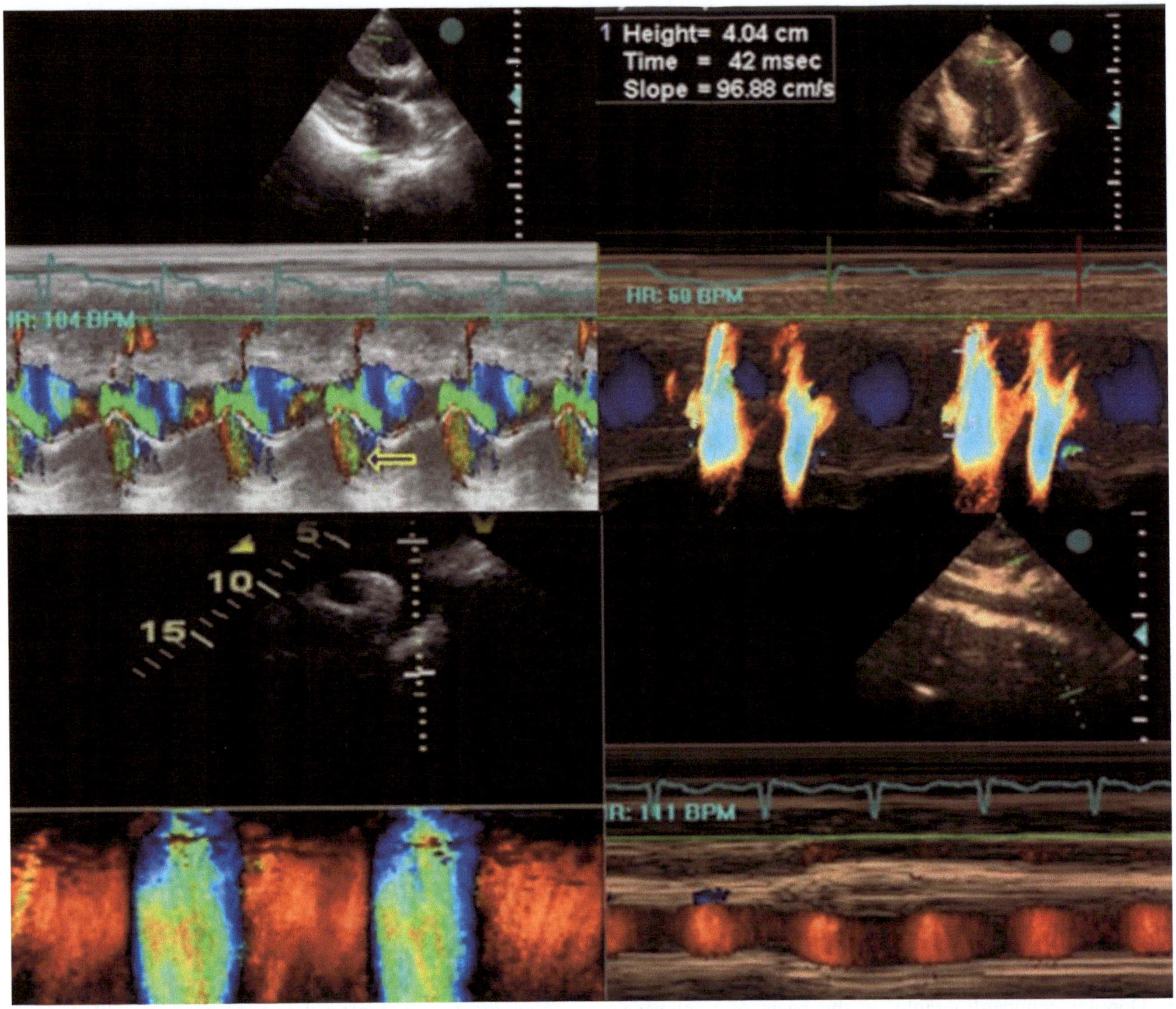

Fig. 1.19 Color M-mode study in different heart diseases. Left upper: Diastolic mitral regurgitation in acute aortic regurgitation (arrow). Left lower (suprasternal view): Holodiastolic flow reversal in severe aortic regurgitation. Right upper: Measurement of the velocity propagation (Vp) of the mitral inflow in a patient with hypertrophic cardiomyopathy (Vp slope = 96 cm/s). Right lower: Absence of diastolic flow reversal in the abdominal aorta in severe coarctation

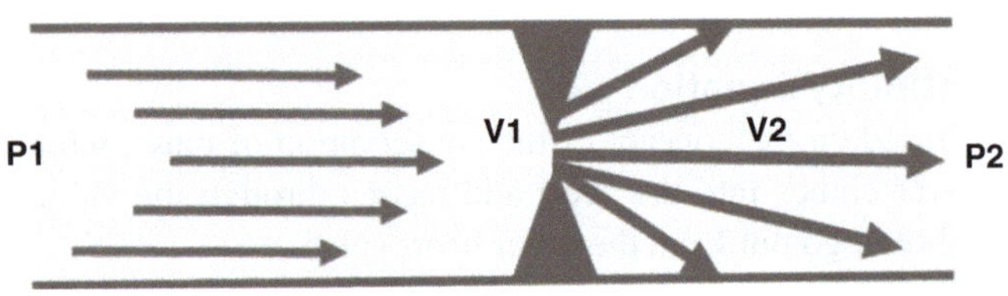

Fig. 1.20 Pressure gradient (P1-P2) between the 2 chambers, separated by a stenotic orifice, can be estimated by the Bernoulli eq. P1 and V1 are the velocity and the pressure at proximal and V2 and P2 are the velocity and the pressure at distal to the orifice. As V1 is much lower than V2, it can be ignored and the equation is further simplified to $\mathbf{\Delta P = 4\,V_2^2}$

- Because the SV across all heart valves is equal, the area of the stenotic or regurgitant valve can easily be calculated using the continuity equation formula (Fig. 1.22).
- Flow measurement is accurate when the flow is laminar and flat. (The blood cells move in the same direction.)
- As the flow velocity varies through the ejection, the integrated velocity during the ejection period, VTI is used to measure the flow rate.
- VTI results from the sum of velocities and is calculated automatically by tracing the Doppler velocity signal. VTI is equal to the stroke distance. The SV is calculated by multiplying the CSA by VTI.

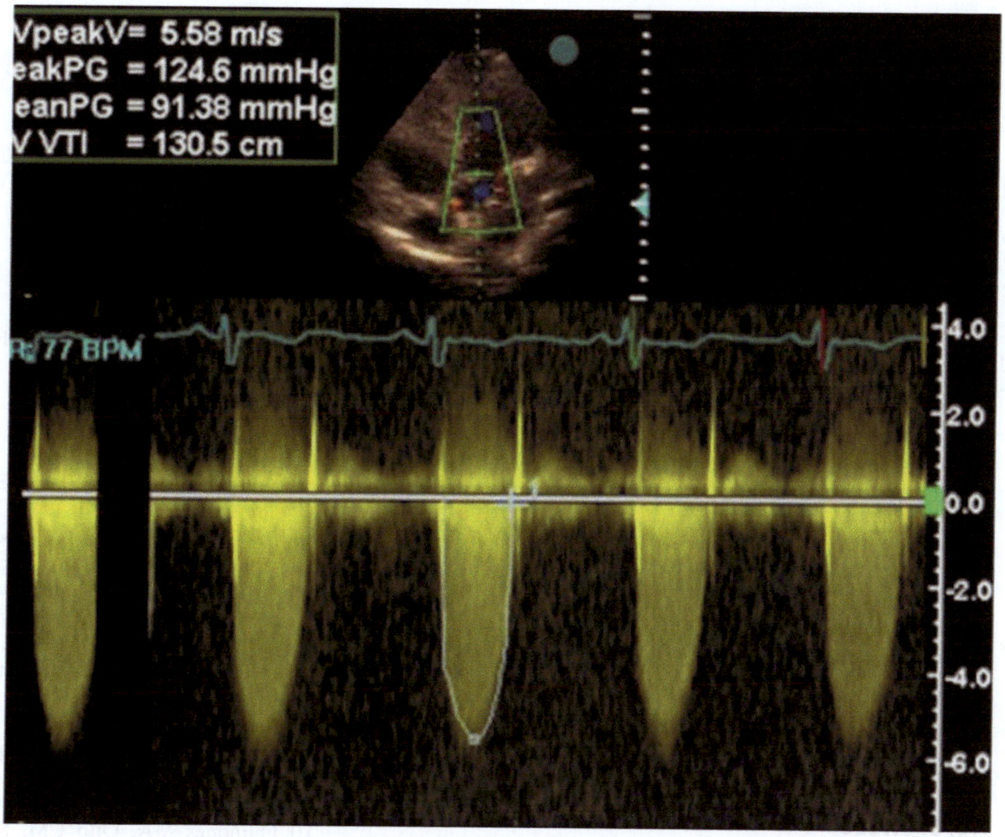

Fig. 1.21 Based on a trans-aortic peak velocity of 5.58 m/s, the maximum pressure gradient is calculated as $4V^2 = 4$ $(5.58 \times 5.58) = 124$ mmHg

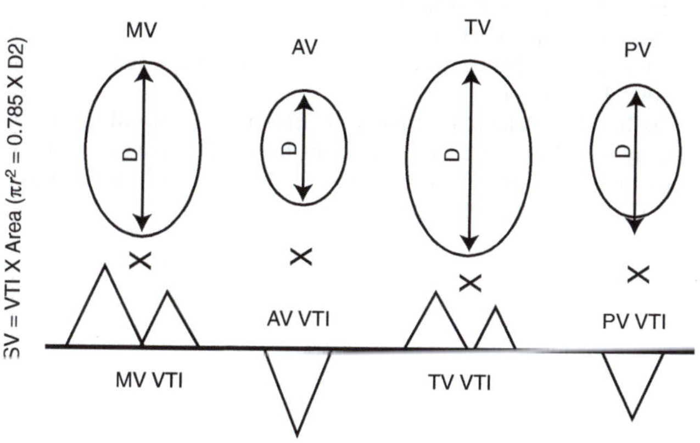

Fig. 1.22 Equal stroke volume across all the heart valves

Common Rules for Flow Measurements

- It is important to match the site of the measurement of the anatomic CSA and the site of velocity recording.
- Preferred sites for the measurement of the annulus and the CSA are those that do not change significantly in the cardiac cycle such as the left ventricular outflow tract (LVOT), aortic annulus, mitral annulus, and pulmonic annulus with an assumed circular annulus.
- Aortic annulus diameter (D) is measured in the parasternal long-axis view in early systole (inner to inner edge) from the junction of the aortic valve leaflets with the mitral valve and septum.
- Largest diameter of 3 to 5 measurements should be selected.
- For tracing VTI, the outer edge of the dense part of the spectral tracing should be traced.
- Usually 3 to 5 cardiac cycles in sinus rhythm and 5 to 10 cycles in atrial fibrillation should be averaged.
- Opening click of the aortic valve should not be seen since it means the sample volume is too close to flow acceleration, whereas the closing click of the aortic valve is often seen (Fig. 1.23).

$$\text{Stroke volume}\,(\mathbf{SV}) = \mathbf{CSA} \times \mathbf{VTI} = \pi \mathbf{r}^2 \times \mathbf{VTI} = \mathbf{0.785} \times \mathbf{D}^2 \times \mathbf{VTI}$$

Commonly the LVOT is used for the measurement of the SV and the stenotic valve area.

$$\mathbf{A_1} \times \mathbf{VTI_1} = \mathbf{A_2} \times \mathbf{VTI_2}$$

$$\mathbf{AV\,area} \times \mathbf{AV\,VTI} = \mathbf{0.785} \times \mathbf{D^2} \times \mathbf{VTI(LVOT)}$$

$$\mathbf{AV\,area} = \frac{\mathbf{0.785} \times \mathbf{D^2} \times \mathbf{VTI(LVOT)}}{\mathbf{AV\,VTI}}$$

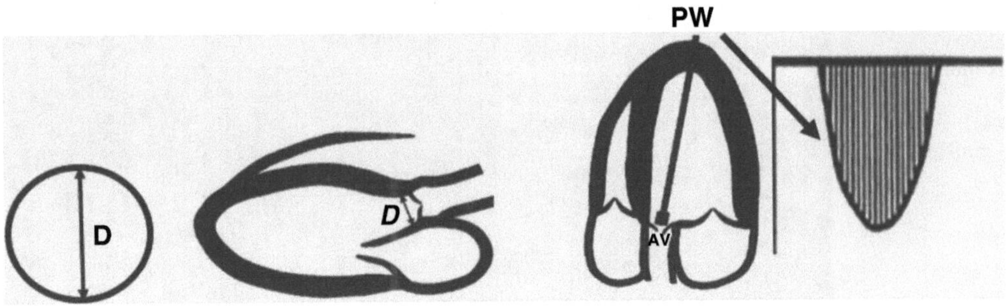

Fig. 1.23 Calculation of the cross-sectional area of the circular shape annulus (D = diameter): area = $\pi r^2 = \pi \times (D/2)^2 = 0.785 \times D^2$; and the velocity time integral (VTI) of the left ventricular outflow tract (LVOT) by placing the pulsed-wave sample volume in the LVOT about 5 mm proximal to the aortic valve in the apical 5-chamber view

Pulmonic annulus is difficult to visualize and measure well. The measurement of the flow across the pulmonic valve is useful for calculating the pulmonic-to-systemic (Qp:Qs) flow ratio in left-to-right intracardiac shunts such as the atrial septal defect.

Flow calculation across the mitral valve needs circular assumption of the mitral valve and measurement of the annulus during early to mid-diastole by positioning the sample volume at the level of the mitral annulus [11].

References

1. Edler I, Henz CH. The use of ultrasonic reflectoscope for the continuous recording of the movements of hean walls. 1954. Clin Physiol Funct Imaging. 2004;24:118–36.
2. Fraser AG. Inge Edler and the origins of clinical echocardiography. Eur J Echocardiogr. 2001;2:3–5.
3. Armstrong WF, Ryan T. Feigenbaum's echocardiography. 7th ed. Philadelphia: Lippincott Williams & Wilkins; 2010.
4. Tajik AJ, Seward IB, Hagler DJ, et al. Two-dimensional real-time ultrasonic imaging of the hean and great vessels: technique, image orientation, structure identification, and validation. Mayo Clin Proc. 1978;53:271–303.
5. Nihoyannopoulos P, Kisslo J. Echocardiography. London: Springer; 2009.
6. Feigenbaum H. Role of M-mode technique in today's echocardiography. J Am Soc Echocardiogr. 2010;23:240–57.
7. Anavekar NS, Oh JK. Doppler echocardiography: a contemporary review. J Cardiol. 2009;54:347–58.
8. Zipes D, Libby P, Bonow R. Braunwald's heart disease: a textbook of cardiovascular medicine. 10th ed. Philadelphia: Saunders, Elsevier Inc.
9. Lancellotti P, Zamorano JL, Habib G, Badano L. The EACVI Textbook of Echocardiography Chapter 3. In: Kasprzak J, Sadeghpour A, Jurcut R, editors. Doppler echocardiography. 2nd ed. Oxford: Oxford University Press; 2017.
10. Quiñones MA, Otto CM, Stoddard M, Waggoner A, Zoghbi W. Recommendations for quantification of Doppler echocardiography: a report from the Doppler Quantification Task Force of the Nomenclature and Standards Committee of the American Society of Echocardiography. J Am Soc Echocardiogr. 2002;15:167–84.
11. Zoghbi WA, Adams D, Bonow R, Enriquez-Sarano M, Foster E, Grayburn P, et al. Recommendations for noninvasive evaluation of native valvular regurgitation, J Am Soc Echocardiogr. 2017. https://doi.org/10.1016/j.echo.2017.01.00.

Transthoracic Echocardiography, Standard Windows and Echocardiographic Views

2

Anita Sadeghpour, Azin Alizadehasl, and Maryam Forouzesh

Abstract

Transthoracic echocardiography (TTE) can provide a comprehensive assessment of the anatomy, function, and hemodynamic of the cardiovascular system. However, it is an operator-dependent technique and requires the expertise of the physician, who should be familiar with the capabilities and limitations (pitfalls and artifacts) of echocardiography. In this chapter we will review the basic principles of TTE, explaining how to perform Adult TTE besides definition and obtaining standard windows and views.

Keywords

Echocardiography · Transthoracic echocardiography · Ultrasonography · Doppler · Imaging planes · Parasternal window · Apical window · 4 chamber view · Subcostal window · Suprasternal view

Abbreviations

AA	Ascending aorta
AO	Aorta
ASE	American society of echocardiography
AV	Aortic valve
HV	Hepatic vein
IVC	Inferior vena cava
IVS	Inter-ventricular septum
LA	Left atrium
LPA	Left pulmonary artery
LV	Left ventricle
LVOT	Left ventrivular outflow tract
MV	Mitral valve
PA	Pulmonary artery
PLAX	Parasternal long-axis
PSAX	Parasternal short axis
PW	Pulse-waved
RA	Right atrium
RV	Right ventricle
RVOT	Right ventricular outflow tract
SVC	Superior vena cava
TTE	Transthoracic echocardiography
TV	Tricuspid valve
V	Vertebra

- Transthoracic echocardiography (TTE) can provide a comprehensive assessment of the anatomy, function, and hemodynamic of the cardiovascular system. However, it is an operator-dependent technique and requires the expertise of the physician, who should be familiar with the capabilities and limitations (pitfalls and artifacts) of echocardiography.
- Many guidelines have been published by the American Society of Echocardiography (ASE) regarding the standards for performing, nomenclature, and measurement of TTE as well as providing a standard echocardiography report [1–3].
- Appropriate use criteria for echocardiography were updated in 2011. Echocardiography is appropriate when the expected incremental data besides clinical judgment exceed the possible negative consequences of the examination [4].

Standard TTE exam and report should include:

1. Demographic and identifying information such as age, gender, indications for TTE, height, weight, and blood pressure

A. Sadeghpour, MD, FACC, FASE
Professor of Cardiology, Echocardiography Research Center, Rajaie Cardiovascular Medical and Research Center, Iran University of Medical Science, Tehran, Iran

A. Alizadehasl, MD, FACC, FASE (✉)
Associate Professor of Cardiology, Echocardiologist, Echocardiography and Cardiogenetic Research Centers, Cardio-Oncology Department, Rajaie Cardiovascular Medical and Research Center, Tehran, Iran

M. Forouzesh
Cardiac Sonographer, Echocardiography Research Center, Rajaie Cardiovascular Medical and Research Center, Vali-Asr St., Tehran, Iran

A. Sadeghpour, A. Alizadehasl (eds.), *Case-Based Textbook of Echocardiography*,
https://doi.org/10.1007/978-3-319-67691-3_2

2. Comprehensive evaluation of the cardiac structure by 2D, M-mode, and spectral and color Doppler imaging of:

- All cardiac chambers:

(a) Left ventricle (LV)
(b) Right ventricle (RV)
(c) Left atrium (LA)
(d) Right atrium (RA)

- All heart valves:

(a) Aortic valve (AV)
(b) Mitral valve (MV)
(c) Tricuspid valve (TV)
(d) Pulmonic valve

- Pericardium
- Aorta
- Pulmonary artery, including the pulmonary artery pressure
- Inferior vena cava (IVC) and pulmonary veins

3. Answering the question of the referring physician
4. Emphasizing the abnormal findings on echocardiography
5. Comparing important differences and similarities between the current TTE and previous echocardiographic studies [1]

Basic Principles

- TTE means performing echocardiography by placing the probe on the anterior chest wall.
- It is important to inspect the patient's color and fingers to look for cyanosis or clubbed fingers.
- It is also important to look at the patient's chest for the presence of the scars of sternotomy.
- Prior to echocardiography, it is important that a brief history taking and a cardiac examination be conducted.
- TTE uses a fan-shaped beam of ultrasound waves sent via a transducer, positioned in the proper window on the chest (Fig. 2.1).
- TTE in adults begins with the parasternal window and in pediatrics from the subxiphoid or subcostal window to allow the determination of visceral situs [5].

How to Perform Adult Transthoracic Echocardiography

- Positioning the patient: In the parasternal and apical windows, the patient should be positioned in the left lateral with the left arm up under his or her head to bring the heart closer to the chest wall and open the rib spaces.
- Transducer is positioned between the ribs on the chest wall.

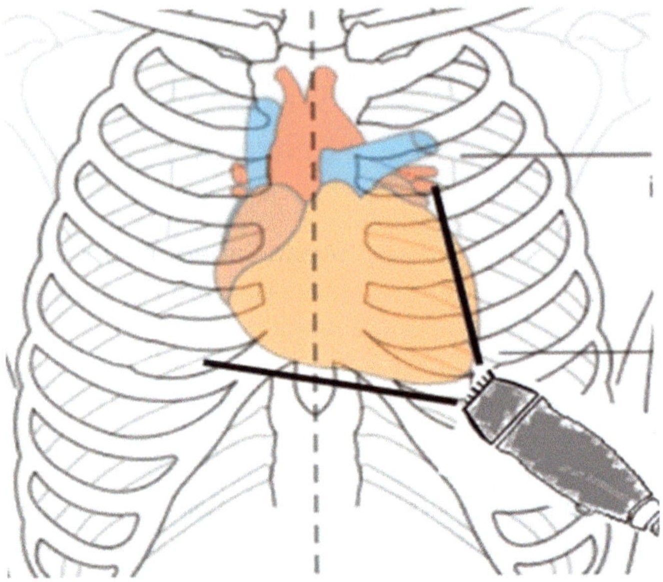

Fig. 2.1 Fan-shaped beam of the ultrasound sent via a transducer, positioned in the apex

- The gel on the probe helps to eliminate the air between the transducer and the patient's chest wall.
- At least 3 chest leads are needed for simultaneous ECG monitoring, which is useful for heart rate and rhythm monitoring and correlating the systolic and diastolic phases of echocardiographic images.
- TTE can be performed by right-handed or left-handed echocardiographers based on the operator's preference.
- Right-handed echocardiographers should sit by the patient's right side and do not bend over the patient to prevent musculoskeletal injury.
  - Probe should be held between the thumb and the 1st and 2nd fingers (Fig. 2.2, left panel).
  - ***Index mark***: The head of all 2D imaging probes is indexed with a notch, ridge, or light placed on the side and correlated with the edge of the imaging plane.
  - Index mark indicates the structure of the imaging plane that will be displayed on the right side of the image screen [1] (Figs. 2.2 and 2.3 middle and right panels).
  - Optimizing the settings (i.e., gain, time gain compensation, depth, velocity scale, and sweep speed) is essential for having the optimal image.

Image Orientation

- By convention, reflected ultrasound signals near the surface of the transducer are displayed at the top of the image and reflecting structures far from the transducer are displayed at the bottom of the screen [1] (Fig. 2.4).
- Four standard windows are used in routine TTE (Fig. 2.5). TTE in adults begins with the parasternal window.

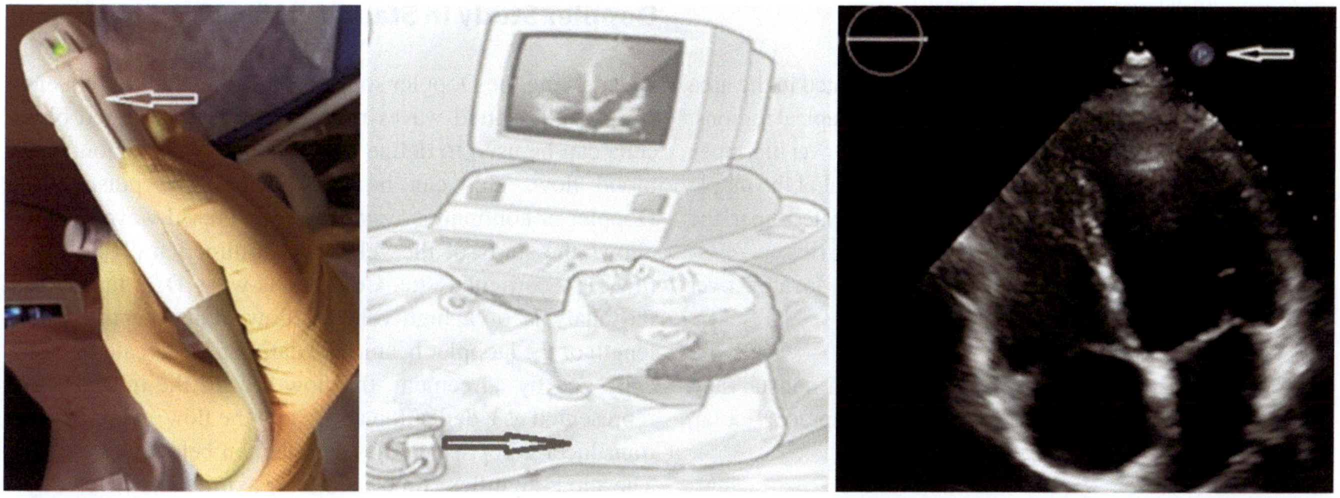

Fig. 2.2 Left: Index marker on the probe (white arrow) is pointed to the patient's left scapulae (black arrow) and is displayed on the right side of the screen (white arrow)

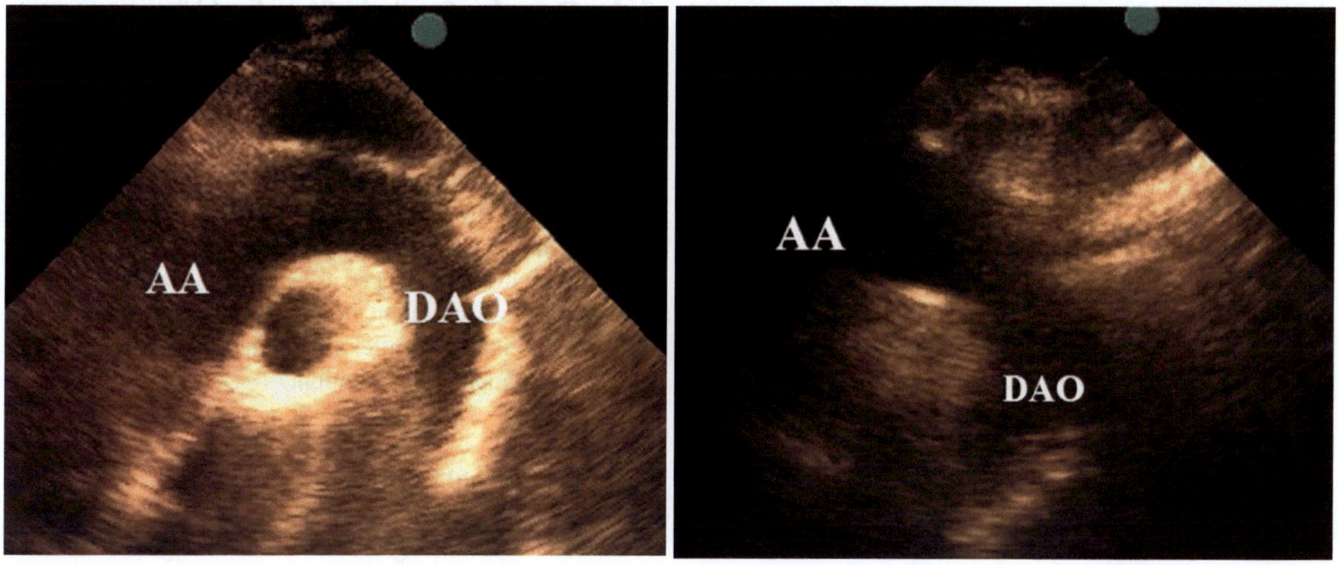

Fig. 2.3 *Left* In the suprasternal window of the normal left aortic arch, when the marker is pointed to the left side of the patient, the long axis of the aorta is displayed on the right side of the image screen. *Right*: In a right-sided aortic arch, pointing the index mark of the transducer to the right side of the patient will show the long axis of the aortic arch on the right side of the image screen

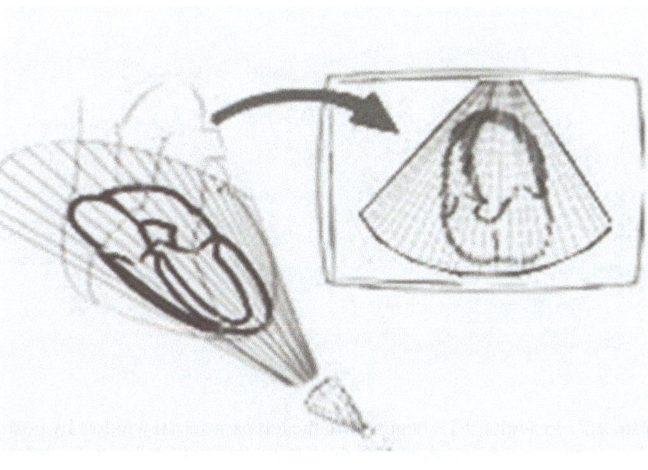

Fig. 2.4 Left ventricular apex, located close to the probe and appearing at the top of the screen, seems to be upside down of the normal position

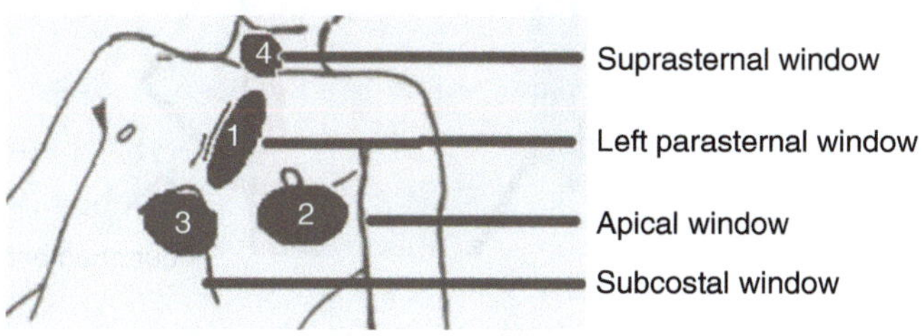

Fig. 2.5 Four standard windows of routine transthoracic echocardiography

A standard window consists of the:

A. **Parasternal window**: The transducer is located in the area surrounded by the left clavicle, sternum, and apical regions.
B. **Apical window:** The transducer is located over the apex impulse, slightly toward the inferior and lateral of the nipple
C. **Subcostal window**: The transducer is located near the midline of the body and beneath the lowest ribs.
D. **Suprasternal window**: The transducer is located over the suprasternal notch

Sometimes, more images are required from nonstandard windows—including the right parasternal, supraclavicular, or right apical window for dextrocardia [1, 2].

Imaging Planes

There are 3 basic imaging planes (long-axis, short-axis, and 4-chamber), which transect the heart not the body (Fig. 2.6).

1. Long-axis plane is parallel to the long axis of the LV (apex to base).
2. Short-axis plane is perpendicular to the LV long axis with a circular cross-section transecting the heart).
3. Four-chamber plane is perpendicular to both long-axis and short-axis views and transect both atria and ventricles.

Each image should be defined based on the acoustic window (position of the transducer) and view (imaging plane). For example, the parasternal long-axis view means a parasternal window with a long-axis plane.

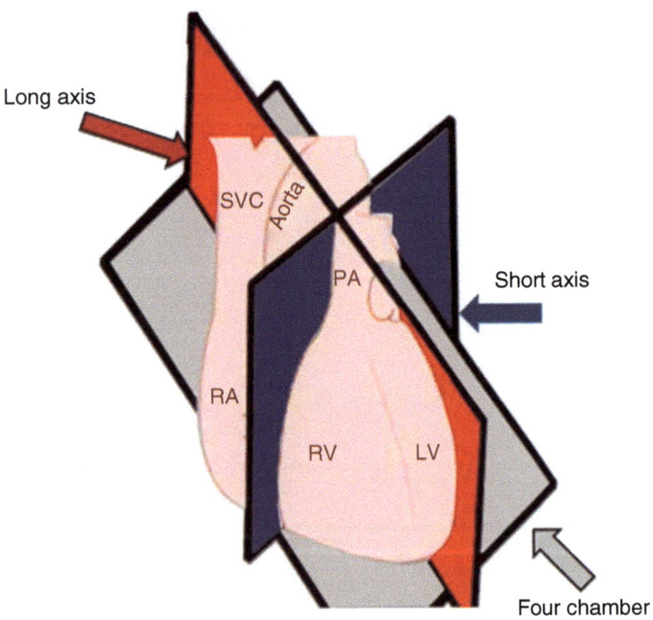

Fig. 2.6 Three basic imaging planes (long axis, short axis, and 4-chamber), which transect the heart

Doppler Study in Standard Views

By applying the Doppler source to ultrasound, the frequency shift of ultrasound waves reflected from moving red blood cells can be used to define the velocity and direction of the blood flow. This can be done with either pulsed-wave Doppler or continuous-wave Doppler. Pulsed-wave Doppler allows the study of the velocity and direction of the blood flow at a particular site. Continuous-wave Doppler permits the analysis of a high-velocity flow alongside the whole length of the Doppler beam. The data can be revealed graphically and by agreement, the flow toward the transducer is represented as a deflection above and the flow away from the transducer is represented as a deflection below the baseline. The x axis signifies "time" and the y axis denotes "velocity". (See Chap. 1).

Color Doppler Study in Standard Views

Color flow mapping also uses the pulsed-wave methodology; it, however, maps the flow velocity at multiple locations within an area and joins this information in color on a black-and-white 2D image. By agreement, and importantly, color coding for the flow velocity toward the transducer is "red" and the flow velocity away from the transducer is "blue". Higher velocities are mapped as brighter shades. A mosaic of color signifies a turbulent flow. A very important point to bear in mind is that parallel alignment to the flow is crucial for accurate Doppler quantitation.

Left Parasternal Window

From this location, long- and short-axis images of the heart may be acquired [6–9] (Fig. 2.7).

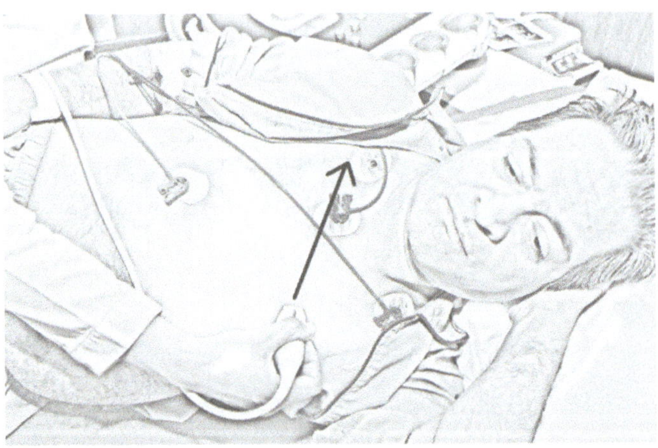

Fig. 2.7 In adults, TTE begins with the left parasternal window by positioning the transducer alongside the left parasternal border at the 3rd or 4th intercostal space with the patient in the left lateral position. The transducer marker should be toward the patient's right (Black arrow)

From the left parasternal window, 3 long-axis views can be obtained:

1. **Left parasternal long-axis view** (Fig. 2.8)
   In the long-axis view, the MV, MV leaflets, and MV chordal apparatus as well as the RV outflow tract, AV, LA, long axis of the LV, and aorta can be assessed.
   In this view, mitral regurgitation is seen as a distinct blue jet in the LA during systole. Small jets may be seen with normal valves. Aortic regurgitation is seen as a blue or red jet emanating from a closed AV. The jet is located in the LVOT and happens in diastole. The presence of this jet represents an abnormal AV.
2. **Left parasternal right ventricular inflow view**
   Right-ward and medial angulation of the probe allows more complete study and imaging of the RV. The RV inflow view allows the evaluation of the RA, proximal portion of the inferior vana cave(IVC), entrance of the coronary sinus, TV, and also the base of the RV (Fig. 2.9, left panel)
   The IVC inflow appears as a red jet at the inferior margin of the RA. It has both systolic and diastolic phases, and the flow velocity is typically less than 1.0 m/s by pulsed-wave Doppler. The TV inflow is seen as a red jet passing the TV. It happens in diastole with velocities less than 0.6 m/s.
   Tricuspid regurgitation is a blue jet in the RA which happens in systole. Small jets are normal. The peak velocity of the regurgitant flow could be quantified by continuous-wave Doppler.
3. **Left parasternal right ventricular outflow view**
   Left-ward angulation of the probe allows more complete study and imaging of the anteriorly placed right ventricular outflow tract (RVOT) and PA (Fig. 2.9, right panel).

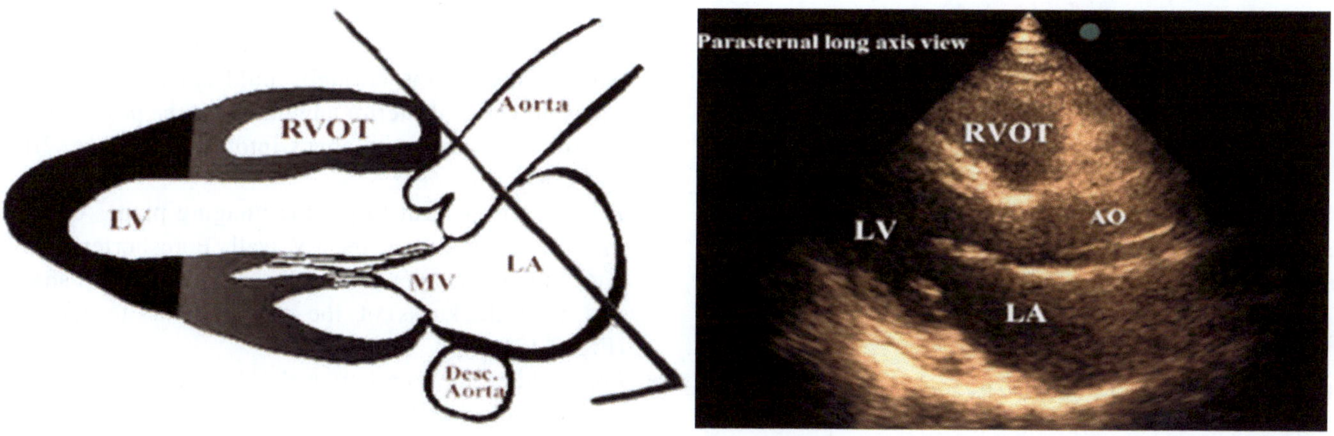

Fig. 2.8 Left parasternal long-axis (PLAX) view. Left ventricle (LV), Right ventricle outflow tract (RVOT), Left atrium (LA), Aortic valve (AV)

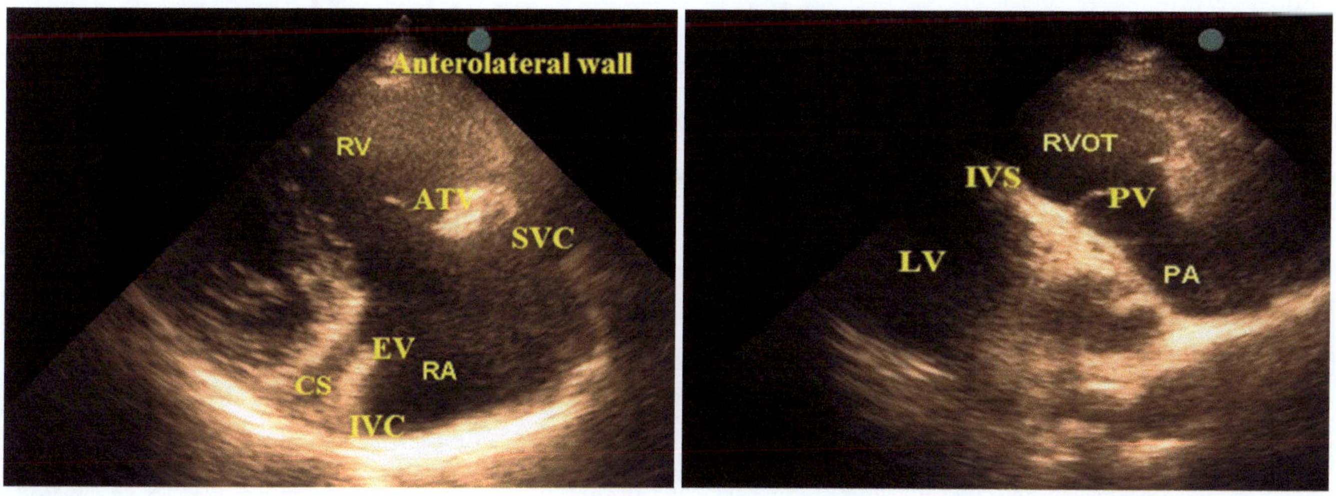

Fig. 2.9 *Left panel*: Left parasternal right ventricular inflow view. *Right panel*: Left parasternal right ventricular outflow view. *RV* right ventricular; *RA* right atrium; *EV* Eustachian valve; *CS* coronary sinus; *ATV* anterior tricuspid leaflet; *PTV* posterior tricuspid leaflet; *RVOT* right ventricular outflow tract; *PA* pulmonary artery; *IVC* inferior vana cave; *SVC* superior vena cava

Parasternal Window (Short-Axis View)

Parasternal short axis **(PSAX)** images are achieved by 90° clockwise rotation from the PLAX window (Fig. 2.10).

- Importantly, a series of cross-sectional images of the LV and the RV are generated by moving the transducer caudally (Figs. 2.11 and 2.12).
- The pulmonary outflow is a systolic blue jet in the pulmonary artery. The normal velocity through the pulmonary outflow tract is 0.6 to 0.9 m/s in adults (Fig. 2.13).

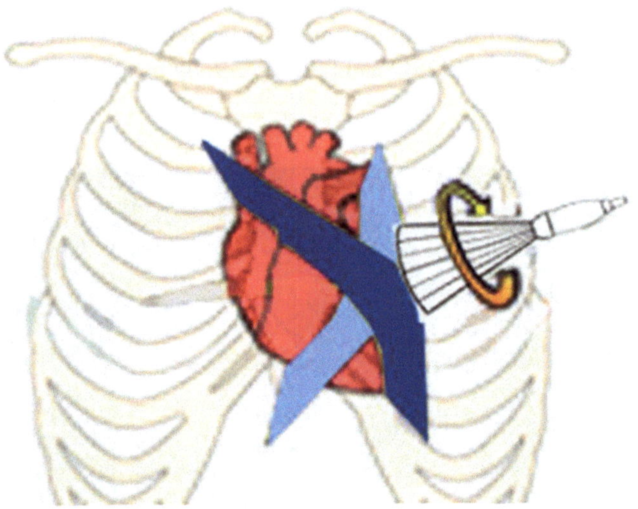

Fig. 2.10 Parasternal short axis images are achieved as the transducer is rotated 90° from the long-axis window

- At the basal level, the fish-mouthed shape of the MV is apparent. At the mid-ventricular level, both anterolateral and posteromedial papillary muscles are seen and the most caudal angulation allows the imaging of the LV apex (Fig. 2.14).

Apical window consists of the:

- **Apical 4 chamber view**
- **Apical 5 chamber view**
- **Apical 2 chamber view**
- **Apical 3 chamber view**

Apical 4 chamber view:

- By placing the echocardiography transducer at the cardiac apex and positioning the imaging sector toward the base of the heart, it is possible to obtain the important apical views of the heart which shows the main four cardiac chambers: the ventricles at the top and atria at bottom since the apex is close to the probe and by convention is shown at top of the image. It is important to look for the normally mild apically displaced tricuspid valve. Posterior angulation of the probe showing the coronary sinus opens into the RA (Figs. 2.15 and 2.16).
- It is very important to get the imaging planes cutting the true LV apex not the LV wall. Foreshortened LV apex is not true apex and is diagnosed by round shape and wall thickness of the apex similar to the LV (Fig. 2.17).
- For avoiding the foreshortened LV apex, the transducer should be displaced to a lower and lateral place.

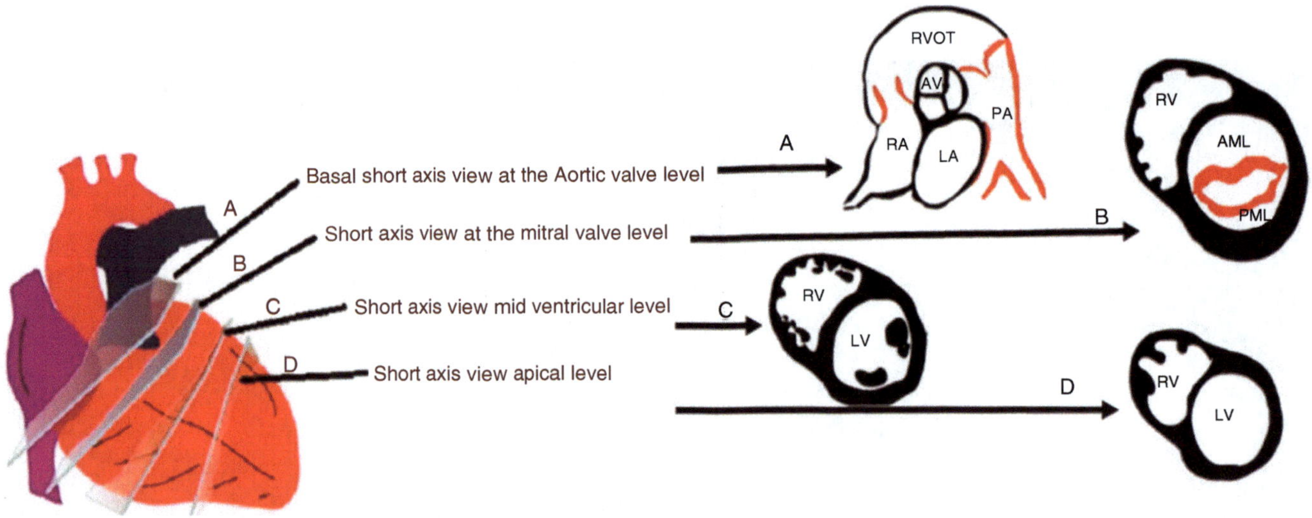

Fig. 2.11 Different imaging plane obtained from parasternal short axis window by sweeping the transducer from the cranial to the caudal position

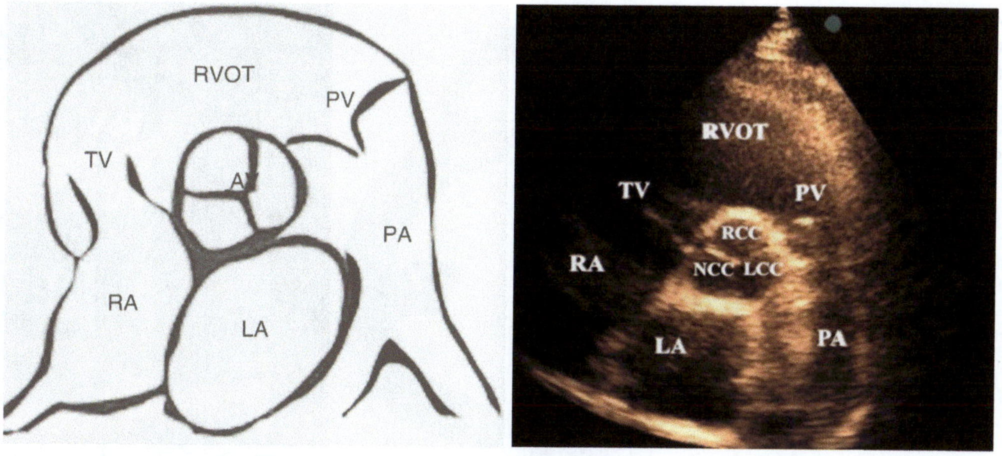

Fig. 2.12 The most cranial view provides the opportunity to image the AV, both atria, RV outflow tract, and proximal portion of the pulmonary arteries. The 3 normal coronary cusps of the AV can be observed with the possible imaging of the proximal portion of the right coronary artery rising from the right coronary cusp at the 10 o'clock site and the left main coronary artery initiating from the left coronary cusp at the 3 o'clock point

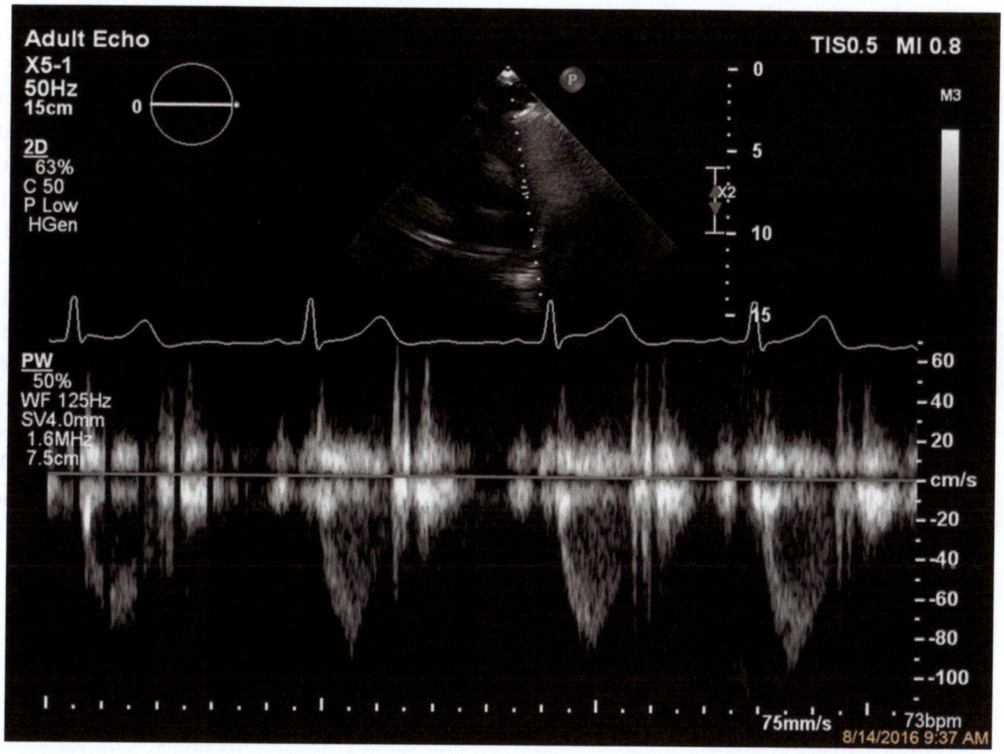

Fig. 2.13 Low velocity flow across the pulmonary valve demonstrated by Pulse-waved (PW) Doppler study

- The trans-MV flow and the TV flow are best assessed in the 4-chamber view thanks to the parallel position of the Doppler beam to the direction of the blood flow. MV inflow blood passing happens in diastole and can be quantified by pulsed-wave Doppler, with the sample volume placed at the MV leaflet tips in the LV cavity (Fig. 2.18).
- Pulmonary vein inflow from the right upper pulmonary vein is seen as a red jet arriving at the LA close to the interatrial septum. It may be quantified by pulsed-wave Doppler, with the sample volume placed 1 to 2 cm into the pulmonary vein. There is a biphasic flow in systole and diastole.

Apical 5 chamber view:

- When the probe is placed in the apical 4 chamber view by slightly anterior angulation, the AV and Ao root appear

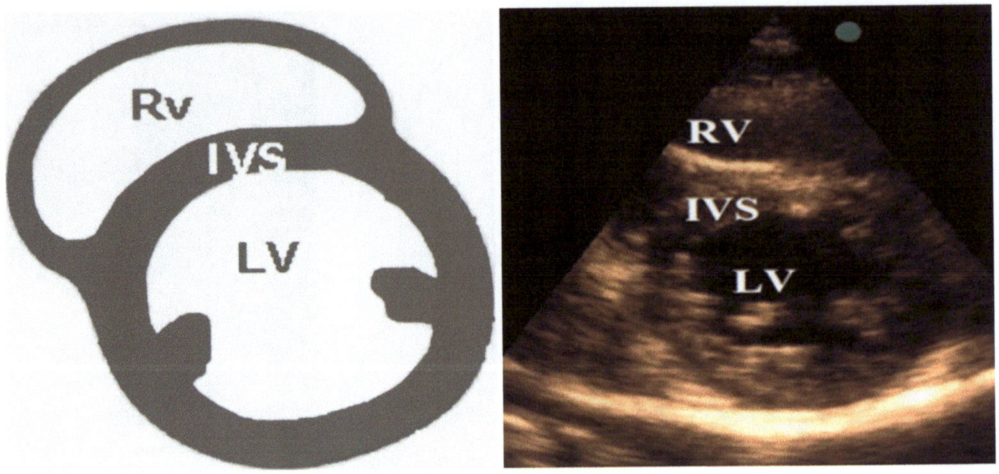

Fig. 2.14 The RV looks like a crescentic structure alongside the right anterior surface of the LV. *RV* Right ventricle, *IVS* Inter ventricular septum, *LV* Left ventricle

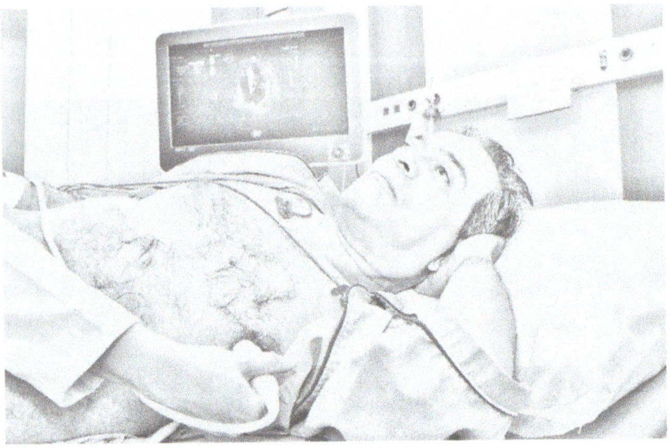

Fig. 2.15 By positioning the patient in the left lateral decubitus, placing the echocardiography transducer at the 5th intercostal space (median axillary line) and pointing toward the patients left an apical 4 chamber view could be obtained

(Fig. 2.19). This view is called apical 5 chamber view. The trans-AV flow can be evaluated in the apical long-axis or 5-chamber view.
- AV and LVOT flows are seen as a blue flow, detected in systole. The Doppler profile resembles a negative, single, uniform systolic contour.

Apical 2 chamber view:

- With the transducer placed in apical 4-chamber view by 60-90° counterclockwise rotation of the probe yields an apical 2-chamber view. 2 Chamber view is used to assess wall motion abnormality and calculating Simpsons' method (Fig. 2.20).

Apical 3 chamber view or apical long axis view:

- Further (another 60 °) counterclockwise rotation of the transducer, placed in apical 2 chamber yields an apical 3-chamber view which is important in evaluating LVOT, Aortic root and true LV apex [7] (Fig. 2.21).

Subcostal view:

- The subcostal window permits ultrasound access to the heart through the solid and homogenous tissue of the liver, which readily conducts sound waves (Fig. 2.22).
- Probe is placed in the midline or slightly to the right pointing down (toward the patient's spine) for better evaluation of the Aorta, inferior vena cava (IVC) and liver which can helps in determining the abdominal situs used in congenital heart disease (Fig. 2.23) [10].
- The alignment of the heart relative to this approach permits better imaging of both interatrial and interventricular septa because the sound beam faces these structures in a perpendicular track (Fig. 2.24).
- Interestingly, in infants and small children, the subcostal window provides excellent images of all cardiac structures.

Suprasternal view:

- The suprasternal view is achieved by placing the transducer in the suprasternal notch. Both longitudinal and transverse planes of the great vessels may be imaged in this view (Fig. 2.25).
- The longitudinal plane orientates through the long axis of the aorta and contains the origins of the innominate, left common carotid, and left subclavian arteries (Figs. 2.26 and 2.27).
- The transverse plane is obtained by 90 ° counterclockwise rotation from long axis view and showing a cross section through the ascending aorta, with the right pulmonary artery passage behind it. Portions of the innominate vein and the superior vena cava (SVC) are observable anterior to the aorta. The LA and the pulmonary veins are posterior to the right pulmonary artery.

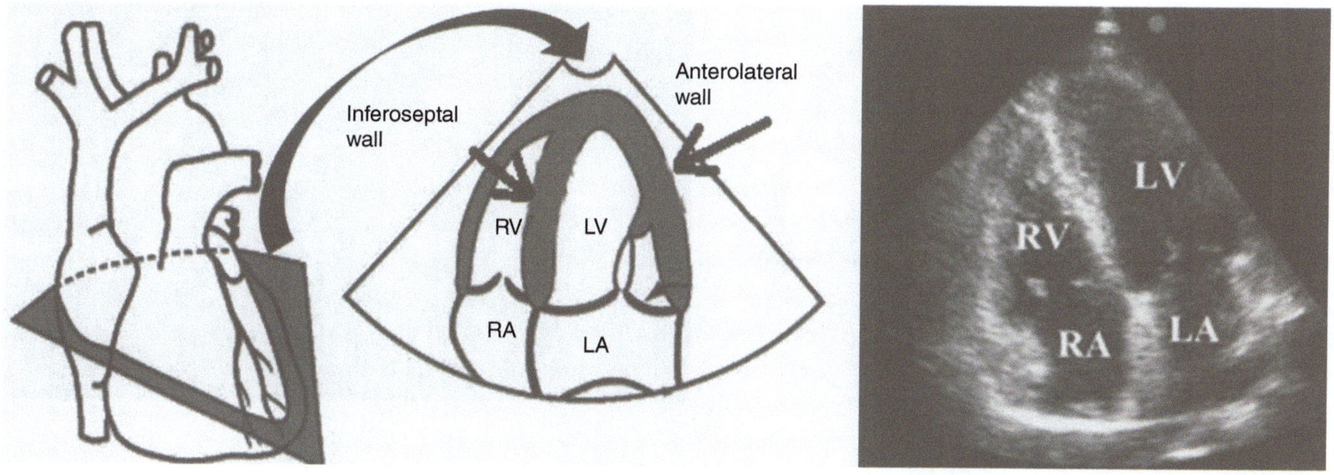

Fig. 2.16 The apical 4-chamber view in TTE permits the imaging of all 4 chambers of the heart and also the TV and the MV. This allows the imaging of all the chambers of the heart and also the TV and the MV and their respective apparatus

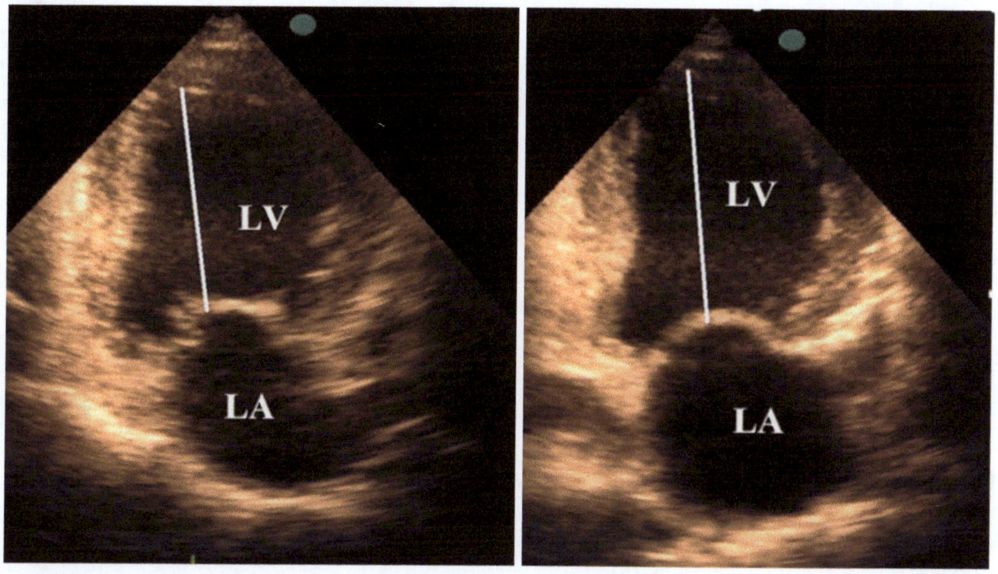

Fig. 2.17 *Left panel*: Foreshortened LV apex that is a false image of apex and thickness is the same as the LV wall. *Right panel* showing thin true apex

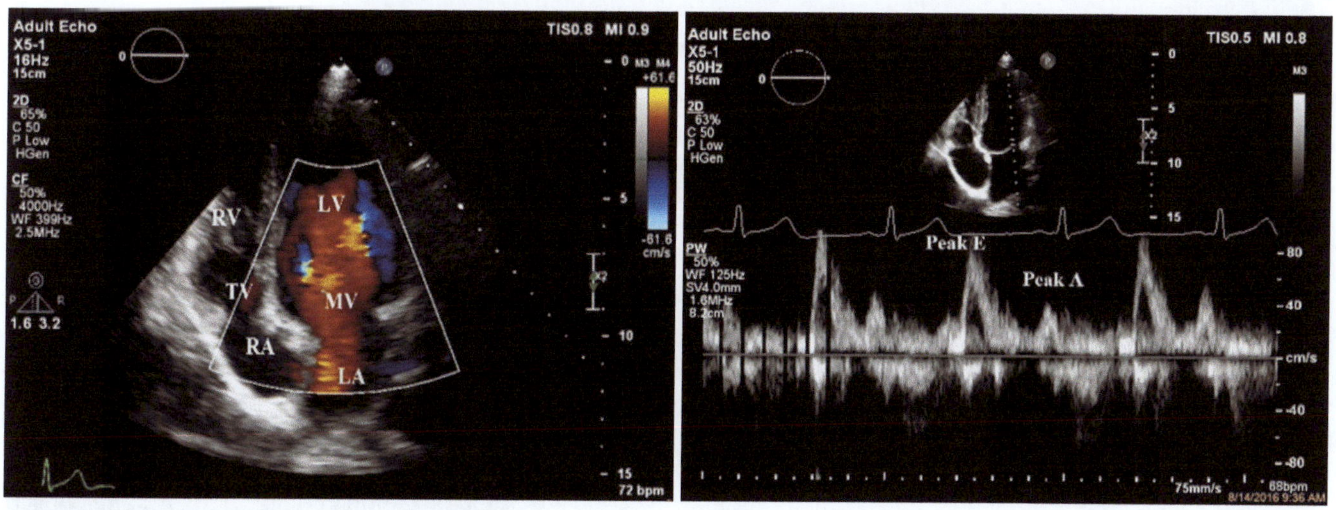

Fig. 2.18 *Left*: Color flow imaging of Mitral inflow showing low velocity red diastolic flow from left atrium to left ventricle. *Right*: First positive deflection (E wave) signifies early passive LV filling, and the consequent deflection (A wave) imitates the late phase of LV filling (LA contraction), Normal E wave velocity is less than 1.2 m/s and for the A wave velocity is less than 0.8 m/s

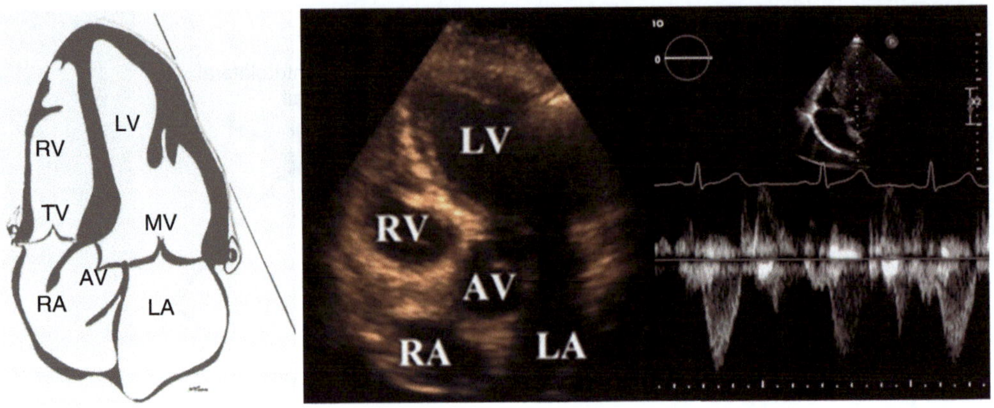

Fig. 2.19 Superficial angulation of the scanning plane from the apical 4-chamber view brings the left ventricular outflow tract (LVOT) and the AV into view and creates a 5-chamber view

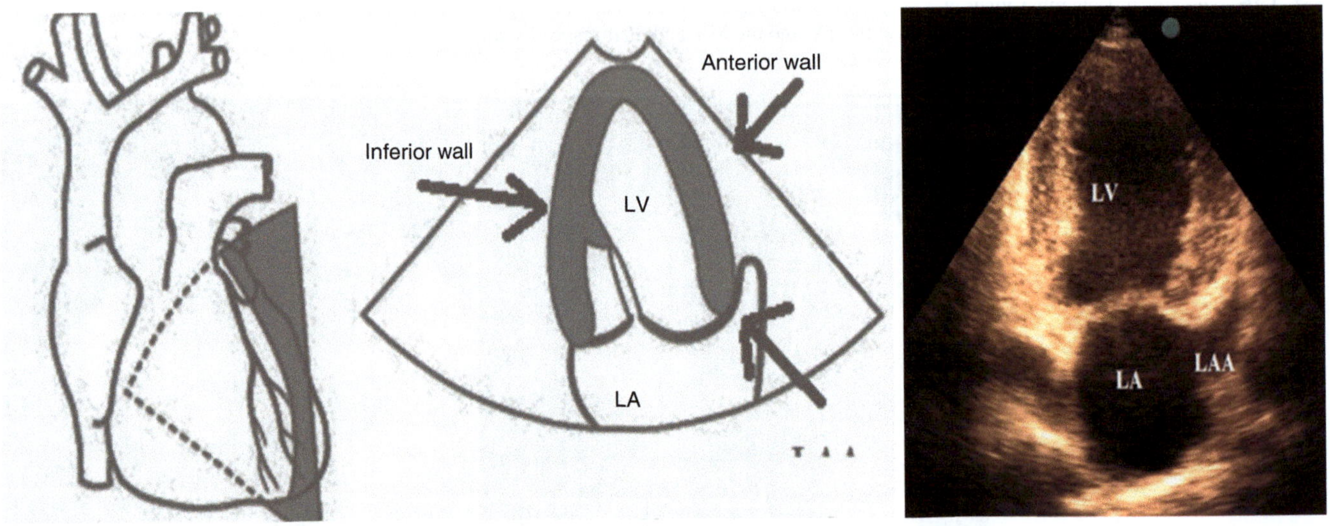

Fig. 2.20 The apical 2-chamber view allows direct imaging of the true inferior and anterior walls of the LV

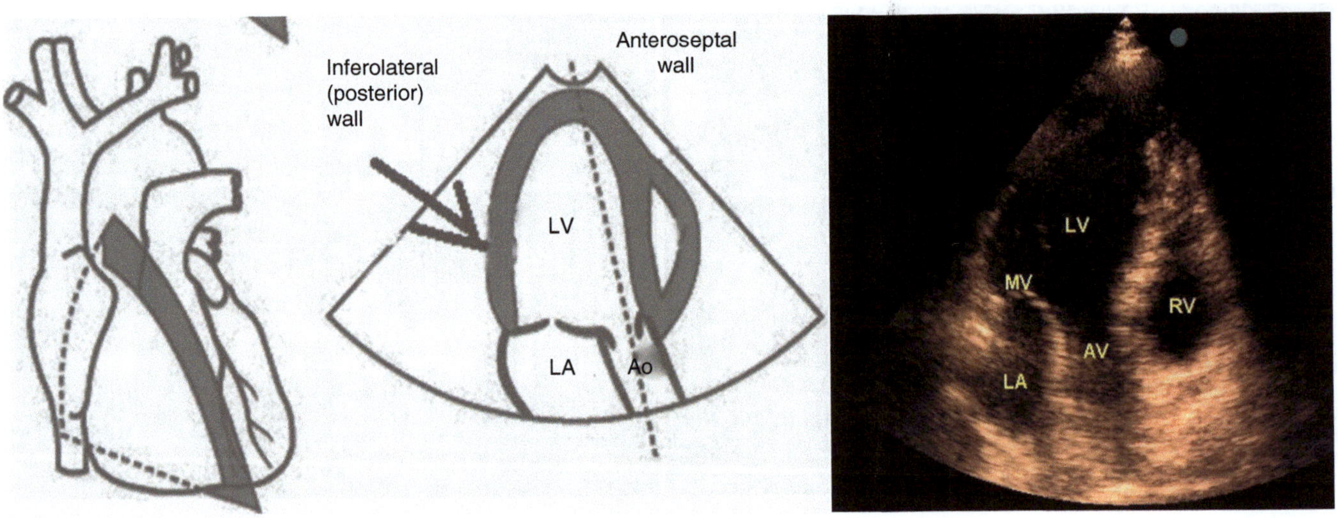

Fig. 2.21 Apical 3 chamber view or apical long axis view allows direct imaging of the inferolateral and anteroseptal walls of the LV

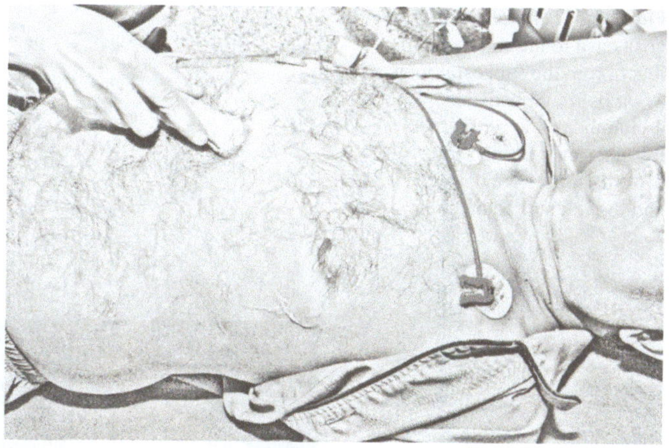

Fig. 2.22 A series of important long- and short-axis images are typically obtained from this chief window. This window can be the only viewpoint to image the heart in a patient with hyperinflated lungs, chest wall injury, or pneumothorax

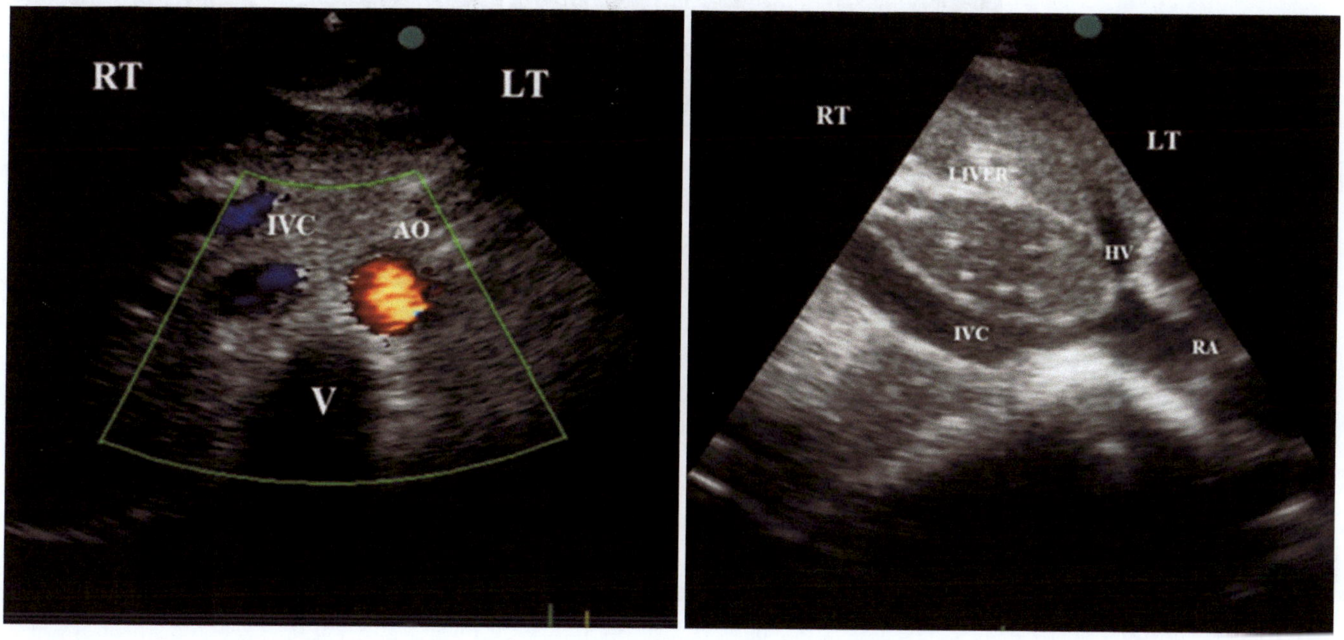

Fig. 2.23 *Left*: Subcostal view Inferior vena cava (IVC) to the right and Aorta (AO) at the left of the vertebra(V). *Right*: IVC continuity to the right atrium (RA), Hepatic vein (HV)

- The suprasternal window is used to record the flow in the ascending and also descending aorta and in the SVC.

Right parasternal view:

- The right parasternal border can also be beneficial for viewing the heart in either longitudinal or transverse orientation. These views are principally helpful with medially positioned hearts as well as in RV enlargement and rightward orientation of the ascending aorta. This view should be examined in all patients with aortic valve and aortic root disease (Fig. 2.28) [7, 8].

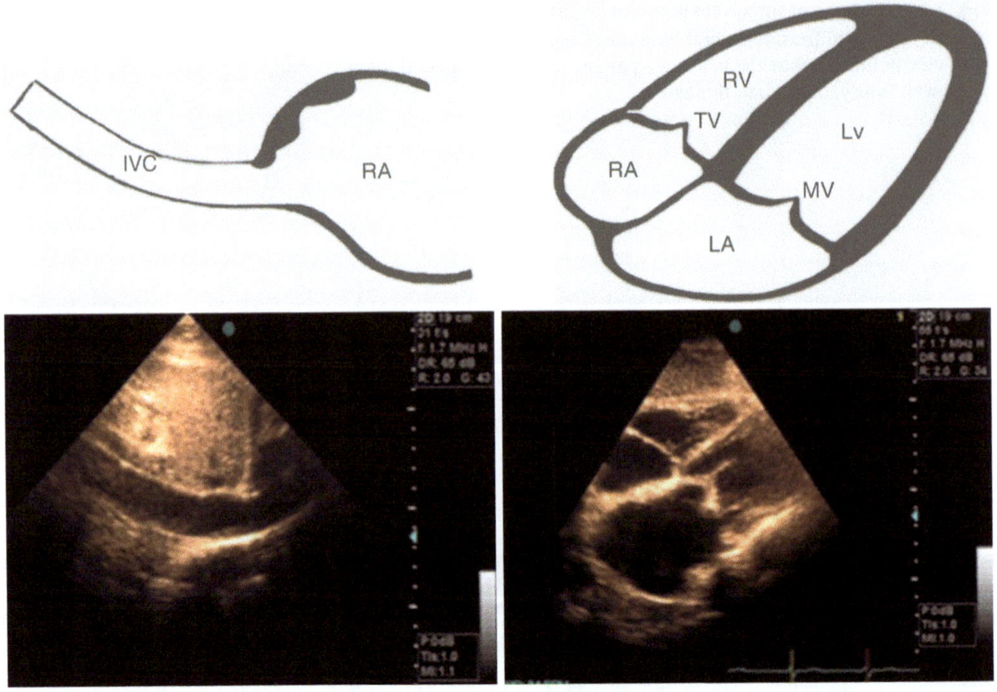

Fig. 2.24 *Left panel*. Inferior vena cava to the right atrium junction in the subcostal view. *Right panel*. Subcostal 4-chamber view is obtained by superiorly tilting probe towards suprasternal notch and the left supraclavicular

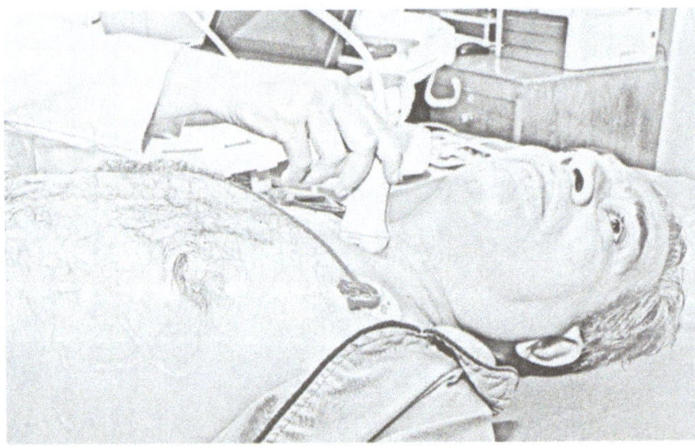

Fig. 2.25 The suprasternal view is achieved by placing the transducer in the suprasternal notch

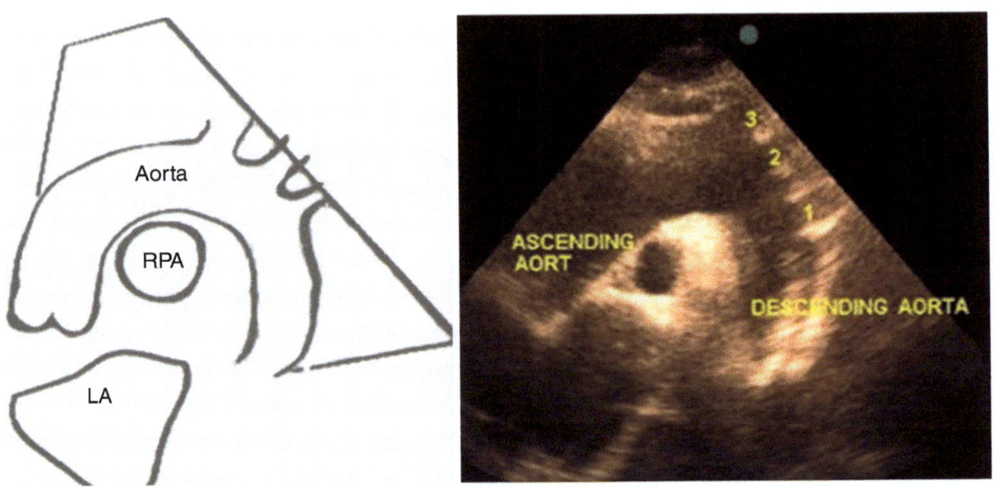

Fig. 2.26 Suprasternal long-axis view, showing the aortic arch and branches besides the short axis of the right pulmonary artery, 1: subclavian artery, 2: Left carotid artery, 3: Innominate artery

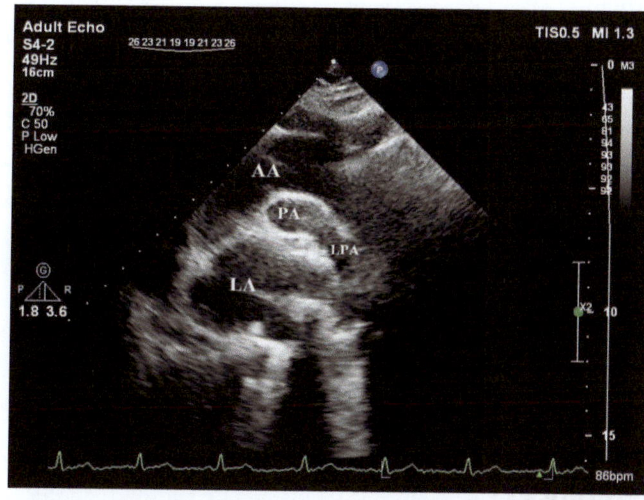

Fig. 2.27 Suprasternal long-axis view, showing the aortic arch and branches besides the short axis of the right pulmonary artery. *AA* Ascending Aorta, *LA* Left atrium, *PA* Pulmonary Artery, *LPA* Left pulmonary artery

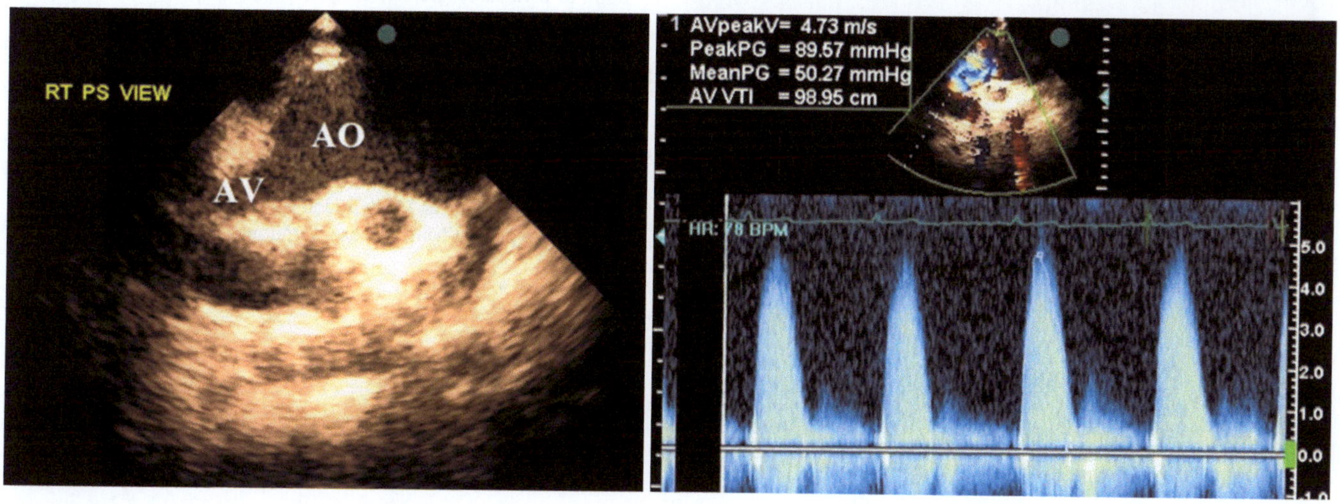

Fig. 2.28 Patient should be positioned in the right lateral and probe pointing toward left arm. The max pressure gradient (89 mmHg) in aortic stenosis obtained in right parasternal view

Questions

1. In the parasternal RV inflow view which structure is shown by question mark and star?

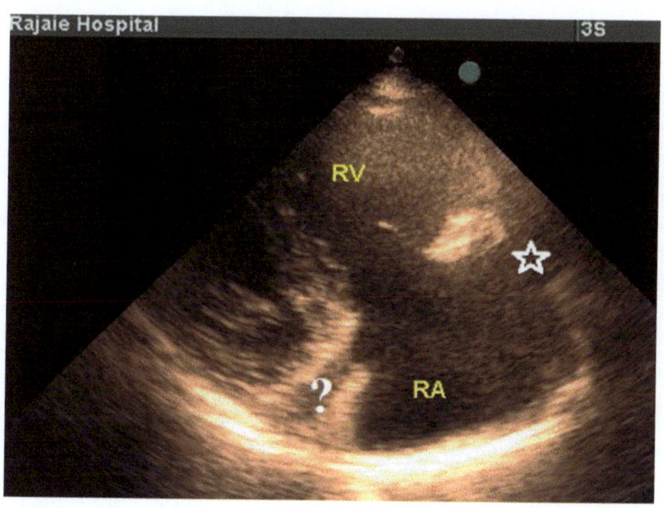

   A. Question mark is IVC and star is SVC
   B. Question mark is CS and star is SVC
   C. Question mark is IVC and star is CS
   D. Question mark is CS and star is IVC

2. Doppler flow study of the Aortic valve in the right parasternal view is shown:
   A. Above the baseline
   B. Below the baseline
   C. Above and below the baseline (mirror image)
   D. This view is not a good view for AV Doppler study

3. For obtaining Apical 3 chamber view from apical 4 chamber view which of the following is correct:
   A. 60°–90° counterclockwise rotation of the transducer, placed in apical 4 chamber yields an apical 3-chamber.
   B. 60°–90° clockwise rotation of the transducer, placed in apical 4 chamber yields an apical 3-chamber.

C. 60°–90° counterclockwise rotation of the transducer, placed in apical 2 chamber yields an apical 3-chamber.
D. 60°–90° clockwise rotation of the transducer, placed in apical 2 chamber yields an apical 3-chamber.

Answers

1. B
2. A
3. C

References

1. Henry W, Demaria A, Raymond G, King D, Kisslo J, Popp R, et al. Report of the American Society of Echocardiography Committee on Nomenclature and Standards in Two-Dimensional Echocardiography. Circulation. 1980;62:2.
2. Gardin JM, Adams D, Douglas PD, Feigenbaum H, Forst DH, Fraser AG et al. Recommendations for a standardized report for adult transthoracic echocardiography. JASE. 2002.
3. Picard M, Adams D, Bierig SM, Dent JM, Douglas PD, Gillam LD et al. Recommendations for quality echocardiography laboratory operations. J Am Soc Echocardiogr. 2011.
4. Douglas PS, Garcia MJ, Haines DE. ACCF/ASE/ACCP/AHA/ASNC/HFSA/HRS/SCAI/SCCM/SCCT/SCMR 2011 Appropriate use criteria for echocardiography. A report of the American College of Cardiology Foundation Appropriate Use Criteria Task Force, American Society of Echocardiography, American Heart Association, American Society of Nuclear Cardiology, Heart Failure Society of America, Heart Rhythm Society, Society for CardiovascularAngiography and Interventions, Society of Critical Care Medicine, Society of Cardiovascular Computed Tomography, and Society for Cardiovascular Magnetic Resonance. J Am Coll Cardiol. 2011;57:1126.
5. Lai W, Geva T, Shirali G, Frommelt P, Humes R, Brook MM, et al. Guidelines and Standards for Performance of a Pediatric Echocardiogram: a Report from the Task Force of the Pediatric Council of the American Society of Echocardiography. J Am Soc Echocardiogr. 2006;19:1413–30.
6. Oh JK, Seward JB, Tajik AJ. The Echo Manual. 3rd ed. Philadelphia: Lippincott Williams & Wilkins.
7. Lancellotti P, Zamorano JL, Habib G, Badano L. The EACVI textbook of echocardiography, Chapter 3. In: Kasprzak J, Sadeghpour A, Jurcut R, editors. Doppler echocardiography. 2nd ed. Oxford: Oxford University Press; 2017.
8. Zipes D, Libby P, Bonow R. Braunwald's heart disease : a textbook of cardiovascular medicine. 10th ed. Philadelphia: Saunders, Elsevier Inc.
9. Armstrong WF, Hyan T. Feigenbaum's echocardiography. 7th ed; 2010.
10. Sadeghpour A, Kiavar M, Alizadehasl A. Comprehensive approach to adult congenital heart disease. London: Springer; 2014.

Transesophageal Echocardiography

3

Azin Alizadehasl, Anita Sadeghpour,
and Fahimeh Khesali

Abstract

Transesophageal echocardiography (TEE) has a key role in evaluation of mitral valve lesions, the left atrium or its appendage, atrial septal defects, intracardiac masses, endocarditis and its complications, and thoracic aortic lesions such as aortic dissection. Patients with atrial fibrillation undergo direct-current cardioversion without chronic anticoagulation if TEE does not show intracardiac thrombi. With ablation procedures, atrial fibrillation has become one of the most common reasons for TEE referrals. The crucial role of TEE in the operating room and the cath lab for the assessment of the result of various valvular repair, and interventional procedures has been proved.

In this chapter, we will review the indications and contraindications of TEE as well as its standard views and necessary preparations.

Keywords

Transthoracic echocardiography · Standard windows · Echocardiographic views · Valvular heart disease · Interventional TEE · Intraoperative TEE

Abbreviations

AV	Aortic valve
IAS	Inter-atrial septum
IE	Infective endocarditis
IVC	Inferior vena cava
IVS	Inter-ventricular septum
LA	Left atrium
LAA	Left atrial appendage
LLPV	Left lower pulmonary vein
LUPV	Left upper pulmonary vein
LV	Left ventricle
LVOT	Left ventrivular outflow tract
MV	Mitral valve
MVLs	Mitral valve leaflets
P	Posterior
RA	Right atrium
RLPV	Right lower pulmonary vein
RUPV	Right upper pulmonary vein
RV	Right ventricle
RVOT	Right ventricular outflow tract
SVC	Superior vena cava
TEE	Transesophageal echocardiography
TTE	Transthoracic Echocardiography
TVLs	Tricuspid valve leaflets

A. Alizadehasl, MD, FACC, FASE
Associate Professor of Cardiology, Echocardiologist, Echocardiography and Cardiogenetic Research Centers, Cardio-Oncology Department, Rajaie Cardiovascular Medical and Research Center, Tehran, Iran

A. Sadeghpour, MD, FACC, FASE (✉) · F. Khesali
Professor of Cardiology, Echocardiography Research Center, Rajaie Cardiovascular Medical and Research Center, Iran University of Medical Science, Tehran, Iran

Preparations for Transesopheageal Echocardiography

- Transesophageal echocardiography (TEE) is a semi-invasive technique that can be very uncomfortable in unprepared patients. Indeed, patients must be cognizant as to why TEE is done. The entire procedure must be explained; this includes even rare side effects (1%) or complications such as laryngospasm, shortness of breath, transient throat pain, methemoglobinemia, aspiration, hypotension, hypertension, tachycardia, esophageal rupture, and even the very rare risk of death. For an elective TEE, the case must fast for at least 6 hours before this procedure. A history of clinically significant dysphagia or any other esophageal disease must be assessed before TEE is done [1, 2].

A. Sadeghpour, A. Alizadehasl (eds.), *Case-Based Textbook of Echocardiography*,
https://doi.org/10.1007/978-3-319-67691-3_3

- If the patient has dentures, they must be removed. Every patient must have a perfect intravenous access for the administration of any contrast agent or necessary medications.
- Closely before intubation with the transesophageal probe, local anesthetic spray in tandem with other anesthetic drugs is used, the details of which are provided in the next chapter.
- Prophylaxis for sub-acute bacterial endocarditis is not necessary or commonly used even in cases with a prosthetic valve [3].
- A nasogastric or endotracheal tube typically does not interfere considerably with esophageal intubation by the TEE probe or hinder the acquisition of desirable images. Esophageal perforation is an infrequent but calamitous complication of TEE. TEE must not be done in cases with dysphagia without further assessment of the esophagus. Also, intubation of a TEE probe must not be forced. Prolonged intubation of the probe, especially during an operation, might increase the risk of perforation. Importantly, when the TEE probe is not used intraoperatively, it can be disconnected from the echo machine to diminish thermal injury. Also, it is important that the TEE probe not be left in the esophagus or stomach in the locked position [1, 4].
- The TEE probe is a changed gastro-esophageal endoscopy probe, classically with a 3- to 7-MHz ultrasound transducer at its tip. It can be manipulated to different positions in the esophagus and stomach, so the heart and other cardiovascular and adjacent structures may be imaged. The diameter of the adult transducer tip is 9–14 mm, and this is scaled down to less than 3 mm for pediatric and neonatal and even fetal use [1–3].
- All adult probes use multi-plane transducers, which can be rotated in 180°. The transducer typically is rotated by a "finger pressure sensitive" switch. The tip of the probe also can be ante-flexed or retro-flexed or moved side to side by larger knobs on the probe. The elective examination starts with the patient in the left lateral decubitus position. The TEE procedure room is furnished with oral suction, pulse oximeter, oxygen supply, and importantly all cardiopulmonary resuscitation abilities. In critically ill cases for whom transfer is difficult and high risk, the examination is done at the bedside. For a mechanically ventilated patient, the TEE probe is frequently introduced with the patient in the supine position [1, 4].
- A bite guard is usually used to protect and keep the TEE probe, except when the patient is edentulous. When the scope is introduced, the sensitive imaging surface of the transducer faces the patient's tongue, which directs the ultrasound beam from the posteriorly located esophagus and anteriorly toward the cardiac system. A digital technique is commonly employed for esophageal intubation. When the probe is introduced, the posterior portion of the tongue is depressed with the left index finger to minimize tongue movement, and the tip of the transducer is placed over the left index finger to a position at the center of the tongue. After the transducer is in the correct position, the left index finger is placed over the distal shaft or tip of the probe and depressed directly and straight downward onto the tongue. This places the tip of the probe in direct alignment with the posteriorly located esophagus and away from the anteriorly located trachea. The tip of the transducer is advanced smoothly and slowly posteriorly toward the esophagus. At this time, the patient is asked to swallow. The tip of the TEE transducer must be advanced into the esophagus without force or notable resistance. The distance from the incisors to the part of the esophagus behind the mid left atrium is nearly 30 cm [1–3, 5].
- Injury by TEE can be from direct trauma to the airway and esophagus, and from indirect effects of TEE. Direct trauma to the airway and esophagus could lead to esophageal bleeding, tearing, dysphagia and laryngeal discomfort. Bacteraemia and transient vocal cord paralysis have also been reported. Airway compression by a biplane pediatric TEE probe in a child has also been reported.
- Absolute contraindications for TEE:

- Perforated viscus
- Esophageal stricture
- Esophageal tumor
- Esophageal perforation, laceration
- Esophageal diverticulum
- Active upper GI bleed

- Relative contraindications:

- History of radiation to neck and mediastinum
- History of GI surgery
- Recent upper GI bleed
- Barrett's esophagus
- History of dysphagia
- Restriction of neck mobility (severe cervical arthritis, atlantoaxial joint disease)
- Symptomatic hiatal hernia
- Esophageal varices
- Coagulopathy, thrombocytopenia
- Active esophagitis
- Active peptic ulcer disease

Principals of Trans-Esopheageal Echocardiography Examination

- TEE is an invaluable imaging modality in patients with suboptimal transthoracic echocardiography (TTE) windows and specific cardiovascular diseases, rendering diagnoses and guiding therapy in the operating room,

Table 3.1 Major applications of transesophageal echocardiography

Valvular heart disease
Aortic, mitral, tricuspid, pulmonic, prosthetic valves
Interventional imaging
Atrial fibrillation ablation; LA appendage/patent foramen ovale/atrial or ventricular septal defect closure; transcatheter aortic and MV procedures
Intraoperative imaging
Cardiac valves and aorta surgeries, congenital heart disease repair
Cardiac thrombus and embolus valuation
Precardioversion in atrial fibrillation, cardiac source of embolus
Endocarditis and cardiac mass investigation
Vegetations, endocarditis-induced valvular complications, thrombus, tumor
Aortic disease
Aortic dissection, dilatation, hematoma
Critically ill cases
Hemodynamic management of cases in intensive care unit

cardiac catheterization laboratory, and critical care areas. TEE uses a specifically designed ultrasound probe, inserted in a gastroscope.

- In contrast to TTE, TEE placement of the transducer in the esophagus allows for improved visualization of relatively posterior cardiac structures and also provides improved acoustic windows in the absence of intervening structures and air. TEE is most often indicated when TTE imaging is likely to be non-diagnostic or when highly detailed images are needed such as imaging prosthetic valves.
- TEE plays an increasingly essential role in cases with valvular heart disease, particularly during transcatheter cardiac interventions in catheterization laboratories and hybrid operating rooms, and afterward in critical care units [6, 7] (Table 3.1).
- Because of the close proximity of the esophagus and the TEE transducer to the heart, TEE probes use high frequency transducers (5.0–7.5 MHz), which allow a better description of the small structures than the lower frequencies used in TTE (2.5–3.5 MHz).
- Currently, TEE probes are multi-plane probes, in which the ultrasound plane is electronically steered over an arc of 180°.
- All the currently available TEE probes employ 5-MHz transducer. The transducer is mounted on the tip of a gastroscope housing. The tip of the probe is flexible. There are two knobs on the proximal handle. One knob controls anterior and posterior movement (ante flexion and retro flexion) while other knob controls side-to-side movements. One electronic switch is available to scan the heart in various axial views and can visualize the heart in 0 to 180°. Various echocardiographic windows are possible because of the ability to advance and withdraw the probe and to rotate it in combination with ante flexion and retroflexion of probe tip. The probes are of various types; monoplane, biplane or multi-plane. The probes are available in two sizes adult and pediatric (Fig. 3.1).
- Ultrasound wave penetration is affected by fat, bone and air-containing images. Trans-thoracic echocardiographic views will be difficult to obtain in patients with obesity, emphysema, or chest wall abnormality. TEE transducer has advantage that sound waves emitted from the transducer have to pass through the esophageal wall and pericardium to reach the heart. Image distortion due to interference with other media is unlikely. As compared to trans-thoracic transducer, esophageal transducer is in the stable position; hence, continuous recording of cardiac activity for extended period is possible during TEE. Another advantage of TEE is that it does not interfere with surgical field.
- Intraoperative TEE is performed in anaesthetized patients; hence TEE probe is inserted after induction of anesthesia and endotracheal intubation. A lubricated TEE probe is inserted into hypopharynx with the patient's neck in extended position. The probe will be advanced into the esophagus with minimal force. During this manoeuvre the control knobs of the probe should be in neutral. If more than minimal resistance is encountered, one should use laryngoscope to guide the probe into esophagus. Bite block is essential to prevent damage to teeth and the transducer during probe manoeuvring.
- In TEE, the anteroposterior orientation of the images from the esophagus is the reverse of the images from the TTE window because the ultrasound beam first meets the more posterior structures close to the esophagus.

Transesophageal Echocardiographic Windows

There are 4 main positions within the esophagus from which the standard TEE scan planes may be acquired. These 4 "windows" are (1) upper esophageal, (2) mid esophageal, (3) transgastric, and (4) deep transgastric. From these 4 positions, in combination with appropriate scan plane angulations, all the aforementioned cross-sectional views of the Society of Cardiovascular Anesthesiologists-20 (SCA-20) may be imaged. An alternative way to organize the scan plane images is by "structure of interest". For example, the mitral valve may be imaged from the mid-esophageal level from multiple scan angles, from the transgastric level, and from the deep transgastric level.

In 1999, a combined taskforce of the SCA and the American Society of Echocardiography (ASE) produced a set of guidelines for a comprehensive intraoperative TEE study. A subset of 20 views was produced, which was termed the "SCA-20 standard views". A comprehensive study should contain (but not limited to) these in conjunction with qualitative and quantitative Doppler studies as

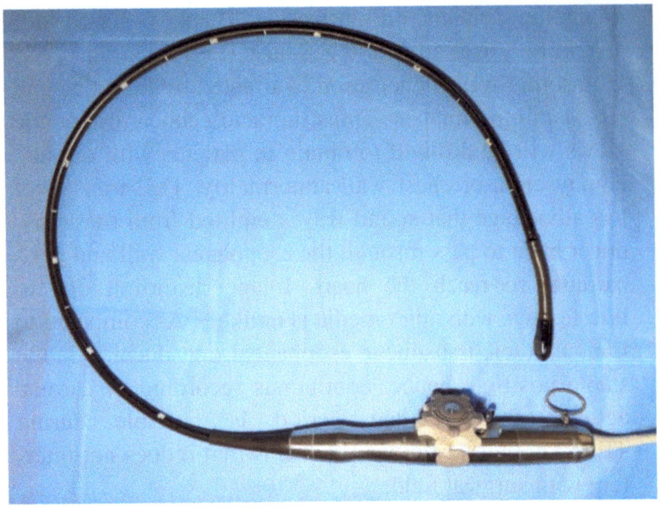

Fig. 3.1 Transesophageal probe. The expansion of the standard imaging set was an attempt to elevate the use of TEE beyond basic intraoperative imaging and to present and refine views that are helpful in certain diagnostic applications and/or catheter-based procedures [6–9]

Table 3.2 Comprehensive TEE examination: the old 20 and new 28 views

The old "20 Views" of TEE	The new "28 Views" of TEE
	1. ME 5 chamber
I. ME 4 chamber	2. ME 4 chamber
II. ME commissural	3. ME commissural
III. ME 2 chamber	4. ME 2 chamber
IV. ME LAX	5. ME LAX
V. ME AV LAX	6. ME AV LAX
VI. ME Asc aorta LAX	7. ME Asc aorta LAX
VII. ME Asc aorta SAX	8. ME Asc aorta SAX
	9. ME RT.PUL vein
VIII. ME AV SAX	10. ME AV SAX
IX. ME RV in—out	11.ME RV in-out
	12. ME modified Bicaval
X. ME Bicaval	13. ME Bicaval
	14. UE right and left Pulmunary veins
	15.ME LAX
XI. TG basal SAX	16. TG basal SAX
XII. TG mid SAX	17. TG mid SAX
	18. TG apical SAX
	19.TG RV basal view
	20. TG RV inflow-outflow
XIII. dTG LAX	21. dTG 5 chamber
XIV. TG 2-chamber	22. TG 2-chamber
XV. TG RV inflow	23. TG RV inflow
XVI. TG LAX	24. TG LAX
XVII. Desc aortic SAX	25. desc aortic SAX
XVIII. Desc aortic SAX	26. desc aortic SAX
XIX. UE aortic arch LAX	27. UE aortic arch LAX
XX. UE aortic arch SAX	28. UE aortic arch SAX

AV aortic valve; *dTG* deep transgastric; *ME* mid-esophageal; *LAV* long axis view; *LAX* long axis view; *RT.PUL* right pulmonary; *RV* right ventricular; *SAX* short axis view; *TG* transgastric; *UE* upper-esophageal

indicated. There were several routinely acquired views omitted from this set. In addition, several structures which should be part of the routine study (i.e., right ventricle, left atrial appendage, left ventricular outflow tract, and pulmonary veins) were either only limitedly represented or omitted completely.

The most recent ASE/SCA document (2013) has incorporated 8 new views. Several are just additions of views commonly used, albeit not incorporated into the original 20 (i.e., mid-esophageal 5-chamber, modified bicaval view and trans-gastric apical short-axis) while the others para-atrial structures (i.e., mid-esophageal right pulmonary veins, upper-esophageal right and left pulmonary veins, and mid-esophageal left atrial appendage) and the right ventricle (transgastric right ventricular basal view and also trans-gastric right ventricular inflow-outflow) (Table 3.2).

Performing a Comprehensive Transesophageal Echocardiography Study (2D)

There are 2 basic schemes for performing a comprehensive study. The underlying principle is to ensure a complete and comprehensive study. This may be achieved by either acquiring images from a given level within the esophagus (e.g., upper, middle, trans-gastric, or deep transgastric) or by organizing the study based upon "structure of interest" (e.g., left ventricle, mitral valve, aortic valve, etc.). Both systems work, each with its strengths and limitations. Esophageal level-focused studies have the advantage of limiting the movement of the probe, which may allow a global or 3D sequential imaging strategy and might be best tolerated in a sedated, if not completely anesthetized, patient. The structure-focused study may facilitate a more comprehensive study of the valves and chambers in question and may allow the interrogation of a particular structure from varying levels or vantage points.

Whichever system is used, the most important point is to document and communicate the findings. This is essential to a complete study [6–8].

Organized by Differing Levels in the Esophagus

In this sequence, the study begins in the upper esophageal level and proceeds distally from the mid-esophageal level, to the transgastric level and then to the deep transgastric level. In this fashion, minimal probe movement up and down the esophagus occurs. This may be better tolerated in a sedated patient; however, it is of little consequence when the TEE study is done under general anesthesia and tracheal intubation. It does need the operator to integrate views of various structures across various scan levels. The structure viewed from the upper esophageal level is the aortic arch in the short- and long-axis views.

Advancing the probe distally, the operator arrives at the level of the left atrium and the mid-esophageal vantage point, usually starting at 0° and retro-flexion and the development of the mid-esophageal 4-chamber view. Typically, the array is advanced form 0- to 120 + °, and full interrogation of the mitral valve, aortic valve, interatrial septum, left atrial appendage, and pulmonary veins is done. At the same time, the walls of the left ventricle are studied as well. Images of the SCA-20 that are acquired at this level are illustrated below.

Color-flow Doppler might be added for better interrogation of the mitral and aortic valves as regards stenosis and regurgitation. More details may be acquired by changing the depth setting to a shallower area when studying the 2 valves when compared to imaging the more distal ventricular walls. Right-side study of the tricuspid valve, pulmonic valve, and right atrial and right ventricular outflow tracts is done by turning the probe to the right side and similarly progressing through the scan plane. The proximal ascending aorta is also imaged form this level in both short- and long-axis views.

Upon the completion of mid-esophageal level imaging, the probe is returned to 0° and advanced more distally to the transgastric level. Here, short- and long-axis view imaging of both ventricles is done and the subvalvular apparatus of the mitral and tricuspid valves is visualized. The descending aorta is then imaged either from the mid-esophageal or transgastric level; however, it needs the counterclockwise turning of the probe ~120°. The final views are completed by further advancement to the deep transgastric level and retro-flexion to acquire the deep transgastric long-axis view. This view is most common for the Doppler flow interrogation of the left ventricular outflow tract and the aortic valve as it affords parallel beam alignment to the blood flow [6, 7, 10, 11].

Structure-Focused TEE Study Sequence

As was previously mentioned, the disadvantage of an esophageal-level study sequence is that the views of the structures must be integrated across different level scan sequences. As an alternative strategy and one typically more easily understood by more inexperienced echocardiographers, the studies now proceed according to "structure of interest". Classically, the sequence will progress from evaluating the left ventricle from both transgastric and mid-esophageal levels with scan planes optimized at these levels to image the ventricular walls. The views incorporate the transgastric short-axis view at the mid papillary, basal, and apical levels. Advancing the multi-plane angle develops the transgastric, 2-chamber, and aortic valve long-axis view as well. Next, the mitral valve is imaged from the transgastric level, followed by the mid-esophageal level. Depth is usually dropped when compared to that utilized for left ventricular interrogation, and sequential views with and without color-flow Doppler are acquired. Thus, the sequence might be the mid-esophageal 4-chamber, commissural 2-chamber, and aortic valve long-axis view. Spectral Doppler is applied to complete the mitral valve study. The aortic valve is next typically imaged in the mid-esophageal aortic valve short-axis and long-axis views and is complemented with color-flow Doppler and finally spectral Doppler from the deep transgastric position. Subsequently, the left atrial structures, including the pulmonary veins, are viewed. Turning the probe to the right helps to image the interatrial septum in the 4-chamber and bicaval views [6].

Right-side study of the tricuspid valve, right atrium, and right ventricle is carried out at both mid-esophageal and transgastric levels. Finally, the probe is returned to the mid-esophageal level and then rotated ~120° counterclockwise to image the descending aorta in the short- and long-axis views before it is withdrawn to complete the study of the aortic arch.

Imaging the descending aorta is possible by turning the probe 120° to 140° counterclockwise, setting the center display on Aorta, decreasing the depth, and maximizing the megahertz. To image the aortic arch, the operator should withdraw the probe as far as the upper-esophageal window. The branches of the aortic arch can be identified via a longitudinal plane examination of the aortic arch. The left subclavian and the left common carotid arteries are positioned more posteriorly and are best visualized by the counterclockwise rotation of the transducer (Tables 3.3, 3.4, 3.5) and (Figs. 3.2, 3.3, 3.4, 3.5, 3.6, 3.7, 3.8, 3.9, 3.10, 3.11, 3.12, 3.13, 3.14, 3.15, 3.16, 3.17, 3.18, 3.19, 3.20, 3.21, 3.22, 3.23, and 3.24) [6–11].

Limitations of TEE in the Evaluation of the Ventricular Systolic and Diastolic Function

The ventricular apex may be foreshortened, unless care is taken to avoid this issue. If unnoticed or unaddressed, apical foreshortening may result in the underestimation of ventricular volumes.

Because Doppler beam alignment may be challenging, particularly of the aortic valve, Doppler-based ventricular function indices might not be as accurate with TEE. Although the evaluation of the diastolic function is accurately and efficiently done by TTE, in technically difficult situations or when TEE is being done for other purposes, TEE may be used to evaluate diastolic parameters. TEE can be used to

Table 3.3 Comprehensive TEE study and the imaged structures

Midesophageal views	
Transducer angle: ~0–10° **Level:** Mid-esophageal **Maneuver** (from prior image)**:** NA	Aortic valve LVOT Left atrium/right atrium Left ventricle/right ventricle/IVS Mitral valve (A_2-A_1-P_1) Tricuspid valve
Transducer angle: ~0–10° **Level:** Mid-esophageal **Maneuver** (from prior image)**:** Advance ± retroflex	Left atrium/right atrium IAS Left ventricle/right ventricle/IVS Mitral valve (A_2A_2-P_2P_1) Tricuspid valve
Transducer angle: ~50–70° **Level:** Mid-esophageal **Maneuver** (from prior image)**:** NA	Left atrium Coronary sinus Left ventricle Mitral valve (P_3-$A_3A_2A_1$-P_1) Papillary muscles Chordae tendinae
Transducer angle: ~80–100° **Level:** Mid-esophageal **Maneuver** (from prior image)**:** NA	Left atrium Coronary sinus Left atrial appendage Left ventricle Mitral valve (P_3-$A_3A_2A_1$)
Transducer angle: ~120–140° **Level:** Mid-esophageal **Maneuver** (from prior image)**:** NA	Left atrium Left ventricle LVOT RVOT Mitral valve (P_2-A_2) Aortic valve Proximal ascending aorta
Transducer angle: ~120–140° **Level:** Mid-esophageal **Maneuver** (from prior image)**:** Withdrawl ± anteflex	Left atrium LVOT RVOT Mitral valve (A_2-P_2) Aortic valve Proximal ascending aorta
Transducer angle: ~90–110° **Level:** Upper-esophageal **Maneuver** (from prior image)**:** Withdrawl	Mid-ascending aorta Right pulmonary artery
Transducer angle: ~0–30° **Level:** Upper-esophageal **Maneuver** (from prior image)**:** CW	Mid-ascending aorta (sax) Main/bifurcation Pulmonary artery Superior vena cava
Transducer angle: ~0–30° **Level:** Upper-esophageal **Maneuver** (from prior image)**:** CW, advance	Mid-ascending aorta Superior vena cava Right pulmonary veins
Transducer angle: ~25–450° **Level:** Mid-esophageal **Maneuver** (from prior image)**:** CCW, advance, Anteflex	Aortic valve Right atrium Left atrium Superior IAS RVOT Pulmonary valve
Transducer angle: ~50–70° **Level:** Mid-esophageal **Maneuver** (from prior image)**:** CW, advance	Aortic valve Right atrium Left atrium Superior IAS Tricuspid valve RVOT Pulmonary valve
Transducer angle: ~50–70° **Level:** Mid-esophageal **Maneuver** (from prior image)**:** CW	Right atrium Left atrium Mid-IAS Tricuspid valve Superior vena cava Inferior vena cava/coronary sinus
Transducer angle: ~90–110° **Level:** Mid-esophageal **Maneuver** (from prior image)**:** CW	Left atrium Right atrium/appendage IAS Superior vena cave Inferior vena cava
Transducer angle: ~90–110° **Level:** Upper-esophageal **Maneuver** (from prior image)**:** Withdraw, CW for the right veins, CCW for the left veins	Pulmonary vein (upper and lower) Pulmonary artery
Transducer angle: ~90–110° **Level:** Mid-esophageal **Maneuver** (from prior image)**:** Advance	Left atrial appendage Left upper pulmonary vein

A anterior; *CCW* counter clockwise; *CW* clockwise; *IAS* interatrial septum; *IVS* interventricular septum; *LAA* left atrial appendage; *LUPV* left upper pulmonary vein; *LVOT* left ventricular outflow tract; *NA* not applicable; *P* posterior; *RVOT* right ventricular outflow tract

acquire mitral inflow velocities, pulmonary vein velocities, and tissue Doppler velocity. Among these, access to all 4 pulmonary veins and an optimal orientation of the Doppler beam constitute particular advantages of TEE. Mitral inflow and annular tissue Doppler velocities are equally well assessed by TTE or TEE, unless the former images are poor quality or the position of the transducer is inaccessible [6, 10, 11].

Table 3.4 Transgastric views and the imaged structures

Transgastric views	
Transducer angle: ~0–20° **Level:** Transgastic **Maneuver (from prior image):** Advance ± Anteflex	Left ventricle (base) Right ventricle (base) Mitral valve (short-axis)
Transducer angle: ~0–20° **Level:** Transgastic **Maneuver (from prior image):** Advance ± Anteflex	Left ventricle (mid) Papillary muscles Right ventricle (mid)
Transducer angle: ~0–20° **Level:** Transgastic **Maneuver (from prior image):** Advance ± Anteflex	Left ventricle (apes) Right ventricle (apes)
Transducer angle: ~0–20° **Level:** Transgastic **Maneuver (from prior image):** Advance ± Anteflex	Left ventricle (mid) Right ventricle (mid) Right ventricular outflow tract Tricuspid valve (SAX) Pulmonary valve
Transducer angle: ~0–20° **Level:** Transgastic **Maneuver (from prior image):** Advance ± Anteflex	Right atrium Right ventricle Right ventricular outflow tract Pulmonary valve Tricuspid valve
Transducer angle: ~0–20° **Level:** Transgastic **Maneuver (from prior image):** Advance ± Anteflex	Left ventricle Left ventricular outflow tract Right ventricle Aortic valve Aortic root Mitral valve
Transducer angle: ~90–110° **Level:** Transgastic **Maneuver (from prior image):** Neutral flexion, withdraw	Left ventricle Left atrium/appendage Mitral valve
Transducer angle: ~90–110° **Level:** Transgastic **Maneuver (from prior image):** CW	Right ventricle Right atrium Tricuspid valve
Transducer angle: ~120–140° **Level:** Transgastic **Maneuver (from prior image):** CCW	Left ventricle Left ventricular outflow tract Right ventricle Aortic valve Aortic root Mitral valve

A anterior; *IAS* interatrial septum; *IVS* interventricular septum; *LAA* left atrial appendage; *LUPV* left upper pulmonary vein; *LVOT* left ventricular outflow tract; *NA* not applicable; *P* posterior; *RVOT* right ventricular outflow tract

Table 3.5 Aortic views

Aortic views	
Transducer angle: ~0–10° **Level:** Transgastric to mid-esophageal **Maneuver** (from prior image): Natural flexion	Descending aorta Left thorax Hemiazygous and Azygous veins Intercostal arteries
Transducer angle: ~90–100° **Level:** Transgastric to mid-esophageal **Maneuver** (from prior image): Neutral flexion	Descending aorta Left thorax
Transducer angle: ~0–10° **Level:** Upper esophageal **Maneuver** (from prior image): withdraw	Aortic arch Innominate vein Mediastinal tissue
Transducer angle: ~70–90° **Level:** Transgastric to mid-esophageal **Maneuver** (from prior image): NA	Aortic arch Innominate vein Pulmonary artery Mediastinal tissue

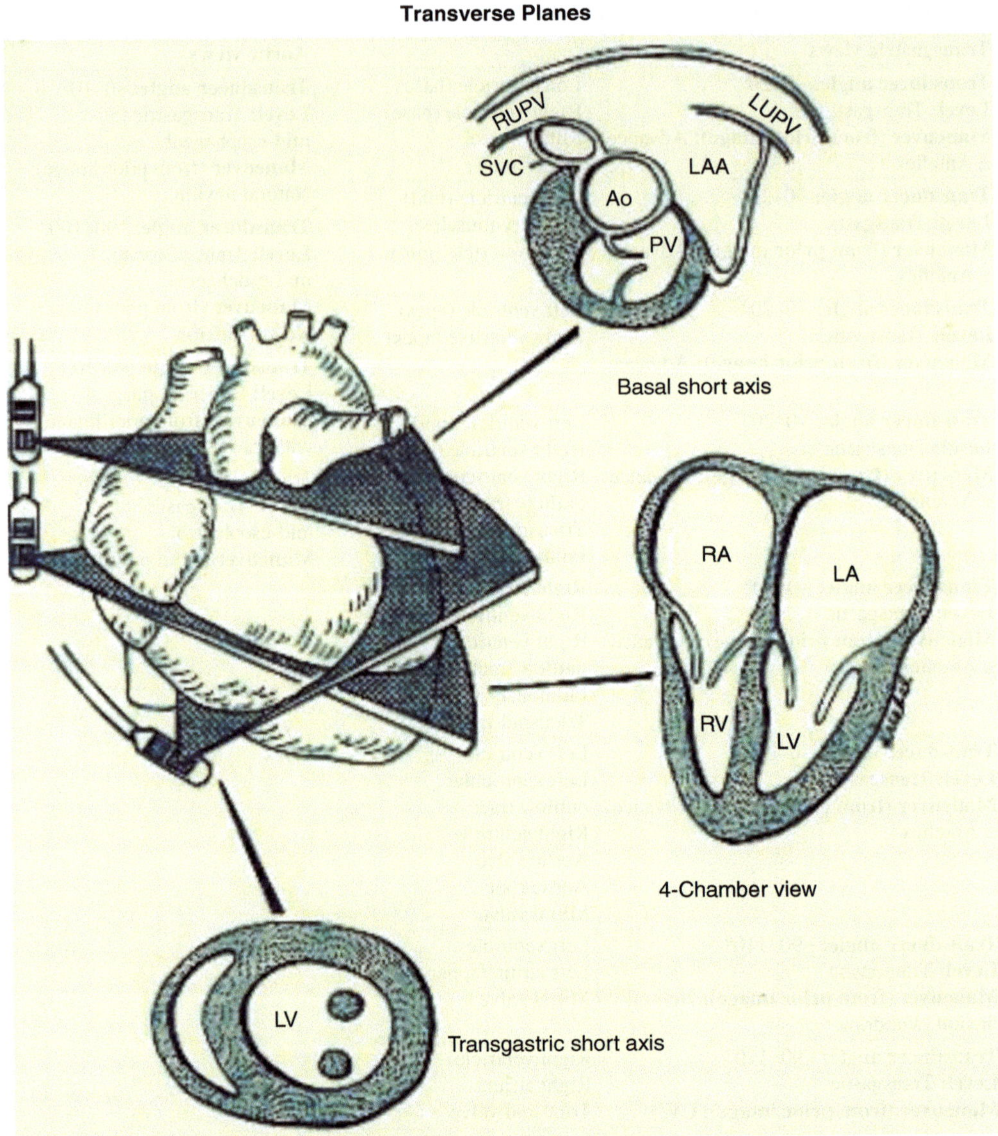

Fig. 3.2 Standard transverse planes perpendicular to the probe shaft

Left Atrium and Left Atrium Appendage

LA and LA appendage imaging has become an increasingly important role for TEE. The most common reason for TEE is cardiac source of embolus, and the LA appendage is a primary target for this assessment. The sensitivity and specificity of TEE to diagnose thrombus in the LA appendage are 100% and 99%, respectively, but cause of the complex nature of this structure, small (<2 mm) thrombi can be missed. Previous and recent support the use of TEE for the assessment of cardiac source of embolus or to facilitate clinical decision making in cases with atrial fibrillation or atrial flutter [6, 11].

Contrast TEE

In many cases, TEE avoids the physical contributors to poor TTE images such as soft tissue and intervening lung. In addition, the close proximity of the probe to the heart allows the use of higher transducer frequencies and thereby higher resolution images, albeit at the cost of far field attenuation. Though overall, endocardial definition must be better with TEE, on occasions, image quality might be limited. In such cases, contrast agents may improve border definition. Contrast administration also is able to augment Doppler signals. And finally, agitated saline contrast via a peripheral venous access is used to rule out atrial shunts [6, 11–13].

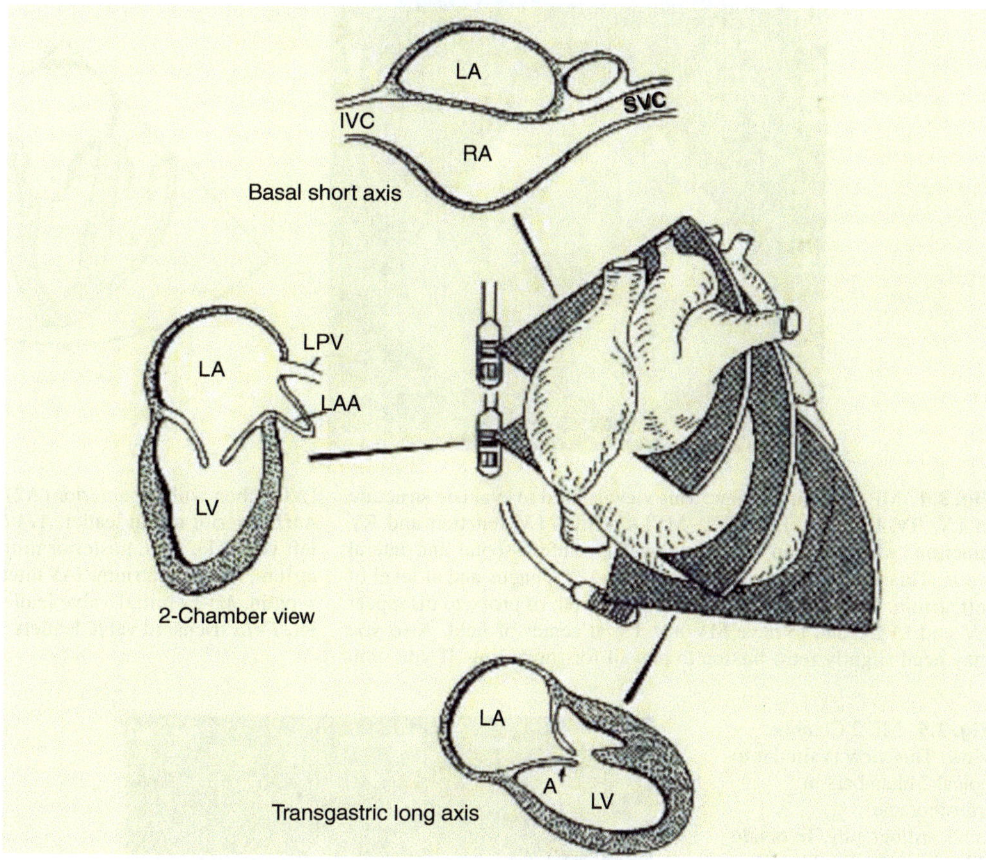

Fig. 3.3 Standard longitudinal planes perpendicular to the transverse planes

Shunt Study

TEE improves the diagnostic accuracy of shunt detection; false positive results on TTE were due to intrapulmonary shunts, and false-negative results were due to inadequate right atrial opacification.

The use of color Doppler alone with TTE reduces the sensitivity for shunt detection to 22% (with specificity, 96%). So, although PFO can be documented with color flow Doppler, the absence of flow across the foramen ovale must not be used to exclude PFO. Normally, cause of their large size (>5 mm), intra-venously injected saline bubbles are trapped in the lungs and do not appear in the left heart unless there is an intra-cardiac or intra-pulmonary shunt. The appearance of more than 3 saline bubbles in the left heart soon after opacification of the right heart (within 3 beats) is most consistent with the PFO. The timing of appearance of bubbles in the LA will depend on the pressure difference between the RA and LA. Some authors have advocated quantifying the relative size of the PFO by the number of microbubbles appearing in the LA: three to 10 microbubbles were defined as a small shunt, 11 to 30 micro-bubbles as a moderate shunt, and >30 micro-bubbles as a large shunt, however others have suggested that a PFO is present if more than one contrast bubble appears in the LA and a large shunt if >10 bubbles can be demonstrated in the LA. The sensitivity of detection of a right-to left shunt through a PFO may vary depending on the site of injection and RA pressure; femoral vein injections have the highest sensitivity, particularly in the setting of a prominent Eustachian valve. Intra-pulmonary shunting happens when there are arterio-venous communications that bypass the capillaries. After intra-venous injection, saline bubbles characteristically appear in the left heart after a delay (more than 3–8 cardiac cycles) [6, 10].

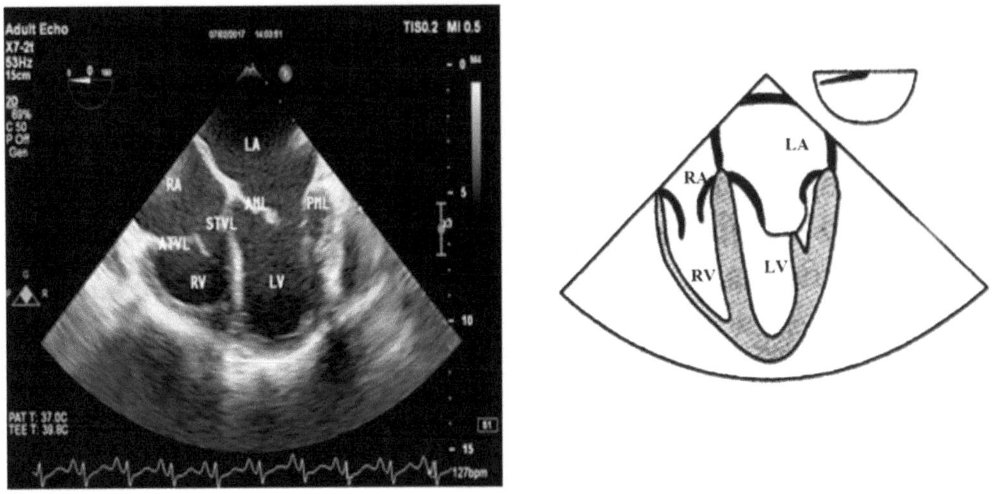

Fig. 3.4 ME 4 Chamber view: This view is used to evaluate structure of LV, RV, LA, RA, IAS, IVS, MVLs, TVLs, LV function and RV function. Also you can assess regional LV infero-septal and lateral walls. This view is obtained with 0° in mid esophagus and at level of left atrium. You should rotate and change depth of probe to disappear AV and LVOT and to have MV and TV at center of field. Also you may need slightly retro-flexion to prevail for-shortening. If you omit LVOT then will see anterior (A2) and posterior (P2) segments of MV. *AML* anterior mitral leaflet, *ATVL* anterior tricuspid valve leaflet, *LV* left ventricle, *PML* posterior mitral leaflet, *RV* right ventricle, *LA* left atrium, *RA* right atrium, *IAS* inter-atrial septum, *IVS* inter-ventricular septum, *MVLs* mitral valve leaflets, *STVL* septal tricuspid valve leaflet, *TVLs* tricuspid valve leaflets

Fig. 3.5 ME 2 Chamber view: This view is similar to apical 2 chambers in transthoracic echocardiography. To obtain this view you should insert probe at level similar ME 4 chamber but in 90° until RV no longer is displayed. Disappeared. You can assess LV, LA, MV and LAA. In this view you determine anterior (A3) and posterior (P3) segments of MV. Also LV anterior and posterior walls are addressed. *CS* coronary sinus

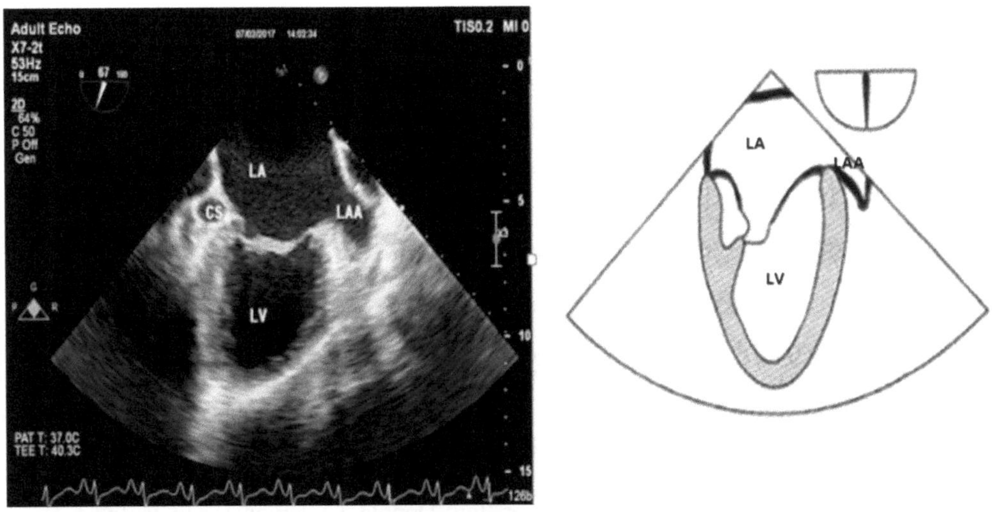

Fig. 3.6 ME Long-axis view: Rotate probe at mid esophageal level from 2 chamber to 120° till you see AV and LVOT to get aortic root horizontally in field and AV and MV in the center, also you see LV. Structures in this view includes LV, LA, MV, AV, LVOT and proximal of ascending aorta and LV antero-septal and posterior walls. MV anterior (A2) and posterior (P2) are displayed too

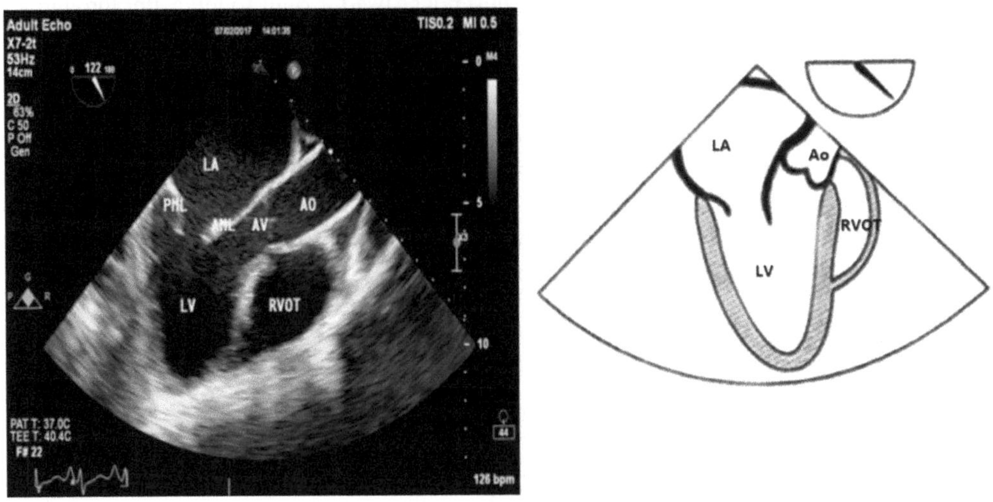

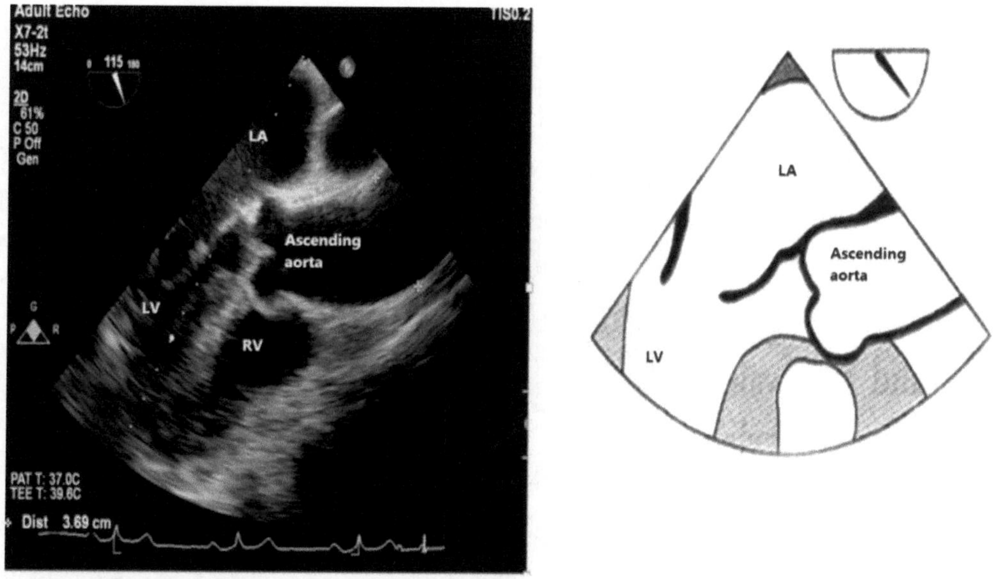

Fig. 3.7 ME, AV LAX View; 120–150° showing LA, LVOT, AV, proximal ascending Aorta line up. For the best view we should optimize the aortic annulus and make the sinuses of Valsalva symmetric

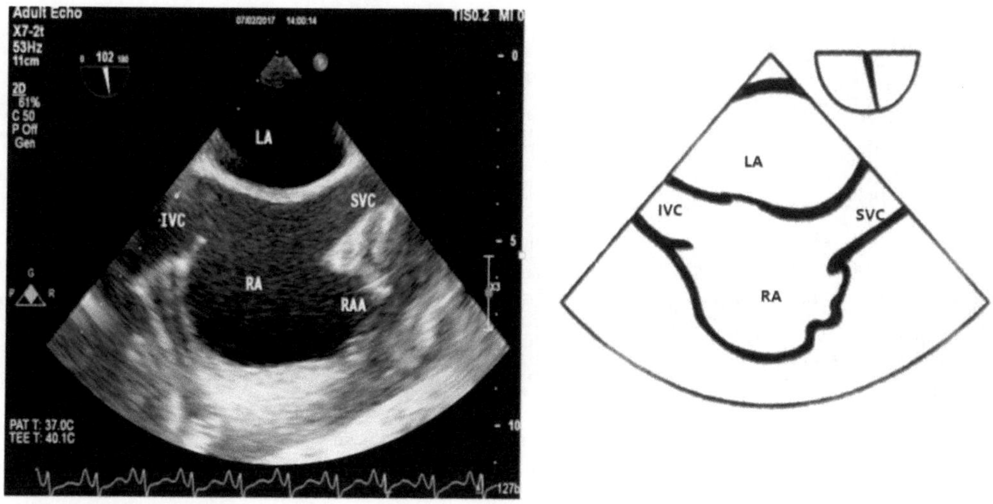

Fig. 3.8 ME Bicaval view: By chaning probe angle to 90–110° and turning clockwise IAS is displayed at center horizontally. This view includes SVC, IVC, LA, RA and IAS

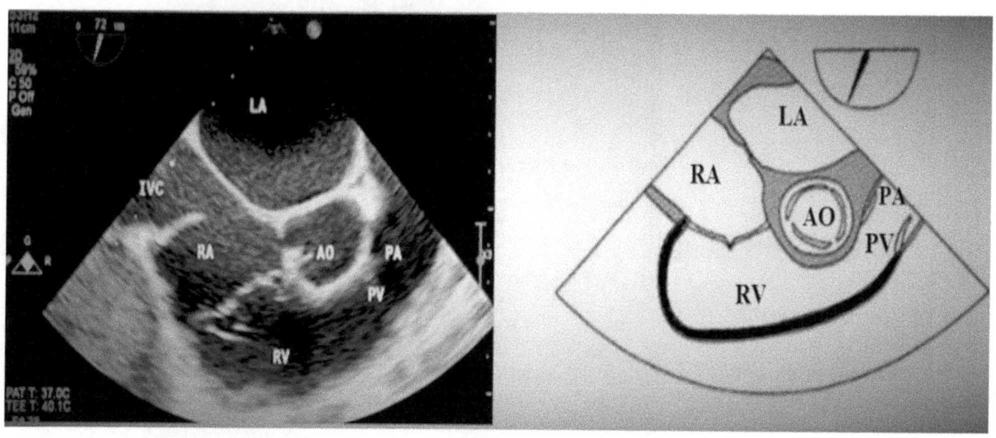

Fig. 3.9 ME RV inflow view: For obtaining this view while probe is in mid esophage level you should rotate probe to 70° and turn clockwise to get AV, TV and PV. LA, RA, IAS, RV, RVOT, proximal of main PA, TV and PV are visualized

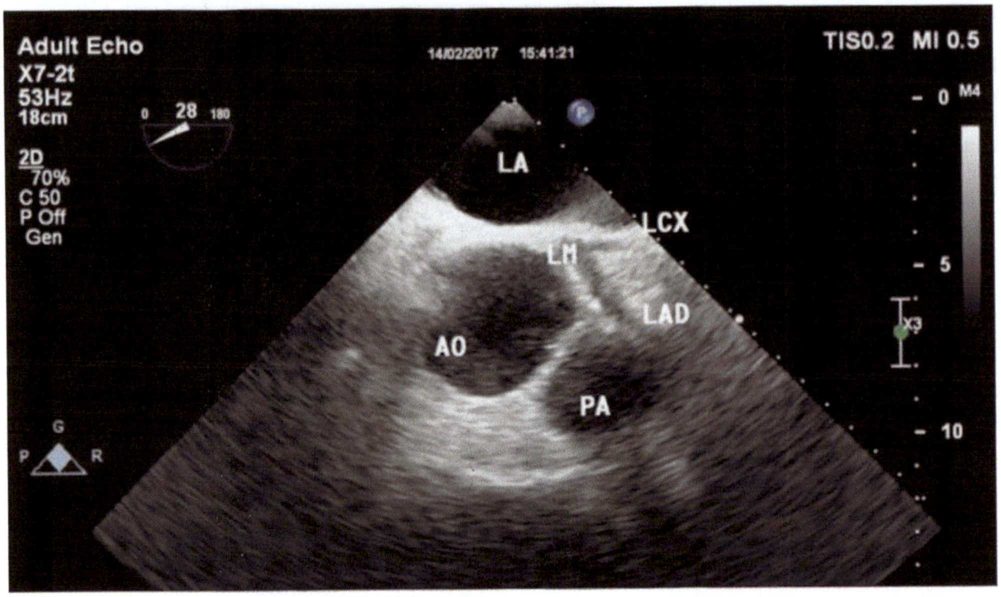

Fig. 3.10 ME 20–45′ view: For obtaining this view you should withdraw the probe slightly and turn it counterclockwise to get proximal part of ascending aorta and origin of left main coronary artery and its branches

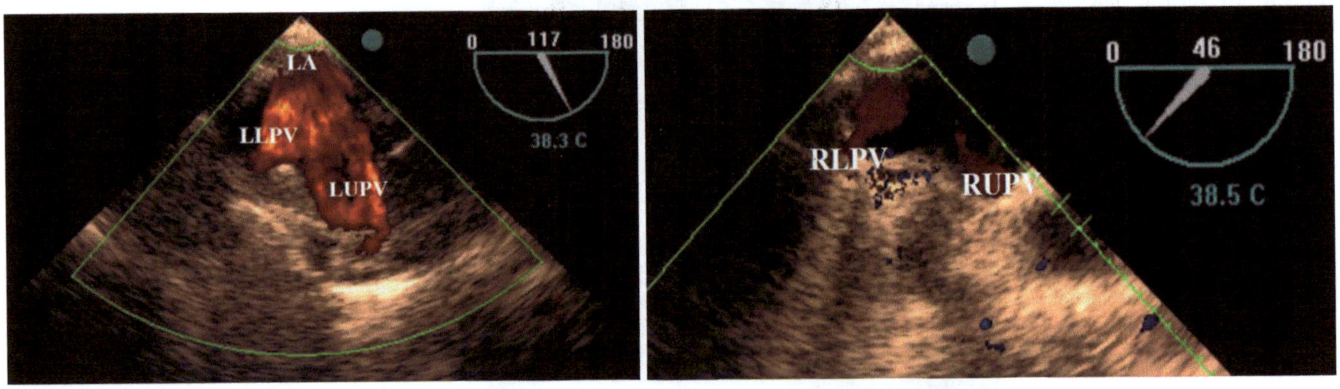

Fig. 3.11 ME, With advancing the probe, 90–110′ and counterclockwise maneuver showing the left upper and lower pulmonary veins (left figure) and in 50–70′ and clockwise maneuver showing the right upper, middle and lower pulmonary veins (right figure)

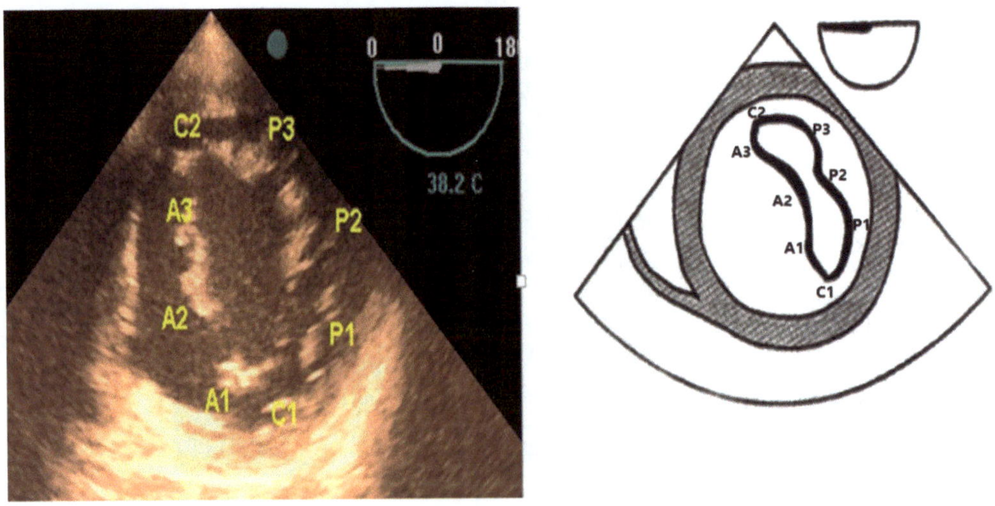

Fig. 3.12 TG, 0–20′, MV scallops, From TG mid SAX view withdraw the probe until MV is seen in SAX, Aim to see symmetric MV scallops and commissures

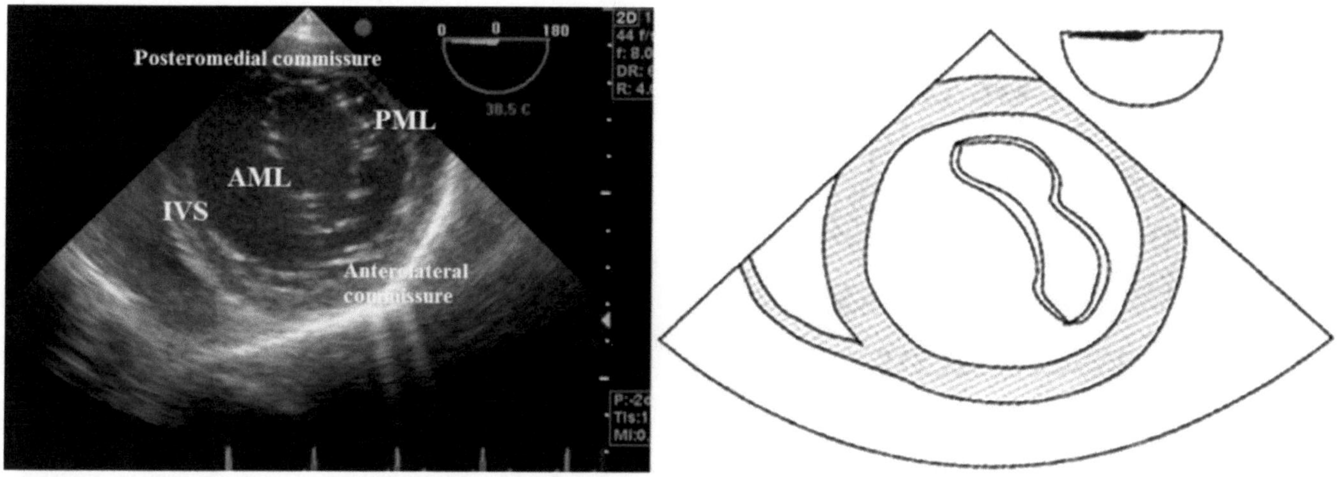

Fig. 3.13 TG, 0–20′, MV scallops and commissures, please see the Fig. 3.12 too

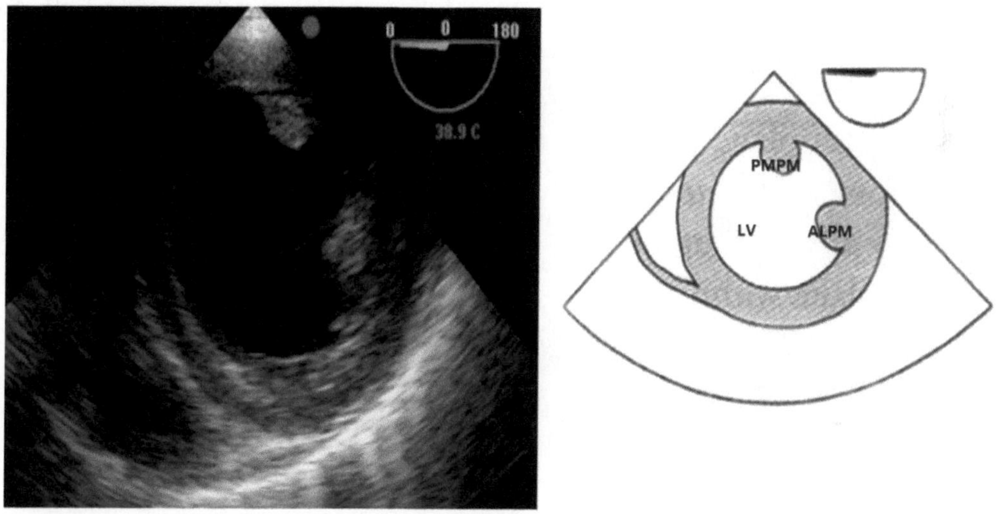

Fig. 3.14 TG mid SAX (0°): Advance probe until you see stomach or liver; Ante-flex to contact stomach wall and inferior wall of heart, Center LV by turning probe R or L, Image both papillary muscles and all 6 mid LV segments viewed at once from the stomach. For: Left Ventricle size, function, IVS motion, VSD, Pericardial effusion

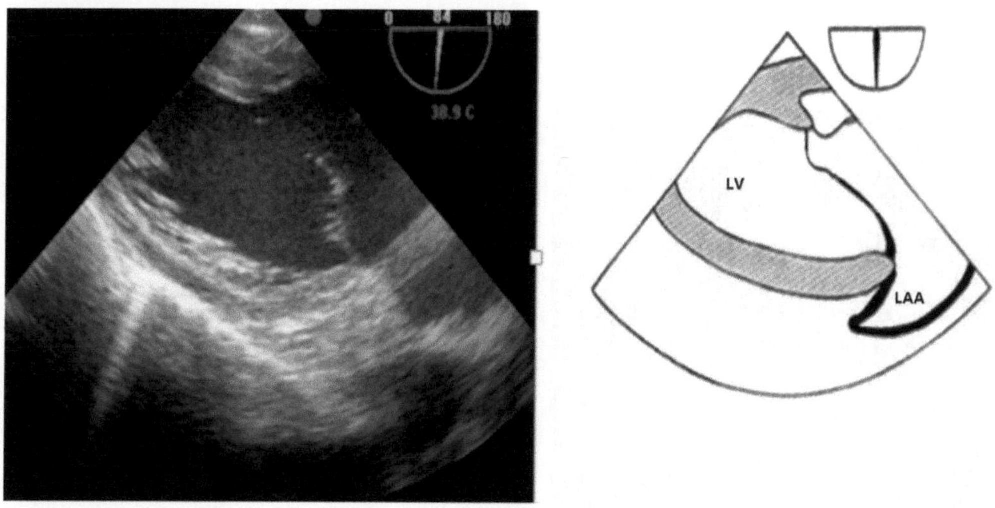

Fig. 3.15 TG, angle 90°. Anteflex until LV is horizontal imaging plane, . showing inferior wall of the LV and subvalvular structures of the mitral valve from the stomach. For: LV function, Mitral Valve subvalvular pathology, MV and LAA

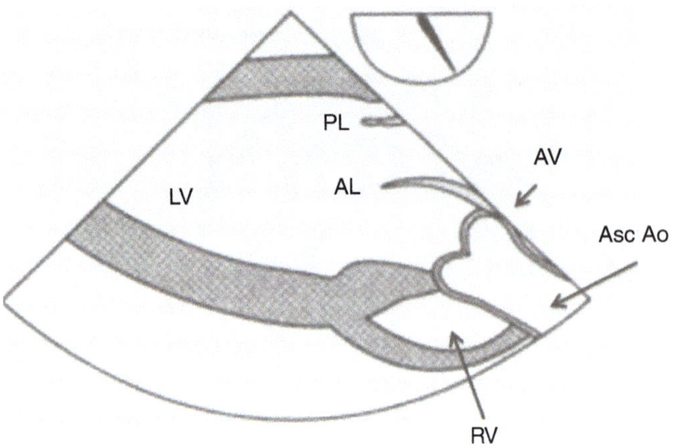

Fig. 3.16 TG LAX (110–120°): Imaging plane is directed longitudinally through the LV to image the aortic root in LAX. For: MV Pathology,VSD, LV systolic function, Aortic Valve: spectral and color doppler, LVOT: spectral and color Doppler

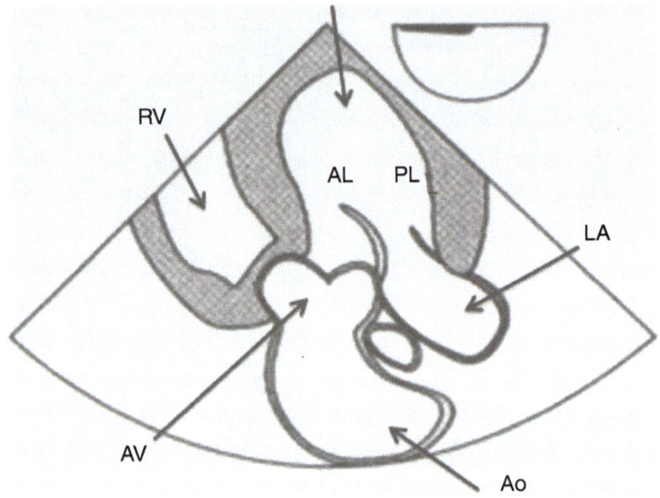

Fig. 3.18 Deep TG LAX(0°): From mid or apical TG SAX view, anteflex and gently advance probe, hugging the stomach mucosa until the LV apex is seen at the top of the display. For: Paravalvular leak prosthetic aortic valve; AV gradient spectral doppler; LVOT gradient spectral Doppler

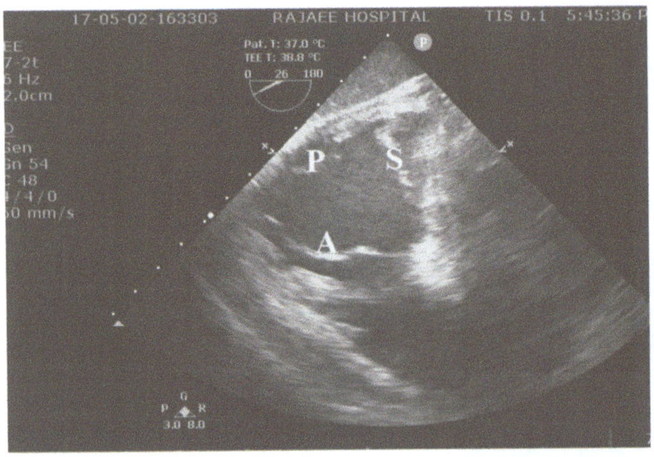

Fig. 3.17 TG RV (0–20°): From mid TG LV SAX (0°) turn probe right to put RV in center and see the tricuspid valve anterior (A), posterior (P) and septal (S) leaflets

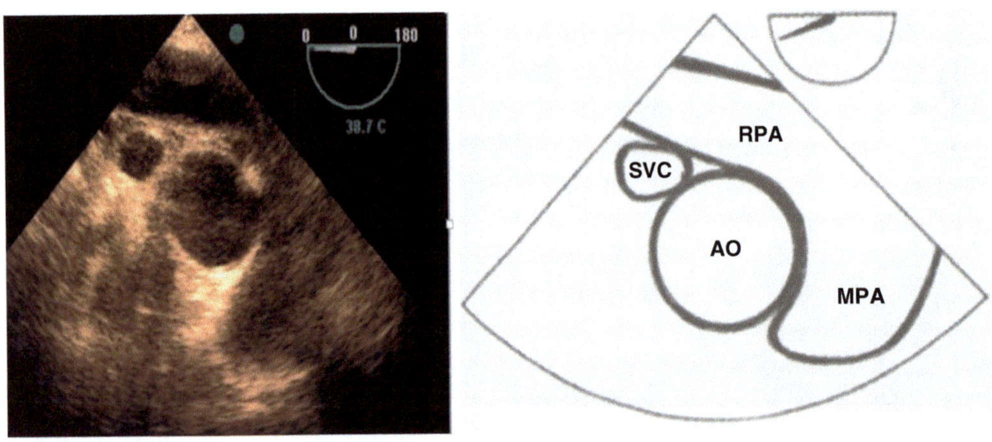

Fig. 3.19 UE, 0′ view, Mid-ascending aorta, Superior vena cava, Right pulmonary vein, RPA and MPA views. Please see the Fig. 3.20

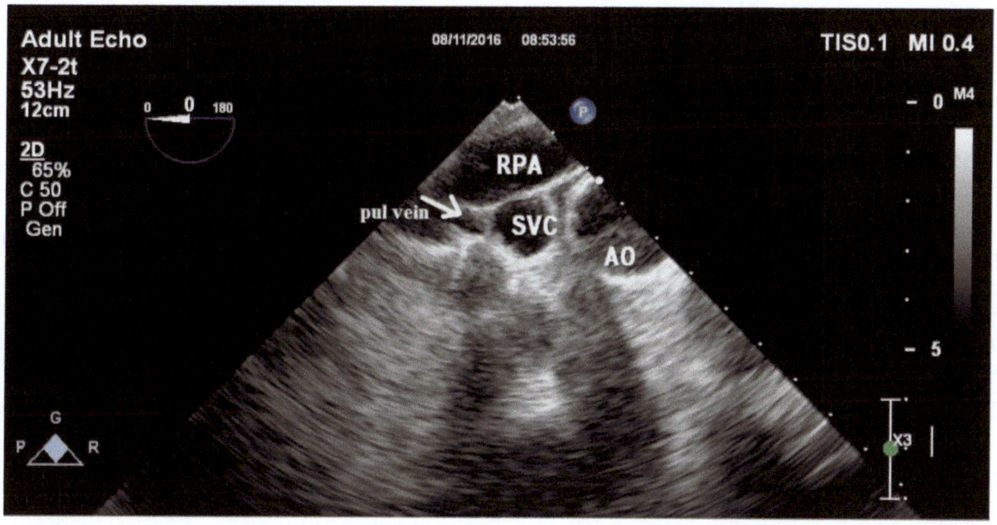

Fig. 3.20 UE, Imaging plane is directed slightly above the aortic valve through the RPA (seen in LAX), ascending aorta (seen in SAX) and SVC (SAX). For: PA pathology, Pulmonary Embolus, Ascending Aorta pathology, PDA, Swan-Ganz in SVC

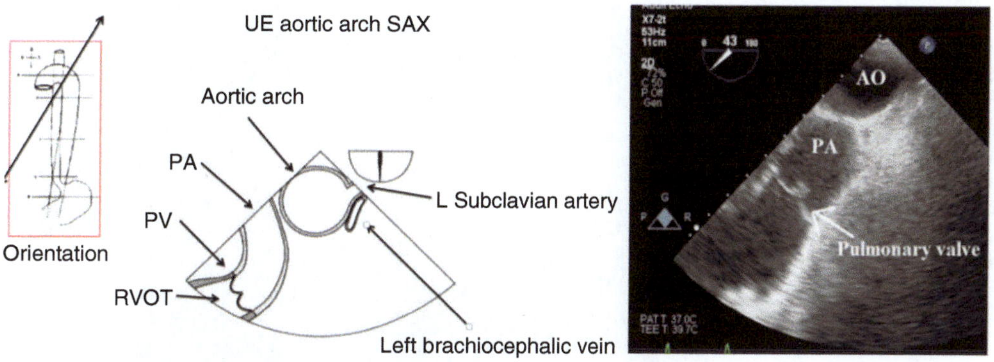

Fig. 3.21 From UE Aortic Arch LAX (0°) view rotate the angle to 60–90, Bring the pulmonic valve and pulmonary artery in view; Imaging plane is directed through the transverse aortic arch in SAX and the pulmonary artery in LAX. For: Aortic Arch pathology, Pulmonic Valve disease, PDA

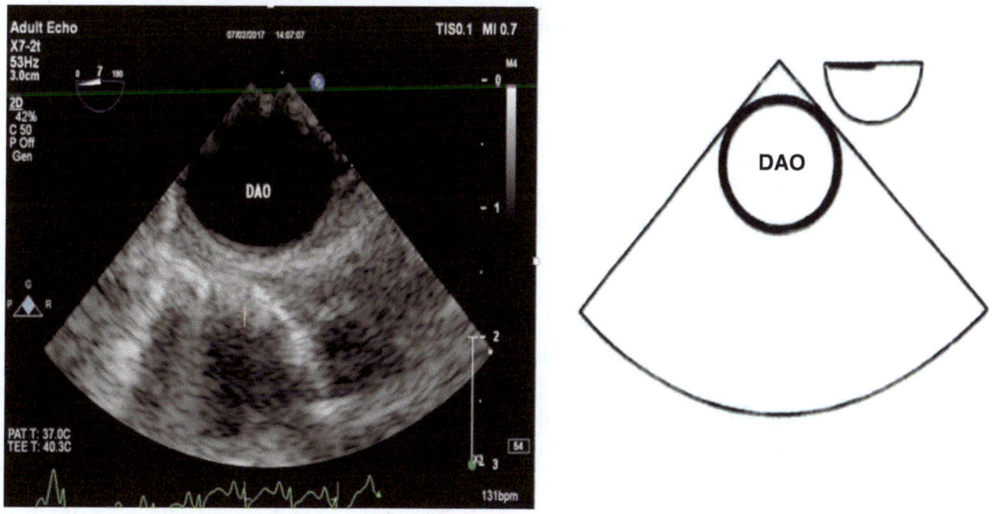

Fig. 3.22 Descending aort, short axis view: Rotate probe to about 0–10° with conter clockwise and slightly withdrawal probe to see aorta in short axis view. You can assess atherosclerothoc plaque, dissection and aortic aneurysm. You can change depth of probe to see more distal or proximal of descending aorta. For lanmarking of lesions in this view you can define them by means of distance from incisors

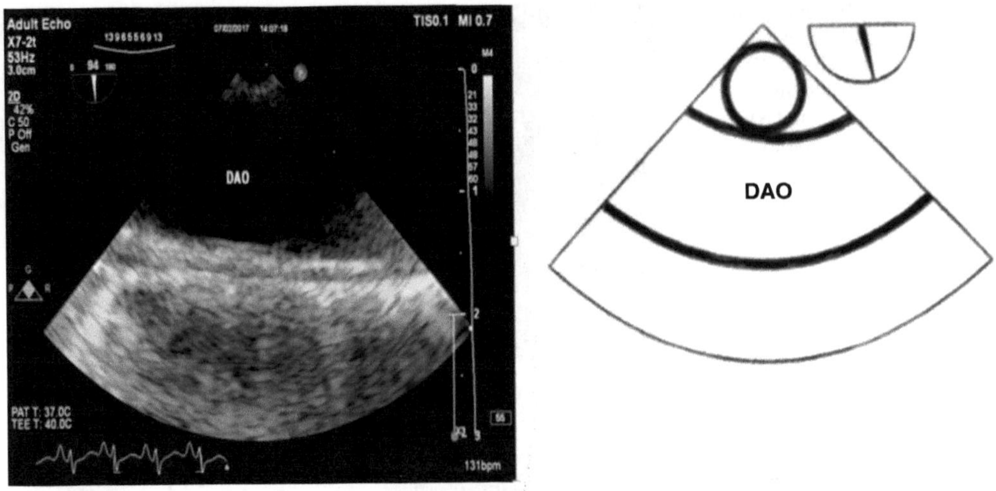

Fig. 3.23 Descending aort, long-axis view: This view is orthogonal to short axis of descending aorta, so by changing angle to 90–100° from short axis of aorta it will appear. By advancing or withdrawal probe you can see entire of descending aorta. Similar to short axis of descending aorta view you can evaluate pathology of aorta and again use distance to incisors to identify location of pathology

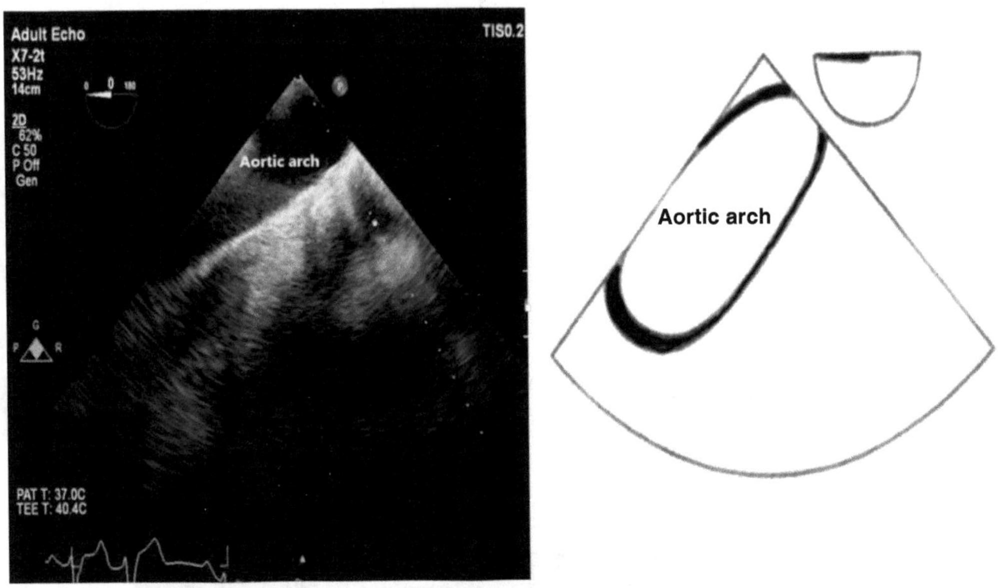

Fig. 3.24 UE Aortic Arch LAX (0°): From ME (0°), ME Descending Aorta SAX (0°) view withdraw probe until aorta changes into oval shape the turn probe slightly to the right; Imaging plane is directed thru the longitudinal axis of the transverse aortic arch. The circular shape of the DA changes to an oblong shape of the transverse aortic arch (0°)

Conclusion

This document presents 28 views in a comprehensive TEE study. A suggested protocol of image acquisition is provided, with the caveat that anatomic variability might require that unconventional imaging planes be used. Though the performance of a comprehensive TEE study is suggested whenever possible, individual patient characteristics, anatomic variations, pathologic features, or time constraints imposed might limit the ability to perform all aspects of the study described in this document. The "Particular Structural Imaging" section of this document contains additional views that may be acquired. The document is not intended to review particular indications for TEE or cover extensively abnormalities seen with this modality. The applications of TEE have increased constantly over the recent years. 3D TEE has added value to this technique. Interventional TEE imaging in structural heart disease is widely expanding. Trans-catheter procedures are emerging techniques that are increasingly guided with TEE. Intraoperative TEE continues to be a valued tool for cardiac surgeons [6, 11–14].

Questions

1. Absolute contraindications for transesophageal echocardiography are as follows, except for:
   A. Perforated viscus
   B. Esophageal stricture
   C. Esophageal tumor
   D. Recent upper gastrointestinal bleeding

2. If you omit the left ventricular outflow tract in midesophageal 4-chamber view at 0°, you will see which of the following scallops of the mitral valve ?
   A. A1, P1
   B. A2, P2
   C. A3, P3
   D. A1, P2

3. In midesophageal bicaval view, by changing the probe angle to 90° to 110° and ……, the interatrial septum is displayed at the center horizontally.
   A. turning it clockwise
   B. turning it counterclockwise
   C. anteflexing it
   D. retroflexing it

4. This figures shows:

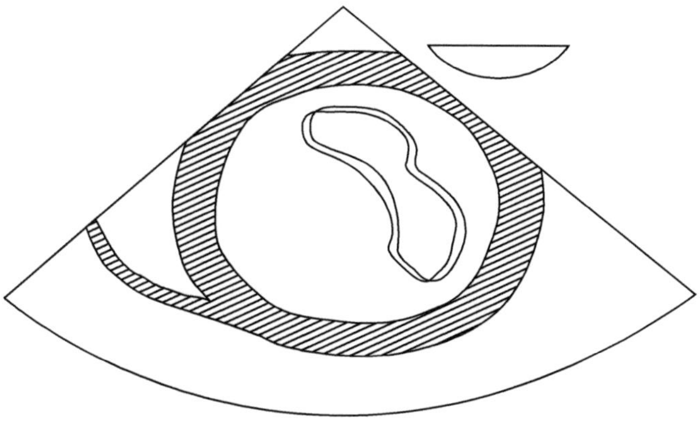

   A. Transgastric view, 0-20'
   B. Mid esophageal view, 0-20'
   C. Transgastric view, 60'
   D. Mid esophageal view, 60'

Answers

1. D
2. B
3. A
4. A

References

1. Hahn RT, Abraham T, Adams MS, Bruce CJ, Glas KE, Lang RM, Reeves ST, Shanewise JS, Siu SC, Stewart W, Picard MH. Guidelines for Performing a Comprehensive Transesophageal Echocardiographic Examination: Recommendations from the American Society of Echocardiography and the Society of Cardiovascular Anesthesiologists. ASE GUIDELINES AND STANDARDS. J Am Soc Echocardiogr. 2013;26:921–64.
2. Min JK, Spencer I, Furlong KT, et al. Clinical features of complications from transesophageal echocardiography: a single-center case series of 10,000 consecutive examinations. J Am Soc Echocardiogr. 2005;18:925–9.
3. Novaro GM, Aronow HD, Militello MA, et al. Benzocaine-induced methemoglobinemia: experience from a high-volume transesophageal echocardiography laboratory. J Am Soc Echocardiogr. 2003;16:170–5.
4. Brinkman WI, Shanewise JS, Clements SO, et al. Transesophageal echocardiography: not an innocuous procedure. Ann Thorac Surg. 2001;72:1725–6.
5. Steckelberg JM, Khandheria BK, Anhalt P, et al. Prospective evaluation of the risk of bacteremia associated with transesophageal echocardiography. Circulation. 1991;84:177–80.
6. Hahn RT, Abraham T, Adams MS, Bruce CJ, Glas KE, Lang BM, et al. Guidelines for Performing a Comprehensive Transesophageal Echocardiographic examination: Recommendations from the American Society of Echocardiography and the Society of Cardiovascular Anesthesiologists. J Am Soc Echocardiogr. 2013;26:921–64.
7. American College of Cardiology Foundation Appropriate Use Criteria Task Force, American Society of Echocardiography, American Heart Association, American Society of Nuclear Cardiology, Heart Failure Society of America, Heart Rhythm Society, et al. ACCF/ASE/AHA/ASNC/HFSA/HRS/SCAI/SCCM/SCCT/SCMR 2011 appropriate use criteria for echocardiography. A report of the American College of Cardiology Foundation Appropriate Use Criteria Task Force, American Society of Echocardiography, American Heart Association, American Society of Nuclear Cardiology, Heart Failure Society of America, Heart Rhythm Society, Society for Cardiovascular Angiography and Interventions, Society of Critical Care Medicine, Society of Cardiovascular Computed Tomography, Society for Cardiovascular Magnetic Resonance American College of Chest Physicians. J Am Soc Echocardiogr. 2011;24:229–67.
8. American College of Cardiology Foundation Appropriate Use Criteria Task Force, Hendel RC, Patel MR, Allen JM, Min JK, Shaw LJ, et al. Appropriate use of cardiovascular technology: 2013 ACCF appropriate use criteria methodology update. J Am Coll Cardiol. 2013;61:1305–17.
9. Intersocietal Accrediation Commission. IAC standards for adult echocardiography accreditation. http://www.intersocietal.org/echo/standards/IACAdultEchocardiographyStandards2012.pdf. Accessed 27 Jul 2013.
10. Skiles JA, Griffin BP. Transesophageal echocardiographic (TEE) valuation of ventricular function. Cardiol Clin. 2000;18:681–97.
11. Flachskampf FA, Badano L, Daniel WG, Feneck RO, Fox KF, Fraser AG, et al. Recommendations for transoesophageal echocardiography: update. Eur J Echocardiogr. 2010;11:557–76.
12. Zamorano JL, Badano LP, Bruce C, Chan KL, Goncalves A, Hahn RT, et al. EAE/ASE recommendations for the use of echocardiography in new transcatheter interventions for valvular heart disease. J Am Soc Echocardiogr. 2011;24:937–65.
13. Hahn R, Abraham T, Adams M, et al. Guidelines for performing a comprehensive transesophageal echocardiographic examination: recommendations from the American Society of Echocardiography and the Society of Cardiovascular Anesthesiologists. J Am Soc Echocardiogr. 2013;9:921–64.
14. Evangelista A, Flachskampf FA, Erbel R, et al. European Association of Echocardiography; Echocardiography in aortic diseases: EAE recommendations for clinical practice. Eur J Echocardiogr. 2010;8:645–58.

Sedation for Transesophageal Echocardiography

4

Rasoul Azarfarin and Ramin Rohanifar

Abstract

Transesophageal echocardiography (TEE) is a minimal invasive diagnostic tool performed for a growing number of patients in echocardiography departments and intensive care units. Such as other semi-invasive procedures, TEE requires some degrees of sedation to achieve better patient safety and comfort and operator convenience. Given the potential minor and rarely major cardio-respiratory complications of TEE, it is essential that a highly skilled person conduct the sedation. Noninvasive blood pressure measurement, ECG, and pulse oximetry are essential monitoring tools, but they cannot replace the clinical examination and observation of the patient thorough the TEE procedure. In this chapter, we offer anesthesiologists and non-anesthesiologist providers practical notes regarding sedation during TEE to guarantee best patient safety.

Keywords

Moderate sedation · Transesophageal echocardiography · Benzodiazepines · Opioid analgesics · Complications

Abbreviations

ASA	American society of anesthesiologists
BIS	Bispectral index
TEE	Transesophageal echocardiography

R. Azarfarin, MD, FACC (✉)
Echocardiography Research Center, Rajaie Cardiovascular, Medical and Research Center, Iran University of Medical Sciences, Tehran, Iran

R. Rohanifar, MD
Anesthesiologist, Pain Medicine Fellow, Tehran Clinic Hospital, Tehran, Iran

Introduction

- The Merriam-Webster dictionary defines *"sedation"* as a relaxed, calm, or sleepy condition that results from taking a drug (called a sedative).
- The aim of sedation and analgesia in medical interventional procedures such as TEE is to provide a situation that reduces the patient's discomfort and anxiety and reduce the patient's memory of the experience [1]. Also, patient sedation by creating a calm and cooperative state improves the cardiologist's satisfaction and improves the outcome of the procedure.
- According to a statement by the American Society of Anesthesiologists (ASA) [2]: "Moderate sedation/analgesia ("conscious sedation") is a drug-induced depression of consciousness during which patients respond purposefully to verbal commands, either alone or accompanied by light tactile stimulation. No interventions are required to maintain a patient airway, and spontaneous ventilation is adequate. Cardiovascular function is usually maintained." "Deep Sedation/Analgesia is a drug-induced depression of consciousness during which patients cannot be easily aroused but respond purposefully following repeated or painful stimulation. The ability to independently maintain ventilatory function may be impaired. Patients may require assistance in maintaining a patent airway, and spontaneous ventilation may be inadequate. Cardiovascular function is usually maintained" [2].
- So, our goal during TEE procedures is to provide "moderate sedation/analgesia ("conscious sedation") to ensure adequate patient safety.

Pre-Procedural Preparation and Assessment

- It is well known that co-existing risk factors have been related with higher mortality and morbidity in the perioperative period [3]. These factors consist of age > 60 years

A. Sadeghpour, A. Alizadehasl (eds.), *Case-Based Textbook of Echocardiography*,
https://doi.org/10.1007/978-3-319-67691-3_4

Table 4.1 List of absolute and relative contraindications to transesophageal echocardiography [4] Guidelines for performing a comprehensive transesophageal echocardiographic examination

Absolute contraindications	Relative contraindications
• Perforated viscus	• History of radiation to the neck and mediastinum
• Esophageal stricture	• History of gastrointestinal surgery
• Esophageal tumor	• Recent upper gastrointestinal bleeding
• Esophageal perforation, laceration	• Barrett's esophagus
• Esophageal diverticulum	• History of dysphagia
• Active upper gastrointestinal bleed	• Restriction of neck mobility (severe cervical arthritis, atlantoaxial joint disease)
	• Symptomatic hiatal hernia
	• Esophageal varices
	• Coagulopathy, thrombocytopenia
	• Active esophagitis
	• Active peptic ulcer disease

old, body mass index >35 kg/m^2, systemic and pulmonary hypertension, heart failure, renal failure, acute coronary syndromes, chronic lung disease, sleep apnea disorders, and mental disorientation. Airway assessment and patency is an essential part of physical examination either for sedation or performing TEE. Mouth opening, temporomandibular joint movement, and thyro-mental distance must be assessed before the procedure.

- The potential presence of both absolute and relative contraindications of TEE should be kept in mind. These contraindications include previous esophagectomy, esophagogastrectomy, esophageal varices, post-radiation therapy stricture, previous bariatric surgery, tracheoesophagea fistulae, and esophageal traumas (Table 4.1). Generally, for patients with a history of any oropharyngolaryngeal and gastroesophageal disease, if the expected benefit outweighs the potential risk, TEE can be used with appropriate caution.
- It is very important to ask the patients whether or not they have recently used drugs effecting on the coagulation system such as aspirin, warfarin, heparin (unfractionated or enoxaparin), nonsteroidal anti-inflammatory drugs, clopidogrel, or thrombolytic drugs and clearly ask the time interval since the cessation of these drugs [3]. Usual laboratory tests should include coagulation tests (e.g., PT, PTT, and INR) and platelet count. During history taking of the patient, special attention should be paid to hereditary and acquired coagulation disorders.

Topical Anesthesia for Transesophageal Echocardiography

- To achieve local anesthesia, 3–5 puffs (each puff containing 10 mg of lidocaine 10%) are applied on the patient's pharynx 2–3 min before TEE.
- Some echocardiologists additionally ask the patient to swallow lidocaine HCl 2% jelly. Lidocaine is well absorbed from the oropharyngeal mucosa, but a small amount of the drug enters the bloodstream due to its biotransformation in the liver. Topical lidocaine has minimal systemic and hemodynamic effects; however, it may cause modest hypotension in some patients when used within the recommended doses.
- The maximum allowable dose of lidocaine is 4.5 mg/kg or 300 mg in normal healthy adults. Topical lidocaine should be used only by trained clinicians who are well experienced in the diagnosis and management of drug toxicity and other acute emergencies.
- Oxygen should be immediately available. Cardiopulmonary resuscitation drugs, equipment, and team are needed for the proper management of toxic reactions and possible emergencies. Any delay in the appropriate management of local anesthetic systemic toxicity, hypoventilation, and hypotension may progress to severe metabolic acidosis, cardiac arrest and, even death.
- When topical lidocaine is used in the oropharyngeal region, the patient should be informed that it may impair swallowing and increase the risk of aspiration; consequently, food and liquid should not be ingested at least for 60 min after TEE.
- Before beginning the examination, the procedure should be explained to the patient. Patient cooperation is needed for the insertion of the probe. In intubated and anesthetized patients in the ICU or the operating room, the pharynx secretions should be suctioned and then the tracheal tube cuff should deflated. After the lubricated probe is passed, the cuff should be re-inflated. The flexion of the patient's neck sometimes facilitates the insertion of the probe. If there is resistance against the passing of the probe, the operator should avoid more force because of the risk of esophageal rupture.

Sedative and Analgesic Agents Used for Transesophageal Echocardiography

Benzodiazepines

- Midazolam is the most commonly used benzodiazepine for sedation during TEE.
- For normal adults, incremental doses of 0.5 mg up to 2 mg in combination with an opioid such as fentanyl (25–50 μg) provide a smooth and pleasant sedation.
- There is high individual variability in the response of patients to benzodiazepines and this feature is unpredictable. Therefore, the best way to reach moderate sedation is the titration of the drug and waiting for 3–5 min to achieve the peak effect of the drug. If the patient is not adequately tranquilized, the dose may be repeated.
- One of the most common errors in sedation with midazolam and/or fentanyl (or other agents) is the failure to

wait for 3–5 min for the adequate drug effect. Indeed, the echocardiographer may hurry to introduce the TEE probe into the mouth of an awake patient and thus induce gag reflex, nausea, and discomfort.

- TEE in an insufficiently sedated patient causes discomfort and can lead to tachycardia and hypertension. It may even prone to myocardial ischemia or arrhythmia. A sedation that is too light in patients with stenotic valvular lesions such as mitral stenosis could progress to pulmonary edema.
- In patients with ASA class 3 or more (Table 4.2) and those with difficult airways, it is recommended to consult with an anesthesiologist to ensure better patient safety.
- As TEE is performed in different cardiovascular patients with various degrees of ventricular dysfunction, pulmonary disease [5], old age, and sometime history of taking neuropsychological drugs and opium addiction, it is emphasized that the response of these patients to sedative/analgesic agents is unpredictable and the practitioner should administer these drugs at incremental doses. Midazolam dosage and some pharmacologic properties are summarized in Table 4.3. In case of midazolam overdose or severe respiratory depression, flumazenil (0.2 mg IV) can be used and if a satisfactory reversal of midazolam fails to occur, a second dose may be administered every 60 s up to a maximum of 4 additional times.

Table 4.2 American Society of Anesthesiologists' physical status classification

Class 1: A normally healthy patient
Class 2: A patient with mild systemic disease
Class 3: A patient with severe systemic disease that is not incapacitating
Class 4: A patient with an incapacitating systemic disease that is a constant threat to life
Class 5: A moribund patient who is not expected to survive for 24 h with or without operation

Anesthesiology. 1963;24:111

Opioids

- Opioids such as fentanyl, remifentanil, and morphine are drugs frequently used for procedural sedation/analgesia.
- **Fentanyl is the most commonly used opioid for analgesia during TEE and is usually used in combination with other hypnotic agents such as midazolam.** The onset of the action of fentanyl is rapid (1–2 min), and its peak effect is reached in 3–5 min (Table 4.3) and lasts for 30–60 min at a dose of 2 μg/kg. Smaller doses (25–50 μg) have a shorter recovery time and are recommended in conjugation with low-dose midazolam (0.5–1 mg).
- Respiratory depression is the most common adverse effect of opioids. It is dose dependent and is more frequent when used with other sedative drugs (midazolam or propofol) and in patients with pulmonary disease and also in the elderly.
- Opioids in combination with other sedatives may cause hypotension. This effect can be more profound in patients who spend a long fasting time with baseline hypovolemia. Fentanyl has minor hemodynamic effects even in the presence of ventricular or hepatorenal dysfunction, so it is the ideal analgesic for sedation during TEE. Morphine may cause some degrees of hypotension (due to vasodilation and histamine release) and is, thus, not deemed first choice for procedural analgesia. Nevertheless, it is the best analgesic agent in the ICU setting and in the postoperative period.
- Some anesthesiologists prefer to use remifentanil with low doses of midazolam for sedation during TEE [7]. Remifentanil is a short-acting opioid with a fast recovery time and is as such an attractive drug for the outpatient setting. However, it should be kept in mind that this opioid agent, if used by a non-anesthesiologist non-skilled person, my rapidly cause apnea and hypotension.

Table 4.3 Commonly used drugs for procedural sedation and analgesia in adults [6]

Drug	Adult dose	Onset of action	Duration of action[a]	Comments
Midazolam	0.02–0.1 mg/kg IV initially; if further sedation is required, may repeat with 25% of initial dose after 3–5 min; not to exceed 2.5 mg/dose (1.5 mg for elderly persons) and 5 mg cumulative dose (3.5 mg for elderly persons)	1–2 min (time to peak =3–5 min)	30–60 min	Respiratory depression or hypotension may occur, particularly when rapidly administered or combined with fentanyl (may need to decrease midazolam dose); does not provide analgesia; action reversed by flumazenil
Fentanyl	1–2 mcg/kg slow IV push (over 1–2 min); may repeat dose after 30 min	1–2 min (time to peak =3–5 min)	30–60 min	May cause chest wall rigidity, apnea, respiratory depression, or hypotension; elicits minimal cardiovascular depression; may cause dysphoria, nausea, vomiting, or electroencephalographic changes; action reversed by naloxone
Propofol	0.5–1 mg/kg IV loading dose; may repeat by 0.5 mg/kg increments q3–5 min	< 1 min	3–10 min	Provides rapid onset and recovery phase, and brief duration of action; has anticonvulsant properties; can rapidly cause deepening sedation; causes cardiovascular depression and hypotension

[a]Duration of action based on normal drug elimination (i.e., nonelderly adults with normal renal and hepatic function)

Furthermore, if the user cannot manage the airway and hemodynamics, it could lead to catastrophic outcomes and patient death.

- In the case of significant respiratory depression or oxygen desaturation due to opium overdose, a starting dose of 0.4 mg IV of naloxone may be given and it may be repeated 2 to 3 times if needed. In patients with coronary artery disease or pulmonary hypertension, opioid effect reversal should be done with caution to avoid myocardial ischemia or hypertension crisis.

Propofol

- Propofol (2, 6-di-isopropyl phenol) is a short-acting hypnotic drug. It delivers hypnotic, sedative, and amnestic properties without any analgesic effects. Propofol quickly crosses the blood-brain barrier and it is thought that its effects are mediated by the positive modulation of the inhibitory function of the GABA receptors in the central nervous system. The drug is highly lipophilic, and its preparations are available in 1 and 2% solutions.
- It seems that sedation with **propofol has some advantages for TEE over sedation with a benzodiazepine/opioid combination given the faster recovery period and better physician and/or patient satisfaction.** In addition, propofol-sedated patients have better scores on psychomotor function, superior near memory, and mental status after sedation.
- However, propofol has powerful cardiorespiratory depressant effects and should not be administered by non-anesthesiologists. The risk of hypotension or apnea by propofol is higher than that by other hypnotics/analgesics and if it is used by a person who is inexperienced in airway management and monitoring patient hemodynamics, the sedation may even lead to patient respiratory and/or cardiac arrest. Propofol loading dose for sedation is 0.5–1 mg/kg IV and can be continued by repeated doses of 0.5 mg/kg each 3–5 min (Table 4.2) or continuous infusions of 25–75 μg/kg/min.

Ketamine

- Ketamine is usually used in the pediatric population for procedural sedation. However, some physicians use it safely in adults. Ketamine is a unique sedation drug and has dissociative effects and causes amnesia and analgesia in patients. This combined sedative/analgesic activity is useful for administration as a single agent for painful procedures.
- Ketamine may cause hypertension and tachycardia and increase intracranial pressure. Some patients may experience unusual dreams, hallucinations, excitation, physical combativeness, delirium, and nightmare after ketamine use. Accordingly, most anesthesiologists do not consider it a first drug for sedation in adults.

Dexmedetomidine

- Dexmedetomidine is a highly selective α 2-adrenergic agonist with dose-dependent sedative, anxiolytic, and analgesic effects via a central mechanism by activating pre-synaptic receptors.
- Dexmedetomidine is a new sedative drug that has been successfully used for procedural sedation in recent years. Its starting dose is 1 μg/kg; it is administered over a 10-min period, followed by 0.2–0.7 μg/kg/h. Generally, dexmedetomidine is similar to other sedatives in achieving sufficient levels of sedation with comparable rates of respiratory depression, oxygen desaturation, and hemodynamic instability [8]. The main drawback of dexmedetomidine is the long infusion time of the starting dose (10 min). Also, an infusion pump must be available for administering this drug.

Monitoring During Transesophageal Echocardiography

- The ASA's guidelines recommend **continuous ECG monitoring** of patients with cardiovascular and pulmonary disease and in old patients during sedation [9].
- In addition, all patients undergoing IV sedation should be monitored with **noninvasive blood pressure measurement**.
- **Continuous pulse oximetry monitoring** efficiently diagnoses oxygen desaturation and hypoxemia in these patients [10]. It should be borne in mind that pulse oximetry is partially insensitive to the early stages of respiratory depression because major changes in arterial partial pressure of oxygen (in ranges >60 mm Hg) may happen with minimal changes in oxygen saturation. This situation usually happens in patients receiving supplemental oxygen. **Thus, observation of the patient's chest movement and maintenance of an open airway during TEE are mandatory**.
- **Capnography is a noninvasive measurement of end-tidal carbon dioxide** and monitoring of real-time respiratory activity. It more readily detects respiratory depression than pulse oximetry and thereby helps with the early recognition of hypoventilation. Adding capnography to patient monitoring tools may improve patient safety. The ASA's guidelines recommend that capnography be performed for all patients undergoing deep sedation. It is

useful during moderate sedation in patients whose ventilation cannot be observed directly [9].

- The bispectral index (BIS) is an electroencephalographic-based technique for evaluating the level of consciousness by using an algorithm to create a weighted index. However, BIS values my not exactly be concomitant or parallel with the clinical level of sedation. In conclusion, the BIS was not associated with any improvement in recovery times or decrease in the propofol dose in a study [11].

Complications

- There are 2 types of complications that may occur during TEE.
- The first type is related to TEE itself and includes complications of the probe insertion into the mouth, pharynx, and esophagus. There are also local anatomic injuries to the mucosa, spasm, bleeding, and/or perforation, as well as general complications consisting of arrhythmia, hypertension, and heat failure (Table 4.4).

Table 4.4 Type and incidence of complications during diagnostic transesophageal echocardiography [4]

Complication	Diagnostic transesophageal echocardiography	Intraoperative transesophageal echocardiography
Overall complication rate	0.18–2.8% (refs 24, 25)	0.2% (ref 7)
Mortality	<0.01–0.2% (refs 24, 25, 27)	0% (ref 7)
Major morbidity	0.2% (ref 27)	0–1.2% (refs 7, 28, 29)
Major bleeding	<0.01% (ref 24)	0.03–0.8% (refs 7, 28)
Esophageal perforation	<0.01% (ref 24)	0–0.3% (refs 7, 28, 29)
Heart failure	<0.05% (ref 28)	
Arrhythmia	0.06–0.3% (refs 7, 28, 30)	
Tracheal intubation	0.02% (ref 30)	
Endotracheal tube malposition		0.03% (ref 7)
Laryngospasm	0.14% (ref 27)	
Bronchospasm	0.06–0.7% (refs 24, 30)	
Dysphagia	1.8% (ref 31)	
Minor pharyngeal bleeding	0.01–0.2% (refs 24, 25, 27)	0.01% (ref 7)
Severe odynophagia		0.1% (ref 7)
Hoarseness	12% (ref 31)	
Lip injury	13% (ref 31)	
Dental injury	0.1% (ref 31)	0.03% (ref 7)

The second type of complications during TEE is associated with sedation. Complications following the administration of sedative drugs can be categorized as cardiovascular and respiratory.

- Regarding the fasting of patients before TEE and some degrees of intravascular volume depletion, after the injection of sedative agent(s), the patient's systemic blood pressure usually drops. If intravascular hypovolemia is significant, even minimal doses of sedative drugs could give rise to severe hypotension by blocking sympathetic tone and vasodilation.
- **Thus, it is recommended to place a peripheral vein access and infuse 200–300 mL of normal saline, Ringer's or 1/3–2/3 (DW5%-normal saline) intravenous solutions to the patient before the administration of sedative drugs and commencement of the examination**. By volume replacement and titration of hypnotic and/or analgesic drugs, the occurrence of hypotension can be minimized even in patients with left ventricular systolic dysfunction.
- Among sedative drugs, propofol has stronger hypotensive effects, followed by midazolam (especially in combination with opioids). Dexmedetomidine, a new sedative drug, has minimal adverse hemodynamic effects (either hypotension or bradycardia). Ketamine via modest sympathetic nervous system stimulation leads to a minimal rise in blood pressure and heart rate. Nonetheless, due to some adverse effects—including psychological reactions, agitation, confusion, and hallucinations—it is not considered first choice in TEE for adults.
- Some sedative drugs—especially opioids—can cause bradycardia, which in patients taking beta-blockers or calcium channel blockers may be severe and dangerous.
- Another type of sedative drug complications is respiratory one. The most common respiratory side effect of sedatives is respiratory depression (<8 breath/min), which occurs after using benzodiazepines in combination with opioids. Older patients and those with coexisting pulmonary and central nervous system disorders are more vulnerable to this complication. Respiratory depression usually presents with desaturation (peripheral oxygen saturation < 90%) and cyanosis. The practitioner can overcome the respiratory depression by ventilating the patient with bag and mask and supplemental oxygen. Rarely, profound respiratory depression—not least with hemodynamic instability—may necessitate endotracheal intubation, which can rapidly rescue the patient.

Key Points

- Sedation providers (either anesthesiologists or echocardiologists) should have a comprehensive knowledge of drugs used for sedation during TEE and the skills essential for the diagnosis and management of cardiopulmonary complications.

- Noninvasive blood pressure, ECG, and pulse oximetry are essential monitoring tools; nonetheless, they cannot replace clinical examination and observation of the patient via TEE with sedation.
- The most common sedative regimen used for TEE is small doses of midazolam in combination with fentanyl. The titration of these drugs is crucial in cardiac patients with various types of coexisting diseases.
- There are 2 types of complications during TEE. The first kind is related to the insertion of the probe and anatomical injuries and the second kind is systemic and is associated with sedative drugs. The practitioner should be fully au fait with the contraindications and complications of TEE and their management.

References

1. Lichtenstein DR, Jagannath S, Baron TH, Anderson MA, Banerjee S, Dominitz JA, Fanelli RD, Gan SI, Harrison ME, Ikenberry SO, Shen B, Stewart L, Khan K, Vargo JJ. Sedation and anesthesia in GI endoscopy, Standards of Practice Committee. Gastrointest Endosc. 2008;68(2):205–16. https://doi.org/10.1016/j.gie.2008.06.002.
2. Statement on Granting Privileges for Administration of Moderate Sedation to Practitioners Who is Not Anesthesia Professionals. http://www.asahq.org/quality-and-practice-management/standards-and-guidelines. Released on 10.19.2011, Downloaded on Oct 12, 2016.
3. Cornelissen H, Arrowsmith JE. Preoperative assessment for cardiac surgery. Contin Educ Anaesth Crit Care Pain. 2006;6(3):109–13. https://doi.org/10.1093/bjaceaccp/mkl013.
4. Hahn RT, Abraham T, Adams MS, Bruce CJ, Glas KE, Lang RM, Reeves ST, Shanewise JS, Siu SC, Stewart W, Picard MH. Guidelines for Performing a Comprehensive Transesophageal Echocardiographic Examination: Recommendations from the American Society of Echocardiography and the Society of Cardiovascular Anesthesiologists. J Am Soc Echocardiogr. 2013;26(9):921–64.
5. Blondheim DS, Levi D, Marmor AT. Mild sedation before transesophageal echo induces significant hemodynamic and respiratory depression. Echocardiography. 2004;21(3):241–5.
6. Orlewicz MC, Schraga ED. Procedural sedation. http://emedicine.medscape.com/article/109695-overview#a7. Accessed 27 Oct 2016.
7. Renna M, Chung R, Li W, Maguire C, Mullen MJ, Chambers J, Henein MY. Remifentanil plus low-dose midazolam for outpatient sedation in transesophageal echocardiography. Int J Cardiol. 2009;136(3):325–9.
8. Cooper L, Candiotti K, Gallagher C, Grenier E, Arheart KL, Barron ME. A randomized, controlled trial on dexmedetomidine for providing adequate sedation and hemodynamic control for awake, diagnostic transesophageal echocardiography. J Cardiothorac Vasc Anesth. 2011;25(2):233–7.
9. American Society of Anesthesiologists Task Force on Sedation and Analgesia by Non-Anesthesiologists. Practice guidelines for sedation and analgesia by non-anesthesiologists. Anesthesiology. 2002;96(4):1004–17.
10. Ziyaeifard M, Azarfarin R. Efficacy and safety of sedation in cardiac imaging. Arch Cardiovasc Imaging. 2014;2(1):e17357. https://doi.org/10.5812/acvi.17357.
11. Drake LM, Chen SC, Rex DK. Efficacy of bispectral monitoring as an adjunct to nurse-administered propofol sedation for colonoscopy: a randomized controlled trial. Am J Gastroenterol. 2006;101:2003–7.

Basic of 3D Echocardiography; Clinical Use in Daily Practice

5

Ahmad S. Omran

Abstract

Three-dimensional echocardiography (3DE) represents a major innovation and revolution in the field of cardiovascular ultrasound. Advances in computer and transducer technologies has permitted real-time 3DE acquisition and presentations of cardiac structures from any spatial point of view. 3D transesophageal echocardiography (3D TEE) creates a "common language" between echo cardiologist, cardiac surgeon, and cardiac interventionist in the operating room and cath lab for appropriate decision-making. In this chapter, technical background and modes of image acquisition are extensively reviewed. Introduction of xMATRIX technology has enabled utilization of more than 3000 fully sampled elements for 360° focusing and steering. With this powerful technology built in echo probes, any plane of the heart can be imaged. Further advancements in computer technology in speedy processing of the acquired data has resulted in creating images with high temporal and spatial resolutions in a single-beat acquisition format. Nowadays 3DE is becoming part of the routine echocardiography modality. Its role in diagnosis and management of valvular heart disease, cardiac chamber quantification, cardiac masses, and congenital heart disease are discussed in this chapter. The emerging and unique role of 3D TEE in guiding surgical and percutaneous interventions are of importance and will be discussed as well. 3DE is a new modality and like any other new techniques has its own limitations and pitfalls. Low spatial and temporal resolutions, motion and stitch artifacts, and lack of direct 3D measurements are the major limitations. Further technical improvements will heighten its role as the first cardiac imaging modality in our daily practice.

A. S. Omran, MD, FACC, FESC, FASE
King Abdulaziz Cardiac Center,
Ministry of National Guard Health Affairs,
Riyadh, Saudi Arabia

Keywords

3D echocardiography · Three-dimensional echocardiography · Transesophageal echocardiography · Mitral valve · Artifacts in imaging

Abbreviations

3DE	Three-dimensional echocardiography
2D	Two-dimensional
ALC	Anterolateral commissure
AoV	Aortic valve
ASE	American society of echocardiography
CHD	Congenital heart disease
CS	Coronary sinus
EACVI	European association of cardiovascular imaging
fps	Frame per second
HVR	High volume rate
IAS	Interatrial septum
IVC	Inferior vena cava
LA	Left atrium
LAA	Left atrial appendage
LAPV	Left upper pulmonary vein
LCC	Left coronary cusp
LUPV	Left upper pulmonary vein
LV	Left ventricle
LVOT	Left ventricular outflow tract
MI	Myocardial infarction
MPA	Main pulmonary artery
MPR	Multiplanar reconstruction
MR	Mitral regurgitation
MS	Mitral stenosis
MV	Mitral valve
MVA	Mitral valve area
NCC	Non-coronary cusp
PISA	Proximal isovelocity surface area
PMC	Posteromedial commissure
PR	Pulmonary regurgitation

A. Sadeghpour, A. Alizadehasl (eds.), *Case-Based Textbook of Echocardiography*,
https://doi.org/10.1007/978-3-319-67691-3_5

PV Pulmonic valve
PVR Pulmonic valve replacement
RA Right atrium
RAA Right atrial appendage
RCC Right coronary cusp
RV Right ventricle
RVOT Right ventricular outflow tract
TAVI Transcatheter aortic valve implantation
TEE Transesophageal echocardiography
TR Tricuspid regurgitation
TS Tricuspid stenosis
TTE Transthoracic echocardiography
TV Tricuspid valve

Introduction

Three-dimensional (3D) echocardiography has a long history with the first 3D-reconstruction of two-dimensional (2D) images in 1974 [1]. However, the equipment was impractical and images were unsuitable for clinical use. Over the subsequent decades, several researchers, primarily in biomedical engineering, worked on overcoming the technical challenges in order to make the equipment smaller yet capable of generating high-resolution images from complex transducers. They developed instruments that acquired a series of 2D scans in a linear, fan-like, or rotational manner and consolidated them into a 3D image. This concept of image production needed both the transducer and the patient to be in a fixed position relative to each other during the acquisition of serial 2D scans. This was a major limitation to the development of real-time 3D imaging.

The first 3D-TEE was performed in 1992 [2]. Initially, this technique was thought to allow a better understanding of both the spatial relationships of cardiac structures and complex morphology of the valves. However, the image quality using early reconstructive techniques was critically dependent on the quality of the 2D images. Minor patient movements or heart translation would result in image artifacts that could render the image not to be suitable for interpretation [3].

Further advances in computer and crystal technology led to the introduction of currently used matrix-array transducer for the use in transthoracic echocardiography (TTE). This transducer uses a large number of elements (more than 3000) and is capable of generating 3D images in real time [4]. Further reduction in transducer size led to the introduction of the first echocardiographic system allowing real-time 3D TTE and TEE (Philips Medical Systems, Andover, MA, Figs. 5.1a–d and 5.2a–d).

Instrumentation, Modes of Image Acquisition

The current 3D TTE and TEE probes provide all conventional modalities of echocardiography such as 2D imaging, M-mode, pulsed and continuous wave Doppler as well as color flow Doppler imaging. The earlier generation of TTE probe was large and bulky (X3-1), but the newer version of this probe is smaller, almost the same size of 2D TTE probe, and is easy to use (X5-1). This single transducer can be used for 2D and 3D imaging for the same view and does not need to be changed. 3D TEE probe is the same size of multiplane

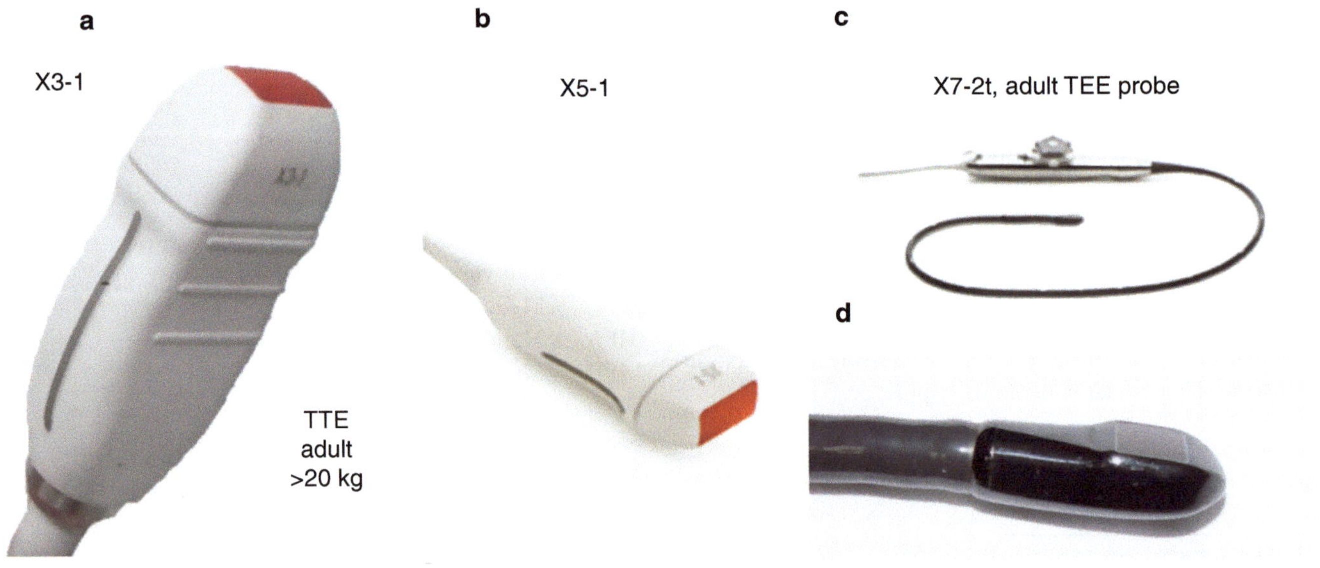

Fig. 5.1 (**a–d**) Philips machines transducers. (**a**) X7-1 transducer with xMATRIX array technology and 2400 elements. This is the first generation transthoracic 3D probe and is used with iE 33 machine. It is a bulky probe and now is replaced by a new generation smaller probe. (**b**) New generation smaller size TTE probe, X5-1 xMATRIX array transducer with pure wave crystal technology. Number of the elements are 3040 and frequency range is 5-1 MHz. Applications of this probe is for adult and pediatric transthoracic 2D and 3D echocardiography. (**c** and **d**) X7-2 t TEE probe with xMATRIX technology. Number of the elements are 2500 and frequency range is 7-2 MHz. Applications of this probe are 2D and 3D TEE

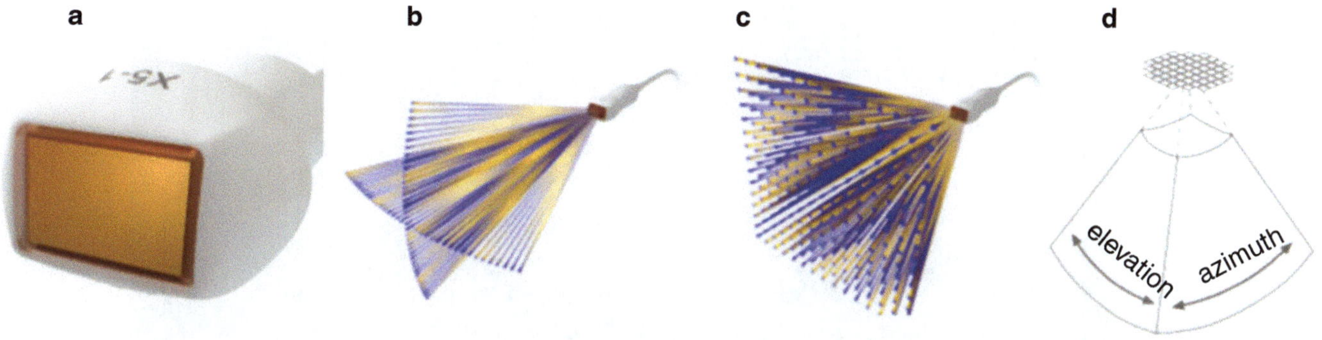

Fig. 5.2 (**a–d**) xMATRIX array technology utilizes more than 3000 fully-sampled elements for 360° focusing and steering. With this modality any planes may be imaged simultaneously

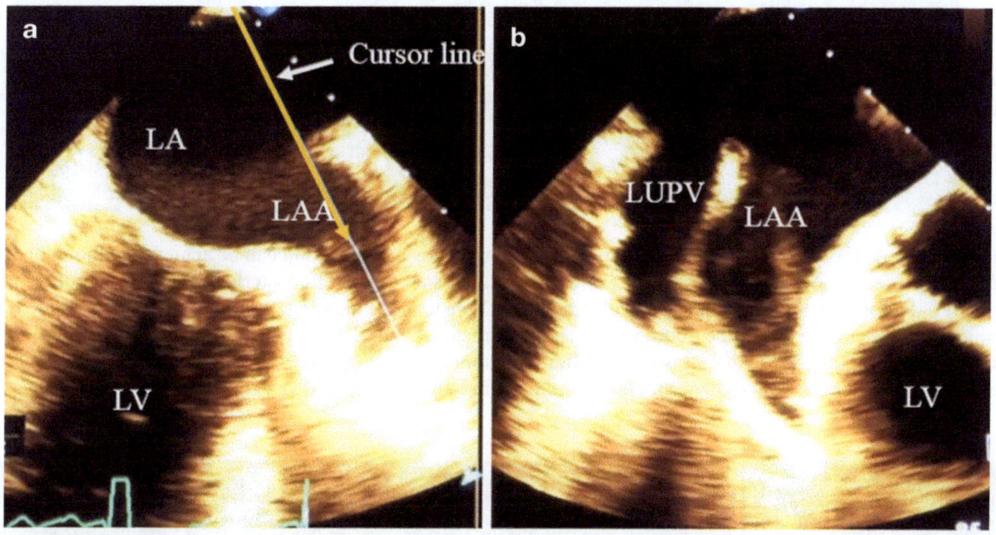

Fig. 5.3 (**a** and **b**) Xplane mode of left atrial appendage (LAA). (**a**) Reference view of the LAA in 3D TEE showing smoke inside the LAA but not clot. (**b**) Aligning cursor line across the appendage shows another orthogonal image of the LAA. This mode is very helpful to confirm the anatomic findings of reference image and its orientation. Note: second orthogonal image in Xplane is right and left inverted as well and this is very important during interpretation. For example, in reference image left upper pulmonary vein (LAPV) was located at the right side of the LAA but in image B appears at the left side. (*LV* left ventricle; *LA* left atrium)

2D TEE probe and is capable of acquiring all 2D echo modalities in addition to 3D. The First Recommendations in 3D echocardiography was published jointly by the European Association of Cardiovascular Imaging (EACVI) and the American Society of Echocardiography (ASE) in 2012 [5]. Currently most vendors are offering the following five modalities of imaging in 3D echocardiography machines [6].

1. **Xplane mode:** is simultaneous multiplane imaging and is a unique modality available in 3D matrix technology. Although these dual or quad- screen images are real-time 2D display, they are available only in echo machines with 3D technology. In Philips echo machine, Xplane mode consists of two orthogonal images with reference view at left side of the screen and the second image is perpendicular to the first and right to left inverted. This mode is very useful in assessment of left atrial appendage (LAA) prior to cardioversion (Fig. 5.3a, b). During monitoring septal puncture for intervention in structural heart diseases such as MitraClip repair or LAA closure, Xplane mode is very helpful (Fig. 5.4a, b). This mode plays a major role in the assessment of mitral leaflet insertion and monitoring of second clip deployment during MitraClip repair. Color Doppler can be superimposed on Xplane mode but the frame rate is very low.
2. **Live 3D:** displays a pyramidal dataset with narrow dimension and can be used to display cardiac structures in near field. Live 3D is a single beat acquisition with high frame rate and good spatial resolution but cannot obtain entire volume of a structure (Fig. 5.5a–c). In newer machines, color Doppler can be added to the image but the frame rate is still very low.
3. **3D Zoom:** this mode provides a focused, wide sector view of a cardiac structure. During applying 3D zoom mode, two boxes appear with reference image at the left and perpendicular view at the right. Sizes of these two boxes should be adjusted to cover the structure. Optimal dimensions of the sector size is important to acquire an image with best possible temporal and spatial resolutions.

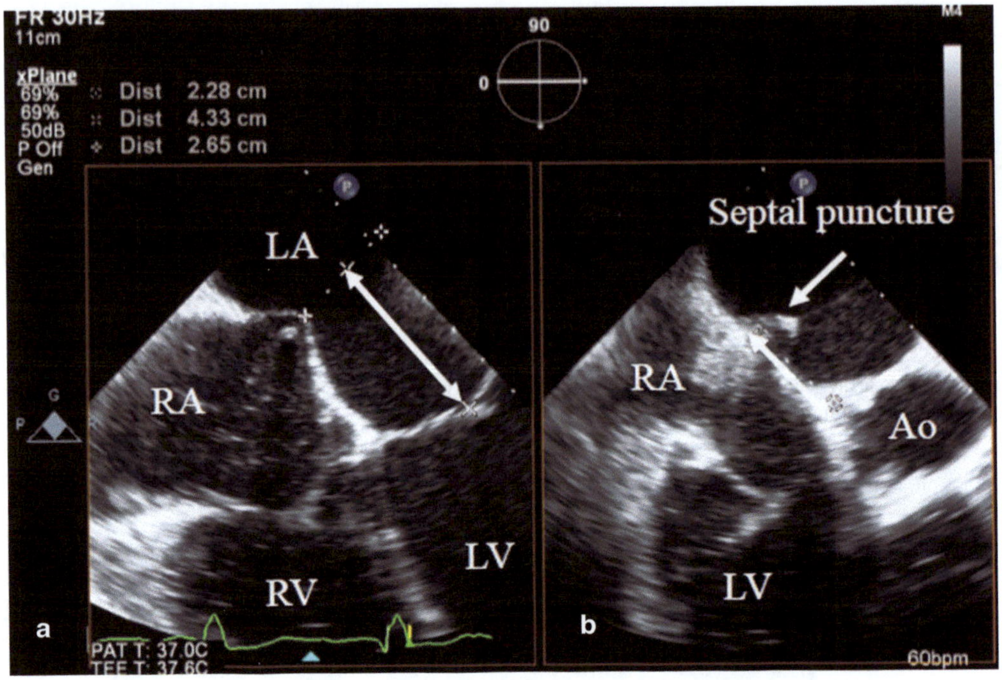

Fig. 5.4 (**a** and **b**) Xplane mode for guiding the interventionist during atrial septal puncture for placement of MitraClip system. (**a**) Septal tenting is seen from RA side. Ideal location of septal puncture should be around 4–5 cm superior to the closure line of the mitral valve leaflets (in this case = 4.3 cm). (**b**) By Xplane mode not only superior-inferior location of the septal puncture can be monitored but an optimal anterior- posterior location can be achieved at the same time. Suitable location is about 2.5 cm posterior to the aortic root (in this case = 2.3 cm). Xplane mode plays a crucial role in guiding MitraClip repair for assessment of mitral leaflets insertion and for second clip placement. This topic will be discussed more in this chapter later. (*LV* left ventricle; *LA* left atrium; *RV* right ventricle; *RA* right atrium)

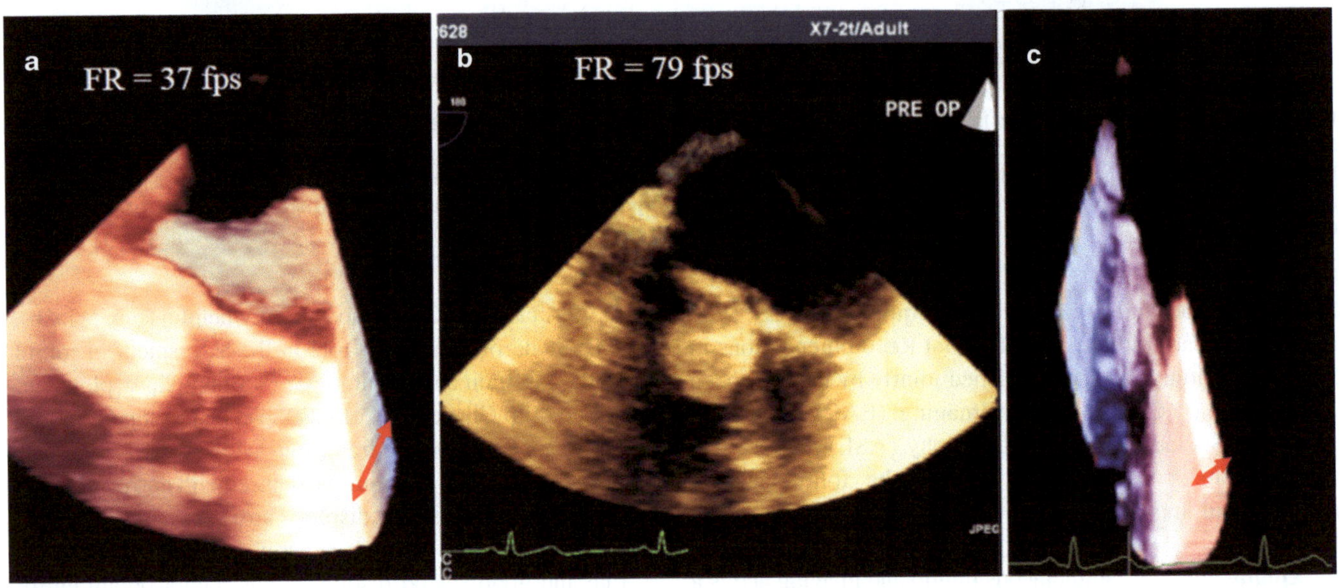

Fig. 5.5 (**a**–**c**) Live 3D TEE acquisition (single beat acquisition) of mitral valve (MV) in a patient with large fibroelastoma. (**a**) Live 3D shows small sector with thin slice (red arrow) but high frame rate (volume rate = 37 Hz). (**b**) Second option available in iE33 with larger sector size can increase the volume rate to 79 Hz with a price of very thin slice. (**c**) Very thin slice is seen in lateral projection (red arrow). In this option live 3D image is like a thicker 2D image

Large size sector of zoom mode will decrease the image resolutions. In older generation of echo machines, zoom mode is a single beat acquisition but in the newer generation 2, 3, or 4 beats can be stitched together to create an image in expense of possibility of stitch artifact. In the newer machines, color Doppler can be added to the zoom mode, but again the low frame rate is a limitation. Zoom mode is suitable for assessment of LAA (Fig. 5.6a, b). The ideal structure to be assessed by zoom mode is mitral valve, whereby it displays an en-face, surgeon's view of

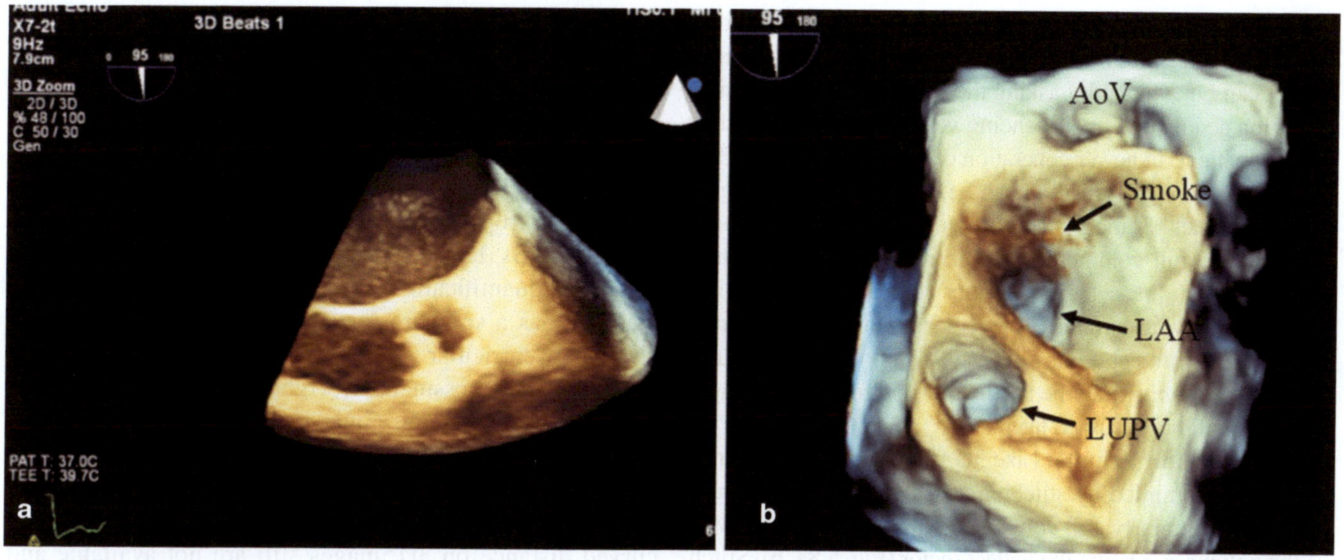

Fig. 5.6 (**a** and **b**) 3D TEE zoom mode acquisition of left atrial appendage (LAA) in a patient with atrial fibrillation, prior to cardioversion. (**a**) Zoom mode creates enlargement of subsegment at the area of the LAA. Appendage is not clear due to very high gain and uncropped image. (**b**) After decreasing the gain and cropping of the image, LAA can be seen with severe smoke due to atrial fibrillation and stagnant blood. Note: this is a surgical view of the LAA when surgeon opens the left atrium for procedures in the left atrium and mitral valve. (*AoV* aortic valve; *LUPV* left upper pulmonary vein)

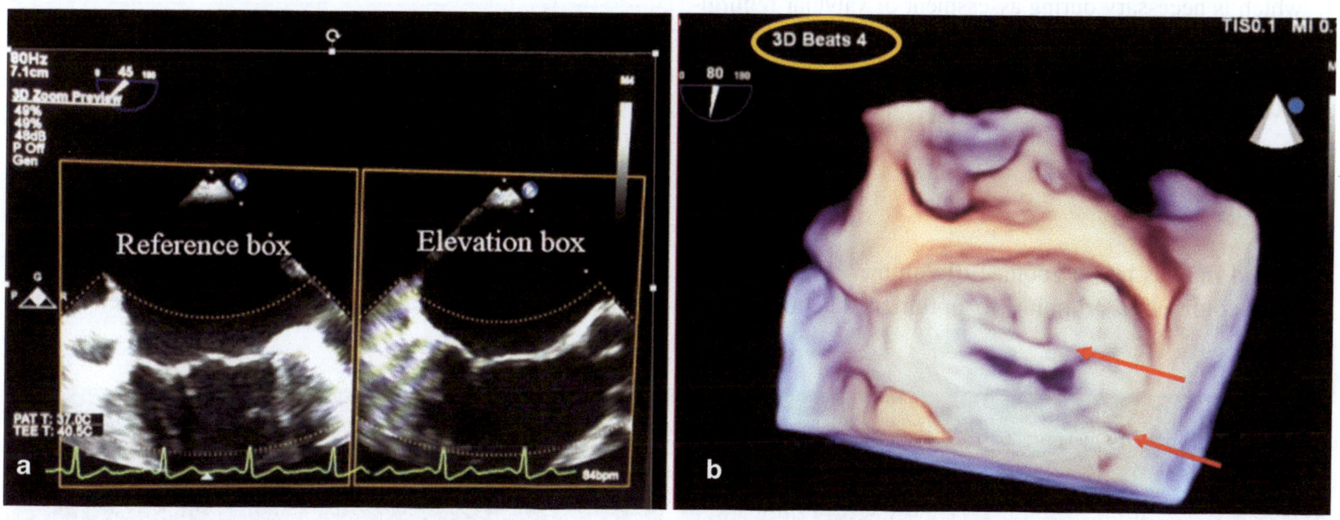

Fig. 5.7 (**a** and **b**) 3D TEE zoom mode acquisition of mitral valve. (**a**) In zoom mode acquisition of any specific structure reference box should cover the entire anatomy of the structure and elevation box should be almost same size of reference box. (**b**) Zoom mode acquisition in Philips iE 33 machine is single beat acquisition with low volume rate (8–10 volumes per second). In this image which was acquired with EPIQ 7 machine, zoom mode of mitral valve is acquired with stitching of 4 beats and volume rate is high (37 Hz). Note: stitch artifacts (*red arrows*)

the valve (Fig. 5.7a, b) in pre- op and post-op evaluations during the mitral valve repair. Aortic, tricuspid, and pulmonic valves can be assessed by 3D zoom mode as well, but images are not optimal due to the limitations in the frame rate and anterior locations of these valves in TEE. In the newer machines, the zoom mode modality has superimposed color Doppler with accepting its low frame rate.

4. **3D Full Volume:** this mode provides a wide pyramidal data set by merging four to seven narrower subvolume wedges obtained over four to seven heartbeats. This mode of acquisition is large enough to include entire left ventricle or both ventricles for assessing volumes and function. Full volume acquisition can also be used for evaluation of the valves with higher frame rate (volume rate) especially if a fast moving structure like vegetation or ruptured chorda are to be investigated. In the older generation of Philips echo machine (iE33), there are three options for full volume acquisition: *volume size* for largest size sector, *frame rate* with narrower sector, and *acquire beat* for patient with tachycardia. Full volume acquisition improves temporal resolution of the image (improves frame rate or volume rate) with the price of

having stitch artifact. Irregular heart rhythm, patient movement, and respiration are the source for artifacts. Stitch artifact can be avoided by asking the patient to stop breathing during acquisition or suspending ventilation in the anesthetized patient. In newer generation of Philips machine (EPIQ 7), full volume acquisition can be obtained by stitching 2, 4, or 6 beats. Some vendors (Siemens Medical Solutions) developed full volume acquisition with single beat, which avoids stitch artifact, and all other companies are working towards having similar achievement. Full volume image is displayed in echo machine as 40% autocropped picture. Further *cropping* may be needed for optimizing the image, which will be discussed later.

5. **3D Color Full Volume:** Like 3D full volume, color acquisition is compiled by stitching seven to 14 heartbeat subvolume. Similarly, full volume color has three options with the *volume size* being the widest sector (Fig. 5.8a, b). Stitch artifact is the main limiting factor in 3D color acquisition. Although in the newer generation of echo machines, color acquisition can be obtained on single beat but volume rate is very low. In EPIQ 7 machine, there is an option of HVR (high volume rate) which can obtain a higher volume rate, which is necessary during assessment of valvular regurgitations. 3D color has several types of color maps and has options for calculation of PISA (proximal isovelocity surface area) in valvular regurgitations.

Cropping

Acquired images in 3D zoom, full volume, and color full volume color need cropping to optimize the images for better visualization and diagnosis. Cropping can be done in the machine on-line during the acquisition of the image or later as off-line by the software installed in the digital storage system. Philips Medical System (Andover, MA) developed a series of QLAB softwares (8, 9, 10, and 10.5) which are built in the machines and can be used as off-line as well for cropping and measurements. Each versions of these QLABs have capability of measuring basic and advanced quantifications. The latest version of EPIQ 7 machine has a software for automated calculation of left atrial and ventricular volumes (Heart Model software), and software for assessment of right ventricular volume is forthcoming. Siemens machines (Siemens Medical Solutions, Mountain View, CA, USA) have software called eSieValve which creates automated model of mitral valve and aortic root with several quantifications. Calculation of curved distance on 3D images still are not available and existing 3D measurement or 3D grid will underestimate the distance compared to 2D measurement. Cropping of the 3D images can be done as icrop, box cropping, and plane cropping (Figs. 5.9a, b and 5.10a, b).

Mitra Valve

Mitral valve (MV) can be assessed by transthoracic and transesophageal echocardiography (TEE). The role of 2D TEE and intraoperative TEE for evaluation of mitral valve and identification of accurate anatomy for reparability have been reviewed in detail in the past 20 years [7]. 2D TEE assessment of the MV needs mental reconstruction to create a "common language" with the cardiac surgeon in the

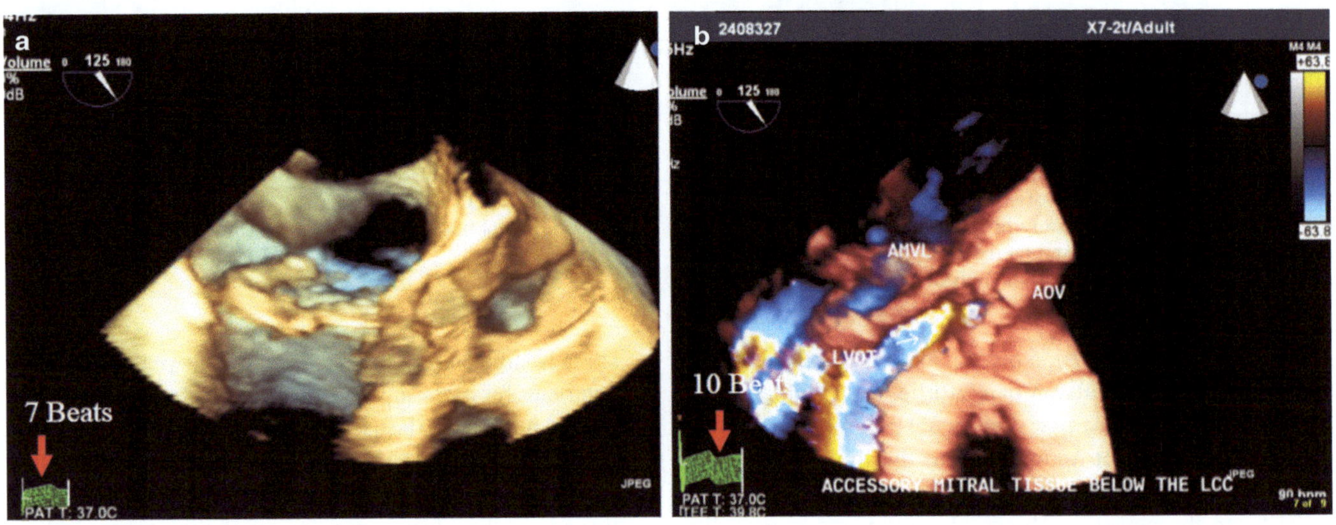

Fig. 5.8 (**a** and **b**) 3D TEE full volume acquisition without and with color Doppler. (**a**) Full volume acquisition of heart in a patient with flail posterior mitral valve leaflet and subaortic accessory tissue. In this image 7 beats (red arrow) are stitched together to create the entire volume of the heart with good spatial and temporal resolution. (**b**) Acquisition of the same view with full volume color. In this acquisition 10 beats (red arrow) are stitched together. Full volume color in iE33 machine has 2 options of 7, 10 beats stitching together with three different sector sizes. Volume size option (with low density) in this machine gives widest sector size which is very helpful to assess the origin of mitral regurgitation during mitral valve repair

operating room. 3D TEE with the en-face, surgeon's view of the MV can create that common language to better communicate with the surgeon and establish a road map for MV repair [8].

Anatomic location and orientation of the MV, which is perpendicular to the ultrasound beam, originating from a TEE transducer inside the esophagus makes it an ideal target for interrogation. Mitral leaflets are thicker than other valves' cusps and opening/closing of the leaflets are relatively slow. Both of these two characteristics of mitral leaflets are in favor of current 3D technology with low spatial and temporal resolutions. Therefore, 3D TEE images of mitral valve are very optimal compared to other valves.

Perioperative 3D TEE assessment of mitral valve and its nomenclature based on Carpentier's classification create an easy way of communication with the cardiac surgeon. Mitral valve images should be acquired at 90° plane perpendicular to the closure line of the valve to create an optimal surgeon's view (Fig. 5.11a, b). MV can be viewed from left atrial (LA) or left ventricular (LV) perspectives; however, the surgeon does not have the privilege to investigate the MV from LV side.

In rheumatic mitral stenosis, thickening of the leaflets, calcification and fusion of the commissures can be evaluated by 3D TEE. Anatomic MV area can be measured by 3D planimetry from the LA or LV side (Fig. 5.12a, b). Moreover, mitral valve area (MVA) can be calculated by basic QLAB software.

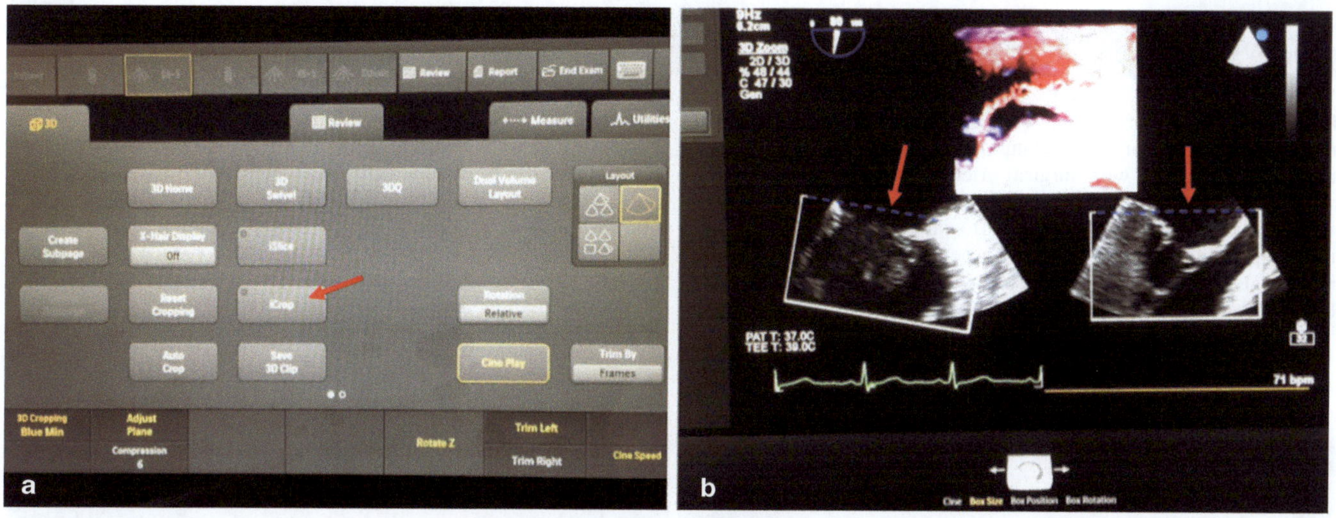

Fig. 5.9 (**a** and **b**) Cropping images in Philips EPIQ 7 machine. (**a**) "icrop" knob in touch screen of the EPIQ 7 machine (red arrow). (**b**) With pressing this knob for any acquired 3D image (zoom mode or full volume), two orthogonal boxes will appear on the screen (red arrows). These boxes can be changed in sizes, location, and orientation. Boxes should be optimized on targeted anatomy. Cropped 3D image within the two boxes appears at the top of the screen looking through the *blue* lines (red arrows)

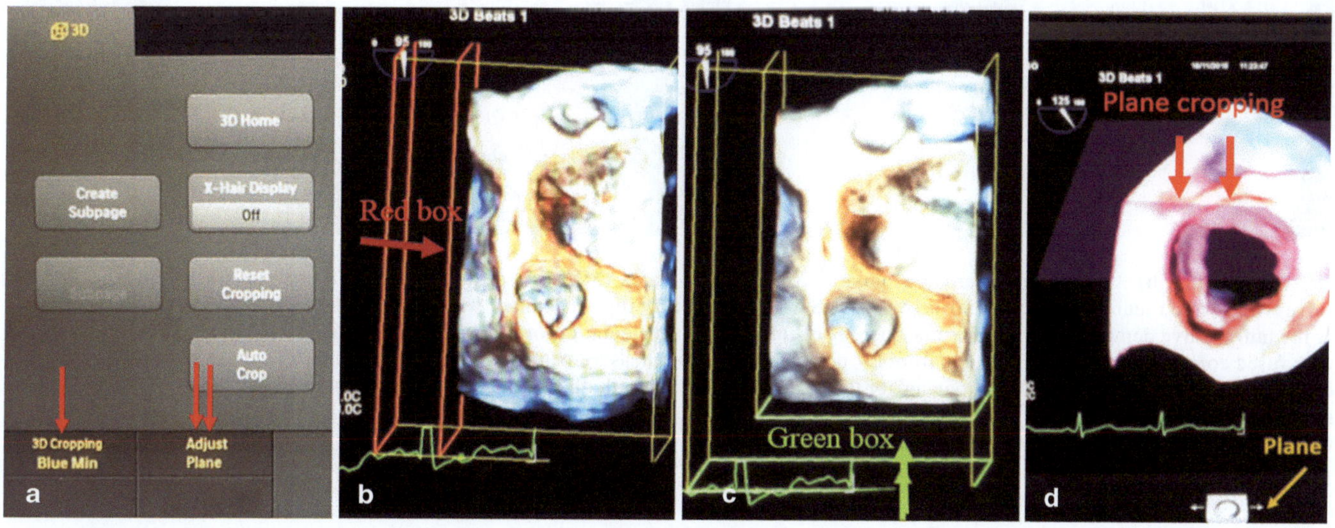

Fig. 5.10 (**a**–**d**) Box cropping and plane cropping in Philips machines. (**a**) Screen of EPIQ 7 machine showing box crop icon (red arrow) and plane crop icon (double red arrows). (**b**) Box cropping by advancing red box (red arrow). (**c**) Box cropping by advancing green box (green arrow). (**d**) Plane cropping by adjusting and advancing an oblique plane. Note: all of the above mentioned modes of cropping are exist in all machines of Philips Company and are almost similar in other vendors

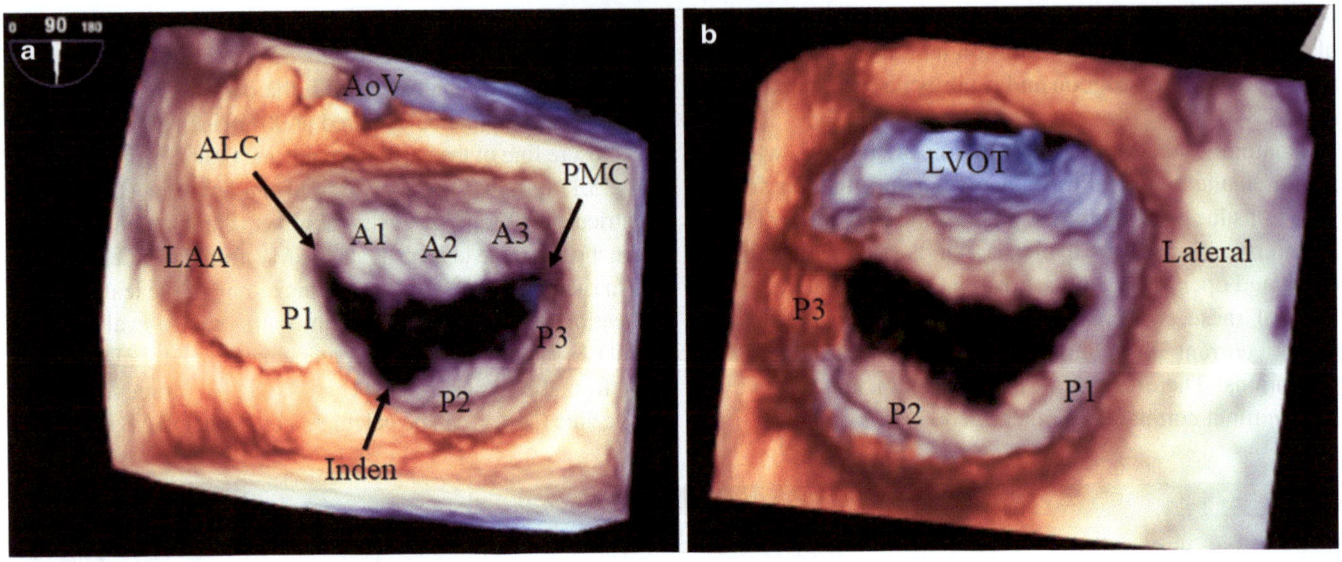

Fig. 5.11 (**a** and **b**) 3D TEE zoom mode acquisition of a normal mitral valve (MV) for nomenclature. (**a**) En-face view of the MV from LA perspective with surgical orientation. Aortic valve (AoV) should be at the top of the image and left atrial appendage (LAA) should be at the left side of the image (towards the head of the patient in the operating room). Based on Carpentier's classification of the mitral valve, posterior mitral valve has three scallops (P1, P2, and P3). There are two natural indentations (inden) between three posterior scallops which sometimes appears very deep and mimicking posterior mitral leaflet cleft. Anterior mitral leaflet has no scallops but arbitrary can be divided in to 3 segments (A1, A2, and A3). There are two commissures between 2 leaflets which are called anterolateral commissure (ALC) and posteromedial commissure (PMC). (**b**) Mitral valve from LV perspective which shows same anatomy but right to left inverted. (*LA* left atrium; *LV*: left ventricle; *LVOT*: left ventricular outflow tract)

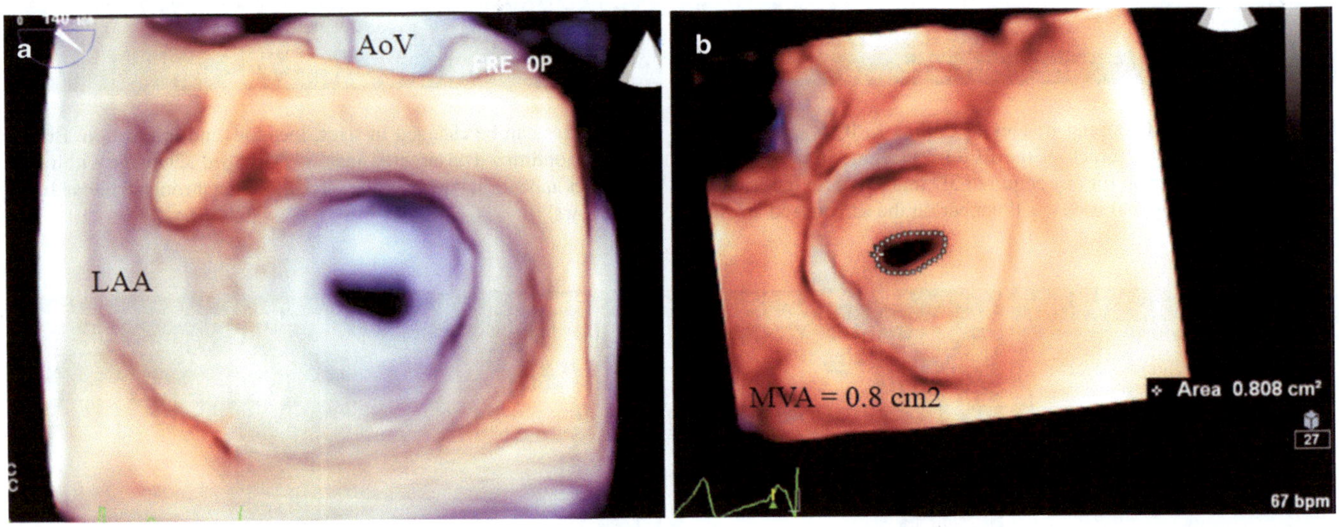

Fig. 5.12 (**a** and **b**) 3D TEE zoom mode acquisition of a mitral valve with severe rheumatic mitral stenosis (MS). (**a**) Surgical view of the mitral valve demonstrates very narrow opening of the leaflets with fused commissures. (**b**) Mitral valve from LV perspective confirms very restricted and "fish-mouth opening" of the valve compatible with severe MS. This study was done by an EPIQ 7 machine which has capability of direct measuring on 3D images. Mitral valve area (MVA) was traced about 0.8 cm^2. In older generation of the Philips machines which do not have direct measurements on 3D, calculation of the MVA can be achieved by 3D grids. Note: direct measurement and 3D grids calculation cannot measure the curved length on 3D images; therefore, underestimates the MVA compared to calculation by pressure half-time method. (*LAA* left atrial appendage; *AoV* aortic valve)

Although these two 3D methods of MVA, which give anatomic area of the mitral valve, underestimate the valve area measured by pressure half-time (physiologic valve area), they are still very useful tools in Cath Lab during percutaneous balloon mitral valvuloplasty.

In degenerative (myxomatous) mitral valve disease, 3D TEE plays a major role in identifying prolapsed or flail segments, shape and the size of mitral annulus, and degree and direction of mitral regurgitation jet (s). Mitral QLAB software in Philips machine (MVQ or MVN) and eSieValve software in Siemens machine are very useful tools for mitral valve quantification assessments [9–13]. Pre-operative 3D TEE can localize the flail scallops or segments and identify the number of ruptured chorda. Immediate post-operative study can show the detail of surgical repair. In case of residual mitral regurgitation (MR), post-operative assessment can evaluate the degree and etiology of the MR and plan for possible re-repair (Figs. 5.13a, b and 5.14a, b).

3D TEE is very useful for assessment of mechanism of ischemic (functional) mitral regurgitation and measuring the annuloplasty ring size prior to operation and evaluate the result of repair [14, 15].

Aortic Valve

Aortic valve (AoV) is not favorable to be assessed by 3D TTE or TEE with current technology. Aortic cusps are paper-thin which makes them not suitable for low spatial resolution of 3D echocardiography. Fast opening/closing of aortic cusps (less than 20 ms) makes this valve unfavorable for low frame rate 3D acquisition. Finally, anterior location and oblique orientation of the AoV in relation to the 3D TEE probe makes it hard to visualize all three cusps in one view. All above-mentioned limitations create artifactual holes in the cusps, which may be mistaken as fenestration. As a general rule, perforation of the cusps should not be reported without confirmation by color Doppler.

3D TEE acquisition of the AoV should be done at long-axis view (120°). Image can be acquired by 3D zoom mode or full-volume mode. Image can be rotated to create surgeon's view as non-coronary cusp locates at the bottom of the picture (Fig. 5.15a–c).

QLAB software in Philips machine can be used to measure the aortic annulus diameter in sagittal and coronal view (CT views) and to calculate aortic annular perimeter for transcatheter aortic valve implantation (TAVI). Anatomic aortic valve area can be calculated accurately by QLAB software. In Siemens echo machine, software of eSieValve is very useful to demonstrate aortic root model for TAVI.

3D color full volume acquisition can show the vena contracta of the aortic regurgitation (AI). Multiplanar reconstruction mode (MPR) in Philips machine can verify the origin of the AI [16].

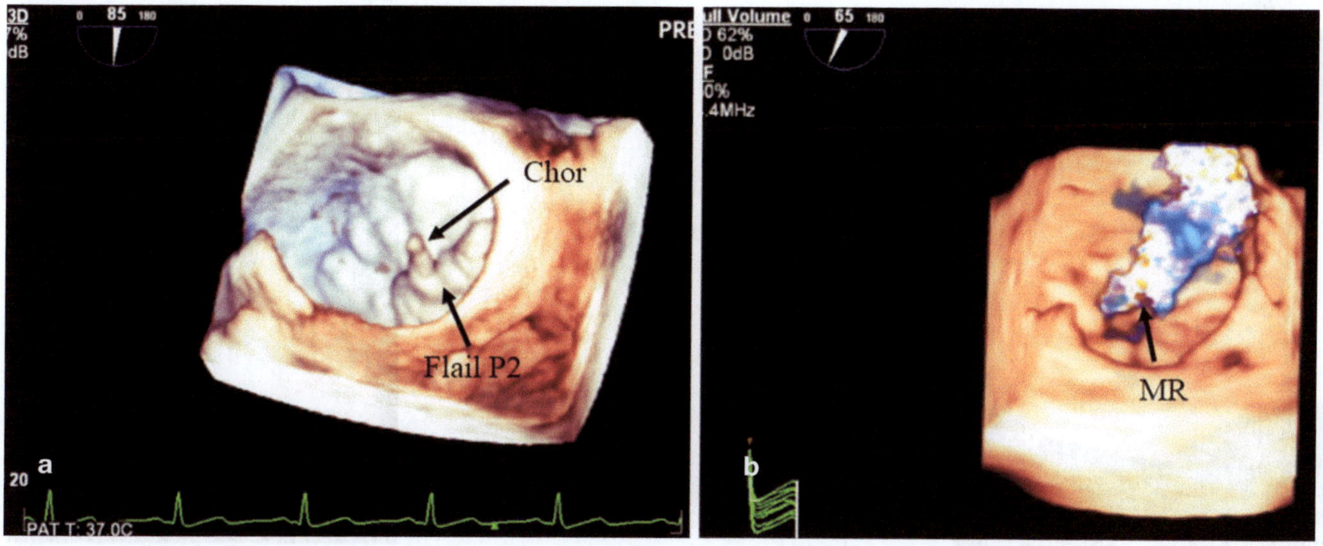

Fig. 5.13 (**a** and **b**) Flail middle scallop of posterior mitral valve leaflet (P2) in a 40-year-old man presented with pulmonary edema. (**a**) 3D TEE zoom mode acquisition in surgical view showing flail P2 with ruptured chorda (chor). (**b**) Full volume color acquisition in same view demonstrates severe anteriorly directed jet of mitral regurgitation (MR)

Tricuspid Valve

In 3D TEE, tricuspid images should be acquired at long-axis view (120°), and then the image can be rotated and displayed as surgeon's view with septal leaflet located at the bottom of the picture (Fig. 5.16a, b).

3D TEE color full volume can show the severity of tricuspid regurgitation and its etiology (lack of leaflets' coaptation or flail cusps).

Tricuspid annular geometry can be evaluated by 3D TEE and appropriate surgical technique can be planned [17].

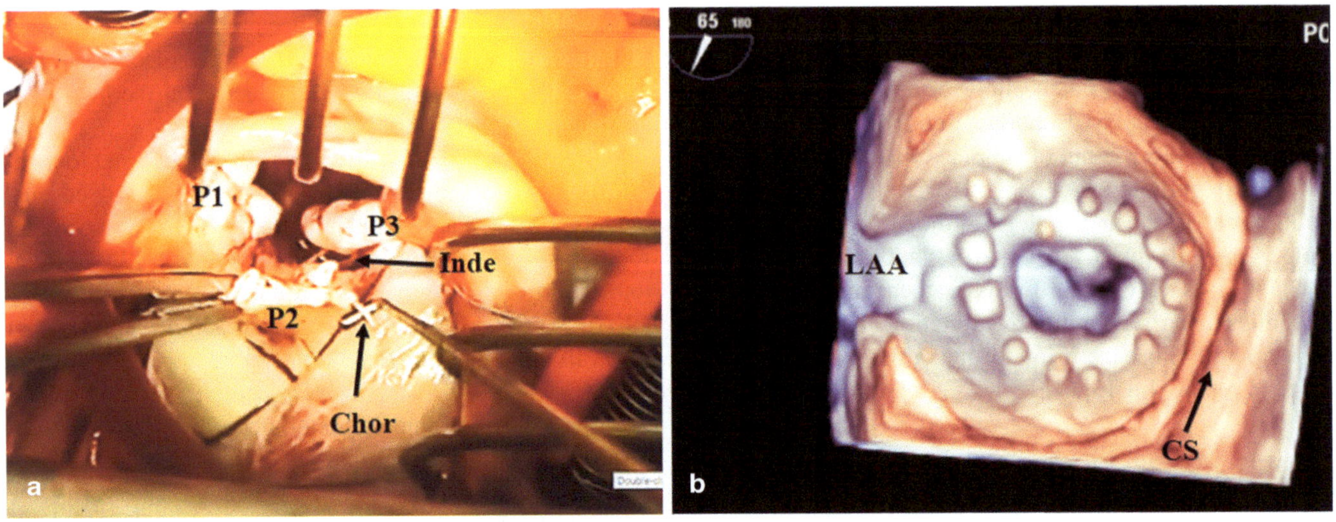

Fig. 5.14 (**a** and **b**) Mitral valve repair in the previous patient. (**a**) Surgical exploration of the mitral valve showing flail middle scallop of the posterior leaflet (P2) with ruptured chorda (chor). Deep indentations (inde) are seen between P2 and two other scallops. These indentations are natural and necessary for physiologic function of the mitral valve and should not be closed during mitral valve repair unless creating mitral regurgitation (otherwise valve will be stenotic). (**b**) Mitral valve repair with quadrangular resection of P2 and insertion of a size 30 Carpentier Physio ring. Mitral valve became competent with no residual leak. (*LAA* left atrial appendage; *CS* coronary sinus)

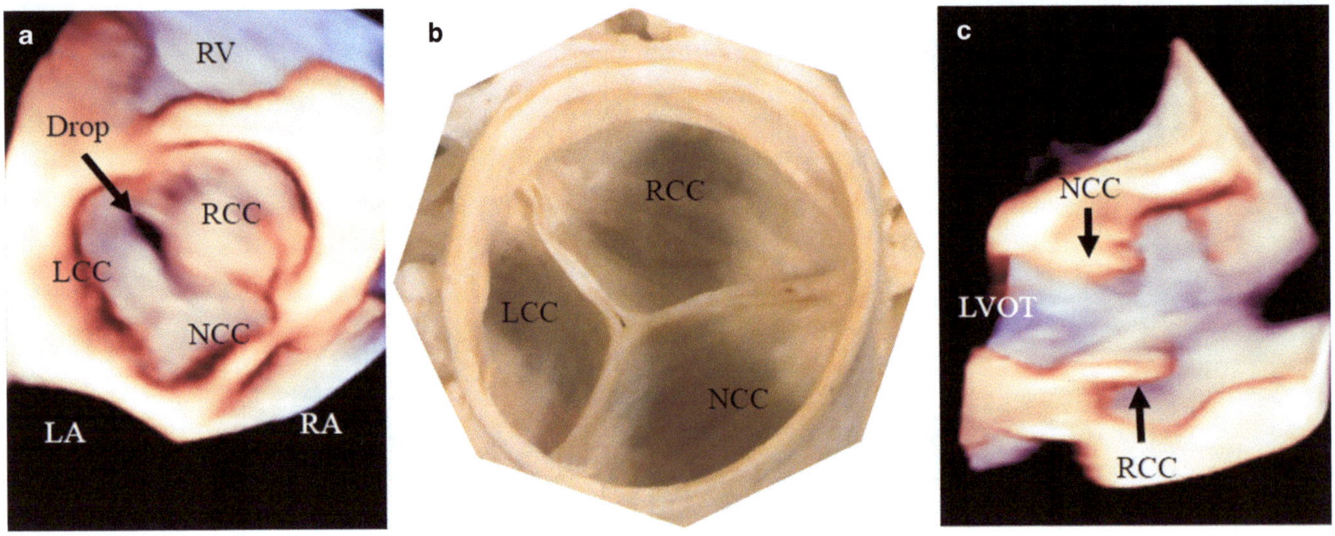

Fig. 5.15 (**a–c**) 3D TEE zoom mode acquisition of the normal aortic valve with surgical correlation. (**a**) Surgical view of the aortic valve (AoV) showing three cusps in diastole. Note: sometimes during 3D zoom mode acquisition of the normal aortic valve, an artifactual echo dropout (drop) is seen at the middle of the cusps. This artifact is due to thin and fast moving nature of the AoV and should not be mistaken as a pathologic fenestration unless proven with a color flow. (**b**) Surgical demonstration of the normal aortic valve. (**c**) Long-axis view of the AoV in same patient. (*RV* right ventricle; *RA* right atrium; *LA* left atrium; *LVOT* left ventricular outflow tract; *RCC* right coronary cusp; *NCC* non-coronary cusp; *LCC* left coronary cusp)

Pulmonic Valve

Pulmonic valve (PV) is rarely assessed by 3D TEE. PV pathologies are part of congenital heart disease in pediatric population. When PV is thickened due to pathologic process, it is easier to be imaged by 3D TEE. Acquisition should be done at 60-70° of TEE probe and can be acquired by zoom mode or full volume mode (Fig. 5.17a, b).

Native Valve Endocarditis

Sensitivity of 3D TEE for detecting vegetations is less than 2D TEE in native valves endocarditis due to lower spatial and temporal resolution.

3D TEE has an advantage over the 2D TEE in showing the entire bulk of the vegetation and its exact location on the valves. In assessment of complications of endocarditis such as peri-annular abscess and its extension, 3D TEE is very useful [18, 19].

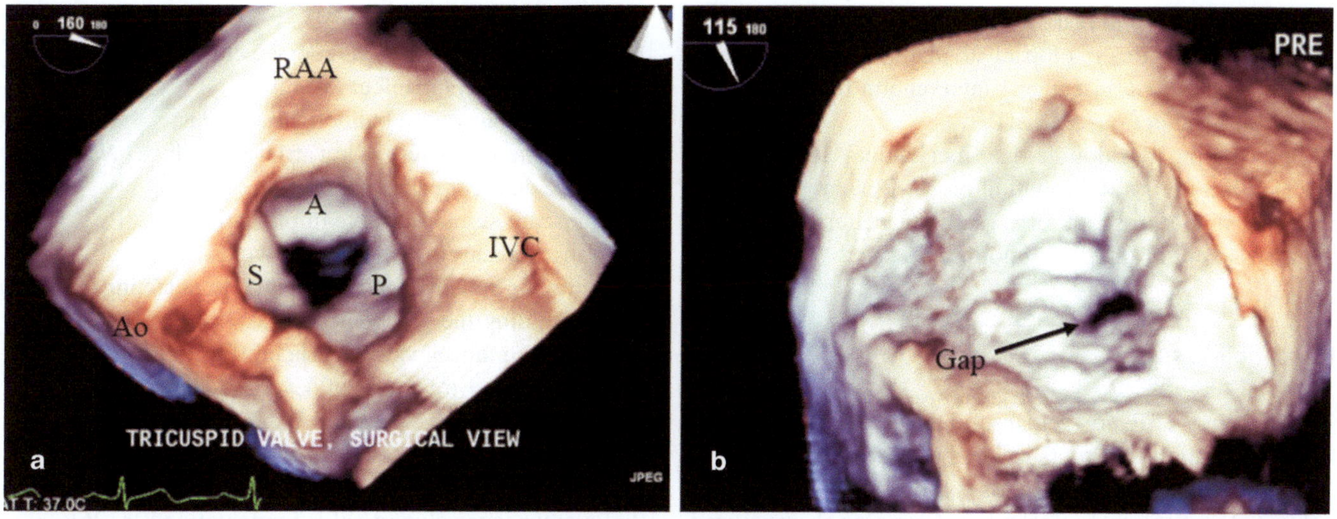

Fig. 5.16 (**a** and **b**) 3D TEE zoom mode acquisition of the tricuspid valve (TV). (**a**) Surgical view of a tricuspid valve in a patient with severe rheumatic mitral stenosis and moderate tricuspid stenosis (TS). Thickening and restricted opening of all three tricuspid valve cups during diastole is demonstrated. In surgical view of the TV, right atrial appendage (RAA) is the landmark for anterior cusp (A), Interatrial septum (IAS) for septal cusp (S), and IVC for posterior cusp (P). (**b**) Surgical view of a tricuspid valve in another patient with secondary severe tricuspid regurgitation (TR). Large gap during systole is shown causing severe TR. (*IVC* inferior vena cava)

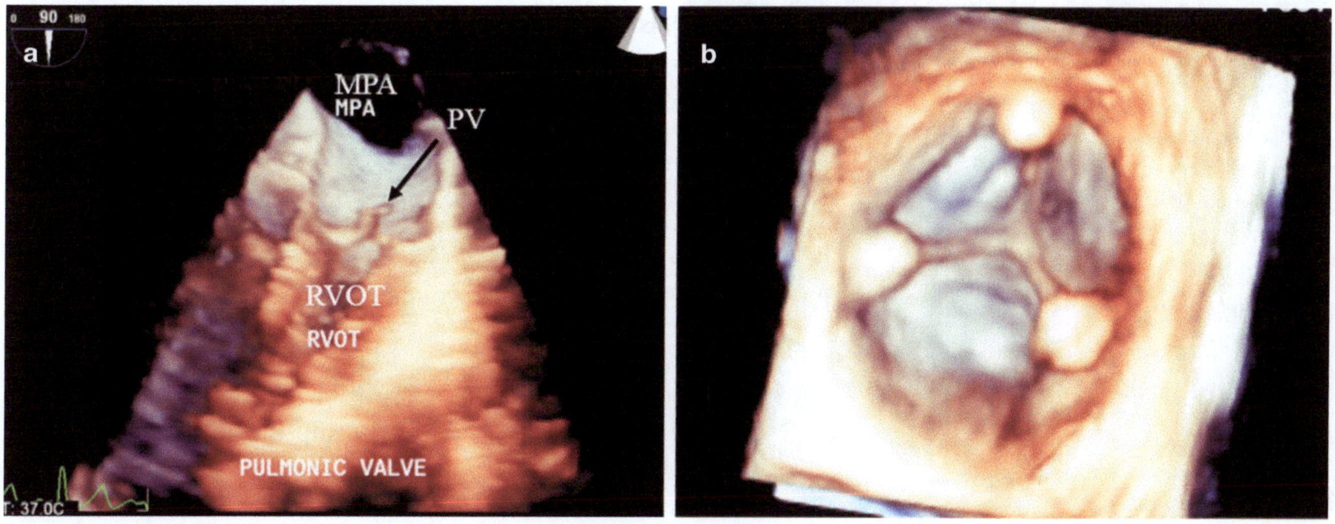

Fig. 5.17 (**a** and **b**) 3D TEE zoom mode acquisition of the pulmonic valve (PV). (**a**) 3D TEE acquisition at RVOT view. Normal pulmonic valve is thin and due to its anterior location is very difficult to obtain a clear image with all three cusps. (**b**) A bioprosthetic PVR in another patient with severe PR. In this 3D TEE zoom mode, all three leaflets are clear during diastole. (*RVOT* right ventricular outflow tract; *MPA* main pulmonary artery; *PVR* pulmonic valve replacement; *PR* pulmonary regurgitation)

Prosthetic Valve Dysfunction

3D TEE is an ideal tool to assess prosthetic mitral valve in en-face view. In the cardiac operating room, intraoperative 3D TEE can show the function of prosthetic mitral valve and the degree of transvalvular regurgitation (MR). In the presence of paravalvular MR, again degree and location of leak can be identified very accurately.

3D TEE has a crucial role in diagnosing a stuck disc, pannus formation on the sewing ring and burden of possible clot on the valve in mitral position.

Prosthetic mitral valve can be assessed by 3D TEE for detecting paravalvular leak. By obtaining a "clock-face" display of the location(s) of paravalvular leak, decision can made for possible transcatheter intervention for device closure or surgical options [20, 21].

In assessing the double-disc mechanical aortic valve, 3D TEE has the same limitation of 2D TEE in visualizing both discs. Fluoroscopy or CT are the better options for the assessment of the discs' motion.

Cardiac Masses

3D TTE and TEE are very useful in assessing clots and benign or malignant tumors inside the heart [22].

3D acquisition of cardiac masses can delineate their entire volume, location, and attachment. Cropping the acquired image can identify necrosis, liquefaction and calcification, which may help in differentiation between the clot, benign or malignant tumors [23].

In left atrial myxoma, which is the most common benign tumor of the heart, 3D TEE acquisition can show the size, pedicle and location of the attachment (Fig. 5.18a, b) This may facilitate the surgical approach (left atriatomy vs. right atriatomy and trans-septal).

Structural Heart Disease Intervention

Transesophageal echocardiography (TEE), especially 3D TEE, plays a major role in guiding and monitoring of the procedures in the Cath Lab as of the following:

1. Atrial septal defect (ASD) device closure
2. Ventricular septal defect (VSD)
3. Percutaneous mitral balloon valvuloplasty
4. Percutaneous closure of left atrial appendage (Watchman device and Amplatzer plug)
5. Transcatheter aortic valve implantation (TAVI)
6. Transcatheter closure of paravalvular leak(s)
7. MitraClip repair- role of 3D TEE in selecting patients and guiding the procedure and assessment of the result in clipping mitral valve is crucial (Fig. 5.19a, b)
8. Transcatheter treatment of severe tricuspid valve regurgitation with the MitraClip system (TricuClip); so far, about 200 cases have been performed worldwide
9. Alcohol septal ablation for hypertrophic cardiomyopathy
10. Percutaneous valve-in-valve implantation [24–26].

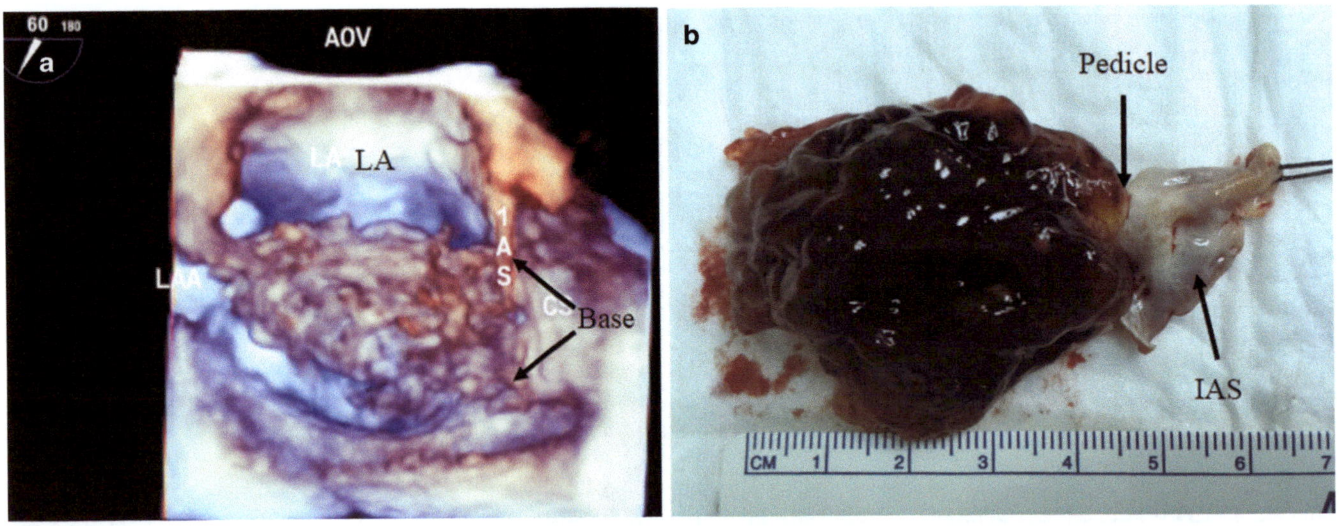

Fig. 5.18 (**a** and **b**) 3D TEE zoom mode acquisition of a left atrial (LA) myxoma in a 36-old-man who presented with acute inferior wall MI. (**a**) 3D TEE acquisition in surgical view showing a large myxoma which is attached to the interatrial septum (IAS) with a broad base pedicle. (**b**) Myxoma was resected via a right atriatomy. Myxoma was taken out with part of the IAS to prevent future possible recurrence. (*MI* myocardial infarction)

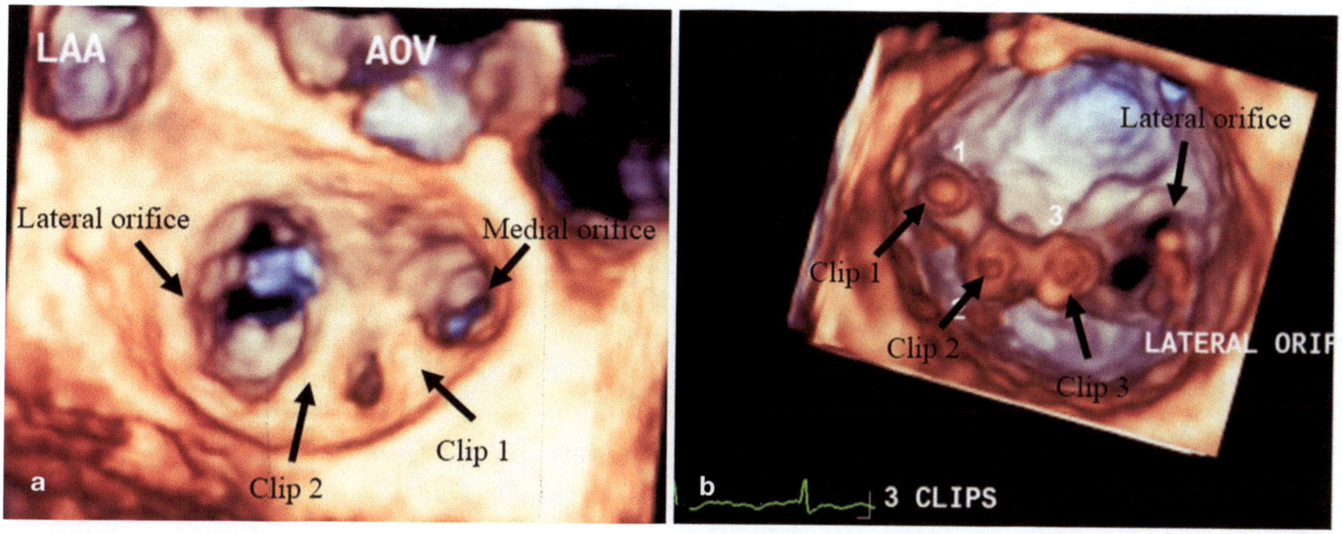

Fig. 5.19 (**a** and **b**) 3D TEE in cath lab. For guiding MitraClip repair. (**a**) 3D TEE zoom mode acquisition after placement of 2 clips on mitral valve (MV). First clip is deployed in medial side of the MV leaflets and second clip more towards the lateral side. Mitral valve became triple- orifice. (**b**) MitraClip repair in another patient who had 3 clips placement. Mitral valve is seen from left ventricular (LV) perspective. Three clips are seated well. 3D zoom mode from LV side is very important view after placement of the clip for confirmation of the leaflets insertion. Gradual cropping in this view can show that both leaflets are equally grasped by the clipper. Partial grasping of the leaflet tissue and inadequate insertion may cause partial or complete detachment of the clip and embolization. This risk was reported in many trials in about 2–4% of patients

Congenital Heart Disease

Three- dimensional echocardiography has become important in the management of patients with congenital heart disease (CHD) [27]. Transthoracic 3D is increasingly used in children because of good acoustic windows and the non-invasive nature of the technique. As mentioned earlier, TEE 3D has important role in the Cath Lab during intervention in CHD such as ASD and VSD device closure. 3D TEE plays an important role in pre-op and post-op assessments of CHD in the operating room (Fig. 5.20a, b).

Chamber Quantification

The full volume mode in 3D TTE or TEE is ideal for assessing left ventricular volumetrics. Recently, various software have been developed to use the on-line or off-line to calculate left atrial and right ventricular volumes as well [28].

In older software, endocardial border is semi-automatically traced at end- diastole and end-systole, and then the system calculates left ventricular (LV) end-systolic and diastolic volumes and ejection fraction. The software also allows a 17-segment motion analysis to demonstrate time to minimum systolic volume of each segment as curves. This segmental analysis may be useful for assessment of LV dyssynchrony in CRT (Figs. 5.21a, b and 5.22a, b).

Recently Philips Healthcare developed a new fully-automated quantification software installed in EPIQ 7 (HeartModel) which is able to calculate LV and LA volumes based on one four-chamber full-volume acquisition of the heart [29, 30].

Limitations, Image Artifacts, Future Directions

Limitations

3D echocardiography (3DE) provides a new dimension in cardiovascular imaging; it is a revolution in the field of echocardiography to assess the pathology and guiding the appropriate intervention. Like any other new technique, 3DE has its own limitations and needs further technical improvements. Followings are some of the limitations in current 3DE:

1. Poor spatial resolution especially in TTE (currently spatial resolution of 3D TTE is worse than that of 2D TTE; therefore, in patients with poor echo window, it is impossible to obtain optimal 3D TTE images)
2. Low temporal resolution (low frame rate or volume rate) (frame rate of 2DE images are usually 50-100 frame per second (fps), while in 3DE with single- beat acquisition it is less than 15 fps)
3. Motion artifact due to the patient's movement or cardiac translation (during 3D TTE, the patient should be instructed to hold in breathing for 10-15 seconds in order to acquire

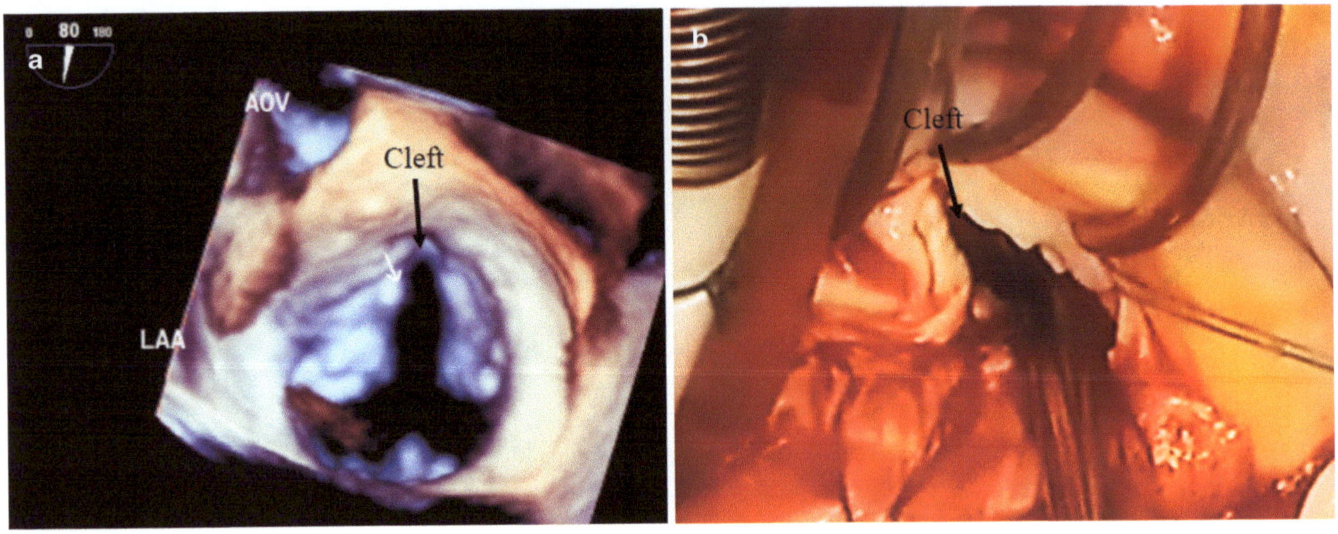

Fig. 5.20 (**a** and **b**) 3D TEE zoom mode acquisition of mitral valve in a 29-year-old woman presented with severe mitral regurgitation (MR). (**a**) Surgical view of the mitral valve demonstrating trifoliate mitral valve with cleft of anterior mitral leaflet. (**b**) Surgical exploration confirmed the diagnosis of cleft anterior leaflet. Patient underwent cleft repair with direct suturing and insertion of an annuloplasty ring. Follow up echo in 5 years showed no residual MR or mitral stenosis

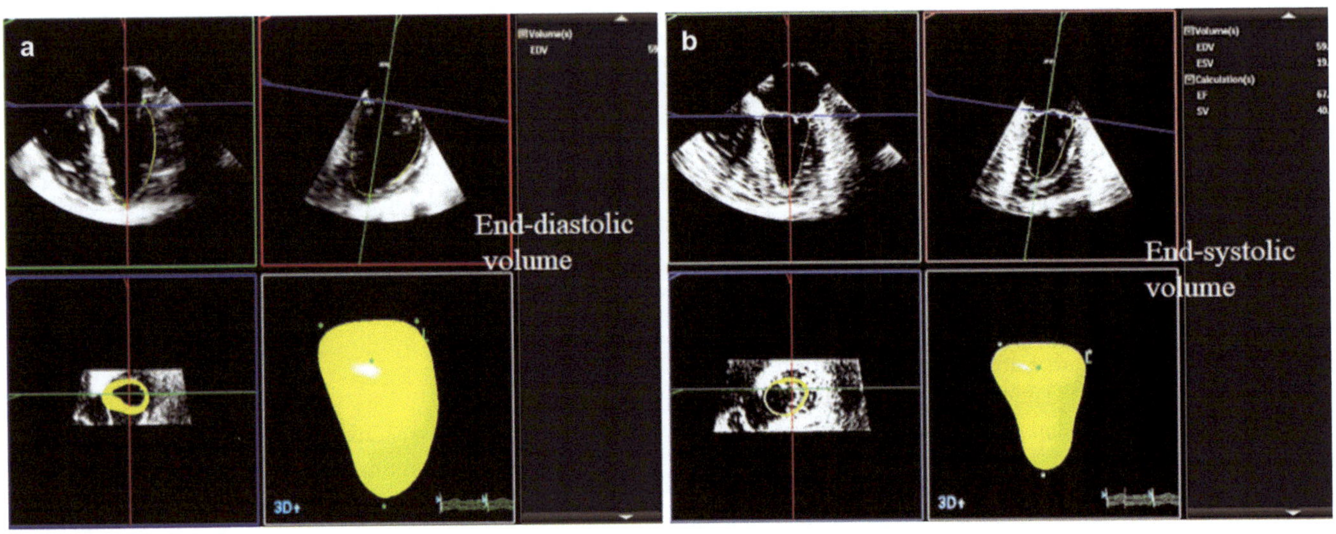

Fig. 5.21 (**a** and **b**) Calculation of left ventricular (LV) volume in Philips EPIQ 7 machine by QLAB 10. (**a**) LV full volume acquired by TEE. Semiautomatic left ventricular (LV) endocardial border tracing at the end of diastole which calculates end-diastolic volume. (**b**) Endocardial border tracing at the end of systole and calculating end-systolic volume. At the end LV ejection fraction is calculated which in this example was 67.3%. In latest generation of Philips machine with HeartModel, LV and LA volume can be calculated in a totally automatic format. (*LA* left atrium)

the image. During 3D TEE, breath holding for patients may be difficult. In intubated patients, use of the breathing machine can be suspended temporarily)

4. Above-mentioned limitations of 3D color Doppler (including narrow sector and a more chance of stitch artifact)
5. No valid direct measurements on 3D echo images (the existing measurements in newer generation machines are not able to measures curved lengths and tend to underestimate the actual dimensions)
6. No 3D screen in echo machines (the existing echo machines lack 3D screen and therefore display the images in 2D screen)

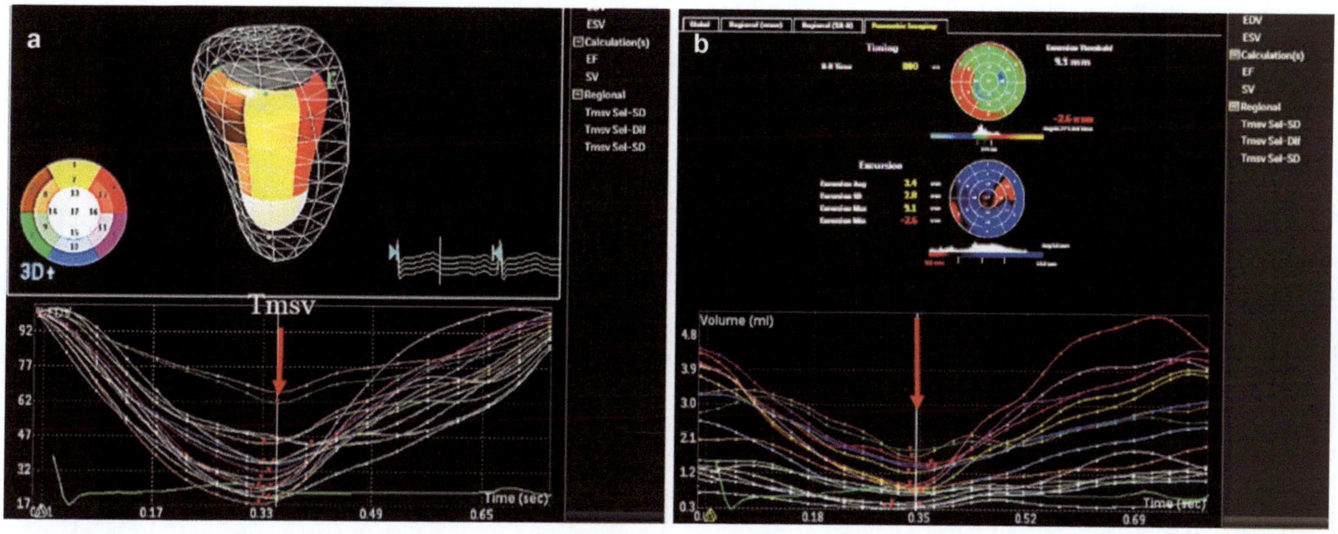

Fig. 5.22 **a** and **b**: Segmental analysis of surface rendering full volume of the left ventricle (LV) by QLAB 10. (**a**) 3D TEE full volume acquisition of the LV. Segmental analysis by 3D Q advance software showing curve of time to minimum systolic volume (Tmsv) for each 17 segment. Tmsv of each segment is marked by a small red triangle. In normal LV, all of the curves representing 17 segments should come to a minimum volume at the middle of the systole almost at the same time (in red arrow time). (**b**) Regional time differences is normalized by heart rate of the patient and is shown as *dyssynchrony index* which is normally below 5% (in this patient = 2.69%). Dyssynchrony index more than 20% is compatible with severe LV intraventricular dyssynchrony and that patient should benefit from a CRT. (*CRT* cardiac resynchronization therapy)

Overall, 3DE is a transitional modality and cannot provide a complete diagnostic study alone without adjunctive 2DE.

Image Artifacts

3D echocardiography is subject to the same types of artifacts encountered in 2D echocardiography. Followings are the most common artifacts in 3D TTE and TEE:

1. Stitching (reconstruction) artifacts during multibeat acquisition in patients with irregular rhythm or due to breathing (Fig. 5.23a, b)
2. Dropout artifacts (creating a hole in the middle of the interatrial septum or aortic cups)
3. Blurring (amplification) artifacts (thin structures may appear thicker)
4. Blooming artifacts (producing fringes extending beyond the borders of mechanical discs)
5. Artifacts in 3D TEE during catheter-based interventions and ablation procedures (blooming artifacts of the guidewires, railroad-shaped artifacts, reverberations and shadowing).
6. Gain (there are no specific recommendations for gain setting, but generally the optimal setting is when the static noises disappear. It is recommended to perform 3D echocardiography or off-line cropping in a room with deem light to avoid excessive gain) [31].

Future Directions

As for the future directions of 3D echocardiography and what it is hoped to achieve, the following is the list of suggestions to see in this new modality in echocardiography:

1. Single-beat acquisition to avoid stitch artifacts
2. Better spatial resolution especially in 3D TTE and a smaller size probe (this will make 3D TTE more favorable and popular in day-to-day use in echocardiography laboratories)
3. Higher frame (volume) rate to make it possible to be used for stress echocardiography and 3D strain imaging
4. Automated cropping
5. Wider color sector to cover the entire structure like multiple jets of mitral regurgitation (this will be very helpful during MitraClip procedure and assessment of paravalvular leak(s) in the post-operative setting and intervention for device closure)
6. Direct valid 3-dimensional measurements
7. Having 3D screen in echo machines and all workstations for 3D image display

Overall, if this technique is to substitute 2D echocardiography, it should become more friendly to use and less time consuming. This transition was seen to occur in M-mode modality to 2DE and is expected to happen in 2D to 3D echocardiography.

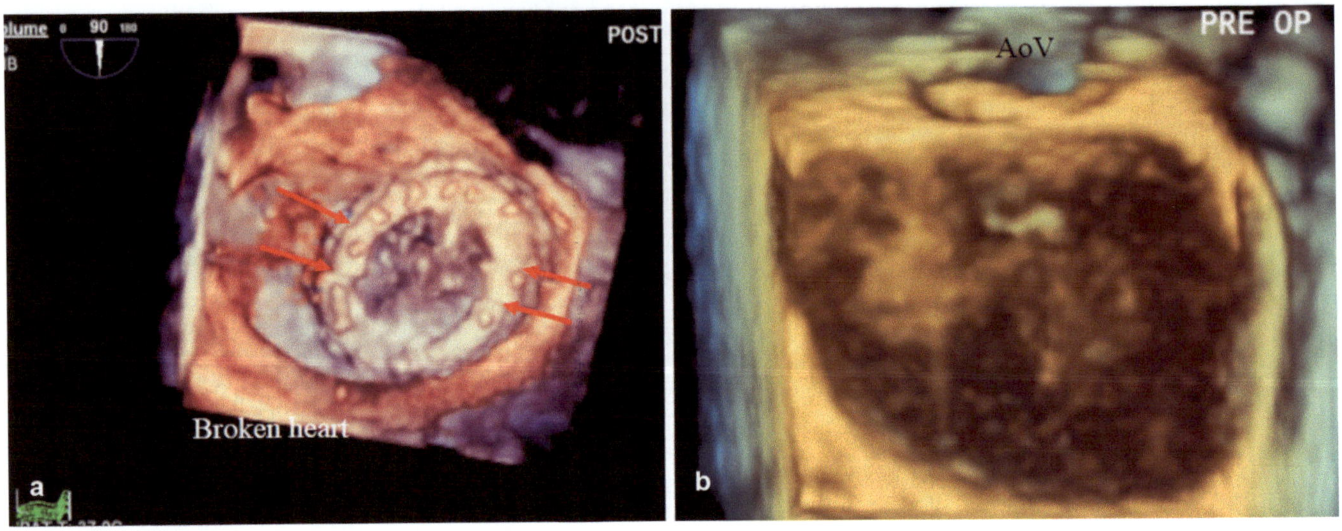

Fig. 5.23 (**a** and **b**) Artifacts in 3D echocardiography. (**a**) Full volume 3D TEE acquisition of a mechanical mitral valve in the operating room (OR). Stitch artifact is seen creating "broken valve". Stitch artifact is due to multiple subvolume stitching together, and happens more often due to arrhythmia, patient's breathing or moving. Solution for this artifact is acquisition with breath holding or suspending the mechanical ventilation in the OR. (**b**) 3D TEE zoom mode acquisition of a mitral valve with severe stenosis and severe smoke in the left atrium. High gain and severe smoke are obscuring the mitral valve. (*AoV* aortic valve)

Questions

1. In modes of image acquisition in 3D echocardiography, which of the following statement IS CORRECT?
   A. Xplane mode with color, provides high frame rate image but spatial resolution is very low
   B. In zoom mode, a particular structure like mitral valve (MV) can be shown with magnification and high frame rate
   C. Zoom mode, en-face view of the MV can be used as a live image during interventional procedures like MitraClip repair
   D. In live 3D with color, temporal resolution is better than full volume color multibeat acquisition

2. In application of 3D TEE during surgical mitral valve repair which of the following statement IS CORRECT?
   A. In pre-operative assessment, 3D full volume color is import to measure the color jet area and define the severity of the mitral regurgitation
   B. In surgical view of the mitral valve, aortic valve should be oriented at the top of the image and left atrial appendage to the left side of the screen
   C. In surgical view of the mitral valve, medial scallops of the mitral leaflets and posteromedial commissure are located at the left side of the screen
   D. Mitral leaflets coaptation and possible vegetations on the mitral leaflets can be assessed by 3D single beat acquisition better than full volume multibeat acquisition

3. In assessment of aortic valve by 3D echocardiography, which of the following IS CORRECT?
   A. 3D QLAB can calculate the aortic valve area at the level of the leaflet tips and this is more accurate than 2D planimetry
   B. In patients with aortic regurgitation, 3D TEE can define the fenestrations and perforations of the aortic cusps for better planning in surgical repair
   C. Calcifications on aortic valve will be overestimated by 3D TEE compared to transthoracic echocardiography
   D. In using of 3D TEE prior to TAVI, aortic annulus dimension measured by 3D TEE, overestimate the dimensions compared to CT measurements

4. In application of 3D TEE in cath lab during structural heart disease intervention, which of the following IS CORRECT?
   A. Intra-operative 3D TEE in the cath lab is mandatory for guiding the TAVI procedure
   B. 3D TEE is better than transthoracic 3D echocardiography for assessment of tricuspid valve (TV), prior to percutaneous intervention for TV repair
   C. 3D en-face view of the atrial septum is necessary for accurate location of the septal puncture during MitraClip repair
   D. Live 3D zoom mode en-face view of the mitral valve is very useful to assess the perpendicularity of the clip during Mitraclip procedure

5. In limitations and image artifacts in 3D echocardiography which of the following IS CORRECT?
   A. In 3D TEE assessment of the atrial septum during intervention, extra hole(s) may be seen in the septum due to dropout artifacts
   B. Stitching artifacts are more common in live 3D mode than full volume acquisition
   C. Due to blooming artifacts, guidewires may look thinner during transcatheter interventions in the cath lab
   D. Currently spatial and temporal resolutions of 3D echocardiography are better than 2D echocardiography

Answers

1. C
2. B
3. A
4. D
5. A

References

1. Dekker DL, Pizaili RL, Dong E Jr. A system for ultrasonically imaging the human heart in three dimensions. Comput Biomed Res. 1974;7(6):544–53.
2. Pandian NG, Nanda NC, Schwarts SL, Fan P, Cao QL, Sanyal R, et al. Three-dimensional and four-dimensional transesophageal echocardiographic imaging of the heart and aorta in humans using a computed tomographic imaging probe. Echocardiography. 1992; 9(6):677–87.
3. Levine RA, Handschumacher MD, Sanfilippo AJ, Hagege AA, Harrigan P, Marshall JE, et al. Three-dimensional echocardiographic reconstruction of the mitral valve, with implications for the diagnosis of mitral valve prolapse. Circulation. 1989;80(3):589–98.
4. Sugeng L, Weinert L, Thiele K, Lang RM. Real-time 3-dimensional echocardiography using a novel matrix array transducer. Echocardiography. 2003;20(7):623–35.
5. Lang RM, Badano PB, Tsang W, Adams DH, Agricola E, Buck T, et al. EAE/ASE recommendations for image acquisition and display using three-dimensional echocardiography. J Am Soc Echocardiogr. 2012;25:3–46.
6. Vegas A. Three-dimensional transesophageal echocardiography: principles and clinical applications. Ann Card Anaesth. 2016;19(Special Issue 1):S35–43.
7. Omran AS, Woo A, David TEE, Feindel CM, Rakowski H, Siu SC. Intraoperative transesophageal echocardiography accurately predicts mitral valve anatomy and suitability for repair. J Am Soc Echocardiogr. 2002;15:950–7.
8. Salcedo EE, Quiafe RA, Seres T, Carroll JD. A framework for systematic characterization of the mitral valve by real-time three-dimensional transesophageal echocardiography. J Am Soc Echocardiogr. 2009;22:1087–99.
9. Apor A, Nagy AI, Kovacs A, Manouras A, Andrassy P, Merkely B. Three-dimensional dynamic morphology of the mitral valve in different forms of mitral valve prolapse-potential implications for annuloplasty ring selection. Cardiovasc Ultrasound. 2016;14(32):1–7.
10. Pierce EL, Pierre J, Rabbah JPM, Thiele K, Wei Q, Vidakovic B, et al. Three-dimensional field optimization method: Gold-standard validation of a novel color Doppler method for quantifying mitral regurgitation. J Am Soc Echocardiogr. 2016;29:917–25.
11. Tan TC, Zeng X, Jiao Y, Wang L, Wei Q, Thiele K, et al. Three-dimensional field optimization method: clinical validation of a novel color Doppler method for quantifying mitral regurgitation. J Am Soc Echocardiogr. 2016;29:926–34.
12. Sardari Nia P, Heuts S, Daemen J, Luyten P, Vainer J, Hoorntje J, et al. Preoperative planning with three-dimensional reconstruction of patient's anatomy, rapid prototyping and simulation for endoscopic mitral valve repair. Interact Cardiovasc Thorac Surg. 2016: 1–6.
13. Jin CN, Salgo IS, Schneider RJ, Kam KKH, Chi WK, So CU, et al. Using anatomic intelligence to localize mitral valve prolapse on three-dimensional echocardiography. J Am Soc Echocardiogr. 2016;29:938–45.
14. Machino-Ohtsuka T, Seo Y, Ishizu T, Sato K, Sugano A, Yamamoto M, et al. Novel mechanistic insights into atrial functional mitral regurgitation. 3-dimentional echocardiography study. Circ J. 2016;80: 2240–8.
15. Owais K, Montealegre-Gallegos M, Jeganathan J, Matyal R, Khabbaz KR, Mahmood F. Dynamic changes in the ischemic mitral annulus: implication for ring sizing. Ann Card Anaesth. 2016;9:15–9.
16. Regeer MV, Kamperidis V, Versteegh MIM, Schalij MJ, Marsan NA, Bax JJ, et al. Three-dimensional transesophageal echocardiography of the aortic valve and root changes in aortic root dilatation. Eur Heart J Cardiovasc Imaging. 2016;13:1–8.
17. Knio Z, Montealegre-Gallegos M, Yeh L, Chaudary B, Jeganathan J, Matyal R, et al. Tricuspid annulus: a spatial and temporal analysis. Ann Card Anaesth. 2016;19:599–605.
18. Han J, He Y, Gu X, Sun L, Zhao Y, Liu W, et al. Echocardiographic diagnosis and outcome of pseudoaneurysm of the mitral-aortic intervalvular fibrosa. Medicine. 2016;95:1–6.
19. Janardhanan R, Umar Kamal M, Riaz IB, Smith MC. Anterior mitral valve aneurysm: a rare sequelae of aortic valve endocarditis. Echores Pract. 2016:K7–K13.
20. Lancelloti P, Pibarot P, Chsambers J, Edvardsen T, Delgado V. Dulgheru, et al. Recommendations for the imaging assessment of prosthetic heart valves: a report from the European Association of Cardiovascular Imaging, the Inter-American Society of Echocardiography, and the Brazilian Department of Cardiovascular Imaging. Eur Heart J Cardiovasc Imaging. 2016;17:589–90.
21. Arribas-Jimenesz A, Rama-Merchan J, Barreiro-Perez M, Merchan-Gomez S, Iscar- Galan A, Martin-Garcia A, et al. Utility of real-time 3-dimensional transesophageal echocardiography in the assessment of mitral paravalvular leak. Circ J. 2016;80:738–44.
22. Saric M, Armour AC, Arnaout MS, Chaudhry FA, Grimm RA, Kronzon I, et al. Guidelines for the use of echocardiography in the evaluation of a cardiac source of embolism. J Am Soc Echocardiogr. 2016;29:1–42.
23. Espinola-Zavaleta N, Lozoya-Del Rosal JJ, Colin-Lizalde L, Lupi-Herrera E. Left atrial cardiac myxoma: two unusual cases studied by 3D echocardiography. BMJ Case Rep. 2014.
24. Hadeed K, Hascoet S, Amadieu R, Karsenty C, Cuttone F, Leobon B, et al. Assessment of ventricular septal defect size and morphology by three-dimensional transthoracic echocardiography. J Am Soc Echocardiogr. 2016;29:777–85.
25. Hammerstingl C, Schueler R, Malasa M, Werner N, Nickenig G. Transcatheter treatment of severe tricuspid regurgitation with the MitraClip system. Eur Heart J. 2016;37:849–53.
26. Nejjari M, Himbert D, Brochet E, Attias D. First-in-man full percutaneous valve-in-valve implantations using Edwards SAPIEN 3 prostheses to treat a patient with degenerated mitral and aortic bioprosthesis. Interact Cardiovasc Thorac Surg. 2016;23: 505–10.

27. Simpson J, Lopez L, Acar P, Friedberg M, Khoo N, Ko H, et al. Three-dimensional echocardiography in congenital heart disease: an expert consensus document from the European Association of Cardiovascular Imaging and the American Society of Echocardiography. Eur Heart J Cardiovasc Imaging. 2016;17:1071–97.
28. Lang RM, Badano LP, Mor-Avi V, Afilalo J, Armstrong A, Emande L, et al. Recommendations for cardiac chamber quantification by echocardiography in adults: an update from the American Society of Echocardiography and the European Association of Cardiovascular Imaging. J Am Soc Echocardiogr. 2015;28:1–39.
29. Tsang W, Salgo I, Medvedofsky D, Takeuchi M, Prater D, Weinert L, et al. Transthoracic left heart chamber quantification using an automated adaptive analytics algorithm. J Am Coll Cardiol Img. 2016;9:769–82.
30. Otani K, Nakazono A, Salgo I, Lang R. Three-dimensional echocardiographic assessment of left heart chamber size and function with fully automated quantification software in patients with atrial fibrillations. J Am Soc Echocardiogr. 2016;29:955–65.
31. Faletra FF, Ramamurthi A, Dequarti MC, Leo LA, Moccetti T, Pandian N. Artifacts in three-dimensional transesophageal echocardiography. J Am Soc Echocardiogr. 2014;27:453–62.

Basic Principles of Fetal Echocardiography

6

Mahmood Ebrahimi

Abstract

Heart defects are among the most common malformations in the developing fetus. Carry the highest mortality among all congenital malformations and are very challenging to detect.

The fetal heart is notoriously difficult to evaluate due to its complex anatomy and physiology. Many obstetrics ultrasound units are able to successfully obtain and correctly interpret views of the heart, including the four chamber and the outflow tracts views. Unfortunately standards for imaging are not uniform, nationally or internationally with a significant variation in detection rates. While experienced tertiary centers report a high level of diagnostic accuracy, the overall detection rate remains low. Meticulous and preferably standardized screening with referral of the patients with abnormal findings to Pediatric Fetal cardiology specialists would be the ideal approach. This brief manuscript is organized in short paragraphs that are accompanied by illustrations made of drawings as well as real fetal echocardiography pictures that have been conveniently labeled to assist the learner. It should be viewed as a brief introduction to the how to of the screening fetal cardiac ultrasound examination.

Our approach goes beyond the four chamber and outflow views. Our screening fetal ECHO consists of five sequential horizontal slices from fetal abdomen and chest. We believe the best time to perform fetal echocardiogram is around 20 weeks of gestation.

Keywords

Fetal echocardiography · Fetal cardiac ultrasound examination · Congenital heart disease · Chromosomal abnormalities · Hydrops fetalis · Teratogenic medications

With special thanks to Ruben J Acherman, MD and Merujan R Uzunyan, MD for their contributions.

M. Ebrahimi, MD, RDCS
Division of Neonatology, LAC+USC Medical Center, Keck School of Medicine of the University of Southern California, Los Angeles, CA, USA
e-mail: ebrahimi@usc.edu

Abbreviations

A.Ao	Ascending aorta
DA	Ductus arteriosus
Dao	Descending aorta
F.O.	Foramen ovale
IVC	Inferior vena cava
LA	Left atrium
LV	Left ventricle
MB	Moderator band
MPA	Main pulmonary artery
MTHFR	Methylene tetrahydrofolate reductase
MV	Mitral valve
RA	Right atrium
RPA	Right pulmonary artery
RV	Right ventricle
RVOT	Right ventricular outflow tract
SVC	Superior vena cava
TV	Tricuspid valve

Practical Approach to Fetal Echocardiography: Prenatal Detection of Congenital Heart Disease

Introduction

- Prenatal diagnosis of congenital anomalies in the fetus is becoming an important part of obstetrics and the management of the pregnant mother and her newborn baby. Ultrasonic evaluation of the fetus is a routine part of every pregnancy for evaluation of fetal growth, gender and age and also detection of different congenital anomalies. Considering cardiac defects are the most frequent malformation of fetal development, fetal echocardiography and cardiac evaluation of the fetus has become an important part of Maternal Fetal Medicine and management of the newborn with critical congenital heart defects.

A. Sadeghpour, A. Alizadehasl (eds.), *Case-Based Textbook of Echocardiography*,
https://doi.org/10.1007/978-3-319-67691-3_6

- Cardiac evaluation of the fetus by ultrasound has been done since the 1960s and 1970s, but the first publication in 1980 [1] by Kleinman and colleagues should be considered the beginning of a new era in fetal echocardiography and fetal cardiology as a new super specialty.
- Visualization of the fetal heart is possible from 9 weeks of gestation transvaginal and 11 weeks transabdominal [2]. By 16 weeks cardiac structures and abnormalities become more recognizable on fetal echocardiogram.
- **The best time to scan for accurate diagnosis is between 16 and 22 weeks of gestation. Early imaging provides enough genetic testing and decision making if is needed** [3]. Nevertheless, some investigators believe early imaging does not have enough accuracy and might miss late developing lesions [3–5]. For different legal and ethical reasons one should decide when to perform fetal echocardiogram on individual bases.
- We routinely perform our scans at 20 weeks of gestation.
- Congenital heart diseases occur at the rate of less than 1% (8/1000 live births), but they have the highest rate of mortality of congenital malformations in infancy. Mortality rate of the cardiovascular system is about 50% vs. 20% for respiratory system. It is very unfortunate that even in developed countries 10% of the infants with congenital heart disease are dying without being diagnosed. These are the infants who die at home or emergency rooms without being diagnosed until after the autopsy shows that the cause of death was critical congenital heart disease, which may have been diagnosed prenatally (if the mother had adequate fetal cardiac evaluation). Prenatal diagnosis of critical congenital heart disease allows for advance planning to have the delivery done in a facility with all necessary equipment and personnel to start immediate evaluation and treatment if necessary. Furthermore, perinatal counseling and interventions could be done if the diagnosis of congenital heart disease was made in advance [6, 7].

Table 6.1 Risk factors for fetal heart disease and current indications for fetal echocardiography

Risk factors for fetal heart disease and current indications for fetal echocardiography
Maternal
• Suspected fetal cardiac anomaly during obstetric ultrasound
• Maternal Diabetes
• Phenylketonuria
• Methylene tetrahydrofolate reductase (MTHFR) gene mutations
• Medications
• Alcohol
• Illicit drugs
• Infections
• Autoimmune diseases
• Maternal congenital heart disease
• Maternal obesity
• Pregnancies of assisted reproductive technology
Familial
• Congenital heart disease
• Nonchomosomal syndromes
Fetal
• Increased nuchal transluscency thickness
• Signle umbilical artery
• Chromosomal abnormalities
• Hydrops fetalis
• Cardiac arrhythmias
• Extracardiac abnormalities
• Monochorionic placentation
• Abnormal first trimester markers

Current Status

- With improvements in ultrasound technology and operator's skill, the diagnosis of critical congenital heart disease is approaching 100% (if a complete fetal echocardiogram is performed by an experienced echocardiographer), but prenatal detection of congenital heart disease remains at about 35%. The low prenatal detection rate is due to the fact that fetal echocardiograms are routinely performed only in high-risk pregnancies (Table 6.1), while most infants with congenital heart disease are born to mothers in low risk population [8].

As part of a routine obstetric ultrasound, obtaining a 4-chamber view of the heart is recommended by the American Institute of Ultrasound in Medicine and the American College of Radiology [9–11]. Recent studies by different investigators have shown 4-chamber view alone, even when right and left ventricular outflow tracts [8, 13] are added, is not sufficient and up to two thirds of serious congenital heart disease remain undiagnosed [14, 15]. Thus Ackerman et al. [14] proposes universal screening with fetal cardiac evaluation as the best method for detecting serious cardiac malformations prenatally.

Screening Fetal Echocardiogram

- Since a comprehensive fetal echocardiogram is costly and not readily available for every pregnancy, in 2007, Acherman group [14] proposed replacing the four chamber view strategy by a universal screening fetal cardiac evaluation, as previously was proposed by Yagel and colleagues in 2001 [16]. Considering obstetricians and perinatologist are the first to evaluate congenital malformations in the fetus and a cardiologist is not always present, screening fetal echocardiography becomes an indispensable part of prenatal ultrasound to establish a sense of normalcy. As soon as any deviation from this normalcy appears, the patient should be referred for further cardiac evaluation and detailed fetal echocardiography by an experienced fetal cardiologist.

- The screening fetal echo consists of five horizontal slices from fetal abdomen and chest. Starting from the upper abdomen, at the level of cord insertion and sliding slowly towards the head (Fig. 6.1).
- In order to determine the situs of the fetus, it is essential to figure out which is the left side of the fetus. This is done by looking at its presentation and position.

Upper Abdominal Slice

By establishing right-left and anterior-posterior position of the fetus, this cut will clearly determine the abdominal situs (Fig. 6.1–1). Spine is located in the back and abdominal aorta is in the front and slightly to the left of the spine. Inferior vena cava sits to the right and in front of the aorta. Stomach is to the left and the liver to the right. Umbilical vein from the insertion takes a right-sided course and drains to the portal sinus. If gallbladder is visualized, it is always on the right side of the umbilical vein (Fig. 6.2).

Apical Four-Chamber View

By moving slightly cephalad from previous cuts the 4-chamber view can be obtained. This slice is a transverse cut of the fetal chest (Fig. 6.1).

In this view, cardiac position, cardiac axis, cardiac size, structures surrounding the heart, and finally intracardiac anatomy should be investigated.

- **Cardiac position.** In the four chamber view, the heart is normally sitting in the left chest which causes the left lung to appear smaller than the right lung. In a normal situatio, the apex of the heart is looking the same direction as the stomach and the free wall of the right ventricle is more anterior and in contact with the chest wall. The Presence

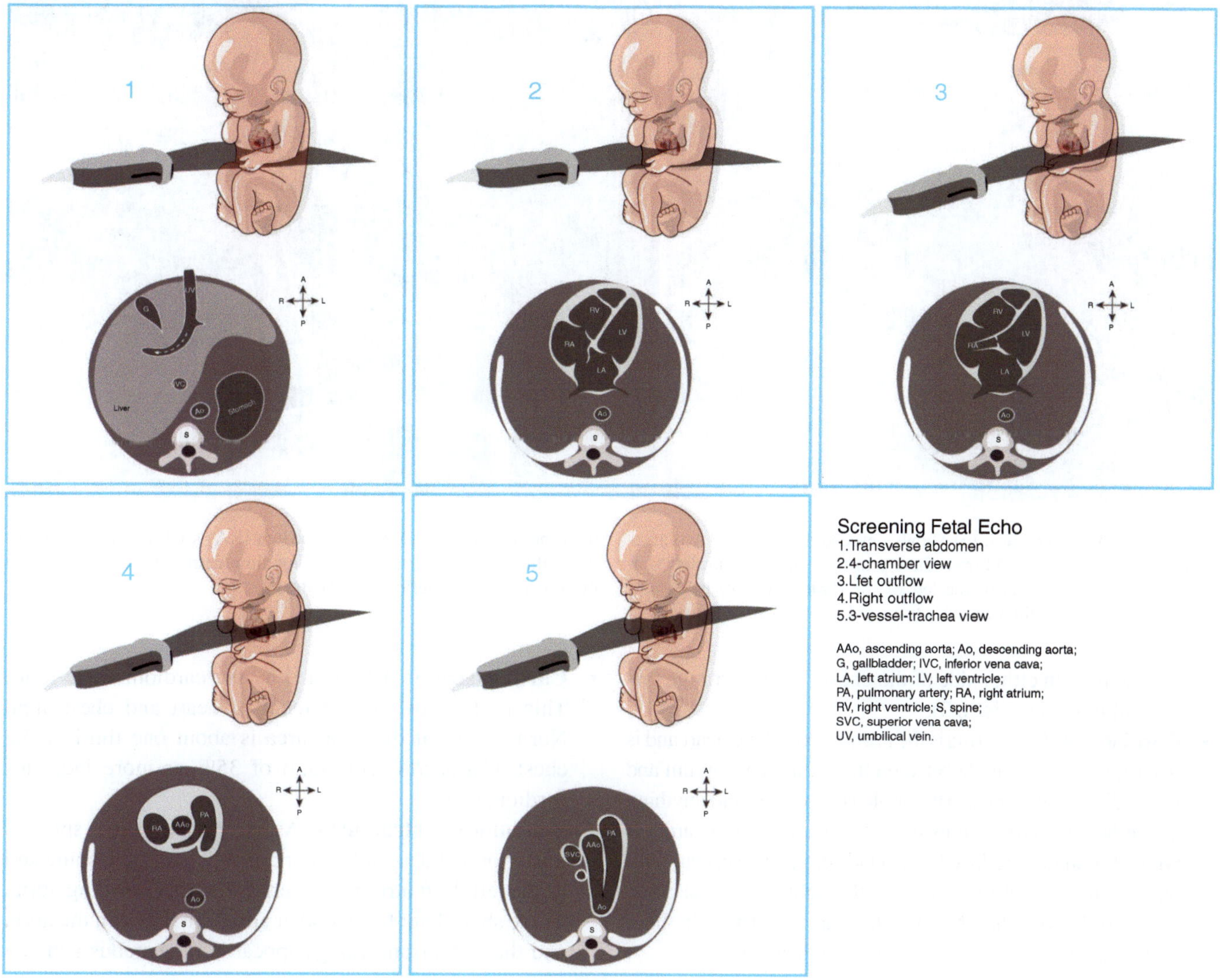

Fig. 6.1 **Screening Fetal Echo.** Courtesy of Ruben J Acherman MD et al.

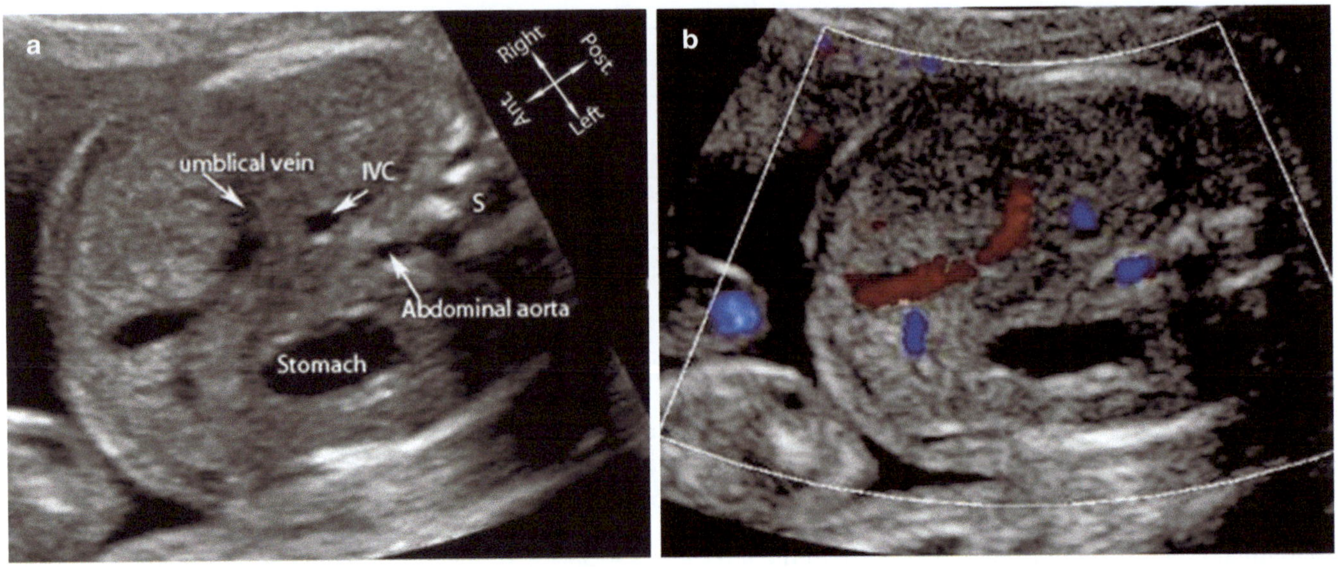

Fig. 6.2 **Upper Abdominal cut.** (**a**) Demonstrating stomach on the left side of the abdomen; Umbilical vein turns to the right; abdominal aorta in front of the spine (S) and to the left; inferior vena cava (IVC) anterior and to the right of the aorta. (**b**) Color flow applied for better visualization of the structures

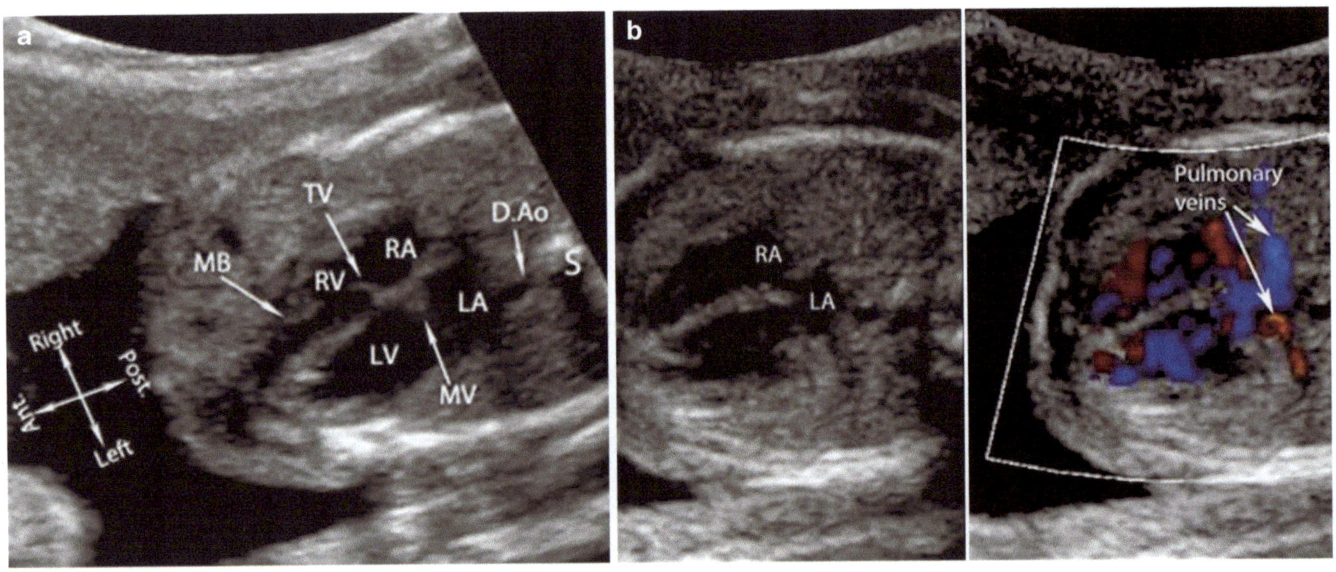

Fig. 6.3 **4-chamber view.** (**a**) Shows descending aorta (D. Ao) anterior spine; left atrium (LA) immediately in front of the aorta; left ventricle (LV) posterior and to the left of the right ventricle; moderator band (MB) in the right ventricle; tricuspid valve (TV) seating lower than the mitral valve (MV); right atrium (RA) slightly anterior and to the right of the left atrium. (**b**) Color flow demonstrates at least two pulmonary veins entering the left atrium

of any mass in either side of the chest could rearrange this normal position (Fig. 6.3).

- **Cardiac axis.** Levocardia is the normal axis of the heart and is determined by the angle between the ventricular septum and the midline of the chest. This angle is about 45° and anything above 50° is considered extreme Levocardia. Mesocardia is when this angle is reduced to around zero and dextrocardia is anytime the axis of the heart is to the right side of the chest. Extreme Levocardia, Mesocardia and Dextrocardia have higher incidence of assaulted congenital heart disease.
- **Cardiac size.** Is determined by the cardiothoracic ratio. This is done by measurement of heart and chest area. Normal size of the heart area is about one third of the chest. Cardiac/thoracic ratio of 35% or more indicates cardiomegaly.
- **Surrounding structures.** As in previous slice, spine is posterior and descending aorta is in front of the spine and to the left. Left atrium is anterior to the descending aorta. There should not be any other structure between the aorta and the left atrium. Lungs appear homogeneous and any

significant increase or decrease in echogenicity could be due to the presence of a mass.

- **Intracardiac anatomy.** In this view the 4-chambers of the heart should be evaluated. 2 atria of almost equal size and very thin atrial septum should be visualized with the flap of foramen ovale opening into the left atrium. The two ventricles are almost the same size with the right ventricle slightly larger and more trabeculated. The right ventricle contains the moderator band. The left ventricle has a smoother interior and does not have moderator band. Normally both ventricles are apex forming. Atrioventricular valves are approximately the same size and the tricuspid valve is normally slightly closer to the apex. The Intraventricular septum is thinner at the level of the atrioventricular valves and becomes thicker and more muscular as it reaches the apex. Visualizing the pulmonary veins entering the left atrium is not easy but is possible, especially if colors flow Doppler is used (Fig. 6.3).

Left Ventricular Outflow

This slice is obtained by tilting the transducer towards the head. This cut will demonstrate the aorta rising from the left ventricle (Fig. 6.1). In a normal situation, the anterior wall of the aorta and intraventricular septum are in continuation. As are the posterior wall of the aorta and anterior leaflet of the mitral valve. Thin aortic valve leaflet appears between the left ventricle and ascending aorta and disappear during the systole (Fig. 6.4).

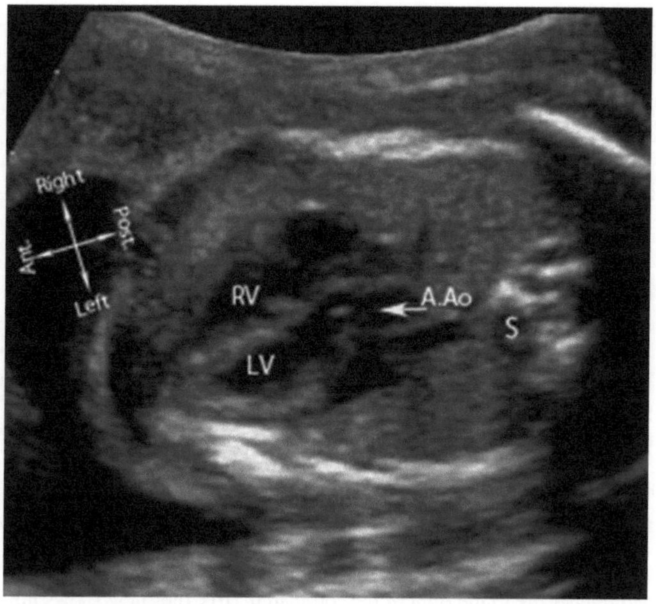

Fig. 6.4 Left ventricular outflow. This image demonstrates left ventricular outflow which gives rise to the ascending aorta (A.Ao) with a very thin aortic valve in between. (RV) right ventricle; (LV) left ventricle

Right Ventricular Outflow Tract

This slice is obtained by moving slightly cephalad from the previous cut. The right outflow is anterior-superior and to the left of the left outflow (Fig. 6.1). In this view usually the right outflow, ascending aorta and superior vena cava are seen together as the **3-vessel view** [12]. The right outflow is to the left of the aorta and slightly larger, superior vena cava immediately to the right of the aorta and slightly smaller (Fig. 6.5).

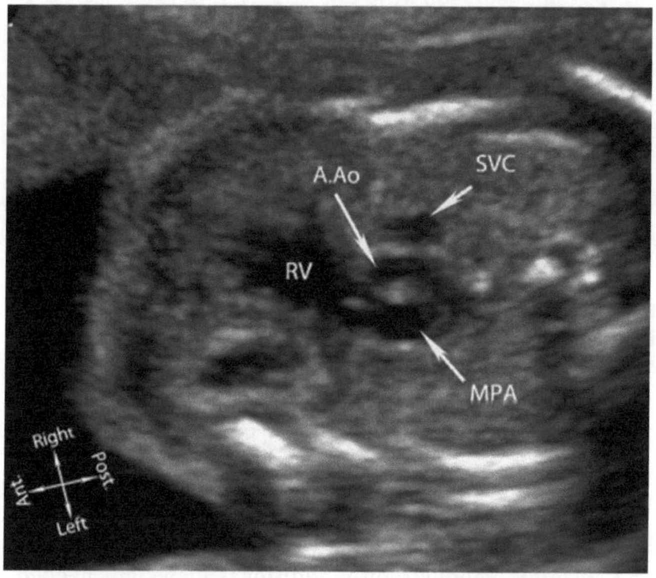

Fig. 6.5 Right ventricular outflow. Main pulmonary artery (MPA) exits the right ventricle (RV) to the left of ascending aorta (A.Ao); superior vena cava (SVC) to the right of the aorta entering the right atrium. Note the pulmonary artery is the largest of the three vessel

Three Vessel and Trachea

By moving slightly cephalad to the previous cut, the position and size of the aortic arch can be evaluated from three vessel and trachea view (Fig. 6.1). At this level the three vessels are: From the left to the right, ductal arch, aortic arch and superior vena cava. Normally, the trachea is to the right of the aortic arch and ductal arch to the left of it (Fig. 6.6a). In the absence of critical congenital heart disease blood flow in both arches is in the same direction (Fig. 6.6b). The presence of the trachea to the left of the aorta indicates a right-sided aortic arch. It is important to know that a right aortic arch and left ductal arch with trachea in between forms a vascular ring.

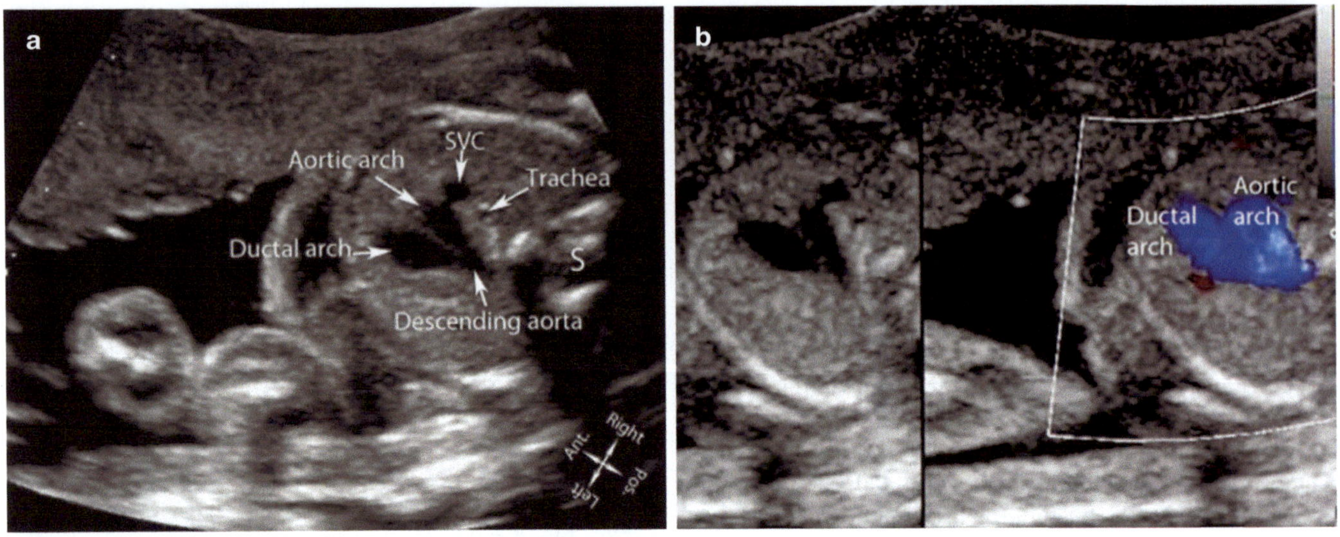

Fig. 6.6 **3 Vessel + Trachea.** (**a**) Left-sided ductal arch and aortic arch entering descending aorta anterior to the spine; superior vena cava (SVC) and trachea are to the right of the aortic arch. (**b**) Color flow shows flow direction into aortic arch and ductal arch are the same

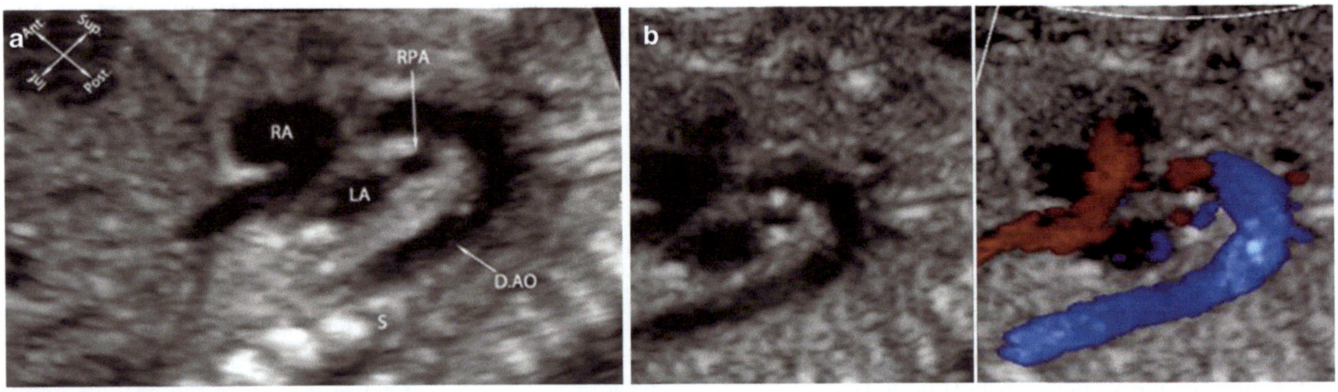

Fig. 6.7 **Aortic arch.** (**a**) Aortic arch is shown with neck vessels arising from the transverse arch. Descending aorta (Dao) anterior to the spine (S); right pulmonary artery (RPA) under the transverse arch; left atrium (LA) posterior to the right atrium (RA). (**b**) Color flow demonstrates the direction of the blood flow

Sagittal Cuts

For further evaluation of the aortic arch, the ductal arch and systemic venous return, additional views are needed. These very important views are obtained from sagittal slices. A 90° rotation from transverse cuts will provide the sagittal cuts. If the position of the fetus permits, sagittal views are obtained from a longitudinally cut of the fetal chest and abdomen. When the cut is done anterior-posteriorly and superior-in inferiorly, the ascending aorta is midline and anterior. By slightly moving to the left, the transverse arch and neck vessels can be visualized (Fig. 6.7). The ductal arch can be viewed as the direct continuation of the main pulmonary artery which arises from the anteriorly situated right ventricle. The ductal arch then runs under the aortic arch in a posterior course to join the descending aorta at the Isthmus, anterior to the spine (Fig. 6.8).

Tilting the probe from midline to the right will demonstrate the systemic venous return. The superior vena cava enters the right atrium just to the right of the ascending aorta. The inferior vena cava and hepatic system enter the right atrium just above their diaphragm. The flap of the foramen ovale opens to the left atrium which is posterior and to the left of the right atrium (Fig. 6.9). If this sagittal cut is performed from the lateral position rather than an anterior-posterior approach, the arches and systemic vessels could be demonstrated in one cut.

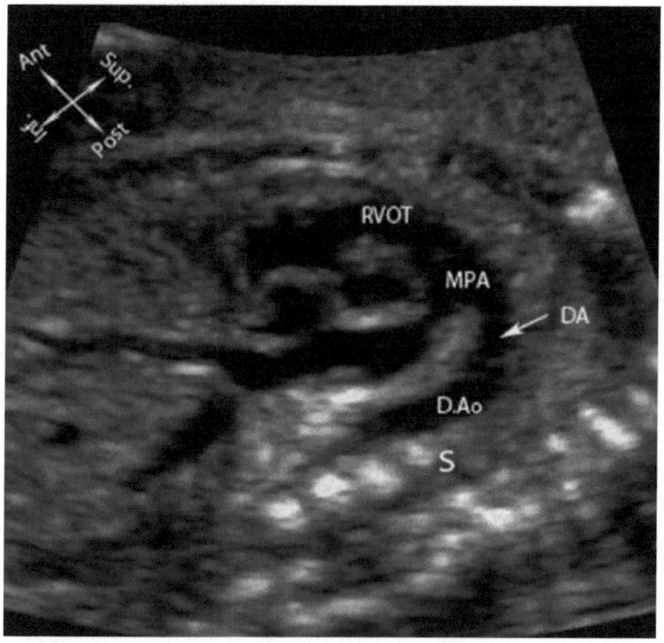

Fig. 6.8 Ductal arch. Right ventricular outflow tract (RVOT) is shown exiting the anterior ventricle with continuation to main pulmonary artery (MPA); ductus arteriosus (DA) connects the MPA to the descending aorta (D.Ao) in anterior to the spine

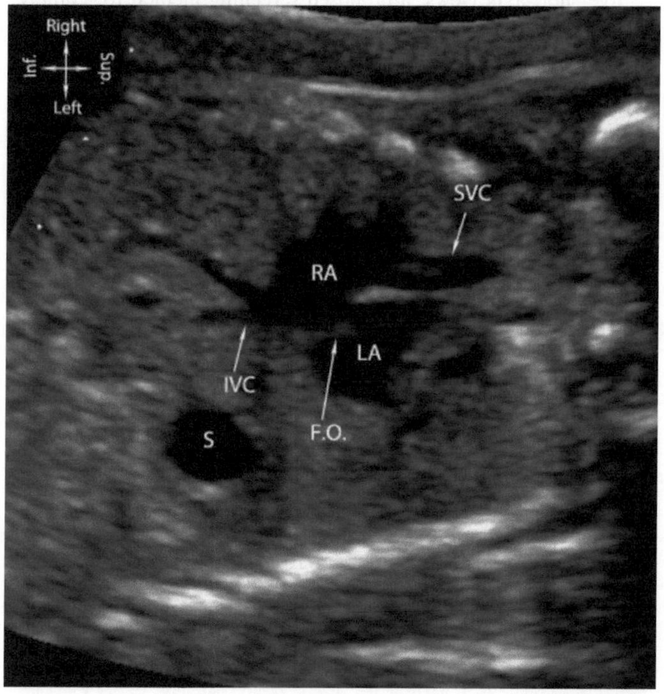

Fig. 6.9 Systemic venous return. Inferior vena cava (IVC) and superior vena cava (SVC) are shown entering the right atrium (RA) anterior and to the right of the left atrium (LA); flap of foramen ovale (F.O.) sitting in the left atrium. *S* stomach

Questions

1. In the US, the prenatal detection of critical congenital heart diseases:
   A. Has improved dramatically over the last 15 years
   B. Remains low
   C. Approaches 100%
   D. Cannot Improve with the current the current technology
   E. Has decreased dramatically over the last 15 years

2. The Best Gestational Age to Perform Timely and Accurate Fetal Echo Is:
   A. 9 weeks
   B. 11 weeks
   C. 16 weeks
   D. 20 weeks
   E. 25 weeks

3. In Fetal Echocardiography the 3 Vessel View Includes:
   A. Main pulmonary artery, pulmonary artery branches, an ascending aorta
   B. Ascending aorta, superior vena cava, and inferior vena cava
   C. Main pulmonary artery, ascending aorta, and superior vena cava
   D. Ascending aorta, subclavian artery, and main pulmonary artery
   E. There is not such a view in fetal echocardiography

4. All the Following Statements Are True **except:**
   A. Congenital heart disease occurs in about 8/1000 live births
   B. Fetal echo diagnosis of critical heart disease approaches 100%
   C. There is no advantage of prenatal diagnosis vs. postnatal diagnosis of critical congenital heart disease
   D. Most congenital heart disease happens in the low risk population

5. All of the following are indication for a fetal echocardiography exam **except:**
   A. History of tuberous sclerosis
   B. Family history of congenital heart disease
   C. Exposure to teratogenic medications
   D. Echogenic foci
   E. Extracardiac abnormality

Answers

1. C
2. D
3. C
4. C
5. D

References

1. Kleinman CS, Hobbins JC, Jaffe CC, Lynch DC, Talner NS. Echocardiographics studies of the human fetus: prenatal diagnosis of congenital heart disease and cardiac dysrhythmias. Pediatrics. 1980;65:1059–67.
2. Souka AP, Pilalis A, Kavalaskia I, et al. Screening for major structural abnormalities at the 11 to 14-week ultrasound scan. Am J Obstet Gynecol. 2006;194:393.
3. Alan LD. Cardiac anatomy screening: What is the best time for screening in pregnancy? Curr Opin Obstet Gynecol. 2003;15:143.
4. Smreck JM, Berg C, Geipel A, et al. Detection rate of early fetal echocardiography and in utero development of congenital heart defects. J Ultrasound Med. 2006;25:187.
5. Guariglia L, Rosati P. Transvaginal sonographic detection of embryonic-fetal abnormalities in early pregnancy. Obstet Gynecol. 2000; 96:328.
6. Tworetzky W, McElhinney DB, Reddy VM, Brook MM, Hanley FL, Silverman NH. Improved surgical outcome after fetal diagnosis of hypoplastic left heart syndrome. Circulation. 2001;103:1269–73.
7. Sklansky M, Tang A, Levy D, Grossfeld P, Kashani I, Shaughnessy R, et al. Maternal psychological impact of fetal echocardiography. J Am Soc Echocardiogr. 2002;15:159–66.
8. Stümpflen I, Stümpflen A, Wimmer M, Bernasheck G. Effect of detailed fetal echocardiography as part of routine prenatal ultrasonographic screening on detection of congenital heart disease. Lancet. 1996;348:854–7.
9. Standards for the Performance of the Antepartum Obstetrical Ultrasound Examination. Copyright 1994, by the American Institute of Ultrasound in Medicine.
10. American College of Radiology Standard for Performance of Antepartum Obstetrical Ultrasound.
11. American Institute of Ultrasound in Medicine. AIUM Practice Guideline for the Performance of Obstetric Ultrasound Examinations. Laurel, MD: American Institute of Ultrasound in Medicine; 2007. http://www.aium.org/publications/guidelines/obstetric.pdf
12. Luna CF, Acherman RJ, Rollins RC, Castillo WJ, Berthoty DP, Evans WN. Laterally displaced superior vena cava on the fetal 3-vessel view from a right diaphragmatic hernia. J Ultrasound Med. 2011;30:1161–2. forms a vascular ring.
13. Carvalho JS, Mavrides E, Shinebourne EA, Campbell S, Thilanganathan B. Improving the effectiveness of routine prenatal screening for major congenital heart defects. Heart. 2002;88:387–91.
14. Acherman RJ, Evans WN, Luna CF, Rollins R, Kip KT, Collazos JC, Restrepo H, Adasheck J, Iriye BK, Roberts D, Sacks AJ. Prenatal detection of congenital heart disease in southern Nevada: the need for universal fetal cardiac evaluation. J Ultrasound Med. 2007;26:1715–9.
15. Friedberg MK, Silverman NH, Moon-Grady AJ, Tong E, Nourse J, Sorenson B, Lee J, Hornberger LK. Prenatal detection of congenital heart disease. J Pediatr. 2009;155:26–31.
16. Yagel S, Cohen SM, Achiron R. Examination of the fetal heart by five short-axis views: a proposed screening method for comprehensive cardiac evaluation. Ultrasound Obstet Gynecol. 2001;17: 367–9.

Handheld Echocardiography

7

Dominika Filipiak-Strzecka, Piotr Lipiec, and Jarosław D. Kasprzak

Abstract

Pocket-size imaging devices, due to their size and weight can be carried around by the physicians and used for bedside monitoring of patients' status and screening for major abnormalities, even if they offer only basic image acquisition and analysis possibilities. The potential clinical implementation of PSID include the evaluation of the left and right ventricle, pericardial effusion assessment, valve disease assessment, estimation of the right atrial pressure based on size and respiratory changes of inferior vena cava, establishing the diagnosis of ascending aortic dilatation, diagnosing pleural effusion and the presence of B-lines. The availability of hybrid cardiac/linear probe can expand the diagnostic capabilities by e.g. assessment of local complications resulting from the punctures preceding the invasive percutaneous procedures or detection of deep vein thrombosis. The agreement between the results of the PSID examination and the test performed by means of the stationary echocardiographs is high. The simplicity of PSID operation allows for their use in extension of physical examination. However, the basic training requirements are consistent with basic level of echocardiographic examination.

Keywords

Handheld echocardiography · PSID · Pocket size imaging device · Mobile echocardiographs · Portable echocardiographs · Pocket ultrasonographs

D. Filipiak-Strzecka (✉) · P. Lipiec · J. D. Kasprzak
Department of Cardiology, Bieganski Hospital, Medical University of Lodz, Lodz, Poland

Abbreviations

2D	Two dimensional
3D	Three dimensional
Ao	Aorta
EF	Ejection fraction
FA	Femoral artery
FV	Femoral vein
ICA	Internal carotid artery
IVC	Internal vena cava
LA	Left atrium
LV	Left ventricular
PSID	Pocket size imaging device
RA	Right atrium
RV	Right ventricle
TEE	Transesophageal echocardiography
TTE	Transthoracic echocardiography

Introduction

Depending on the size, portability, image acquisition and analysis capabilities modern echocardiographs can be divided into four groups:

- The most advanced group consists of **stationary high-end systems** offering full range of diagnostic feasibilities including transthoracic and transoesophageal echocardiography and advanced digital analysis of recorded images. Despite the fact that their architecture does not exclude the possibility of transportation it is not desired course of action due to the equipment size, cost and fragility.
- **Mobile echocardiographs** are smaller than high-end systems and thus are easier to move; moreover they offer full

A. Sadeghpour, A. Alizadehasl (eds.), *Case-Based Textbook of Echocardiography*,
https://doi.org/10.1007/978-3-319-67691-3_7

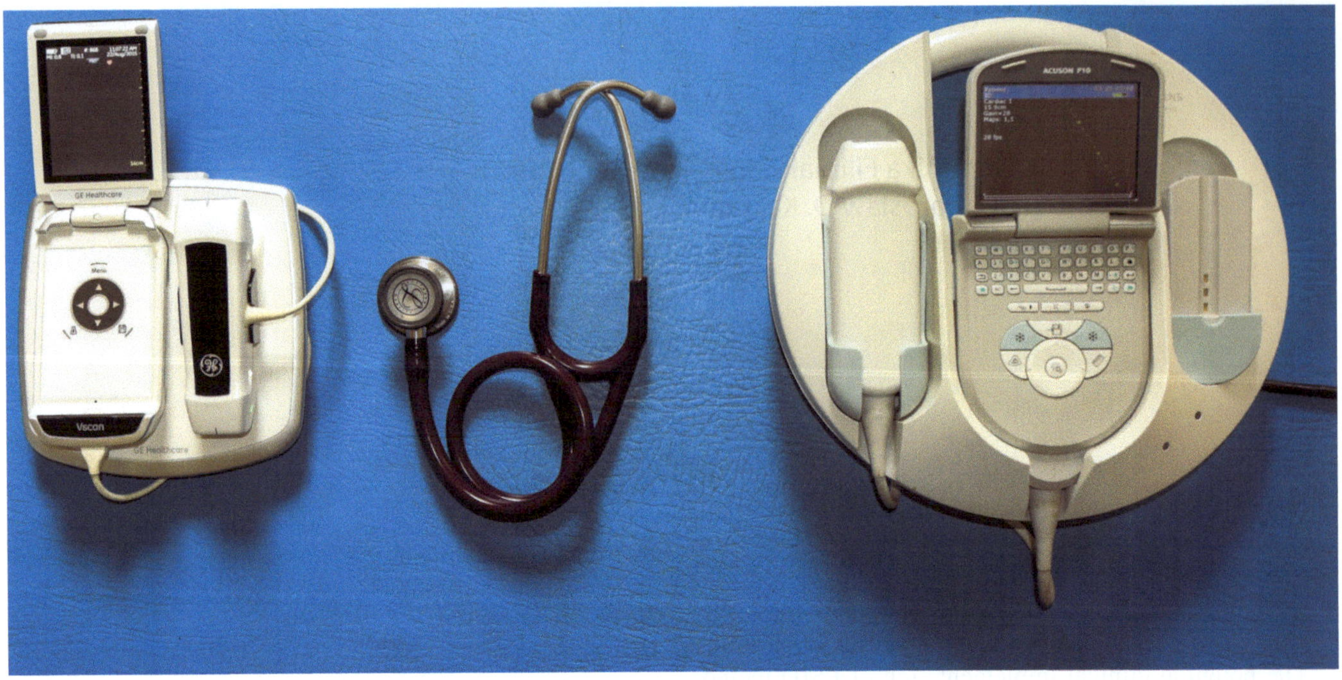

Fig. 7.1 The size of PSIDs (fitted on the docking stations) compared side by side with the stethoscope

range of standard imaging modalities. Usually they are not equipped with the tools needed for the most advanced image acquisition and analysis (e.g. 3D—echocardiography techniques).

- The third group of devices includes the laptop-sized **portable echocardiographs**. The range of imaging modalities varies depending on the specific model but with the few exceptions it does not transcend the basic diagnostic functions. Built-in battery enables bedside echocardiographic examinations.
- The fourth group of echocardiographs are novel **pocket-size imaging devices** (PSID, or **handheld ultrasonographs**, HHU) small enough to fit in the whitecoat pocket. Even though only basic greyscale and colour Doppler image acquisition is possible, they can accompany a clinician during the everyday clinical routine or virtually anywhere where cardiac imaging may be needed (Fig. 7.1) [1, 2].

Diagnostic Capabilities

- PSIDs are equipped with broad-bandwidth, phased-array probe; a model with dual probe combining the advantages of sector and linear probe is also available
- 2-Dimensional grayscale imaging (Fig. 7.2)
- Sector width does not exceed 75° and sector depth is not greater than 25 cm

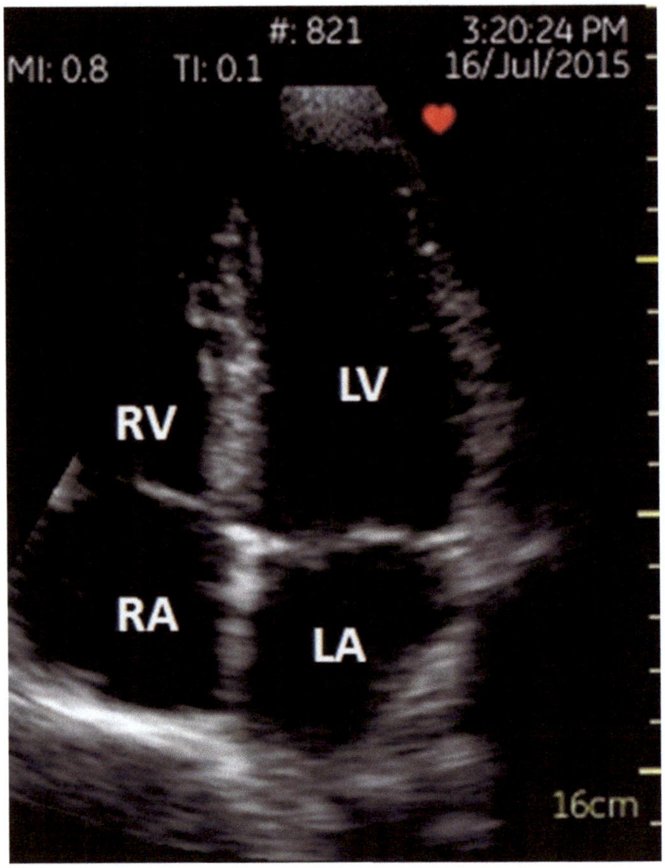

Fig. 7.2 The 4-chamber apical view obtained with the use of PSID

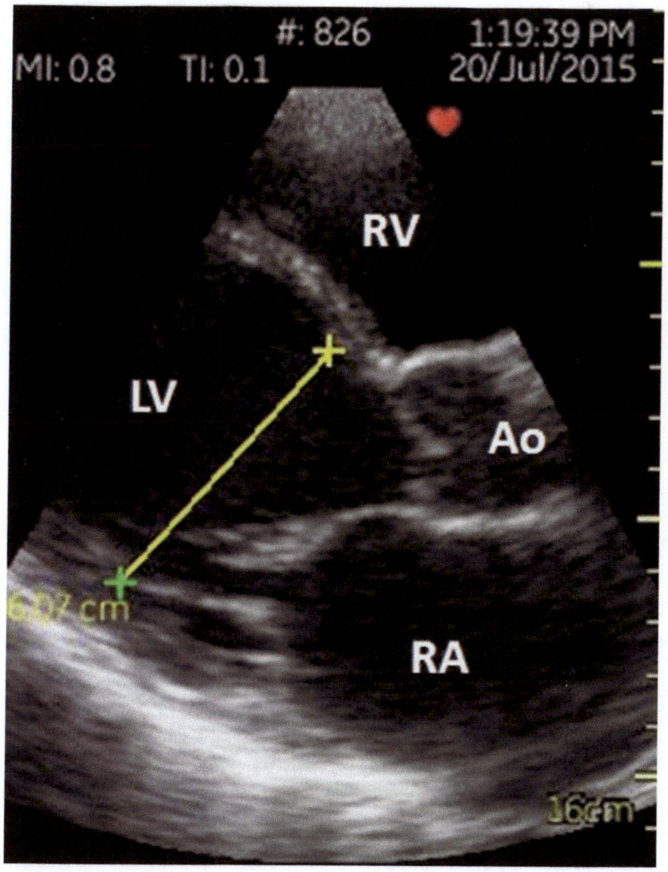

Fig. 7.3 Linear measurement of the left ventricle diastolic diameter performed with PSID; the parasternal long axis view

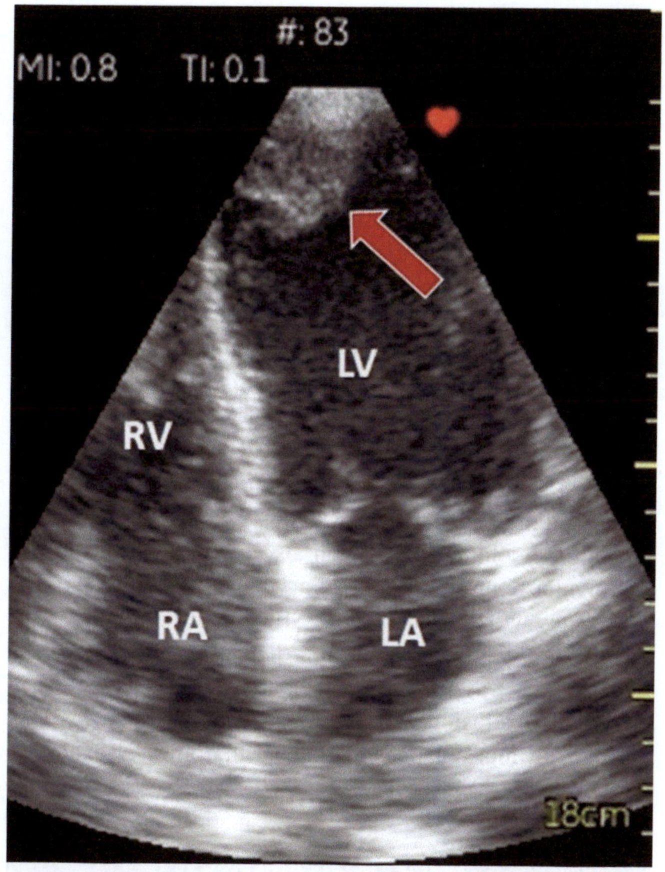

Fig. 7.4 Bedside monitoring of the thrombus present in the apical part of the left ventricle during the intensive anticoagulation therapy

- Measuring capabilities: all devices support linear measurements; in case of one device area calculation is also possible (Fig. 7.3)
- Color Doppler imaging modality
- Acquired images can be stored and archived (automated cycle length, without ECG gating)
- Stock battery allows for 60–75 min of examination and full battery recharge lasts for 1.5–2 h.
- Recorded patient's examination can be identified on the basis of the assigned ID number, voice notes regarding the examination can also be created and stored.

Clinical Applications

- Portable and pocket ultrasonographs are best suited for the examination serving the purpose of the supplement of physical examination performed in the point of care. The concordance between the results of the PSID examination and the test performed by means of the stationary echocardiographs is high. PSID should serve principally for the examination aimed at specific pathology (bedside screening of previously identified dysfunction or screening oriented at specific type of dysfunction) (Fig. 7.4)

General assessment of cardiac morphology and function does not replace full echocardiogram [1].

The concordance between the results of the PSID examination and the test performed by means of the stationary echocardiographs is high. Technical capabilities of pocket ultrasonographs allow for:

- The evaluation of the left ventricle. The feasibility of visual assessment of left ventricular ejection fraction with PSID and diagnosing LV enlargement is well confirmed. Good agreement has been obtained in cases of LV sectional wall motion abnormalities, also in patients with the established diagnosis of acute coronary syndrome [3–5].
- The evaluation of the right ventricle. Fewer studies attempted to verify the reliability of PSID in RV assess-

ment. Nevertheless, the detection of RV enlargement and visual global function evaluation with PSID has been reported. This, along with the possibility of the inspection of lower limbs deep veins system makes PSID an appropriate tool for the purpose of pulmonary embolism screening [6, 7].

- Pericardial effusion assessment. PSIDs enable a quick confirmation or the exclusion of the presence pericardial effusion with high sensitivity and specificity [6, 8].
- Assessment of valvular disease. All PSIDs allow for visual detection of abnormal valve morphology or color Doppler flow abnormalities, without quantification in the absence of spectral Doppler module. 2-dimensional imaging is sufficient to set a qualitative suspicion of aortic or mitral stenosis (based on thickening or calcification and limited movement of valve leaflets) and devices equipped with the colour Doppler can also aid in identification of valvular regurgitation. Grading the severity of the insufficiency with the support of PSID remains doubtful as the tendency to overestimate the degree of regurgitation is observed [8]. An important benefit of PSID use lies in reliable exclusion of valve regurgitation or stenosis as a cause of murmur detected during the physical examination (Fig. 7.5) [8].

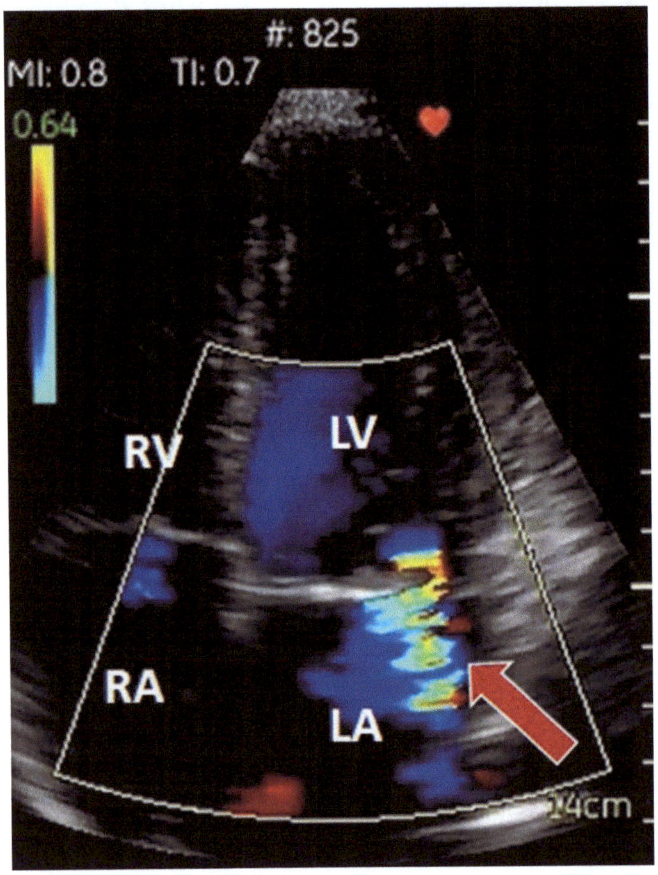

Fig. 7.5 Moderate mitral regurgitation recognised during the screening with the use of PSID; 4-chamber apical view, colour Doppler imaging

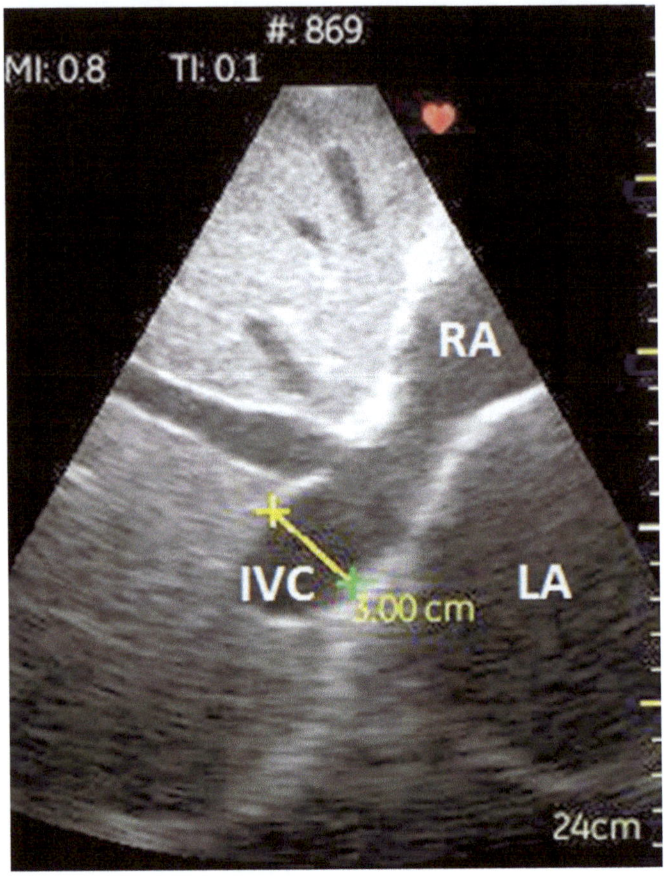

Fig. 7.6 IVC dilatation observed in the patient with the severe mitral regurgitation

- Estimation of the right atrial pressure based upon the evaluation of size and respiratory changes of inferior vena cava (certain studies suggested the difficulties in reliable assessment when performed by inexperienced researchers) (Fig. 7.6) [3].
- Establishing the diagnosis of ascending aorta dilatation [9]. Certain limited clinical data suggest, that PSID can aid in detecting the aortic dissection [10].
- Pleural effusion and the presence of B-lines perceived as the markers of fluid retention in the interstitial lung space [11, 12].

The presence of the linear probe can expand the diagnostic capabilities by fulfilling the following clinical tasks:

- Assessment of local complications resulting from the punctures preceding the invasive percutaneous procedures [13]
- Detection of deep vein thrombosis (Fig. 7.7)
- Screening of the carotid arteries regarding the significant stenosis despite the limited reliability of intima media complex measurement (Fig. 7.8)

European and American Cardiac Imaging Societies agree that the examination with the use of portable echocardiographs

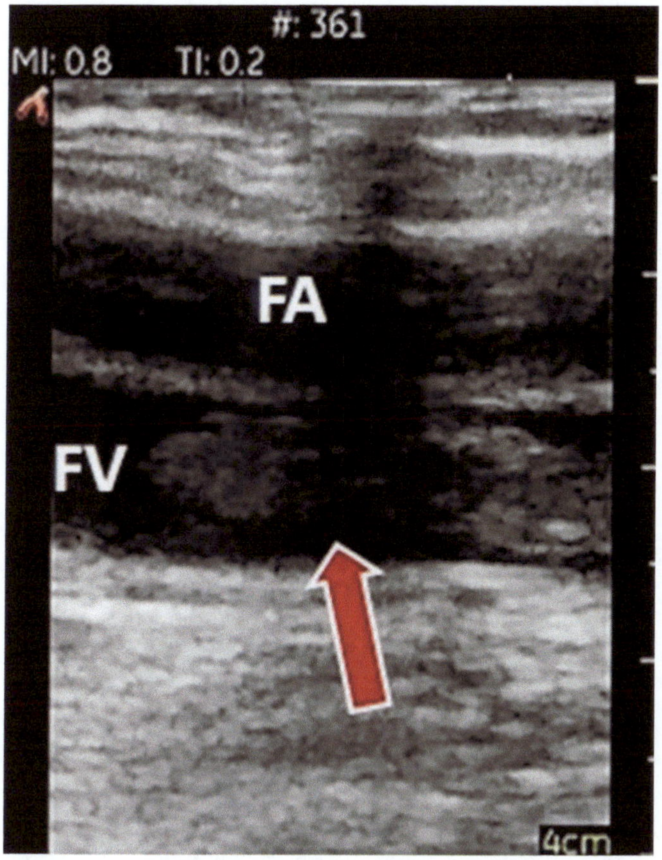

Fig. 7.7 Proximal deep vein thrombosis diagnosed during the 4-point compression ultrasound test performed with the use of PSID. Thrombus in femoral vein marked with an arrow

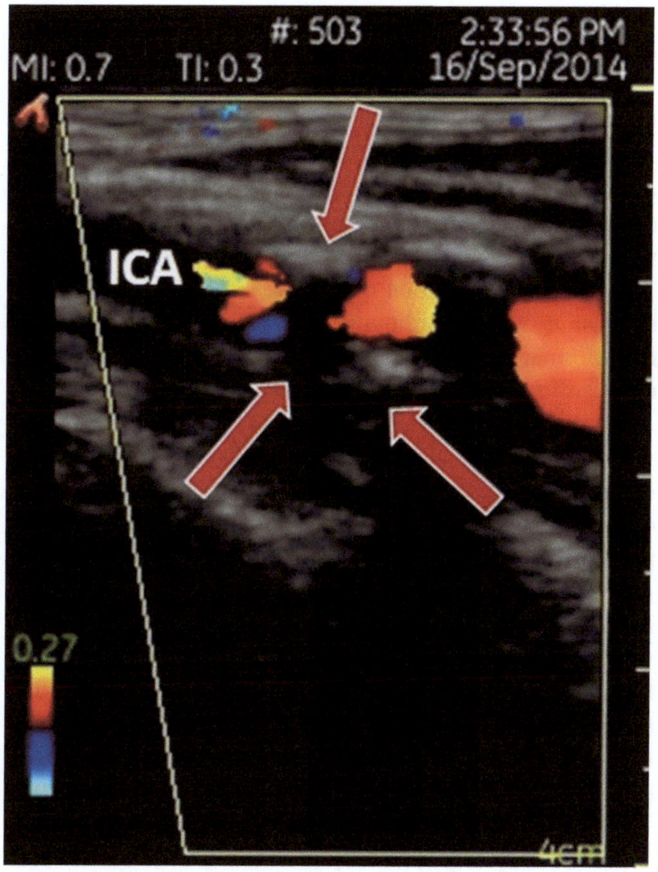

Fig. 7.8 Screening of the carotid artery performed with PSID. The stenosis causing the turbulent blood flow indicated with arrows

should not be perceived as a substitute for the full echocardiographic examination—the fact about which patient needs to be aware of. The choice regarding the visualised structures, the acquired projections and performed measurements is fully operator-dependent. Results of such test ought to be reported as a part of the physical examination [1, 14, 15].

Apart from the bedside screening of patients' status in the conditions of the cardiology ward, the European Association of Echocardiography mentions the following implementations of portable echocardiographs:

- Portable echocardiographs could become the tools used in the primary assessment of the cardiologic status in the ambulance or ER. The environment of both is not well-suited for the conventional auscultation and swift establishing of the diagnosis plays a vital role.
- As a supplementation of the physical examination in the intensive care unit
- During the cardiologic consultations, both inside and outside the hospital
- As a tool for primary assessment of patient conditions in cases when full echocardiographic examination is mulled over
- During the social campaigns and screening programs in organised schools and work places.
- In the teaching process of the medical students during the clinical classes [1].

Training and Certification

Even though scientific data suggest that augmenting the conventional physical examination with the PSID increases its diagnostic value, less experienced practitioners should be fully aware of the increased risk of erroneous interpretation and the fact that they are burdened with the responsibility of further diagnostic proceedings either confirming or excluding the detected pathologies.

Cardiologists/experienced echocardiographers do not need any additional training in order to efficiently take advantage of the features of the PSID [1] and should ideally operate PSID themselves [15]. Notably, existing evidence suggests that even medical students after completion of a brief training could achieve higher diagnostic accuracy than experienced specialists if their examination was supplemented with the elements of echocardiographic imaging acquired with PSID [16, 17].

Trained nurses had good success rate in detecting pleural effusion or the interstitial fluid [18].

When used by the specialist in the outpatient's clinic, the PSID may decrease the number of cases in which full echocardiographic examination is required. By doing so, PSID might introduce significant financial savings as the cases directed to the full-echocardiographic examinations are well-justified [19].

European Association of Echocardiography suggests the expansion of echocardiographic certification training with the information regarding the possible usage of the portable echocardiographs in everyday practice [1].

Cardiology residents, other medical specialities and nurses willing to use PSID during the clinical chores absolutely need to undergo proper training and revision of basic cardiac physiology and pathology knowledge as well as the operation of the particular device [1]. The requirements concerning the program of such training in Europe are yet to be determined. Interestingly, the American Society of Echocardiography mentions the minimum threshold of 150 single-handedly performed examinations and 300 interpreted recordings. Although studies have described the steep learning curve associated with the use of PSID, they have also emphasized the role of echocardiography experience in both acquisition and interpretation of PSID examination findings. The significant differences in both sensitivity and specificity of the diagnostic accuracy of PSID examination between trainees and expert operators were shown in one study [12].

It is vital to bear in mind that diagnostically reliable echocardiography is to very significant extent operator—dependent. Hopefully, the growing accessibility to the devices capable of performing echocardiographic examination by the constantly widening group of medical professionals will be connected with the increase of both practical and theoretical skills regarding rapidly progressing field of echocardiography.

Test

1. PSID enables:

- 2-D greyscale imaging
- Linear measurements
- 3D imaging
- Wireless operation (due to the built-in battery)

2. The main advantages of PSID are:

- The size—they can accompany clinicians during the everyday clinical routine
- The broad range of diagnostic feasibilities
- They are extremely easy to operate
- The possibility of advanced digital analysis of recorded images

3. The best documented clinical implementation of PSID are:

- left ventricle ejection fraction visual assessment
- right ventricle evaluation by TAPSE measurement
- pericardial effusion assessment
- grading of the aortic stenosis

4. Experienced echocardiographers:

- Should complete the special training program in order to efficiently take advantage of the features of the PSID.
- Can increase the diagnostic value of conventional physical examination by augmenting it with short PSID assessment
- Achieved a high agreement between the PSID and stationary echocardiographs examinations results
- According to European Association of Echocardiography the echocardiographic certification training should be expanded with the information regarding the possible usage of PSID in everyday practice.

5. The following implementations of portable echocardiographs are suggested by the European Association of Echocardiography:

- Bedside monitoring of the patient status
- The primary assessement of the cardiologic status in the ambulance or ER.
- During the cardiologic consultations
- In the teaching process of the medical students during the clinical classes

References

1. Sicari R, Galderisi M, Voigt JU, Habib G, Zamorano JL, Lancellotti P, Badano LP. The use of pocket-size imaging devices: a position statement of the European Association of Echocardiography. Eur J Echocardiogr. 2011;12(2):85–7.
2. Seward JB, Douglas PS, Erbel R, Kerber RE, Kronzon I, Rakowski H, Sahn LD, Sisk EJ, Tajik AJ, Wann S. Hand-carried cardiac ultrasound (HCU) device: recommendations regarding new technology. A report from the Echocardiography Task Force on New Technology of the Nomenclature and Standards Committee of the American Society of Echocardiography. J Am Soc Echocardiogr. 2002; 15(4):369–73.
3. Liebo MJ, Israel RL, Lillie EO, Smith MR, Rubenson DS, Topol EJ. Is pocket mobile echocardiography the next-generation stethoscope? A crosssectional comparison of rapidly acquired images with standard transthoracic echocardiography. Ann Intern Med. 2011; 155:33–8.
4. Fukuda S, Shimada K, Kawasaki T, Fujimoto H, Maeda K, Inanami H, Yoshida K, Jissho S, Taguchi H, Yoshiyama M, Yoshikawa J. Pocket-sized transthoracic echocardiography device for the measurement of cardiac chamber size and function. Circ J. 2009;73(6):1092.
5. Culp BC, Mock JD, Chiles CD, Culp WC Jr. The pocket echocardiograph: validation and feasibility. Echocardiography. 2010;27: 759–64.

6. Andersen GN, Haugen BO, Graven T, et al. Feasibility and reliability of point-of-care pocket-sized echocardiography. Eur J Echocardiogr. 2011;12:665–70.
7. Biais M, Carrie C, Delaunay F, et al. Evaluation of a new pocketechoscopic device for focused cardiac ultrasonography in an emergency setting. Crit Care. 2012;16:R82.
8. Prinz C, Voigt JU. Diagnostic accuracy of a hand-held ultrasound scanner in routine patients referred for echocardiography. J Am Soc Echocardiogr. 2011;24(2):111–6.
9. Filipiak-Strzecka D, John B, Kasprzak JD, Michalski B, Lipiec P. Pocket-size echocardiograph—a valuable tool for nonexperts or just a portable device for echocardiographers? Adv Med Sci. 2013; 58:67–72.
10. Mancuso FJ, Siqueira VN, Moisés VA, Gois AF, Paola AA, Carvalho AC, Campos O. Focused cardiac ultrasound using a pocket-size device in the emergency room. Arq Bras Cardiol. 2014;103(6):530–7.
11. Mirabel M, Celermajer D, Beraud AS, Jouven X, Marijon E, Hagège AA. Pocket-sized focused cardiac ultrasound: strengths and limitations. Arch Cardiovasc Dis. 2015;108(3):197–205.
12. Seraphim A, Paschou SA, Grapsa J, Nihoyannopoulos P. Pocket-sized echocardiography devices: one stop shop service? J Cardiovasc Ultrasound. 2016;24(1):1–6.
13. Filipiak-Strzecka D, Michalski B, Kasprzak JD, Lipiec P. Pocket-size imaging devices allow for reliable bedside screening for femoral artery access site complications. Ultrasound Med Biol. 2014;40(12):2753–8.
14. Panoulas VF, Daigeler AL, Malaweera AS, Lota AS, Baskaran D, Rahman S, Nihoyannopoulos P. Pocket-size hand-held cardiac ultrasound as an adjunct to clinical examination in the hands of medical students and junior doctors. Eur Heart J Cardiovasc Imaging. 2013;14:323–30.
15. Michalski B, Kasprzak JD, Szymczyk E, Lipiec P. Diagnostic utility and clinical usefulness of the pocket echocardiographic device. Echocardiography. 2012;29(1):1–6.
16. Silverman B. Handheld ultrasound is a valuble bedside tool which can supplement the bedside cardiac exam but not replace it. JACC Cardiovasc Imaging. 2015;8(5):621–2.
17. Decara JM, Kirkpatrick JN, Spencer KT, Ward RP, Kasza K, Furlong K, Lang RM. Use of hand-carried ultrasound devices to augment the accuracy of medical student bedside cardiac diagnoses. J Am Soc Echocardiogr. 2005;18(3):257–63.
18. Strömberg A, Wodlin P. Pocket-sized ultrasound—a new tool for heart-failure nurses in daily clinical practice? Eur J Cardiovasc Nurs. 2015;14(4):284–5.
19. Kini V, Mehta N, Mazurek JA, Ferrari VA, Epstein AJ, Groeneveld PW, Kirkpatrick JN. Focused cardiac ultrasound in place of repeat echocardiography: reliability and cost implications. J Am Soc Echocardiogr. 2015;28(9):1053–9.

8 Artifacts and Pitfalls of Echocardiography

Anita Sadeghpour and Azin Alizadehasl

Abstract

Pitfalls and artifacts of imaging are common and inevitable; they are products of the physical principles of ultrasound. We should, therefore, be familiar with the potential pitfalls and artifacts and try to minimize them.

Since many therapeutic plans and surgical interventions are based on cardiac imaging findings, knowledge of artifacts and pitfalls is critical. A pitfall is a danger or problem that is hidden or not obvious at first and an artifact is an accidental effect that falsifies the true anatomy of physiology and leads to incorrect results.

This section aims to categorize and elucidate common undesired artifacts of imaging in everyday practice of echocardiography that influence either the anatomy or the function of cardiac structures. Some of these conditions are easily recognized (e.g., shadowing), while others could create significant misunderstanding and misinterpretation of the final display and potentially compromise the diagnostic potential of a study. These phenomena are due to ultrasound physics or the operator's interference.

Keywords

Artifacts · Pitfalls · Echocardiography · Reverberation · Shadowing · Side lobes artifact · Near field and beam width artifact · Mirror image artifact

A. Sadeghpour, MD, FACC, FASE
Professor of Cardiology, Echocardiography Research Center, Rajaie Cardiovascular Medical and Research Center, Iran University of Medical Science, Tehran, Iran

A. Alizadehasl, MD, FACC, FASE (✉)
Associate Professor of Cardiology, Echocardiologist, Echocardiography and Cardiogenetic Research Centers, Cardio-Oncology Department, Rajaie Cardiovascular Medical and Research Center, Tehran, Iran

Abbreviations

LA	Left atrium
LV	Left ventricle
PISA	Proximal isovelocity surface area

Artifacts

There are 3 definitions for artifacts:

1. Structures that are imaged in the ultrasound beam and have no corresponding anatomic structures (at least at that location), resulting from extraneous signals
2. Failure in accurately recognizing the present structures
3. Imaging the structure that is different from the actual structure

Artifacts have been described as the Achilles' heel of cardiac imaging as they may lead to improper concern or intervention and even inappropriate surgery [1–3].

Types of Artifacts

Reverberations

It is relatively common artifact that limits the interpretation and diagnosis of the final imaging. This phenomenon is due to continuing repetitive echoes among anatomic interfaces which are strong reflectors. Commonly, reverberation are repeated reflection that produce signals at twice the distance from the primary targets. Gradually the signal of the sound decays till it is beyond the range of detection of the transducer. As time passes, the reflected volume of echoes is decreased and the fact ceases. Reverberations are always seen away from a mechanical prosthetic valve or the inter-

A. Sadeghpour, A. Alizadehasl (eds.), *Case-Based Textbook of Echocardiography*,
https://doi.org/10.1007/978-3-319-67691-3_8

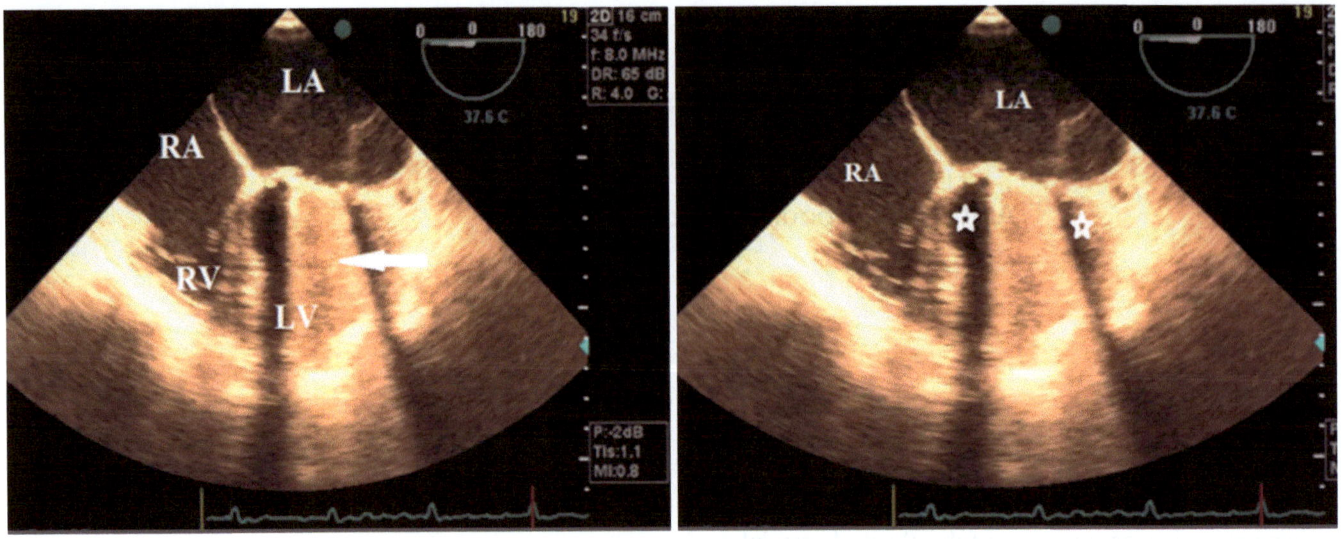

Fig. 8.1 Left: Reverberation (white arrow) are repeated reflections from a mechanical prosthetic valve. Right: Acoustic Shadowing (star) happens with high-density structures (Prosthetics valves and highly calcified structures) so no signal penetrates beyond the shadowing structure .The shape of shadow follows the ultrasound pathway

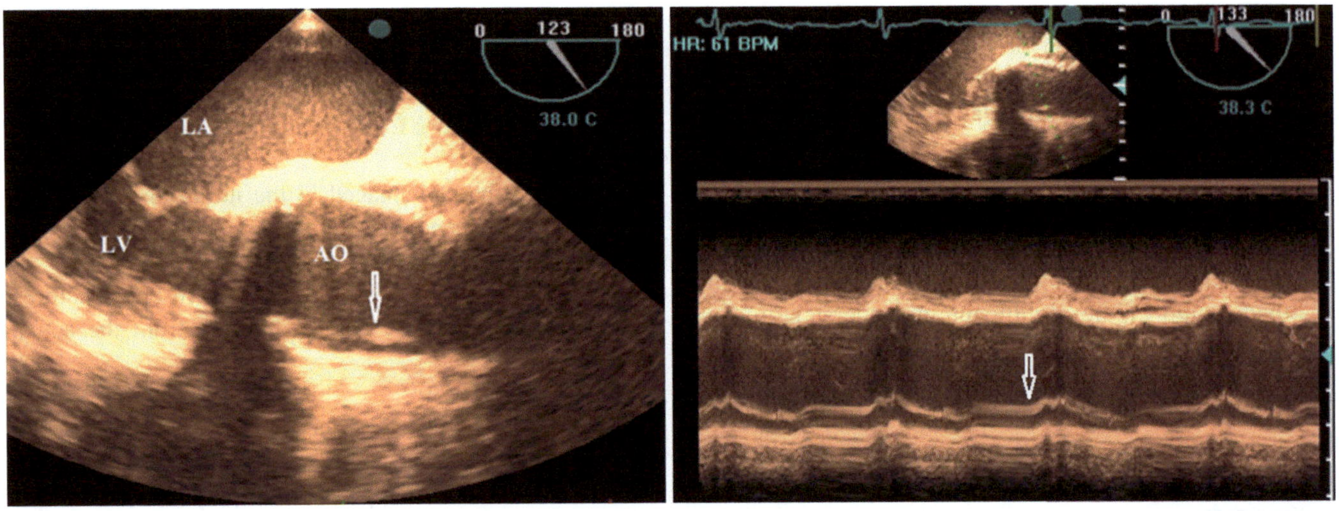

Fig. 8.2 Multiple linear high amplitude echo signals originating from two strong specular reflectors resulting in back-and-forth reflection of the ultrasound signal before it returns to the transducer mimicking dissecting flap. To distinguish an intimal flap definitively from such artifacts, the flap should be identified in more than one view, It should have motion independent of that of the aortic walls or other cardiac structures, and a differentiate color Doppler flow patterns noted between the two lumen

face between the parietal pleura or pericardium and the lung parenchyma. Reverberation which are caused by internal reflections is the persistence of sound in an enclosed space after its generation (Figs. 8.1 and 8.2) [2, 3].

Shadowing

- This so common artifact might be characterized as the "Achilles heel" of echocardiography and happens when the transmitted ultrasound beam encounters a medium of significantly different acoustic impedance and as a result is reflected back to the transducer.
- This artifact is anticipated in highly reflecting artificial or biologic structures such as mechanical valves and calcium accumulation. Also sometimes the color Doppler flow is reflected back by high-density structures such as prosthetic valves or heavily calcified structures such that no signal penetrates distal to the shadowing structure. By using an alternate window or echocardiography mode such as transesophageal echocardiography (Figs. 8.1 and 8.3) [2, 3].

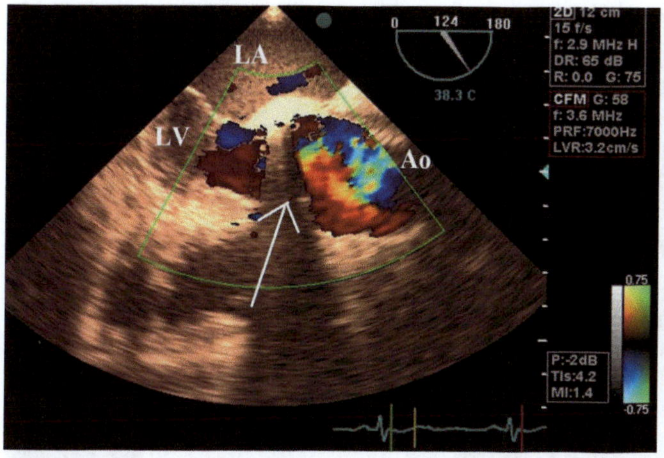

Fig. 8.3 There is an absence of the color flow signals distal to the strong reflector and shadowing (arrow)

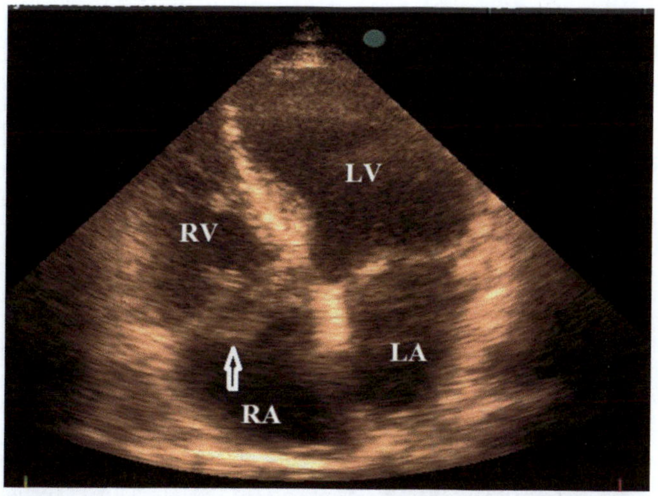

Fig. 8.4 Calcified aortic valve in right atrium (arrow) in apical four-chamber view misinterpreted as a mass. It Occurs due to the strong reflect of the calcified AV in side lobes of the beam that is displayed in the tomographic section corresponding to the main beam

Side Lobe Artifacts

Side lobe artifacts happen when structures reflected from the side lobes of the ultrasound beam are erroneously mapped onto the image. Side lobes are 3D artifacts.

The creation and transmission of the ultrasound beam from the transducers displays a pattern of "lobes" at various directions. The central ultrasound beam (main lobe) has the greatest energy and contributes mainly to the final imaging. The other lobes are called "side lobes" and propagate to the side of the central fundamental beam in undesired directions, producing the phenomenon of "edge effect". Although the power density of the side lobes is usually much less than that of the central main beam, it can be adequate to create artifacts. These artifacts, which are produced by the emitted side lobes, reflect to laterally positioned targets and are erroneously displayed and interpreted as though they originated from the central main ultrasound beam. Since a requirement for the emerging side lobe artifact is a strong reflecting object, common sources of this significant problem in the interpretation of imaging are the atrioventricular groove and also the fibrous skeleton of the heart (Fig. 8.4) [3–6].

Near-Field and Beam-Width Artifacts

This form of artifact is produced by the high amplitude-oscillations of the piezoelectric crystals of the transducers. It has been practically vanished with the use of new echo systems with harmonic imaging, but in case it appears might mimic a probable LV apical thrombus.

Lateral resolution refers to the ability to distinguish 2 or more structures side-by-side on the monitor as separate. When the ultrasound beam widens distal to the focal zone, the 2 separate side-by-side structures may appear as 1 continuous structure on the image display. Poor lateral resolution may be the result of beam-width artifacts. These artifacts occur when the assumption that ultrasound waves are infinitely thin throughout is violated. Adjusting the focal zone with the focus knob may help to eliminate these artifacts. Beam-width artifacts have been attributed to false positives for thrombi in the left atrial appendage for patients undergoing transesophageal echocardiography with atrial fibrillation (Fig. 8.5) [3–6].

Indeed in the near field, the pair of targets is displayed as separate objects. The pair of targets in the far field is imaged at a depth where the ultrasound beam is wide. It is not clear in the displayed image if there are 2 targets or a single wide one.

Mirror-Image Artifacts

Mirror-image artifacts create the appearance of additional structures on the monitor display. Typically, the duplicated structure is deeper, equidistant, and occasionally lateral to the reflector. Similar to reverberation artifacts, mirror-image artifacts happen when the assumption that the ultrasound echo returns to the transducer after only a single reflection is violated. Instead, the ultrasound beam first hits a large, smooth (mirror-like) reflector during the transmission phase, which directs it to a second reflector (i.e., target). The beam then bounces from the target back to the mirror-like surface on its return to the probe (Fig. 8.6). Identifying the smooth reflector using multiple imaging planes will help to differentiate true extra structures from mirror-image artifacts [4–6].

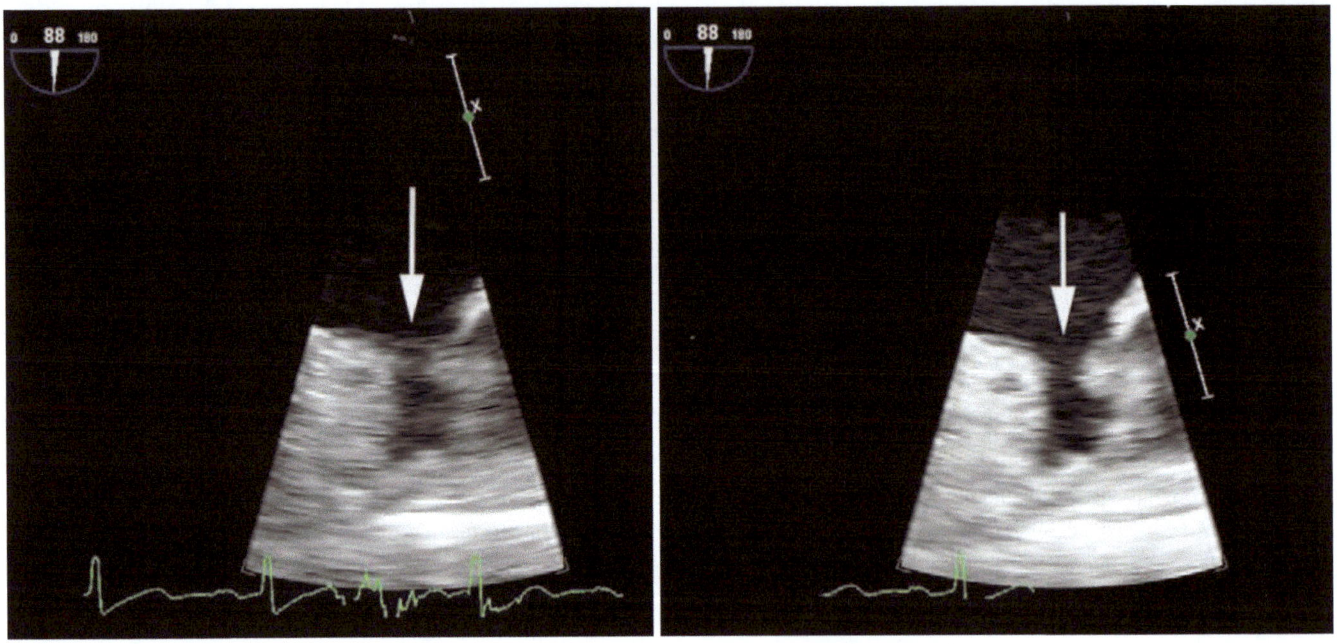

Fig. 8.5 Shows how beam width artifacts might be misdiagnosed as a thrombus in the LA appendage. The area of interest (white arrow) is in the far field of the ultrasound beam (Left panel). As a result, the LA appendage might appear blurred and thrombus cannot be excluded. When the beam is narrowed by repositioning the focus to the level of the appendage, the echogenic material disappears (Right panel, white arrow)

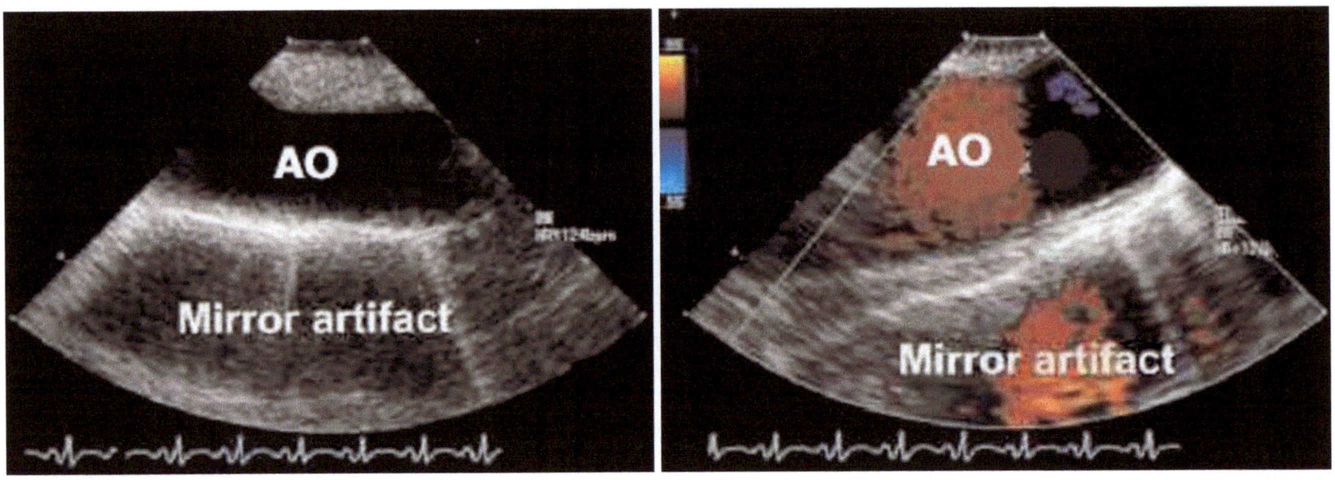

Fig. 8.6 Mirror Image Artifact of Aorta

Doppler Artifacts

Since many therapeutic plans and surgical interventions are based on Doppler hemodynamic findings, knowledge of the capabilities and limitations of echocardiography is critical. Artifacts are deemed the Achilles' heel of echocardiography and result from acoustics principles and the physical interaction between ultrasound and tissue. Artifacts are common and inevitable (Table 8.1).

"Doppler artifact" means recording the signals that falsify the true anatomy of physiology; for instance, detecting the signals with no corresponding anatomic structure or flow in the correct location or failing to recognize signals that are present. These artifacts might lead to improper diagnosis and even treatment. Artifacts in general differ from true flow signals in that the latter have correct anatomical origin and destination, appropriate duration, laminar component, and convergence zone, whereas the former are anatomically incorrect with signals that are too brief to be real. Artifacts appear and disappear when the view is changed and can be usually eliminated with corrective steps [3, 4, 7–9].

Artifacts originate from inappropriate equipment settings such as incorrect gain, velocity, and angle beam and might be overcome by taking appropriate steps such as altering the power, gain, and window. The 2 most important Doppler artifacts are velocity underestimation, which happens with either pulsed wave or continuous-wave Doppler, and signal aliasing, which is inherent to pulsed-wave (and color) Doppler study [4–6].

Doppler Gain

The most important Doppler control is the total gain. Rotating between higher and lower settings will alter the power of the Doppler signals from the audible output and will be perceived by the operator as a change in the volume of the sound. As with any ultrasound system, it is practical to use the lowest gain or power setting that permits the recording of adequate signals. The practical use of a correct gain setting is shown in Fig. 8.7. In this continuous-wave examination from the Apical 4 chamber view. Tricuspid insufficiency is encountered as a systolic velocity spectrum away from the

Table 8.1 Doppler imaging artifacts

Types of Doppler artifacts	Origination	Elimination
Signal aliasing Doppler signal wraps around the baseline, creates confusion to the flow direction, and precludes accurate measurement of maximal velocity (Fig. 8.8)	It happens when pulsed-wave Doppler is applied to flow velocities greater than the Nyquist limit in a non-laminar disturbed flow or a high-velocity laminar flow	• By applying a lower-frequency transducer • By decreasing the depth • By using the continuous-wave Doppler mode
Nonparallel intercept angle It leads to velocity underestimation (Fig. 8.9)	It happens with the malalignment of the interrogating beam and the blood flow direction	By placing the ultrasound beam parallel to the blood flow direction (0° to less than 20°*intercept angle)*
Beam width Superimposition of the 3D volume of the ultrasound beam on a single plane. Even the side lobe image merges with the main beam (Fig. 8.10)	It happens when there is simultaneous recording of different flows (eg, simultaneous recording of the left ventricular inflow and outflow in the apical 4-chamber view). It is sometimes useful and permits measurement of the isovolumic relaxation time	By decreasing the power output or gain
Mirror-image (or "cross-talk) Appearance of the symmetric Doppler signal, both above and below the baseline (Fig. 8.11)	It happens when there is interrogation of a flow (especially turbulent) at a perpendicular angle. Usually, the intensity is less than that of the actual signal	• By decreasing the power output • By optimizing the alignment of the Doppler beam
Electronic interference A band-like signal interfering with the Doppler flow	It is common during intraprocedural echocardiography and is a result of the inadequate shielding of electrical instruments	By shielding and avoiding electrical instruments (if possible) or strong magnetic fields nearby

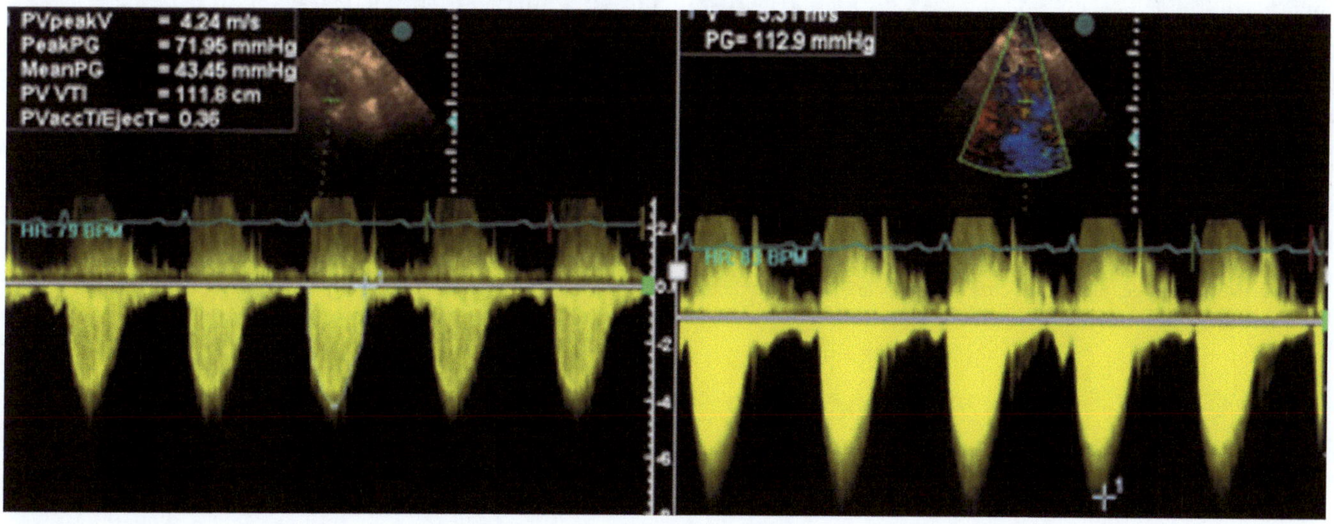

Fig. 8.7 Correct gain in Doppler study in the left panel and overestimation of the Doppler velocity in right panel due to the over gain.

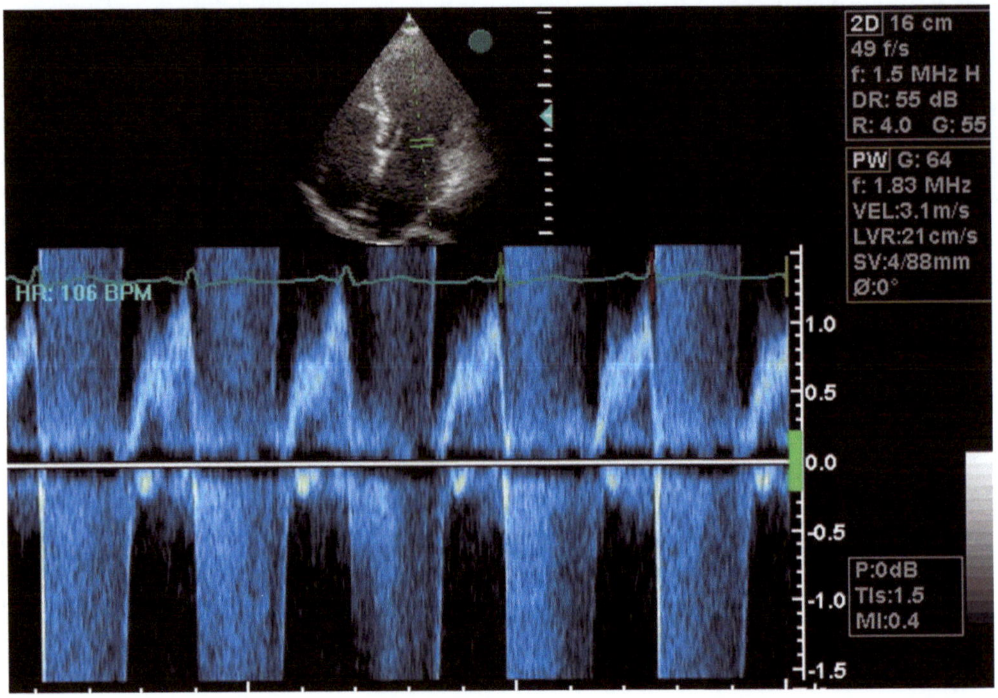

Fig. 8.8 Signal aliasing Doppler signal wrap around the baseline, creates confusion to the flow direction and precludes accurate measurement of maximal velocity

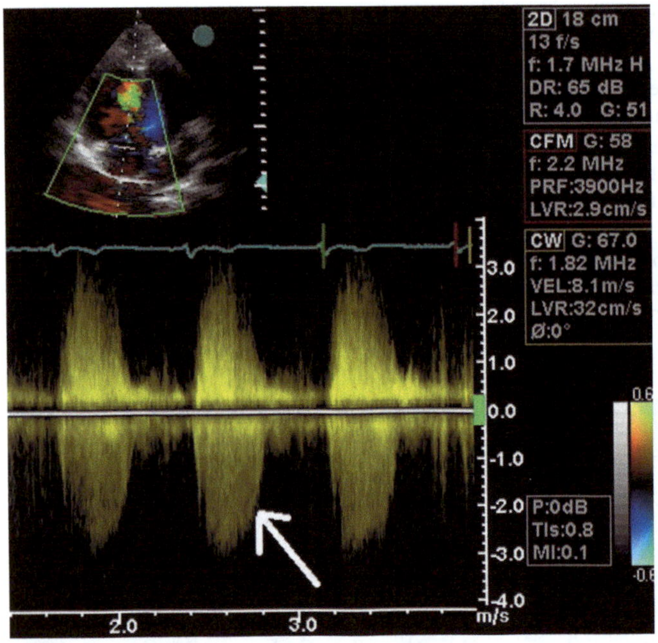

Fig. 8.9 Mirror image (also called crosstalk) appearance of symmetric Doppler signal both above and below the baseline

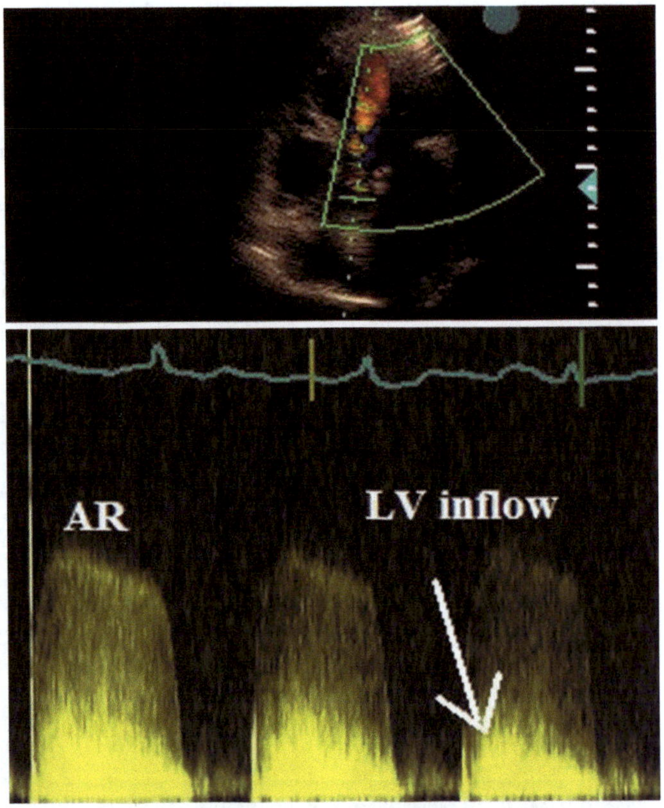

Fig. 8.10 Beam width artifact in Doppler study of the Left Ventricular inflow and outflow in the apical four-chamber view

transducer. In the signals without adequate gain, the full velocity profile is not seen well until the gain is increased to an adequate level that true spectral broadening and the true peak velocity are noted. A beginner should first detect some flow signal and then run through all of the possible gain settings to become familiar with the effect of too much or too little gain [3, 5–7] (Table 8.2).

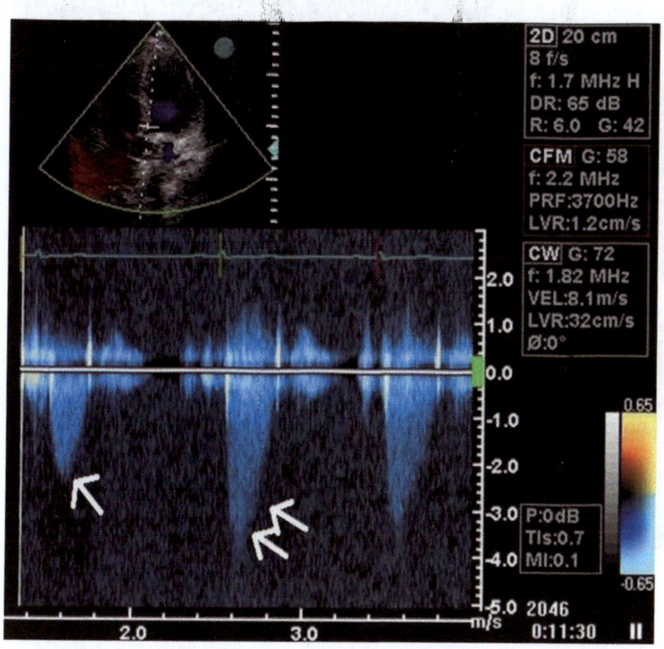

Fig. 8.11 Shows the effect of nonparallel intercept angle which leads to velocity underestimation (misalignment of the interrogating beam and the direction of blood flow that beyond 20 degrees, becomes significant)

3D Artifacts

Stitching Artifacts

This particular form of artifacts has emerged recently and is related to 3D imaging. Three-dimensional imaging has revolutionized echocardiography often by means of computer and circuit processing power; nevertheless, it has a major disadvantage coming from the relatively low speed of sound in soft tissues.

Well-known artifacts are listed in Table 8.3 [4, 6, 7].

Pitfalls

Pitfalls can be define as misinterpretation of normal structure as pathologic structure (Fig. 8.13).

Erroneous Settings Related to Echo Machine

In this context, after the appropriate position of the patient and transducer several prerequisite decisions in the adjustment of the numerous imaging settings should be undertaken that might contribute to an improvement in quality of the display.

Table 8.2 Color Doppler imaging artifacts

Color Doppler artifacts	Origination	Elimination
Shadowing Absence of the color flow signals distal to the strong reflector (Fig. 8.3)	Ultrasound beam is reflected back by high-density structures such as prosthetic valves or heavily calcified structures such that no signal penetrates distal to the shadowing structure	By using an alternate window or echocardiography mode such as transesophageal echocardiography
Ghosting There are brief flashes (usually 1–2 frames) of a large color with no corresponding anatomical flow pattern. It is usually red or blue and is inconsistent beat to beat (Fig. 8.12)	It is caused by the motion of strong reflectors such as prosthetic valve disks	By knowing this artifact and avoiding its misinterpretation as an abnormal flow
Overgain Mosaic pattern of color Doppler signals throughout the image, resulting in background noise	It happens at inappropriately high gain setting	By adjusting the gain setting until the background noise disappears and by making sure that the real flow information is not over suppressed
Undergain There is inadequate gain, leading to the absence of the color flow signals and jet area	It happens at inappropriately low-gain setting	By increasing the gain setting just below the level at which the noise appears
Aliasing There is a wrap-around color flow or an opposite color in spectral display	It is caused by flow velocities exceeding the Nyquist limit Aliasing in color Doppler imaging is very common and even useful as the quantification of the flow in the PISA (proximal isovelocity surface area) is based on aliasing	Reducing the depth of imaging and decreasing the frequency
Intercept angle There is a change in the color flow or absence of the color Doppler signal	It happens when the interrogating beam crosses the image plane at 90°	By changing the interrogating beam direction

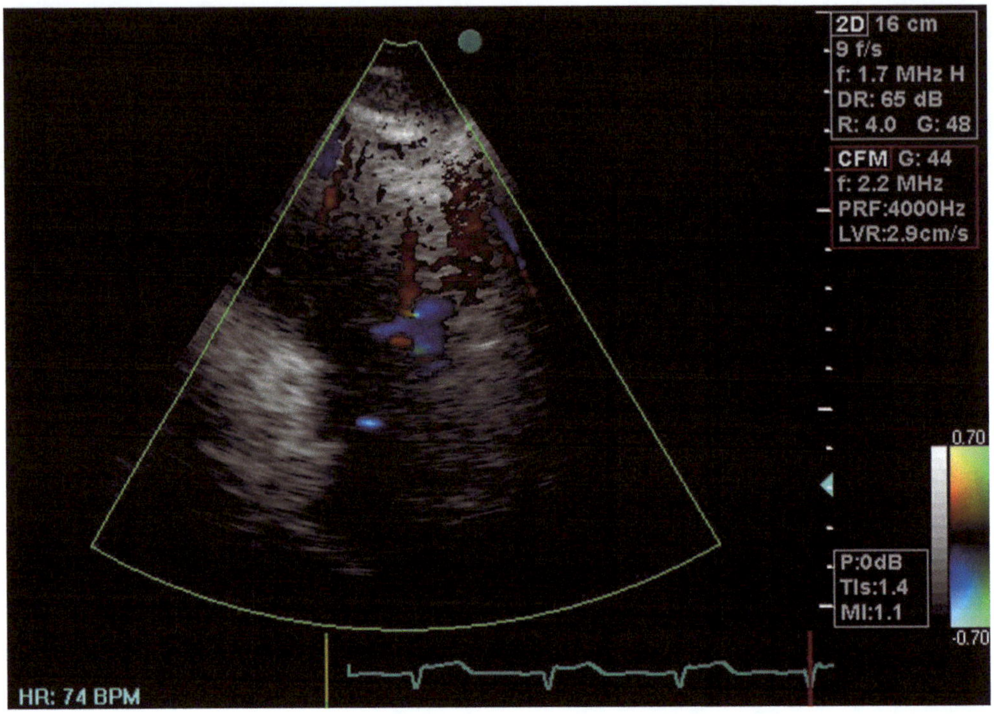

Fig. 8.12 Ghosting Appearance of brief (usually 1-2 frame) large color pattern that overlay anatomic structure with no corresponding underlying flow pattern. Caused by strong moving reflectors (PVs) It is usually red or blue and is inconsistent beat to beat. By knowing this artifact and avoiding its misinterpretation as an abnormal flow

Table 8.3 Three-dimensional artifacts

Artifacts	Characteristics	How to eliminate
Stitching	Presence of demarcation lines within the image, making the image appear "sliced" and shifted	Minimize the heart's out-of-plane movement during the ECG-gated image acquisition period (ie, eliminate dysrhythmias, cease ventilation or patient or probe movement, or cease electrocautery). High volume rates (high volume rate mode) might minimize stitching
Dropout	Missing data from image structures that are parallel to the ultrasound pulse	Increase the gain. Change the probe position to move the area of interest from the position parallel to the ultrasound beam
Railroad	Objects with wide lumens displayed as if they have a railroad track appearance	Optimize the spatial and temporal resolution. Change the probe position to move the ultrasound beam to 90° of the area of interest
Blurring	Objects appear thicker than they are in reality	Optimize the spatial and temporal resolution

Modified table from: Huong T. Le, Nicholas Hangiandreou, Robert Timmerman, Mark J. Rice, W. Brit Smith, Lori Deitte, Gregory M. Janelle. Imaging artifacts in echocardiography. Anesth Analg. 2016;122:633–46

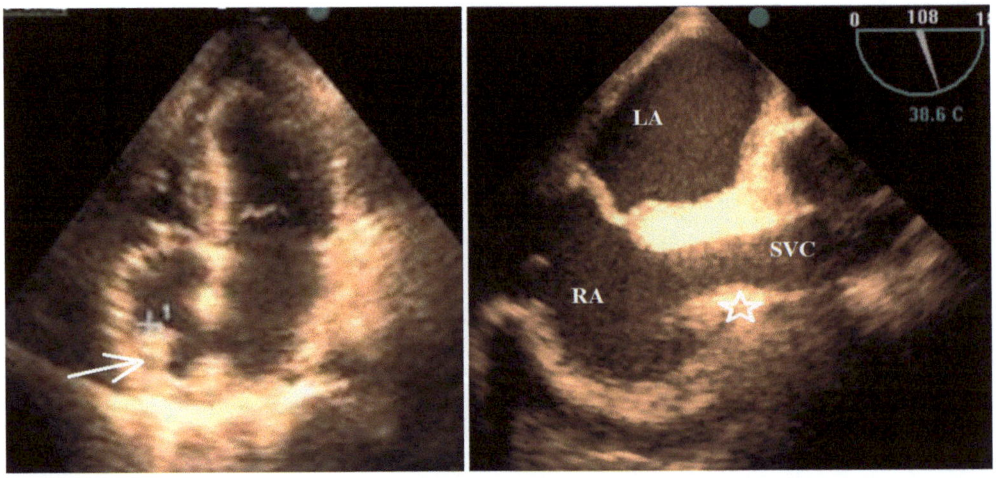

Fig. 8.13 Crista terminalis Misinterpretation as RA tumor or thrombus. Prominent muscular ridge originate at junction of RA and SVC and runs toward IVC. CT separate trabeculated and smooth portion of RA

The following table depicts some common problems encountered in daily practice and their suggested solutions Table 8.4 [2–4, 6].

Errors in Measurements

Quantification of cardiac chamber size and function along with valvular heart disease study are the central and most frequently requested indications of echocardiography. However non-standardized measurements have been mostly contradictory and less successful compared to other imaging modalities and therefore echocardiographically measurements are sometimes perceived as inconsistent. These special types of errors are the common encountered cases even in modern echocardiography labs equipped with new advanced ultrasound technology devices such as foreshortened LV apex (Fig. 8.14). The imaging planes should cut the true LV apex not the LV wall as in the foreshortened LV apex and is diagnosed by round shape and wall thickness of the apex which is similar to the LV. The foreshortened LV apex can be corrected by re-positioning the transducer to a lower and lateral point.

Lack of standardization usually heralds great variation regarding the reliability of measurements. Once guidelines have been established, good reproducibility and reliability has been achieved and used in different clinical settings [3, 6–8].

Table 8.4 Common problems and the suggested solutions

Difficulties and pitfalls	Solutions
Obese patients with suboptimal imaging	Decrease the transmission frequency of the ultrasound beam
Potentially 2 small structures lying along the axis of the beam cannot be differentiated	Increase the transmission frequency of the ultrasound beam
In the apical 4-chamber projection, the inter-atrial septum cannot be seen clearly and might mimic a patent foramen ovale or an atrial septal defect	1. Use modified views. 2. Increase the gain of the received signal. 3. Inject agitated saline as a contrast with the Valsalva maneuver
Moving cardiac structures in real-time scanning are aesthetically of rather low quality	Lower the sector width of the display and/or the depth of the field
Chronic mitral regurgitation that seems to be severe, though the left ventricle is not dilated	Adjust properly the color gain settings of the machine, Using more quantitative data
	Decreasing
Patients with no history of myocardial infarction and abnormal perfusion of the apex in rest images	The focus button should be adjusted to the level of the interest

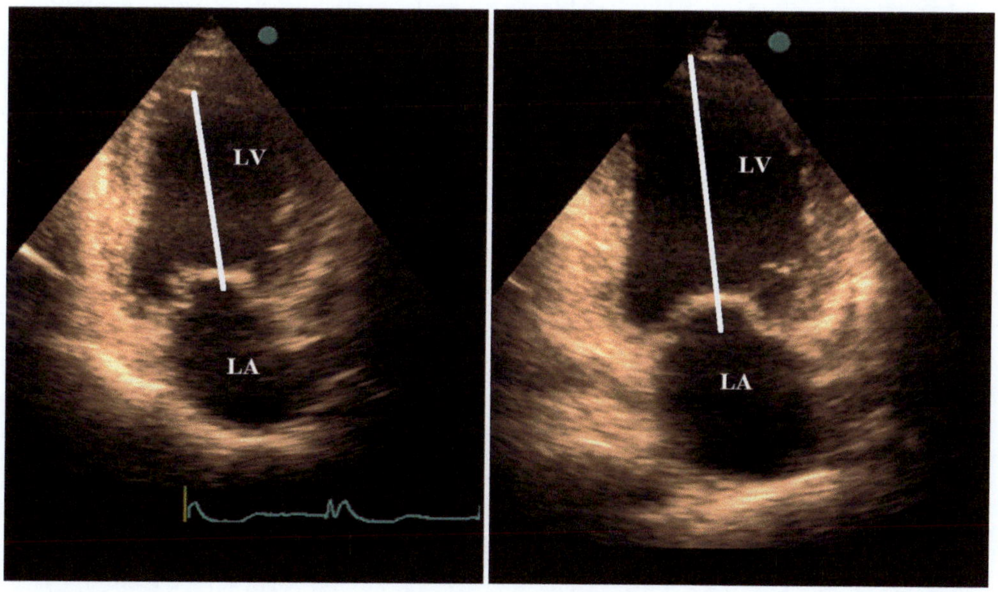

Fig. 8.14 Foreshortened left ventricle at left panel and corrected one at right sided panel (White lines)

References

1. Mann DL, Zipes DP, Libby P, Bonow R. Braunwald's heart disease. A textbook of cardiovascular medicine. 10th ed. Amsterdam: Elsevier; 2017.
2. Anderson B. Echocardiography. 2nd ed. Manly, QLD: MGA Graphics; 2007.
3. Feigenbaum's H. Echocardiography. 6th ed. Philadelphia: Lippincott Williams & Wilkins; 2005.
4. Vegas A, Meineri M. Three-dimensional transesophageal echocardiography is a major advance for intraoperative clinical management of patients undergoing cardiac surgery: a core review. Anesth Analg. 2010;110:1548–73.
5. Lang R, Bierig M, Devereux R, et al. Recommendations for chamber quantification. Eur J Echocardiogr. 2006;7:79–108.
6. Le HT, Hangiandreou N, Timmerman R, Rice MJ, Smith WB, Deitte L, Janelle GM. Imaging artifacts in echocardiography. Anesth Analg. 2016;122:633–46.
7. Rudski LG, Picard MH. Artifacts, truths, and consequences. Am J Med. 2000;108:589–91.
8. Sharma V, Fletcher SN. A review of echocardiography in anaesthetic and peri-operative practice. Part 2: training and accreditation. Anaesthesia. 2014;69:919–27.
9. The EACVI Textbook of Echocardiography, Chaptert 3 "Doppler Echocardiography" Kasprzak J, Sadeghpour A, Jurcut R. 2nd edition. Oxford university press 2017.

Contrast Echocardiography

9

Farimah Aminian and Harald Becher

Abstract

Contrast echocardiography is an enhanced ultrasound imaging technique utilizing a contrast agent to increase blood echogenicity in cardiac chambers or myocardial microvessels. This technique can improve image quality and provide interpretable recordings in cases with suboptimal acoustic window like ventilated or obese patients. Contrast enhancement can be used during transthoracic, transesophageal and stress echocardiography.

Clinical applications for contrast echocardiography are classified into four main categories: Left ventricular opacification, Detection of intracardiac shunt, Doppler signal enhancement and assessment of myocardial perfusion.

Keywords

Echocardiography · Contrast · imaging

Abbreviations

CAD	Coronary artery disease
EBD	Endocardial border delineation
EF	Ejection fraction
IV	Intravenous
LV	Left ventricle
LVO	Left ventricular opacification
MBF	Myocardial blood flow
MCE	Myocardial contrast echocardiography
PFO	Patent foramen ovale
TEE	Transesophageal echocardiography
UCA	Ultrasound contrast agent

Introduction

Suboptimal images are defined as the inability to detect endocardial borders of two or more contiguous segments in any three of the apical windows [1]. Suboptimal images are important issues in echocardiography even when new machines with harmonic tissue modality are used. Good endocardial definition is particularly important in stress echocardiography, where reliable assessment of LV wall motion and thickening are crucial for obtaining reproducible results [1–4].

Contrast administration improves image quality through enhanced endocardial border definition. Enhancement of image quality by contrast can overcome LV apical artifacts like near field clutter so facilitates identification of apical abnormalities (Fig. 9.1).

- Clinical indications for contrast echocardiography are: (A) Left ventricular opacification, (B) Detection of intracardiac shunt, (C) Doppler signal enhancement, (D) Assessment of myocardial perfusion [1, 3, 4].

A. LV opacification enhances endocardial border visualization that is a key factor for LV structural abnormalities, accurate LV volume, regional and global systolic measurements.

- The following LV structural abnormalities can be confirmed or excluded by contrast enhancement [5–8]:
  Apical hypertrophic cardiomyopathy
  LV non-compaction
  LV thrombus and intracardiac mass
  LV aneurysm versus pseudoaneurysm

B. Contrast injection is indicated to rule out an intrapulmonary or intracardiac right-to-left shunt or to detect residual shunts after defect closure [9].

C. Enhancement of inadequate Doppler flow signals and pressure gradients with contrast echocardiography could be performed on rest or stress studies.

F. Aminian, MD (✉) · H. Becher
Echocardiography Department, Razavi Hospital, Mashhad, Iran

A. Sadeghpour, A. Alizadehasl (eds.), *Case-Based Textbook of Echocardiography*,
https://doi.org/10.1007/978-3-319-67691-3_9

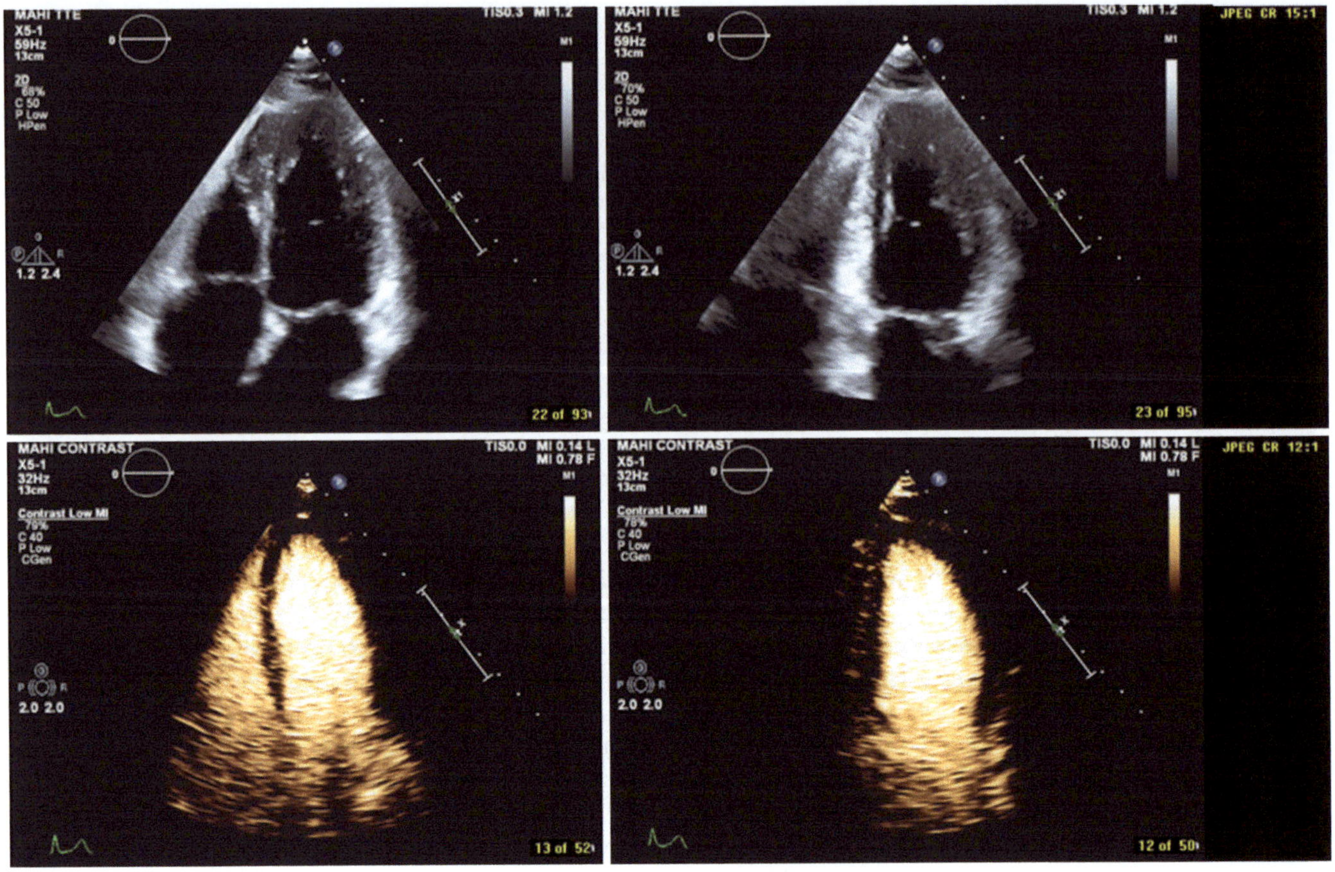

Fig. 9.1 Native and contrast-enhanced 4 and 2-chamber views. Note the good endocardial delineation of the contrast recordings

D. Myocardial contrast echocardiography (MCE) is used for detection of myocardial ischemia, myocardial viability and coronary flow reserve [10].

Attention: No indication exists yet for contrast study in pediatric group [2].

Contrast Agents

Contrast echocardiography can be performed by agitated saline or left heart contrast agents that are named as ultrasound contrast agents (UCA).

Agitated saline contrast: is air-microbubbles contrast and administered intravenously to opacify right heart. These microbubbles are short-lived and can't pass pulmonary circulation, so microbubbles can't be visualized in the left heart unless there is a right to left intracardiac or pulmonary arteriovenous shunt [1, 9] (Fig. 9.2).

- The clinical application of saline microbubbles is identification of cardiac shunts or residual shunts after device closure and enhancing right heart image.
- Early appearance of bubbles in the left heart (within three to five beats) suggests an intracardiac shunt whereas later appearance of bubbles in the left heart suggests pulmonary arteriovenous shunt. Pitfalls of this method are mentioned in Table 9.1.

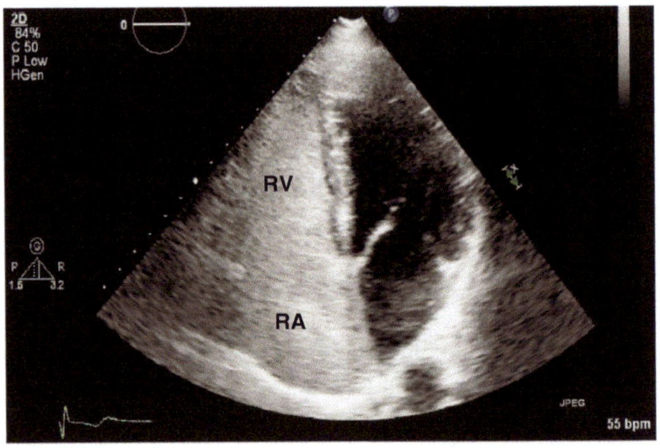

Fig. 9.2 Opacification of right heart by intravenous agitated saline

Ultrasound contrast agents (UCA): are high molecular-weight gases, surrounded by an elastic coating. After intravenous injection, microbubbles can transverse pulmonary circulation and appear in the left heart [11]. Contrast microbubbles are able to resonate in the sound field, they reflect the ultrasound and produce non-linear signals which can be detected with harmonic imaging or newer contrast specific imaging modalities.

- The new second generation of UCAs have advantages over the first generation as the thicker outer shell and high molecular-weight inner gas (instead of air that used in first generation) make the bubbles more stable, so more durable in clinical practice [11, 12] (Table 9.2).

Contrast administration: UCA can be administrated as IV bolus injection or infusion and each method has its cons & pros (Table 9.3). Bolus injection can be easily used for LV opacification, endocardial enhancement and intensification of Doppler signals. Bolus UCA has short enhancing effect and can be repeated safely.

Infusion technique provides continuous contrast enhancement and can be utilized in all clinical applications of contrast study. Contrast infusion reduces the likelihood of acoustic artifacts, commonly encountered after bolus injection. Myocardial contrast echocardiography is merely performed via contrast infusion as it is necessary to have constant concentration of contrast.

Table 9.1 Pitfalls during saline contrast study: difficulty in diagnosis of PFO or differentiation between pulmonary atriovenous shunt and intra-cardiac shunt

Pitfalls in saline contrast study	Possible reasons
Early appearance of bubbles in the left heart in the absence of pulmonary arterio-venous shunt (< 5 beats)	High output state
Late appearance of bubbles in the left heart in the presence of PFO (>3–5 beats)	Delayed Valsalva maneuver or coughing
False negative study for PFO	Insufficient saline agitation, weak cough, persistent right bowing of IAS

Contrast Safety and Side Effects

Safety of contrast administration has been emphasized in many studies and critical cardiopulmonary reactions and fatalities were noted uncommon during or after contrast administration [16–22]. However, all patients should be monitored for cardio-respiratory instability after UCA injection esp. those patients with acute coronary syndrome or other unstable cardiopulmonary conditions [13–15].

- IV contrast injection is contraindicated to use in patients with bidirectional or right to left shunt (PFO is not included in this category and UCAs can be used in patients with PFO) [1].
- Corrected or uncorrected congenital heart disease is not a contraindication for contrast administration by itself [19].
- Contrast can be cautiously administrated in a patient with pulmonary hypertension if it is needed to enhance right or left ventricular visualization [21, 22].
- SonoVue should not be administered in patients with severe pulmonary hypertension (>90 mmHg) and acute respiratory distress syndrome (ARDS) [15].

UCAs should not be administrated in patients with history of contrast hypersensitivity; Optison and Definity are contraindicated in patients with perflutren hypersensitivity. Moreover, Optison is contraindicated in patients who have allergy to blood products or Albumin [13–15].

Side effects with contrast agents are often transient and tolerable (Table 9.2). Hypersensitivity reactions to UCA are pos-

Table 9.2 2nd generation UCAs: Definity, Optison and SonoVue

UCA 2nd generation	Optison [13]	Definity (Luminity) [14]	SonoVue [15]
Inner gas	Perfluoropropane	Perfluoropropane	Sulphur hexafluoride
Shell	Human albumin	Phospholipid	Surfactant
More frequent side effects	Headache, nausea, flushing, dizziness	Headache, flushing, Back pain	Headache, nausea, chest pain
Safety approved in clinical trials [16–22]	Safe	Safe	Safe

Table 9.3 Methods of intravenous UCA administration; pros & cons of bolus vs. infusion technique

Method of UCA administration	Pros	Cons
Bolus	Easy	Short contrast effect
	Rapid contrast effect and wash out	Artifacts
Infusion	Less artifacts (e.g. attenuation, swirling)	Usually needs infusion pump with syringe rotation
	Continuous contrast effect is beneficial in patients with suboptimal images during stress echocardiography	Contrast stability (contrast clearance needs a burst of high power ultrasonic energy)
	Mandatory for evaluation of myocardial perfusion or coronary flow reserve	

sible and Allergy kit should be easily accessible. The reactions are usually mild, including skin rashes and wheezing but rarely can be life threatening, resulting in severe hypotension or laryngeal edema.

Machine Setting

Mechanical Index

Harmonic imaging or newer contrast specific imaging modalities are used for contrast echocardiography. The power of the ultrasound which is transmitted from the transducer determines the tissue features and bubble behavior. The power of the ultrasound is reported as mechanical index (MI). By definition, MI values are classified to: very low (< 0.2), low (< 0.3), intermediate (0.3–0.5), and high (>0.5) [1].

- For contrast echocardiography of the left heart, harmonic imaging or a newer contrast specific imaging modality should be used with a mechanical index <0.3 (low power)

Low ultrasound power reduces the intensities of myocardial and valvular signals as well as apical noise artifacts and prolongs the duration of the contrast effect. This enhances the display of the blood within the LV and the myocardial vessels.

Because of attenuation of the ultrasound in the far field (basal LV segments in apical views), microbubbles do not resonate as well as microbubbles in the near field (apex) which can lead to poor contrast in the basal LV cavity (which is defined as attenuation artifact). This can be compensated by increasing the transmit power.

- The mechanical index needs to be individually adjusted to avoid attenuation and bubble destruction in the nearfield.
- High MI imaging can be used Intermittently to clear contrast from myocardium and masses [10, 11].

Gain and Compression

Optimum machine setting improves detection of contrast signals by changing the display characteristics.

Gain is an ultrasound control to adjust the amplification of the backscattered ultrasound. It is different from the ultrasound power which is the amount of ultrasound energy transmitted from the transducer [23].

- For contrast LV opacification, gain should be adjusted to provide optimal endocardial border enhancement in all segments
- For myocardial perfusion imaging it is usually beneficial to use higher gain than for LV opacification

Focus

In the image focus area, the ultrasound power is highest. This provides better tissue image quality in non contrast high power imaging. In contrast echocardiography for which low ultrasound power is used; there could be increased microbubble destruction or better contrast effect in the focal area depending on the precordial attenuation of the ultrasound beam.

- It is recommended to set the image focus at mitral annular level. In myocardial contrast echocardiography additional recording may be performed with the focus near the apex when a perfusion defect is observed with the regular focus position at the mitral valve level.

Artifacts

Contrast echocardiography encounters acoustic artifacts which can be avoided.

Inappropriate setting of machine and/or the way of contrast administration are the main reasons for artifacts [13, 14].

- It is recommended to use the contrast presets of the echocardiography scanner, which are provided by the manufacturers.

Attenuation artifact: increased echogenicity especially in the near field resulting in shadowing of the farfield and incomplete LV opacification (Fig. 9.3). Attenuation artifacts usually occur early after injection of contrast bolus. To reduce attenuation artifacts, perform the recordings later after the bolus injection or decrease bolus dose.

- Attenuation artifact is also possible with continuous infusion instead. In this case the infusion rate has to be reduced.

Swirling artifact: Low contrast bolus dosage, high MI (microbubble destruction), or too low contrast infusion rate can lead to contrast turbulence instead of a homogeneous contrast distribution in the near field (Fig. 9.4). Swirling can be overcome by decreasing MI and increasing contrast dose and infusion rate.

- Swirling artifact is more common in patients with LV dysfunction or LV aneurysm.

Rib/lung artifacts: Filling defects (especially in the lateral wall) due to shadowing from ribs or lung tissue (Fig. 9.5). Rib artifacts reduce by adjusting the probe position. Lung artifacts eliminate by breath holding during image acquisition.

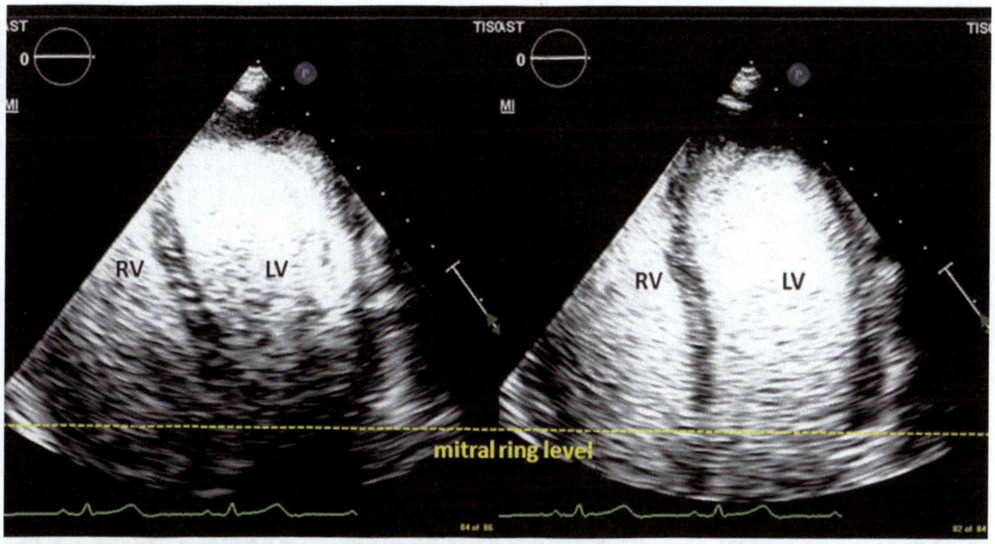

Fig. 9.3 Incomplete LV opacification due to attenuation artifact

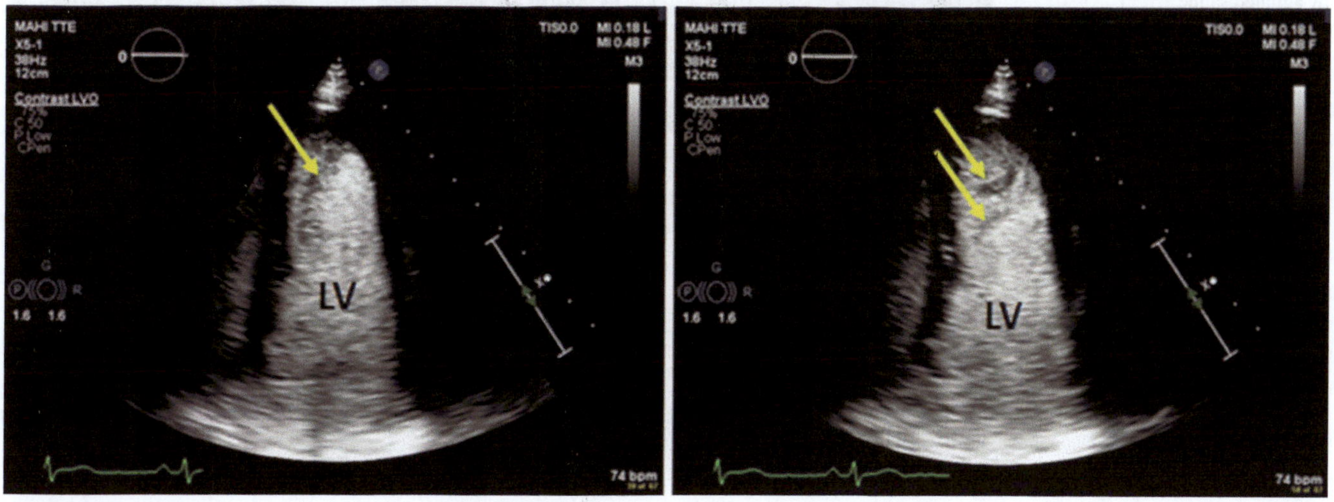

Fig. 9.4 Inhomogeneous contrast distribution in LV due to swirling artifact (arrows)

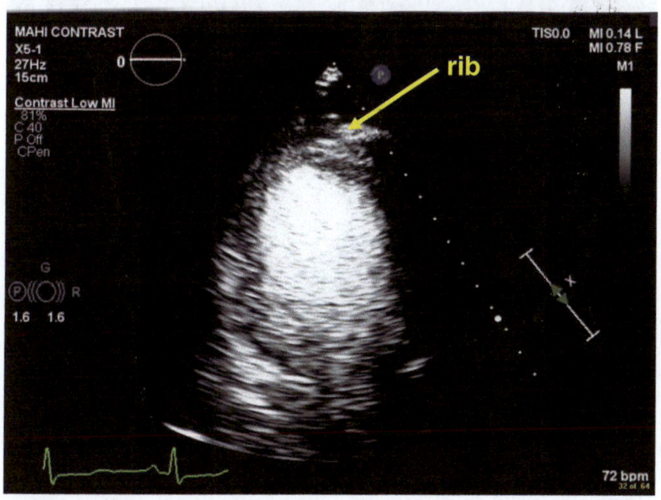

Fig. 9.5 Rib artifact; Shadowing from rib during LV contrast echocardiography

Role of -UCAs in Clinical Echocardiography

A. Doppler signal enhancement
B. Left ventricular opacification
C. Assessment of myocardial perfusion

A. Doppler signal enhancement

UCAs are commonly used for augmentation of weak Continuous wave (CW) Doppler signals and measurement of peak transvalvular velocity. Contrast agents can also enhance flow detection by color flow mapping.

- Trans-aortic pressure gradient can be effectively measured by using UCAs in patients with poor Doppler signals. The severity of aortic stenosis can be assessed noninvasively by this echocardiography technique [24, 25] (Fig. 9.6a, b).

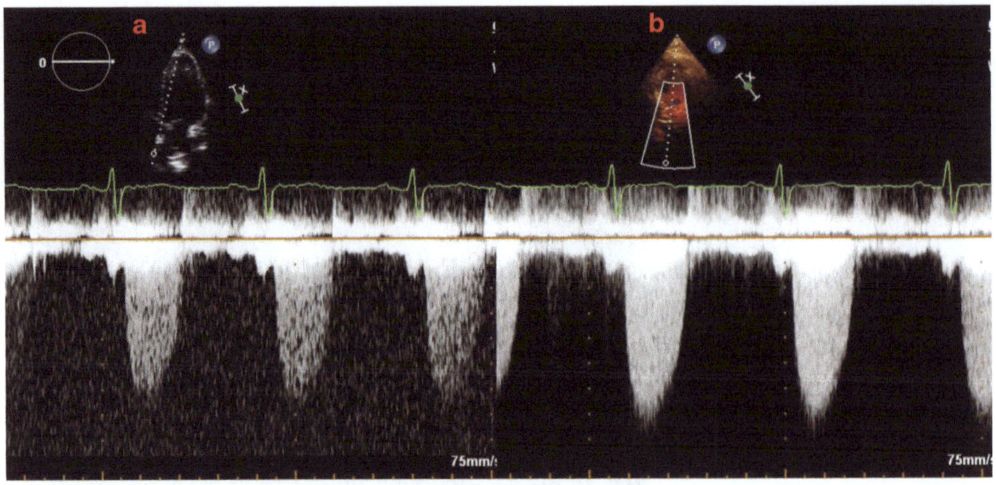

Fig. 9.6 Enhanced spectral Doppler envelope of aortic valve by contrast. The severity of aortic stenosis was revealed after using UCA (**a**,**b**)

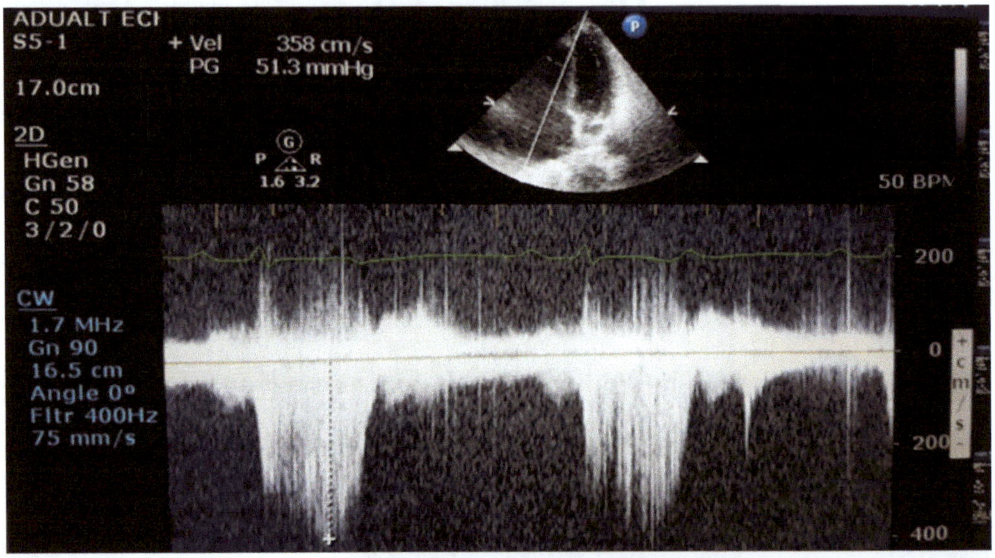

Fig. 9.7 Measurement of TR peak velocity after enhancement by agitated saline

- UCAs and agitated saline contrast can be used to augment weak CW envelope of tricuspid regurgitation (TR). This technique provides reliable measurement of TR peak velocity thus accurate estimation of pulmonary pressure [26] (Fig. 9.7).

B. LV opacification (LVO)

LVO by contrast agents enhances endocardial border delineation (EBD) in suboptimal images and helps to make certainty about LV geometry, structural abnormality or segmental wall motion. EBD facilitates assessment of regional and global LV systolic function.

- Accurate measurement of LVEF is crucial in cancer patients undergoing chemotherapy and this technique can provide reliable results in serial echocardiographic measurements of LVEF [27, 28].

In patients referred to emergency department for acute chest pain, echocardiography has diagnostic role and normal segmental wall thickening is enough to rule out an acute ischemic event.

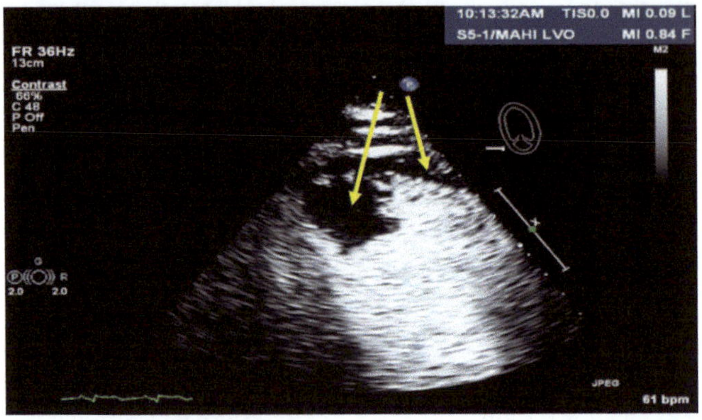

Fig. 9.8 LV apical thrombus is seen after UCA administration. Filling defect (arrows) estimates the size and extent of thrombus

- Contrast-enhancement yields optimal sensitivity for detecting small regional wall motion abnormality during echocardiography.

LVO improves detection of intra-cardiac thrombus (Fig. 9.8) & structural abnormalities including: apical hyper-

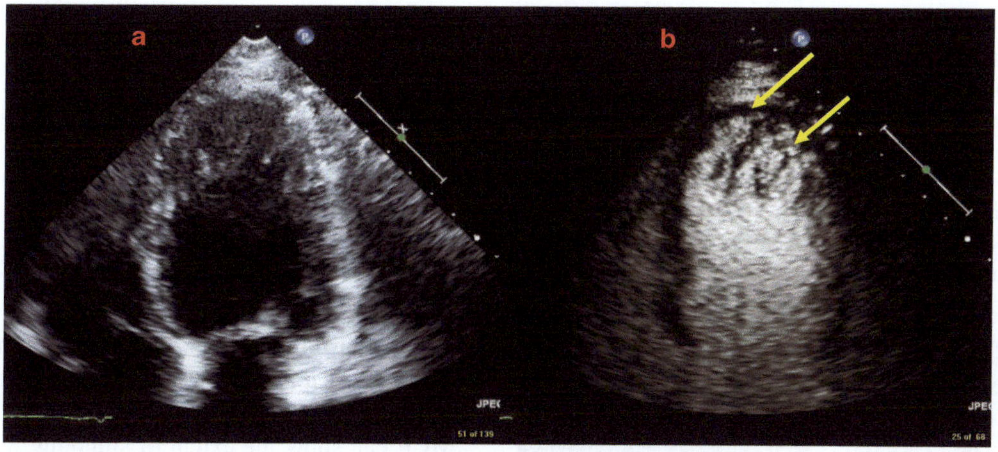

Fig. 9.9 (**a**) LV noncompaction. Apical 4-chamber view is nondiagnostic. (**b**) After contrast LV opacification, multiple deep trabeculations of the LV myocardium are seen

trophic cardiomyopathy, LV non-compaction (Fig. 9.9) and pseudo-aneurysms [5–8].

UCAs can be also used during TEE for better delineation of a thrombus in left atrial appendage and differentiating between spontaneous contrast and thrombus [29].

LVO in stress echocardiography: The efficacy of contrast has been pointed out during both exercise and pharmacological stress echocardiography in patients with inadequate ultrasound images [22, 30].

- Contrast enhancement can improve visual assessment of systolic wall thickening at stress phase and facilitate the detection of new regional wall motion abnormality.

The protocols and image acquisition are the same for contrast-enhanced and non- enhanced stress echocardiography. Contrast is administered at rest, at low level of stress and prior to acquisition of the peak stress loop via continuous or bolus injection. With infusion of contrast it is easier to obtain good recordings than after bolus injection; the infusion can be stopped and resumed when needed [3].

In summary, contrast administration increases the diagnostic accuracy of stress echocardiography and decreases interobsever variability.

C. Assessment of myocardial perfusion

myocardial blood flow (MBF) can be assessed noninvasively by myocardial contrast echocardiography (MCE). An infusion of the contrast agent is recommended for assessment of myocardial perfusion. This technique is based on myocardial enhancement by displaying the microbubbles in the myocardial vessels and evaluation of signal intensity that denotes capillary blood volume. Moreover, after depletion of microbubbles, the rate of contrast replenishment can be assessed [10].

- MCE adds prognostic information over wall motion in stress echocardiography [31]. Reduced contrast density (decreased capillary blood volume) and delayed contrast appearance (reduced blood flow velocity) are the key diagnostic findings for coronary artery disease.

Low MI imaging is the preferred method for two reasons: It provides continuous real-time assessment of both wall motion and perfusion and total contrast dose is less than what should be used in high MI imaging (less bubble destruction at low MI). Brief high-MI flashes (three to 10 frames) is used to destroy microbubbles and clear contrast from the myocardium in order to analyze the rate of contrast replenishment [10].

- This technique can be also used for intracardiac masses to evaluate its vascularity; contrast enhancement of the mass after a burst of high MI flashes indicates a vascular tumor [32].

MCE can be performed in rest or stress phases for: (1) Detection of myocardial ischemia, (2) Myocardial viability, (3) Assessment of myocardial Flow Reserve.

MCE for Detection of Myocardial Ischemia

This technique can help to detect abnormal myocardial perfusion in patients with coronary artery disease even in the acute or chronic setting (Table 9.4).

In patients with acute coronary syndromes, resting MCE can detect myocardial perfusion abnormality that is a finding earlier than troponin elevation.

- A new wall motion abnormality in parallel with a perfusion defect suggests coronary artery disease. A new wall motion abnormality without a perfusion defect can be a consequence of myocardtitis [3]. (please note about artifacts in myocardial perfusion imaging, therefore a new clear wall motion abnormality still may be caused by coronary artery disease)

Table 9.4 Interpretation of resting and stress MCE (modified from the EAE recommendations [3])

Resting MCE	Normal wall motion + Normal MCE	Abnormal wall motion + Abnormal MCE	Abnormal wall motion + Normal MCE	Normal wall motion + Abnormal MCE
	Normal	Ischemia	Stunning, hibernation	Artifact
Stress MCE	Normal wall motion + Normal MCE	New WMA + Abnormal MCE	New WMA + Normal MCE	Normal wall motion + Abnormal MCE
	Normal	Ischemia	Artifact, Cardiomyopathy[a]	Ischemia

WMA: wall motion abnormality
[a]In patients with cardiomyopathy especially those with myocardtitis, WMA can be present with normal MCE study

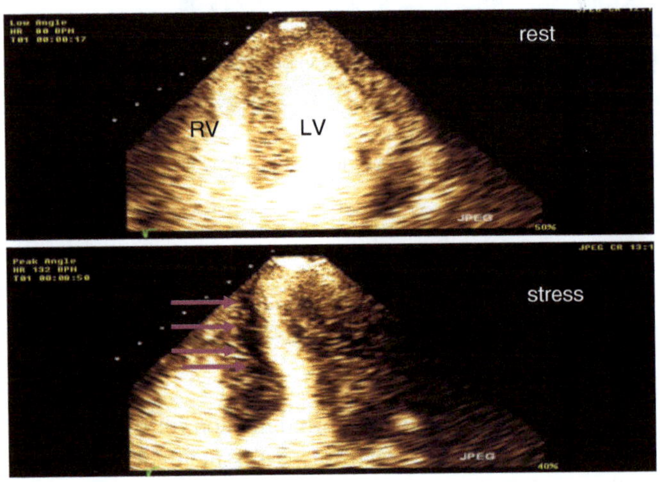

Fig. 9.10 Dobutamine stress echocardiography, 4 chamber view: Normal perfusion at rest (top), septal ischemia with subendocardial perfusion defect in the septum (arrows)

MCE is a useful imaging tool for detection of residual perfusion abnormality after thrombolytic therapy, a consequence of significant residual infarct-related coronary stenosis or multivessel disease [33].

The clinical advantages of MCE have been also highlighted in patients with chronic stable angina. Stress MCE can help to determine the hemodynamic significance of an intermediate coronary stenosis on coronary angiography (Fig. 9.10). Normal perfusion and wall motion in the territory of the coronary artery, will obviate the need for interventional procedure [3, 34].

- A contrast defect is usually seen first in the subendocardium and does not extend over myocardial full thickness; In patients with chronic CAD Full thickness defects are more likely artifacts [35].

MCE for Evaluation of Myocardial Viability

MCE can differentiate between viable myocardium and nonviable necrotic or scar tissue and is based on the correlation of viable myocardium with microvascular integrity [36]. It was proven that peak contrast intensity in MCE is correlated well with capillary density, so the extent of nonviable myocardium (transmural vs. non transmural) can be recognized by evidence of a perfusion defect after contrast administration [37].

MCE can show the extent of stunning myocardium after myocardial infarction, so LV contractile reserve can be predicted [37].

- Bright and thin myocardium (thickness $\leq$ 5 mm) indicates scar tissue thus it is unnecessary to assess perfusion in these segments [3].

MCE can also identify hibernating myocardium in patients with chronic CAD. Good contrast enhancement in resting perfusion study indicates preserved myocardial blood flow and viability, although the segment is severely hypokinetic or akinetic [38].

MCE for Assessment of Myocardial Flow Reserve

Myocardial flow reserve is the ratio of the maximal myocardial blood flow (MBF) at stress to the myocardial blood flow at rest. The capillary blood velocity is 1 mm/s and myocardial contrast replenishment happens within 4–5 s at rest, while during stress imaging, it should occur within 2 s. Any decrease in MBF prolongs replenishment time in proportion to the reduction in MBF [39].

- Stress imaging is preferentially performed by vasodilators for assessment of coronary flow reserve (e.g. adenosine, dipyridamole).

The normal increase in myocardial and coronary flow after vasodilator is reduced or absent in territories with significant coronary stenosis or microvessel disease. Therefore, less contrast intensity is observed during MCE in areas supplied by stenotic coronary arteries whereas we see a marked enhancement of signal intensity in the myoacardium supplied by normal coronary arteries. By using special computer programs (for example Qlab), the signal intensity in a myocardial region of interest is measured.

- The maximum intensity reached after the replenishment (A) and the speed of replenishment (beta) are measured and myocardial blood flow is calculated by multiplying A x beta

- Abnormal myocardial flow reserve can also occur in microvascular disease which is common in patients with hypertensive heart disease. MCE has specific advantage in small vessel disease especially in the absence of concomitant epicardial coronary artery disease [40, 41].

Myocardial blood flow reserve correlates well with coronary blood flow reserve. Coronary flow reserve can be assessed by measuring the peak diastolic velocity of coronary flow, using coronary Doppler at rest and during adenosine or dipyridamole infusion.

- LAD flow often can be detected with transthoracic colour Doppler and quantified with PW Doppler. Weak or noisy Doppler signals can be enhanced by injection of UCA

Conclusion

UCA are safe and serious side effects are uncommon (rate of death: 1 in 500,000) [42]. Contrast echocardiography improves early diagnosis and reduces the risk of missing a potentially fatal complication like pseudoaneurysm. Contrast enhanced imaging reduces the variability of echocardiographic measurements in patients with suboptimal acoustic window and can obviate the subsequent need for further invasive investigation [43].

Questions

1. A False positive diagnosis of PFO can be made in:
   A. Delayed Valsalva maneuver
   B. Delayed coughing
   C. High cardiac output state
   D. Weak coughing

2. Which statement is correct for different methods of intravenous UCA administration during contrast echocardiography?
   A. Bolus injection results in less attenuation artifacts
   B. Infusion administration results in less swirling artifact
   C. Bolus injection is more useful for evaluation of myocardial perfusion
   D. A burst of high power ultrasonic energy isn't needed for contrast clearance after infusion administration

3. Optison is contraindicated in patients with:
   A. Uncorrected congenital heart disease
   B. Pulmonary hypertension
   C. Known Allergy to blood products
   D. Acute coronary syndrome

4. Contrast echocardiography is less useful in:
   A. Differentiation between Apical HCM and endomyocardial fibrosis
   B. Enhancement of Doppler envelope for evaluation of AS severity
   C. Differentiation between LAA spontaneous contrast and thrombosis during TEE
   D. Imaging of new regional wall motion abnormality during dobutamine stress echocardiography

5. Assessment of myocardial perfusion by contrast echocardiography is indicated in:
   A. Detection of residual perfusion abnormality after thrombolytic therapy
   B. Evaluation of hemodynamic significance of a moderate coronary stenosis
   C. Evaluation of LV tumor vascularity
   D. All

Answers

1. C
2. B
3. C
4. A
5. D

References

1. Porter TR, Abdelmoneim S, Belcik JT, McCulloch ML, Mulvagh SL, Olson JJ, et al. Guidelines for the cardiac sonographer in the performance of contrast echocardiography: a focused update from the American society of echocardiography. J Am Soc Echocardiogr. 2014;:797–810.
2. Mulvagh SL, Rakowski H, Vannan MA, Abdelmoneim SS, Becher H, Bierig M, et al. ASE consensus statement on the clinical applications of ultrasonic contrast agents in echocardiography. J Am Soc Echocardiogr. 2008;21:1179–201.
3. Senior R, Becher H, Monaghan M, Agati L, Zamorano J, Vanoverschelde JL, Nihoyannopoulos P. Contrast echocardiography: evidence-based recommendations by European Association of Echocardiography. Eur J Echocardiogr. 2009;10:194–212.
4. Olszewski R, Timperley J, Szmigielski C, Monaghan M, Nihoyannopoulos P, Senior R, et al. The clinical applications of contrast echocardiography. Eur J Echocardiogr. 2007;8:S13–23.
5. Thanigaraj S, Schechtman KB, Perez JE. Improved echocardiographic delineation of left ventricular thrombus with the use of intravenous second-generation contrast image enhancement. J Am Soc Echocardiogr. 1999;12(12):1022–6.
6. Soman P, Swinburn J, Callister M, Stephens NG, Senior R. Apical hypertrophic cardiomyopathy: bedside diagnosis by intravenous contrast echocardiography. J Am Soc Echocardiogr. 2001;14(4):311–3.
7. Koo BK, Choi D, Ha JW, Kang SM, Chung N, Cho SY. Isolated noncompaction of the ventricular myocardium: contrast echocardiographic findings and review of the literature. Echocardiography. 2002;19(2):153–6.

8. Moreno R, Zamorano JL, Almeria C, Rodrigo JL, Villate A, Serra V, et al. Usefulness of contrast agents in the diagnosis of left ventricular pseudoaneurysm after acute myocardial infarction. Eur J Echocardiogr. 2002;3(2):111–6.
9. Soliman OII, Geleijnse ML, Meijboom FJ, Nemes A, Kamp O, Nihoyannopoulos P, et al. The use of contrast echocardiography for the detection of cardiac shunts. Eur J Echocardiogr. 2007;8:S2–12.
10. Kaul S. Myocardial contrast echocardiography: a 25-year retrospective. Circulation. 2008;118(3):291–308.
11. McCulloch M, Gresser C, Moos S, Odabashian J, Jasper S, Bednarz J, et al. Ultrasound contrast physics: a series on contrast echocardiography. J Am Soc Echocardiogr. 2000;13:959–67.
12. Stewart MJ. Contrast echocardiography. Heart. 2003;89(3):342–8.
13. GE Healthcare. OPTISON prescribing information. 2012.
14. Luminity Summary of Product Characteristics. 2011.
15. EMEA. Scientific discussion. SonoVue: European Public Assessment Report; 2016.
16. Main ML, Ryan AC, Davis TE, Albano MP, Kusnetzky LL, Hibberd M. Acute mortality in hospitalized patients undergoing echocardiography with and without an ultrasound contrast agent. Am J Cardiol. 2008;102(12):1742–6.
17. Shaikh K, Chang SM, Peterson L, Rosendahl-Garcia K, Quinones MA, Nagueh SF, et al. Safety of contrast administration for endocardial enhancement during stress echocardiography compared with noncontrast stress. Am J Cardiol. 2008;102:1444–50.
18. Wei K, Mulvagh SL, Carson L, Davidoff R, Gabriel R, Grimm RA, et al. The safety of Definity and Optison for ultrasound image enhancement: a retrospective analysis of 78,383 administered contrast doses. J Am Soc Echocardiogr. 2008;21(11):1202–6.
19. Parker JM, Weller MW, Feinstein LM, Adams RJ, Main ML, et al. Safety of ultrasound contrast agents in patients with known or suspected cardiac shunts. Am J Cardiol. 2013;112:1039–45.
20. Abdelmoneim SS, Bernier M, Scott CG, Dhoble A, Ness SAC, Hagen ME, et al. Safety of contrast agent use during stress echocardiography in patients with elevated right ventricular systolic pressure: a cohort study. Circ Cardiovasc Imaging. 2010;3(3):240–8.
21. Wever-Pinzon O, Suma V, Ahuja A, Romero J, Sareen N, Henry SA, et al. Safety of echocardiographic contrast in hospitalized patients with pulmonary hypertension: a multi-center study. Eur Heart J Cardiovasc Imag. 2012;13:857–62.
22. Dolan MS, Gala SS, Dodla S, Abdelmoneim SS, Xie F, Cloutier D, et al. Safety and efficacy of commercially available ultrasound contrast agents for rest and stress echocardiography a multicenter experience. J Am Coll Cardiol. 2009;53(1):32–8.
23. Becher H, Burns PN. Assessment of left ventricular function by contrast echo. Handbook of contrast echocardiography. Berlin: Springer; 2000. p. 47–79.
24. Nakatani S, Imanishi T, Terasawa A, Beppu S, Nagata S, Miyatake K. Clinical application of transpulmonary contrast-enhanced Doppler technique in the assessment of severity of aortic stenosis. J Am Coll Cardiol. 1992;20(4):973–8.
25. Nakatani S, Satoshi T. Contrast-enhanced Doppler in the assessment of aortic stenosis. In: Nanda NC, Schleif R, Goldberg BB, editors. Advances in echo imaging using contrast enhancement. Dordrecht: Springer; 1997. p. 253–61.
26. Dubourg O, Delorme G, Jondeau G, Chikli F, Clavier H, Valtier B, et al. Simultaneous measurement of systolic pulmonary artery pressure by catheterization and contrast enhancement doppler echocardiography. Arch Mal Coeur Vaiss. 1993 Dec;86(12):1721–7.
27. Kurt M, Shaikh KA, Peterson L, Kurrelmeyer KM, Shah G, Nagueh SF, et al. Impact of contrast echocardiography on evaluation of ventricular function and clinical management in a large prospective cohort. J Am Coll Cardiol. 2009;53(9):802–10.
28. Thavendiranathan P, Grant AD, Negishi T, Plana JC, Popovic ZB, Marwick TH. Reproducibility of echocardiographic techniques for sequential assessment of left ventricular ejection fraction and volumes: application to patients undergoing cancer chemotherapy. J Am Coll Cardiol. 2013;61:77–84.
29. Jung PH, Mueller M, Schuhmann C, Eickhoff M, Schneider P, Seemueller G, et al. Contrast enhanced transesophageal echocardiography in patients with atrial fibrillation referred to electrical cardioversion improves atrial thrombus detection and may reduce associated thromboembolic events. Cardiovasc Ultrasound. 2013; 11:1–5.
30. Plana JC, Mikati IA, Dokainish H, Lakkis N, Abukhalil J, Davis R, et al. A randomized cross-over study for evaluation of the effect of image optimization with contrast on the diagnostic accuracy of dobutamine echocardiography in coronary artery disease The OPTIMIZE Trial. JACC Cardiovasc Imaging. 2008;1(2):145–52.
31. Gaibazzi N, Reverberi C, Lorenzoni V, Molinaro S, Porter TR. Prognostic value of high-dose dipyridamole stress myocardial contrast perfusion echocardiography. Circulation. 2012;126(10): 1217–24.
32. Lepper W, Shivalkar B, Rinkevich D, Belcik T, Wei K. Assessment of the vascularity of a left ventricular mass using myocardial contrast echocardiography. J Am Soc Echocardiogr. 2002;15(11): 1419–22.
33. Janardhanan R, Senior R. Accuracy of dipyridamole myocardial contrast echocardiography for the detection of residual stenosis of the infarct-related artery and multivessel disease early after acute myocardial infarction. J Am Coll Cardiol. 2004;43(12):2247–52.
34. Arnold JR, Karamitsos TD, Pegg TJ, Francis JM, Olszewski R, Searle N, et al. Adenosine stress myocardial contrast echocardiography for the detection of coronary artery disease: a comparison with coronary angiography and cardiac magnetic resonance. JACC Cardiovasc Imaging. 2010;3(9):934–43.
35. Zamorano JL, García-Fernández MA. Contrast echocardiography in clinical practice, vol 1. Mailand: Springer; 2004. p. 241.
36. Shimoni S, Frangogiannis NG, Aggeli CJ, Shan K, Quinones MA, Espada R, et al. Microvascular structural correlates of myocardial contrast echocardiography in patients with coronary artery disease and left ventricular dysfunction: implications for the assessment of myocardial hibernation. Circulation. 2002;106(8):950–6.
37. Janardhanan R, Moon JC, Pennell DJ, Senior R. Myocardial contrast echocardiography accurately reflects transmurality of myocardial necrosis and predicts contractile reserve after acute myocardial infarction. Am Heart J. 2005;149:355–62.
38. Shimoni S, Frangogiannis NG, Aggeli CJ, Shan K, Verani MS, Quinones MA, et al. Identification of hibernating myocardium with quantitative intravenous myocardial contrast echocardiography: comparison with dobutamine echocardiography and thallium-201 scintigraphy. Circulation. 2003;107:538–44.
39. Wei K, Jayaweera AR, Firoozan S, Linka A, Skyba DM, Kaul S. Quantification of myocardial blood flow with ultrasound-induced destruction of microbubbles administered as a constant venous infusion. Circulation. 1998;97:473–83.
40. Abdelmoneim SS, Basu A, Bernier M, Dhoble A, Abdel-Kader SS, Pellikka PA, et al. Detection of myocardial microvascular disease using contrast echocardiography during adenosine stress in type 2

diabetes mellitus: prospective comparison with single-photon emission computed tomography. Diab Vasc Dis Res. 2011;8(4):254–61.
41. Madua EC, Potua C, Baugh D, Tulloch-Reid E. Myocardial contrast echocardiography in the evaluation of hypertensive heart disease. Cardiol Res. 2011;2(6):259–68.
42. Main ML, Goldman JH, Grayburn PA. Thinking outside the "Box"—the ultrasound contrast controversy. J Am Coll Cardiol. 2007;50(25):2434–7.
43. Lindner JR. Microbubbles in medical imaging: current applications and future directions. Nat Rev Drug Discov. 2004;3(6):5–32.

Summary of Cardiac Chamber Quantification in Adults by Echocardiography

10

Nehzat Akiash

Abstract

The evaluation of cardiac chamber size and function remains the key role of the echocardiography which is the most commonly used cardiac imaging modality.

As the size and function of the cardiac chamber is important for clinical decision making, these method of quantification should be standard and be based on the latest recommendations.

In this chapter we have summarized the correct measurement of the size and function of the cardiac chambers, Aorta and Inferior Vena Cava.

Keywords

Cardiac chamber quantification · Echocardiography Body surface area · Doppler tissue imaging · End-diastolic volume · Ejection fraction · End-systolic volume Fractional area change · Global longitudinal strain

Abbreviations

2D	Two-dimensional
2DE	Two-dimensional echocardiography
3D	Three-dimensional
3DE	Three-dimensional echocardiography
BSA	Body surface area
CMR	Cardiac magnetic resonance
DTI	Doppler tissue imaging
EDV	End-diastolic volume
EF	Ejection fraction
ESV	End-systolic volume
FAC	Fractional area change
GLS	Global longitudinal strain
I-I	Inner edge–to–Inner edge
IVC	Inferior vena cava
LA	Left atrial
L-L	Leading edge–to– Leading edge
LV	Left ventricular
M-mode	Motion mode
RA	Right atrial
RIMP	Right ventricular index of myocardial performance
RV	Right ventricular
TAPSE	Tricuspid annular plane systolic excursion
TTE	Transthoracic echocardiography

N. Akiash, MD
Atherosclerosis Research Center, Ahvaz Jundishapur University of Medical Sciences, Ahvaz, Iran

The evaluation of cardiac chamber size and function remains the key role of the echocardiography which is the most commonly used cardiac imaging modality.

As the size and function of the cardiac chamber is important for clinical decision making, these method of quantification should be standard and be based on the latest recommendations.

In this chapter we have summarized the correct measurement of the size and function of the cardiac chambers, Aorta and Inferior Vena Cava.

The Left Ventricle

- ***Measurement of the LV Size***
- We use linear internal dimensions and volumes for evaluation of LV cavity size.

Linear Measurements. Values should be derived in the parasternal long-axis view just below the level of the mitral valve leaflets in perpendicular position to the LV long axis and interventricular septum with two-dimensional echocardiography (2DE) (Fig. 10.1a) and M-mode approach [1] (Fig. 10.1b).

Volumetric Measurements. Recommended approach for evaluation of the Volumetric measurements with 2D echocardiography is the biplane method of disks summation technique (modified Simpson's rule), which is tracings the

A. Sadeghpour, A. Alizadehasl (eds.), *Case-Based Textbook of Echocardiography*,
https://doi.org/10.1007/978-3-319-67691-3_10

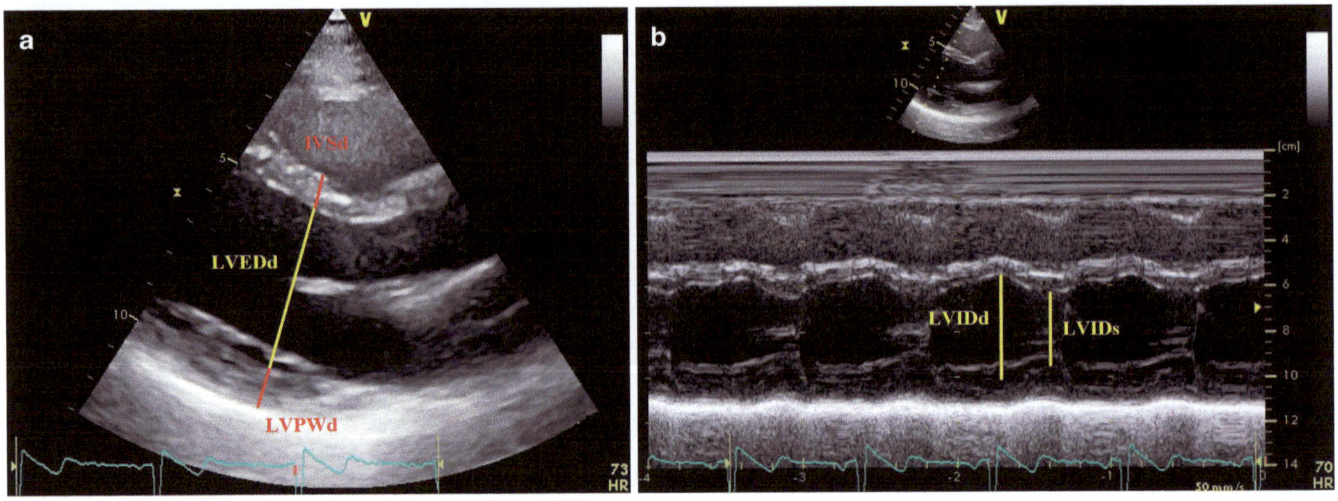

Fig. 10.1 Left Ventricular Linear Measurement using two-dimensional echocardiography (2DE) (**a**) and M-mode (**b**) approach. *LVIDd* left ventricular internal dimension in diastole, *LVIDs* left ventricular internal dimension in systole, *IVSd* interventricular septum in diastole, *LVPWd* left ventricular posterior wall in diastole

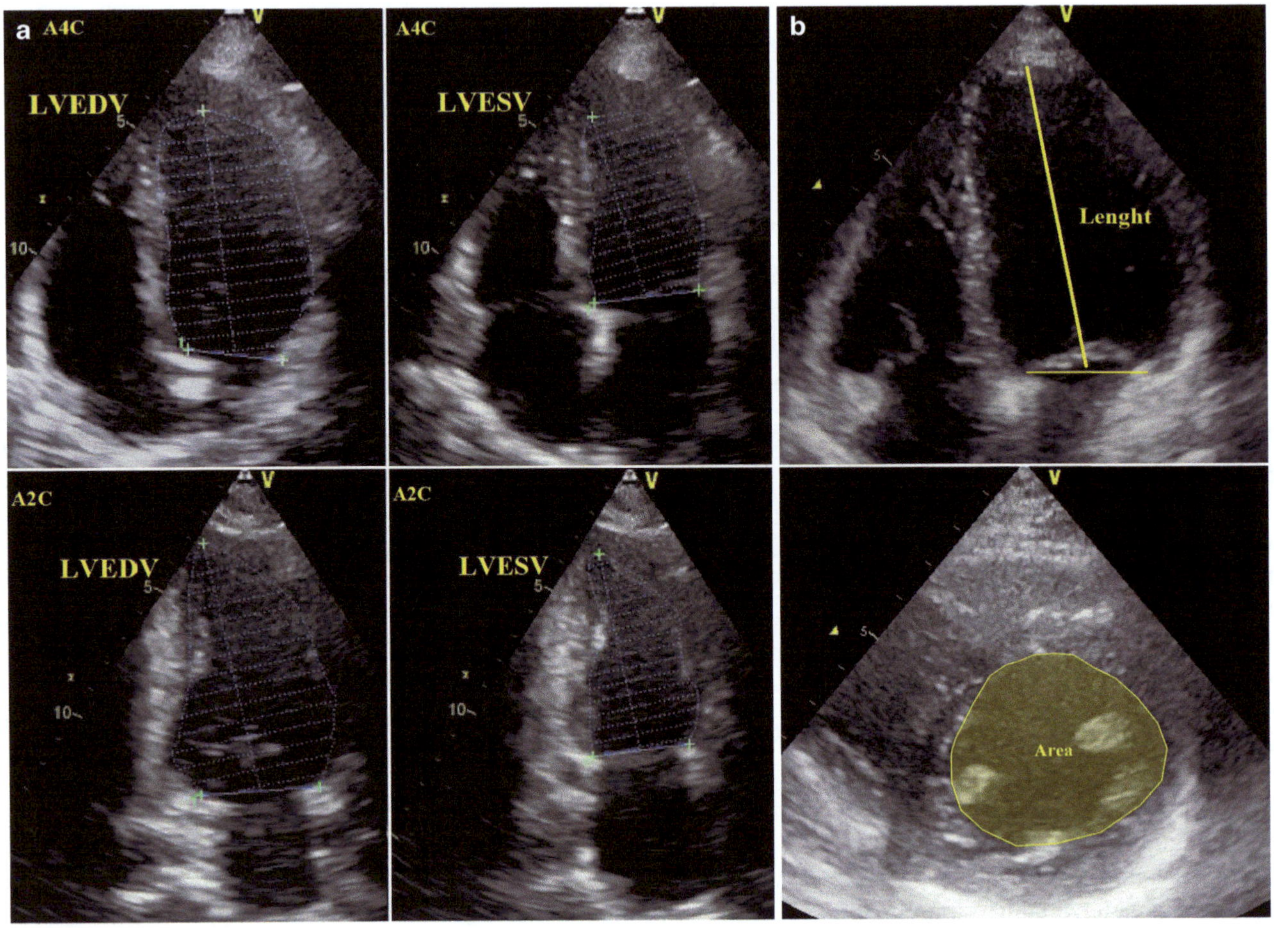

Fig. 10.2 Area-Length approach (**a**) and Volumetric Measurement of Left Ventricle by modified Simpson's method (**b**). *LVEDV* left ventricular end diastolic volume, *LVESV* left ventricular end systolic volume, *A2C* apical 2-chamber, *A4C* apical 4-chamber

endocardial border of LV cavity in the apical four and two-chamber views [2]. In this regard, it is important to avoid foreshortening of the left ventricle which underestimates the volumes (Fig. 10.2).

Area-length method is the other volumetric method that assumes LV as a bullet and is useful when LV apex is not visualize well. The area of the mid LV is traced in short axis view and the length is measured in apical four chamber view

(Fig. 10.2a). Normal values for LV measurements are shown in Table 10.1.

- ***LV Global Systolic Function***
- Global LV function is obtained by evaluation of the end-diastolic and end-systolic values with two and Three-dimensional echocardiography (Fig. 10.3) and final ejection fraction [3] is calculated by using the formula (2):

$$\mathrm{EF} = \frac{(\mathrm{EDV} - \mathrm{ESV})}{\mathrm{EDV}}$$

Table 10.1 Normal values for 2D echocardiographic of LV size and function

Parameter	Male		Female	
	Mean ± SD	2-SD range	Mean ± SD	2-SD range
LV internal dimension (LVID)				
Diastolic dimension (mm)	50.2 ± 4.1	42.0–58.4	45.0 ± 3.6	37.8–52.2
Systolic dimension (mm)	32.4 ± 3.7	25.0–39.8	28.2 ± 3.3	21.6–34.8
LV volumes (biplane)				
LV EDV (mL)	106 ± 22	62–150	76 ± 15	46–106
LV ESV (mL)	41 ± 10	21–61	28 ± 7	14–42
LV volume normalized by BSA				
LV EDV (mL/m²)	54 ± 10	34–74	45 ± 8	29–61
LV ESV (mL/m²)	21 ± 5	11–31	16 ± 4	8–24
LV EF (biplane)	62 ± 5	52–72	64 ± 5	54–74

Body surface area (BSA), End-diastolic volume (EDV), End-systolic volume (ESV), Ejection fraction (EF), Left Ventricular (LV), Standard deviation (SD). Modified from Lang RM, Badano LP, Mor-Avi V, et al. Recommendations for cardiac chamber quantification: A report from the American Society of Echocardiography and the European Association of Cardiovascular Imaging. J Am Soc Echocardiogr. 2015;28:1–39

- ***Global Longitudinal Strain (GLS)***

Deformation imaging provides valuable information about regional and global ventricular function. Strain (S) describes deformation from its baseline length. The rate of deformation is Strain rate (SR). Lagrangian Strain can be calculated using following formula:

$$\mathrm{S}(\%) = \frac{L_t - L_0}{L_0}$$

Where L_t is the length at time t, and L_0 is the initial length at the reference time t_0 [4, 5].

Peak GLS shows the relative changes of the LV myocardium length in end-diastolic and end-systolic periods on 2-dimensional echocardiography (2DE). GLS should be measured in the end-systolic frame of the 2D images by endocardial borders tracing from the three standard apical views. Finally, GLS is evaluated as the mean strain of all cardiac segments [6] (Fig. 10.4).

- ***LV Regional Function***

Left ventricle is divided in to 16, 17 or18 segments for evaluation of regional function. The Segmentations represent coronary perfusion territories and are applicable

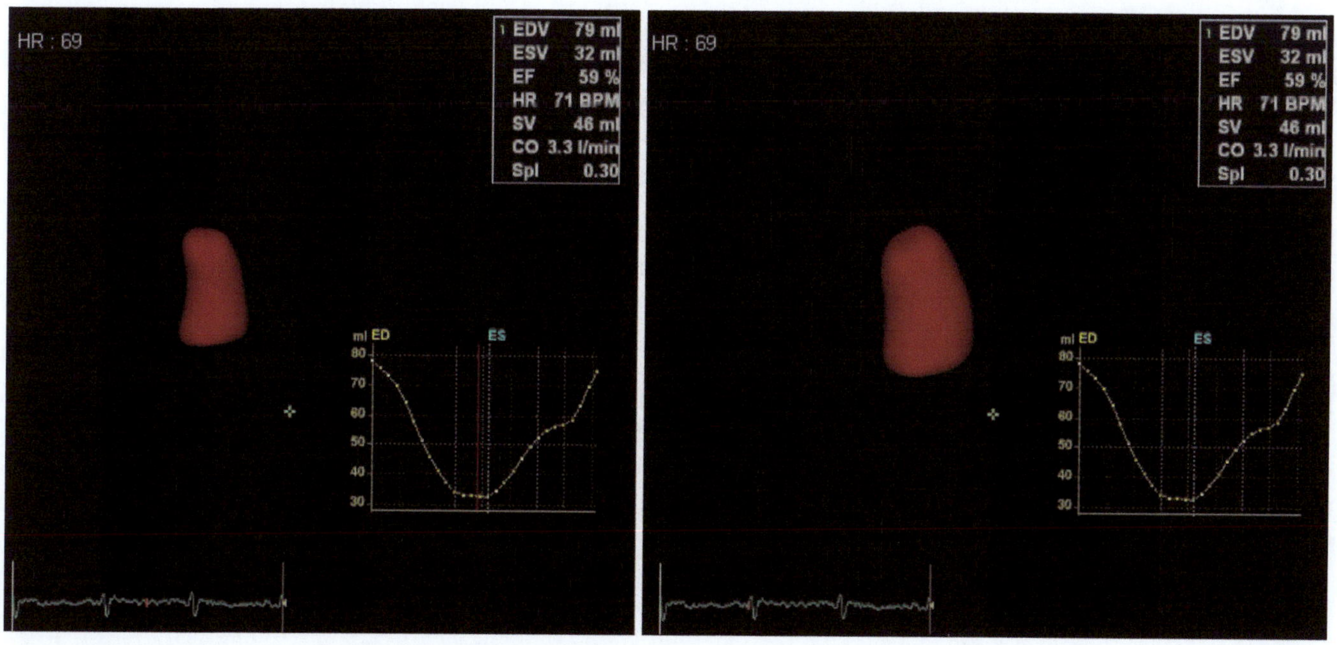

Fig. 10.3 Left Ventricular End Diastolic Volume, End Systolic Volume and Global Systolic Function assessment using 3-dimentional echocardiography

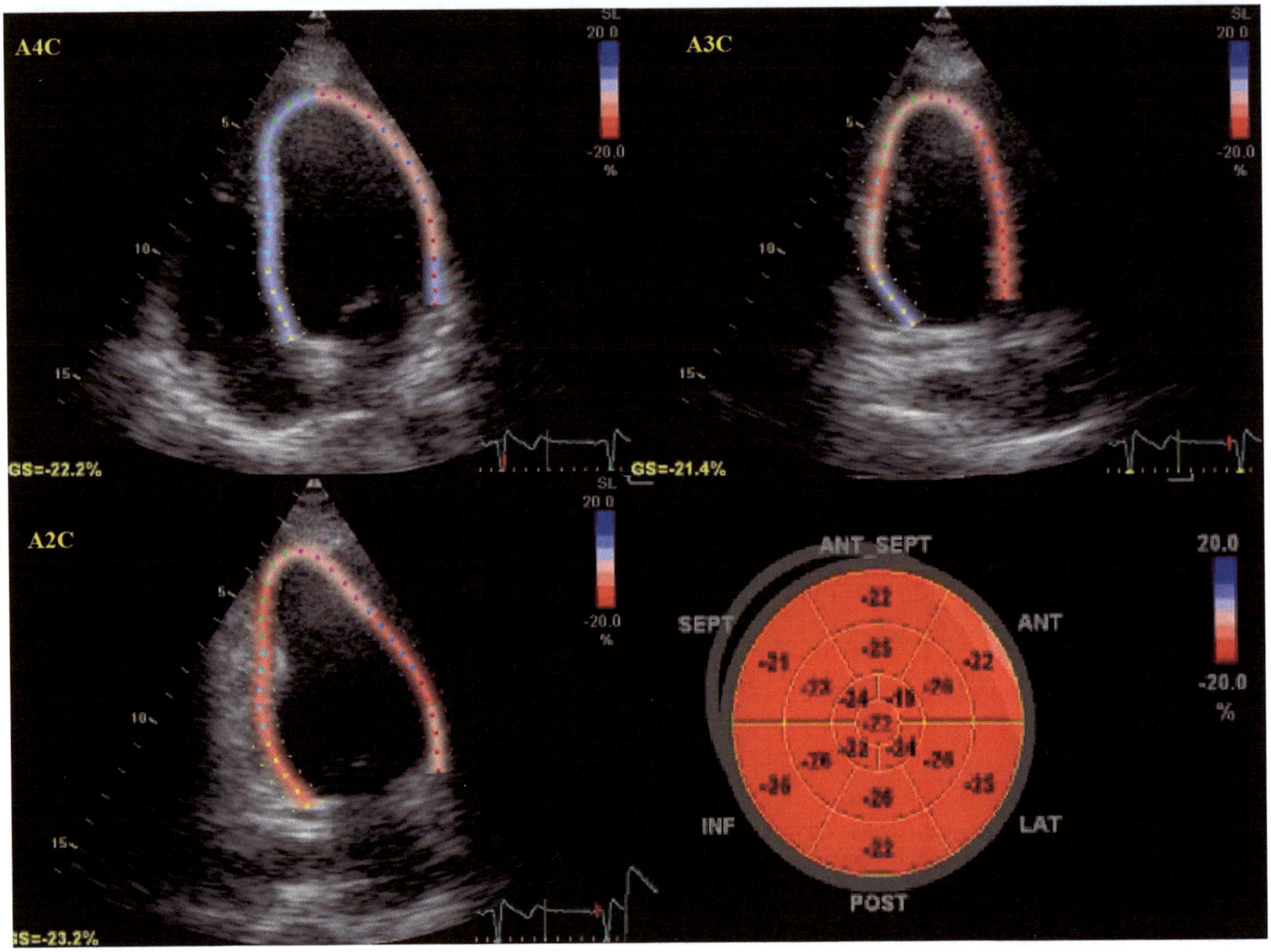

Fig. 10.4 Myocardial Strain Measurement With 2-Dimensional Speckle-Tracking Echocardiography from each apical view with bull's eye plot

for analysis of left ventricular wall motion abnormality and perfusion of myocardial tissue. The 17-segment model is widely used. In 17-segment model (Figs. 10.5, 10.6 and 10.7), segments 1 and 7, show basal anterior and mid-anterior segments. The names of Segments 2 and 3 are basal anteroseptal and basal inferoseptal. The segment 4, 5, 6 are the basal inferior, the basal inferolateral, and the basal anterolateral respectively. The names of 7 to 12 are similar 1 to 6 segments at mid-ventricular levels. 13 to 16 segments are related to apical anterior, apical septal, apical inferior and apical lateral and the final segment is apical cap and represents segment 17 [7].

Each segment should be examined in 2, 3 and 4-chamber views for evaluation of regional wall motion abnormality, and the wall motion score in each segment is assessed as semi-quantitative LV wall motion score index according to a four-point scale in Table 10.2 and eventually, the mean or average value of the scores of all segments, is obtained [8].

Two-dimensional strain can achieve left ventricular wall-motion analysis [9]. Strain imaging has an important role in the detection of ischemic cardiomyopathy. In patient with subclinical LV systolic dysfunction due to obstructive coronary artery disease at rest, longitudinal systolic strain is abnormal; therefore in patients with normal ejection fraction with increased atherosclerotic risk, a progressive abnormal result of the 2D global strain is compatible with severity of coronary disease [4].

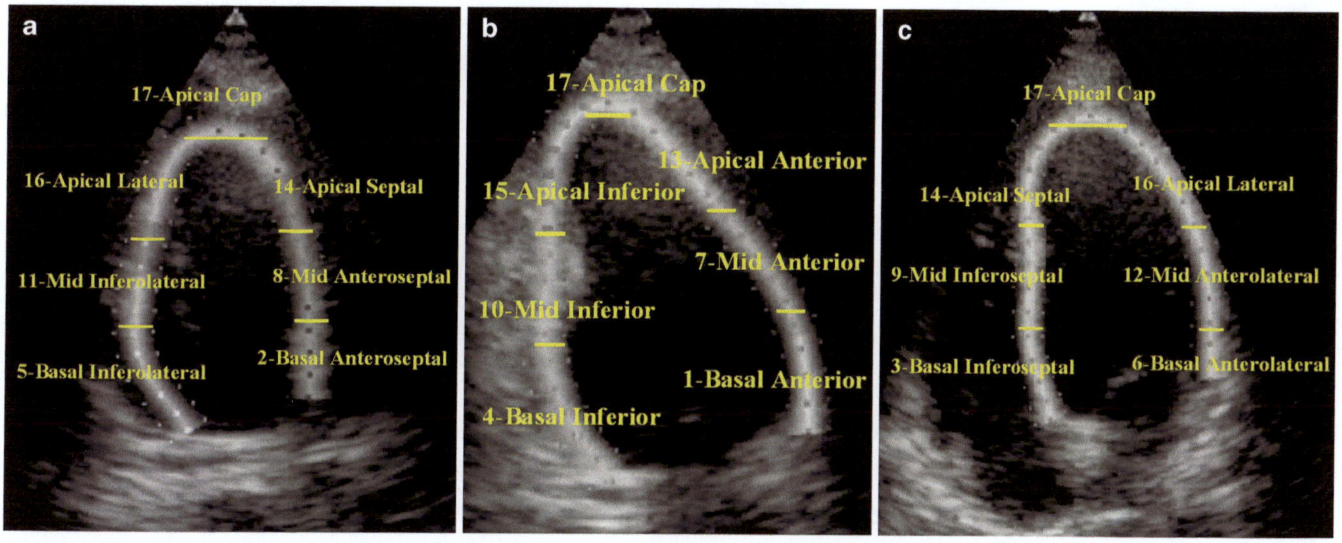

Fig. 10.5 Diagram of 17-segment model in each view. Apical long-axis (**a**), Apical two-chamber (**b**) and Apical four-chamber (**c**) views

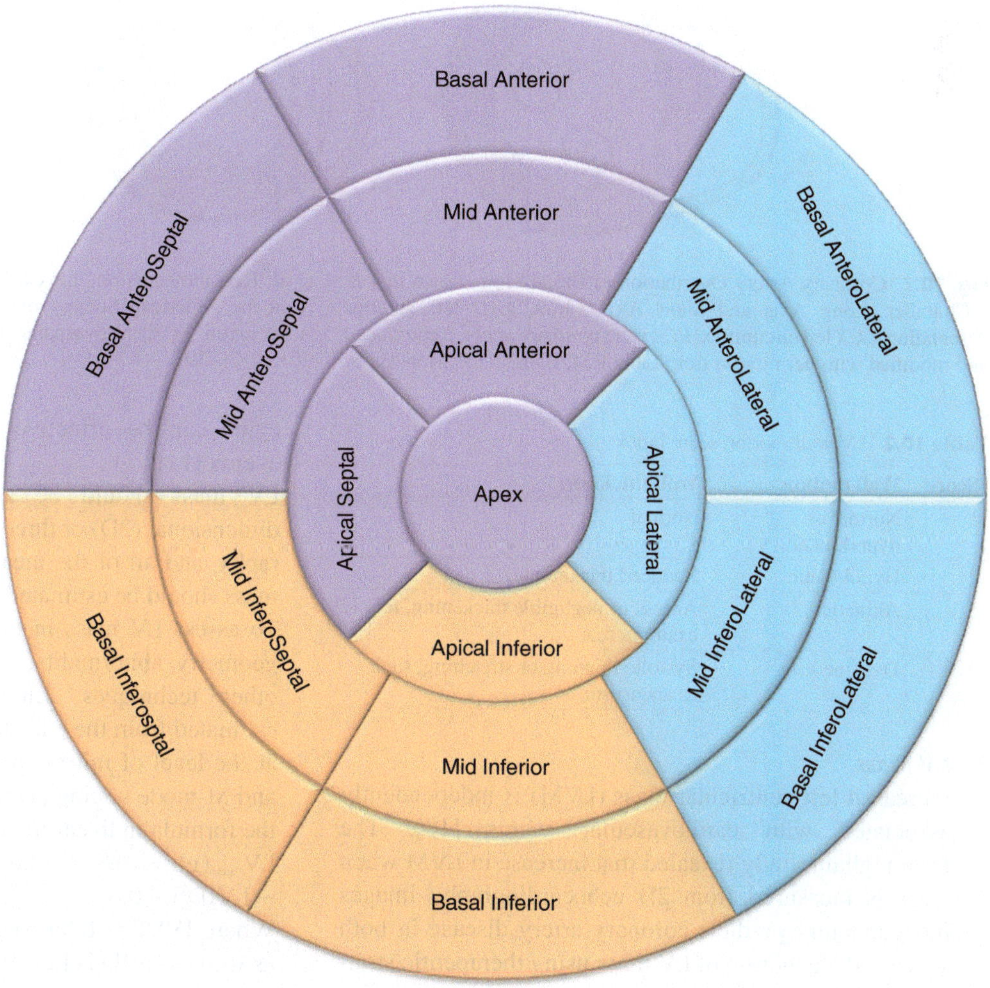

Fig. 10.6 17-Segment myocardial modeling on a bull's eye map

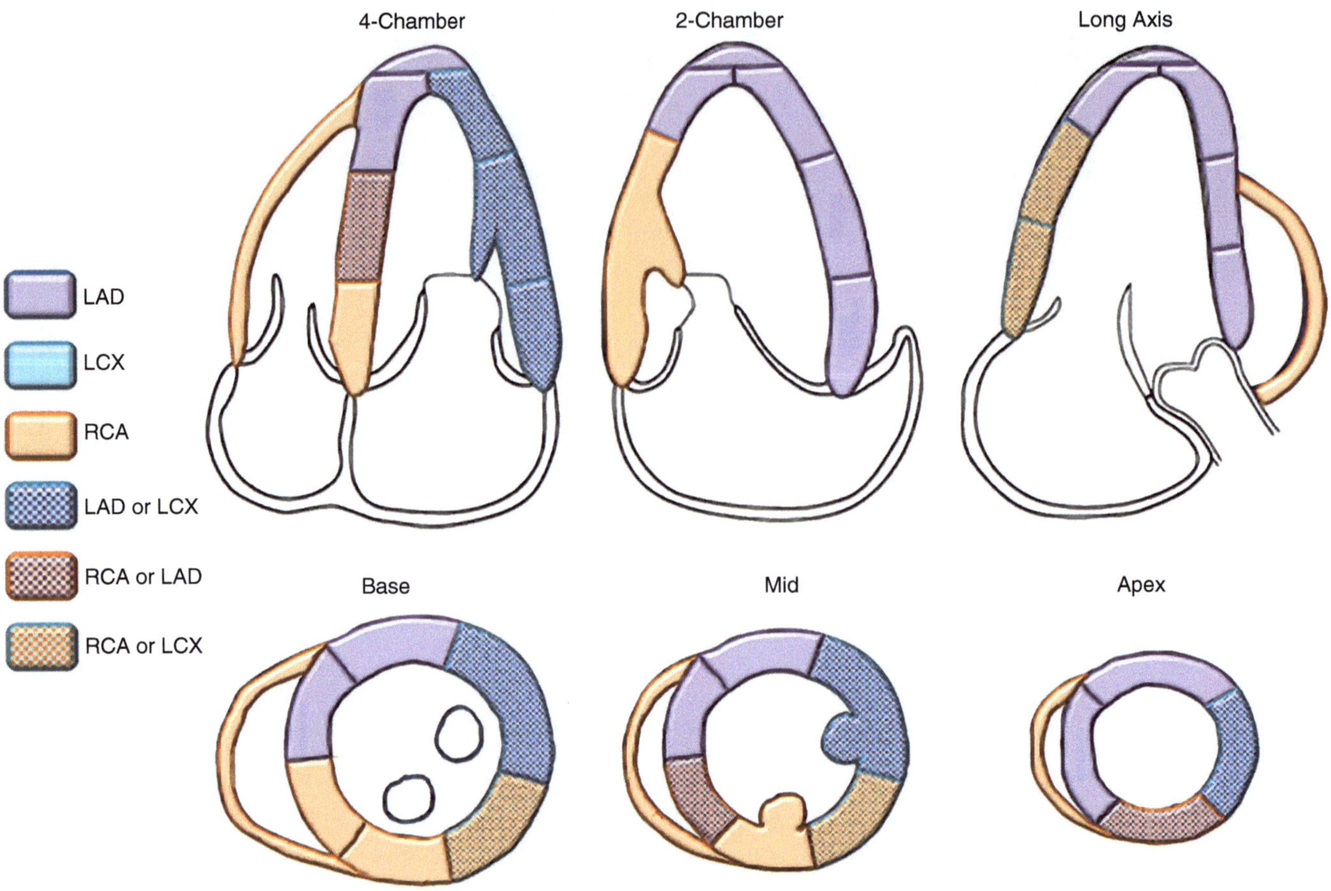

Fig. 10.7 Coronary Artery Distribution of Blood Flow shown in 4 & 2-Chamber, Long Axis and Short Axis views. *LAD* left anterior descending, *LCX* left circumflex, *RCA* right coronary artery. Reproduced and modified with permission from Lang RM, Badano LP, Mor-Avi V, et al. Recommendations for cardiac chamber quantification: A report from the American Society of Echocardiography and the European Association of Cardiovascular Imaging. J Am Soc Echocardiogr. 2015;28:1–39

Table 10.2 LV wall motion score index

Score	Wall motion	Wall thickness
1	Normal or hyperkinetic	Normal
2	Hypokinetic	Reduced thickening
3	Akinetic	Absent or negligible thickening, for example scar
4	Dyskinetic	Systolic thinning or stretching, such as aneurysm

- ***LV Mass***

  Increased left ventricular mass (LVM) is independently associated with cardiovascular events [10]. The Framingham Study revealed that increase in LVM when mass is measured from 2D echocardiography images independently predicts coronary artery disease in both sexes and Reduction of LV mass using therapeutic strategies can be effective to reduce the cardiovascular events [11].

  LV mass should be assessed using M-mode, two-dimensional (2D) or three-dimensional (3D) echocardiography, and all of the measurements for evaluation of LV mass should be estimated at the end of diastole.

  To assess LV mass in individual without major cardiac geometry abnormality, linear method is preferred over other techniques. Linear measurements should be estimated from the parasternal view at the end of diastole at the level of mitral valve leaflet tips using 2D images and M-mode tracing [12]. LV mass is calculated by using the formula in linear method [13]:

  $LV_{mass}(g) = 0.8 \cdot 1.04 \cdot [(IVST + LVID + PWT)^3 - LVID^3] + 0.6$

  Where IVST is Interventricular Septum wall Thickness, as well as LVID is Left Ventricular Internal Diameter and

PWT is Posterior Wall Thickness, The formula assumes the LV as a prolate ellipse [14].

Truncated ellipsoid methods for estimating left ventricular mass by 2DE is assessed using following formula:

$$LV_{mass} = 1.05\pi\left\{(b+t)^2\left[\frac{2}{3}(a+t)+d-\frac{d^3}{3(a+t)^2}\right]-b^2\left[\frac{2}{3}a+d-\frac{d^3}{3a^2}\right]\right\}$$

Where "b" is left ventricular minor axis measured at the level of the papillary muscles. LV Length, "L", is divides into "a" and "b". The "a" is distance from the minor axis to the endocardium at the LV apex and "d" is the distance from minor axis to mitral annular plane. The "t" is the average wall thickness (Fig. 10.8) [14, 15].

3-dimensional echocardiography evaluation of LV mass remove geometrical assumptions about left ventricular cavity shape in patient with cardiac disease (Fig. 10.9) [16]. Table 10.3 shows the normal ranges for LV mass indices.

The Right Ventricle

As part of the heart structure, the right ventricle (RV) has long received less attention than the left ventricle (LV). Nevertheless, technological advances in the assessment of the RV have proved this part of the heart to be a strong predictor of cardiac events in ischemic heart diseases, cardiomyopathy, congenital heart diseases and pulmonary diseases [17, 18].

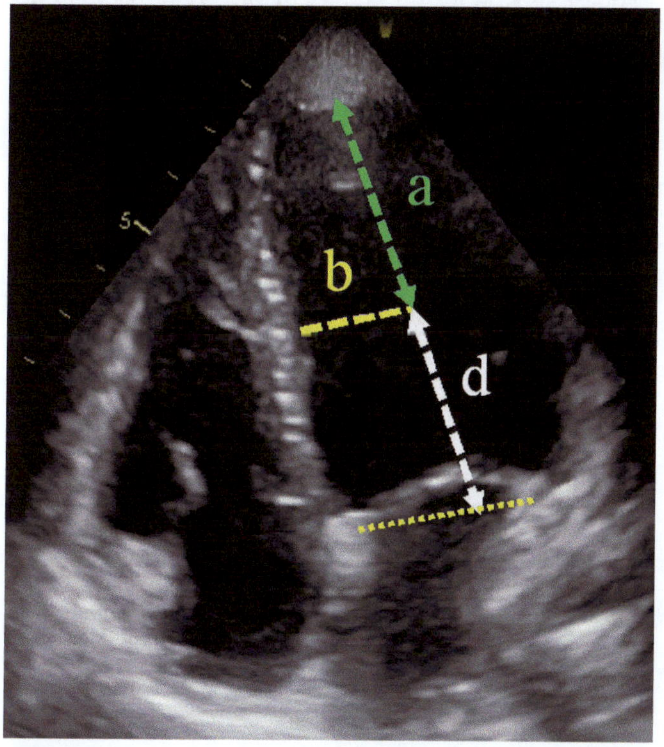

Fig. 10.8 Left Ventricular Mass measurement based on the Truncated Ellipsoid Model

Different dimensions of the RV are evaluated in echocardiography and it is preferable to examine all the dimensions in the apical 4 chamber view with a sharp focus on the RV [18]. The apex of the RV should be placed in the middle of the scanning sector. Nonetheless, the parasternal Long axis and short axis views are also used for the comprehensive assessment of the RV.

In the apical 4-chamber view, inflow part of RV is measured at 1/3 of the base of RV. Mid cavity dimension is assessed in the middle part of the RV cavity at the level of the papillary muscles (Fig. 10.10a) and the longitudinal dimension assessment is performed from the middle of the tricuspid valve to the RV apex. The proximal part of the RV outflow tract is measured in the parasternal long axis (Fig. 10.10b) and short axis view at end-diastole [17, 18].

The distal right ventricular outflow tract (RVOT) is measured at the junction of the pulmonary valve [19]. Normal values for RV chamber size are reported in Table 10.4.

RV function can be assessed with respect to different components, including:

- ***Fractional Area Change***
  Fractional Area Change (FAC) is an independent predictor of outcomes following Myocardial Infarction (MI) that shows a valuable relationship with the Right Ventricular Ejection Fraction (RVEF) measured by Cardiovascular Magnetic Resonance Imaging (CMR) and can be assessed using the following formula (Fig. 10.11) [17–20]:

$$FAC(\%) = 100\cdot\frac{(EDA-ESA)}{EDA}$$

- ***Tricuspid Annular Plane Systolic Excursion (TAPSE)***
  The TAPSE is another factor to assess the right ventricular function; this important and repeatable parameter does not depend on angles in high-quality imaging [18]. TAPSE indicates the excursion of the tricuspid annulus,

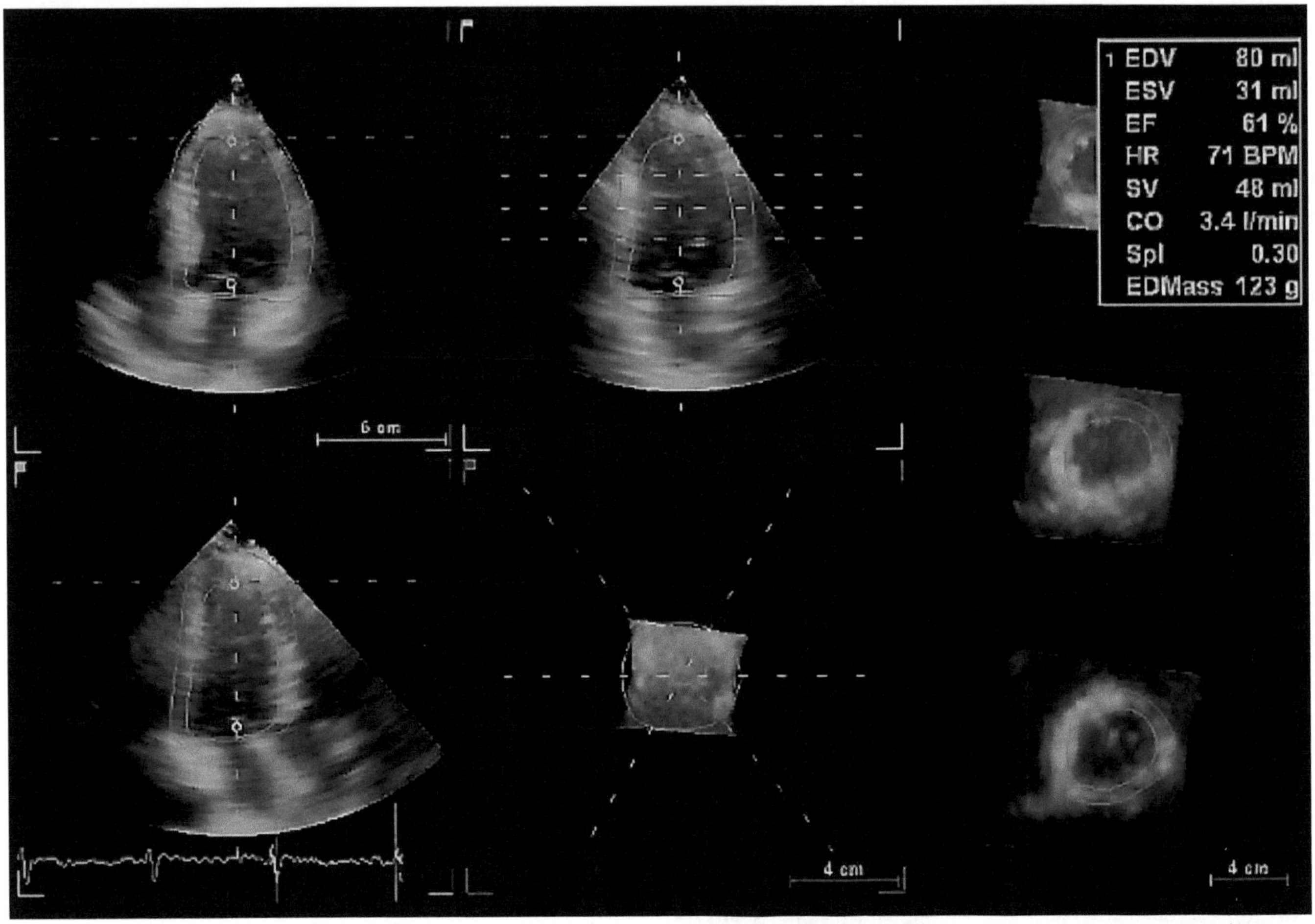

Fig. 10.9 LV mass measurement using 3-dimentional echocardiography

Table 10.3 Normal ranges of LV mass parameters

	Women	Men
Linear method		
LV mass (g)	67–162	88–224
LV mass/ BSA (g/m^2)	**43–95**	**49–115**
Relative thickness (cm)	0.22–0.42	0.24–0.42
Septal thickness (cm)	**0.6–0.9**	**0.6–1.0**
Posterior wall thickness (cm)	**0.6–0.9**	**0.6–1.0**
2D method		
LV mass (g)	66–150	96–200
LV mass/ BSA (g/m^2)	**44–88**	**50–102**
Bold values are more validated.		

Modified from Lang RM, Badano LP, Mor-Avi V, et al. Recommendations for cardiac chamber quantification: A report from the American Society of Echocardiography and the European Association of Cardiovascular Imaging. J Am Soc Echocardiogr. 2015;28:1–39

in which changes are assessed from the end of diastole to the end of the systole (Fig. 10.12a, b). It is preferable to assess the TAPSE in the tissue color M-mode (Fig. 10.12b), because in this way, the end of the systole and diastole are clearly visible [18].

- ***Peak Tissue Doppler Velocity***
  Peak Tissue Doppler Velocity (S′) is calculated using the Doppler based method and assesses the longitudinal function of the RV and is taken in the 4-chamber view where the cursor is placed on the free wall of the RV (Fig. 10.13) and it is preferable to be measured in at least three cycles. S′ is a reliable method with a high reproducibility [21].

- ***Right Ventricular Index of Myocardial Performance (RVIMP)***
  The Right Ventricular Index of Myocardial Performance is a global index for assessing the right ventricular function that represents the systolic and diastolic function of the RV. The RVIMP is load-dependent and calculated using the following formula based on tissue Doppler study (Fig. 10.14) [17, 19, 20]:

$$\text{RIMP} = \frac{(\text{IVRT} + \text{IVCT})}{\text{ET}} = \frac{(\text{TCO} - \text{ET})}{\text{ET}}$$

Normal values for parameters of RV function are listed in Table 10.5.

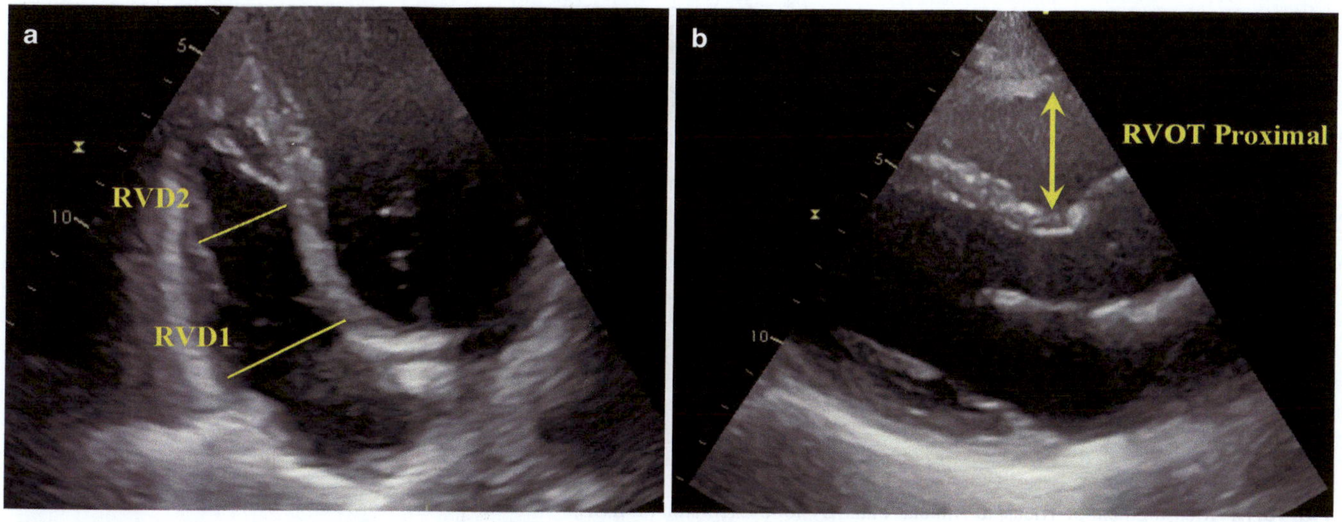

Fig. 10.10 Right Ventricular Measurements. *RVD* right ventricular diameter, *RVOT* right ventricular outflow tract

Table 10.4 Normal values for RV

Parameter	Mean ± SD	Normal range
RV basal diameter (mm)	33 ± 4	25–41
RV mid diameter (mm)	27 ± 4	19–35
RV longitudinal diameter (mm)	71 ± 6	59–83
RVOT PLAX diameter (mm)	25 ± 2.5	20–30
RVOT proximal diameter (mm)	28 ± 3.5	21–35
RVOT distal diameter (mm)	22 ± 2.5	17–27
RV wall thickness (mm)	3 ± 1	1–5

PLAX parasternal, Long-axis view; *RVOT* RV outflow tract. Modified from Lang RM, Badano LP, Mor-Avi V, et al. Recommendations for cardiac chamber quantification: A report from the American Society of Echocardiography and the European Association of Cardiovascular Imaging. J Am Soc Echocardiogr. 2015;28:1–39

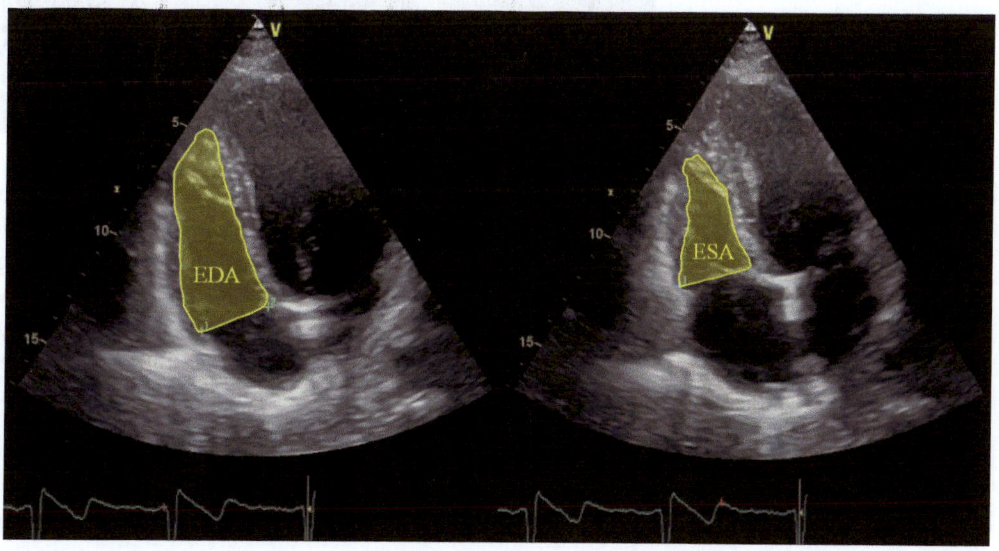

Fig. 10.11 Example of fractional area change measurement. *EDA* end diastolic area, *ESA* end systolic area

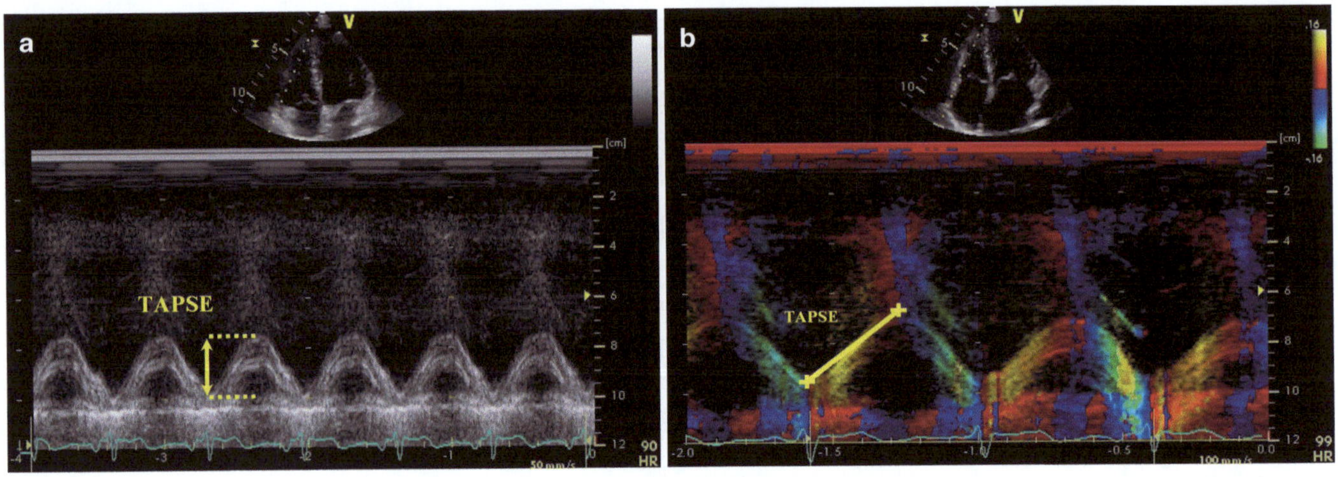

Fig. 10.12 Measurement of Tricuspid Annular Plane Systolic Excursion (TAPSE)

Fig. 10.13 Peak systolic velocity of tricuspid annulus (S′) by pulsed-wave

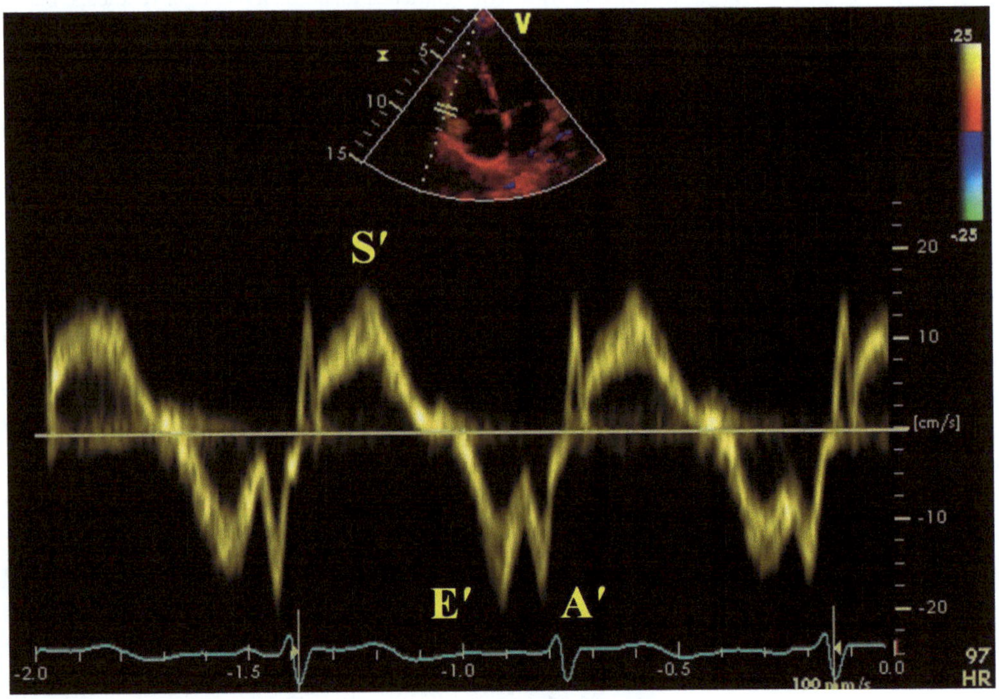

The Left Atria

The left atrial (LA) function in close contact with the LV plays an important role in the LV function and is considered a conduit and reservoir that is responsible for booster pump [22]. The LA function has an important role in maintaining a normal cardiac output. LA contraction increases the left ventricular stroke volume by approximately 20–30% in normal people [23].

Foreshortening should be avoided as much as possible in assessing the LA.

- ***Linear Assessment of the LA***
  Standard method for LA size measurement is anteroposterior linear dimension using M-mode or 2DE obtained from the parasternal long-axis view [24, 25] (Fig. 10.15a), Assessing the surface of the LA is performed in the 4 chamber view (Fig. 10.15b) and one frame before the opening of the mitral valve.
  It should also be noted that the area under the mitral valve and the entrance of the pulmonary veins should be excluded in this measurement [8].

- ***LA Volume***
  There are two methods for measuring the LA volume such as area-length technic and biplane method of discs. In the biplane method of discs, which is similar to Simpson's method of LV volume assessment, LA is

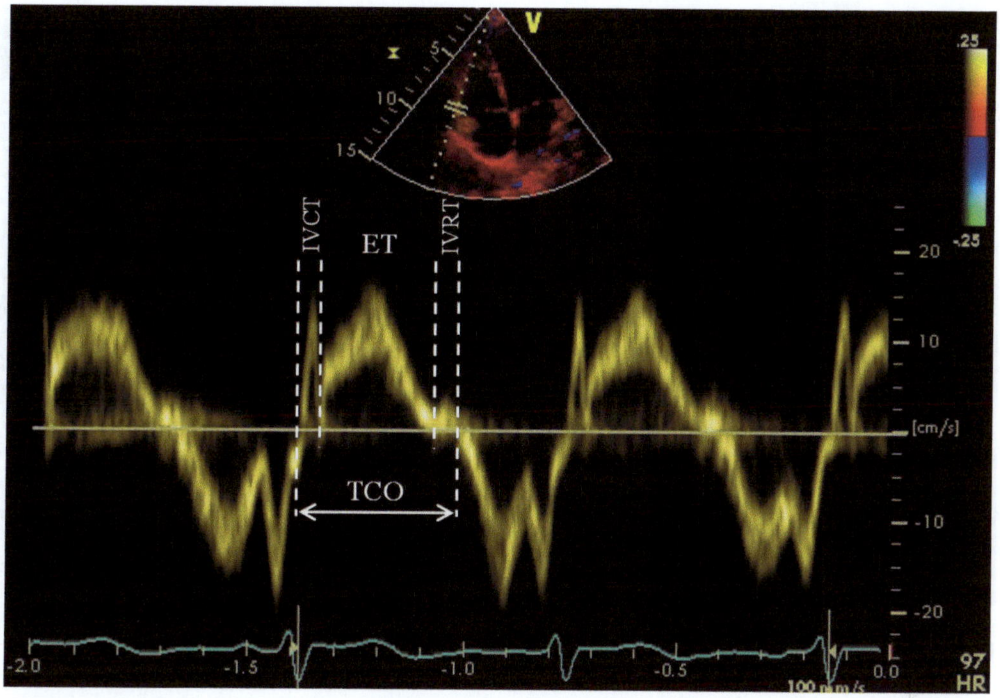

Fig. 10.14 Calculation of Myocardial Performance Index (MPI) base on pulsed Doppler study. *TCO* tricuspid closure opening, *IVCT* isovolumic contraction time, *IVRT* isovolumic relaxation time, *ET* ejection time

Table 10.5 Normal values for parameters of RV function

Parameter	Mean ± SD	Abnormality threshold
TAPSE (mm)	24 ± 3.5	< 17
Pulsed Doppler S wave (cm/s)	14.1 ± 2.3	< 9.5
Color Doppler S wave (cm/s)	9.7 ± 1.85	< 6.0
RV fractional area change (%)	49 ± 7	< 35
RV free wall 2D strain * (%)	−29 ± 4.5	> −20 (20 in magnitude with the negative sign)
RV 3D EF (%)	58 ± 6.5	< 45
Pulsed Doppler MPI	0.26 ± 0.085	> 0.43
Tissue Doppler MPI	0.38 ± 0.08	> 0.54
E wave deceleration time (ms)	180 ± 31	< 119 or >242
E/A	1.4 ± 0.3	< 0.8 or >2.0
e′/a′	1.18 ± 0.33	< 0.52
e′	14.0 ± 3.1	< 7.8
E/e′	4.0 ± 1.0	> 6.0

MPI myocardial performance index

* *Limited data; values may vary depending on vendor and software version*

Modified from Lang RM, Badano LP, Mor-Avi V, et al. Recommendations for cardiac chamber quantification: a report from the American Society of Echocardiography and the European Association of Cardiovascular Imaging. J Am Soc Echocardiogr. 2015;28:1–39

divided into a series of stacked oval disks, the following formula is ultimately used for calculation [24]:

$$\frac{\pi}{4}(h)\sum(D_1)(D_2)$$

Where "h" is height and the major and minor orthogonal axes are D1 and D2, respectively.

A method used for calculation of LA volume is area-length method that is evaluated in 4-chamber and 2-chamber views. This method are based on tracing the inner surface of LA in both 2-chamber and 4-chamber views. It should be noted that the LAA should be excluded when calculating the area of LA. The length of LA should be obtained at both 2-chamber and 4-chamber views (Fig. 10.16), and the shortest length is used to calculate LA volume. However, it must be noted that the length of LA in 2-chamber view should not be more than 5 mm different from that in 4-chamber view in order to calculate the LA volume reliably. Volume can be estimate using the following formula [8, 24]:

$$LAvolume = \frac{8}{3\pi}\left[\frac{A_1 \cdot A_2}{L}\right]$$

Where "L" is Length of LA and the "A" is the area of LA in 4-chamber and 2-chamber views.

The Right Atria

Few studies have evaluated the clinical outcomes of Right Atrial (RA) size assessment. One of the most common methods of RA assessment is in the 4-Chamber view, in which a line is drawn from the lateral wall of the RA perpendicular to the longitudinal axis of the RA toward the interatrial septum (Fig. 10.17). The length of this line

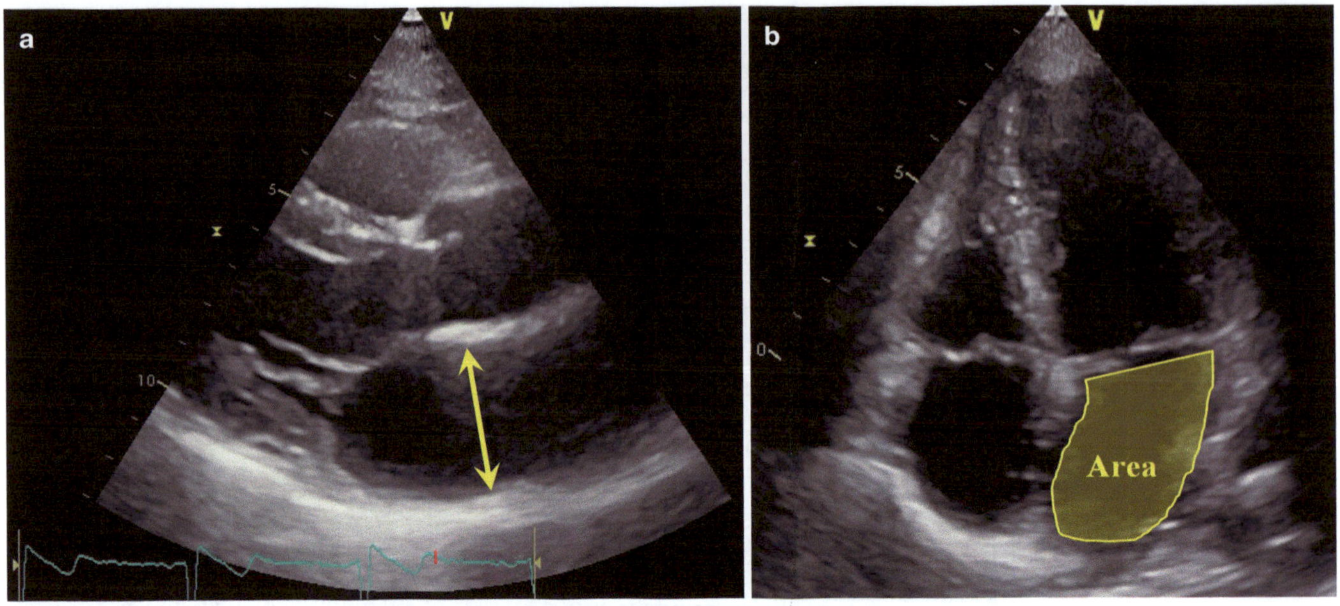

Fig. 10.15 Linear Anteroposterior Dimension (**a**) and Area Measurement (**b**) of Left Atrium

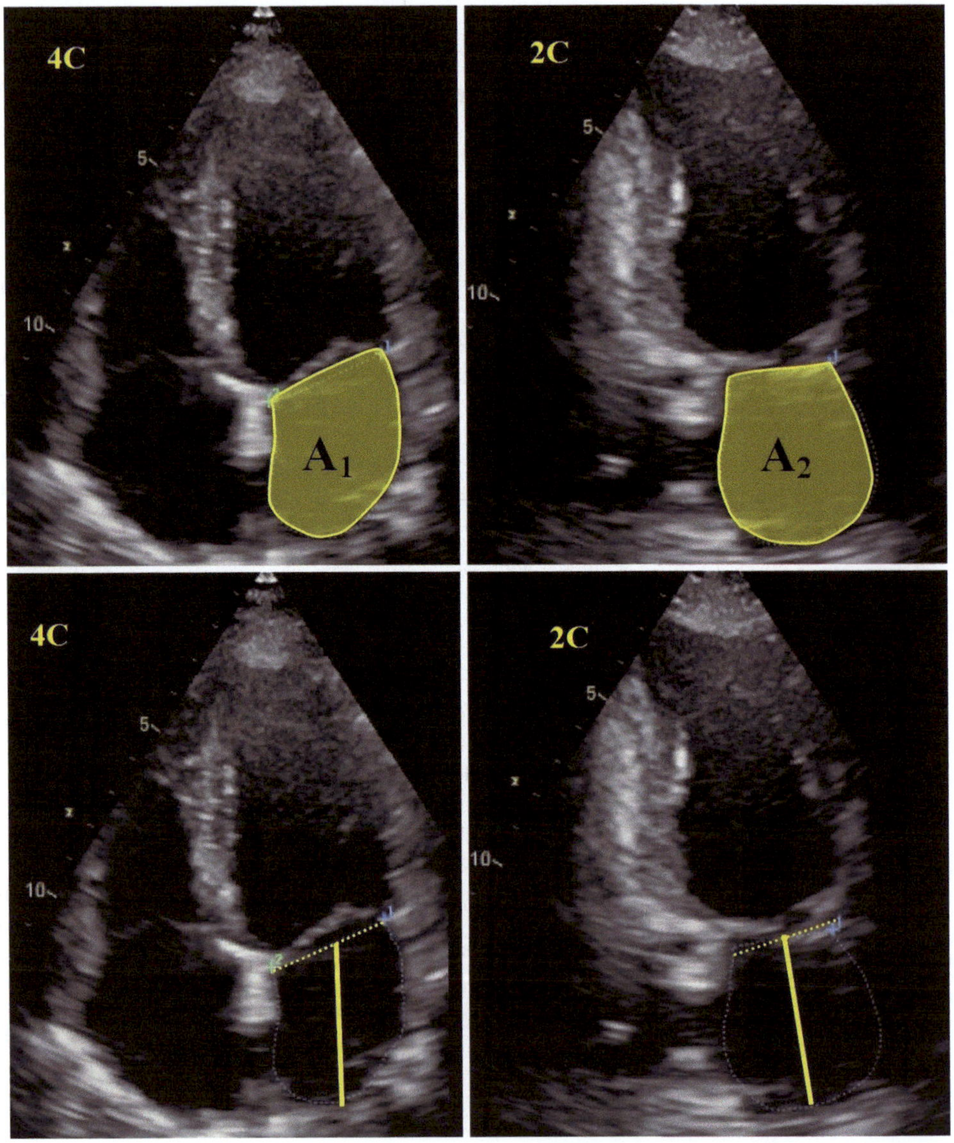

Fig. 10.16 Volumetric Measurement of Left Atrium by Area-Length. *2C* 2-Chamber, *4C* 4-Chamber

represents the size of the minor-axis of the RA [8, 24]. The normal range of RA minor axis dimension is 1.9 ± 0.3 cm/m^2 in male and female [8].

Although there are limited findings about RA volume assessment, assessing the RA volume yields a better strength and accuracy than the linear measurement.

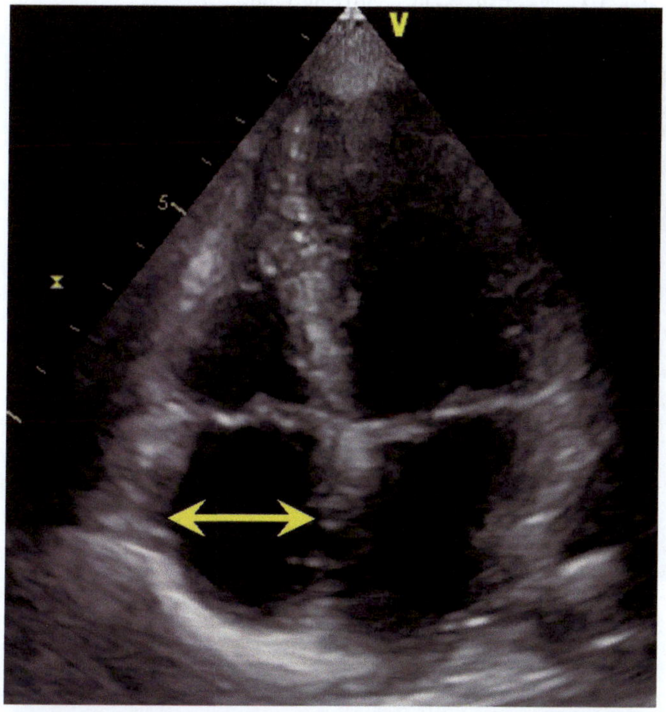

Fig. 10.17 Linear Dimension of Right Atrium (Minor Axis)

The Aortic Annulus, Aortic Root and Ascending Aorta

The aortic root provides a protection for the aortic valve leaflets, which extends from the base of the leaflets' junction in the ventricle to the Sino-Tubular junction [26]. The aortic root and the LVOT are seen in the 2DE images in the parasternal view. The following measurements should often be performed in this view, 1: Aortic Valve Annulus, 2: the Sinuses of Valsalva, 3: the Sino-Tubular Junction (Fig. 10.18a) and 4: Ascending Aorta (Fig. 10.18b).

It should be noted that the discussed measurements can be performed in the parasternal long axis and right parasternal views. The measurements must be perpendicular to the longitudinal axis of the aortic [8, 24, 27].

In all the cases, the views should be taken in a way that the largest diameter of the aortic root is recorded.

Aortic root dimensions in normal adults are shown in Table 10.6.

The aortic annulus should be assessed in the mid-systole using the Inner edge–to–Inner edge (I-I) method and the other measurements should be performed at the end diastole using the Leading edge–to–Leading edge (L-L) approach [28].

The Inferior Vena Cava

The Inferior Vena Cava (IVC) assessment is performed statically and dynamically. Respiratory variation is measured in the dynamic assessment and the IVC diameter in the static assessment (Fig. 10.19a, b).

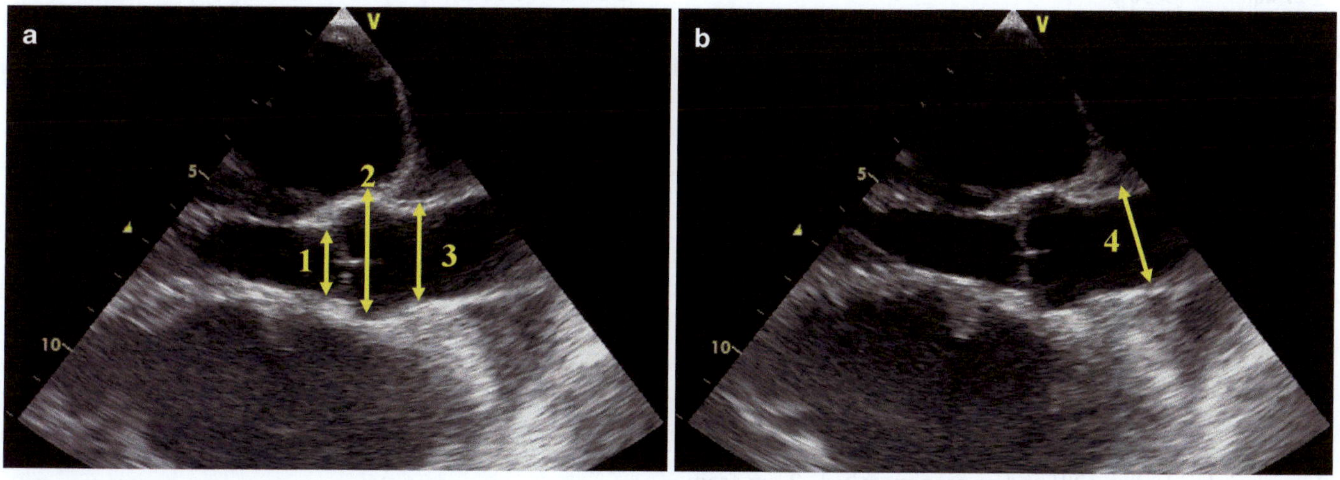

Fig. 10.18 Measurements of the Aortic Root (**a**) and Ascending Aorta (**b**). 1: Aortic Valve Annulus, 2: the Sinuses of Valsalva, 3: the Sino-Tubular Junction, and 4: Ascending Aorta

Table 10.6 Aortic root dimension in normal adults

	Absolute values (cm)		Indexed values (cm/m²)	
Aortic root	Men	Women	Men	Women
Annulus	2.6 ± 0.3	2.3 ± 0.2	1.3 ± 0.1	1.3 ± 0.1
Sinuses of Valsalva	3.4 ± 0.3	3.0 ± 0.3	1.7 ± 0.2	1.8 ± 0.2
Sinotubular junction	2.9 ± 0.3	2.6 ± 0.3	1.5 ± 0.2	1.5 ± 0.2
Proximal ascending aorta	3.0 ± 0.4	2.7 ± 0.4	1.5 ± 0.2	1.6 ± 0.3

Modified from Lang RM, Badano LP, Mor-Avi V, et al. Recommendations for cardiac chamber quantification: A report from the American Society of Echocardiography and the European Association of Cardiovascular Imaging. J Am Soc Echocardiogr. 2015;28:1–39

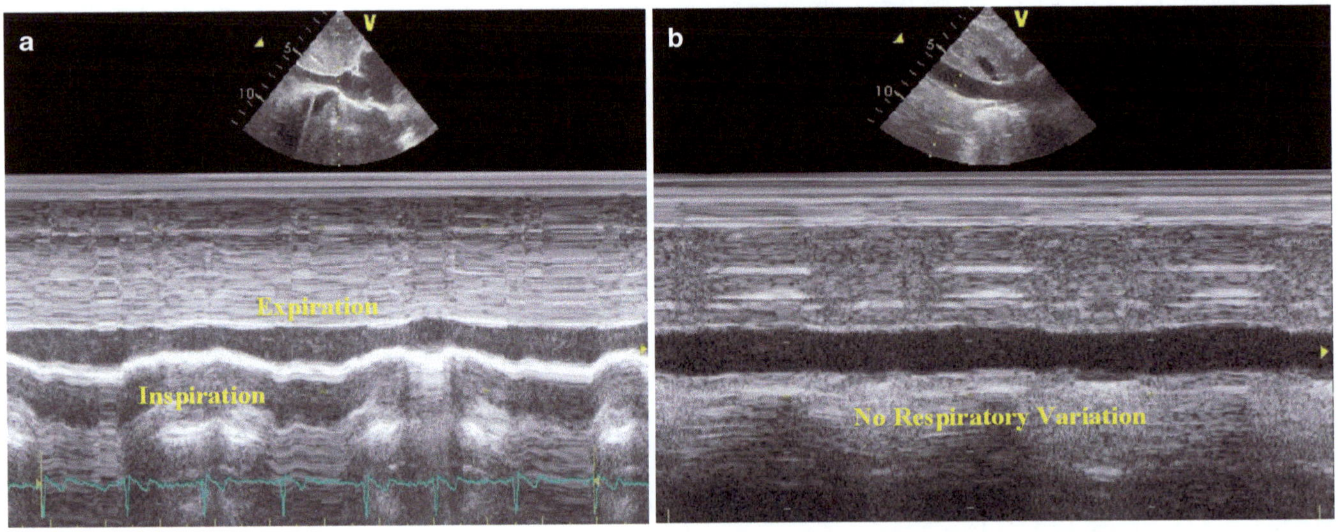

Fig. 10.19 Respiratory variation in inferior vena cava diameter

Table 10.7 Echocardiographic estimation of right atrial pressure on bases of IVC diameter and collapse

IVC diameter	IVC respiratory variation	RA pressure (mmHg)
≤ 21 mm	> 50%	5
≤ 21 mm	< 50%	10
> 21 mm	> 50%	10
> 21 mm	< 50%	15
> 21 mm	None	20

IVC inferior vena cava, *RA* right atrium. Modified from Otto CM. The practice of clinical echocardiography, 4th ed. Elsevier Health Sciences; 2012, p 618

A negative pressure is produced in the chest during spontaneous inhalation that results to move the blood from the IVC to the RA and RV and various degrees of IVC collapse.

In most studies, the best way to measure the IVC is in the subxiphoid view [28] and approximately 1–2 cm from the junction of the IVC to the RA. The best time to measure respiratory variation is during the sniff maneuver. IVC size and respiratory variation are used in RA pressure estimation (Table 10.7). Pulmonary artery pressure assessment is performed with TR jet velocity and RA pressure [8, 24, 26–28].

Questions

1. A male patient presents with Chronic Obstructive Pulmonary Disease (COPD). Given the results below, which one of the following items is the pulmonary arterial pressure?
   - TR velocity: 3 m/s
   - IVC Diameter: > 21 mm
   - IVC Respiratory Variation: < 50%

   A. 60–65 mmHg
   B. 50–55 mmHg
   C. 40–45 mmHg
   D. 30–35 mmHg

2. Calculate the Right Ventricular Index of Myocardial Performance (RVIMP) regarding the results in the figure below (Fig. 10.20)

   A. $\frac{a+b}{d}$
   B. $\frac{a-b}{d}$
   C. $\frac{a+b}{c}$
   D. $\frac{a-b}{c}$

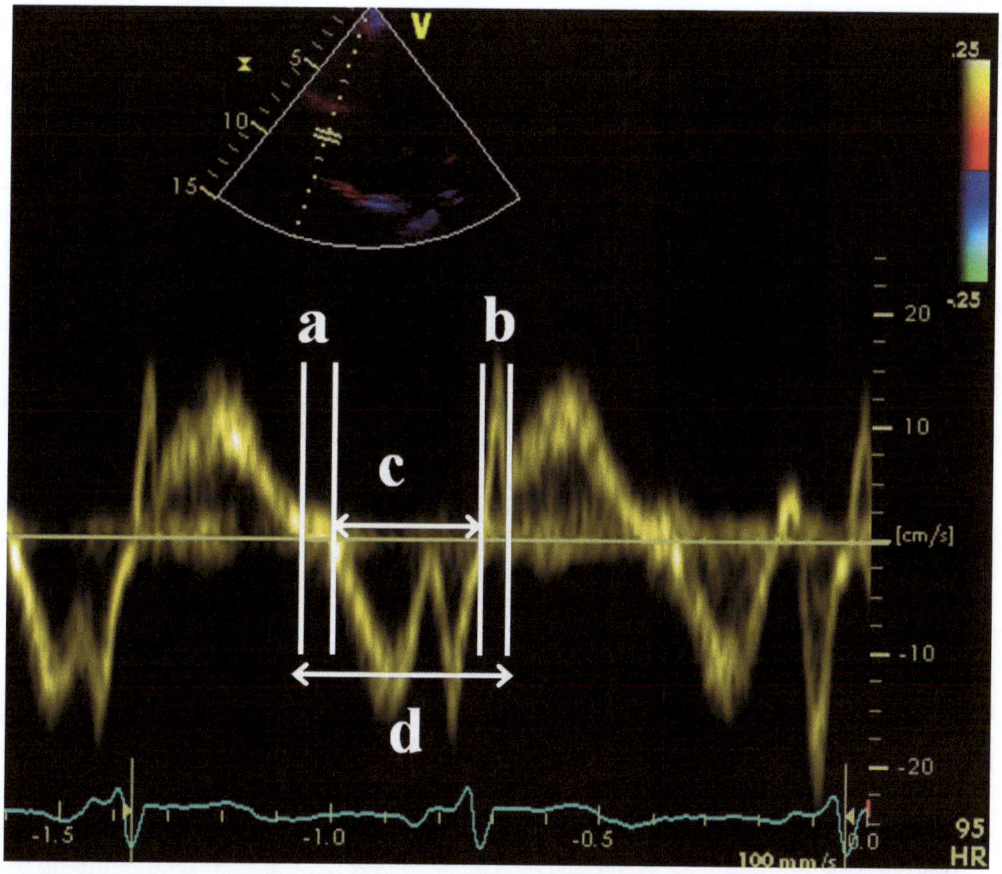

Fig. 10.20 Pulsed-wave tissue Doppler measurements of tricuspid valve annulus

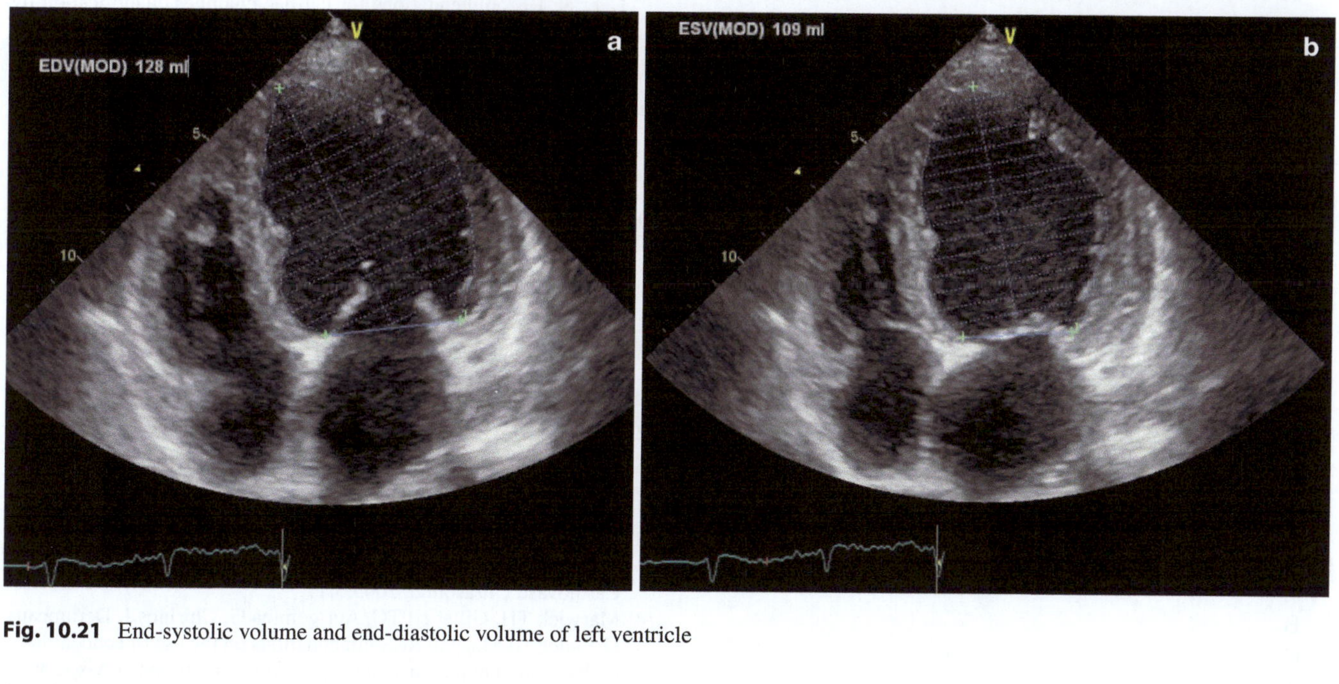

Fig. 10.21 End-systolic volume and end-diastolic volume of left ventricle

3. The patient is a 52-year old man with exertional dyspnea for the past 3 months. Dyspnea has exacerbated over the past 3 days. The following results were obtained through the echocardiography (Fig. 10.21). Calculate the patient's EF.
   A. 15%–20%
   B. 20%–25%
   C. 30%–35%
   D. 40%–45%

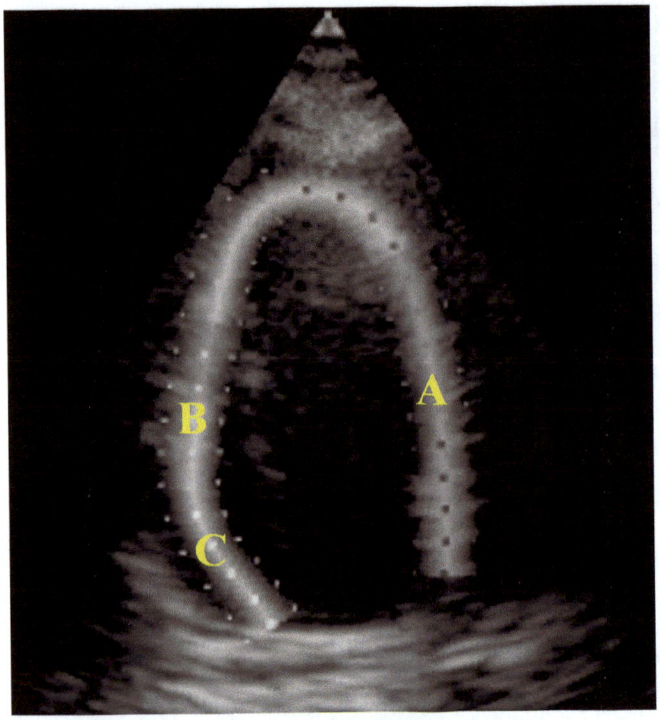

Fig. 10.22 3-Chamber view of the Left ventricle

4. Match the specified segments in the Fig. 10.22 with their respective option.
   A. A: Mid Anterior, B: Mid Inferolateral, C: Basal Inferolateral
   B. A: Mid Anteroseptal, B: Mid Inferior, C: Basal Inferior
   C. A: Mid Anterior, B: Mid Inferior, C: Basal Inferior
   D. A: Mid Anteroseptal, B: Mid Inferolateral, C: Basal Inferolateral

5. What is the best phase of the cardiac cycle and the most preferable method for evaluation of the size of the ascending aorta, respectively?
   A. End diastole, Inner edge–to–Inner edge
   B. End diastole, Leading edge–to–Leading edge
   C. Mid-systole, Inner edge–to–Inner edge
   D. Mid-systole, Leading edge–to–Leading edge

Answers

1. B
2. C
3. A
4. C
5. B

References

1. Kutty S, Russell D, Li L, Hasan R, Peng Q, Frommelt PC, et al. Echocardiographic measurement methods for left ventricular linear dimensions in children result in predictable variations in results. Int J Cardiovasc Imaging. 2014;30(2):305–12.
2. Bellenger NG, Burgess MI, Ray SG, Lahiri A, Coats AJ, Cleland JG, et al. Comparison of left ventricular ejection fraction and volumes in heart failure by echocardiography, radionuclide ventriculography and cardiovascular magnetic resonance; are they interchangeable? Eur Heart J. 2000;21(16):1387–96.
3. Dorosz JL, Lezotte DC, Weitzenkamp DA, Allen LA, Salcedo EE. Performance of 3-dimensional echocardiography in measuring left ventricular volumes and ejection fraction: a systematic review and meta-analysis. J Am Coll Cardiol. 2012;59(20):1799–808.
4. Hoit BD. Strain and strain rate echocardiography and coronary artery disease. Circ Cardiovasc Imaging. 2011;4(2):179–90.
5. Stanton T, Leano R, Marwick TH. Prediction of all-cause mortality from global longitudinal speckle strain: comparison with ejection fraction and wall motion scoring. Circ Cardiovasc Imaging. 2009;2(5):356–64.
6. Voigt JU, Pedrizzetti G, Lysyansky P, Marwick TH, Houle H, Baumann R, et al. Definitions for a common standard for 2D speckle tracking echocardiography: consensus document of the EACVI/ASE/industry task force to standardize deformation imaging. J Am Soc Echocardiogr. 2015;28(2):183–93.
7. Cerqueira MD, Weissman NJ, Dilsizian V, Jacobs AK, Kaul S, Laskey WK, et al. Standardized myocardial segmentation and nomenclature for tomographic imaging of the heart. A statement for healthcare professionals from the cardiac imaging Committee of the Council on clinical cardiology of the American Heart Association. Circulation. 2002;105(4):539–42.
8. Lang RM, Badano LP, Mor-Avi V, Afilalo J, Armstrong A, Ernande L, et al. Recommendations for cardiac chamber quantification by echocardiography in adults: an update from the American Society of Echocardiography and the European Association of Cardiovascular Imaging. J Am Soc Echocardiogr. 2015;28(1):1–39.e14.
9. Leitman M, Lysyansky P, Sidenko S, Shir V, Peleg E, Binenbaum M, et al. Two-dimensional strain-a novel software for real-time quantitative echocardiographic assessment of myocardial function. J Am Soc Echocardiogr. 2004;17(10):1021–9.
10. Kishi S, Magalhaes TA, George RT, Dewey M, Laham RJ, Niinuma H, et al. Relationship of left ventricular mass to coronary atherosclerosis and myocardial ischaemia: the CORE320 multicenter study. Eur Heart J Cardiovasc Imaging. 2015;16(2):166–76.
11. Bluemke DA, Kronmal RA, Lima JA, Liu K, Olson J, Burke GL, et al. The relationship of left ventricular mass and geometry to incident cardiovascular events: the MESA (multi-ethnic study of atherosclerosis) study. J Am Coll Cardiol. 2008;52(25):2148–55.
12. Armstrong AC, Gidding S, Gjesdal O, Wu C, Bluemke DA, Lima JALV. Mass assessed by echocardiography and CMR, cardiovascular outcomes, and medical practice. JACC Cardiovasc Imaging. 2012;5(8):837–48.
13. Foppa M, Duncan BB, Rohde LE. Echocardiography-based left ventricular mass estimation. How should we define hypertrophy? Cardiovasc Ultrasound. 2005;3:17.
14. Marwick TH, Gillebert TC, Aurigemma G, Chirinos J, Derumeaux G, Galderisi M, et al. Recommendations on the use of echocardiography in adult hypertension: a report from the European Association of Cardiovascular Imaging (EACVI) and the American Society of Echocardiography (ASE)dagger. Eur Heart J Cardiovasc Imaging. 2015;16(6):577–605.

15. Collins KA, Korcarz CE, Lang RM. Use of echocardiography for the phenotypic assessment of genetically altered mice. Physiol Genomics. 2003;13(3):227–39.
16. Badano L, Lang RM, Zamorano JL. Textbook of real-time three dimensional echocardiography. London: Springer; 2010.
17. Kossaify A. Echocardiographic assessment of the right ventricle, from the conventional approach to speckle tracking and three-dimensional imaging, and insights into the "right way" to explore the forgotten chamber. Clin Med Insights Cardiol. 2015;9:65–75.
18. Valsangiacomo Buechel ER, Mertens LL. Imaging the right heart: the use of integrated multimodality imaging. Eur Heart J. 2012;33(8):949–60.
19. Rudski LG, Lai WW, Afilalo J, Hua L, Handschumacher MD, Chandrasekaran K, et al. Guidelines for the echocardiographic assessment of the right heart in adults: a report from the American Society of Echocardiography endorsed by the European Association of Echocardiography, a registered branch of the European Society of Cardiology, and the Canadian Society of Echocardiography. J Am Soc Echocardiogr. 2010;23(7):685–713. quiz 86-8
20. Sadeghpour A, Alizadehasl A. The right ventricle: a comprehensive review from anatomy, physiology, and mechanics to hemodynamic, functional, and imaging evaluation. Arch Cardiovasc Imaging. 2015;3(4).
21. Bigdelu L, Azari A, Fazlinezhad A. Assessment of right ventricular function by tissue doppler, strain and strain rate imaging in patients with left-sided valvular heart disease and pulmonary hypertension. Arch Cardiovasc Imaging. 2014;2(1).
22. Hoit BD. Left atrial size and function: role in prognosis. J Am Coll Cardiol. 2014;63(6):493–505.
23. Rosca M, Lancellotti P, Popescu BA, Pierard LA. Left atrial function: pathophysiology, echocardiographic assessment, and clinical applications. Heart. 2011;97(23):1982–9.
24. Lang RM, Bierig M, Devereux RB, Flachskampf FA, Foster E, Pellikka PA, et al. Recommendations for chamber quantification. Eur J Echocardiogr. 2006;7(2):79–108.
25. Rusinaru D, Tribouilloy C, Grigioni F, Avierinos JF, Suri RM, Barbieri A, et al. Left atrial size is a potent predictor of mortality in mitral regurgitation due to flail leaflets: results from a large international multicenter study. Circ Cardiovasc Imaging. 2011;4(5):473–81.
26. Anderson RH. The surgical anatomy of the aortic root. Multimedia manual of cardiothoracic surgery. MMCTS. 2007;2007(102):mmcts 2006 002527.
27. Kim M, Roman MJ, Cavallini MC, Schwartz JE, Pickering TG, Devereux RB. Effect of hypertension on aortic root size and prevalence of aortic regurgitation. Hypertension. 1996;28(1):47–52.
28. Stone MB, Huang JV. Inferior vena cava assessment: correlation with CVP and plethora in Tamponade. Glob Heart. 2013;8(4):323–7.

Echocardiography Evaluation of Left Ventricular Systolic Function, Systolic Dysfunction, and Ventricular Dyssynchrony

11

Nehzat Akiash, Azin Alizadehasl, and Anita Sadeghpour

Abstract

The ejection fraction (EF) is the most widely used measure and popular method in evaluating left ventricular (LV) systolic function and is considered a critical prognostic factor in all types of heart diseases.

Precise evaluation of LV volume and systolic function is necessary for defining the optimal timing of surgery in patients with valvular heart diseases such as severe mitral regurgitation and aortic regurgitation.

This section attempts to introduce the different findings that can be obtained from echocardiography in patients with systolic heart failure.

Keywords

Echocardiography · Left ventricular systolic function · Systolic dysfunction · Ventricular dyssynchrony · Speckle-tracking echocardiography · Stroke volume · Cardiac resynchronization therapy · Global longitudinal strain

Abbreviations

CRT	Cardiac resynchronization therapy
EF	Ejection fraction
GLS	Global longitudinal strain
HR	Heart rate
IVC	Inferior vena cava
LV	Left ventricle
LVOT	Left ventricular outflow tract
PAP	Pulmonary arterial pressure
PVR	Pulmonary vascular resistance
RA	Right atrium
RV	Right ventricle
STE	Speckle-tracking echocardiography
SV	Stroke volume
TDI	Tissue Doppler imaging
TRV	Tricuspid regurgitation velocity
VTI	Velocity time integral

Left Ventricular Systolic Function

- LV systolic function is affected by preload, afterload, and myocardial contractility. Indeed, systolic function has a complex mechanism including contraction of the helical arrangement of the LV myocardial fibers.
- Stroke volume (SV) has been introduced as a measure of LV pump performance and when it is assessed relative to end-diastolic volume, ventricular systolic function can be defined.
- That was the reason why the EF has been used as an index of myocardial contractility and systolic function. It is calculated via the following formula:

$$EF = \frac{(EDV - ESV)}{EDV}$$

where EDV stands for end-diastolic volume and ESV for end-systolic volume.

Electronic Supplementary Material The online version of this chapter (https://doi.org/10.1007/978-3-319-67691-3_11) contains supplementary material, which is available to authorized users.

N. Akiash, MD
Assistant Professor of Cardiology, Atherosclerosis Research Center, Ahvaz Jundishapur University of Medical Sciences, Ahvaz, Iran

A. Alizadehasl, MD, FACC, FASE
Associate Professor of Cardiology, Echocardiologist, Echocardiography and Cardiogenetic Research Centers, Cardio-Oncology Department, Rajaie Cardiovascular Medical and Research Center, Tehran, Iran

A. Sadeghpour, MD, FACC, FASE (✉)
Professor of Cardiology, Echocardiography Research Center, Rajaie Cardiovascular Medical and Research Center, Iran University of Medical Science, Tehran, Iran

A. Sadeghpour, A. Alizadehasl (eds.), *Case-Based Textbook of Echocardiography*,
https://doi.org/10.1007/978-3-319-67691-3_11

- It is noteworthy that acute loading conditions can have a major influence on the EF. However, in chronic heart disease, the EF can be an important index of contractile function.
- Normally, the LV ejects more than half of its end-diastolic volume [1].

Routine visual assessment of the EF with 2D echocardiography is highly operator-dependent and, thus, susceptible to errors. New modalities in the evaluation of the LVEF and the LV function assessment have, therefore, enhanced the value of echocardiography as a diagnostic tool [2].

- The LV function is routinely assessed by visual assessment, and the evaluation of the LV contractility and wall motion is performed in all standard 2D echocardiography views [3].

M-Mode, 2D, and 3D Echocardiography

Measurement of the Left Ventricular Volumes and Evaluation of the Left Ventricular Function

- EF can be measured via M-mode, 2D, or 3D echocardiography (See Chap. 10). Each method has its own advantages and limitations.
- Endocardial border definition is required for the evaluation of the LVEF through measuring volumes and M-mode. Sometime, ultrasound contrast agents may be required for the detection of the LV endocardial border, particularly in obese patients or those with pulmonary diseases [4].
- In 2-D-guided M-mode, the linear internal dimensions are recorded by placing the beam perpendicular to the LV in the parasternal long-axis view, just below the mitral valve leaflets. The end-systolic diameter, end-diastolic diameter of the LV cavity, and the end-systolic and end-diastolic interventricular septum diameters as well as the end-systolic and end-diastolic posterior wall diameters of the LV are measured. Changes in the LV diameter are easily measurable by recording the posterior and septal wall motions [5]. Although the evaluation of the LVEF is widely used on the strength of its simplicity, reproducibility of its data, and its predictive value, it has certain technical limitations [6, 7].
- The Teichholz and Quinones methods calculate the LVEF (Fig. 11.1) by linear diameters [8].
- Prolate- ellipsoid method is based on the model of the left ventricle as a prolate ellipse and use the cubed method, which simply assumes the following:

$$LV\,Volume = 4/_3\,\pi\,\frac{L}{2}\,\frac{D_1}{2}\,\frac{D_2}{2}$$

where L is long axis(2D), D_1 and D_2 are orthogonal minor axis and $D_1 = D_2$. Consequently:

$LV\ Volume \cong D^3$

- Area-length method is the other method for evaluation of LV volume when precise tracing of LV apex is

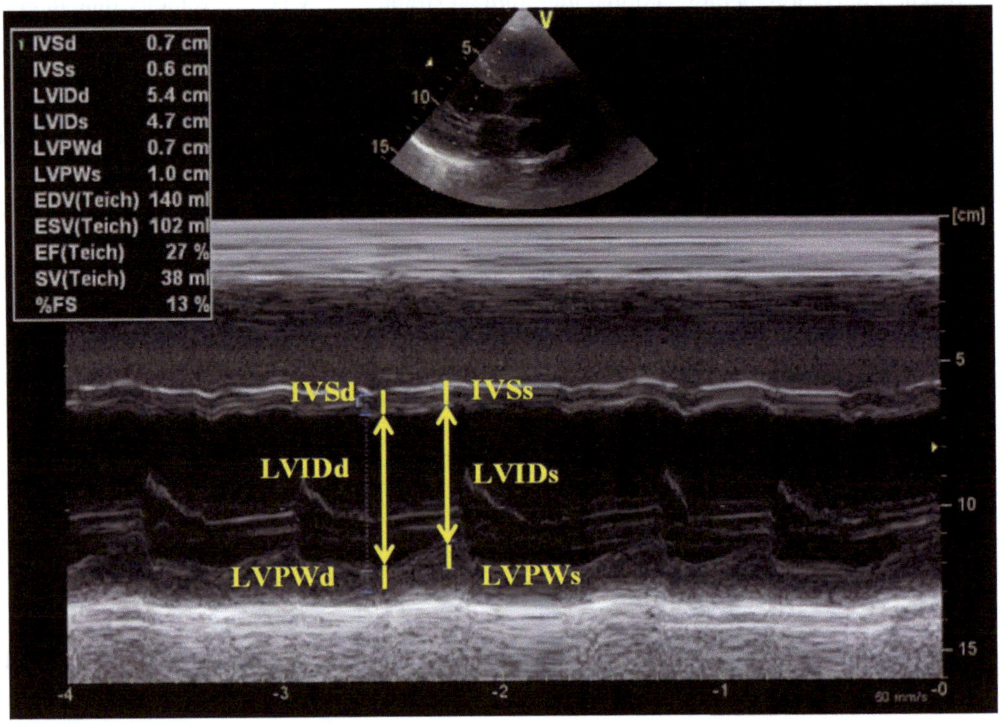

Fig. 11.1 Left ventricular ejection fraction measurement using the M-mode approach by 2D. *LVIDd* left ventricular internal dimension in diastole, *LVIDs* Left ventricular internal dimension in systole, *IVSd* interventricular septum in diastole, *IVSs* interventricular septum in systole, *LVPWd* left ventricular posterior wall in diastole, *LVPWs* left ventricular posterior wall in systole

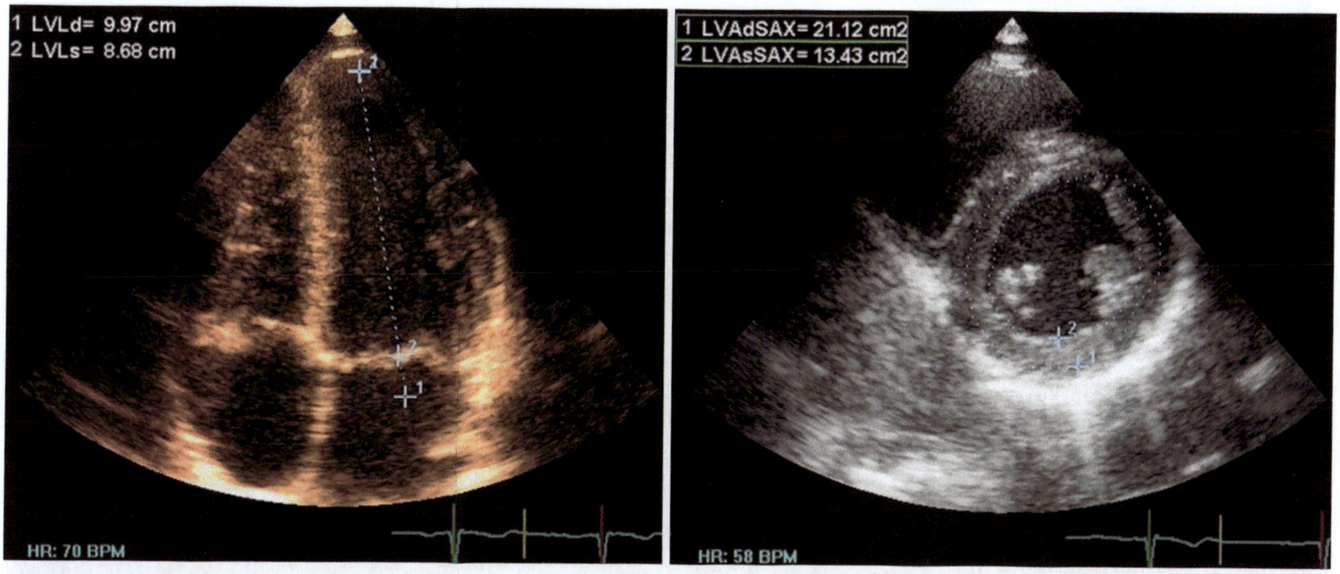

Fig. 11.2 Left ventricular volume measurement using the Area-length method by 2DE. *LVLd* left ventricular length in diastole, *LVLs* left ventricular length in systole, *LVAd* left ventricular area in diastole, *LVAs* left ventricular area in systole

not possible. The area of the mid-LV is traced in short axis view at the level of papillary muscles and the length is measured in apical four chamber view (Fig. 11.2).

- These methods are based on the assumption of a fixed geometric shape of the LV and may be inaccurate especially in the distortion of the LV geometry [9, 10].
- Biplane Simpson method: It is used for the EF assessment and volume measurement in 2D echocardiography. In this method, the end-systolic and end-diastolic endocardial surface is traced in the apical 4-chamber (Fig. 11.3) and apical 2-chamber views. The papillary muscles should not be included in endocardial tracing, and foreshortening should also be avoided in measuring the LVEF. Based on ECG, the end-diastolic and end-systolic phases are measured, respectively, from the start of the Q wave and near the end of the T wave [11]. The use of echocardiography for the evaluation of the EF can have a prognostic value and is also helpful in evaluating patients with systolic heart failure after treatment [12].

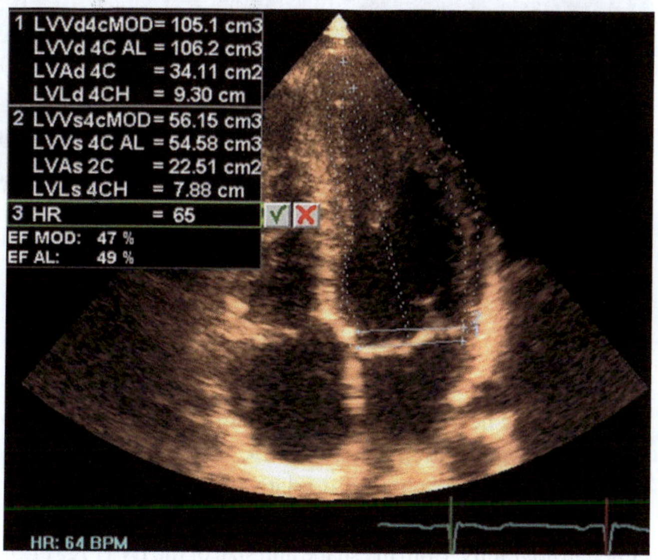

Fig. 11.3 End-systolic and end-diastolic endocardial surface is traced in the apical 4-chamber view

3D echocardiography: 3D echocardiography has the advantages of direct measurement of the LV cavity without geometrical assumptions. 3D echocardiography is superior to 2D echocardiography in terms of reproducibility and the accuracy (Fig. 11.4, Movie 11.1), particularly in patients with asymmetric LV volume and ventricular aneurysms [13].

There are certain limitations that need to be taken into account in the EF evaluation, including geometrical assumptions (in some methods) and load and heart rate (HR) dependency [14].

- ***Left ventricular size and shape***

The LV remodeling occurs after myocardial infraction in heart failure patients with a low EF and is considered a prognostic factor.

The LV diameter plays a key role in the management of valvular heart diseases. The LVEF assessment, using exclusively diameter evaluation, is not accurate in heart failure

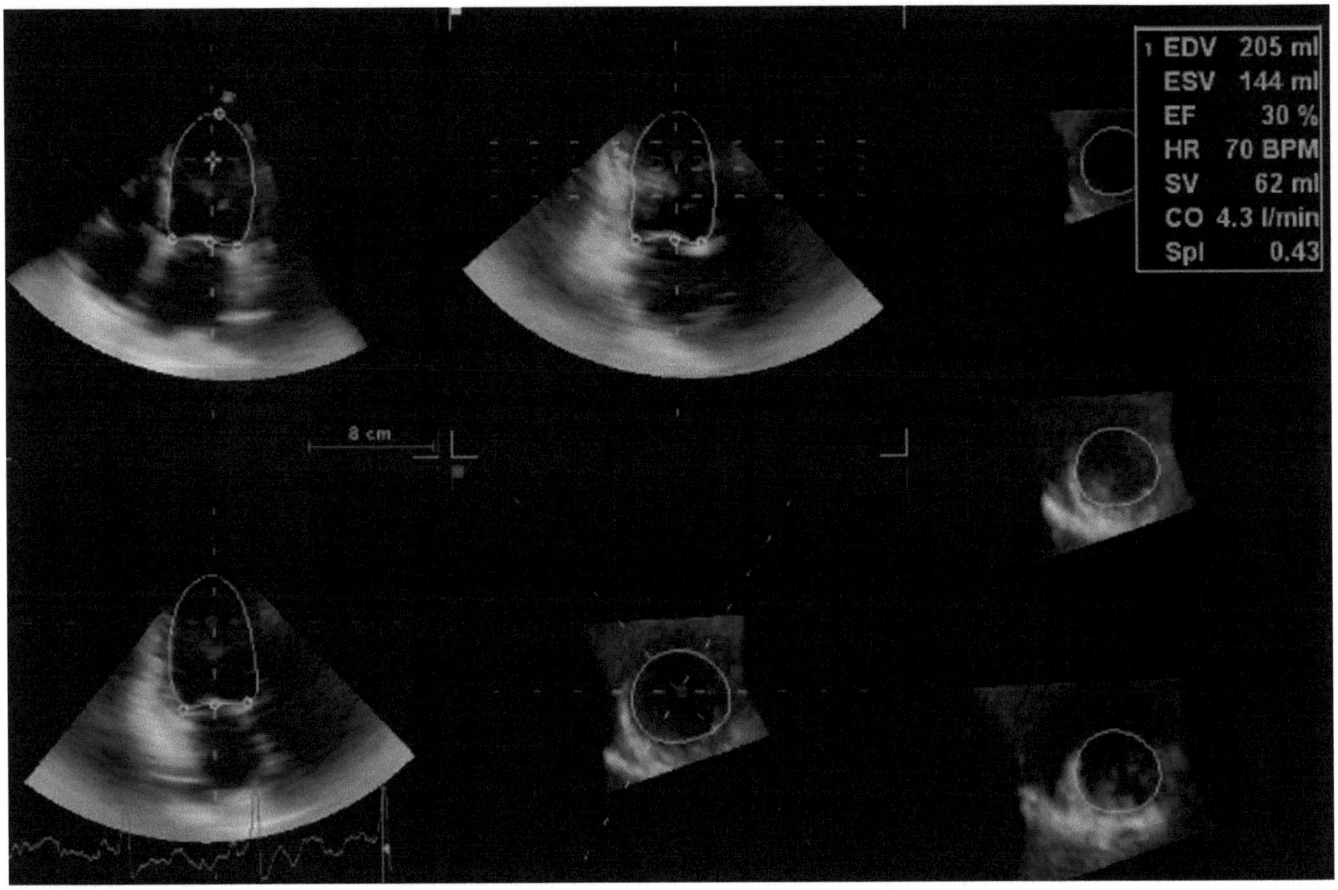

Fig. 11.4 (Movie) Left Ventricular ejection fraction measurement using 3D echocardiography

with ischemic heart disease and myocardial infarction due to ventricular wall motion abnormalities.

3D echocardiography has a relatively high sensitivity for the evaluation of remodeling and is more accurate than 2D echocardiography. Both the shape and size of the LV (Fig. 11.5, Movies 11.2 and 11.3) play a key role in the evaluation of heart failure.

Since the LV shape is influenced by the LV wall motion abnormalities, 3D echocardiography can be more helpful than 2D echocardiography in this evaluation [15, 16].

- ***Regional left ventricular function evaluation***

Stress Echocardiography

The differentiation of myocardial scare tissues from the hibernating and stunned myocardium and the detection of the residual viable tissues with contractile dysfunction have great applications for the treatment, outcome, and long-term prognosis of patients with ischemic cardiomyopathy.

Low-dose dobutamine is used in stress echocardiography to investigate contractile reserve. (See Chap. 27.) Improvement in the LV wall motion during dobutamine infusion can affect management approaches in patients with ischemic cardiomyopathy [17, 18].

- ***Pulmonary edema***

Increase in extravascular water in the lung tissue in heart failure can be detected through the appearance of lung comets in 2D echocardiography. It is examined in emergency departments using portable devices and is a low-cost and simple method to distinguish the causes of shortness of breath. Lung comets consist of multiple comet tails that extend from the lung surface and originate from the thickened inter-lobular septa; they are referred to as "Kerley B" lines in radiology [19, 20].

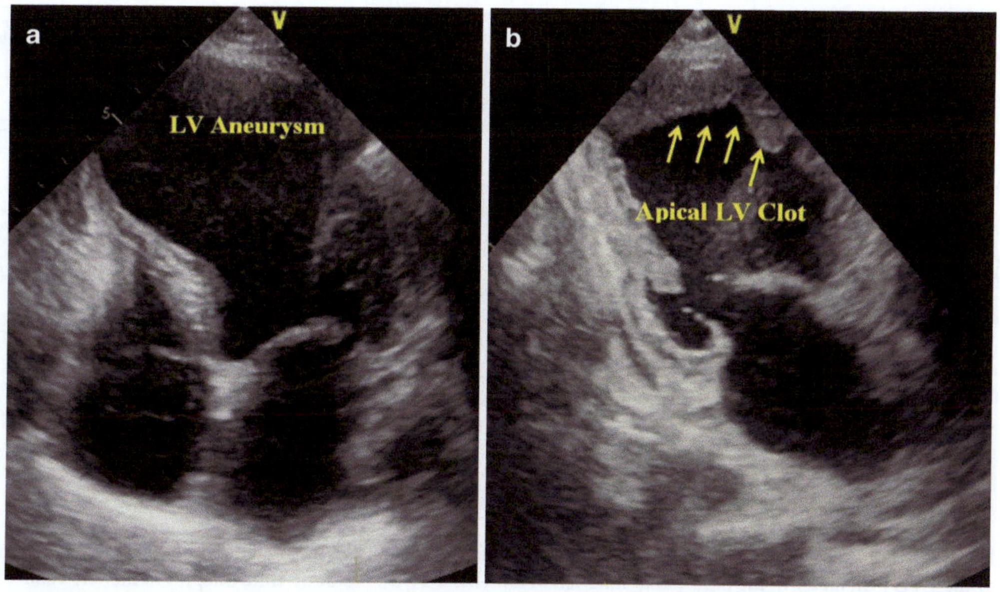

Fig. 11.5 (Movie). 2D echocardiography, showing an aneurysm of the LV apex in the 4-chamber view (**a**). Large thrombus into the LV apex (**b**). *LV* left ventricle

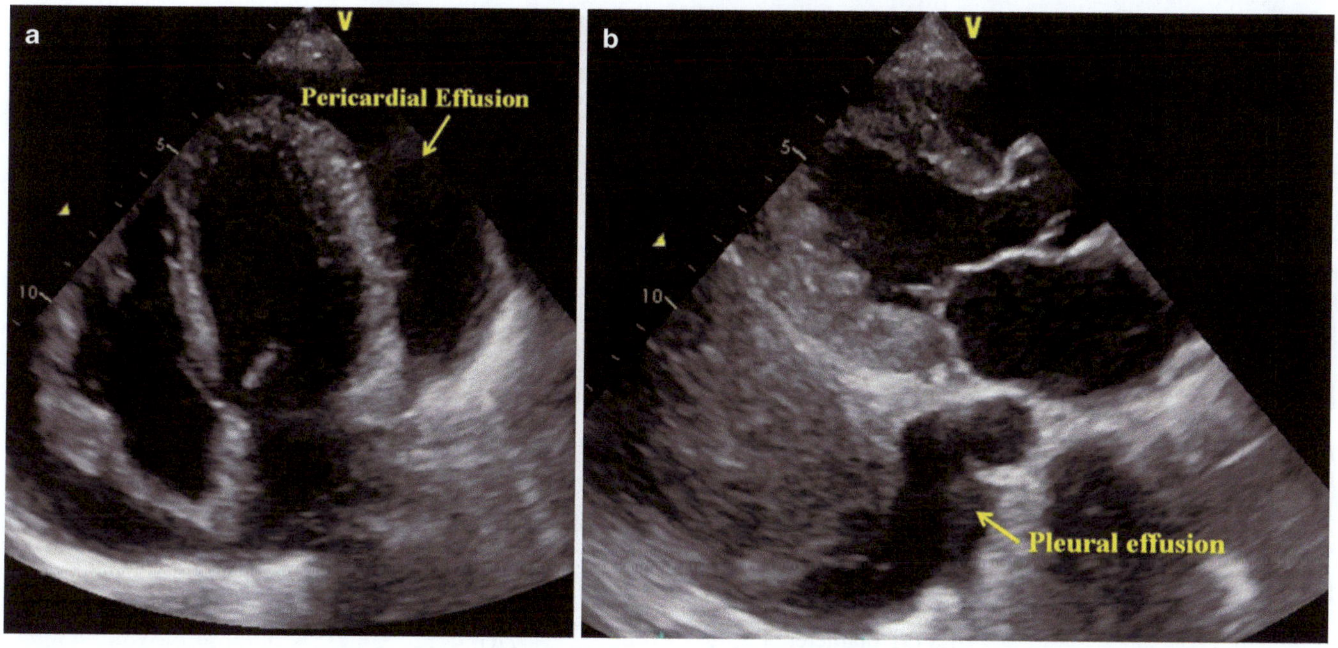

Fig. 11.6 2D echocardiography, showing a large amount of pericardial effusion (**a**) and pleural effusion (**b**) in the 4-chamber and parasternal long-axis views, respectively movie

- ***Pericardial and pleural effusion***

The accumulation of fluid in the pericardial and pleural spaces (Fig. 11.6, Movies 11.4 and 11.5) is a common complication of congestive heart failure [21]. Echocardiography can be employed as a primary assessment for the diagnosis of pericardial effusion with nearly 100% accuracy.

Echocardiography is also very helpful in the evaluation of the physiological and hemodynamic effects of pericardial effusion [22].

Doppler Echocardiography

- ***Cardiac output and stroke volume***

The cardiac output is a factor for determining the global performance of the cardiovascular system and is calculated by multiplying the SV by the HR. The cardiac output can be assessed by obtaining the velocity time integral (VTI) of the LVOT through Doppler echocardiography (Fig. 11.7a), and the LVOT diameter can be assessed in the parasternal long-axis

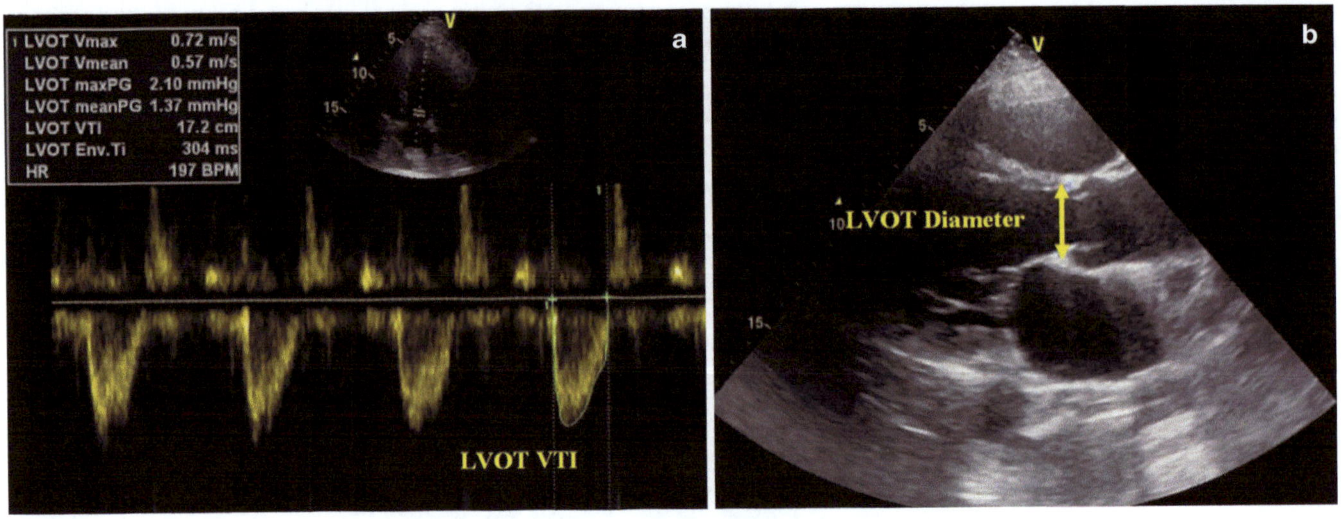

Fig. 11.7 Measurement of the VTI_{LVOT} in the apical 5-chamber view and tracing the pulsed-wave Doppler obtained in the LVOT (**a**). Measurement of the LVOT diameter in the parasternal long-axis view (**b**). VTI_{LVOT}, Velocity-time integral in the left ventricular outflow tract

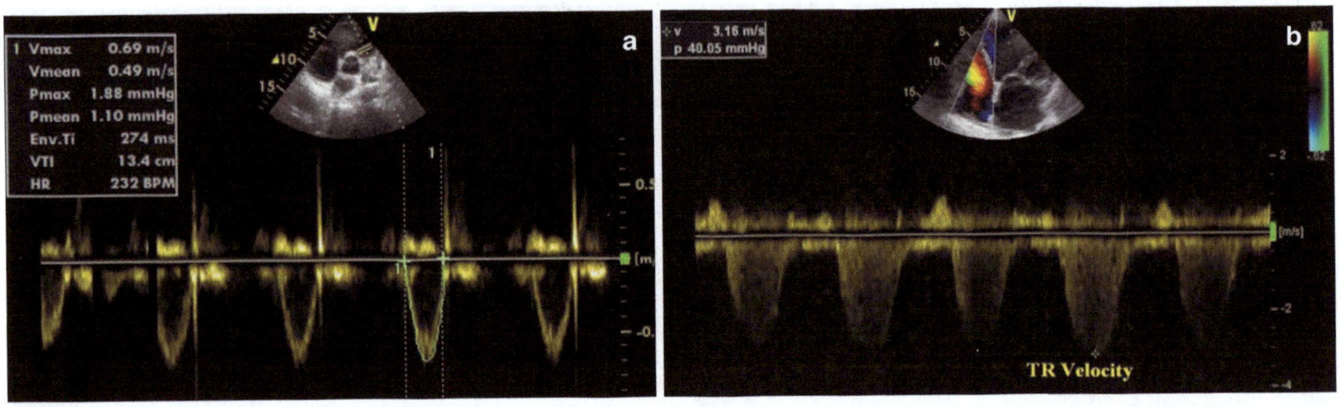

Fig. 11.8 Measurement of the right ventricular outflow tract velocity-time integral in the parasternal short-axis view and tracing the pulsed-wave Doppler obtained in the right ventricular outflow tract (**a**). Measurement of the tricuspid valve regurgitation jet velocity (**b**)

view using 2D echocardiography (Fig. 11.7b). The cardiac output is then calculated from the following formula [23, 24]:

$$\text{Cardiac Output} = \text{HR} \cdot VTI_{LVOT} \cdot \left(\frac{\text{LVOT diameter}}{2}\right)^2 \cdot 3.14$$

where VTI_{LVOT} is velocity-time integral in the left ventricular outflow tract (LVOT).

- ***Pulmonary vascular resistance and pulmonary arterial pressure***

The pulmonary vascular resistance (PVR) and the PVR index constitute some of the findings of Doppler echocardiography in patients with advanced heart failure. An irreversible elevation in the PVR is a contraindication for heart transplantation alone. Moreover, a high pulmonary capillary wedge pressure (PCWP) is an important factor that contributes to poor prognosis in patients with advanced heart failure [25]. The PVR is estimated using the following equation:

$$\text{PVR} = \frac{TRV}{VTI_{RVOT}} \cdot 10 + 0.16$$

where TRV is the tricuspid regurgitation jet velocity and VTI_{RVOT} is velocity-time integral in the right ventricular outflow tract(Fig. 11.8a) [26].

Doppler echocardiography is used to assess pulmonary arterial pressure (PAP) by calculating the gradient between the right ventricular (RV) and the right atrial (RA) pressures. The tricuspid regurgitation jet velocity (TRV) signifies the difference between the RA and RV pressures (Fig. 11.8b). The tricuspid regurgitation (TR) jet is obtained from continuous wave Doppler in the apical 4-chamber view.

$PAP_{Systolic}$ is calculated using the following formula:

$PAP_{Systolic} = 4 \cdot TRV^2 + \text{RA pressure}$

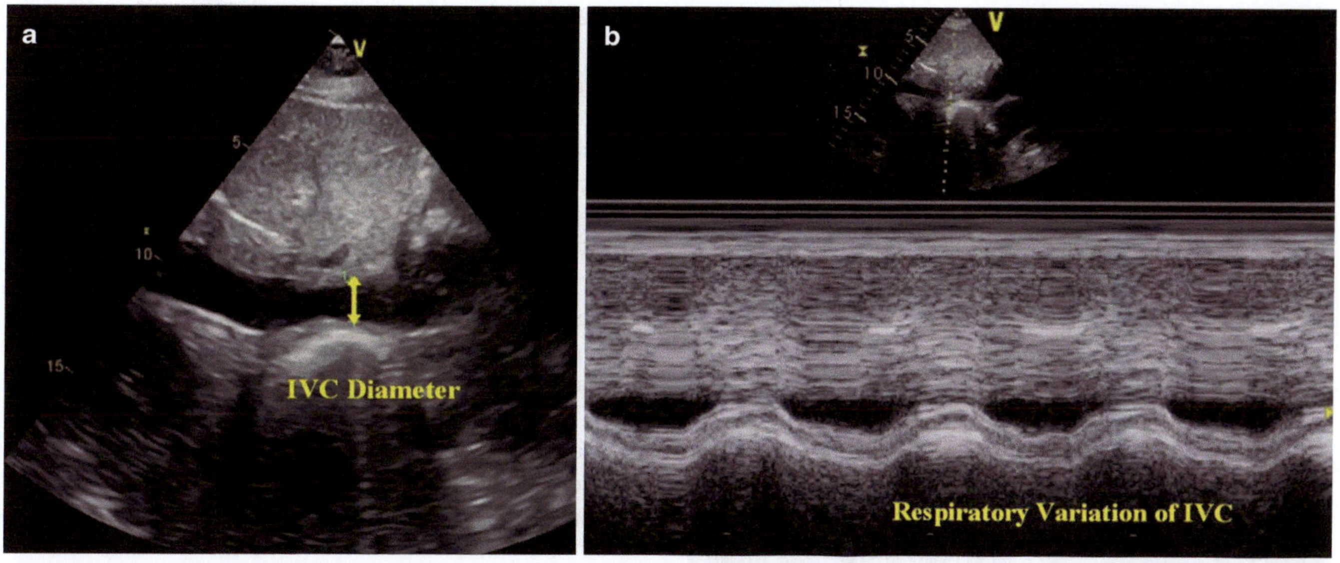

Fig. 11.9 2D echocardiographic measurement of the IVC diameter (**a**). Respiratory variations in the IVC diameter via the M-mode approach (**b**). *IVC* inferior vena cava

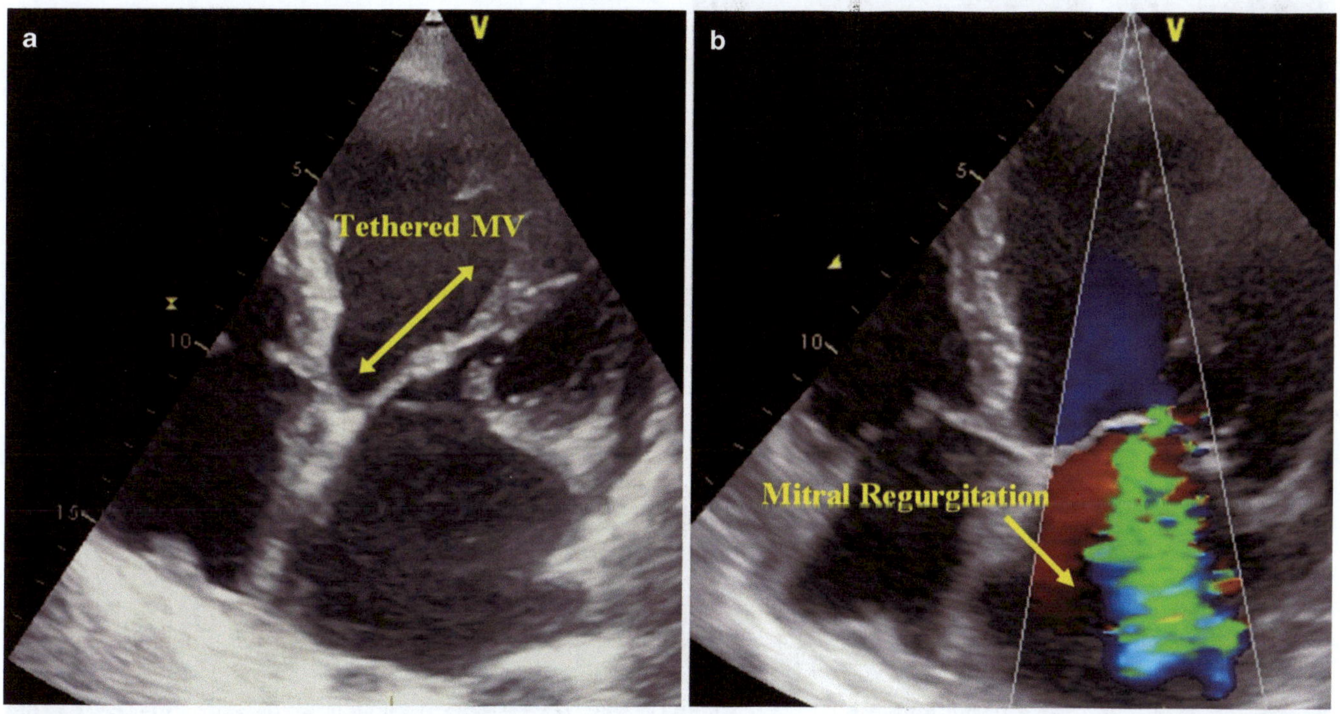

Fig. 11.10 (Movie) Significant tethering of the mitral valve leaflets (**a**) with severe mitral regurgitation in the apical 4-chamber view (**b**)

The RA pressure is calculated using the inferior vena cava (IVC) diameter (Fig. 11.9a) and the respiratory variation of the IVC (Fig. 11.9b) [27].

- ***Mitral regurgitation***

Functional mitral regurgitation is a complication of ischemic heart failure that is caused by changes in the ventricular geometry and the tethering of the mitral leaflets (Fig. 11.10a, Movie 11.6) in the presence of structurally normal mitral leaflets. The severity of mitral regurgitation is an indicator of the prognosis of systolic heart failure. It is worth noting that ischemic mitral regurgitation is dynamic [28].

In heart failure with a low EF, geometrical changes in the LV displace the papillary muscles toward the apex, thereby reducing the coaptation between the anterior and posterior mitral valve leaflets: This gives rise to mitral valve regurgitation (Fig. 11.10b, Movie 11.7) [29, 30].

The degree of mitral regurgitation in systolic heart failure is not associated with the severity of the LV dysfunction. Regional LV remodeling may increase the tenting area (Fig. 11.11) of the mitral valve, reduce the mitral annulus contraction, and therefore increase mitral valve regurgitation [31, 32].

- ***Diastolic function assessment (See Chap. 13)***

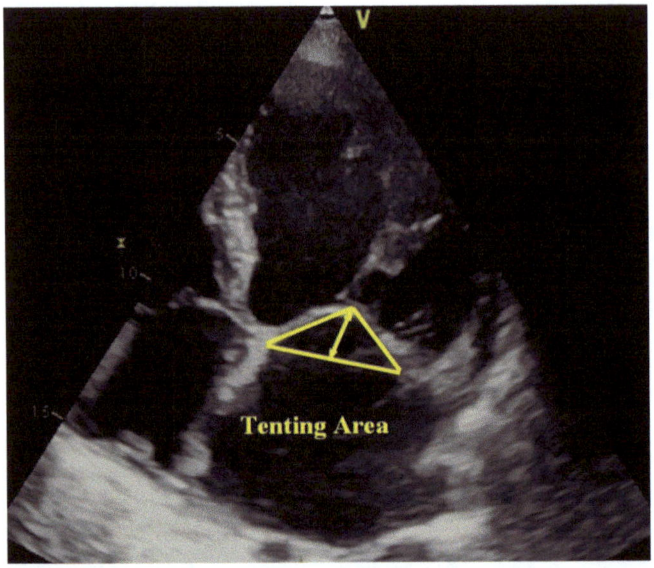

Fig. 11.11 Apical displacement of the mitral valve leaflets and measuring the tenting area and the coaptation depth (double-headed yellow arrow) in the apical 4-chamber view

Tissue Doppler Study

- ***Tissue Doppler velocity***

Tissue Doppler imaging (TDI) can be used to evaluate the systolic and diastolic functions, regional wall motion abnormalities, LV filling pressures, and LV synchrony [33].

TDI is a simple, reproducible, and highly accurate method for the assessment of systolic and early diastole velocities. Reduced peak systolic and early ventricular diastole velocities (Fig. 11.12) have prognostic values and indicate reduced ventricular systolic and diastolic functions.

The reduced mean systolic velocity and the mean early diastolic velocity derived from the mitral annulus area are consistent with a globally reduced systolic and diastolic function [34].

- ***Speckle-tracking echocardiography***

Speckle-tracking Echocardiography (STE) enables the assessment of deformations in the radial, circumferential, and longitudinal planes. This method is preferred due to its dependency on the angle of insonation.

One of the applications of STE is its prognostic value in patients with dilated cardiomyopathy, which can be evaluated by both 2D and 3D echocardiography (Fig. 11.13).

The LVEF assessment has low sensitivity in the LV dysfunction, while the assessment of the strain rate and the longitudinal strain can provide high sensitivity and specificity in the assessment of the LV function because it is less dependent on load and the operator's skills than the LVEF. The assessment of the strain using STE is, therefore, far more preferred over all the other methods [35–37].

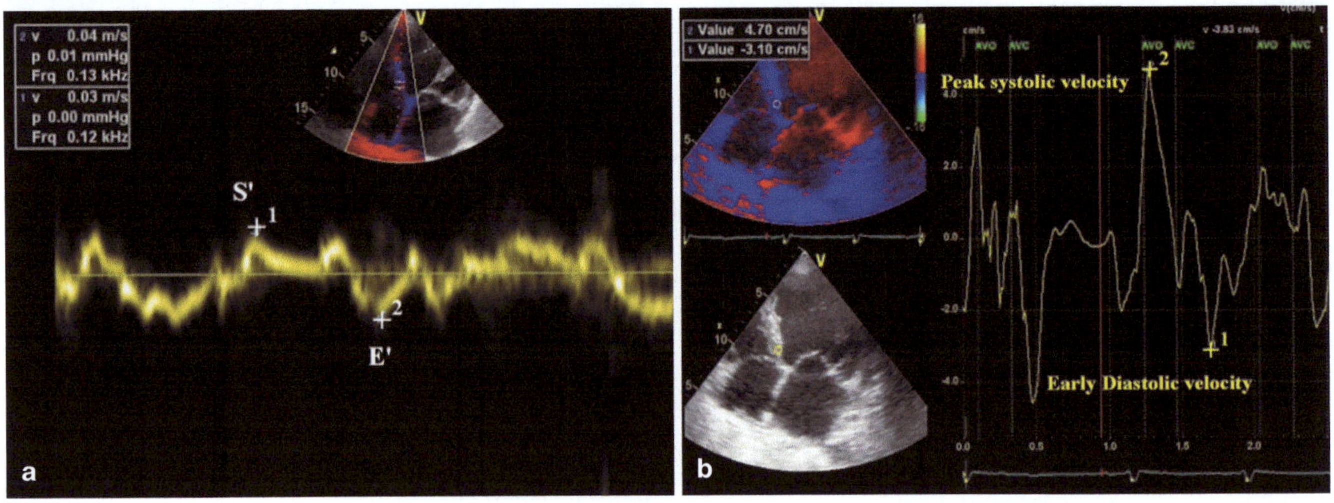

Fig. 11.12 Pulsed-wave tissue Doppler imaging myocardial velocity, measured at the basal septal part of the mitral valve annulus. Reduced peak systolic (S′) and early diastolic myocardial velocity (E′) (**a**). Color-encoded tissue Doppler imaging myocardial velocity obtained at the basal inferoseptal wall. Reduced peak systolic and early diastolic velocity (**b**). *AVO* aortic valve opening, *AVC* aortic valve closure

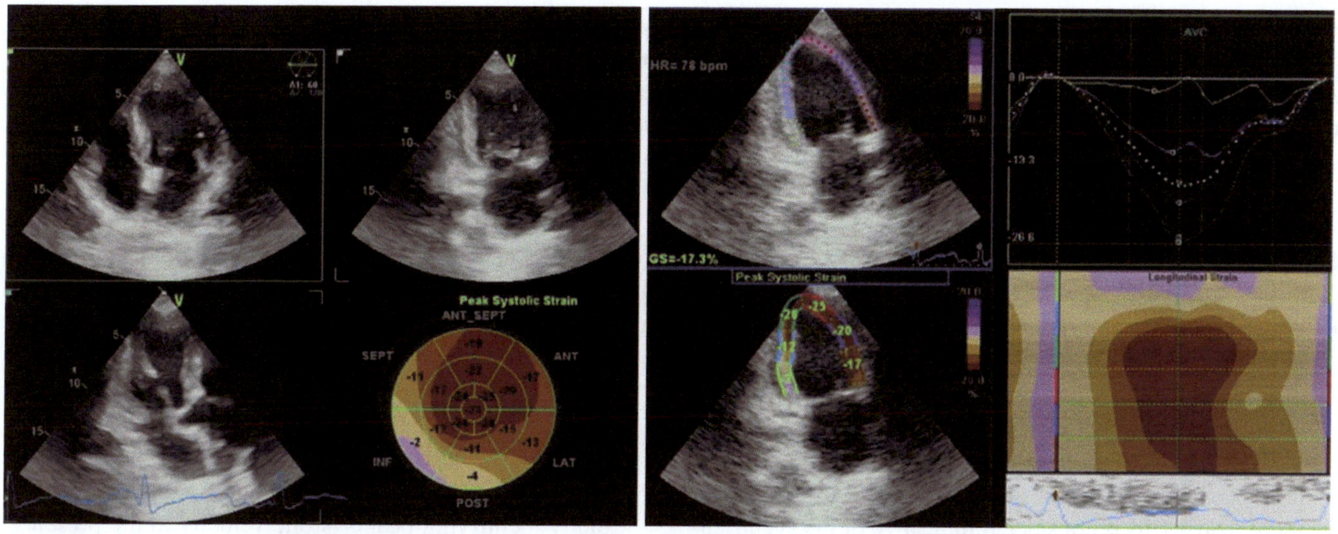

Fig. 11.13 2D left ventricular speckle-tracking multiplane view, showing global and regional left ventricular longitudinal strain

Longitudinal strain assessment using STE can predict the infarct size after acute myocardial infarction and can, thus, play an important role in myocardial viability assessment by evaluating the regional myocardial function [35].

Echocardiographic Study of Cardiac Dyssynchrony in Heart Failure

- Heart failure is a major health issue, with as many as 10% of those older than 65 years affected. Even though the medical management of heart failure has improved substantially in recent years, morbidity and mortality still remain high—particularly for cases with a poor functional class, despite optimal medical therapy.
- Deleterious effects of intraventricular conduction abnormalities have been known for several years. Cardiac resynchronization therapy (CRT) helps to improve the ventricular contraction by simultaneous pacing of right and left ventricle, thereby decreasing morbidity and mortality according to large-scale, prospective clinical studies. Indeed, patients with heart failure who have both electrical dyssynchrony (widened QRS) and mechanical dyssynchrony are the optimal cases for CRT.
- So far, case selection has focused on ECG criteria. According to the current guidelines, CRT is recommended in patients with the following conditions:
  - Symptomatic heart failure (New York Heart Association functional class III or IV) despite optimal medical management
  - Prolonged QRS duration (≥120 ms)
  - LVEF of equal to or less than 35%
- Benefits of CRT in patients with non-left bundle branch block morphology and intermediate QRS duration (120–149 ms) are more unpredictable. Further, the absence of response in up to 30% of cases in most studies highlights the need for improved selection criteria [38–42].

Dyssynchrony Evaluation

- Basic assessment of dyssynchrony begins with a standard, comprehensive echocardiographic examination, including precise evaluation of the LV (the biplane method of discs or the Simpson rule) and RV systolic functions, LV diastolic function, and filling pressures. Alternatively, the LV volumes and the EF can be assessed by full-volume 3D study.
- Specific attention should be paid to the presence, mechanism, and severity of mitral regurgitation.
- Presence of viable tissue increases the likelihood of a favorable response to CRT implantation.
- Though not an indication for CRT in itself, the presence of substantial mitral regurgitation lends additional support to an indication for biventricular pacing. Indeed, a decrease in the mitral regurgitation grade has consistently been shown in cases undergoing CRT [39, 43–45].
- A more improvement attributed to the LV reverse remodeling has also been reported.
- LV dyssynchrony can occur in three levels:

1. Atrioventricular dyssynchrony
2. Interventricular dyssynchrony
3. Intraventricular dyssynchrony

- Although the echocardiographic evaluation of the LV dyssynchrony is not necessary for patient selection for CRT, the presence or absence of the LV dyssynchrony has prognostic effects [39].

Atrioventricular Dyssynchrony

Atrioventricular dyssynchrony is measured by the ratio of the diastolic filling time to the cardiac cycle (Fig. 11.14). A diastolic filling time less than 40% is abnormal [46, 47].

Interventricular Dyssynchrony

- Presence of interventricular dyssynchrony is easily studied by measuring the difference of the left and right pre-ejection intervals. These intervals are measured from the onset of the QRS complex to the onset of the corresponding Doppler ejection signal. While values of 20 ± 10 ms have been measured in healthy control subjects, a delay of more than 40 ms is considered indicative of interventricular dyssynchrony [46].
- Measurement of the delayed mid peak systolic velocity of the RV free wall and the LV by TDI has also been used to study interventricular dyssynchrony. The presence of interventricular dyssynchrony, however, appears to be faintly associated with morbidity, mortality, and response to CRT—thereby limiting its clinical usefulness [39].

Intraventricular Dyssynchrony

The study of intraventricular dyssynchrony should first and foremost rely on qualitative visual valuation. This essential first step constitutes a screening evaluation and is also beneficial to support information obtained by purely quantitative methods. In cases of dilated cardiomyopathy, an undulating systolic movement may be observed beginning at the level of the interventricular septum and extending to the other LV segments—typically with the late activation of the LV lateral wall. Quantitative evaluation based on quantitative criteria is major in establishing the diagnosis and studying the severity of the LV dyssynchrony [48, 49].

A septal-to-posterior wall delay longer than 130 ms was found to be a good predictor of reverse remodeling after CRT initiation (63% specificity, 100% sensitivity and 85% accuracy) [48], with responders defined as cases having a 15% or more decrease in the LV end-systolic volume [50].

- This criterion was later found to be associated with fewer clinical events during long-term follow-up. Though easily applied, this method is again limited by the difficulty in exactly identifying peak systolic velocity in the presence of tethering effect in ischemic cardiomyopathy. Most importantly, septal-to-posterior wall delay did not predict clinical or echocardiographic response to CRT [51]. Lastly, the aortic pre-ejection interval, measured from the onset of the QRS to the onset of the aortic flow, has been recommended as a marker of the LV dyssynchrony. Values ranging more than 140 ms have been used as indicators of dyssynchrony [52, 53].

Tissue Doppler Imaging

- Previously, TDI was more widely applied for dyssynchrony assessment. Afterward, the PROSPECT study showed that it cannot be considered the gold standard for dyssynchrony assessment [52].
- TDI permits regional myocardial velocity measurement. Precise determination of the amplitude, timing of onset,

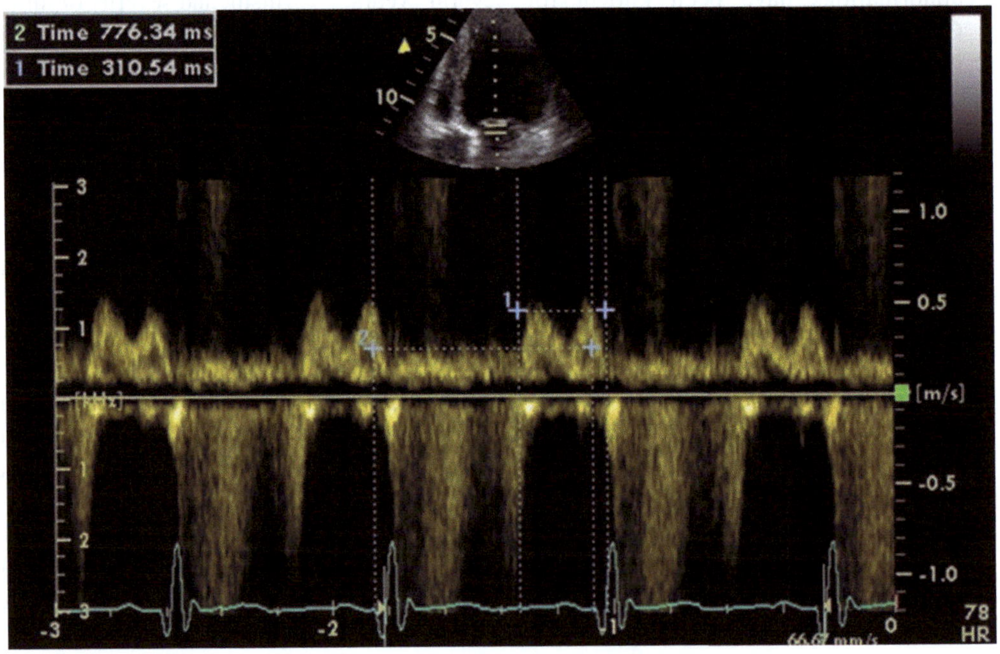

Fig. 11.14 Pulsed-wave Doppler study of the mitral inflow, showing no significant atrioventricular dyssynchrony (310.5/776 = 40%)

and peak systolic and diastolic velocities may be obtained in relation to the ECG signal. Several new methods have been derived from TDI that yield a quantitative and detailed evaluation of the LV dyssynchrony. Pulsed-wave TDI, a standard TDI recording, with the sample volume placed in the center of a myocardial segment (rather than on the mitral valve annulus as for diastolic function evaluation), typically demonstrates two systolic and two diastolic deflections [54–56].

- Closely after the QRS onset, a first positive low-amplitude systolic signal, corresponding to the isovolumic contraction time, is observed. The second positive systolic deflection, the S wave, is frequently of a higher amplitude than the first one. In diastole, two negative deflections are noted—namely the Ea and Aa waves, corresponding to early rapid filling and atrial contraction, respectively.

The limitations of pulsed-wave TDI include the restriction of measurements to single points during one cardiac cycle and the occasionally hard identification of low-amplitude systolic waves, particularly in the presence of interfering motion artifacts. Therefore, a comparison of different myocardial segments requires multiple, non-simultaneous acquisitions with the inherent limitation of variations due to changes in the heart rate, loading situations, or respiration [56, 57].

Reconstructed TDI analysis: To overcome some of the limitations of pulsed-wave TDI, the operator should record color TDI loops and analyze them off-line as reconstructed signals [58].

Strain and Strain Rate

- Noninvasive evaluation of the regional function can be done by measuring myocardial strain or deformation. Strain is a dimensionless index, expressed as a percentage of change in the length of the myocardial fibers from their original length.
- By convention, lengthening or expansion has a positive value, while shortening or compression is assigned a negative value. The strain rate, the time derivative of strain, represents the rate of myocardial deformation. Derived from TDI velocity data, these parameters have the benefit of differentiating active contraction from passive motion caused by the tethering of the adjacent myocardial regions [58, 59].
- Data can be expressed either as 2D color maps or tracings that depict strain/strain rate variations according to time. The parametric imaging of the LV wall displacement or tissue tracking is also derived from color TDI data. Tissue tracking offers a simple visual evaluation of the regional myocardial function and timing, thereby permitting rapid study of the LV dyssynchrony. Otherwise, the data may be expressed as tracings of the LV wall displacement as a function of time [60]. Despite its theoretical benefits, the clinical application of TDI-derived strain imaging remains limited—mainly because of its variable reproducibility and substantial angle dependency [58].

Tissue Synchronization Imaging

- Tissue synchronization imaging is another method to study dyssynchrony. Tissue synchronization imaging consists of an automated analysis of electro-systolic delay data, with color coding of this delay with reference to the QRS.

An automated color-coding algorithm assigns a different color according to the timing of the peak velocity—with green for earliest activation, followed by yellow/orange for intermediate activation and red for latest activation (Fig. 11.15). Reconstructed as a color map, tissue synchronization imaging confers direct and rapid visualization of segments with asynchrony [46, 61].

- Association between mechanical dyssynchrony and arrhythmia in heart failure and syncope in patients with hypertrophic cardiomyopathy has also been suggested [62].

Speckle-Tracking Echocardiography (2D Strain Echocardiography)

- STE tracks the movement of the speckles and assess myocardial deformation in longitudinal, radial, and circumferential directions.

In a recent study on a large series of patients who received CRT, Delgado et al. found that the baseline global circumferential strain and the global longitudinal strain (GLS) could add more prognostic value than the ECG criteria selection and the LVEF value. They showed that the cutoff value of −9% for both global longitudinal strain and global circumferential strain was associated with long-term outcomes. Indeed, a global longitudinal strain greater than −9% and a global circumferential strain greater than −9% were associated with increased risk and unfavorable events [63].

3D Echocardiography

3D echocardiography, initially as reconstructed images and more recently as real-time acquisition, provides reproducible study of the LV volumes, dimensions, and systolic function. Using dedicated reconstruction software, semi-automated border detection permits continuous volume calculation of all 16 myocardial segments instantaneously. Represented as regional volumetric curves during the cardiac cycle, the timing of the minimal volume for each segment may be analyzed. The systolic dyssynchrony index, which is the time to the minimal regional volume, is a marker of the LV dyssyn-

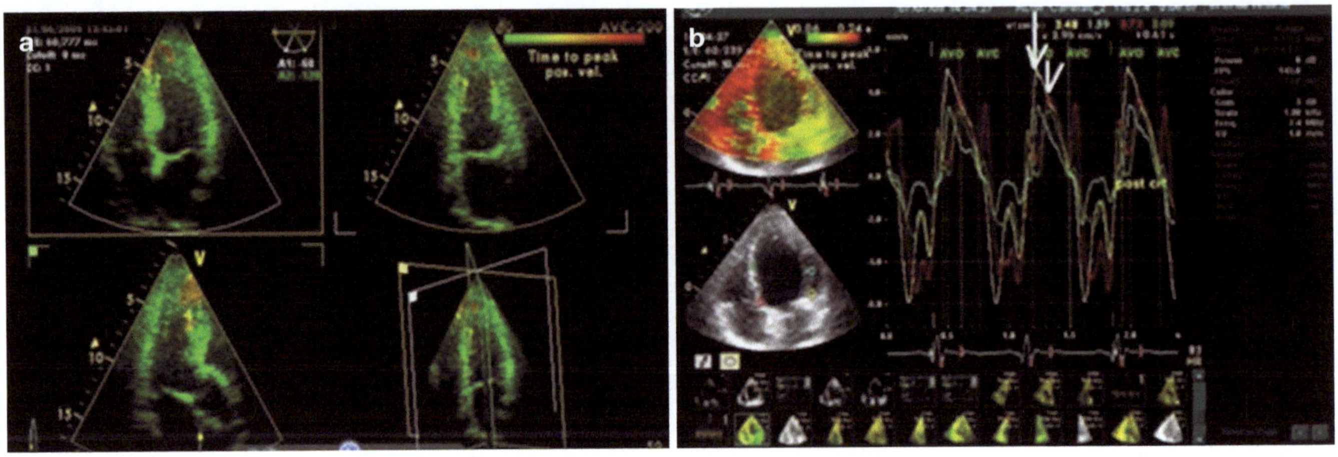

Fig. 11.15 Left: Color-coded tissue Doppler imaging or tissue synchronization imaging of three apical views, showing normal synchronous contraction as green color (**a**). Right: Significant dyssynchrony between the septal and lateral walls (**b**) (white arrow and arrow head)

chrony and a cutoff value of 6.4% has been suggested with sensitivity of 88% and specificity of 85% to predict CRT responders [64, 65].

- With normal homogeneous activation, the different LV segments reach their minimal volume at the same time, while in the presence of dyssynchrony, minimal volumes are achieved at different time points. Displayed as a polar color map, real-time 3D imaging offers instantaneous imagining of all the segments—with easy documentation of the dyssynchrony [65].
- Limitations of the present software include suboptimal imaging in cases with poor acoustic windows and time-consuming offline analysis [66].

Conclusions

CRT is now considered a standard therapeutic strategy for refractory heart failure. Although echocardiographic evaluation of the LV dyssynchrony is not necessary for patient selection for CRT, the presence or absence of the LV dyssynchrony has prognostic effects. New methods such as real-time 3D echocardiography, which are still under active evaluation, may prove to be worthwhile.

Questions

1. Which of the following equation is echocardiography based estimation of pulmonary vascular resistance?
   A. $PVR = \frac{TRV}{VTI_{RVOT}} \cdot 0.16$
   B. $PVR = \frac{VTI_{RVOT}}{TRV} \cdot 0.16 + 10$
   C. $PVR = \frac{TRV}{VTI_{RVOT}} \cdot 10 + 0.16$
   D. $PVR = \frac{TRV}{VTI_{RVOT}} + 0.16$

2. All of the following statements about mitral regurgitation in systolic heart failure are true EXCEPT
   A. Regional LV remodeling increases valve regurgitation
   B. The degree of MR is associated with the severity of the LV dysfunction
   C. The severity of MR is an indicator of the prognosis
   D. MR occurs in the presence of structurally normal mitral leaflets

3. Which of the following statement regarding speckle-tracking echocardiography in heart failure is not true?
   A. Plays an important role in myocardial viability assessment
   B. Can provide high sensitivity in the assessment of the LV function
   C. Can predict the infarct size after MI
   D. Is dependent on the angle of insonation

4. Which of the following method can be used to estimate LV volumes and ejection fraction without geometrical assumptions?
   A. Teichholz and Quinones
   B. Prolate- ellipsoid
   C. Area-length
   D. 3D echocardiography

Answers

1. C
2. B
3. D
4. D

References

1. Otto CM. The practice of clinical echocardiography. 5th ed. Philadelphia: Saunders; 2017. p. 107–27.
2. Kumar N, Oommen R, Thomson VS, Jose JV. Assessment of left ventricular systolic function by velocity vector imaging. Indian Heart J. 2012;64(2):146–9.
3. Wang TJ, Evans JC, Benjamin EJ, Levy D, LeRoy EC, Vasan RS. Natural history of asymptomatic left ventricular systolic dysfunction in the community. Circulation. 2003;108(8):977–82.
4. Mulvagh SL, DeMaria AN, Feinstein SB, Burns PN, Kaul S, Miller JG, et al. Contrast echocardiography: current and future applications. J Am Soc Echocardiogr. 2000;13(4):331–42.
5. Gutgesell HP. Echocardiographic assessment of cardiac function in infants and children. J Am Coll Cardiol. 1985;5(1 Suppl):95s–103s.
6. Cameli M, Mondillo S, Solari M, Righini FM, Andrei V, Contaldi C, et al. Echocardiographic assessment of left ventricular systolic function: from ejection fraction to torsion. Heart Fail Rev. 2016;21(1):77–94.
7. Quinones MA, Waggoner AD, Reduto LA, Nelson JG, Young JB, Winters WL Jr, et al. A new, simplified and accurate method for determining ejection fraction with two-dimensional echocardiography. Circulation. 1981;64(4):744–53.
8. Wandt B, Bojo L, Tolagen K, Wranne B. Echocardiographic assessment of ejection fraction in left ventricular hypertrophy. Heart. 1999;82(2):192–8.
9. Gottdiener JS, Bednarz J, Devereux R, Gardin J, Klein A, Manning WJ, et al. American Society of Echocardiography recommendations for use of echocardiography in clinical trials. J Am Soc Echocardiogr. 2004;17(10):1086–119.
10. Lang RM, Badano LP, Mor-Avi V, Afilalo J, Armstrong A, Ernande L, et al. Recommendations for cardiac chamber quantification by echocardiography in adults: an update from the American Society of Echocardiography and the European Association of Cardiovascular Imaging. J Am Soc Echocardiogr. 2015;28(1):1–39. e14.
11. Otterstad JE, Froeland G, St John Sutton M, Holme I. Accuracy and reproducibility of biplane two-dimensional echocardiographic measurements of left ventricular dimensions and function. Eur Heart J. 1997;18(3):507–13.
12. Senni M, Rodeheffer RJ, Tribouilloy CM, Evans JM, Jacobsen SJ, Bailey KR, et al. Use of echocardiography in the management of congestive heart failure in the community. J Am Coll Cardiol. 1999;33(1):164–70.
13. Dorosz JL, Lezotte DC, Weitzenkamp DA, Allen LA, Salcedo EE. Performance of 3-dimensional echocardiography in measuring left ventricular volumes and ejection fraction: a systematic review and meta-analysis. J Am Coll Cardiol. 2012;59(20):1799–808.
14. Marwick TH. Methods used for the assessment of LV systolic function: common currency or tower of Babel? Heart. 2013;99(15):1078–86.
15. Mannaerts HF, van der Heide JA, Kamp O, Stoel MG, Twisk J, Visser CA. Early identification of left ventricular remodelling after myocardial infarction, assessed by transthoracic 3D echocardiography. Eur Heart J. 2004;25(8):680–7.
16. Marwick TH. The role of echocardiography in heart failure. J Nucl Med. 2015;56(Suppl 4):31s–8s.
17. Bax JJ, Poldermans D, Schinkel AF, Boersma E, Elhendy A, Maat A, et al. Perfusion and contractile reserve in chronic dysfunctional myocardium: relation to functional outcome after surgical revascularization. Circulation. 2002;106(12 Suppl 1):I14–8.
18. Schinkel AF, Bax JJ, van Domburg R, Elhendy A, Valkema R, Vourvouri EC, et al. Dobutamine-induced contractile reserve in stunned, hibernating, and scarred myocardium in patients with ischemic cardiomyopathy. J Nucl Med. 2003;44(2):127–33.
19. Jambrik Z, Monti S, Coppola V, Agricola E, Mottola G, Miniati M, et al. Usefulness of ultrasound lung comets as a nonradiologic sign of extravascular lung water. Am J Cardiol. 2004;93(10):1265–70.
20. Picano E, Frassi F, Agricola E, Gligorova S, Gargani L, Mottola G. Ultrasound lung comets: a clinically useful sign of extravascular lung water. J Am Soc Echocardiogr. 2006;19(3):356–63.
21. Natanzon A, Kronzon I. Pericardial and pleural effusions in congestive heart failure-anatomical, pathophysiologic, and clinical considerations. Am J Med Sci. 2009;338(3):211–6.
22. Klein AL, Abbara S, Agler DA, Appleton CP, Asher CR, Hoit B, et al. American Society of Echocardiography clinical recommendations for multimodality cardiovascular imaging of patients with pericardial disease: endorsed by the Society for Cardiovascular Magnetic Resonance and Society of Cardiovascular Computed Tomography. J Am Soc Echocardiogr. 2013;26(9):965–1012. e15.
23. Ayuela Azcarate JM, Clau Terre F, Ochagavia A, Vicho Pereira R. Role of echocardiography in the hemodynamic monitorization of critical patients. Med Intensiva. 2012;36(3):220–32.
24. Stein JH, Neumann A, Preston LM, Costanzo MR, Parrillo JE, Johnson MR, et al. Echocardiography for hemodynamic assessment of patients with advanced heart failure and potential heart transplant recipients. J Am Coll Cardiol. 1997;30(7):1765–72.
25. St John Sutton M. A comprehensive noninvasive hemodynamic assessment of systolic heart failure. Circ Heart Fail. 2010;3(3):337–9.
26. Abbas AE, Fortuin FD, Schiller NB, Appleton CP, Moreno CA, Lester SJ. A simple method for noninvasive estimation of pulmonary vascular resistance. J Am Coll Cardiol. 2003;41(6):1021–7.
27. Howard LS, Grapsa J, Dawson D, Bellamy M, Chambers JB, Masani ND, et al. Echocardiographic assessment of pulmonary hypertension: standard operating procedure. Eur Respir Rev. 2012;21(125):239–48.
28. Lancellotti P, Gerard PL, Pierard LA. Long-term outcome of patients with heart failure and dynamic functional mitral regurgitation. Eur Heart J. 2005;26(15):1528–32.
29. Lamas GA, Mitchell GF, Flaker GC, Smith SC Jr, Gersh BJ, Basta L, et al. Clinical significance of mitral regurgitation after acute myocardial infarction. Survival and Ventricular Enlargement Investigators. Circulation. 1997;96(3):827–33.
30. Yiu SF, Enriquez-Sarano M, Tribouilloy C, Seward JB, Tajik AJ. Determinants of the degree of functional mitral regurgitation in patients with systolic left ventricular dysfunction: a quantitative clinical study. Circulation. 2000;102(12):1400–6.
31. Ciampi Q, Villari B. Role of echocardiography in diagnosis and risk stratification in heart failure with left ventricular systolic dysfunction. Cardiovasc Ultrasound. 2007;5:34.
32. Sadeghpour A, Abtahi F, Kiavar M, Esmaeilzadeh M, Samiei N, Ojaghi SZ, et al. Echocardiographic evaluation of mitral geometry in functional mitral regurgitation. J Cardiothorac Surg. 2008;3(1):54.
33. Schwarzwald CC, Schober KE, Bonagura JD. Methods and reliability of tissue Doppler imaging for assessment of left ventricular radial wall motion in horses. J Vet Intern Med. 2009;23(3):643–52.
34. ur Rahman H, Khan SB, Noor L, Hadi A, Nawaz T, Shah ST, et al. Assessment of left ventricular systolic and diastolic function by tis-

sue Doppler imaging after acute myocardial infarction. J Ayub Med Coll Abbottabad. 2011;23(2):108–11.
35. Abduch MC, Alencar AM, Mathias W Jr, Vieira ML. Cardiac mechanics evaluated by speckle tracking echocardiography. Arq Bras Cardiol. 2014;102(4):403–12.
36. Mondillo S, Galderisi M, Mele D, Cameli M, Lomoriello VS, Zaca V, et al. Speckle-tracking echocardiography: a new technique for assessing myocardial function. J Ultrasound Med. 2011;30(1):71–83.
37. Nahum J, Bensaid A, Dussault C, Macron L, Clemence D, Bouhemad B, et al. Impact of longitudinal myocardial deformation on the prognosis of chronic heart failure patients. Circ Cardiovasc Imaging. 2010;3(3):249–56.
38. Bajraktari G, Henein MY. The clinical dilemma of quantifying mechanical left ventricular dyssynchrony for cardiac resynchronization therapy: segmental or global? Echocardiography. 2015;32(1):150–5.
39. Bax JJ, Bleeker GB, Marwick TH, Molhoek SG, Boersma E, Steendijk P, et al. Left ventricular dyssynchrony predicts response and prognosis after cardiac resynchronization therapy. J Am Coll Cardiol. 2004;44(9):1834–40.
40. Brignole M, Auricchio A, Baron-Esquivias G, Bordachar P, Boriani G, Breithardt OA, et al. 2013 ESC guidelines on cardiac pacing and cardiac resynchronization therapy: the task force on cardiac pacing and resynchronization therapy of the European Society of Cardiology (ESC). Developed in collaboration with the European Heart Rhythm Association (EHRA). Europace. 2013;15(8):1070–118.
41. Cleland J, Freemantle N, Ghio S, Fruhwald F, Shankar A, Marijanowski M, et al. Predicting the long-term effects of cardiac resynchronization therapy on mortality from baseline variables and the early response a report from the CARE-HF (Cardiac Resynchronization in Heart Failure) Trial. J Am Coll Cardiol. 2008;52(6):438–45.
42. Parameswaran AC, Purushottam B, Amanullah A, Figueredo VM. Distribution of dyssynchrony in subjects with no known cardiac disease and comparison of velocity vector imaging to color-coded tissue Doppler imaging. Echocardiography. 2013;30(2):180–9.
43. Solomon SD, Foster E, Bourgoun M, Shah A, Viloria E, Brown MW, et al. Effect of cardiac resynchronization therapy on reverse remodeling and relation to outcome: multicenter automatic defibrillator implantation trial: cardiac resynchronization therapy. Circulation. 2010;122(10):985–92.
44. Verbrugge FH, Verhaert D, Grieten L, Dupont M, Rivero-Ayerza M, De Vusser P, et al. Revisiting diastolic filling time as mechanistic insight for response to cardiac resynchronization therapy. Europace. 2013;15(12):1747–56.
45. Wu VC-C, Takeuchi M. Three-dimensional echocardiography: current status and real-life applications. Acta Cardiol Sin. 2017;33(2):107–18.
46. Edner M, Kim Y, Hansen KN, Nissen H, Espersen G, La Rosee K, et al. Prevalence and inter-relationship of different Doppler measures of dyssynchrony in patients with heart failure and prolonged QRS: a report from CARE-HF. Cardiovasc Ultrasound. 2009;7:1.
47. van der Hulst AE, Delgado V, Blom NA, van de Veire NR, Schalij MJ, Bax JJ, et al. Cardiac resynchronization therapy in paediatric and congenital heart disease patients. Eur Heart J. 2011;32(18):2236–46.
48. Galderisi M, Cattaneo F, Mondillo S. Doppler echocardiography and myocardial dyssynchrony: a practical update of old and new ultrasound technologies. Cardiovasc Ultrasound. 2007;5:28.
49. Pitzalis MV, Iacoviello M, Romito R, Massari F, Rizzon B, Luzzi G, et al. Cardiac resynchronization therapy tailored by echocardiographic evaluation of ventricular asynchrony. J Am Coll Cardiol. 2002;40(9):1615–22.
50. Delgado V, Ypenburg C, van Bommel RJ, Tops LF, Mollema SA, Marsan NA, et al. Assessment of left ventricular dyssynchrony by speckle tracking strain imaging: comparison between longitudinal, circumferential, and radial strain in cardiac resynchronization therapy. J Am Coll Cardiol. 2008;51(20):1944–52.
51. Marcus GM, Rose E, Viloria EM, Schafer J, De Marco T, Saxon LA, et al. Septal to posterior wall motion delay fails to predict reverse remodeling or clinical improvement in patients undergoing cardiac resynchronization therapy. J Am Coll Cardiol. 2005;46(12):2208–14.
52. Chung ES, Leon AR, Tavazzi L, Sun JP, Nihoyannopoulos P, Merlino J, et al. Results of the predictors of response to CRT (PROSPECT) trial. Circulation. 2008;117(20):2608–16.
53. Gorcsan J 3rd. Echocardiographic assessment of ventricular dyssynchrony. Curr Heart Fail Rep. 2008;5(1):31–7.
54. Cho EJ, Caracciolo G, Khandheria BK, Steidley DE, Scott R, Abhayaratna WP, et al. Tissue Doppler image-derived measurements during isovolumic contraction predict exercise capacity in patients with reduced left ventricular ejection fraction. JACC Cardiovasc Imaging. 2010;3(1):1–9.
55. De Backer J, Matthys D, Gillebert TC, De Paepe A, De Sutter J. The use of Tissue Doppler Imaging for the assessment of changes in myocardial structure and function in inherited cardiomyopathies. Eur J Echocardiogr. 2005;6(4):243–50.
56. Kadappu KK, Thomas L. Tissue Doppler imaging in echocardiography: value and limitations. Heart Lung Circ. 2015;24(3):224–33.
57. Mundigler G, Zehetgruber M. Tissue Doppler Imaging: myocardial velocities and strain—are there clinical applications? J Clin Basic Cardiol. 2002;5(2):125–32.
58. Dandel M, Lehmkuhl H, Knosalla C, Suramelashvili N, Hetzer R. Strain and strain rate imaging by echocardiography – basic concepts and clinical applicability. Curr Cardiol Rev. 2009;5(2):133–48.
59. Marwick TH. Measurement of strain and strain rate by echocardiography: ready for prime time? J Am Coll Cardiol. 2006;47(7):1313–27.
60. Marwick TH, Yu C-M, Sun JP, editors. Myocardial imaging: tissue Doppler and speckle tracking. Malden: Wiley-Blackwell; 2007.
61. Van de Veire NR, Bleeker GB, De Sutter J, Ypenburg C, Holman ER, van der Wall EE, et al. Tissue synchronisation imaging accurately measures left ventricular dyssynchrony and predicts response to cardiac resynchronisation therapy. Heart. 2007;93(9):1034–9.
62. Sadeghpour A, Kyavar M, Behzadnia N, Maddadi S, Parsaei M, Maleki M, et al. Left ventricular systolic dyssynchrony in patients with hypertrophic cardiomyopathy: the prevalence and its relation to syncope. Iran Cardivasc Res J. 2010;4(4):152–8.
63. Delgado-Montero A, Tayal B, Goda A, Ryo K, Marek JJ, Sugahara M, et al. Additive prognostic value of echocardiographic global longitudinal and global circumferential strain to electrocardiographic criteria in patients with heart failure undergoing cardiac resynchronization therapy. Circ Cardiovasc Imaging. 2016;9(6):e004241.
64. Badano LP, Lang RM, Zamorano JL. Textbook of real-time three dimensional echocardiography. New York: Springer; 2011.
65. Marsan NA, Bleeker GB, Ypenburg C, Van Bommel RJ, Ghio S, Van de Veire NR, et al. Real-time three-dimensional echocardiography as a novel approach to assess left ventricular and left atrium reverse remodeling and to predict response to cardiac resynchronization therapy. Heart Rhythm. 2008;5(9):1257–64.
66. Rabben SI. Technical principles of transthoracic three-dimensional echocardiography. In: Badano L, Lang RM, Zamorano JL, editors. Textbook of real-time three dimensional echocardiography. London: Springer; 2010. p. 9–24.

Echocardiographic Assessment of Myocardial Mechanics: Velocity, Strain, Strain Rate and Torsion

12

Hoorak Poorzand, Anita Sadeghpour, Azin Alizadehasl, and Samir Saha

Abstract

Echocardiography has been routinely used for assessment of cardiac mechanics. M-Mode and two dimensional echocardiography provide semi-quantitative data in the context of ventricular function and have limited ability in defining subtle changes in the function. Doppler tissue imaging (DTI) and Speckle tracking echocardiography (STE), two newer techniques, have emerged greater concerns for their role in quantification of ventricular systolic and diastolic function. These methods are more objective and provide more reproducible results. This chapter focuses on the technical properties of DTI, STE and tortional parameters and their clinical implication.

Keywords

Tissue Doppler imaging · Ventricular mechanics · Atrial mechanics · Strain · Velocity · Torsion

Abbreviations

2D	Two-dimensional
3D	Three-dimensional
DT	Doppler tissue
DTI	Doppler tissue imaging
ET	Ejection time
GCS	Global circumferential strain
GLS	Global longitudinal strain
GRS	Global radial strain
IVA	Isovolumic acceleration
IVCT	Isovolumic contraction time
IVRT	Isovolumic relaxation time
MPI	Myocardial performance index
ROI	Region of interest
RV	Right ventricular
SR	Strain rate
STE	Speckle-tracking echocardiography

H. Poorzand, MD, FASE
Cardiovascular Department, Faculty of Medicine, Imam Reza Hospital, Mashhad University of Medical Sciences, Mashhad, Iran

A. Sadeghpour, MD, FACC, FASE (✉)
Professor of Cardiology, Echocardiography Research Center, Rajaie Cardiovascular Medical and Research Center, Iran University of Medical Science, Tehran, Iran

A. Alizadehasl, MD, FACC, FASE
Associate Professor of Cardiology, Echocardiologist, Echocardiography and Cardiogenetic Research Centers, Cardio-Oncology Department, Rajaie Cardiovascular Medical and Research Center, Tehran, Iran

S. Saha
Cardiac Imaging Lab, Sundsvall, Sweden

Introduction

Myocardial tissue imaging and Speckle tracking have been introduced as methods to study global and regional systolic and diastolic (left and right) ventricular and atrial function. The first report appeared in 1972 which used the Doppler principle to measure myocardial velocities from the posterior left ventricular (LV) wall [1]. Development in tissue Doppler imaging in the 1990s allowed for imaging the myocardial velocity and the analysis of the segments independently of each other [2, 3].

These improvements facilitated the use of tissue Doppler imaging in evaluation of LV diastolic function and in the measurement of strain and strain-rate of each myocardial segments. Due to the limitations posed by the angle dependence of the Doppler beam, techniques based on real time, 2D echocardiography such as speckle tracking imaging were then provided [4]. This technique has been improved and is used to calculate twist and torsion [5].

Definition of the Main Parameters of Myocardial Mechanics [6, 7]:

– **Displacement (d):** The distance that a cardiac structure or myocardial element (e.g., a speckle) moves between

A. Sadeghpour, A. Alizadehasl (eds.), *Case-Based Textbook of Echocardiography*, https://doi.org/10.1007/978-3-319-67691-3_12

two consecutive frames. Displacement is measured in centimeters.

- **Velocity (v):** Displacement per unit of time or speed of a cardiac structure or speckle. It is measured in centimeters per second.
- **Strain (ε):** The fractional change in the length of a myocardial segment. Strain is unitless, usually expressed as a percentage. It is reported as positive or negative values (which reflect lengthening or shortening, respectively). It can be measured in longitudinal, circumferential and radial directions.
- **Strain rate (SR):** Rate of change in strain. It is usually expressed as 1/s or s^{-1}.
- **Segmental strain:** Strain values which can be expressed for each myocardial segment
- **Global strain:** Average value for the strain in all myocardial segments.
- **Territorial strain:** Strain value for each of the theoretical vascular distribution areas.
- **Rotation:** Rotational displacement of myocardium around the long axis of LV. It is expressed in degrees.
- **LV twist angle**: The absolute apex-to-base difference in LV rotation; also expressed in degrees.
- **Torsion:** base-to-apex gradient in the rotation angle along the long axis of the left ventricle, expressed in degrees per centimeter

Doppler Tissue Imaging (DTI)

Doppler tissue imaging is a Doppler echocardiographic technique that directly measures myocardial velocities. The intensity of the signals generated by the myocardium is higher than that generated by blood. Blood velocity usually exceeds that of the myocardium. These differences allow separation of myocardial signals from those of blood flow, using a low-pass filter.

The typical velocity of myocardium ranges from 0 to 20 cm/s and Doppler gain setting must be increased to adequately visualize DT wave forms [8].

DTI includes both color tissue Doppler and spectral pulsed Doppler (Fig. 12.1).

Spectral Pulsed Doppler

In this approach pulsed Doppler is activated and applied to measure mitral and tricuspid annulus velocities. Peak velocities, slopes, and time intervals are measured directly on the spectral display.

The Doppler velocities show systolic motion of the myocardium toward the apex which is the apical motion of the annulus in systole (Sm) (Fig. 12.2a). At diastolic phase, there is an early-diastolic motion away from the apex (Em), occurring at early phase of diastolic filling, and there is a late diastolic motion away from the apex, corresponding to the atrial phase of ventricular filing (Am).

Time intervals (ejection, isovolumic relaxation and isovolumic contraction time) could also be measured (Fig. 12.2b).

Some points are important to keep in mind while using spectral Doppler. Both sample volume and gain could influence the signal amplitudes and corresponding image quality. A sample volume should be set as 4–5 mm and position so that it remains within the region of interest inside the myocardium throughout the cardiac cycle. Excessive gain should be avoided, as this causes spectral broadening and may cause overestimation of peak velocity (Fig. 12.3).

The ultrasound beam should be aligned with the direction of the interrogated myocardial wall. The angle of incidence should not exceed 15°. So, the probability of velocity underestimation would be less than 4% (Fig. 12.4).

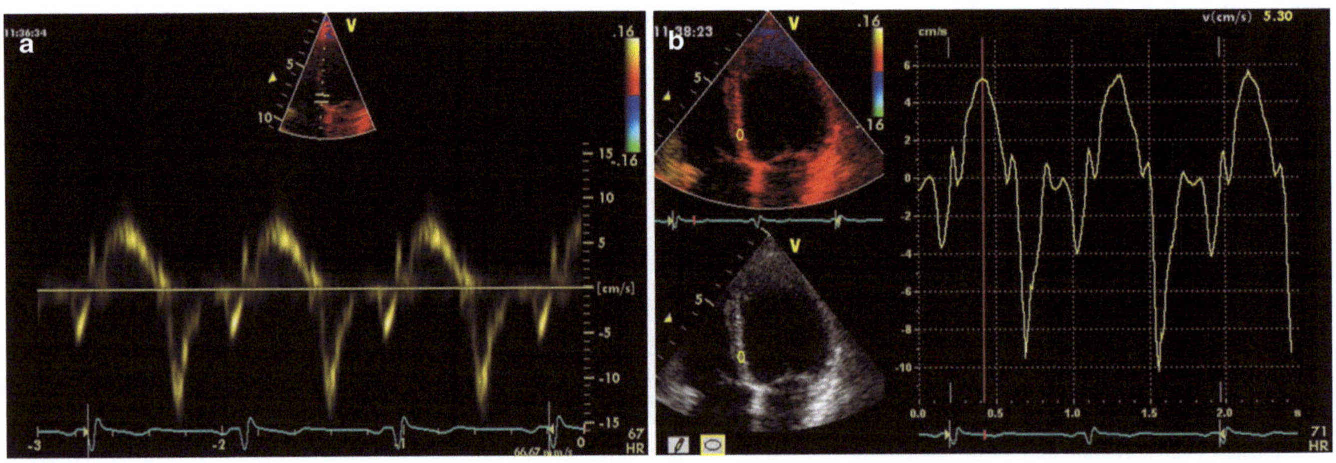

Fig. 12.1 Normal myocardial velocity obtained by spectral pulsed (**a**) and color tissue (**b**) Doppler modes

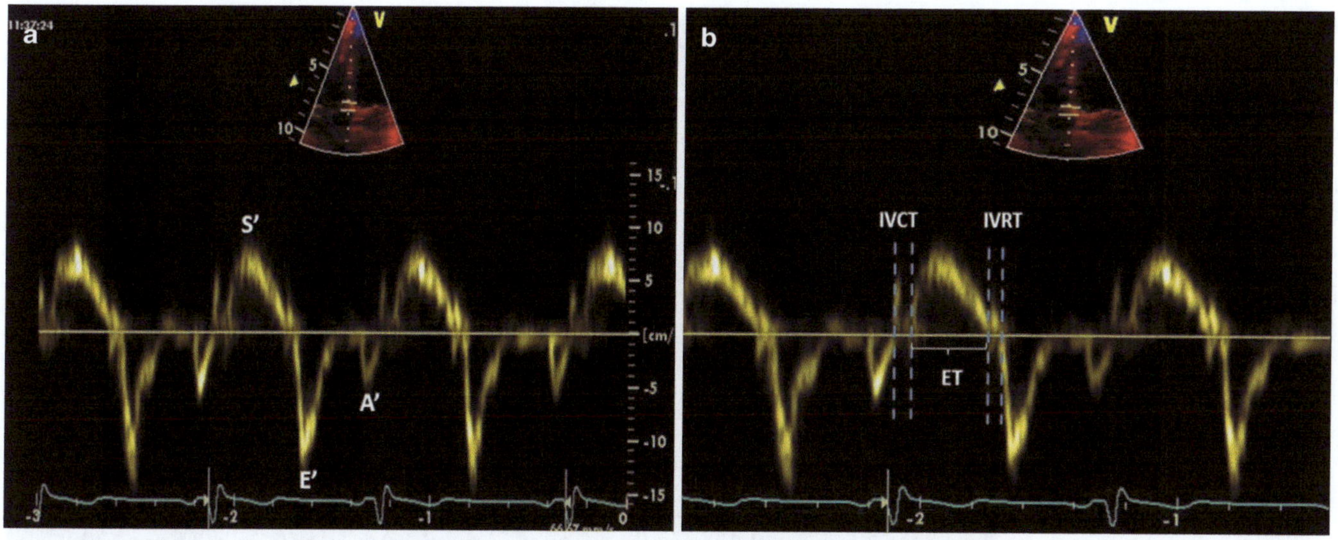

Fig. 12.2 Spectral Doppler obtained from septal side of mitral annulus, representing peak velocities (S′, E′ and A′) in A and time intervals (ET, IVCT and IVRT) in B

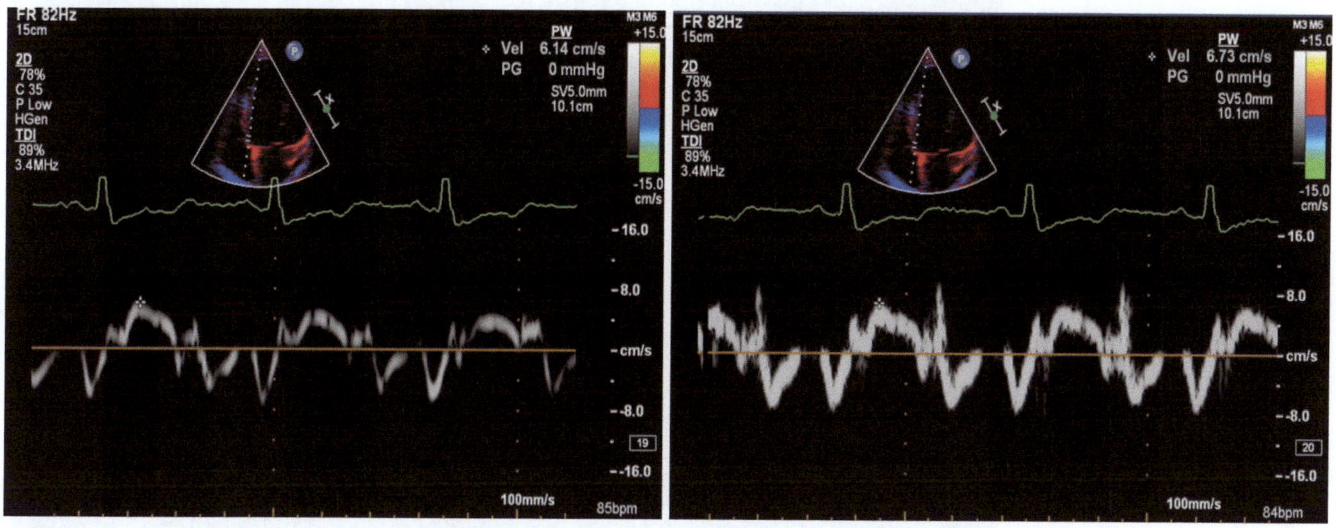

Fig. 12.3 Myocardial velocities by pulsed Doppler mode. The image in the right is obtained with a higher gain than for the left image. Consequently, the estimated S′ is higher (6.7 vs. 6.1 cm/s)

Color Tissue Doppler

In this approach, the myocardial motion is imaged as color-coded velocities superimposed on a 2D gray-scale image in real time (Fig. 12.5). At systolic phase, the base of ventricle moves toward the apex and in the diastole, moves back, while the apex is relatively stationery. These events are interrogated as red-encoded velocities in systolic phase and blue one in the diastole, in apical views.

The image should be optimized in the grayscale display before switching to the color mode and acquiring images [6]. Data can be displayed in three ways (Fig. 12.6):

1. Color coding with a straight M-mode.
2. Color coding with a curved M-mode.
3. Reconstructed curves of regional function.

This permits to track the changes in regional velocities and myocardial motion over the defined time course. Various function parameters can be derived from a selected region of interest (Fig. 12.7) within the same color Doppler data set, including velocity, displacement, SR, and strain.

To optimize the images, gain and depth adjustment, narrowing 2-D sector width (visualizing only the adjacent LV

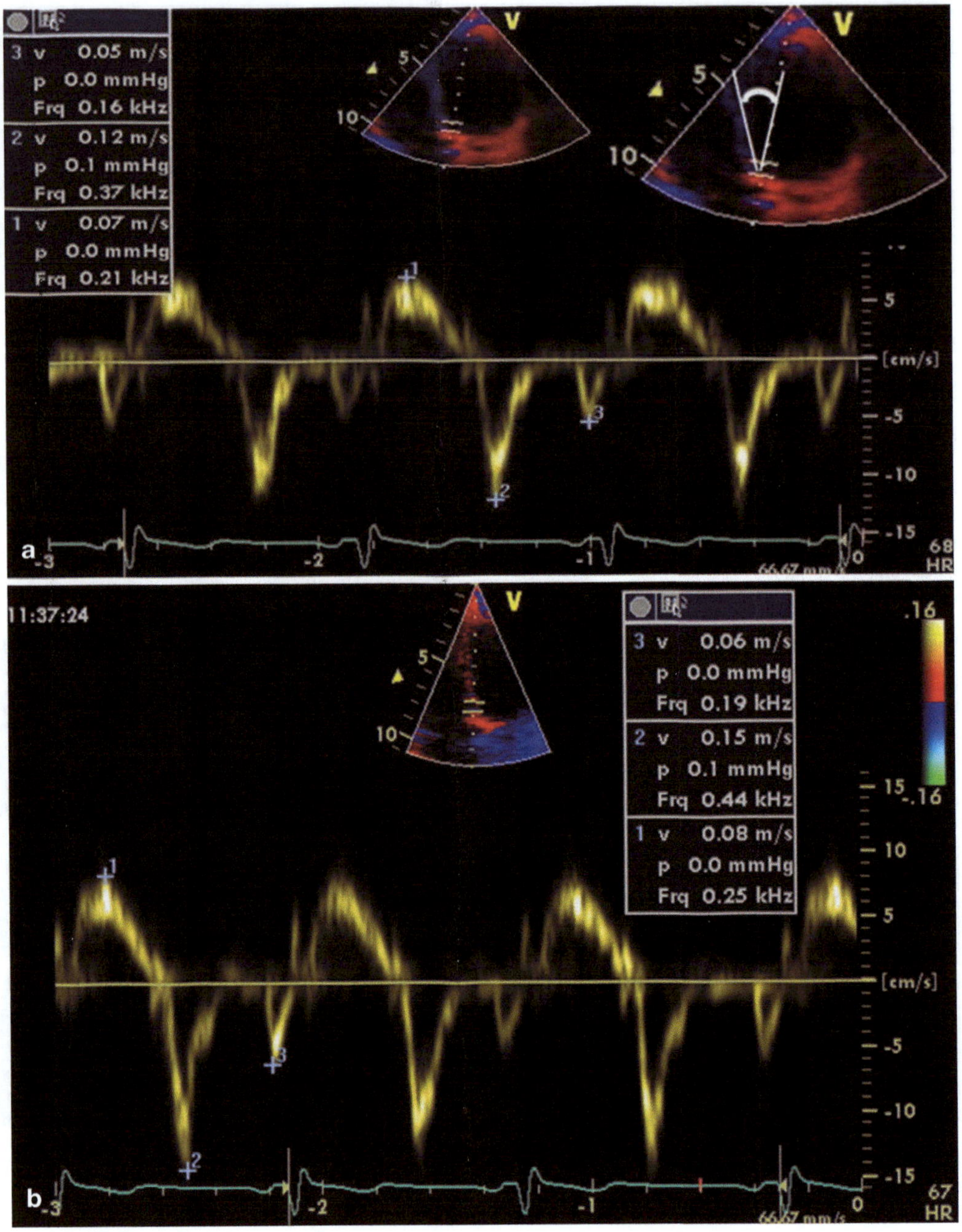

Fig. 12.4 Alignment of the ultrasound beam with the myocardila wall is important, otherwise the measurement could be inaccurate and underestimated. Note the lower velocities in A vs. B in same patient

wall segments to be assessed) are necessary. Higher frame rate (as more than 100 and ideally at least 140) is suggested which could be achieved by reducing depth and sector width. The optimal sample size would be 10 mm × 5 mm. ROI placement should be positioned within the myocardium in such a way that doesn't move away the ventricular wall through the cardiac cycle.

Systolic and diastolic velocity curves (Sm, Em and Am) and the related time intervals could be reached, the same as spectral Doppler (Fig. 12.8).

There is a velocity gradient from the base to the apex with highest velocity at the base (Fig. 12.9).

Key Points

- The fundamental difference between Color Tissue and Spectral Pulsed Doppler is that the former provides the mean velocity in the region of interest, whereas PW Doppler provides the peak velocity at a given site. So that reported pulsed Doppler peak velocity is typically 20–30% higher than that measured by color Doppler.

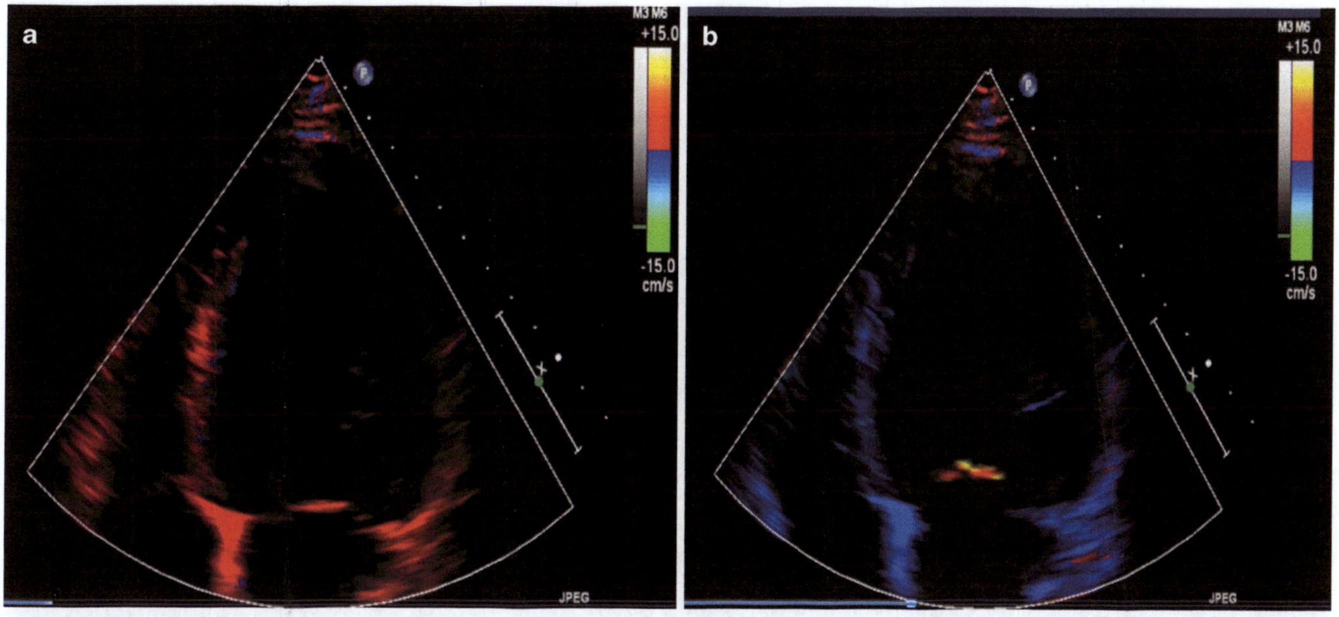

Fig. 12.5 Color coded TDI, in systole (**a**) vs. diastole (**b**); Note the red color in systolic phase in which the base of LV moves toward the apex (transducer) and blue color in diastole due to opposite motion

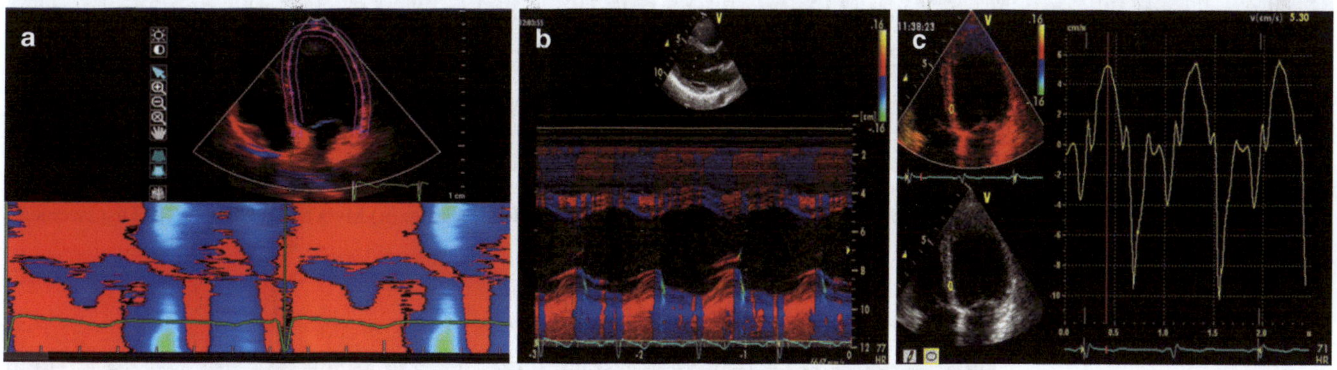

Fig. 12.6 Display of myocardial velocity in Color- coded DTI: (**a**) Curved M mode. (**b**) Straight M-Mode. (**c**) Reconstructed curves of regional function

– In Color Doppler, post processing is possible (adjusting the sample volume, not moving away the ventricular wall throughout a cardiac cycle and achieving multiple parameters of cardiac mechanics) and also we can sample different myocardial regions in the same time [6]. But in spectral Doppler, the data cannot be further processed.

Color Doppler Measurements of Cardiac Mechanics

Color DTI can provide displays of motion (velocity and displacement) and deformation (strain and strain rate) (Fig. 12.10). The relation between these parameters is shown in Fig. 12.11.

The definition, formula and the way for obtaining the data of these four parameters are as follows:

1. Velocity (v):

Doppler imaging provides velocity information. So, velocity at any site and any time can be achieved directly from the color Doppler data.

2. Displacement (d):

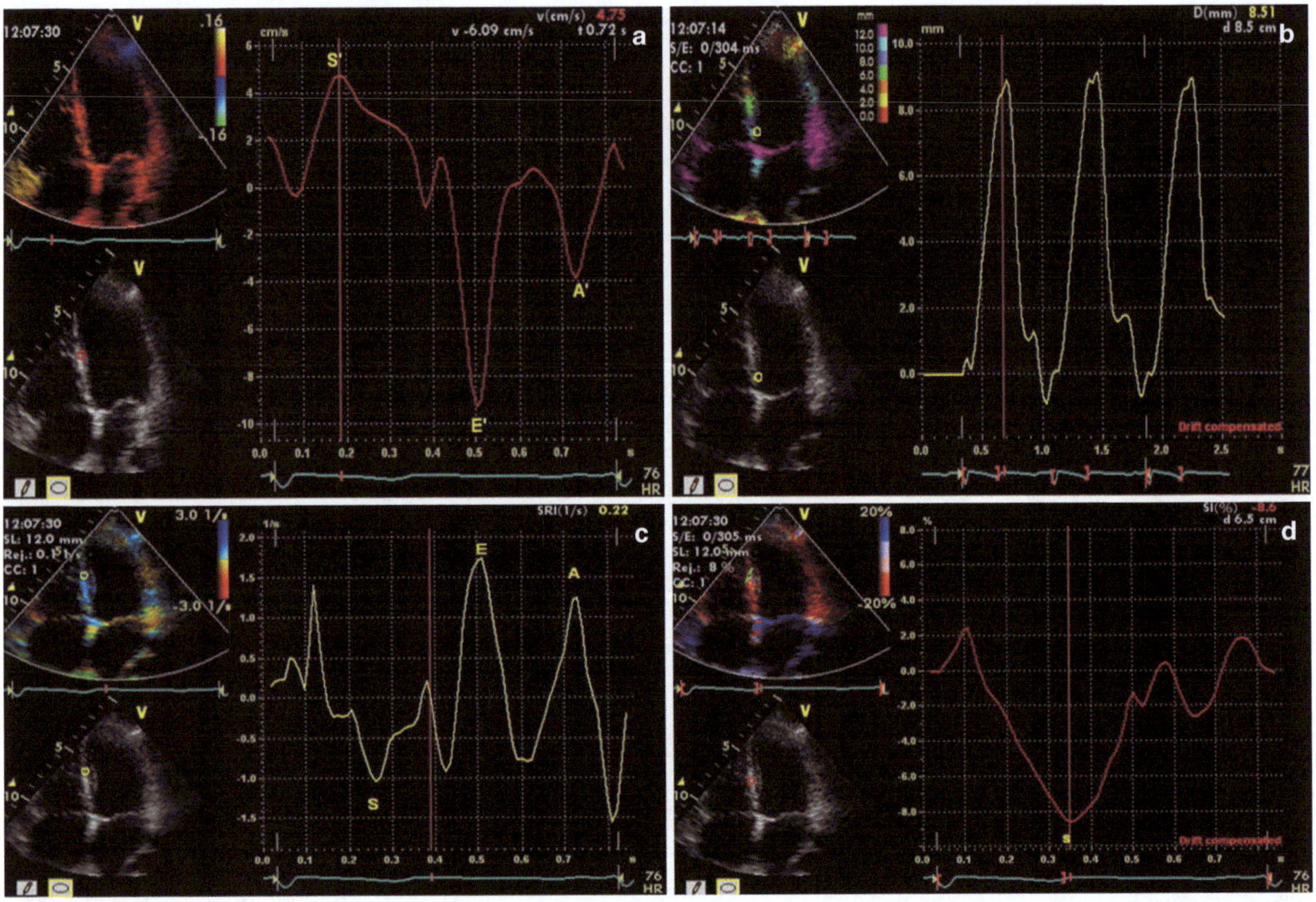

Fig. 12.7 Four parameter of myocardial function obtained from a single ROI in color coded imaging: (**a**) Myocardial velocity, (**b**) Displacement, (**c**) Strain Rate, (**d**) Strain

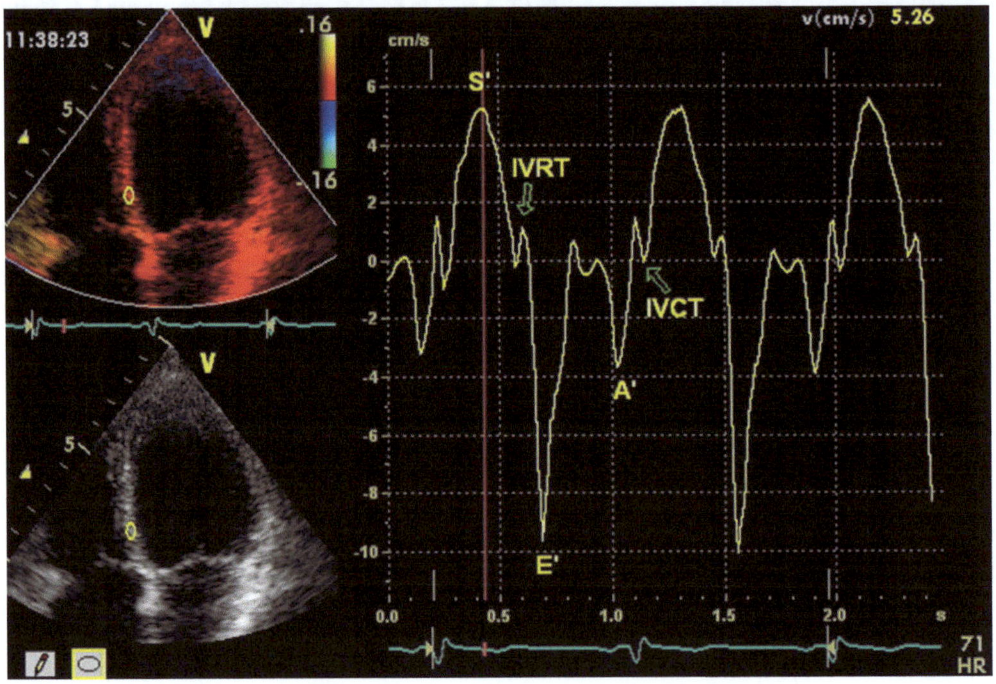

Fig. 12.8 Color Doppler wave form with ROI selected in septal segment of inferoseptum of LV; Peak velocities (S′, E′ and A′) and time intervals (IVRT, IVCT) could be derived

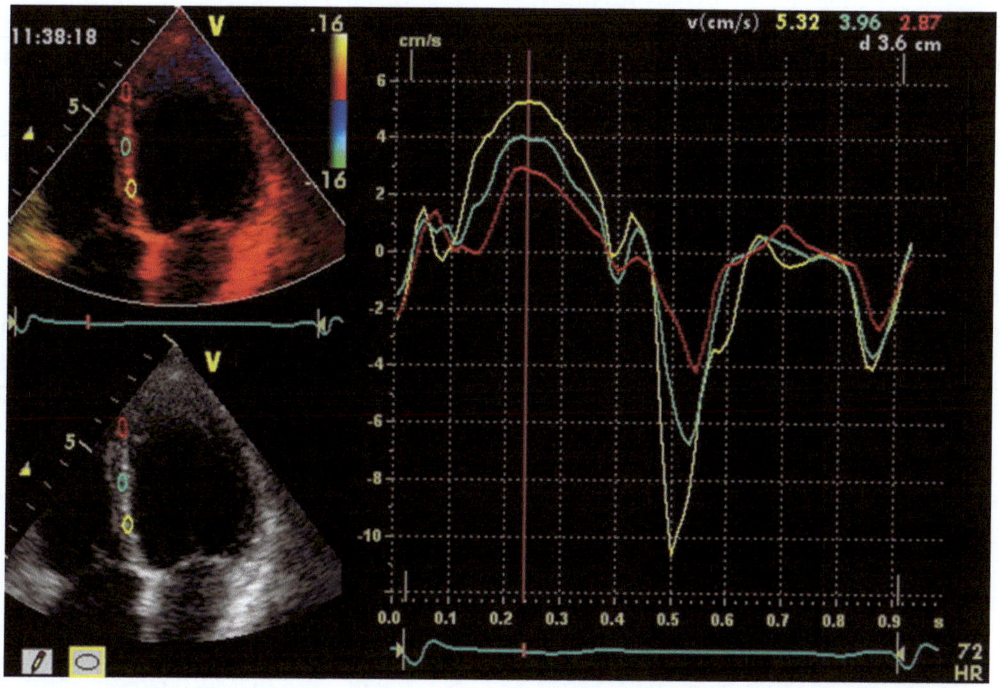

Fig. 12.9 Velocity curves obtained by color-coded DTI; Note the velocity gradient from the base to the apex

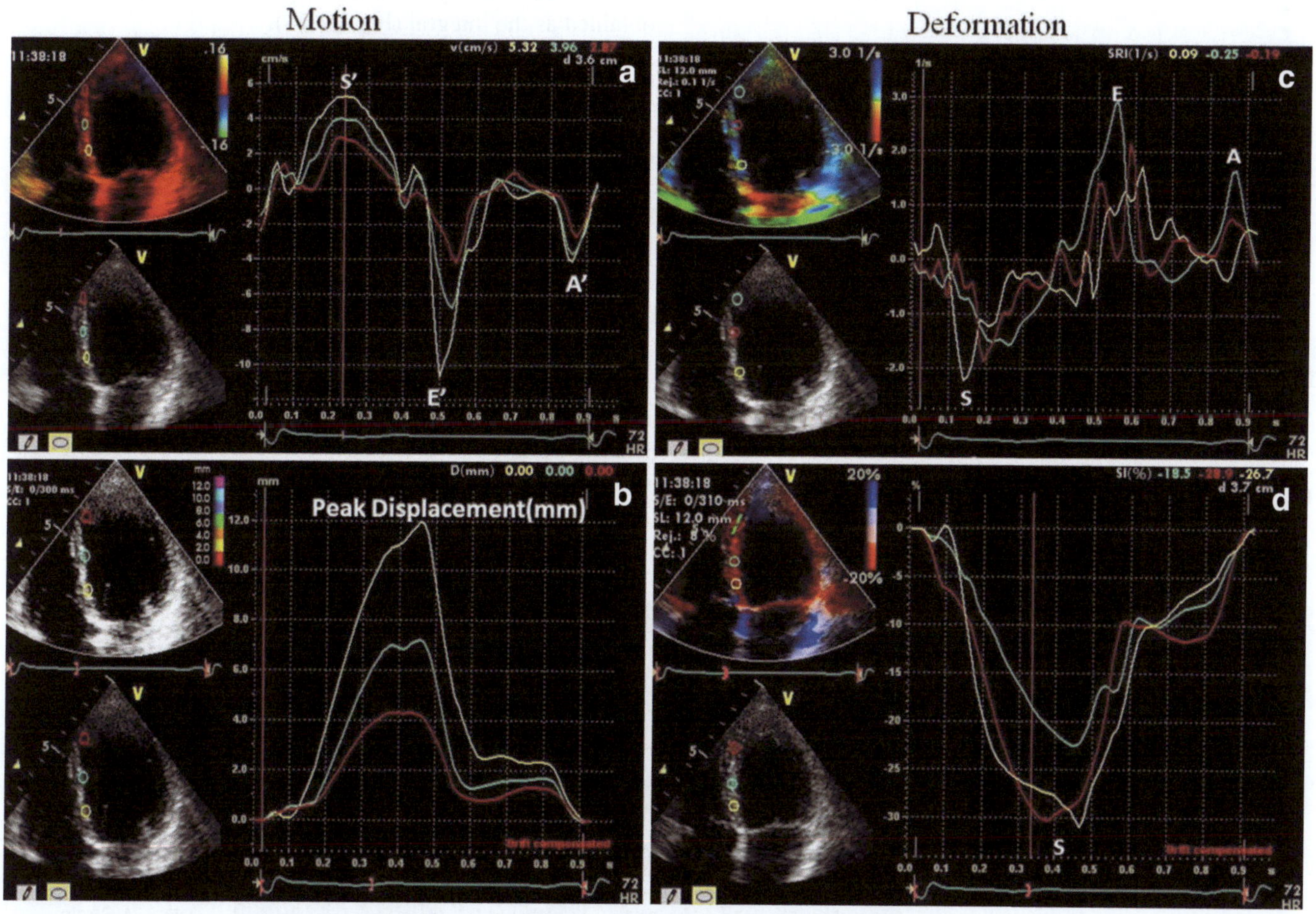

Fig. 12.10 Display of parameters of myocardial function defined as: (**a**) myocardial velocity, (**b**) Displacement, (**c**) Strain Rate, (**d**) Strain. Note the greater velocity and displacement in the base relative to the apex. Such gradient is relatively absent for deformation indices (strain/strain rate)

Displacement is obtained by calculating the temporal integral of the myocardial velocity (v):

$$d = \int v\,dt.$$

"d" describes the motion component of the myocardium in the sample volume (toward or away from the transducer).

Tissue tracking provides a color-coded display of myocardial displacement allowing for easy visualization of LV dyssynchrony and the region of latest activation.

3. Strain rate (SR) or rate of deformation (Fig. 12.12) equals the velocity gradient calculated as the difference of two instantaneous velocities (Velocity A and Velocity B) normalized for the distance (d) between the two velocity locations (A) and (B) as follows [6, 9]:

$$SR = \frac{Va - Vb}{d}$$

The strain rate signal displays compression in systole (expressed as negative value) and expansion (positive value)

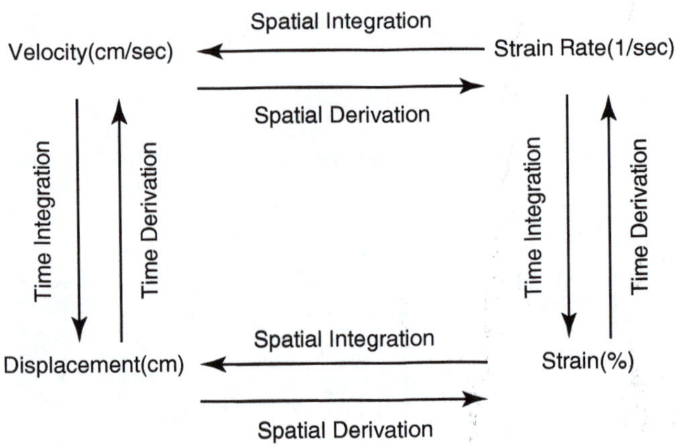

Fig. 12.11 The relation between four parameters of myocardial function

during diastole with three peaks that occur during isovolumetric relaxation and early and late diastole (Fig. 12.7c).

4. Strain (ε): Strain is a change in length between two locations from an initial length (L_0) to a new length (L).

Normalized to L_0 (Fig. 12.13). Thus strain can be expressed as: [10, 11]:

$$\varepsilon = (L - L_0) / L_0.$$

When deformation analysis is based on the initial length L_0, it is referred to as the Lagrangian strain, whereas when deformation is based on an previous time instance(and not original length), then so-called Eulerian (natural) strain is measured [12–14] such as by temporal integration of instantaneous strain rates in TDI (Fig. 12.11).

$$\varepsilon = \int SR\,dt$$

Natural strain is more relevant to cardiac imaging. At low strain (<10%), Lagrangian and natural strain can be used interchangeably [15].

For simplicity, in DTI, strain rate was derived from the gradient of velocity over a sampling distance, and strain obtained as the integral (Fig. 12.11).

Another method for measuring deformation indices is 2D-Speckle tracking echocardiography. In that technique, strain is derived from excursion of the speckles, and SR is derived from differentiation of the strain curve [15].

Key Points

Tissue Doppler velocities may be influenced by global heart motion (translation, torsion, and rotation), by movement of adjacent structures, and by blood flow. To minimize such effects, precise tracking of the myocardial segments and smaller sample size are suggested. However, the latter could result in noisier curves. The patient is asked to hold breathing for several heartbeats to reduce the effects of respiratory

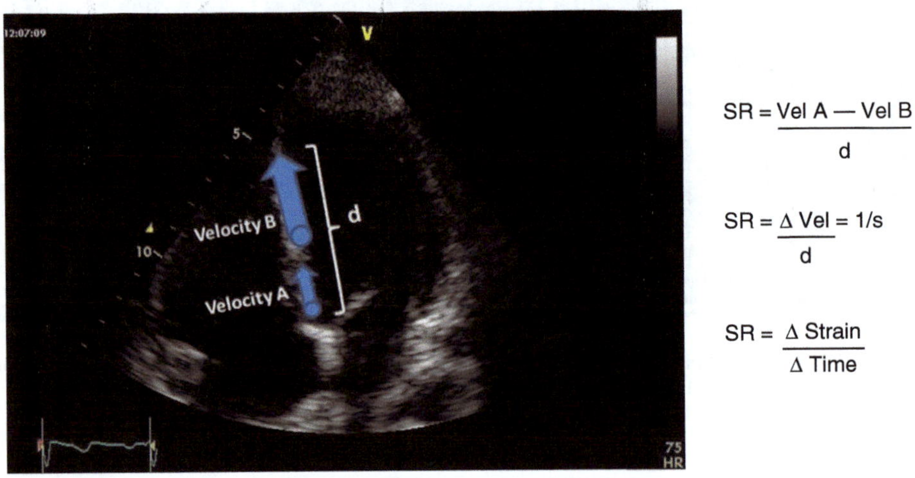

Fig. 12.12 Strain rate is the ratio between the difference in the velocities to the distance

variation. The width of the imaging beam should be adjusted as narrow as possible [6].

Advantages and Disadvantages of DTI

It is readily available and allows objective quantitative evaluation of regional myocardial function.

Data of peak myocardial velocities are reproducible, which is essential for serial evaluations. Also, spectral pulsed DTI has excellent temporal resolution. Online measurements of velocities and time intervals are possible, which is crucial in evaluation of myocardial ischemia and diastolic function.

The major weakness of DTI is its angle dependency. It only measures velocities along the ultrasound beam, while velocities perpendicular to the beam remain undetected. In addition, only one segment can be examined at a time.

Color Doppler-derived strain and SR are noisy. Its temporal resolution is not as good as spectral Doppler (due to its lower frame rate). Training and experience are needed for proper interpretation and detecting artifacts.

In principle, strain/strain rate is not influenced by overall motion of the heart (translation) or by motion caused by contraction in adjacent segments (in contrast to velocity within a myocardial segment that cannot distinguish active from passive deformation.)

Two-Dimensional Speckle-Tracking Echocardiography (2D–STE)

STE is a relatively new, largely angle-independent method for the evaluation of myocardial function. The speckles seen in gray scale images are the result of interference of ultrasound backscattered from structures smaller than the ultrasound wavelength (Fig. 12.14).

Blocks or kernels of speckles can be tracked from frame to frame (simultaneously in multiple regions within an image plane) using block matching, and provide local displacement

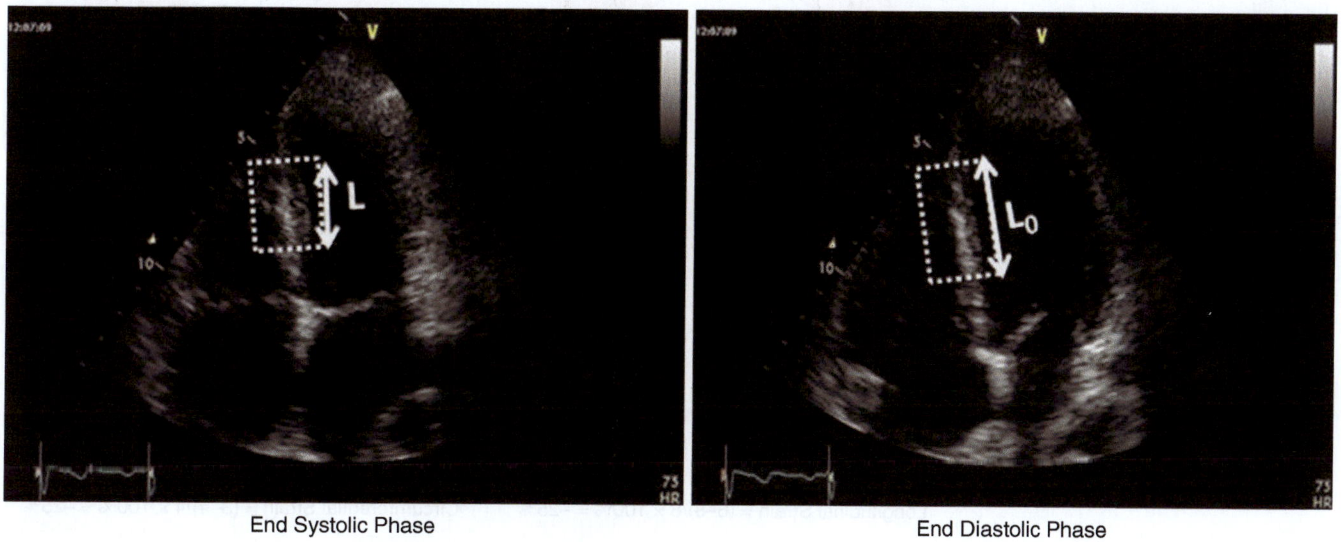

Fig. 12.13 Strain is calculated by the changes in length normalized to the initial length

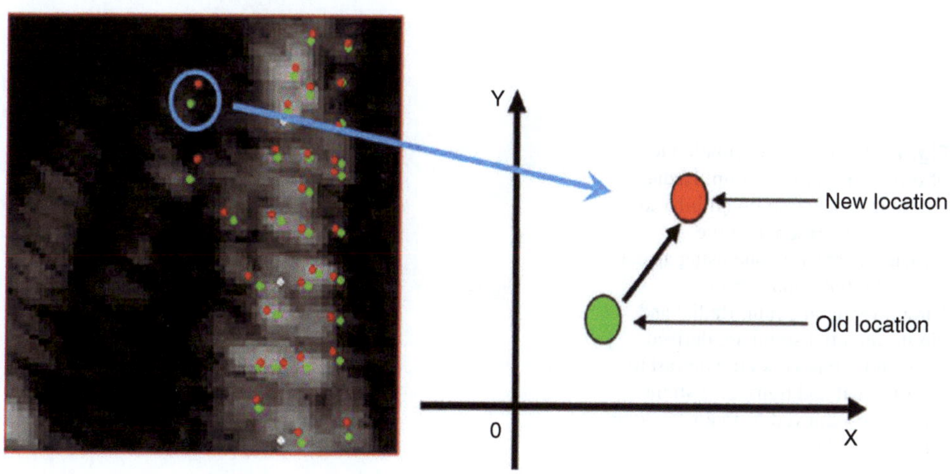

Fig. 12.14 The principle of STE. Myocardial speckles in a gray-scale image are tracked frame-by-frame. So, the myocardial deformation in different directions could be achieved [53, 54]

information, from which parameters of myocardial function such as velocity, strain, and SR can be derived [6].

How to Optimize the Images in 2D-STE?

Frame rates of 40–80 frames/s is used in normal sinus rhythm [16] but higher frame rates are advisable to avoid under-sampling in tachycardia [17]. The focus is placed at an intermediate depth, and sector depth and width should be adjusted to include as little as possible outside the region of interest. Any artifact that resembles speckle patterns will influence the quality of speckle tracking, and thus care should be taken to avoid these.

Types of Strain

LV contraction involves myocardial motion along three-dimensional (3D; *x*, *y*, and *z*) coordinates and results in a variety of strain parameters that can be derived for each myocardial segments.

Consequently, different type of strain could be achieved [18] (Fig. 12.15):

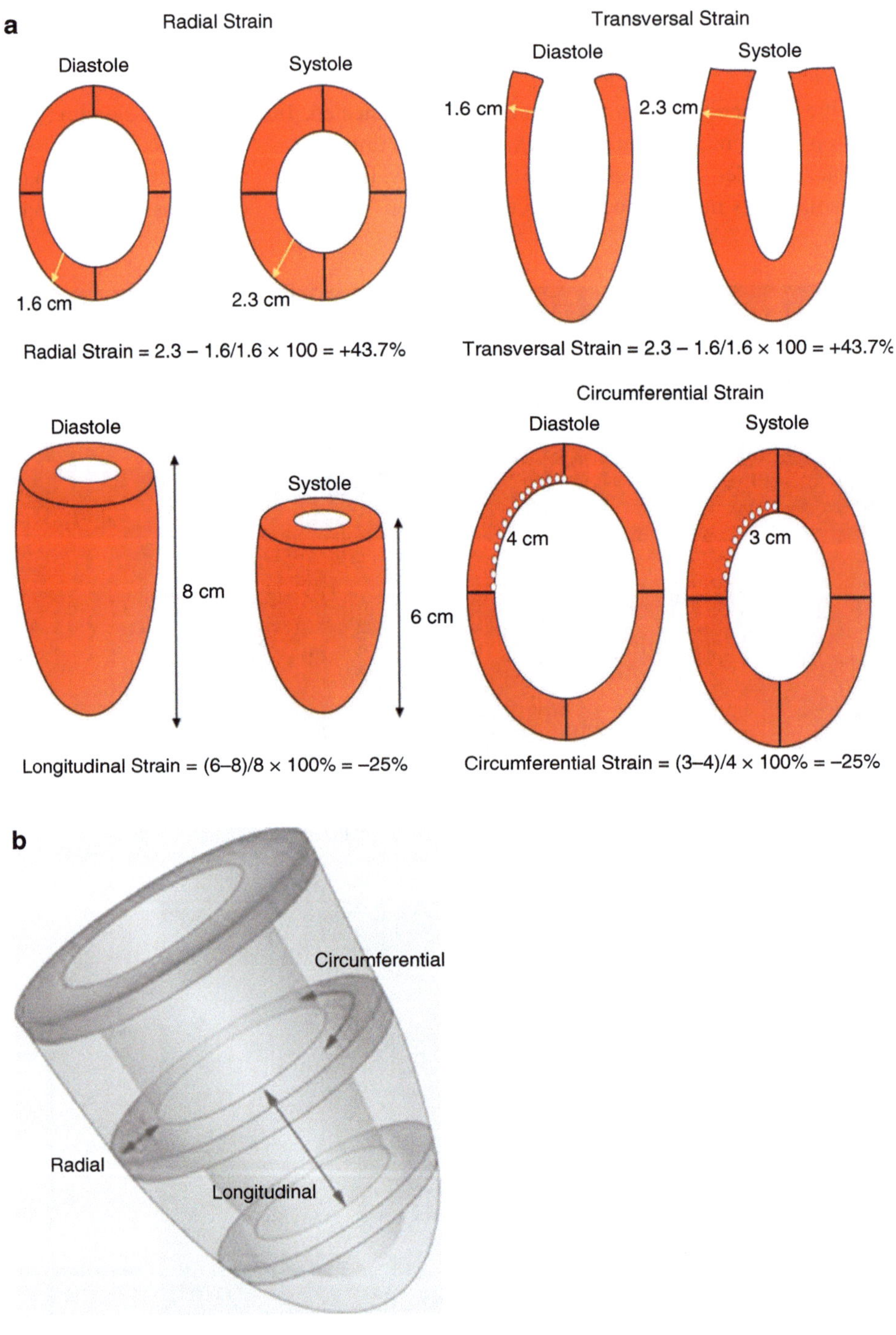

Fig. 12.15 (**a**, **b**) Schematic views of different types of strain: Radial strain; transverse strain (similar to radial strain, except that the measurements are done using apical views. Longitudinal strain. Circumferential strain. Radial and circumferential strain are derived from short axis views in contrast to longitudinal and transverse strain which are achieved from apical, long axis views [33]

1. Longitudinal strain: Changes in the longitudinal length of myocardium (negative value during systole).
2. Radial Strain: changes in myocardial thickness in short axis, e.g., myocardial thickening with inward motion of LV in systole presenting as positive value at this phase.
3. Transverse Strain: Changes in myocardial thickness in apical view, e.g., myocardial thickening with inward motion of LV in the systole, presenting as positive value.
4. Circumferential Strain: Changes in the length measured circumferentially around the perimeter of LV (presented as negative value in the systole).
5. Rotational Strain: Rotational myocardial motion along the long axis of LV (with clockwise rotation represented as negative value and vice versa.)
6. Twist and untwist: Difference in rotation between apex and base. Twist is used for systole and untwist for the diastolic phase.

Other type of strain not routinely used in echocardiography is shear strain [11].

The timing at which peak strain is measured is not uniform across publications. Peak strain can be measured as peak systolic strain (positive or negative), peak strain at end-systole (at time of aortic valve closure, AVC), or peak strain regardless of timing (in systole or early diastole).

End systolic strain, may be exceeded by peak strain, and the difference normalized to the peak strain is usually measured as post systolic index (PSI) (Fig. 12.16).

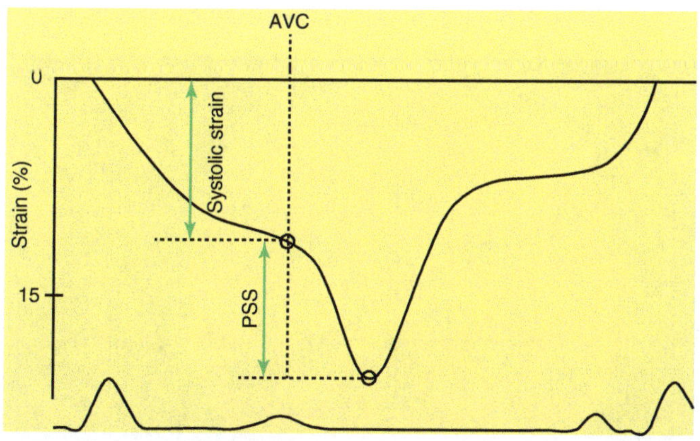

Fig. 12.16 PSS is higher than end systolic strain (measured at aortic valve closure) in this image. Difference in the magnitude of strain and also the time interval have been used in myocardial ischemia (Reduced systolic strain, PSS exceeding 20% of total strain or occurring more than 90 milliseconds after AVC signify pathologic state). *AVC* Aortic valve closure; *PSS* postsystolic shortening. Adapted from Voigt et al. Incidence and characteristics of segmental postsystolic longitudinal shortening in normal, acutely ischemic, and scarred myocardium. J Am Soc Echocardiogr. 2003

Global Strain

Segmental strain is calculated in the three apical views (segmental strain in the apical four- and two-chamber and long axis views) and then averaged as GLS, combined in a polar map (Figs. 12.17, 12.18, 12.19, 12.20, 12.21, 12.22, 12.23, and 12.24).

2D-STE Analysis of Myocardial Mechanics

Two-dimensional STE allows measurements of the above four parameters of myocardial mechanics by tracking groups of intramyocardial speckles (d or v) or myocardial deformation (ε or SR) in the imaging plane. When automated tracking does not fit with the visual impression of wall motion, regions of interest need to be adjusted manually until optimal tracking is achieved.

For the left ventricle, because end-systole can be defined by aortic valve closure as seen in the apical long-axis view, this view should be analyzed first.

Assessment of 2D strain by STE can be applied to both ventricles and atria. However, because of the thin wall of the atria and right ventricle, signal quality may be suboptimal. In contrast, all LV segments can be analyzed successfully in most patients. Feasibility is best for longitudinal and circumferential strain and is more challenging for radial strain.

Pitfalls of 2D STE

1. Suboptimal tracking of the endocardial border.
2. Sensitivity to acoustic shadowing or reverberations.

Both of them could result in under -estimation of the true deformation or non-physiologic traces [19].

Advantages and Disadvantages of 2D- STE

Although both DTI and STE measure myocardial motion against a fixed external point in space (i.e., the transducer), STE is able to measure this motion in any direction within the image plane. In contrast, DTI is just capable to define the velocity component toward or away from the probe. So, STE could measure circumferential and radial components irrespective of the direction of the beam (Table 12.1).

- STE is not completely angle independent. It works better for measuring deformation along the ultrasound beam than in other directions.
- STE relies on good image quality. The details can be tracked from one frame to the next and when out of plane motion does not occur.

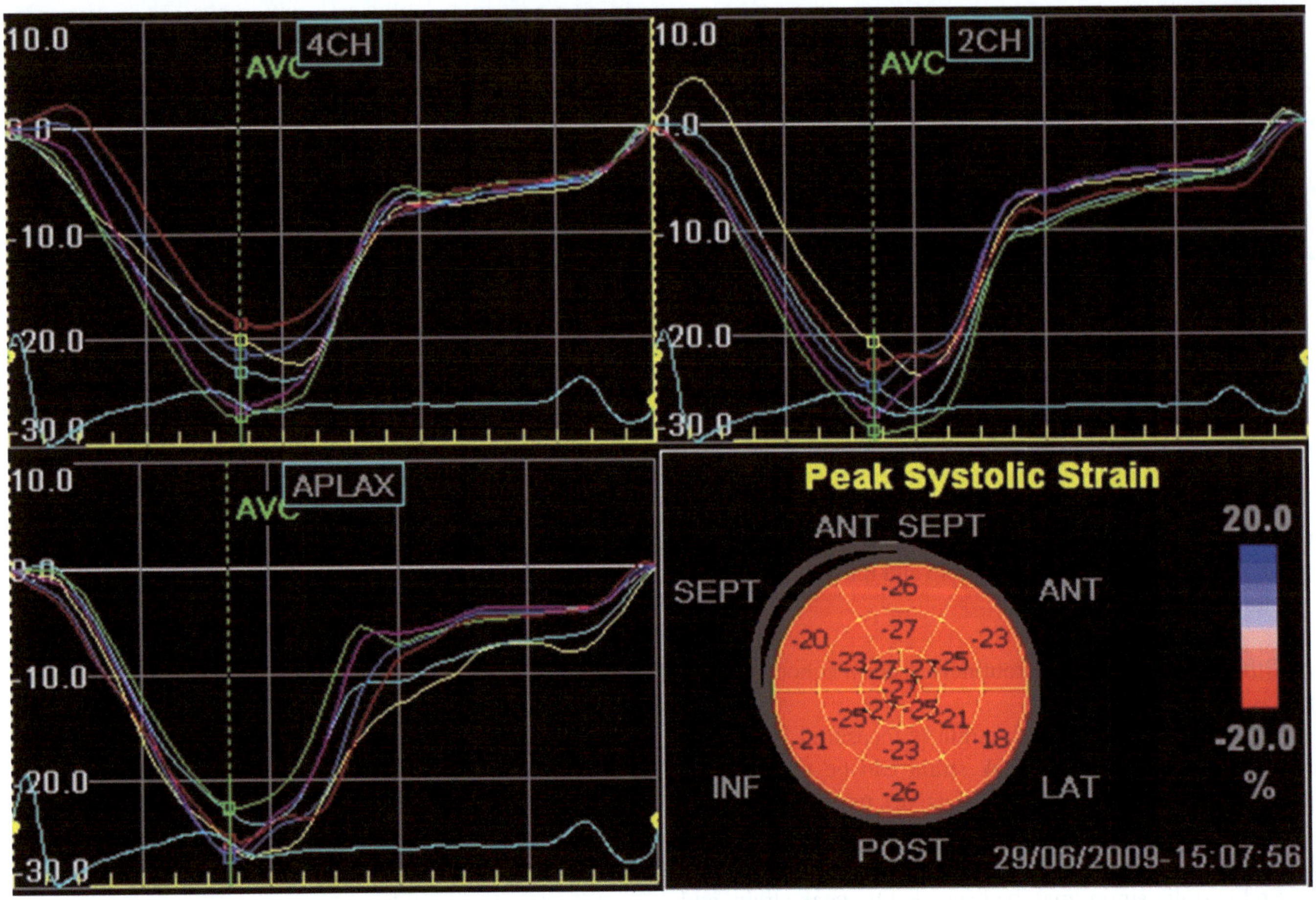

Fig. 12.17 Segmental longitudinal systolic strain curves derived from three apical views

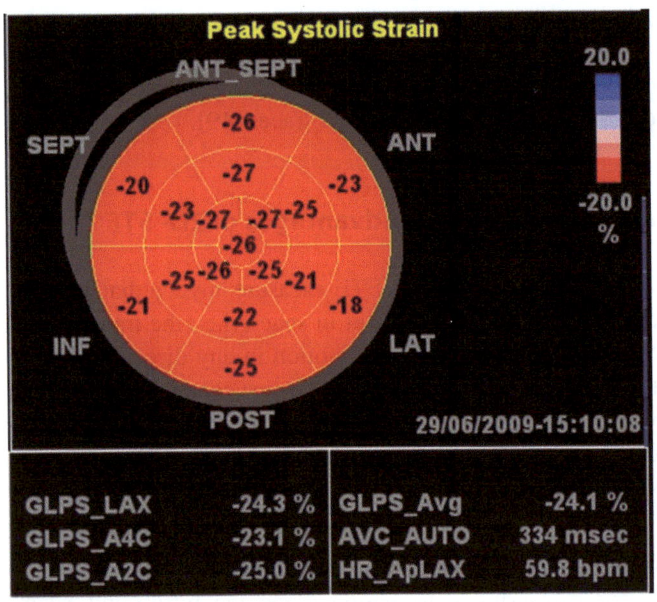

Fig. 12.18 Normal 17-segments Bull's eye template showing myocardial longitudinal strain in each myocardial region. Global longitudinal strain was presented as −24.1% in this case

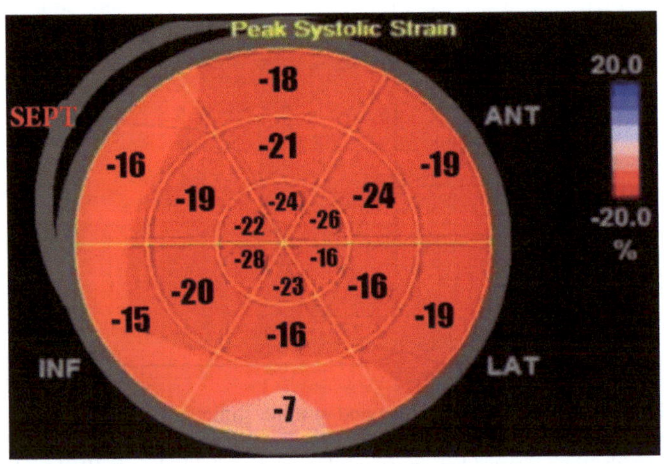

Fig. 12.19 17-segments Bull's eye template showing myocardial longitudinal strain in a case with infero-posterior MI and reduced strain in related segments. Global longitudinal strain was presented as −16.1% in this case

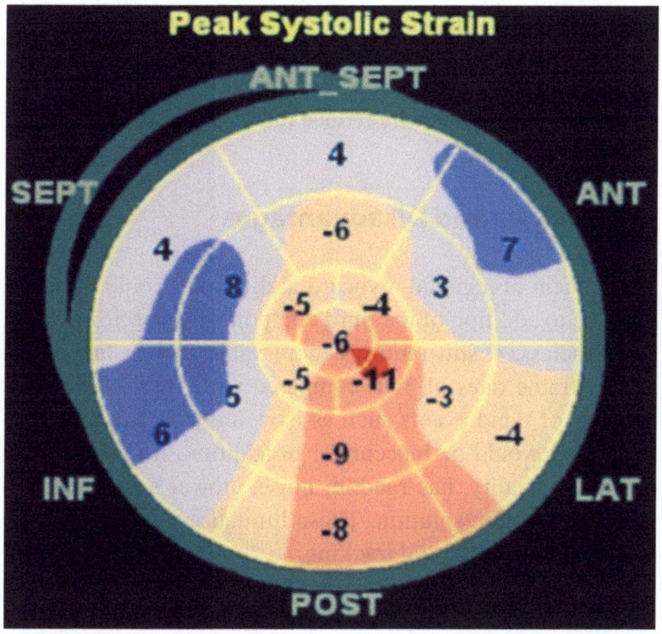

Fig. 12.20 17-segments Bull's eye template showing myocardial longitudinal strain in a case with end stage Dilated Cardiomyopathy and severely reduced strain in all segments. Global longitudinal strain was presented as −6.3% in this case

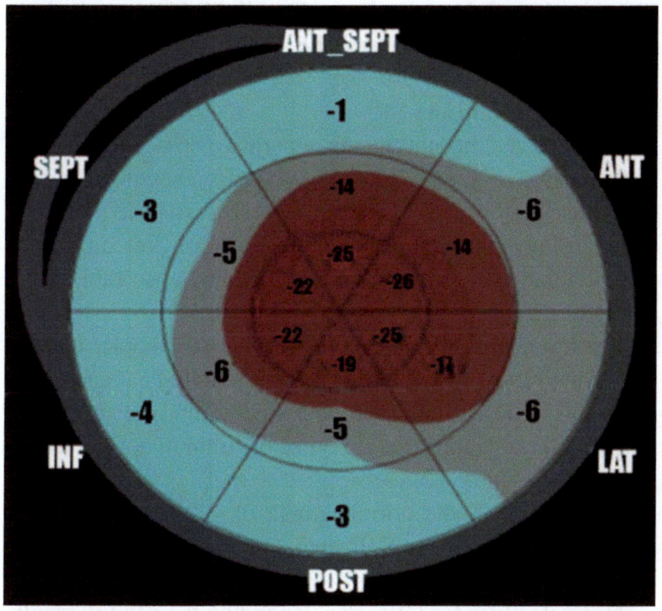

Fig. 12.21 17-segments Bull's eye template showing myocardial longitudinal strain in a case with Hypertrophic Cardiomyopathy and reduced strain in basal and mid hypertrophied segments. Global longitudinal strain was presented as −10.1% in this case

- In higher rate or while measuring short living time intervals (e.g., IVRT), DTI prove to be more useful (due to its higher temporal resolution).
- A significant limitation of the current implementation of 2D STE is the differences among vendors.

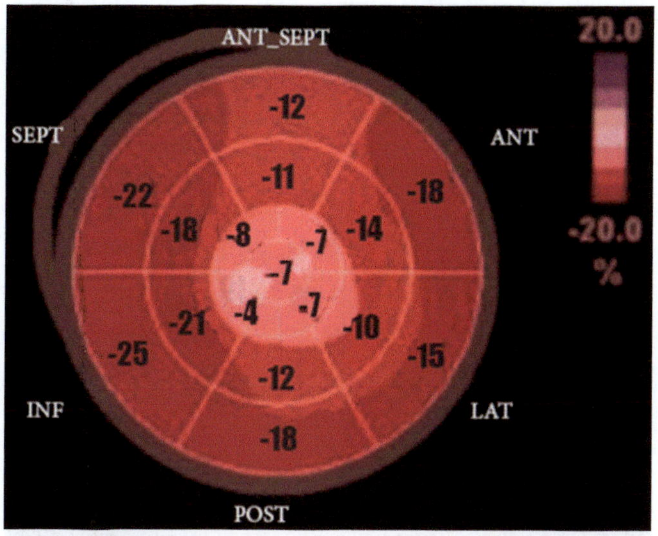

Fig. 12.22 17-segments Bull's eye template showing myocardial longitudinal strain in a case with apical Hypertrophic Cardiomyopathy and reduced strain in apical hypertrophied segments. Global longitudinal strain was presented as −16.8% in this case

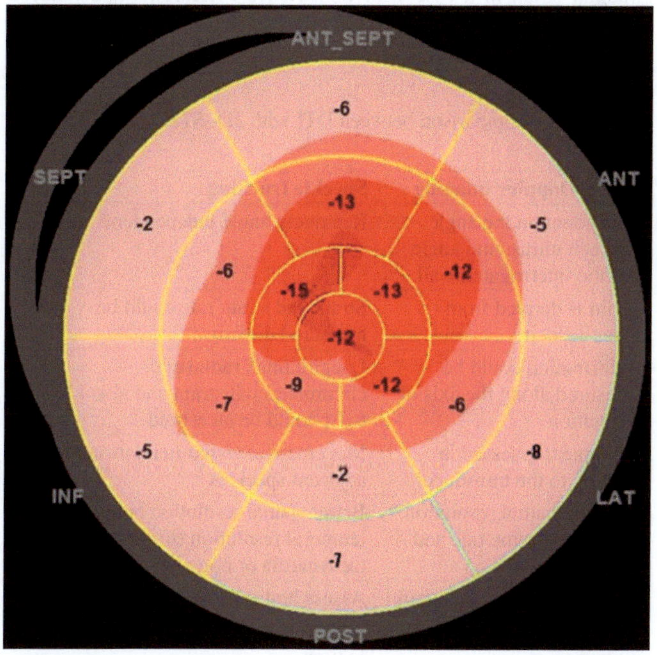

Fig. 12.23 17-segments Bull's eye template showing myocardial longitudinal strain in a case with Restrictive Cardiomyopathy and reduced strain in basal segments and preserved red color apical segments. Global longitudinal strain was presented as −7.8% in this case

Three-Dimensional STE

The entire left ventricle can be analyzed from a single volume of data obtained from the apical transducer position. So, its use was found to considerably reduce the examination time to one third of that for 2D STE [6]. In contrast to 2D

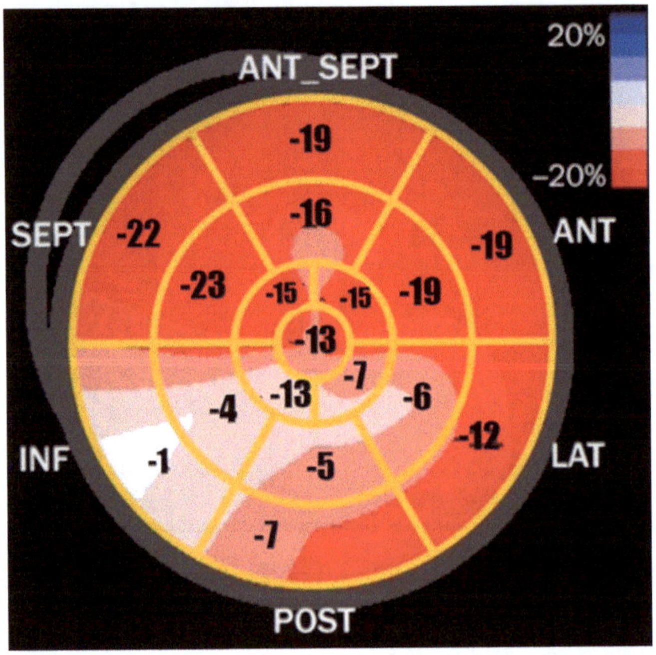

Fig. 12.24 17-segments Bull's eye template showing myocardial longitudinal strain in a case with Constrictive Pericarditis and reduced strain in inferior, posterior and lateral segments. Global longitudinal strain was presented as −14% in this case

Table 12.1 Comparison between DTI with 2D–STE for evaluation of strain

Tissue Doppler imaging	Speckle tracking
Dependent on the angle between ultrasound angle and the interrogated wall	Relatively angle independent
Strain is derived from tissue velocity	Strain and strain rate could be measured directly
Deformation could be measured along the axis of insonation	Longitudinal, radial and circumferential strain and also LV twist could be measured
Movement assessed in relation to the transducer	Movement assessed in relation to the adjacent speckles
Limited Spatial resolution but higher frame rate and temporal resolution	Better spatial resolution but poor temporal resolution (limited utility in tachycardia or non-sinus rhythm)
Assess only regional strain	Assess both regional and global strain
Influenced by translational motion	Less influenced by translational motion
Less reproducibility	Less inter- and intra -observer variability

Modified table from Biswas M et al. Two- and three-dimensional speckle tracking echocardiography: clinical applications and future directions. Echocardiography. 2013;30(53):88–105

STE, which cannot track motion in and out of the imaging plane and measure only one of the three components of the local displacement vector, the recently developed 3D STE can track motion of speckles irrespective of their direction, as long as they remain within the selected scan volume.

3D STE based measurements of LV volumes were found to be in close agreement with magnetic resonance-derived reference values. The agreement were higher than those of 2D STE measurements [20, 21]. It can be applied using full volume mode, including the entire LV cavity within the pyramidal volume. This could obviously reduce the temporal resolution.

Advantages and Disadvantages

Assessment of regional myocardial dynamics could be accurate due to addition of the third component of motion vector. Nevertheless, it still requires more validation. It has much slower frame rates of 3DE compared with 2D STE. So, the analysis of rapid events such as isovolumic contraction and relaxation would be inaccurate. In addition, it is dependent on image quality, has random noise, lower spatial and as noted temporal resolution. These limitations could result in sub-optimal myocardial tracking.

Normal Values of LV Myocardial Mechanics

The normal values vary depending on the specific LV wall and the specific 3D component of each index. Longitudinal velocities in the lateral wall are higher than in the septum. There is also a base-to-apex gradient (with higher velocities recorded at LV base than near the apex).

Minor differences are seen between LV segments for DTI-derived strain and SRs.

STE-derived measurements generally show higher values in the apical segments than DTI. Within a segment, higher velocities and strains are usually recorded from the sub-endocardium than from the sub-epicardium. Velocities and deformation parameters are also affected by age (Table 12.2) and loading conditions.

The lower limits of normal range with the Doppler method were found to be –18.5 and 44.5% for longitudinal and radial strain and –1.00 and 2.45 s^{-1} for longitudinal and radial SR [22].

Normal range for different types of strain in normal adults are shown in Table 12.3.

In Table 12.4, the normal range of strain rate (in three phase of cardiac cycle: S, E and A) and displacement have been provided.

Normal values for GLS also depend on the vendor, resulting in considerable heterogeneity in the published literature (Table 12.5).

To provide some guidance, a peak GLS in the range of –20% can be expected in a healthy person [6, 23].

Clinical Use of LV Displacement, Velocity, Strain, and SR

The following is a brief summary of parameters of myocardial function in multiple disease states, gathered as Table 12.6.

Table 12.2 Normal Values for mitral andtricuspid annulus velocity by TDI in healthy volunteer

	LV (mean of four walls)				RV (free wall)		
	S'(pwTDI)	S'(cTDI)	E'(pwTDI)	A'(pwTDI)	S'(pwTDI)	E'(pwTDI)	A'(pwTDI)
Female	8.2 ± 1.3	6.6 ± 1.1	11.8 ± 3.2	9.7 ± 2	12.5 ± 1.9	13.3 ± 3.0	14.4 ± 3.7
Male	8.6 ± 1.4	6.9 ± 1.3	10.8 ± 3.0	10.3 ± 1.7	12.8 ± 3.3	12.5 ± 3.3	14.2 ± 3.9

Modified table from Dalen H, Thorstensen A, Vatten LJ, et al.: Reference values and distribution of conventional echocardiographic Doppler measures and longitudinal tissue Doppler velocities in a population free from cardiovascular disease. *Circ Cardiovasc Imaging* 3(5):614–622, 2010

Table 12.3 Normal values of different type of strain, considering the interrogated wall or segment

	Interrogated segment	Apicoseptal	Mid septal	Basal septal	Apical lateral	Mid lateral	Basal lateral
Longitudinal strain	Value	–21 ± 4	–19 ± 4	–17 ± 4	–21 ± 7	–19 ± 6	–19 ± 6
Circumferential strain	Interrogated wall	Anterior	Lateral	Posterior	Inferior	Septal	Anteroseptal
	Value	–24 ± 6	–22 ± 7	–21 ± 7	–22 ± 6	–24 ± 6	–26 ± 11
Radial strain	Interrogated segment	Anterior	Lateral	Posterior	Inferior	Septal	Anteroseptal
	Value	39 ± 16	37 ± 8	37 ± 17	37 ± 17	37 ± 19	39 ± 15

Modified table from: Hurlburt HM, Aurigemma GP, Hill JC. Direct ultrasound measurement of longitudinal, circumferential, and radial strain using two-dimensional strain imaging in normal adults. Echocardiography. 2007; 24:723–31

Table 12.4 Normal ranges of SR and displacement have been defined at each phase of the cardiac cycle in four LV walls

	Septum	Lateral	Inferior	Anterior
Peak systolic wave (Ssr)				
Basal	–0.99 ± 0.49	–1.5 ± 0.74	–0.88 ± 0.39	–1.64 ± 0.9
Mid	–1.25 ± 0.73	–1.29 ± 0.58	–0.95 ± 0.54	–0.98 ± 0.68
Apical	–1.15 ± 0.5	–1.09 ± 0.59	–1.38 ± 0.45	–1.05 ± 0.63
Early diastolic wave (Esr)				
Basal	1.95 ± 0.89	1.92 ± 1.11	1.85 ± 0.89	2.03 ± 0.99
Mid	1.94 ± 0.97	1.71 ± 0.66	1.92 ± 1.2	1.7 ± 0.82
Apical	1.91 ± 0.66	1.81 ± 0.87	2.29 ± 0.88	1.76 ± 0.98
Late diastolic wave (Asr)				
Basal	1.54 ± 0.93	0.93 ± 0.59	1.18 ± 0.78	1.49 ± 0.96
Mid	1.29 ± 0.86	1.48 ± 0.77	0.78 ± 0.62	1.04 ± 0.57
Apical	0.95 ± 0.54	1.07 ± 0.68	1.68 ± 0.76	0.68 ± 0.65
Displacement (D)				
Basal	1.2 ± 0.19	0.93 ± 0.22	1.33 ± 0.22	1.05 ± 0.27
Mid	1.13 ± 0.27	0.91 ± 0.18	0.62 ± 0.22	1.04 ± 0.19
Apical	0.65 ± 0.24	0.82 ± 0.27	0.55 ± 0.18	0.41 ± 0.25

Modified table from: Gillam LD, Otto CM. Advanced Approaches in Echocardiography. Philadelphia, PA: Elsevier Saunders; 2012, p 85 (Table 6.1)

Table 12.5 Normal LV strain using specific vendors

Vendor	Software	Mean ± SD	LLN (%)
GE	EchoPAC BT 12	−21.5 ± 2.0%	−18
		−21.5 ± 2.0%	−18
		−21.2 ± 2.4%	−17
	EchoPAC 110.1.3	−21.3 ± 2.1%	−17
Philips	QLAB 7.1	−18.9 ± 2.5	−14
Toshiba	Ultra Extend	−19.9 ± 2.4%	−15
Siemens	WI	−19.8 ± 4.6	−11
	WI	−17.3 ± 2.3	−13
Esoate	Mylab 50	−19.5 ± 3.1	−13

LLN lower limit of normal

Modified table from: Lang RM, Badano LP, Mor-Avi V, Afilalo J, Armstrong A, Ernande L, et al. Recommendations for Cardiac Chamber Quantification by Echocardiography in Adults: An Update from the American Society of echocardiography and the European Association of Cardiovascular Imaging. J Am Soc Echocardiogr. 2015;28:1–39

Twist, Rotation and Torsion

Rotation describes the wringing motion of the heart from contraction of its obliquely oriented muscle bundles. This deformation can be quantified by both tissue Doppler imaging and speckle tracking. Adequate short axis images of the LV apex and base are essential for this measurement. From the view of the apex, the apex rotates counterclockwise in systole (during ejection) and the base rotates clockwise [31].

In late systole and early diastole (the isovolumetric relaxation period and briefly during early LV filling), the apex and base reverse-rotate at the same speed and to the same degree as in systole [32].

By convention, clockwise rotations carry a negative value and counterclockwise rotations are assigned a positive value.

LV systolic twist is defined as the difference between the apical and basal rotations.

$$\text{Twist} = \text{Apex} - (\text{Base}),$$

In normal controls [33], apical rotation is 6° and basal rotation is –6°, producing a twist of 12°.

LV torsion is twist normalized to the distance between the apex and base (degrees/cm) (Fig. 12.25).

Table 12.6 Brief review of some clinical implications of parameters of LV mechanics

Estimation of LV filling pressures	Average E/e' ≥14 is correlated with elevated LV filling pressure [24]
Detection of subclinical diseases/ early myocardial involvement	Reduction in strain/strain rate may occur before changes in LVEF in systemic hypertension, diabetes mellitus, systemic sclerosis or lupus Erythematosus amyloidosis, muscular dystrophy, or changes in LV function after cancer treatment [6, 25–27]
Constrictive vs. restrictive physiology	In the absence of myocardial disease, e′ velocities typically remain normal in constrictive pericarditis (usually >8 cm/s). Deformation (longitudinal and radial) are impaired in RCM and the GCS may remain normal. In CP, only circumferential strain shows abnormalities [28, 29]
Athlete's heart vs. HCM	The reduced e′ velocities could be in favor of HCM [30]
	Subjects with HCM had lower global longitudinal strain but higher dispersion when compared with hypertensive LVH [6]
Myocardial ischemia	Reduction in strain by 2D STE more objective and accurate than assessment of WMA
	Longitudinal, radial, and circumferential strain reduced in ischemic areas in coronary artery disease
	Post-systolic thickening (deformation), detected by radial strain correlates with the severity of ischemia
Myocardial infarction	Global peak systolic strain rate $-0.9\ S^{-1}$ are highly sensitive and specific for the identification of patients with prior myocardial infarction
	2D STE successful in differentiating transmural from subendocardial infarction by showing lower circumferential strain in the former
	Decreased LV segmental longitudinal strain predicts progressive LV dilatation after myocardial infarction
Myocardial viability	Strain measurements by 2D STE more objective and accurate than visual WMA for assessment of myocardial viability during low-dose dobutamine stress echocardiography
	2D STE differentiates active contraction from passive motion due to tethering
Cardiac resynchronization therapy (CRT)	Combining longitudinal strain from TDI velocity with 2D STE radial strain may help in predicting response to CRT
	Longitudinal strain delay index (calculated from the difference between peak and endsystolic strain) of >25% predicts response to CRT (sensitivity 95%, specificity 83%)
	Speckle Tracking and Resynchronization (STAR) study showed that radial and transversal strain were better than longitudinal and circumferential strain in predicting
	LVEF response and long-term survival after CRT
	Lack of dyssynchrony before CRT by 2D STE radial strain associated with death or hospitalization for heart failure
Valvular heart disease	Decreased radial, circumferential, and longitudinal strain in patients with severe aortic stenosis and normal LVEF. Long-term follow-up after valve replacement showed significant improvement with no change in EF
	Reduced preoperative 2D STE longitudinal strain in the ventricular septum (apical four-chamber view) predicts a postoperative LVEF decrease of ≥10% in patients with chronic severe mitral regurgitation
Congenital heart disease	Atrial septal defect—basal clockwise rotation during systole is reduced
	Tetralogy of Fallot—right ventricular global longitudinal strain and strain rate is decreased significantly
Detection of rejection and coronary stenosis in heart transplant patients	Sudden reduction of ≥15% in global radial strain associated with acute rejection
	Decrease in strain and strain rate at rest and with dobutamine stress echo also useful to detect significant coronary stenosis

Normal Rotation values in young adults are shown in Table 12.7.

LV torsion is a sensitive marker to assess impaired LV function, which has many clinical implications.

Apical rotation has been proved to be an indicator of myocardial ischemia, heart failure with preserved EF, hypertrophic cardiomyopathy, and valvular heart disease. In mitral regurgitation, torsion and untwisting usually normal when EF is normal, and decrease with decline in systolic function. It remains to be seen whether the changes in LV torsion can help determine the timing of surgical repair.

In early stages of cardiac amyloidosis, amyloid proteins are deposited in the subendocardium. Accordingly, longitudinal deformation is reduced but circumferential deformation is preserved. Twist and untwisting are normal. With advanced disease, circumferential deformation is affected and peak twist and untwisting rate are reduced [15] (Figs. 12.26, 12.27, and 12.28).

In Table 12.8, some of the clinical implication of twist/untwist have been shown.

Despite the growing evidence in support of clinical implications of LV twist measurements using 2D STE, routine clinical use of this methodology is not recommended at this time [6].

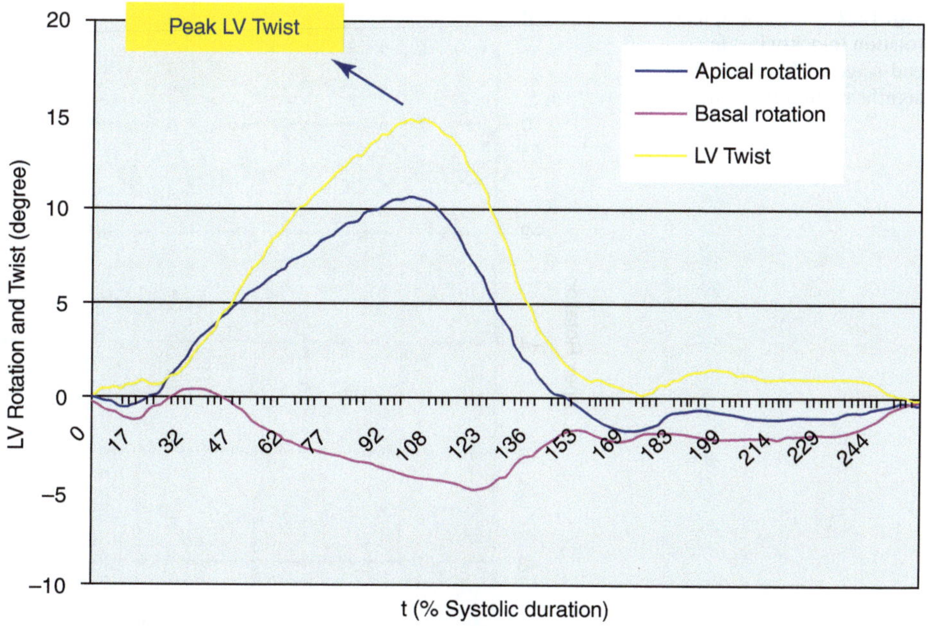

Fig. 12.25 Apical rotation in degrees of rotation (y axis) vs. time in seconds (x axis). Notice the presence of an initial small clockwise rotation (deflection below baseline, followed by counterclockwise rotation. Basal rotation in degrees (y axis) vs. time (x axis). Notice the presence of an initial small counterclockwise rotation (deflection above baseline), followed by clockwise rotation

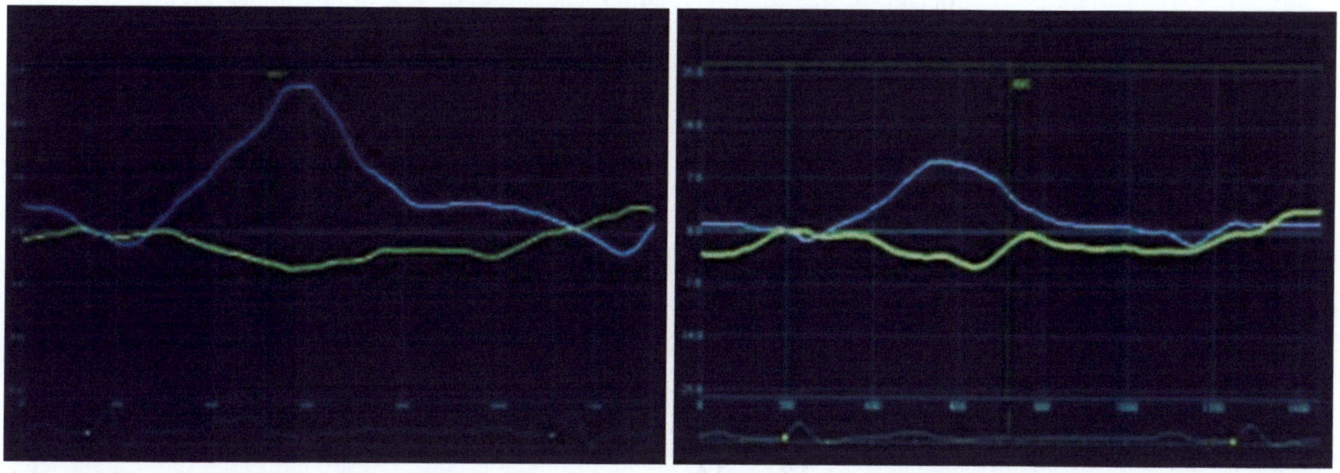

Fig. 12.26 Significantly reduced apical rotation in DCM patient (right panel) in compared with normal subject (left panel). There is no important difference in basal rotation between two cases

Table 12.7 Normal values for parameters of rotation

Parameter	Mean ± SD
Peak apical rotation (°)	10.1 ± 1.9
Peak apical rotation rate (°/s)	61.6 ± 25.3
Peak basal rotation (°)	4.9 ± 2
Peak basal rotation rate (°/s)	44.2 ± 17.8

Modified table from Reproduced from Takahashi K, Al Naami G, Thompson R. Normal rotational, torsion and untwisting data in children, adolescents and young adults. J Am Soc Echocardiogr. 2010;23:286–93

Right Ventricle

DTI and STE both provide indices of RV function. DTI (Pulsed wave and color- coded) allows quantitative assessment of RV systolic and diastolic longitudinal motion (Fig. 12.29) by means of measurement of myocardial velocities from the apical four- chamber view.

DTI of tricuspid annulus provides assessment of systolic (systolic velocity) and diastolic function (Early and late diastolic velocities and the ratio of tricuspid inflow early velocity to early diastolic annulus velocity).

Isovolumic myocardial acceleration (IVA; calculated by dividing the maximal isovolumic myocardial velocity by the time to peak velocity; unit: m/s^2) have also been used for assessment of RV systolic function (less affected by RV shape or loading conditions compared to Systolic velocity) [34] (Fig. 12.30).

At the level of the tricuspid annulus, in the RV free wall, normal systolic velocity by pulsed DTI is >12 cm/s. A peak systolic velocity <10 cm/s should raise the suspicion of abnormal RV function, especially in younger adults [35]. Another parameter of RV function is right ventricular index

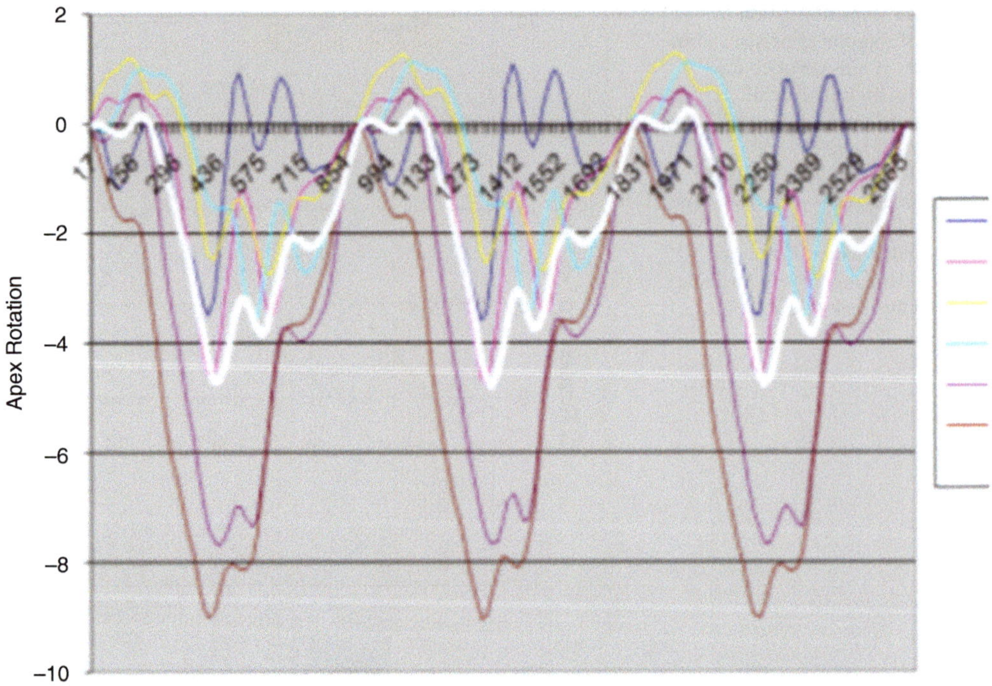

Fig. 12.27 Reverse apical rotation (clock-wise) in end-stage DCM patient with significant fibrotic tissue

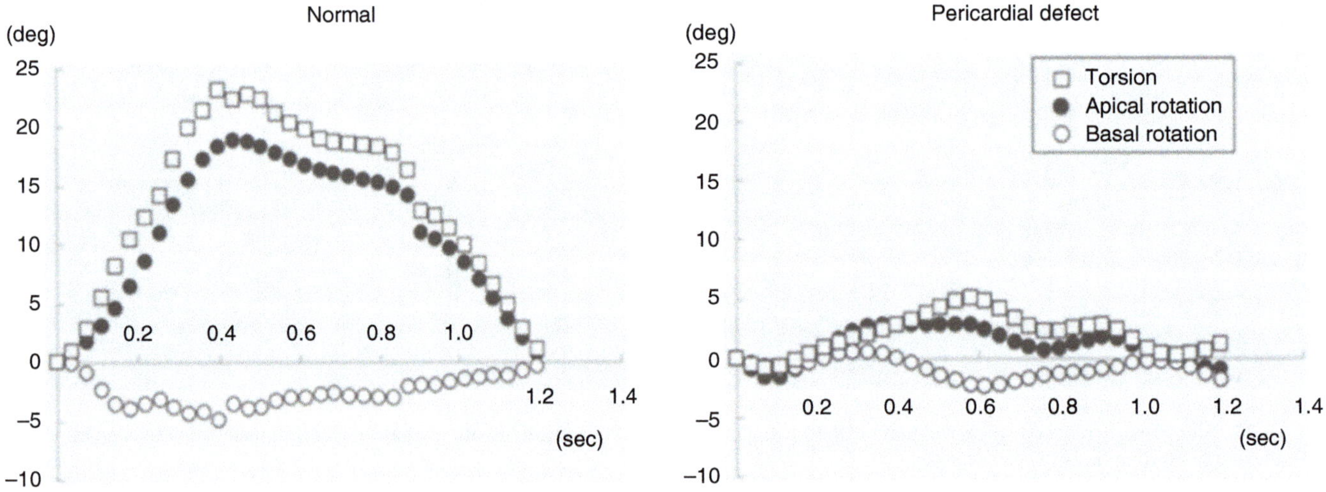

Fig. 12.28 Lack of Twist in patient constrictive Pericarditis

of myocardial performance (RIMP). It is an index of global RV performance. The isovolumic contraction time, the isovolumic relaxation time, and ejection time intervals should be measured in a same cycle (Fig. 12.31). RIMP >0.54 denotes to RV dysfunction. In conditions with elevated RA pressures, RIMP can be falsely low (due to probable association with IVRT shortening).

In healthy individuals, RV longitudinal velocities demonstrate a typical base-to-apex gradient with higher velocities at the base (Fig. 12.32) as in LV. With RV dysfunction, RV longitudinal velocities decrease and the base-to-apex gradient tends to disappear.

In addition, RV velocities are consistently higher compared with the left ventricle. This can be explained by the differences in loading conditions and compliance with a lower afterload in the right ventricle and the dominance of longitudinal and oblique myocardial fibers in the RV free wall [6].

Table 12.8 LV twist in different pathologies

	LV Twist	Untwisting	Time to peak untwisting
Heart failure			
With preserved LVEF	→ or ↑	→ or ↑	Delayed
With reduced LVEF	↓	↓	Delayed
Coronary artery disease			
Subendocardial MI	→	→	Delayed
Transmural MI	↓	↓	Delayed
LV hypertrophy			
Hypertension	→ or ↑	↓	Delayed
HCM	Variable	Variable	Delayed
Aortic stenosis	↓	→ or ↑	Delayed
Dilated cardiomyopathy	↓	↓	Delayed
Pericardial disease	↓	↓	No data
Restrictive CMP	↓[a]	↓[a]	No data

HCM hypertrophic cardiomyopathy, *MI*, myocardial infarction; ↓ reduced;, ↑ elevated; → unchanged
Modified table from: Mor-Avi V, Lang RM, Badano LP, Belohlavek M, Cardim NM, Derumeaux G, Galderisi M, Marwick T, Nagueh SF, et al. Current and Evolving Echocardiographic Techniques for the Quantitative Evaluation of Cardiac Mechanics: ASE/EAE Consensus Statement on Methodology and Indications Endorsed by the Japanese Society of Echocardiography. Eur J Echocardiogr. 2011;12:167–205
[a]In RCM, the subendocardial fiber dysfunction will be associated with depressed GLS and GRS, whereas the spared epicardial fibers will lead to normal or increased GCS, left ventricular (LV) torsion, and LV torsional rate. With disease progression the torsion/torsion rate will decrease

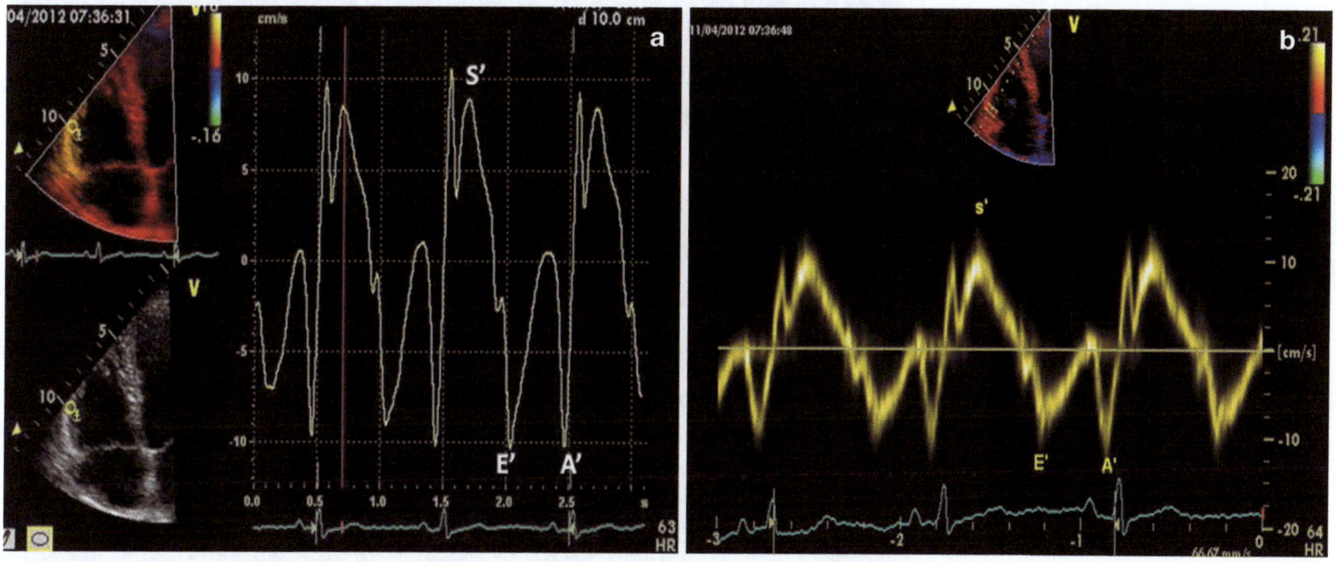

Fig. 12.29 Right ventricle Myocardial velocity, provided by Color Doppler (**a**) and Spectral Doppler (**b**). S′ denotes to systolic velocity and E′ and A′ are related to the diastolic phase

Myocardial Deformation

In RV, like LV, Strain/strain rate imaging could be used for assessment of myocardial function (Figs. 12.33 and 12.34).

In the right ventricle, there is a reverse base-to-apex gradient, reaching the highest values in the apex.

Cutoff points of systolic strain and SR at the basal RV free wall of −25% and $-4\ s^{-1}$ with sensitivities of 81 and 85% and specificities of 82% and 88%, respectively, to predict RV EF >50% [6].

In patients with RV disease or dysfunction, peak systolic strain and SR are significantly reduced and delayed compared

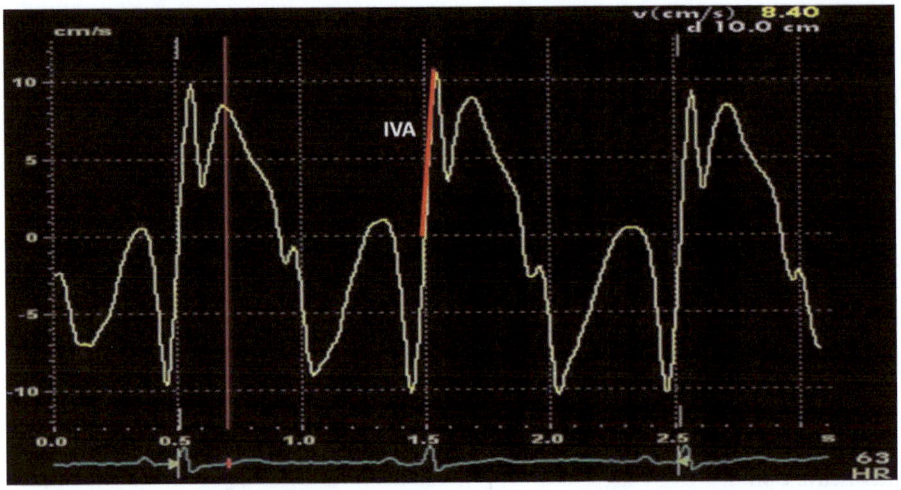

Fig. 12.30 The velocity waveform obtained from color Doppler of RV free wall (with ROI in the basal part). IVA (red line) is measured as isovolumic contraction wave rises from zero line, reaching to its peak point

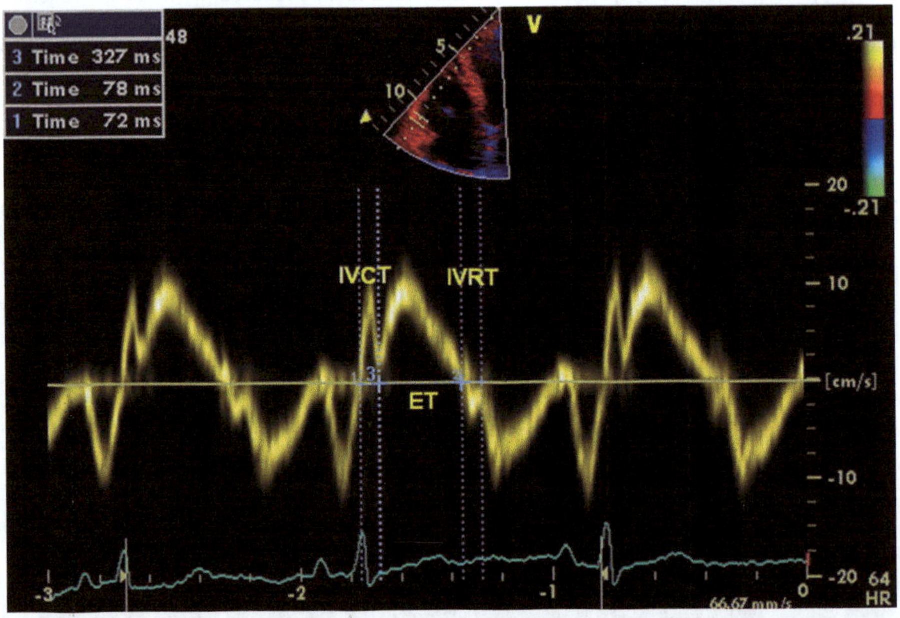

Fig. 12.31 Spectral Doppler of tricupsid annulus, used for measurement of RV MPI ((IVCT + IVRT/ET) which was about 0.45 in this case

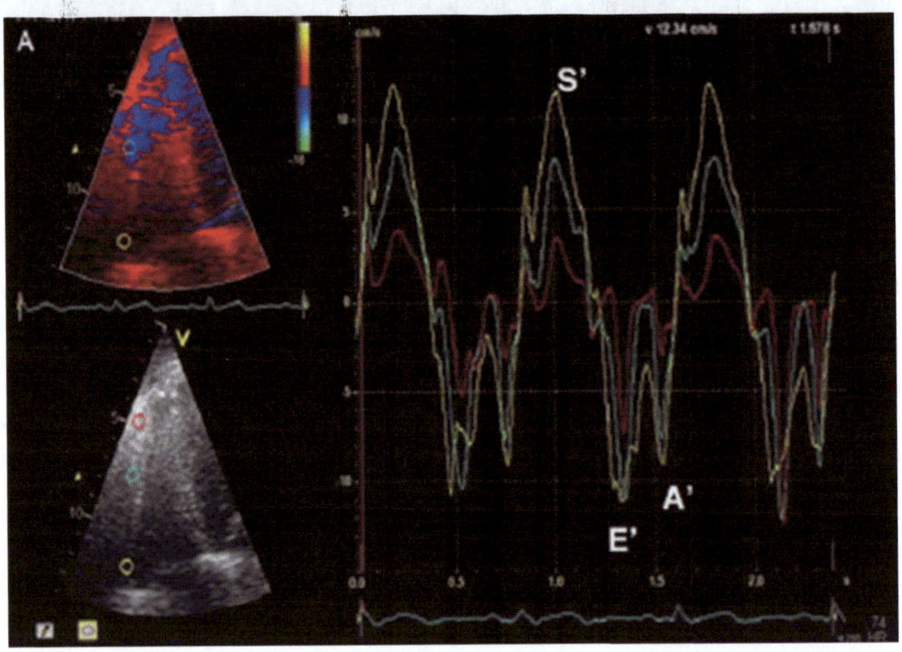

Fig. 12.32 Color coded DTI for assessment of RV myocardial velocity, showing a base to apex gradient

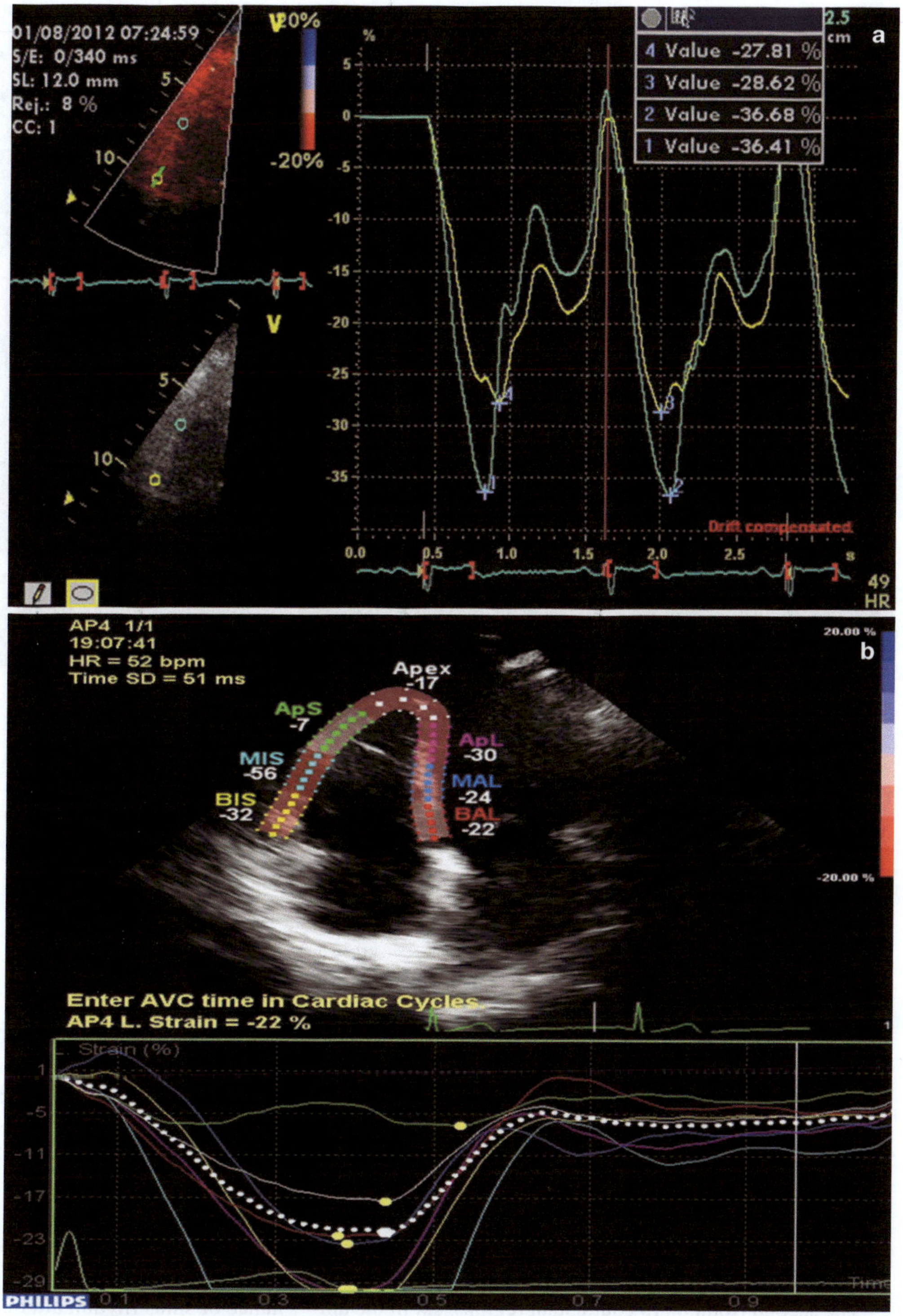

Fig. 12.33 Strain Analysis of RV by Tissue Doppler derived Strain (**a**) and 2d–STE (**b**). In panel b, global strain as average of strain in RV free wall and the septum has been provided (−22%)

with healthy normal. Normal values of multiple parameters of RV function are presented in Table 12.9.

Left Atrium

Myocardial imaging can be used to evaluate left atrial (LA) function. Both DTI and 2D -STE allow noninvasive assessment of global and regional LA function [6]. The mitral annulus late diastolic velocity is easy to measure, has a high reproducibility. It can be affected by LA contractility as well as LA afterload [36]. 2d–STE successfully provides LA volume curves during one cardiac cycle, from which various LA mechanical indices can be obtained [37–42].

The first (total of 12 equidistant regions, six in the apical four-chamber view and six in the apical two-chamber view) takes as a reference point the QRS onset and measures the positive peak atrial longitudinal strain (corresponding to

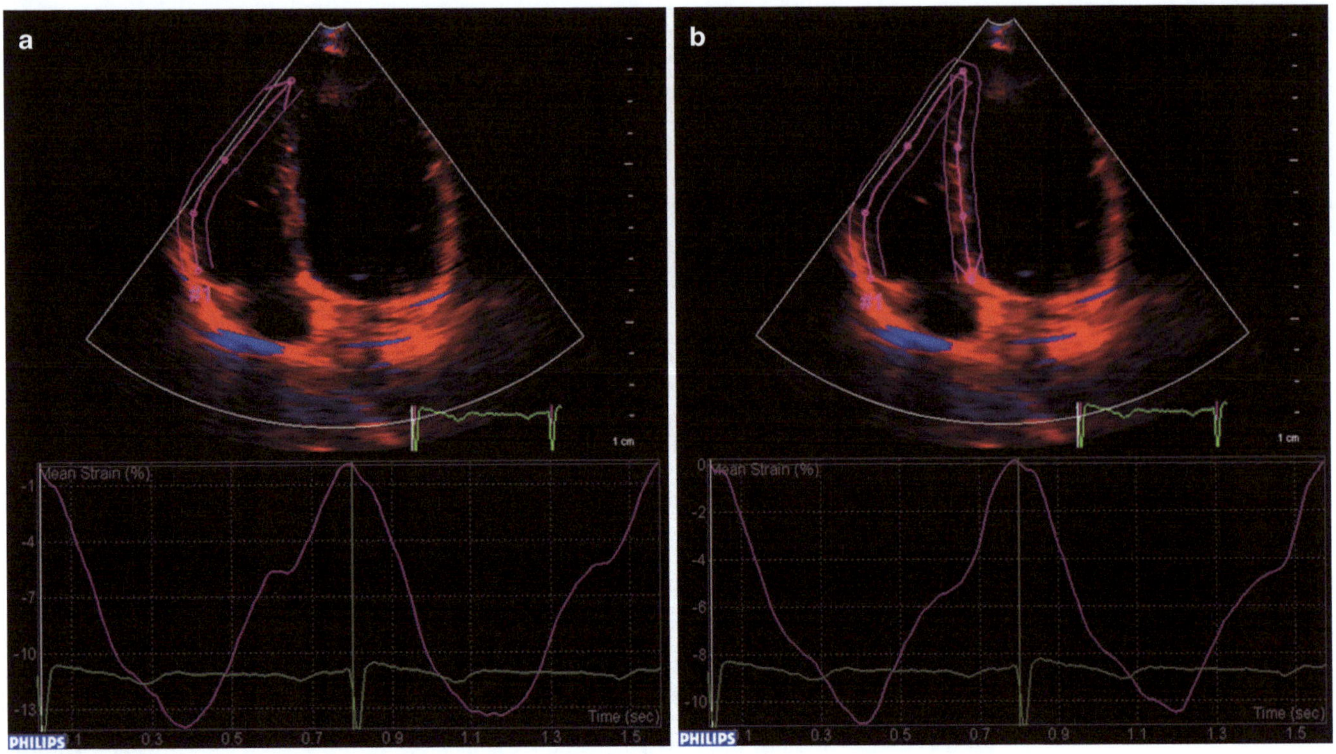

Fig. 12.34 Mean strain in RV free wall and RV free wall + septum (using SQ application)

Table 12.9 Normal values for DTI and 2D–STE related parameters of RV function

Parameter	Mean ± SD	Abnormality threshold
Pulsed Doppler S wave (cm/s)	14.1 ± 2.3	<9.5
Color Doppler S wave	9.7 ± 1.85	<6.0
RV free wall 2D strain (%)	−29 ± 4.5	Cut off point: −20
Tissue Doppler MPI	0.38 ± 0.08	>0.54
E′/A′	1.18 ± 0.33	<0.52
E′	14.0 ± 3.1	<7.8
E/E′	4.0 ± 1.0	>6.0

Modified table from Lang RM, Badano LP, Mor-Avi V, Afilalo J, Armstrong A, Ernande L, Flachskampf FA, et al. Recommendations for Cardiac Chamber Quantification by Echocardiography in Adults: An Update from the American Society of Echocardiography and the European Association of Cardiovascular Imaging. J Am Soc Echocardiogr. 2015;28:1–39

atrial reservoir) [37–41]. The mean peak atrial longitudinal strain was 42.2 ± 6.1% (Fig. 12.35).

The second (total of 15 equidistant regions, six in the apical four-chamber view, six in the apical two- chamber view, and three in the inferoposterior wall in long axis) uses the P wave as the reference point, enabling the measurement of a first negative peak atrial longitudinal strain (corresponding to atrial systole), a second positive peak atrial strain (corresponding to LA conduit function), and their sum [37, 39–44] (Fig. 12.28b).

The average values of positive and negative peak strain were 23.2 ± 6.7% and 14.6 ± 3.5%, respectively.

Utility of LA strain in daily practice is still limited. It has been used in those of atrial fibrillation to predict maintenance of sinus rhythm after cardioversion.

Right Atrium

Similar to left atrium, RA have a passive and active phase of contraction which could be a target for assessment. But clearly there is no validated data on RA strain measurement in such a way that to be considered for routine clinical use [37, 39–41, 45–47] (Figs. 12.36 and 12.37).

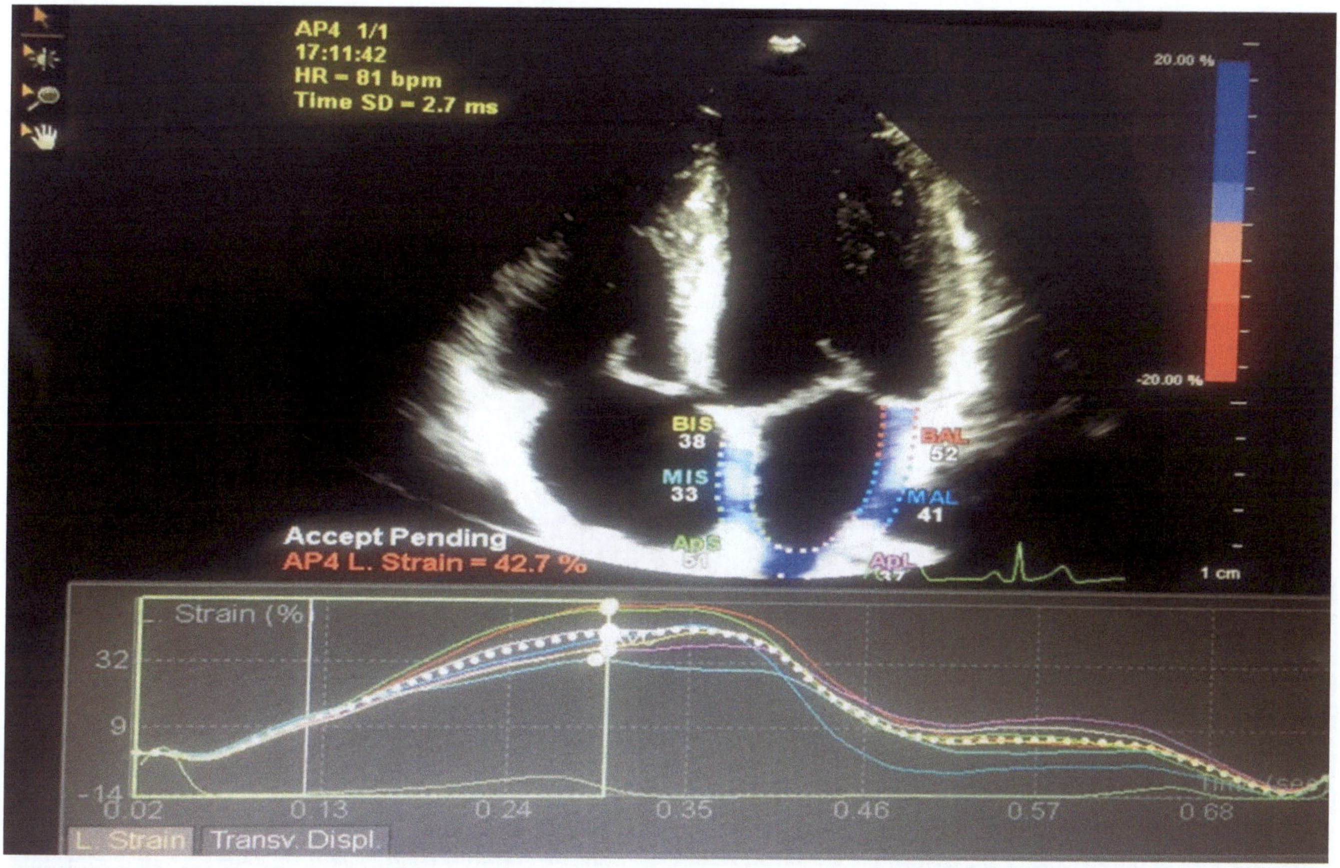

Fig. 12.35 Global and longitudinal LA strain four chamber apical view (with QRS as the reference point)

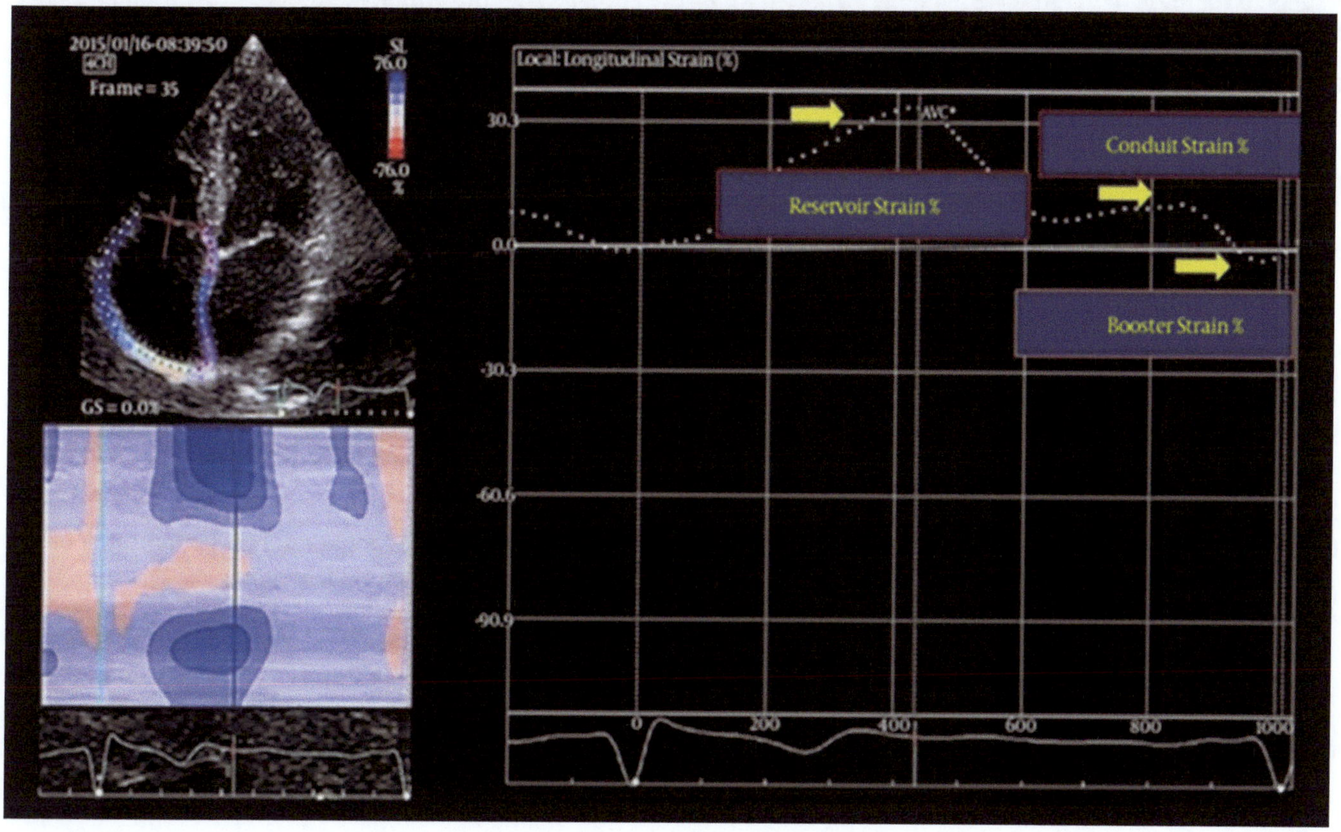

Fig. 12.36 Right atrial strain (%) imaging, showing three mechanical phases in a normal subject

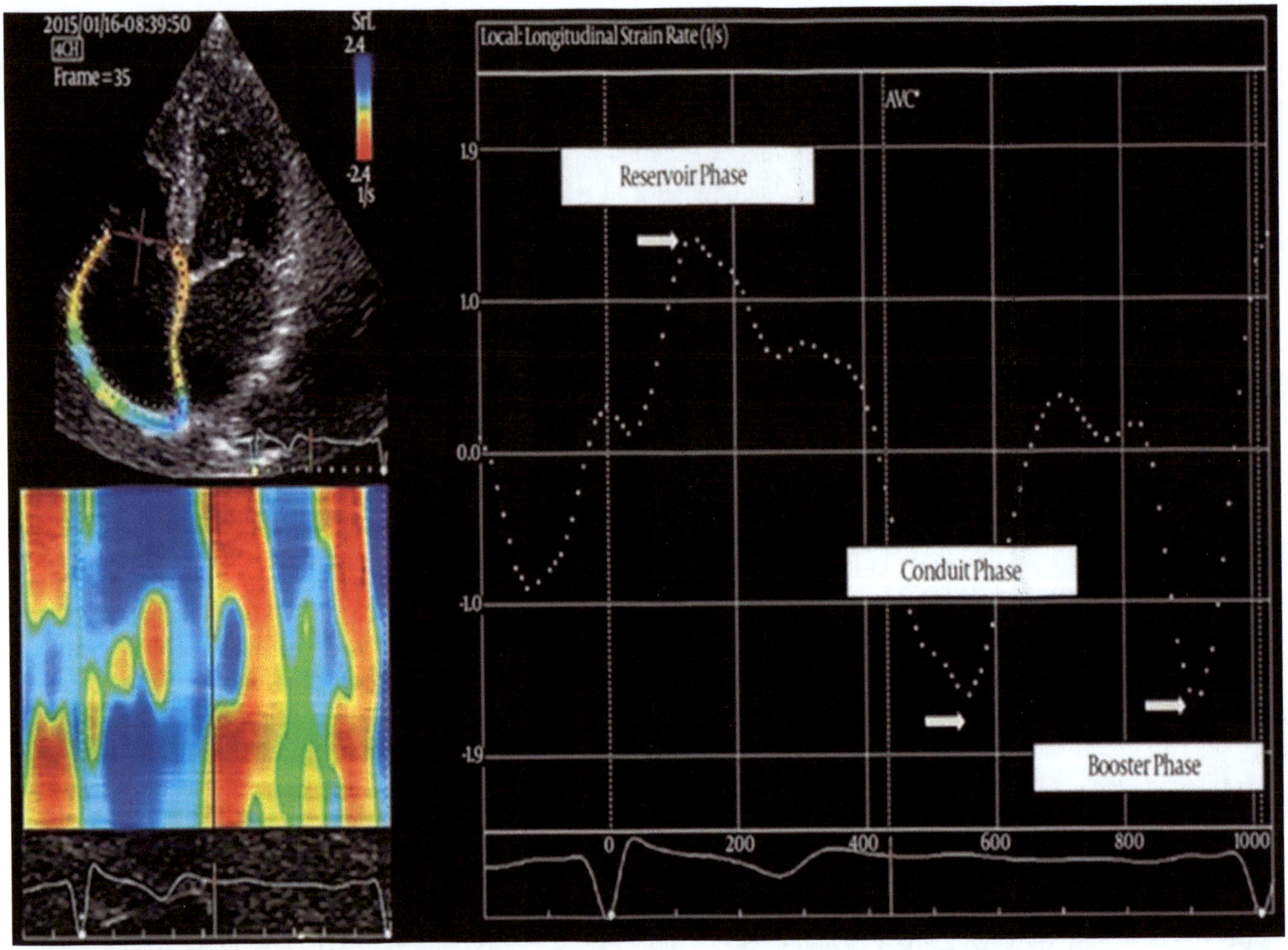

Fig. 12.37 Right atrial strain rate imaging, showing three mechanical phases in a normal subject

Conclusion

DTI and STE and tortional parameters provided objective diagnostic tools in cardiac mechanics. Although their use have been expanded in daily practice, standardization is needed for both the method of measurement and also among the different vendors. On the other hand, additional testing are still necessary to validate the data of parameters of myocardial function [6, 45–51].

Questions

1. All the following statements are the advantages of 2D-Specke tracking (relative to the tissue Doppler imaging) except:
   A. Better Temporal Resolution
   B. Angle Independency
   C. Not influenced by translational motion
   D. Better spatial resolution

2. Which parameter of LV mechanics does not change in constrictive pericarditis?
   A. Longitudinal strain
   B. Circumferential strain
   C. Twisting
   D. Untwisting

3. All following changes could result in optimization of the images in Color Coded DTI, except:
   A. Reducing sector width
   B. Increasing Depth
   C. Gain adjustment
   D. Optimize gray scale display

4. Which one of the following statements is correct about Spectral Pulsed Doppler:
   A. It has excellent temporal resolution.
   B. Mean velocities at a given site could be achieved.
   C. Multiple segments can be examined at a time.
   D. Gain setting has no effect on the results.

5. Which type of strain could be obtained in apical long-axis views:
   A. Radial strain
   B. Circumferential strain
   C. Transverse strain
   D. Shear strain

Answers

1. A
   2d-STE had lower frame rate and poor temporal resolution. Consequently, it has limited utility in tachycardia or non-sinus rhythm)
2. B
   In CP, circumferential strain is reduced but both longitudinal and radial strain are not affected. In RCM, longitudinal, radial are reduced and circumferential strain might be preserved.
3. B
   Narrow sector and reduced depth result in higher frame rate and better images.
4. A
   In spectral Doppler (in contrast to color DTI), peak velocities could be obtained. Excessive gain should be avoided, because can result in over-estimating the velocities. Only one segment can be examined at a time.
5. C
   Transverse strain-, though it is the changes in myocardial thickness- needs long axis apical views.

References

1. Kostis JB, Mavrogeorgis E, Slater A, et al. Use of a range gated, pulsed ultrasonic Doppler technique for continuous measurement of velocity of the posterior heart wall. Chest. 1972;62(5):597–604.
2. McDicken WN, Sutherland GR, Moran CM, et al. Colour Doppler velocity imaging of the myocardium. Ultrasound Med Biol. 1992;18(6–7):651–4.
3. Miyatake K, Yamagishi M, Tanaka N, et al. New method for evaluating left ventricular wall motion by color-coded tissue Doppler imaging: in vitro and in vivo studies. J Am Coll Cardiol. 1995;25(3):717–24.
4. Geyer H, Caracciolo G, Abe H, et al. Assessment of myocardial mechanics using speckle tracking echocardiography: fundamentals and clinical applications. J Am Soc Echocardiogr. 2010;23(4):351–69.
5. Notomi Y, Setser RM, Shiota T, et al. Assessment of left ventricular torsional deformation by Doppler tissue imaging: validation study with tagged magnetic resonance imaging. Circulation. 2005;111:1141–7.
6. Mor-Avi V, Lang RM, Badano LP, Belohlavek M, Cardim NM, Derumeaux G, Galderisi M, Marwick T, Nagueh SF, et al. Current and evolving echocardiographic techniques for the quantitative evaluation of cardiac mechanics: ASE/EAE consensus statement on methodology and indications endorsed by the Japanese Society of Echocardiography. Eur J Echocardiogr. 2011;12:167–205.
7. Otto CM. Advanced echocardiographic modalities. In: Textbook of clinical echocardiography. 5th ed. Philadelphia, PA: Elsevier Saunders; 2013. p. 98–103.
8. Sutherland GR, Bijnens B, McDicken WN. Tissue Doppler echocardiography: historical perspective and technological considerations. Echocardiography. 1999;16(5):445–53.
9. Abraham TP, Dimaano VL, Liang HY. Role of tissue Doppler and strain echocardiography in current clinical practice. Circulation. 2007;116:2597–609.
10. Gilman G, Khandheria BK, Hagen ME, et al. Strain rate and strain: a step-by-step approach to image and data acquisition. J Am Soc Echocardiogr. 2004;17:1011–20.
11. D'Hooge J, Heimdal A, Jamal F, et al. Regional strain and strain rate measurements by cardiac ultrasound: principles, implementation and limitations. Eur J Echocardiogr. 2000;1:154–70.
12. Lang RM, Goldstein SA, Kronzon I, Khandheria BK, Mor-Avi V. ASE's comprehensive echocardiography. 2nd ed. Philadelphia, PA: Elsevier Saunders; 2016. p. 13–6.
13. Heimdal A, Stoylen A, Torp H, Skjaerpe T. Real-time strain rate imaging of the left ventricle by ultrasound. J Am Soc Echocardiogr. 1998;11:1013–9.
14. Urheim S, Edvardsen T, Torp H, Angelsen B, Smiseth OA. Myocardial strain by Doppler echocardiography. Validation of a new method to quantify regional myocardial function. Circulation. 2000;102:1158–64.
15. Gillam LD, Otto CM. Advanced approaches in echocardiography. Philadelphia, PA: Elsevier Saunders; 2012. p. 84–114.
16. Brown J, Jenkins C, Marwick TH. Use of myocardial strain to assess global left ventricular function: a comparison with cardiac magnetic resonance and 3-dimensional echocardiography. Am Heart J. 2009;157:102–5.
17. Amundsen BH, Helle-Valle T, Edvardsen T, Torp H, Crosby J, Lyseggen E, et al. Noninvasive myocardial strain measurement by speckle tracking echocardiography validation against sonomicrometry and tagged magnetic resonance imaging. J Am Coll Cardiol. 2006;47:789–93.
18. Biswas M, Sudhakar S, Nanda NC, Buckberg G, Prradhan M, Roomi AU, et al. Two- and three-dimensional speckle tracking echocardiography: clinical applications and future directions. Echocardiography. 2013;30(1):88–105.
19. Gjesdal O, Hopp E, Vartdal T, Lunde K, Helle-Valle T, Aakhus S, et al. Global longitudinal strain measured by two-dimensional speckle tracking echocardiography is closely related to myocardial

infarct size in chronic ischaemic heart disease. Clin Sci (Lond). 2007;113:287–96.
20. Nesser HJ, Mor-Avi V, Gorissen W, Weinert L, Steringer-Mascherbauer R, Niel J, et al. Quantification of left ventricular volumes using three- dimensional echocardiographic speckle tracking: comparison with MRI. Eur Heart J. 2009;30:1565–73.
21. Maffessanti F, Nesser HJ, Weinert L, Steringer-Mascherbauer R, Niel J, Gorissen W, et al. Quantitative evaluation of regional left ventricular function using three-dimensional speckle tracking echocardiography in patients with and without heart disease. Am J Cardiol. 2009;104:1755–62.
22. Kuznetsova T, Herbots L, Richart T, D'hooge J, Thijs L, Fagard RH, et al. Left ventricular strain and strain rate in a general population. Eur Heart J. 2008;29:2014–23.
23. Lang RM, Badano LP, Mor-Avi V, Afilalo J, Armstrong A, Ernande L, Flachskampf FA, et al. Recommendations for cardiac chamber quantification by echocardiography in adults: an update from the American Society of Echocardiography and the European Association of Cardiovascular Imaging. J Am Soc Echocardiogr. 2015;28:1–39.
24. Nagueh SF, Smiseth OA, Appleton CP, Byrd BF, Dokainish H, Edvardsen T, et al. Recommendations for the Evaluation of left ventricular diastolic function by echocardiography: An update from the American Society of Echocardiography and the European Association of Cardiovascular Imaging. J Am Soc Echocardiogr. 2016;29:277–314.
25. Marwick TH. Measurement of strain and strain rate by echocardiography ready for prime time? J Am Coll Cardiol. 2006;47: 1313–27.
26. Jurcut R, Wildiers H, Ganame J, D'hooge J, De BJ, Denys H, et al. Strain rate imaging detects early cardiac effects of pegylated liposomal Doxoru- bicin as adjuvant therapy in elderly patients with breast cancer. J Am Soc Echocardiogr. 2008;21:1283–9.
27. Poorzand H, Mirfeizi SZ, Javanbakht A, Alimi H. Comparison of echocardiographic variables between systemic lupus erythematosus patients and a control group. Arch Cardiovasc Imag. 2015;3(2):eee30009.
28. Sengupta PP, Mohan JC, Mehta V, Arora R, Pandian NG, Khandheria BK. Accuracy and pitfalls of early diastolic motion of the mitral annulus for diagnosing constrictive pericarditis by tissue Doppler imaging. Am J Cardiol. 2004;93:886–90.
29. Claus P, Salem Omar AM, Pedrizzetti G, Sengupta PP, Nagel E. Tissue tracking technology for assessing cardiac mechanics principles, normal values, and clinical applications. J Am Coll Cardiol Img. 2015;8:1444–60.
30. Cardim N, Oliveira AG, Longo S, Ferreira T, Pereira A, Reis RP, et al. Doppler tissue imaging: regional myocardial function in hypertrophic cardiomyopathy and in athlete's heart. J Am Soc Echocardiogr. 2003;16:223–32.
31. Narula J, Vannan M, DeMaria AN. Of that waltz in my heart. JACC. 2007;49:917–20.
32. Notomi Y, Lysyansky P, Setser RM, et al. Measurement of ventricular torsion by two-dimensional ultrasound speckle tracking imaging. J Am Coll Cardiol. 2005;45:2034–41.
33. Nanda NC. Comprehensive textbook of echocardiography. New Delhi: Jaypee Brothers Medical Publishers; 2014, p.363.
34. Tigen MK, Karaahmet T, Gurel E, Dundar C, Pala S, Cevik C, Akcakoyun M, Basaran Y. The role of isovolumic acceleration in predicting subclinical right and left ventricular systolic dysfunction in hypertensive obese patients. Turk Kardiyol Dern Ars. 2011;39(1):9–15.
35. Rudski LG, Lai WW, Afilalo J, Hua L, Handschumacher M, Chandrasekaran K, et al. Guidelines for the echocardiographic assessment of the right heart in adults: a report from the American Society of Echocardiography. J Am Soc Echocardiogr. 2010;23:685–713.
36. Nagueh SF, Sun H, Kopelen HA, et al. Hemodynamic determinants of the mitral annulus diastolic velocities by tissue Doppler. J Am Coll Cardiol. 2001;37:278–85.
37. Saraiva RM, Demirkol S, Buakhamsri A, Greenberg N, Popovic ZB, Thomas JD, et al. Left atrial strain measured by two-dimensional speckle tracking represents a new tool to evaluate left atrial function. J Am Soc Echocardiogr. 2010;23:172–80.
38. Cameli M, Caputo M, Mondillo S, Ballo P, Palmerini E, Lisi M, et al. Feasibility and reference values of left atrial longitudinal strain imaging by two-dimensional speckle tracking. Cardiovasc Ultrasound. 2009;7:6.
39. Ojaghi Z, Alizadehasl A, Maleki M, Naderi N, Esmaeilzadeh M, Noohi F, Azarfarin R. Echocardiographic assessment of right atrium deformation indices in healthy young subjects. Arch Cardiovasc Imaging. 2013;1(1):2–7.
40. Ojaghi-Haghighi Z, Alizadehasl A, Hashemi A. Reverse left ventricular apical rotation in dilated cardiomyopathy. Arch Cardiovasc Imaging. 2015;3(2):e28112.
41. Naderi N, Ojaghi Z, Pezeshki S, Alizadehasl A. Quantitative assessment of right atrial function by strain imaging in adult patients with totally corrected tetralogy of fallot. Arch Cardiovasc Imaging. 2013;1(1):8–12.
42. Sadeghpour A. Incremental value of left atrium two-dimensional strain in patients with heart failure. Arch Cardiovasc Image. 2013;1(2):49–50. https://doi.org/10.5812/acvi.15896.
43. Ojaghi Haghighi Z, Mostafavi A, Anita S, Peighambari MM, Alizadehasl A, Moladoust H, Ojaghi Haghighi H. Echocardiographic assessment of left ventricular twisting and untwisting rate in normal subjects by tissue Doppler and velocity vector imaging: comparison of two methods. Arch Cardiovasc Imaging. 2013;1(2):63–71. https://doi.org/10.5812/acvi.14289.
44. Zahra Ojaghi Haghighi S, Alizadehasl A, Ardeshiri M, Peighambari MM, Moladust H, Sameie N, et al. The torsional parameters in patients with nonischemic dilated cardiomyopathy. Arch Cardiovasc Imaging. 2015;3(1):e26751. https://doi.org/10.5812/acvi.26751.
45. Alizadehasl A, Sadeghpour A, Hali RR, Bakhshandeh H, Badano L. Assessment of left and right ventricular rotational interdependence: a speckle tracking echocardiographic study. Echocardiogr J. 2017;34(3):415–21.
46. Saha SK. Pulmonary arterial hypertension: a two-dimensional echocardiographic approach from screening to prognosis. Arch Cardiovasc Imaging. 2016;4(2):e41818. https://doi.org/10.5812/acvi.41818.
47. Mihaila S, Cucchini U, Marzaro A, Muraru D, Andras K, Altiok E, Vinereanu D, Sadeghpour A, Alizadehasl A, Badano LP, Becker M. Fully automated measurements of left atrial volume are highly feasible and accurate compared to expert manual measurements: a comparative multi-center study using a novel automated analysis algorithm. In: Abstract presentation. ESC; 2017.
48. Salehi R, Alizadehasl A. Tissue Doppler imaging values in hypertrophic cardiomyopathy according to left ventricular outflow gradient. J Cardiovasc Thorac Res. 2011;2(4):19–22.
49. Alizadehasl A, Haghighi SZO, Sadeghpour A, Bezanjani FN. Echocardiographic assessment of left ventricle torsional parameters by tissue Doppler and velocity vector imaging: comparison of the two Methods. J Am Coll Cardiol. 2013;1(2):63–71.
50. Alizadehasl A, Azarfarin R. Tissue Doppler imaging findings including Prominent S wave in patients with mitral valve prolapse. Arch Cardiovasc Imaging. 2014;1(3):e17123.
51. Kyavar M, Sadeghpour A, Hashemi A, Alizadehasl A, Sanati HR, Hashemi A. The prognostic value of mitral annulus velocities by

tissue Doppler imaging after first anterolateral myocardial infarction. Iranian Heart J. 2013;13(4):(Scopus).

52. Voigt JU, Lindenmeier G, Exner B, Regenfus M, Werner D, Reulbach U, Nixdorff U, Flachskampf FA, Daniel WG. Incidence and characteristics of segmental postsystolic longitudinal shortening in normal, acutely ischemic, and scarred myocardium. J Am Soc Echocardiogr. 2003;16(5):415–423.
53. Manish B, Ravi R. Kasliwal. How do I do it? Speckle-tracking echocardiography. Indian Heart J. 2013;165:117–23.
54. Blessberger H, Binder T. Non-invasive imaging: two dimensional speckle tracking echocardiography: basic principles. Heart. 2010;96:716–722.

13 Echocardiographic Evaluation of the Diastolic Function and Dysfunction

Anita Sadeghpour, Azin Alizadehasl, and Samaneh Pourhosseinali

Abstract

Assessment and study of the diastolic function should be an integral part of the cardiac function evaluation. At present, echocardiography is the best noninvasive way to study and evaluate the diastolic function and to estimate filling pressures. M-mode, 2D, and Doppler (blood flow, tissue, and color) echocardiographic examinations are all useful in evaluating the diastolic function. The left ventricular diastolic filling encompasses a series of events that are affected by numerous factors such as myocardial relaxation, myocardial compliance, cardiac rhythm, and pericardial compliance.

Classification of the diastolic filling pattern (or diastolic dysfunction) is based on several parameters, which will be explained in this chapter.

Keywords

Diastolic dysfunction · Mitral inflow pattern · Tissue Doppler imaging · Pulmonary venous flow · Grading of diastolic function

Abbreviations

A	Peak A-wave velocity of the mitral valve (cm/s)
A′	TDI of the mitral annulus
AF	Atrial fibrillation
AR	Pulmonary valve atrial reversal
AV	Aortic valve
CW	Continuous wave
DT	Deceleration time
E	Peak E-wave velocity of the mitral valve (cm/s)
E′	TDI of the mitral annulus
EF	Ejection fraction
GLS	Global longitudinal strain
HR	Heart rate
IVCT	Isovolumic contraction time
IVRT	Isovolumic relaxation time
LA	Left atrium
LAP	Left atrial pressure
LV	Left ventricle
LVEDP	Left ventricular end-diastolic pressure
MHz	Megahertz
MV	Mitral valve
PCWP	Pulmonary capillary wedge pressure
PV AR	Pulmonary valve atrial reversal
PVs	Pulmonary veins
PVs1	First systolic component of the pulmonary vein
PVs2	Second systolic component of the pulmonary vein
PVd(D)	Diastolic component of the pulmonary vein
PW	Pulsed wave
RV	Right ventricle
SR	Strain rate
TDI	Tissue Doppler imaging
TEE	Transesophageal echocardiography
TTE	Transthoracic echocardiography
TV	Tricuspid valve
VP	Velocity of propagation
VTI	Velocity of time integral

Doppler echocardiography is routinely used noninvasive imaging modality for the assessment of diastolic function. Left ventricular (LV) diastolic function and changes should be included in all Echocardiography reports, particularly in patients with signs and symptoms of dyspnea. The status of diastolic function can guide treatment options and is a prognostic factor for future events [1–3].

A. Sadeghpour, MD, FACC, FASE
Professor of Cardiology, Echocardiography Research Center, Rajaie Cardiovascular Medical and Research Center, Iran University of Medical Science, Tehran, Iran

A. Alizadehasl, MD, FACC, FASE (✉)
Associate Professor of Cardiology, Echocardiologist, Echocardiography and Cardiogenetic Research Centers, Cardio-Oncology Department, Rajaie Cardiovascular Medical and Research Center, Tehran, Iran

S. Pourhosseinali
Echocardiography Research Center, Rajaie Cardiovascular Medical and Research Center, Iran University of Medical Sciences, Tehran, Iran

A. Sadeghpour, A. Alizadehasl (eds.), *Case-Based Textbook of Echocardiography*,
https://doi.org/10.1007/978-3-319-67691-3_13

Definition

- Normal diastolic function is defined as adequately filling ventricle in the setting of normal LA pressure at rest or during exercise.
- LV diastolic dysfunction is the result of impaired LV relaxation with or without reduced restoring forces and increased LV stiffness.

- **LV diastole is divided into four phases**:
  1. Isovolumic relaxation time (IVRT): It is a time period after aortic valve (AV) closure to mitral valve (MV) opening. At this time, LV relaxation occurs with no change in the volume [4].
  2. Early rapid filling: It begins after MV opening and is resulted from the elastic recoil and normal relaxation of the myocardial fibers [5] and ends after the equalization of ventricular and atrial pressures [6]. Over 70% of LV filling occurs during this time [7].
  3. Diastasis: It is a period between early rapid filling and late atrial contraction without a positive driving gradient due to the equilibration of LV and left atrial (LA) pressure [6]. During this time, a small amount of blood is pushed into the LV. In a faster heart rate (HR), diastasis may be absent, in contrast to a slower HR with a longer duration of diastasis.
  4. Atrial contraction: This period contributes to a positive transmitral pressure gradient and accounts for 25% of LV filling (Fig. 13.1).

- Right ventricular (RV) diastolic phases are similar to those of the LV, but the diastolic duration is slightly shorter due to a longer ejection period.

- LV diastolic dysfunction is usually the result of impaired LV relaxation with or without reduced restoring forces (and early diastolic suction), and increased LV chamber stiffness, which increase cardiac filling pressures. when performing an echocardiographic study in patients with potential diastolic dysfunction, one should search for

- The term LV filling pressure refers to the mean pulmonary capillary wedge pressure (PCWP), mean LA pressure,

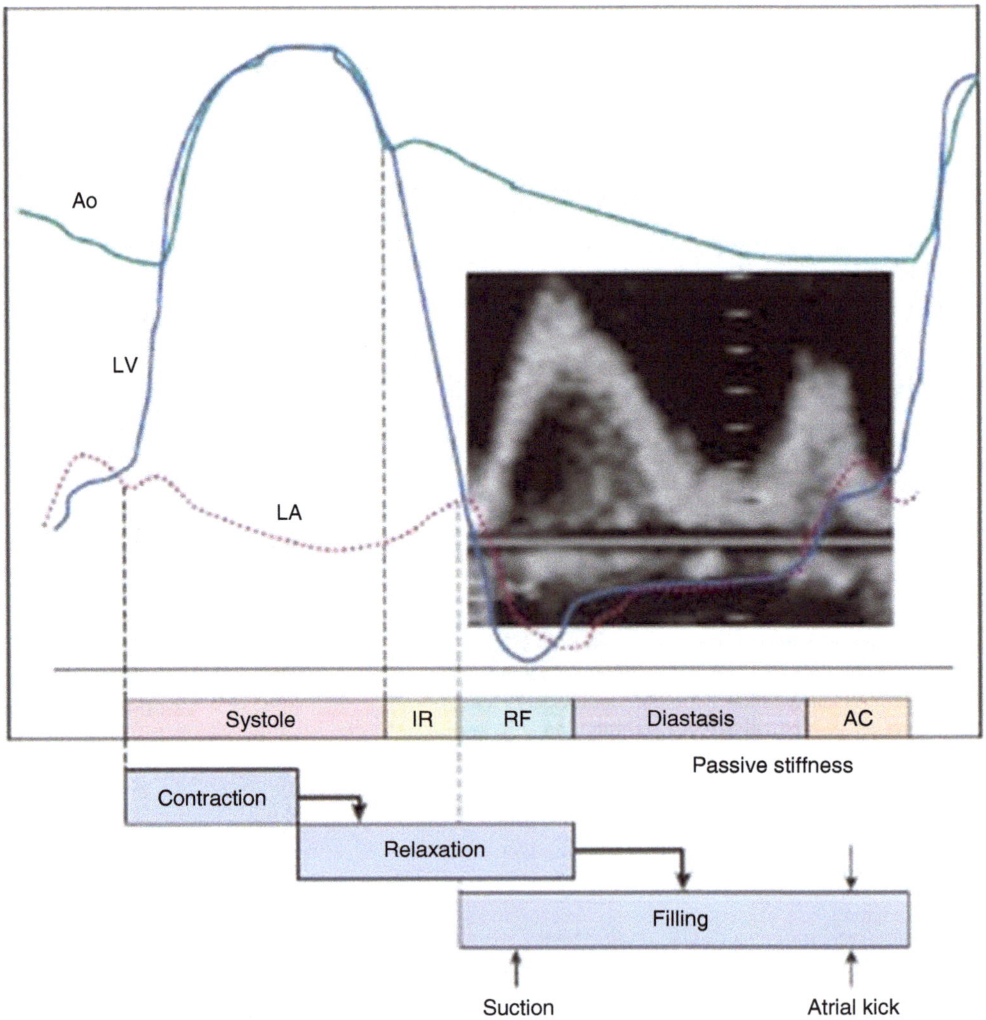

Fig. 13.1 Phases of the cardiac cycle and the relation between the pressure tracing of the Ao, LA, and LV and the transmitral flow. Ao, Aorta; *LA* left atrium, *LV* left ventricle, *AC* atrial contraction, *IR* isovolumic relaxation, *RF* rapid filling

mean LV diastolic pressure, and left ventricular end-diastolic pressure (LVEDP). In the early stage of diastolic dysfunction, only LVEDP is elevated, while the mean PCWP and LA pressure remain normal.

Echocardiographic Parameters for the Assessment of Diastolic Function

- **Doppler techniques** such as transmitral flow velocities, pulmonary vein (PV) flow pattern, tricuspid regurgitation systolic jet velocity, tissue Doppler, and color M-mode are practical parameters for the estimation of the filling pressure.
- **Clinical data, blood pressure, HR, ejection fraction (EF), LV wall thickness, LA volume, presence and severity of MV disease**, and rhythm disturbance should be recorded before the evaluation of diastolic function.
- There is not an isolated index as the sole data in drawing conclusions about LV diastolic function.
- Traditionally diastolic function has been classified based on the Mitral inflow pattern. The rational behind that is that trans mitral flow velocity at the tip of mitral leaflet reflects the pressure gradient between LA and LV. Therefore, E wave velocity is related to the LA pressure and ventricular compliance and A wave shows the strength of atrial contraction (Fig. 13.2).

Grading of Diastolic Dysfunction

- The principal variables for the assessment of diastolic function are:
  - Mitral inflow velocities,
  - e′ velocity,
  - E/e′
  - Peak tricuspid regurgitation jet velocity
  - Indexed LA volume
- Supplementary variables are the PV flow velocity and LV global longitudinal strain (GLS) by speckle-tracking echocardiography.
- Integrated approaches for the assessment of diastolic dysfunction in patients with a normal EF (≥50%) differ from those in patients with a reduced EF
- Consider that aging accounts for impaired relaxation and decreased E/A and e′ velocities. (Less age dependent parameters are E/e′, AR-A duration, pulmonary artery systolic pressure, and LA volume and changes during the Valsalva maneuver.)

- In subjects with a normal EF, four parameters should be evaluated. The following constitute abnormal cutoff values:
  - Annular e′ velocity (septal e′<7)
  - Average E/e′ greater than 14 (lateral E/e′ >13 or septal E/e′ >15)
  - Peak tricuspid regurgitation jet velocity greater than 2.8 m/s
  - Indexed LA volume greater than 34 mL/m^2
- If more than half of the available parameters are within the normal range, LV diastolic function is normal. However, if more than half of the available parameters are abnormal, the presence of diastolic dysfunction is confirmed. If just half of the parameters are present, the grade of diastolic function is not conclusive (Fig. 13.3) [1].

- **In patients with a reduced EF, start with assessing the mitral inflow velocity.** Exclude patients with AF rhythm, mitral stenosis, moderate or severe mitral regurgitation, significant mitral annular calcification , prosthetic MVs, MV repair, pace rhythm, or left bundle branch block, as well as patients with left ventricular assisted devices. Mitral inflow patterns in evaluating diastolic function include:
  - Normal pattern
  - Impaired LV relaxation
  - Pseudonormal pattern
  - Restrictive filling pattern (Fig. 13.4)

- In subjects with E/A less than or equal to 0.8 along with peak E velocity less than or equal to 50 cm/s, the mean LA pressure is normal and the corresponding diastolic dysfunction is grade I (Fig. 13.5).
- In subjects with E/A greater than or equal to 2, the mean LA pressure is elevated so diastolic dysfunction is grade III. Exceptions: There are two conditions with E/A greater than or equal to two despite a normal LV filling pressure:
  1. Recent cardioversion to sinus rhythm, resulting in LA stunning and reduced mitral A velocity
  2. Young subjects (40 years old) (E/A >2 may be normal.)
- **In subjects with E/A less than or equal to 0.8 and peak E velocity greater than 50 cm/s or E/A greater than 0.8 and smaller than 2, the following three parameters should be sought:**
  1. Peak tricuspid regurgitation jet velocity
  2. Average E/e′ ratio
  3. Indexed LA volume
     - If these main parameters are not available, the S/D ratio or S fraction should be assessed.
     - If there is just one parameter available or just two parameters available with opposite information, do not interpret diastolic function.
     - If all the three main parameters are available but only one-third of the positive criteria are present, LA pressure is normal and diastolic dysfunction is grade I.

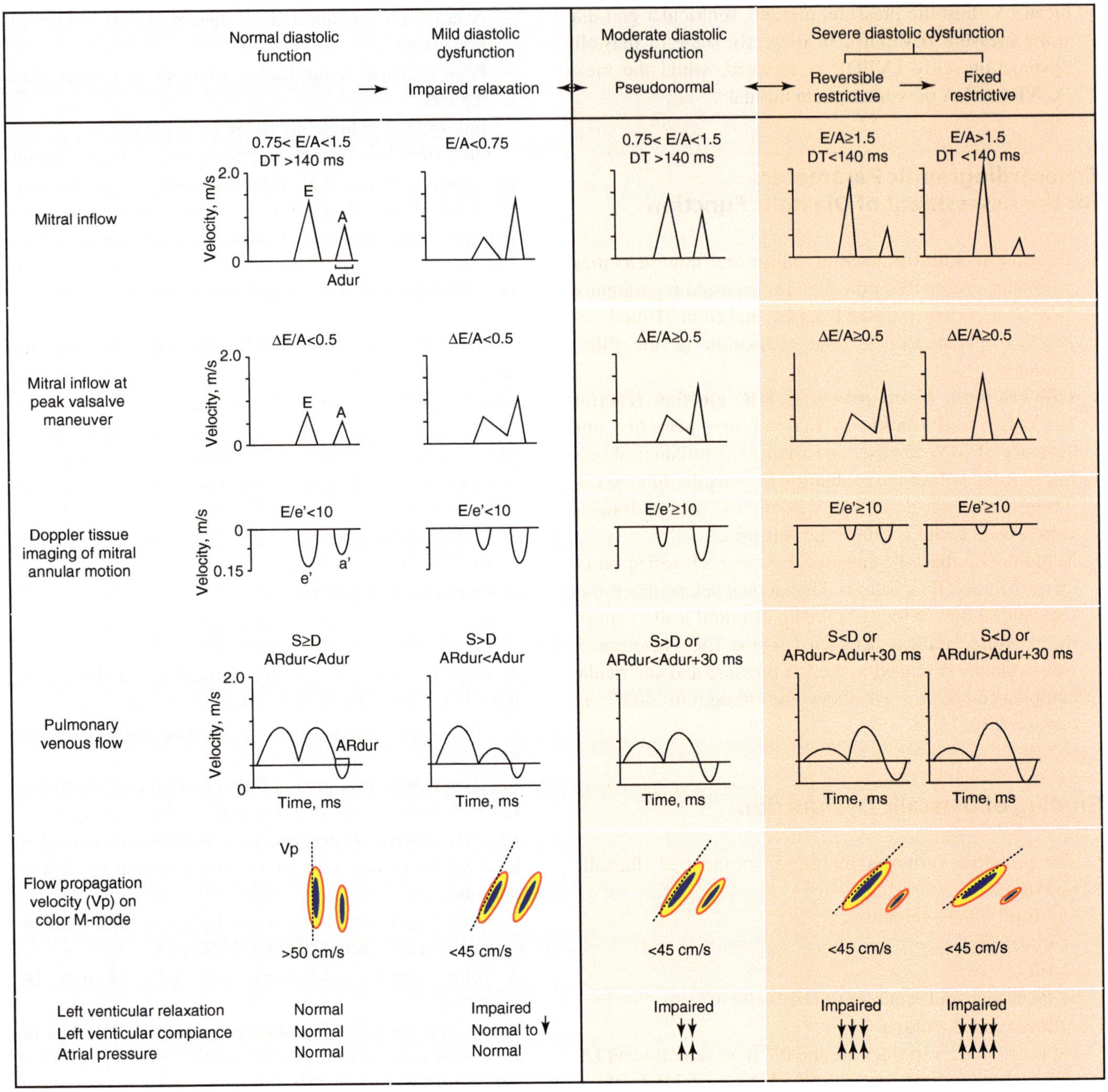

Fig. 13.2 Stages of diastolic dysfunction based on various echocardiographic parameters

– If at least two-thirds of the positive criteria are present, LA pressure is elevated and diastolic dysfunction is grade II.

Mitral Inflow with the Valsalva Maneuver

- Valsalva Maneuver is a forceful expiration against a closed nose and mouth consists of four hemodynamic phases [8]
- Strain phase (phase II) results in a decreased venous return and decreased preload and stroke volumes.
- A decrease of 20 cm/s in mitral E velocity or a 40-mmHg intrathoracic pressure for 10 s is usually considered an adequate effort in a patient without restrictive filling.
- Valsalva maneuver has clinical value in distinguishing normal from pseudonormal patterns and also whether or not the restricted LV filling pressure is reversible. The pseudonormal pattern changes to the impaired relaxation pattern in response to the strain phase (E↓, A↑, DT↑, E/A↓); nonethe-

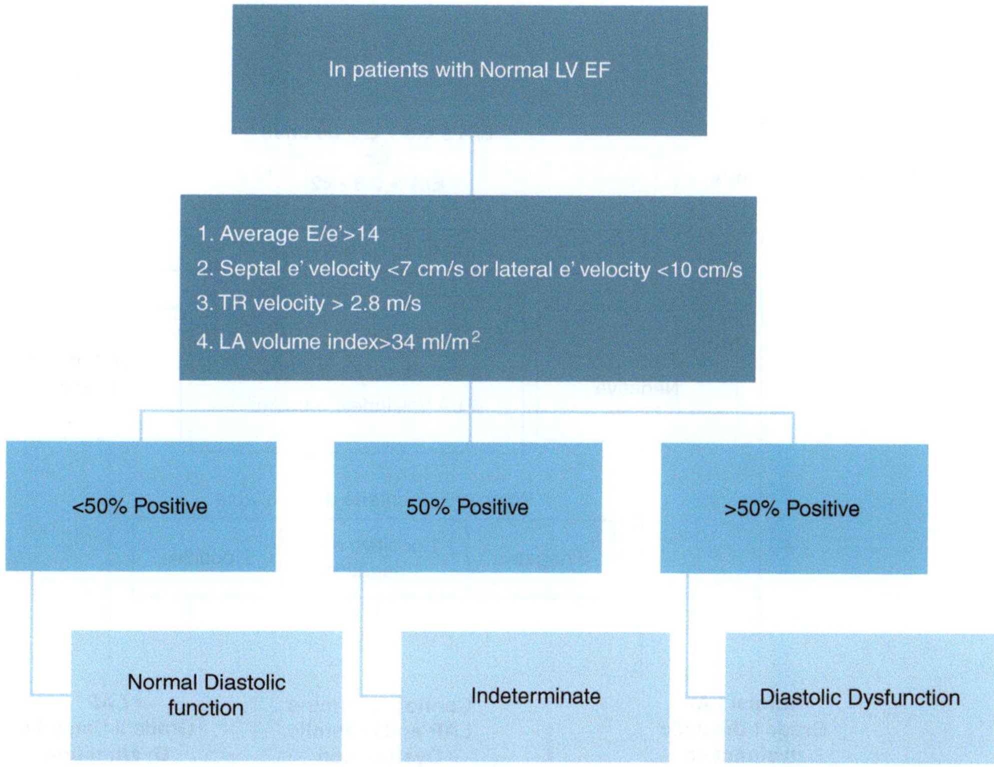

Fig. 13.3 Approach in diastolic dysfunction in patients with a normal ejection fraction. Nagueh S et al. Recommendations for the Evaluation of left ventricular diastolic function by echocardiography: an update from the american society of echocardiography and the European Association of Cardiovascular Imaging. ASE/EACVI Guidelines and standards. J Am Soc Echocardiogr 2016;29:277–314

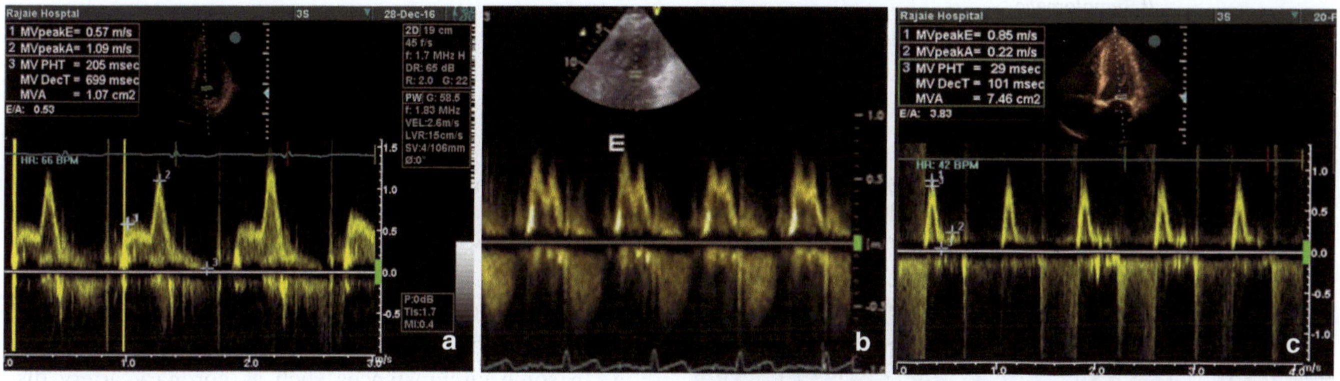

Fig. 13.4 Mitral inflow patterns in different grades of diastolic dysfunction. (**a**) Impaired LV relaxation. (**b**) Pseudonormal pattern. (**c**) Restrictive filling pattern

less, in normal subjects, E and A decrease proportionally (so E/A↔).

- Decrease greater than 50% in the E/A ratio is a clue for an elevated LV filling pressure (Fig. 13.6) [9].

In Mitral inflow Doppler study care should be taken to perform the following steps:

1. Place pulsed-wave (PW) Doppler sample volume (1–3 mm) at the tip of the MV.
2. PW sample volume at the level of the annulus is applied only to calculate the atrial filling duration (A duration).
3. Doppler beam should be aligned parallel to the inflow stream.
4. Color Doppler can be a guide for optimal alignment.
5. Optimize the sweep speed (100 cm/s).
6. Low wall filter setting (100–200 MHz) and a low signal gain.
7. Flow should be recorded at end expiration [1].

- Three parameters should be evaluated via PW at the tip of the MV leaflet:
  1. Early diastolic filling velocity (E velocity in cm/s)
  2. Atrial filling velocity (A velocity in cm/s)
  3. Deceleration time (DT in ms) of the early filling velocity
  4. E/A ratio

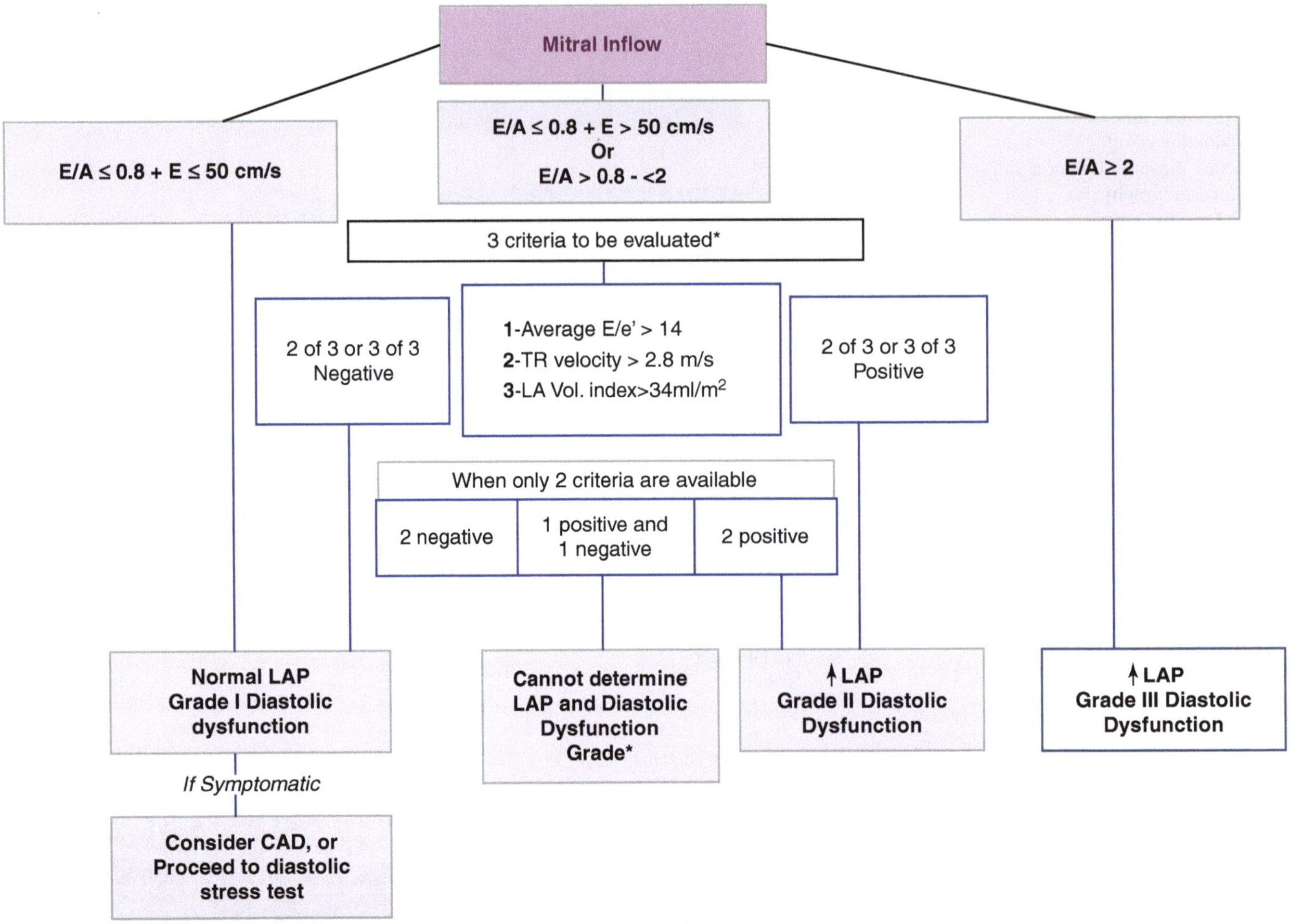

Fig. 13.5 Approach in diastolic dysfunction in patients with a reduced ejection fraction. Nagueh S et al. Recommendations for the evaluation of left ventricular diastolic function by echocardiography: an update from the American Society of Echocardiography and the European Association of Cardiovascular Imaging. ASE/EACVI Guidelines and standards. J Am Soc Echocardiogr 2016;29:277–314

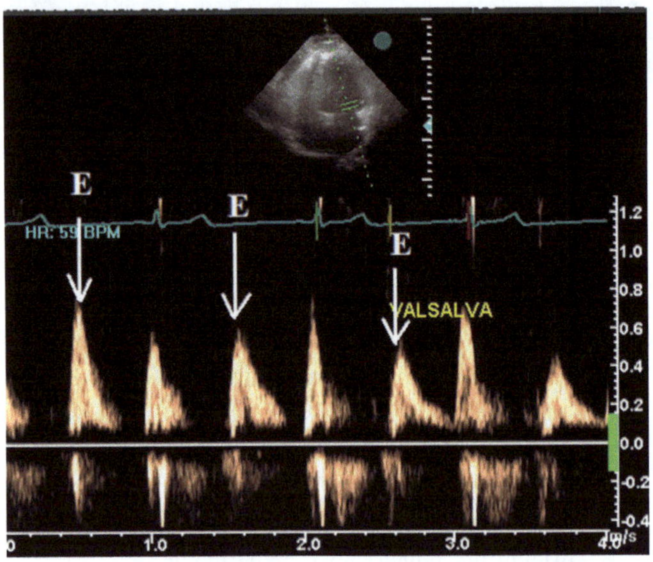

Fig. 13.6 Valsalva maneuver is useful in distinguishing normal from pseudonormal pattern by decreasing greater than 50% in the E/A ratio

- Limitations of the MV inflow recording

  a. In some circumstances such as coronary artery disease, hypertrophic cardiomyopathy with a normal EF, mitral stenosis, and mitral annular calcification, mitral velocities correlate poorly with LV filling pressures.
  b. In arrhythmias and in settings with fused E and A waves
  c. Load and age dependency

- Low velocity mid-diastolic flow (<20 cm/s) may be detected in the MV inflow pattern in normal subjects during bradycardia, but a higher velocity (>20 cm/s)—termed " L velocity"—is a marker of the ongoing LV filling in mid diastole and indicates an elevated LV filling pressure and delayed LV relaxation. This parameter has low sensitivity for elevated filling pressures (Fig. 13.7) [1, 10].

Fig. 13.7 Mid-diastolic flow in the mitral valve inflow, indicative of an elevated filling pressure (arrow)

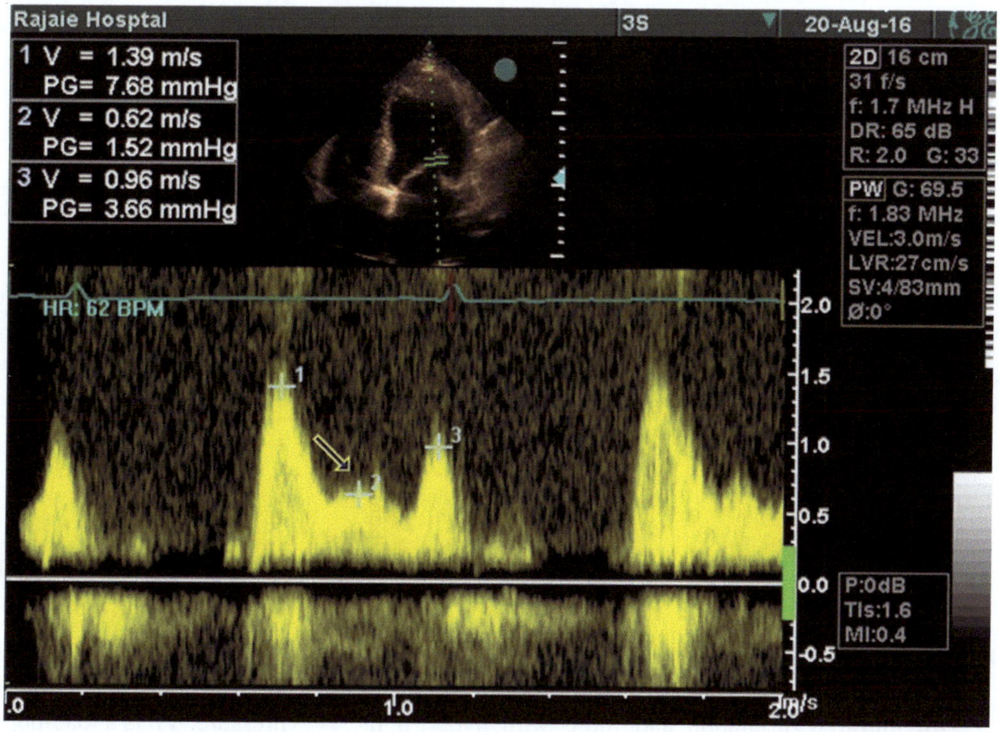

Pulmonary Venous Flow

1. Image acquisition in the apical four-chamber view
2. PW Doppler sample volume (1–3 mm) should be placed between 1 and 2 cm into the right upper PV.
3. Color Doppler can be used to guide optimal position.
4. Sweep speed of 50–100 mm/s, a low signal gain, and a low wall filter setting (100–200 MHz)
5. Recording in end expiration

The PV flow could be recorded in more than 80% of patients [11]. The PV flow profile is triphasic or quadriphasic and comprises the first systolic component of the pulmonary vein (PVs1) (in early systole coincident with atrial relaxation), second systolic component of the pulmonary vein (PVs2) (in mid to late systole and represents the reservoir function of the LA), diastolic component of the pulmonary vein (PVd) (reflects transmitral E velocity and LA conduit function), and pulmonary valve atrial reversal (PV AR) (occurs in late diastole and shows the booster function of the LA) (Fig. 13.8).

- Measurement of the PV waves includes:
  1. Peak systolic velocity (S in cm/s)
  2. Peak antegrade diastolic velocity (D in cm/s)
  3. S/D ratio
  4. Systolic filling fraction (systolic velocity of time integral [VTI]/total forward flow VTI)
  5. Peak pulmonary valve atrial reversal (AR) velocity in late diastole
  6. Duration of the AR velocity (ms)
  7. Time difference between AR velocity and mitral A wave duration (AR-A duration, a parameter independent of the EF and age) (A prolonged time >30 ms indicates a higher filling pressure.)
  8. Deceleration time of the D component

- Normally PVs2 is greater than PVd and S/D is greater than 1.

- One limitation of the PV flow is age dependency. The PV flow in subjects aged below 40 years has a predominant D velocity and in elderly subjects, S/D ratio ↑ and also AR velocity ↑ but it does not exceed 35 cm/s.
- S/D ratio smaller than 1 and S fraction (S VTI/S VTI + D VTI) below 40% indicate an elevated filling pressure in patients with a reduced LVEF (but not in patients with a normal EF, MV disease, hypertrophic cardiomyopathy, and AF rhythm).
- In AF rhythm, blunted S wave and absent AR velocity are seen and the DT of diastolic velocity (D) in the PV flow can be used to estimate the filling pressure.
- AR velocity greater than 35 cm/s and AR-A duration above 30 ms are predictors of an elevated filling pressure [1, 12, 13].

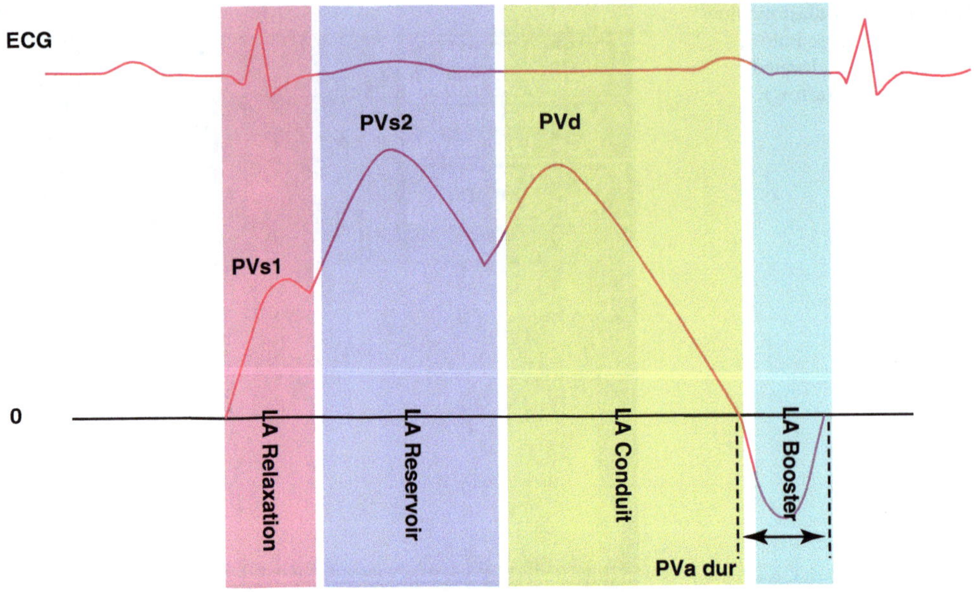

Fig. 13.8 Components of the pulmonary vein (PV) flow: PVs1, PV flow in early systole; PVs2, PV flow in late systole; PVd, PV flow in diastole; PVa dur, PV flow during atrial contraction

- AR-A duration is an age-independent and reliable parameter for the estimation of the filling pressure in patients with mitral regurgitation and those with hypertrophic cardiomyopathy.
- Other limitations of the PV flow velocity are difficulty in recording high quality images, impact of the LA wall motion artifact on the AR velocity, and circumstances with rhythm abnormalities.

Tricuspid Regurgitation Systolic and Pulmonary Valve Insufficiency Diastolic Jet Velocity

- Systolic and diastolic pulmonary artery pressures estimated consecutively by tricuspid regurgitation and pulmonary valve insufficiency end-diastolic jet (in the absence of pulmonary disease) are indicators of LA pressure.
- However, full enveloped tricuspid regurgitation and pulmonary insufficiency jets should be recorded.

Color M-Mode Flow Velocity of Propagation

- Basic concept is derived from the intraventricular pressure gradient from the ventricular suction effect in early diastole. The pressure gradient is generated from the mitral annulus to the LV apex and produces fluid acceleration [14].
- In normal subjects, a faster rate of ventricular relaxation leads the blood flow quickly from the annulus toward the apex, resembling the vertical color M-mode pattern [15].
- PW Doppler recording of the velocity of propagation (VP) in conjugation with mitral E can predict LV filling pressure. VP is a load-dependent parameter.
- Technical points for recording the VP

1. Acquisition in the apical four-chamber view
2. Placement of the color flow with a narrow sector and at a minimum depth to image the LV from the mitral leaflet to the apex
3. M-mode scan line parallel to the mitral inflow
4. Shifting of the color baseline in the direction of the MV inflow
5. Fast sweep speed (100–200 mm/s)

- VP is measured as the slope of the first aliasing flow from the MV plain to 4 cm into the LV chamber during the early rapid filling phase at a four-cm distance [16]. Alternatively, the slope of the transit from no color to color is measured (Fig. 13.9) [15].
- Value greater than 50 cm/s is considered normal [17].

- VP has clinical utility in patients with a reduced EF and a dilated ventricle but not in those with a normal EF and a normal LV volume.
- In patients with a reduced EF, a reduced intraventricular pressure gradient contributes to lower driving pressures and slower mitral-to-apical flow propagation [18].

- Peak E/VP ratio correlates with LV filling pressure. A value greater than 2.5 denotes an LVEDP greater than 15 mmHg [1, 19, 20]

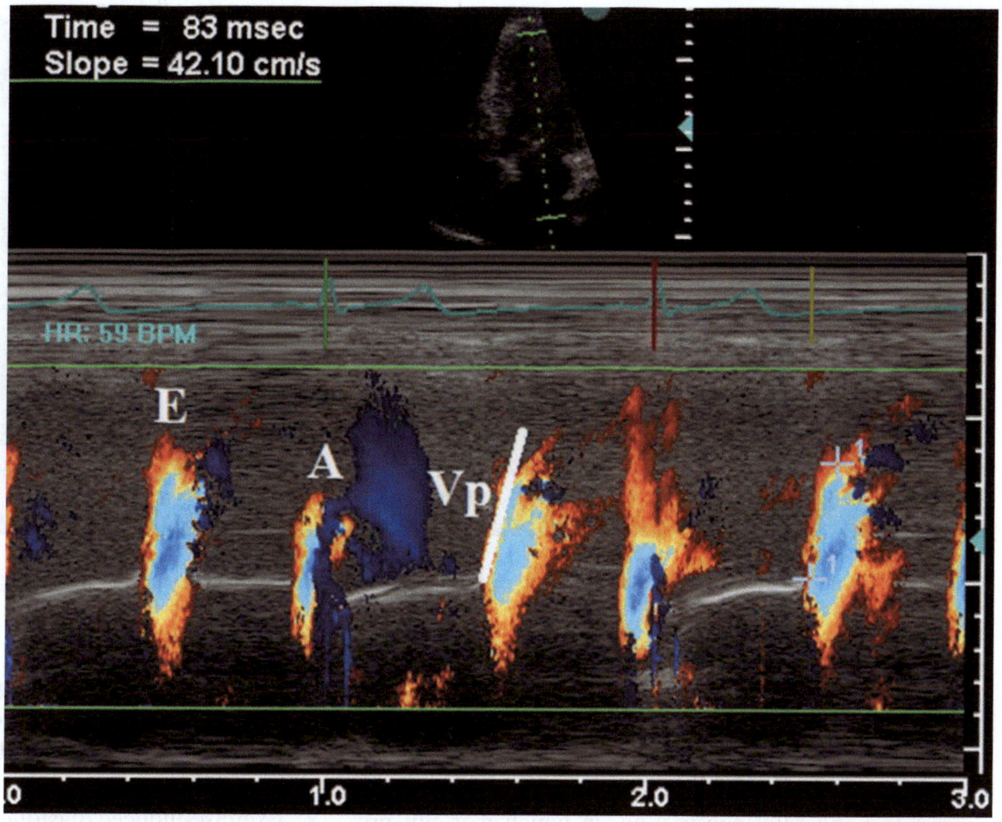

Fig. 13.9 Color M-mode velocity of propagation (VP) <45 cm/s is suggestive for diastolic dysfunction

Tissue Doppler Annular Velocity

- Longitudinal excursion of the MV annulus during systole and diastole can be investigated by pulse tissue Doppler. This parameter is less preload dependent than transmitral flow velocities.

- Points for better recording
  1. In the apical four chamber view, place the sample volume within 1 cm of the septal and lateral sides of the MV annulus and average the velocities [21].
  2. Optimize the Doppler spectral gain and set the velocity scale at 20 cm/s. (Lower settings may be needed in severe LV dysfunction and when there is a markedly reduced annular velocity.)
  3. Parallel Doppler beam is required (<20° angulation).
  4. Sweep speed should be set at 50–100 mm/s.
  5. Set acquisition at end expiration [22].

- Variables that should be recorded
  1. Primary measurements: systolic (S), early diastolic (e′), and late diastolic (a′) velocities (Fig. 13.10) [23]
  2. Secondary measurement: annular e′/a′ and E/e′ ratio. The time interval between the QRS complex and the onset of mitral E velocity is subtracted from the time interval between the QRS complex and e′ onset to derive TE-e′ [23].

- Septal e′ is usually smaller than the lateral one. Septal e′ greater than 10 cm/s and lateral e′ greater than 12 cm/s are considered normal values. In patients with any grades of diastolic dysfunction, e′ velocity decreases [24].
- Tissue Doppler imaging (TDI) parameters are age dependent. By age, e′ velocity drops, whereas a′ velocity and the E/e′ ratio rise [25].
- Average E/e′ ratio smaller than 8 indicates a normal LV filling pressure, whereas a value greater than 14 is in favor of an increased LV filling. (When the value is 8< and <15, other echocardiographic indices should be used.) [26]
- In subjects with a normal EF, it is preferable to record lateral E/e′ because of its better correlations with LV filling pressure [27].
- E/e′ ratio should not be used in patients with constrictive pericarditis and MV disease (mitral stenosis, significant mitral regurgitation, and mitral annular calcification), and post MV surgery (prosthetic MVs and ring annuloplasty) [28].
- Time interval between the onset of E and e′ is prolonged with diastolic dysfunction [29].

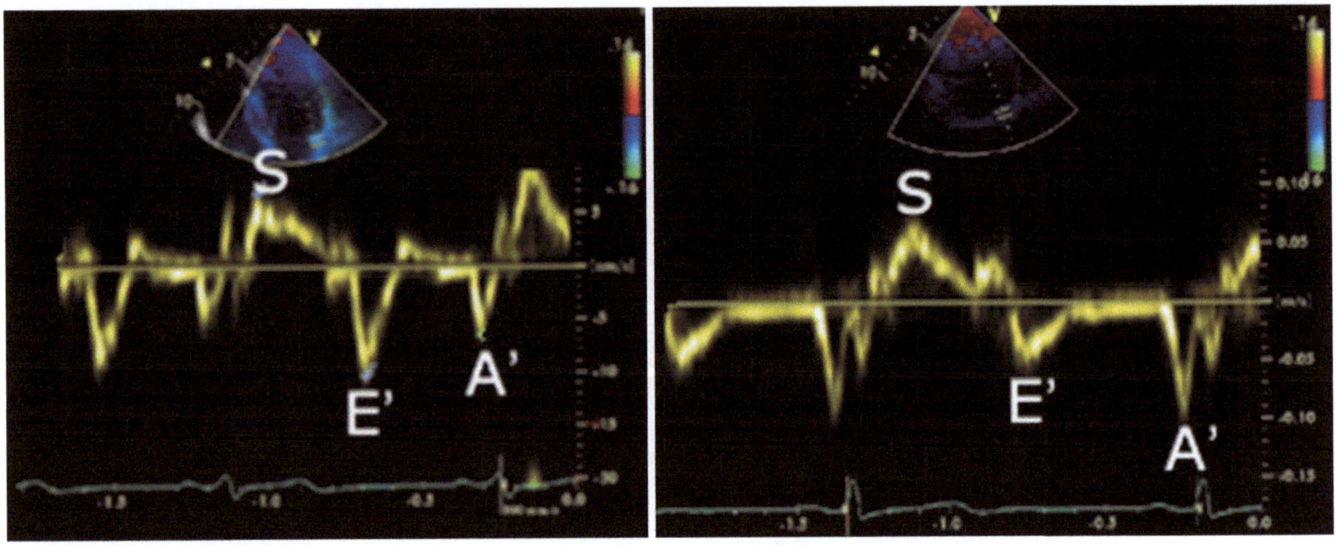

Fig. 13.10 Tissue Doppler imaging in normal (left) and diastolic dysfunction with a reduced E′ velocity (right)

- IVRT/TE-e′ ratio is practical in patients in the gray zone of values (8< E/e′<15), in those with MV disease, and in normal subjects [30].
- TE-e′ is prolonged in restrictive cardiomyopathy, in contrast to pericardial constriction, in which it is not prolonged [31].

Diastolic Stress Echocardiography

- Basis for this test is a rise in LA pressure and PCWP due to tachycardia and increased LV afterload.
- It can be performed using the supine bicycle or treadmill. Dobutamine infusion is discouraged [32].
- It can be applied in patients with mild diastolic dysfunction and normal filling pressures at rest who suffer unexplained exertional dyspnea.

- What parameters in which intervals should be recorded?
  1. E velocity
  2. e′ velocity
  3. Peak tricuspid regurgitation jet velocity

a. At rest
b. During exercise
c. 1–2 min after the cessation of exercise

Response to Exercise Stress Echocardiography in Normal Subjects and in Those with Heart Disease

- In normal subjects, E and e′ velocities rise proportionally so the E/e′ ratio is reversible or drops (<10) [1, 33].
- In patients with underlying heart disease, mitral E velocity rises and stays increased within a few minutes after the cessation of exercise. In addition, e′ drops, E/e′ ratio rises, and DT decreases [34].
- Exercise-induced diastolic dysfunction is considered if all the following parameters are present:
  1. Average E/e′ greater than 14 or septal E/e′ ratio greater than 15
  2. Septal e′ velocity less than 7 cm/s
  3. Peak TR velocity greater than 2.8 m/s

Estimation of LV Filling Pressures in Specific Cardiovascular Diseases [1]

- In subjects with atrial arrhythmias, abnormal cardiac structure, valvular heart disease (in the absence of pulmonary vascular or parenchymal disease), a reliable parameter for estimating LA pressure is the tricuspid regurgitation jet.
- Increased LA volume in the absence of atrial arrhythmia and MV disease could be a powerful clue for an elevated LA pressure.

AF

- Variable cycle length, absent atrial contraction, and the presence of LA enlargement regardless of filling pressures interfere with precise assessment of diastolic function in AF rhythm.
- The following comprise clues for an elevated filling pressure [35–38]:
  1. Peak tricuspid regurgitation jet velocity greater than 2.8 m/s

2. Acceleration rate of mitral E velocity (≥900 cm/s^2)
3. IVRT (≤65 ms)
4. DT of pulmonary venous diastolic velocity (≤220 ms)
5. E/Vp ratio (≥1.4)
6. Septal E/e′ ratio (≥11)

- Keep in mind to match RR interval (measure E and e′ velocities with the same RR interval) or average several cardiac cycles. Patients with lower beat-to-beat variability in mitral inflow velocities have an elevated filling pressure [36].

Sinus Tachycardia

- Parameters with high specificity for elevated filling pressure are as follows:
  1. IVRT less than or equal to 70 ms
  2. PV systolic filling fraction less than or equal to 40%
  3. Average E/e′ greater than 14 (highest specificity)
- In patients with sinus tachycardia, fused E and A waves are misleading. Therefore, find premature beats which can separate E and A velocities [39, 40].

Atrioventricular Block

- In patients with first-degree atrioventricular block, routine parameters for the evaluation of diastolic function are feasible due to the absence of fused E and A waves.
- In patients with cardiac resynchronization therapy, paced rhythm, left bundle branch block, RV pacing, and measurement of mitral inflow velocities and E/e′ are not reliable [41, 42].

Hypertrophic Cardiomyopathy (Irrespective of the Presence or Absence of Dynamic Obstruction and Less-than-moderate Mitral Regurgitation) [1, 43, 44]

- Average E/e′ ratio (>14)
- Indexed LA volume (>34 mL/m^2)
- PV AR velocity (AR-A duration ≥30 ms)
- Peak velocity of the tricuspid regurgitation jet (>2.8 m/s)

In patients with significant mitral regurgitation, the AR-A duration and peak velocity of the tricuspid regurgitation jet can be applied.

- If fewer than two parameters meet the cutoff value, LA pressure is normal and grade I diastolic dysfunction should be considered.
- If more than two parameters meet the cutoff value, elevated LA pressure and grade II diastolic dysfunction are present.
- If a restrictive filling pattern and a reduced mitral annular e′ velocity (septal <7 cm/s and lateral <10 cm/s) are recorded, grade III diastolic dysfunction is present.
- Septal E/e′ ratio is a predictor of adverse outcomes in children with hypertrophic cardiomyopathy [45]. Enlarged LA and diastolic dysfunction are predictors of poor outcomes in adults with hypertrophic cardiomyopathy [1, 46–48].
- Association between LV and LA strain and LV diastolic function and exercise intolerance has been investigated in recent studies [49, 50].

Restrictive Cardiomyopathy

- Diastolic function ranging from grade I in the early stage of the disease to grade III diastolic dysfunction in later stages is associated with a poor prognosis [51].
- Criteria for grade III diastolic dysfunction are as follows [52–55]:

1. E/A ratio greater than 2.5
2. DT less than 150 ms
3. IVRT less than 50 ms
4. Average E/e′ greater than 14

- Restrictive LV filling in restrictive cardiomyopathy may be mistaken with other cardiomyopathies. Apical sparing in longitudinal strain is a discriminative guide [56].

Valvular Heart Disease

Mitral Stenosis

- In the absence of myocardial disease, patients with mitral stenosis have normal or reduced LV filling pressures.
- In patients with mitral stenosis or other obstructive LV inflow lesions (prosthetic MVs, large and protruding LA tumors, or cor triatriatum), mitral inflow velocities and E/e′ are not reliable parameters for the assessment of LV filling pressure.
- Clues for elevated LV filling pressures are as follows [28]:
  IVRT less than 60 ms
  prolonged TE-e′
  IVRT/TE-e′ smaller than 4.2
  higher peak E velocity
  higher peak A velocity greater than 1.5 m/s

Mitral Regurgitation

- Average E/e′ greater than 14 corresponds to an elevated LA pressure in patients with a depressed EF [57, 58]. Nonetheless, in patients with a normal EF, it has limited value.

Clues for an elevated LV filling pressure are as follows:

1. Time interval AR-A greater than/30 ms [59]
2. IVRT less than 60 ms
3. Prolonged TE-e′
4. IVRT/TE-e′ less than 5.6 [1, 28]

Mitral Annular Calcification

- Small MV area, increased mitral inflow velocities, and small e′ velocity can be seen in moderate-to-severe mitral annular calcification as a result of annular calcification [60]
- Underlying diseases like hypertension, coronary artery disease, aortic valve stenosis, and chronic kidney disease may cause diastolic dysfunction, but annular calcification may confounds the interpretation of diastolic function in these circumstances.

Aortic Valve Disease

- In patients with aortic regurgitation, the opening of the MV may be affected by the aortic regurgitation jet, confounding the Doppler recording.
- Clues for an elevated filling pressure in severe aortic regurgitation are as follows:

Acute aortic regurgitation

1. Premature MV closure
2. Diastolic mitral regurgitation

Chronic aortic regurgitation

1. LA enlargement
2. Average E/e′ ratio greater than 14
3. Tricuspid regurgitation peak velocity greater than 2.8 m/s

- In patients with aortic stenosis, guideline-based criteria are applicable but care should be taken for the presence of significant mitral annular calcification.
- In cases with severe AR be it acute or chronic, premature closure of MV, diastolic MR, LA enlargement, average E/e ratio > 14, and TR peak velocity >2.8 m/s are consistent with high LV filling pressures.

Newer Parameters for the Assessment of Diastolic Function (LV Strain and Stain Rate and Untwist and LA Systolic Strain in Diastolic Function)

- Myocardial strain and strain rate are unique parameters for the assessment of myocardial deformation and may help diagnose diastolic function [61]. In heart failure with a preserved EF, LV GLS may be reduced and a reduced GLS correlates with LVEDP.
- Strain rate during early diastole (SR_E) and global strain rate during isovolumetric relaxation time (SR_{IVR}) correlate with LV relaxation, and E/global strain rate during IVRT (E/SR_{IVR}) and also E/SR_E correlate with LVEDP and LV stiffness.
- Global longitudinal diastolic strain rate of LV during IVRT and strain rate during early diastole (E) are correlated with LV filling pressure and prognosis.
- Reduced SR_{IVR} has been shown in patients with heart failure with a preserved EF.
- E/SR_{IVR}
- (ratio <236 cm = PCWP < 15; ratio > 300 cm = PCWP > 15; and 236< ratio <300 = 75% increased PCWP) (It is helpful in patients with borderline data, 8< E/e′ <15, and normal LVEF) [61–63].
- LV untwist rate and the timing of the peak untwist rate are used as the markers of LV relaxation [64, 65]. The correlation between the timing of the peak untwisting rate and the state of diastolic function in subjects with a normal LV volume and a normal EF has been shown in recent studies. Delayed peak of LV untwisting rate in subjects with a normal LVEF is a marker of delayed relaxation [64, 65].
- Decrease in LA systolic strain is related to an elevated mean PCWP [66, 67].
- There is a reverse correlation between the mean PCWP and LA systolic strain, although the measurement of LA strain may be technically challenging in some circumstances. This relation has been demonstrated in both heart failure with a reduced EF and heart failure with a preserved EF [68, 69].

Questions

1. Principal variables for the assessment of the diastolic function are all of the following, except for:
   A. Mitral inflow velocities
   B. a′ velocity
   C. E/e′
   D. Peak tricuspid regurgitation jet velocity

2. In mitral inflow Doppler study, care should be taken to perform the following steps, except for:
   A. Place the pulsed-wave Doppler sample volume (1–3 mm) at the tip of the mitral valve.
   B. Doppler beam should be aligned parallel to the inflow stream.
   C. Color Doppler can be a guide for optimal alignment.
   D. Optimize the sweep speed (20 cm/s).

3. Peak E/VP ratio correlates with the left ventricular filling pressure. A value greater than…denotes a left ventricular end-diastolic pressure greater than 15 mmHg.
   A. 1.5
   B. 2.5
   C. 3.5
   D. 4.5

4. Which parameter is suggestive of diastolic dysfunction in hypertrophic cardiomyopathy (with less-than-moderate mitral regurgitation)?
   A. average E/e' ratio (>8)
   B. indexed left atrial volume (>34 cm^2/m^2)
   C. pulmonary vein AR velocity (AR-A duration ≥30 ms)
   D. peak velocity of the tricuspid regurgitation jet (>1.8 m/s)

Answers

1. B
2. D
3. B
4. C

References

1. Nagueh SF, Smiseth OA, Appleton CP, Byrd BF, Dokainish H, Edvardsen T, et al. Recommendations for the evaluation of left ventricular diastolic function by echocardiography: an update from the American Society of Echocardiography and the European Association of Cardiovascular Imaging. ASE/EACVI GUIDELINES AND STANDARDS. J Am Soc Echocardiogr. 2016;29:277–314.
2. Traversi E, Pozzoli M, Cioffi G, Capomolla S, Forni G, Sanarico M, et al. Mitral flow velocity changes after 6 months of optimized therapy provide important hemodynamic and prognostic information in patients with chronic heart failure. Am Heart J. 1996;132:809–19.
3. Aljaroudi W, AlraiesMC, Halley C, Rodriguez L, Grimm RA, Thomas JD, et al. Impact of progression of diastolic dysfunction on mortality in patients with normal ejection fraction. Circulation. 2012;125:782–8.
4. Thomas JD, Flachskampf FA, Chen C, et al. Isovolumic relaxation time varies predictably with its time constant and aortic and LA pressure: implications for the noninvasive evaluation of ventricular relaxation. Am Heart J. 1992;124:1305–13.
5. Klein AL, Asher CR. Disease of the pericardium, restrictive cardiomyopathy, and diastolic dysfunction. In: Topol EJ, Califf RM, Prystowsky EN, editors. Textbook of cardiovascular medicine. Philadelphia: Lippincott Williams & Wilkins; 2007. p. 420–59.
6. Little WC, Downes TR. Clinical evaluation of left ventricular diastolic performance. Prog Cardiovasc Dis. 1990;32:273–90.
7. Thomas JD, Weyman AE. Echo-Doppler evaluation of ventricular diastolic function: physics and physiology. Circulation. 1991;77:977–90.
8. Nishimura RA, Tajik AJ. The Valsalva maneuver—3 centuries later. Mayo Clin Proc. 2004;79:577–8.
9. Hurrell D, Nishimura RA, Ilstrup DM, Appleton CP. Utility of preload alteration in assessment of left ventricular filling pressure by Doppler echocardiography: a simultaneous catheterization and Doppler echocardiographic study. J Am Coll Cardiol. 1997;30:459–67.
10. Ha JW, Oh JK, Redfield MM, Ujino K, Seward JB, Tajik AJ. Triphasic mitral inflow velocity with middiastolic filling: clinical implications and associated echocardiographic findings. J Am Soc Echocardiogr. 2004;17:428–31.
11. Jensen JL, Williams FE, Beilby BJ, Johnson BL, Miller LK, Ginter TL, et al. Feasibility of obtaining pulmonary venous flow velocity in cardiac patients using transthoracic pulsed wave Doppler technique. J Am Soc Echocardiogr. 1997;10:60–6.
12. Klein AL, Tajik AJ. Doppler assessment of pulmonary venous flow in healthy subjects and in patients with heart disease. J Am Soc Echocardiogr. 1991;4:379–92.
13. Dini FL, Michelassi C, Micheli G, et al. Prognostic value of pulmonary venous flow Doppler signal in left ventricular dysfunction: contribution of the difference in duration of pulmonary venous and mitral flow at atrial contraction. J Am Coll Cardiol. 2000;36:1295–302.
14. Courtois M, Kovacs SJ Jr, Ludbrook PA. Transmitral pressure-flow velocity relation. Importance of regional pressure gradients in the left ventricle during diastole. Circulation. 1988;78:661–71.
15. Brun P, Tribouilloy C, Duval AM, et al. Left ventricular flow propagation during early filling is related to wall relaxation: a color M-mode Doppler analysis. J Am Coll Cardiol. 1992;20:420–32.
16. Garcia MJ, Ares MA, Asher C, Rodriguez L, Vandervoort P, Thomas JD. An index of early left ventricular filling that combined with pulsed Doppler peak E velocity may estimate capillary wedge pressure. J Am Coll Cardiol. 1997;29:448–54.
17. Takatsuji H, Mikami T, Urasawa K, Teranishi J, Onozuka H, Takagi C, et al. A new approach for evaluation of left ventricular diastolic function:spatial and temporal analysis of left ventricular filling flow propagation by color M-mode Doppler echocardiography. J Am Coll Cardiol. 1996;27:365–71.
18. Stugaard M, Smiseth OA, Risoe C, Ihlen H. Intraventricular early diastolic filling during acute myocardial ischemia. Assessment by multigated color M-mode Doppler echocardiography. Circulation. 1993;88:2705–13.
19. Steine K, Stugaard M, Smiseth OA. Mechanisms of retarded apical filling in acute ischemic left ventricular failure. Circulation. 1999;99:2048–54.
20. Rivas-Gotz C, Manolios M, Thohan V, Nagueh SF. Impact of left ventricular ejection fraction on estimation of left ventricular filling pressures using tissue Doppler and flow propagation velocity. Am J Cardiol. 2003;91:780–4.
21. Waggoner AD, Bierig SM. Tissue Doppler imaging: a useful echocardiographic method for the cardiac sonographer to assess systolic and diastolic left ventricular function. J Am Soc Echocardiogr. 2001;14:1143–52.
22. Nagueh SF, Appleton CP, Gillebert TC, et al. Recommendations for the evaluation of left ventricular diastolic function by echocardiography. J Am Soc Echocardiogr. 2009;22:107–33.
23. Nagueh SF, Middleton KJ, Kopelen HA, Zoghbi WA, Quinones MA. Doppler tissue imaging: a non-invasive technique for evaluation of left ventricular relaxation and estimation of filling pressures. J Am Coll Cardiol. 1997;30:1527–33.
24. Mogelvang R, Sogaard P, Pedersen SA, et al. Tissue Doppler echocardiography in persons with hypertension, diabetes, or ischaemic heart disease: the Copenhagen City Heart Study. Eur Heart J. 2009;30:731–9.
25. De Sutter J, De Backer J, Van de Veire N, Velghe A, De Buyzere M, Gillebert TC. Effects of age, gender, and left ventricular mass on septal mitral annulus velocity (E') and the ratio of transmitral early peak velocity to E' (E/E'). Am J Cardiol. 2005;95:1020–3.

26. Ommen SR, Nishimura RA, Appleton CP, Miller FA, JK O, Redfield MM, et al. Clinical utility of Doppler echocardiography and tissue Doppler imaging in the estimation of left ventricular filling pressures: a comparative simultaneous Doppler-catheterization study. Circulation. 2000;102:1788–94.
27. Kasner M, Westermann D, Steendijk P, Gaub R, Wilkenshoff U, Weitmann K, et al. Utility of Doppler echocardiography and tissue Doppler imaging in the estimation of diastolic function in heart failure with normal ejection fraction: a comparative Doppler-conductance catheterization study. Circulation. 2007;11:637–47.
28. Diwan A, McCulloch M, Lawrie GM, Reardon MJ, Nagueh SF. Doppler estimation of left ventricular filling pressures in patients with mitral valve disease. Circulation. 2005;111:3281–9.
29. Rivas-Gotz C, Khoury DS, Manolios M, Rao L, Kopelen HA, Nagueh SF. Time interval between onset of mitral inflow and onset of early diastolic velocity by tissue Doppler: a novel index of left ventricular relaxation experimental studies and clinical application. J Am Coll Cardiol. 2003;42:1463–70.
30. Min PK, Ha JW, Jung JH, Choi EY, Choi D, Rim SJ, et al. Incremental value of measuring the time difference between onset of mitral inflow and onset of early diastolic mitral annulus velocity for the evaluation of left ventricular diastolic pressures in patients with normal systolic function and an indeterminate E/E'. Am J Cardiol. 2007;100:326–30.
31. Sohn DW, Kim YJ, Park YB, et al. Clinical validity of measuring time difference between onset of mitral inflow and onset of early diastolic mitral annulus velocity in the evaluation of left ventricular diastolic function. J Am Coll Cardiol. 2004;43:2097–101.
32. Voigt JU, Exner B, Schmiedehausen K, Huchzermeyer C, Reulbach U, Nixdorff U, et al. Strain-rate imaging during dobutamine stress echocardiography provides objective evidence of inducible ischemia. Circulation. 2003;107:2120–6.
33. Ha JW, Lulic F, Bailey KR, Pellikka PA, Seward JB, Tajik AJ, et al. Effects of treadmill exercise on mitral inflow and annular velocities in healthy adults. Am J Cardiol. 2003;91:114–5.
34. Ha JW, JK O, Pellikka PA, Ommen SR, Stussy VL, Bailey KR, et al. Diastolic stress echocardiography: a novel noninvasive diagnostic test for diastolic dysfunction using supine bicycle exercise Doppler echocardiography. J Am Soc Echocardiogr. 2005;18:63–8.
35. Sohn DW, Song JM, Zo JH, Chai IH, Kim HS, Chun HG, et al. Mitral annulus velocity in the evaluation of left ventricular diastolic function in atrial fibrillation. J Am Soc Echocardiogr. 1999;12:927–31.
36. Nagueh SF, Kopelen HA, MA Q~n. Assessment of left ventricular filling pressures by Doppler in the presence of atrial fibrillation. Circulation. 1996;94:2138–45.
37. Chirillo F, Brunazzi MC, Barbiero M, Giavarina D, Pasqualini M, Franceschini-Grisolia E, et al. Estimating mean pulmonary wedge pressure in patients with chronic atrial fibrillation from transthoracic Doppler indexes of mitral and pulmonary venous flow velocity. J Am Coll Cardiol. 1997;30:19–26.
38. Li C, Zhang J, Zhou C, Huang L, Tang H, Rao L. Will simultaneous measurement of E/e' index facilitate the non-invasive assessment of left ventricular filling pressure in patients with non-valvular atrial fibrillation? Eur J Echocardiogr. 2010;11:296–301.
39. Nagueh SF, Mikati I, Kopelen HA, Middleton KJ, Quinones MA, Zoghbi WA. Doppler estimation of left ventricular filling pressure in sinus tachycardia. A new application of tissue Doppler imaging. Circulation. 1998;98:1644–50.
40. Sohn DW, Kim YJ, Kim HC, Chun HG, Park YB, Choi YS. Evaluation of left ventricular diastolic function when mitral E and A waves are completely fused: role of assessing mitral annulus velocity. J Am Soc Echocardiogr. 1999;12:203–8.
41. Nagueh SF, Bhatt R, Vivo RP, Krim SR, Sarvari SI, Russell K, et al. Echocardiographic evaluation of hemodynamics in patients with decompensated systolic heart failure. Circ Cardiovasc Imag. 2011;4:220–7.
42. D'Souza KA, Mooney DJ, Russell AE, MacIsaac AI, Aylward PE, Prior DL. Abnormal septal motion affects early diastolic velocities at the septal and lateral mitral annulus, and impacts on estimation of the pulmonary capillary wedge pressure. J Am Soc Echocardiogr. 2005;18:445–53.
43. Nagueh SF, Lakkis NM, Middleton KJ, Spencer WH III, Zoghbi WA, Quinones MA. Doppler estimation of left ventricular filling pressures in patients with hypertrophic cardiomyopathy. Circulation. 1999;99:254–61.
44. Kitaoka H, Kubo T, Okawa M, Takenaka N, Sakamoto C, Baba Y, et al. Tissue Doppler imaging and plasma BNP levels to assess the prognosis in patients with hypertrophic cardiomyopathy. J Am Soc Echocardiogr. 2011;24:1020–5.
45. McMahon CJ, Nagueh SF, Pignatelli RH, Denfield SW, Dreyer WJ, Price JF, et al. Characterization of left ventricular diastolic function by tissue Doppler imaging and clinical status in children with hypertrophic cardiomyopathy. Circulation. 2004;109:1756–62.
46. Biagini E, Spirito P, Rocchi G, Ferlito M, Rosmini S, Lai F, et al. Prognostic implications of the Doppler restrictive filling pattern in hypertrophic cardiomyopathy. Am J Cardiol. 2009;104:1727–31.
47. Nagueh SF, Bierig SM, Budoff MJ, Desai M, Dilsizian V, Eidem B, et al. American Society of Echocardiography, American Society of Nuclear Cardiology, Society for Cardiovascular Magnetic Resonance, Society of Cardiovascular Computed Tomography. American Society of Echocardiography clinical recommendations for multimodality cardiovascular imaging of patients with hypertrophic cardiomyopathy: endorsed by the American Society of Nuclear Cardiology, Society for Cardiovascular Magnetic Resonance, and Society of Cardiovascular Computed Tomography. J Am Soc Echocardiogr. 2011;24:473–98.
48. Cardim N, Galderisi M, Edvardsen T, Plein S, Popescu BA, D'Andrea A, et al. Role of multimodality cardiac imaging in the management of patients with hypertrophic cardiomyopathy: an expert consensus of the European Association of Cardiovascular Imaging endorsed by the Saudi Heart Association. Eur Heart J Cardiovasc Imag. 2015;16:380.
49. Chang SA, Kim HK, Kim DH, Kim JC, Kim YJ, Kim HC, et al. Left ventricular twist mechanics in patients with apical hypertrophic cardiomyopathy cardiomyopathy: assessment with 2D speckle tracking echocardiography. Heart. 2010;96:49–55.
50. Wang J, Buergler JM, Veerasamy K, Ashton YP, Nagueh SF. Delayed untwisting the mechanistic link between dynamic obstruction and exercise tolerance in patients with hypertrophic obstructive cardiomyopathy. J Am Coll Cardiol. 2009;54:1326–34.
51. Klein AL, Hatle LK, Burstow DJ, Seward JB, Kyle RA, Bailey KR, et al. Doppler characterization of left ventricular diastolic function in cardiac amyloidosis. J Am Coll Cardiol. 1989;13:1017–26.
52. Koyama J, Ray-Sequin PA, Falk RH. Longitudinal myocardial function assessed by tissue velocity, strain, and strain rate tissue Doppler echocardiography in patients with al (primary) cardiac amyloidosis. Circulation. 2003;107:2446–52.
53. Sallach JA, Klein AL. Tissue Doppler imaging in the evaluation of patients with cardiac amyloidosis. Curr Opin Cardiol. 2004;19:464–71.
54. Appleton CP, Hatle LK, Popp RL. Demonstration of restrictive ventricular physiology by Doppler echocardiography. J Am Coll Cardiol. 1988;11:757–68.
55. Cohen GI, Pietrolungo JF, Thomas JD, Klein AL. A practical guide to assessment of ventricular diastolic function using Doppler echocardiography. J Am Coll Cardiol. 1996;27:1753–60.
56. Phelan D, Collier P, Thavendiranathan P, Popovic ZB, Hanna M, Plana JC, et al. Relative apical sparing of longitudinal strain using

two dimensional speckle-tracking echocardiography is both sensitive and specific for the diagnosis of cardiac amyloidosis. Heart. 2012;98:1442–8.
57. Bruch C, Stypmann J, Gradaus R, Breithardt G, Wichter T. Usefulness of tissue Doppler imaging for estimation of filling pressures in patients with primary or secondary pure mitral regurgitation. Am J Cardiol. 2004;93:324–8.
58. Bruch C, Klem I, Breithardt G, Wichter T, Gradaus R. Diagnostic usefulness and prognostic implications of the mitral E/E0 ratio in patients with heart failure and severe secondary mitral regurgitation. Am J Cardiol. 2007;100(5):860.
59. Rossi A, Cicoira M, Golia G, Anselmi M, Zardini P. Mitral regurgitation and left ventricular diastolic dysfunction similarly affect mitral and pulmonary vein flow Doppler parameters: the advantage of end-diastolic markers. J Am Soc Echocardiogr. 2001;14:562–8.
60. Soeki T, Fukuda N, Shinohara H, Sakabe K, Onose Y, Sawada Y, et al. Mitral inflow and mitral annular motion velocities in patients with mitral annular calcification: evaluation by pulsed Doppler echocardiography and pulsed Doppler tissue imaging. Eur J Echocardiogr. 2002;3:128–34.
61. Dokainish H, Sengupta R, Pillai M, Bobek J, Lakkis N. Usefulness of new diastolic strain and strain rate indexes for the estimation of left ventricular filling pressure. Am J Cardiol. 2008;101:1504–9.
62. Ersbøll M, Andersen MJ, Valeur N, Mogensen UM, Fahkri Y, Thune JJ, et al. Early diastolic strain rate in relation to systolic and diastolic function and prognosis in acute myocardial infarction: a two-dimensional speckle tracking study. Eur Heart J. 2014;35:648–56.
63. Wang J, Khoury DS, Thohan V, Torre-Amione G, Nagueh SF. Global diastolic strain rate for the assessment of left ventricular relaxation and filling pressures. Circulation. 2007;115:1376–83.
64. Notomi Y, Lysyansky P, Setser RM, Shiota T, Popovic ZB, Martin-Miklovic MG, et al. Measurement of ventricular torsion by two dimensional ultrasound speckle tracking imaging. J Am Coll Cardiol. 2005;45:2034–41.
65. Helle-Valle T, Crosby J, Edvardsen T, Lyseggen E, Amundsen BH, Smith HJ, et al. New noninvasive method for assessment of left ventricular rotation: speckle tracking echocardiography. Circulation. 2005;112:3149–56.
66. Ersbøll M, Andersen MJ, Valeur N, Mogensen UM, Waziri H, Møller JE, et al. The prognostic value of left atrial peak reservoir strain in acute myocardial infarction is dependent on left ventricular longitudinal function and left atrial size. Circ Cardiovasc Imag. 2013;6:26–33.
67. Antoni ML, ten Brinke EA, Atary JZ, Marsan NA, Holman ER, Schalij MJ, et al. Left atrial strain is related to adverse events in patients after acute myocardial infarction treated with primary percutaneous coronary intervention. Heart. 2011;97:1332–7.
68. Kurt M, Wang J, Torre-Amione G, Nagueh SF. Left atrial function in diastolic heart failure. Circ Cardiovasc Imag. 2009;2:10–5.
69. Wakami K, Ohte N, Asada K, Fukuta H, Goto T, Mukai S, et al. Correlation between left ventricular end-diastolic pressure and peak left atrial wall strain during left ventricular systole. J Am Soc Echocardiogr. 2009;22:847–51.

Echocardiographic Evaluation of the Right Heart

14

L. Rudski and J. Deschamps

Abstract

There is one consensus Guideline for the Echocardiographic Assessment of the Right heart in adults in 2010, with a recent update ASE/EACVI in 2015. The RV is particularly prone to inaccurate measurements due to its triangular/crescentic shape, and requires modification of some views, including the RV focused four chamber apical view. Complete assessment requires a combination of qualitative and quantitative measurements of the RH chamber size, two RV regional and one global systolic function measurements, and estimation of systolic pulmonary artery pressure. Additional measurements are optional and disease or situation specific.

RH measurements are not corrected for body surface area, age or ethnicity, although there are increasing data aiming to provide these stratifications.

Most causes of RV dysfunction are secondary to either pressure overload, volume overload, or acute myocardial contractility dysfunction. A minority of cases are congenital or secondary intrinsic wall dysfunction. Conditions associated with pressure overload pattern include acute and chronic PE, Pulmonary Arterial Hypertension, Left Heart Disease and Lung disease. Conditions associated with volume overload include Tricuspid Regurgitation, Left Heart Disease, Intrinsic myocardial disorders.

Keywords

2DE: Two dimensional echo · 3DE: Three dimensional echo · CHFpEF: CHF with preserved EF · CHFrEF: CHF with reduced EF · Mean pulmonary artery pressure · Right heart disease

L. Rudski, MD, FRCPC, FACC, FASE (✉)
J. Deschamps, MD, FRCPC
Azrieli Heart Center Division of Cardiology, Department of Medicine, Jewish General Hospital, McGill University, Montreal, QC, Canada

Abbreviations

2DE	Two dimensional echo
3DE	Three dimensional echo
4C	Four chamber
AMI	Acute myocardial infarction
BSA	Body surface area
CHFpEF	CHF with preserved EF
CHFrEF	CHF with reduced EF
CTED	Chronic thromboembolic disease
CTEPH	Chronic thromboembolic PH
DTI	Doppler tissue imagine
EF	Ejection fraction
ET	Excursion time
FAC	Fractional area change
HF	Heart failure
IVC	Inferior vena cava
LHD	Left heart disease
LV	Left ventricle
MPAP	Mean pulmonary artery pressure
PADP	Pulmonary artery diastolic pressure
PE	Pulmonary embolus
PH	Pulmonary hypertension
PLAX	Parasternal long axis
POCUS	Point of care ultrasound
PSAX	Parasternal short axis
PW	Power wave
RA	Right atrium
RH	Right heart
RV	Right ventricle
RVOT	Right ventricular outflow tract
RVSP	Right ventricular systolic pressure
SPAP	Systolic pulmonary artery pressure
STE	Speckle tracking echocardiography
TA	Tricuspid annulus
TCO	Tricuspid closure-opening time
TR	Tricuspid regurgitation
TV	Tricuspid valve

A. Sadeghpour, A. Alizadehasl (eds.), *Case-Based Textbook of Echocardiography*,
https://doi.org/10.1007/978-3-319-67691-3_14

Introduction

- This chapter will briefly review the physiology of the right heart followed by measurements needed for the echocardiographic assessment of the right heart. A review of specific conditions and their echocardiographic particularities will include right heart dysfunction secondary to thromboembolic disease, left heart disease, valvular heart disease, intrinsic myocardial dysfunction and coronary disease. It will not cover pulmonary arterial hypertension and congenital disease—please refer to appropriate chapters.
- The only current consensus guideline that specifically details right heart measurements is the Guidelines for the Echocardiographic Assessment of the Right Heart in Adults in 2010, under the American Society of Echocardiography (ASE) [1], though the recommendations included in this document were updated in a recent ASE/EACVI document on recommendations for chamber quantification [2].

Physiology

- The morphology of the right ventricle differs from the left ventricle and is more in keeping with a triangular/crescentic shape, resulting in a shape that resembles a pyramid that wraps around the left ventricle. It additionally differs in the absence of a third spiral layer present in the LV, and consists only of a layer of circumferential fibers and a layer of longitudinal fibers [3–5]. Its contraction is thus principally in a base to apex and less so an inwards motion, rather than towards the center of the cavity in the case of the LV [6]. Its limited contractility potential, as a consequence of the thinner free wall [3] leads to a higher end-diastolic volume, and a reduced RV ejection fraction as compared to the LV [3–5]. The stroke volume is however similar, as the RV is essentially in series with the LV, and obligated to pump the same stroke volume [3, 7]. The RV thus operates at higher volumes than the LV.
- The right heart is adapted to a low afterload state, pumping against a pulmonary vascular system with low vascular resistance, and greater pulmonary artery distensibility than in the systemic circulation [3, 7]. The RV is thus prone to dysfunction in acute pressure overload due to a thinner RV free wall and smaller overall RV mass adapted to a low pressure system.
- In terms of adaptation to chronic stress states, it reacts similarly to the left ventricle. Chronic volume overload states lead to cavity dilatation in order to preserve stroke volume; chronic pressure overload leads to RV hypertrophy [3, 6].

Right Heart Measurements

General Statements

- Assessment of RV size and function requires a combination of qualitative and quantitative measurements. Additionally, the more extensive study of the LV has led to standardized imaging planes for evaluation that are not as well established for RV evaluation [1].
- It is important to recognize that most measures of RV size and function are NOT indexed to body surface area, age or ethnicity. There are few data to support these classifications, but some data has emerged in a few areas. Most notably, RV volumes and ejection fraction by 3D have been stratified [8]. Accordingly, when evaluating and reporting right heart parameters, the interpreting physician needs to use clinical judgment in determining normal from abnormal, particularly at the extremes of body size and age.
- Essential views and which measurements should be obtained are listed below [2].

View/window	Measurement
Standard apical four-chamber view	(Relative RV:LV size ratio), RA dimensions/volume
Right ventricle focused apical four chamber view	RV basal dimension, RV EDA and RV ESA to calculate % FAC
Left parasternal long	Proximal RVOT, RV free wall thickness
Left parasternal short	Proximal RVOT, distal RVOT
Subcostal	RV free wall thickness

- Measurements in RV assessment include mandatory and optional elements [2].

Mandatory	Optional	Preferable(experience/equipment)
Chamber size • RV, RA, • RVOT • IVC	**Chamber size** • RV wall thickness • RVOT	
RV systolic function—Global • Fraction area change (FAC)	**RV systolic function—Global** • RIMP • RV dP/dT	**RV systolic function—Global** • 3DE RV volume • 3DE EF
RV systolic function—Regional • Tricuspid annular plane systolic excursion (TAPSE) • Free wall velocity of excursion (S′)	**RV systolic function—Regional** • 2D strain	

Pulmonary artery • Systolic pulmonary Artery Pressure (SPAP)	**Pulmonary artery** • Pulmonary Artery diastolic pressure (PADP) • Mean PA pressure (MPAP)	
	Others • RV diastolic dysfunction	

RV Apical Views

- There are two views used for RV assessment: the **standard apical four chamber (4C) view** and the **RV focused apical 4C view** (Figs. 14.1, 14.2).
- The standard apical 4C view is used in RV assessment, but has limitations secondary to the pyramidal geometry of the RV. Different cut planes may result in variable dimensions of the cavity, which may affect measurements, so it is used mostly for systolic function and qualitative assessment of RV (Fig. 14.3) [1, 2].
  - If the RV apex displaces the LV apex as the "apex-forming" ventricle, this suggests RV enlargement, even in the presence of "normal" measurements [1].
  - If the RV is more than 2/3rd to 3/4th of the LV size, this suggests enlargement (Fig. 14.2) [1]. This is especially true if the LV appears underfilled.
- The RV focused apical 4C view is obtained by
  - focusing on the RV;
  - having the LV apex at the center of the scanning sector, displaying the largest basal RV diameter—to avoid foreshortening;
  - rotating the transducer until the maximal plane is obtained for the minor distance;
  - avoiding apical 5 chamber view (LVOT in plane) and avoid postural angulation (coronary sinus in plane)

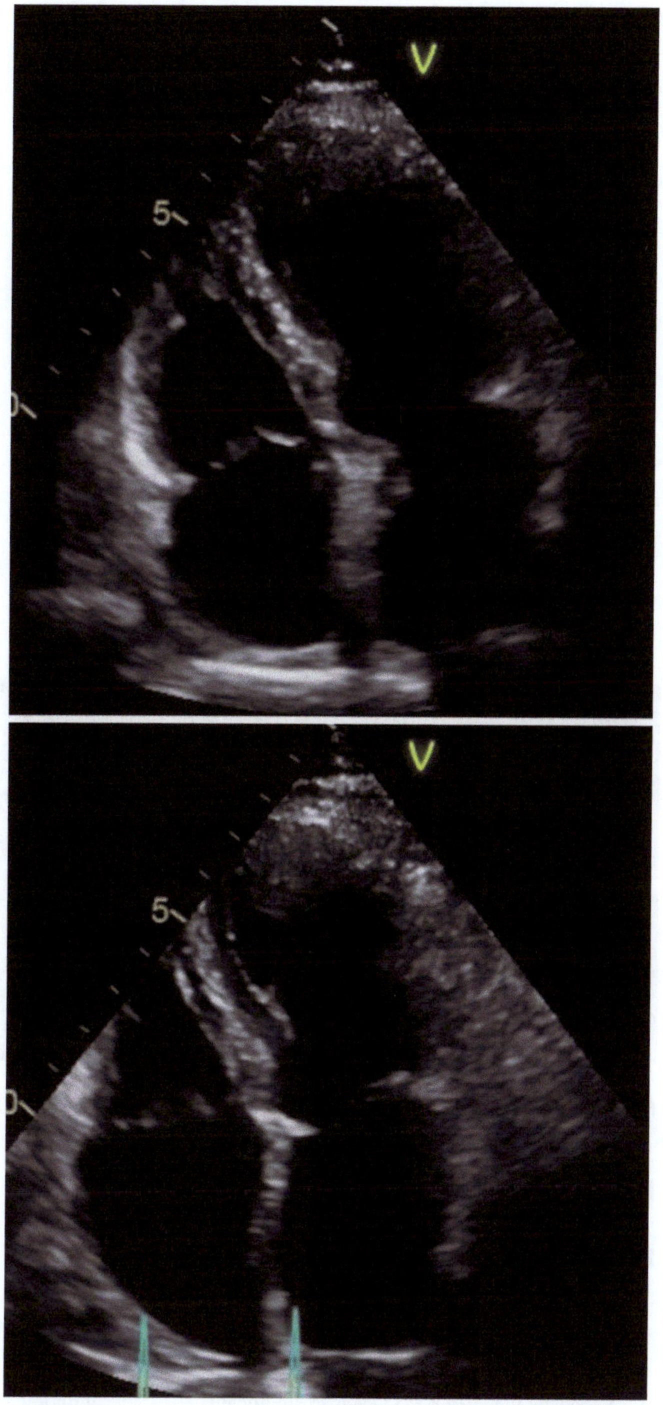

Fig. 14.1 Top: RV focused apical 4C view; Bottom: standard 4C apical view

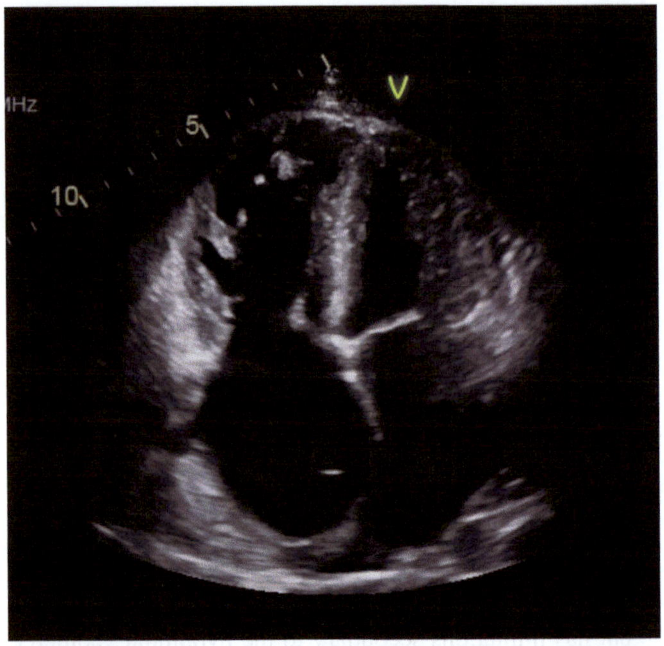

Fig. 14.2 RV enlargement: notice that the RV exceeds 2/3rd of the LV size

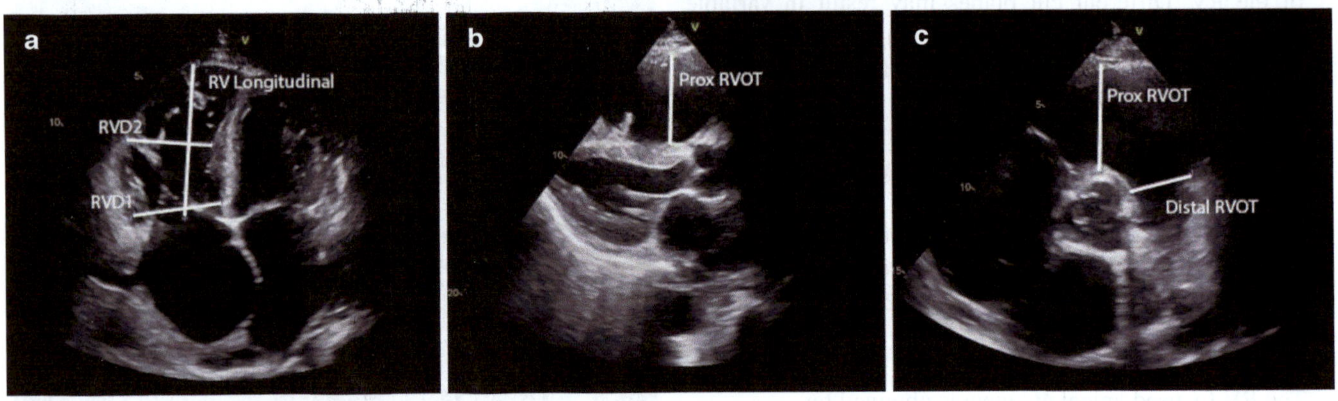

Fig. 14.3 Image 1: Measurements of the RV dimensions; Image 2: RVOT proximal in PLAX; Image 3 and 4: RVOT proximal and distal in PSAX

RV Chamber Size

Linear Measurements

RV basal dimension [1, 2]—Abnormal: Base >41 mm; Mid >35 mm; Longitudinal >83 mm		
Recommended view • **RV focused view—best standardization** • Subcostal view (POCUS) leads to significant translational movement into and out of the imaging plane and is significantly affected by probe angulation, so should not be used to estimate size	**Importance** • Correlation of RV linear dimensions with RV end-diastolic volumes appears to worsen with increased preload/afterload	**Limitations** • Unrealistic to expect a single linear dimension to represent a complex 3-D shape • Possible RV size underestimation due to crescent RV shape • RV linear dimensions dependent on probe rotation • Not BSA indexed
Measures—obtained at end-diastole: • Basal RV linear dimensions (RVD1): maximal transversal dimension in the basal 1/3 of RV inflow • Mid-Cavitary RV linear dimensions (RVD2: transversal RV diameter in the middle 1/3 of RV inflow [1], approximately ½ between maximal basal diameter and apex, at level of papillary muscles • Longitudinal dimension: plane of tricuspid annulus to RV apex		

RV outflow tract dimensions [1, 2]—Abnormal: Proximal RVOT >35 mm; Distal RVOT >27 mm
Recommended view: PSAX or PLAX [2]; Alternate: subcostal short axis or standard apical 4C view anteriorly angulated—thin/large rib space

Importance	Limitations
• First segment of the RV to show diastolic inversion in the setting of tamponade • Report proximal and distal RVOT in congenital heart disease or arrhythmia involving RVOT	• Off axis RV view in respect to RVOT leads to under/ overestimation • Endocardial definition often suboptimal, particularly distal • Limited data

Measures—at end-diastole on QRS deflection:

- PSAX—**Preferred view**
  - **Distal RVOT—Preferred measurement**
    Linear transversal dimension just proximal to pulmonary valve at end-diastole
    Facilitates calculation for regurgitant fraction when significant AR present, or to calculate Qp/Qs when shunt present; most reproducible
  - Proximal RVOT—Linear dimension from anterior RV wall to aortic valve; or anterior aortic wall to the RV free wall above aortic valve
- PLAX
  - Proximal RVOT—Linear dimension from anterior RV wall to IV septal-aortic junction
  - Particularity: best standardized view for evaluation of arrhythmogenic RV cardiomyopathy (Fig. 14.4)

RV wall thickness—Abnormal ≥5 mm [1, 2]

Recommended views: Subcostal or left parasternal window (PLAX)

Importance:	**Limitations**:
• Wall thickness may increase in chronic RV pressure overload, hypertrophic and infiltrative CMP, and in significant LV Hypertrophy even in absence of PH • Wall thickness may decrease focally in arrhythmogenic RV CMP	• Thickened visceral pericardium may lead to overestimation • Challenging when heavily trabeculated

Measures—at end-diastole:

- M-Mode or 2DE
- Measure at a distance below tricuspid annulus approximating fully opened anterior tricuspid leaflet parallel to RV free wall and in subcostal view, at level of tip of anterior tricuspid leaflet
- Exclude trabeculae, papillary muscles and epicardial fat—overestimation may occur otherwise
- Improve imaging by: Using zoomed imaging, decreasing depth and adjusting focus, using fundamental imaging to avoid thickness seen with harmonics (Fig. 14.5)

RA measurements—Abnormal values [1, 2]
RA Volume: Male >25 ± 7 mL/m^2-Upper limit—39 mL/m^2; Women >21 ± 6 mL/m^2-Upper limit 33 mL/m^2
RA Area >18 cm^2; RA major axis >53 mm, RA minor axis >44 mm

Recommended views: Standard apical 4C view

Importance	**Limitations**
• The RA area was a predictor of mortality or transplant in a study of 25 patients with primary PH [1] • RA dilatation was documented in atrial arrhythmias, and showed reversed remodeling after RF ablation	• RA volume is preferred measurement at time of 2015 ASE guidelines; RA dimensions may be preferred if RA volume is not feasible • RA size are gender dependent (as compared to LA)—there is now data available regarding this

RA linear measurements	**RA area measurements**	**RA volume—Preferred measurement**
• End of ventricular systole • Long axis dimension—distance from center of tricuspid annulus to center of superior RA wall, parallel to IA septum • Minor axis dimension—Plane perpendicular to long axis, extending from lateral border of RA to IA septum, at mid level	• End of ventricular systole • Traced from lateral aspect of tricuspid annulus to septal aspect • Exclude area between leaflets and annulus, IVC, SVC and RA appendance	• There are currently no standard orthogonal RA views to use for an apical biplane calculation, so a single plane area-length and/or disk summation (Simpson's) has been proposed

Clinical commentary: Note that using two standard deviations results in an upper limit of 39 mL/m^2 in men. This value, while statistically sound, often appears elevated in a significant number of patients, when reviewing individual echo studies. As such, visual assessment of the RA size relative to other chamber sizes is critical in deciding if the RA size is within normal limits (Fig. 14.6)

RA pressure/IVC dimensions [1]:

Recommended view: Subcostal view

Importance	**Limitations**
• RA pressure is required to have adequate assessment of PA pressures, as it is added to measured TR and PR gradients • IVC diameter dilatation or collapse is an important part of volume status assessment and a sensitive marker of tamponade	• IVC diameter and inspiratory collapse is adequate for Low vs. High pressure measurements but has decreased performance for intermediate values • PPV leads to inaccurate measurements, invasive monitoring preferred

IVC dimensions and collapsibility measurements • Maximal size usually is seen at end expiration • Proximal to junction of hepatic veins (0.5–3.0 cm from ostial-RA junction) • Longitudinal view – check in cross-sectional first to ensure true perpendicularity for adequate assessment • Test collapsibility with quiet respiration and a sniff – Rule out plane translation (i.e. lateral movement during inspiration) as a cause of change in size. Sometimes a short-axis image of the IVC may clarify if translation is present	**Hepatic vein flow measurements:** • With Low/normal RA pressures, there is systolic predominance in hepatic vein flow: the Velocity systolic wave (Vs) is greater than Velocity diastolic wave (Vd) – Elevated Ra pressure may be present if Vs/Vd <1 • **Calculating Hepatic vein systolic filling fraction (Vs/(Vs + Vd)) <55% is the most sensitive/specific sign of elevated RA pressure** – This has been validated in mechanically ventilated patient—average of five consecutive beats + > =1 respiratory cycle
Normal values and interpretation • Normal RA pressure 3 mmHg (0–5 mmHg)—IVC diameter ≤2.1 cm + collapse >50% with sniff • High RA pressure 15 mmHg (10–20 mmHg)—IVC diameter >2.1 cm + collapse <50% with sniff. • Secondary indices of RA pressure – E/E' ratio >0.6 – Diastolic flow predominance in hepatic veins (systolic filling fraction <55%)	**Indeterminate cases** • Specific situations – IVC diameter ≤2.1 cm + collapse <50% – IVC diameter >2.1 cm + collapse >50% • Presence of secondary indices— – upgrade to high RA pressure – in doubt, leave at intermediate (8 mmHg). • If unable to do a sniff, use quiet respiration, in which case a IVC collapse <50% suggests elevated RA pressures

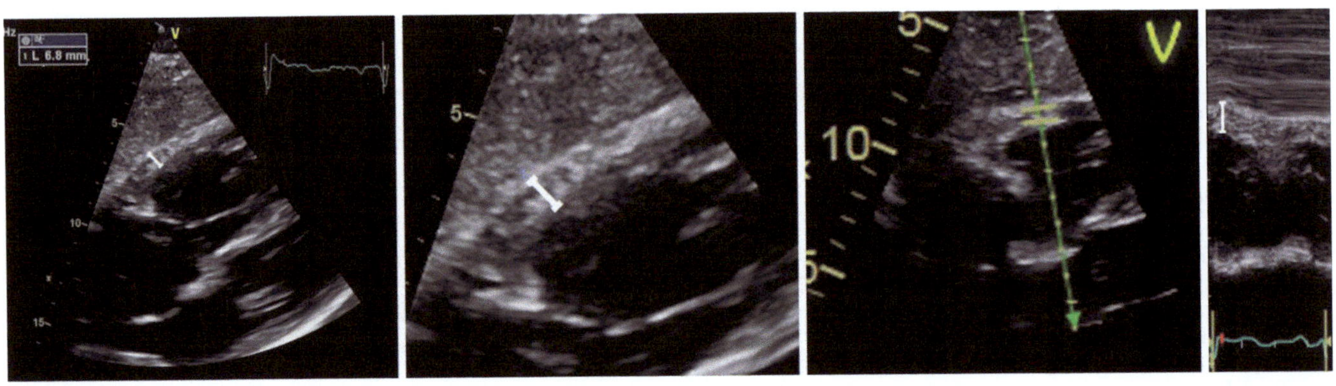

Fig. 14.4 Image 1 and 2 demonstrate target area and delimitation of RV free wall assessment; Image 3 and 4 demonstrate M-mode evaluation of RV free wall dimension

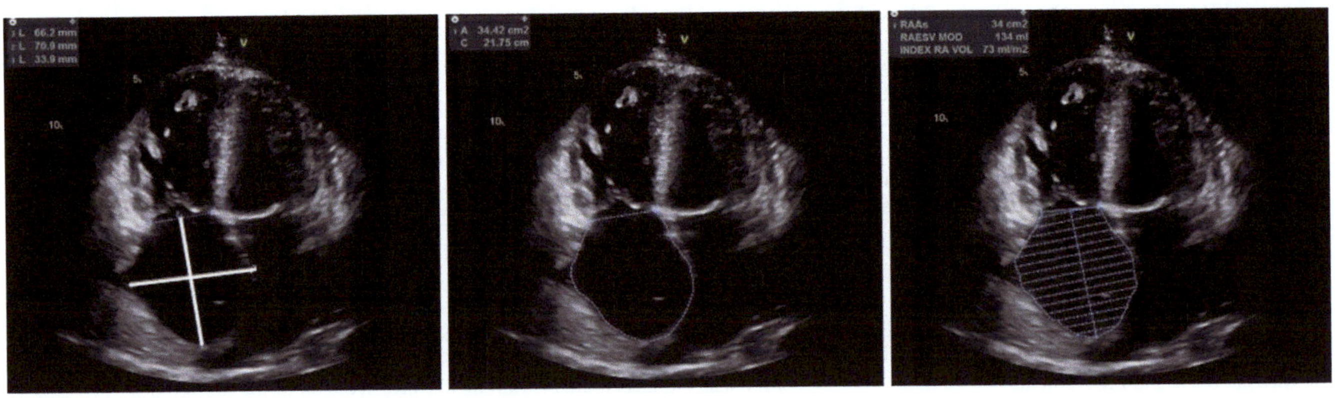

Fig. 14.5 Left image represents linear dimensions acquisition for RA; Middle and right image represents automated RA area and volume calculation based on RA cavity tracing, in apical 4C view

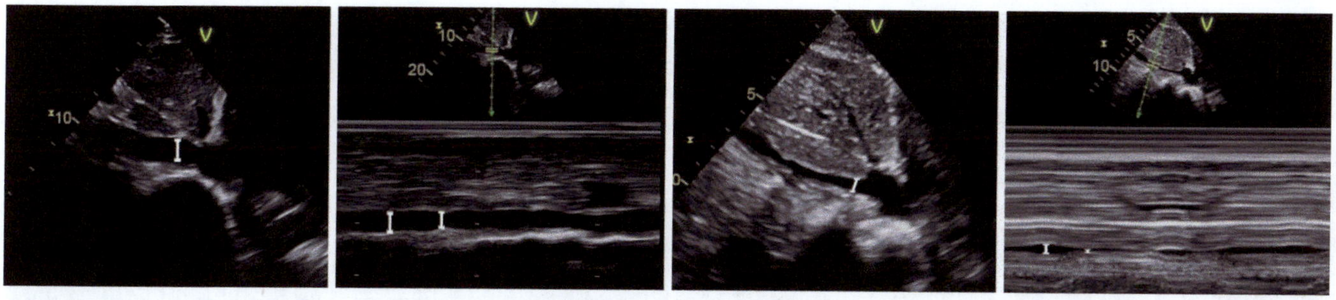

Fig. 14.6 Left to Right: Image 1 and 2 represent full IVC without collapse on M-Mode; Image 3 and 4 represent collapsed IVC with collapse on M-Mode

Volumetric Measurements

3DE RV measurements—normal values [1] RV volume—EDV men 35–87 mL/m^2, women 32–74 mL/m^2; ESV men 10–44 mL/m^2, women 8–36 mL/m^2 RV EF >45%	
Recommended views: Dedicated multibeat 3D acquisition	
Importance • Independent of geometric assumptions • Validated against CMR • EF evaluation by 3D echo includes contribution of RVOT to function. Correlates with CM	**Limitations** • Dependent on image quality, regular rhythm • Needs specific equipment and training • Reference values limited • EF prognostic value not established
Measurements: • Ensure minimal depth and sector angle. Limiting this enables better resolution with a target of >20–25 volumes/seconds for optimal interpretation • Ensure entire RV cavity capture • Verify automatic identification of the end-diastole and end-systole for further analysis • Myocardial trabeculae and moderator band should be included in the cavity • Calculation of RV Ejection Fraction (see below), an excellent measure of global systolic function obtained by – **RV EF (%) = 100 × (EDV−ESV)/EDV**	

RV Systolic Function

- General statements
  - Quantitative measures are required in the standard exam, however these should be combined with the visual assessment of the expert reader. The combination has demonstrated very good inter-reader concordance [9].
  - For S′ and TAPSE, regional velocities or displacement of the myocardium in a single segment may not be representative of global RV function [1] in certain conditions.
  - Clinical utility demonstrated for RIMP, TAPSE, 2D FAC, S′, Longitudinal speckle-tracking echocardiographic strain [2].
  - Presence of significant TR may lead to RV EF not representing RV contractility [1].
  - Different conditions result in different patterns of RV adaptation and remodeling. Since the recommended cut-off values are derived from normal populations, these values may not correlate with presence of a disease or associated outcome (Fig. 14.7)

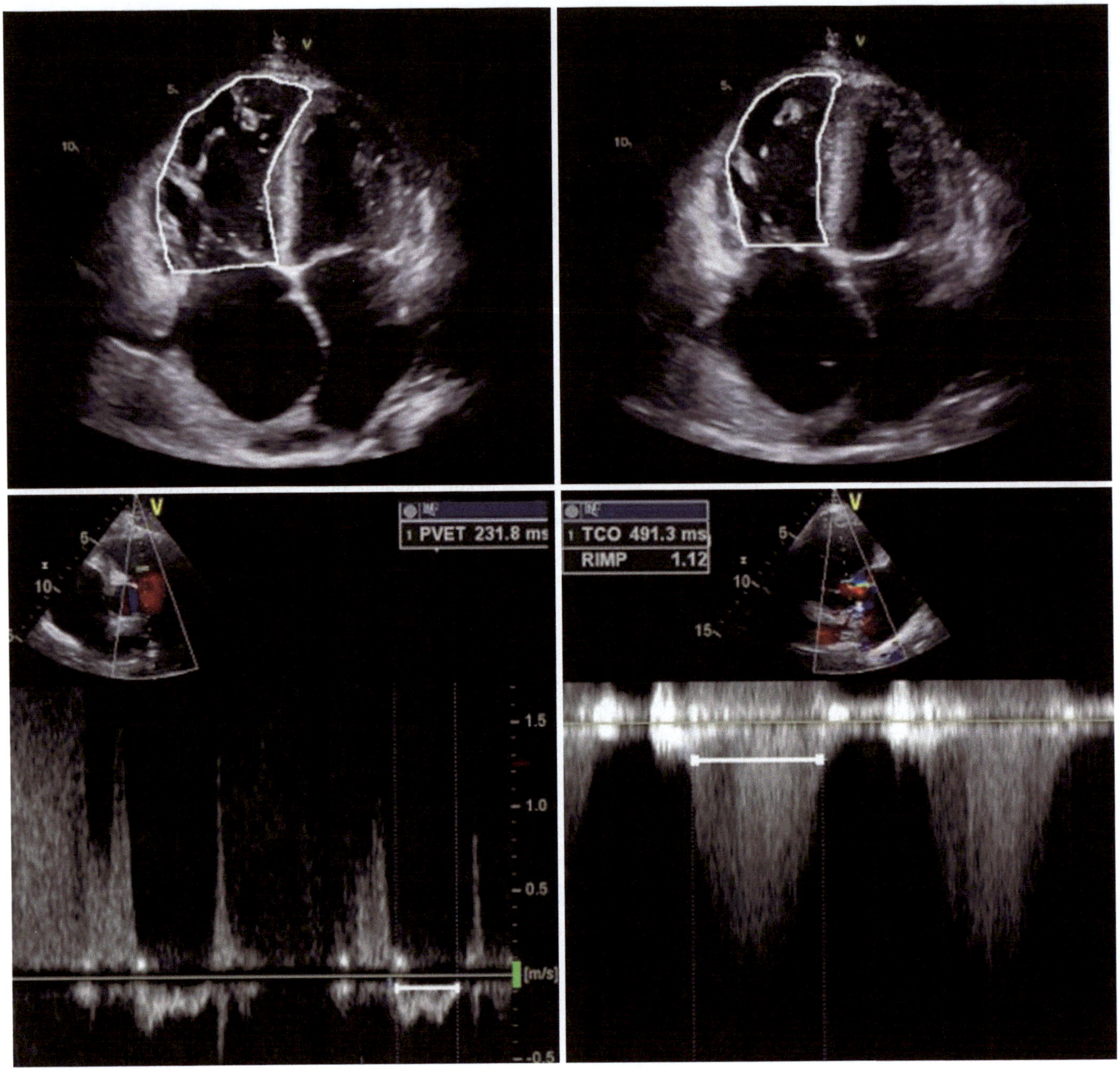

Fig. 14.7 Top: RV 4C view with FAC measurement tracing; Bottom: RIMP by DTI/Tissue Doppler, with ET and TCO measurement location, left and right respectively

Global Assessment

RV 2D Fractional Area Change (FAC) [1]—Abnormal <35%	
Recommended views: RV focused 4C view	
Importance: • RV FAC independent predictor of HF, sudden death, stroke, and mortality in PE and AMI	**Limitations** • Difficult in case of suboptimal image quality of free wall • Difficult with trabeculations—if not included, underestimation of areas. This is more problematic in diastole and with thinner myocardium • Occasionally difficult to have same tomographic plane in end-diastole due to heart movement

Measurements:

- At end-systole (End-systolic area [ESA]) and end-diastole (end-diastolic area [EDA])
- Trace RV endocardial border from
  - Lateral tricuspid annulus to apex along free wall
  - From apex to medial tricuspid annulus along IV septum
- Include trabeculations, papillary muscles and moderator band in the cavity (trace the compacted myocardium).
- Ensure entire RV contained in imaging sector including apex and free wall. This is particularly important when dealing with a dilated RV

RV index of myocardial performance (RIMP)/Tei index [1, 2]—Abnormal RIMP PW Doppler >0.43; RIMP DTI Doppler >0.54
Recommended views: Standard apical 4C or RV focused apical 4C view, with PSAX if using pulsed Doppler technique

Importance	Limitations
• Index of both systolic and diastolic performance • It was studied in pulmonary hypertension, hypertrophic cardiomyopathy, congenital heart disease and RV infarction, with correlation between changes in index and clinical status • It can be used for initial and serial measurements of RV function • Calculation still reliable for wide range of **regular** HR (50–100)	• Increased RA pressures lead to rapid equilibration of pressures between RV and RA, and shortened isovolumetric relaxation time, due to early opening of the tricuspid. The result is a falsely low (pseudo-normal) RIMP • Pulsed Doppler method should not be used with irregular HR

Measurements:
- Two methods can be used—Pulsed Doppler RIMP and Tissue Doppler RIMP
- Obtained by calculation the ratio of the sum of isovolumic contraction and relaxation times (IVCT + IVRT) and the ejection time through the pulmonary valve (ET)
- Since the tricuspid closing to opening time (TCO) is the same duration as the sum of isovolumic contraction times and the ejection time, this can be measured instead to be used in a reorganized equation
  - RIMP = (TCO—ET)/ET

Pulsed Doppler	Tissue Doppler
• ET measured at the RV outflow: time from onset to cessation of the flow. • TCO measured: – Pulsed wave Doppler of tricuspid inflow as time from end of transtricuspid A wave to beginning of transtricuspid E wave – Or Continuous wave Doppler of TR jet, from onset to cessation of flow • Measures from different locations, so requires similar RR interval to ensure adequate ratio calculation: may underestimate or overestimate	• Lateral tricuspid annulus pulsing • Ejection time is from beginning to end of S′, and TCO is from end of A' to beginning of E' • Measures all obtainable from same location, hence a single-beat recording is sufficient

RV dP/dT [1, 2]—Abnormal values <400 mmHg/s

Recommended views: Standard apical 4C; RV focused apical 4C

Importance:	Limitations
• Rate of pressure rise in ventricles is an invasive measurement validated in both LV and RV • **Not recommended for routine use**	• RV dP/dt is load dependent • In severe TR, the rise of RA pressure, and the simplified Bernoulli equation that ignores the inertia component leads to inaccuracies • limited data in both normal subjects and pathologic conditions

Measurements:
- Single measurement done using a continuous-wave Doppler signal of TR jet
  - Time required for the TR jet to increase in velocity from 1 to 2 m/s
- Using a Simplified Bernoulli equation, the change in velocity is equivalent to a change of pressure of 12 mmHg
  - Alternatively, the best correlation detailed is for a change of 0.5 to 2 m/s which is equivalent to 15 mmHg
- The calculation can be done as follows:
- RV dP/dt = 12 mmHg/time in seconds

RV Ejection Fraction (RV EF) >45%. Slightly higher in women

Recommended views: RV focused view—apical window—Dedicated multi-beat acquisition

Importance:	Limitations
• **Most "global" assessement of right heart function** • **Recommended in laboratories with appropriate equipment and expertise**	• RV EF is load dependent and may be overestimated in the setting of significant TR • Challenging image acquisition • Analysis is fully dependent on algorithm designed to contour and analyze RV volumes. Changes in algorithms and multiple techniques result in a paucity of normal data for some newer methods. • Significant learning curve of approximately 120 datasets

Measurements:
- Fully dependent on machine-integrated or stand-alone algorithms which are either automated or semi-automated. Contours are traced after certain landmarks are identified and the user can manually correct these contours. End-diastolic and end-systolic volumes are generated
- The calculation can be done as follows:
- RV EF = 100 × (RV EDV − RV ESV)/RV EDD (Fig. 14.8)

Regional Assessment

Tricuspid annular plane excursion (TAPSE) or Tricuspid annular motion (TAM) [1, 2]—Abnormal <17 mm

Recommended views: Standard apical 4C

Importance:	Limitations
• Single location measurement of the distance of the excursion of the RV annular segment • There is good correlation with parameters estimating RV global function. This may be not valid in disease states with regional abnormalities • It also has established prognostic value, and validation against radionuclide EF	• It may be difficult to have good alignment, and this is very angle-dependent • It may not fully represent RV global function, especially in disease states with RMWA

Measurements:
- M-Mode
- Align the beam in direction of the lateral tricuspid annulus, for parallel beam in regards to motion of the tricuspid annulus
- Measured between end-diastole and peak systole

DTI-derived lateral annular systolic velocity (S′)—Abnormal <9.5 cm/s on free wall [1, 2].

Recommended views: Standard apical 4C

Importance:
- Despite being a regional measurement, there is good correlation with parameters estimating RV global function
- There is good data on specific age-related cut-off values
- It should be used as an indicator for additional workup if below normal, but should not be used alone

Limitations
- It may difficult to obtain adequate alignment, and it is prone to underestimation
- In certain disease states, including post thoracotomy, pulmonary endarterectomy and heart transplant, it may not be fully representative of RV global function

Measurements:
- Two methods can be used—Pulsed Tissue Doppler, or Color Tissue Doppler (not recommended—insufficient data)
- Ensure alignment of basal segment and annulus to limit underestimation
- There are often two peaks—the first being isovolumetric contraction, and the second being actual systolic motion of the annulus. The latter peak is the one measured (see figure above)
- Use either the tricuspid annulus, or the middle of the basal segment of the RV free wall
  - Avoid the apical or mid ventricular free wall as it leads to more variability
  - Do not use the IV septum

Pulsed Doppler
- It was validated against radionuclide EF, has established prognostic value.

Color Doppler
- The sampling is performed after image acquisition, which allows multiple sampling on the same beat. Additionally, analysis can be done offline
- Measures mean velocities since uses color Doppler (Fig. 14.9)
- **Not recommended**

Global and Regional

RV strain and strain rate [2]—Abnormal Global longitudinal free wall strain <20% in absolute value; Not standardized for strain rate

Recommended views: RV focused apical 4C view

Importance:
- The principle is that the system tracks the speckle pattern to assess for degree and rate of shortening of muscle fibers
- It is the only method that does both global and regional assessment
- Studies have been done that have shown use in Heart Failure, Acute MI, Pulmonary HTN and amyloidosis, and additional data is coming

Limitations
- Values depend on RV loading conditions, shape and size
- It is limited by image quality: reverberation, attenuation and other artifacts may lead to inability to do proper tracking, which should be taken into consideration
- The thin RV may make it difficult to setup region of interest easily
- Measurements are not standardized across machines
- Absence of definite references ranges at the moment

Measurements:
- There exist two types: STE derived, and DTI derived (rarely used clinically)
- The STE derived is angle independent; the DTI derived is angle dependent
- The measurement is dependent on the machine, and the algorithm is borrowed from LV measurements
  - As such, the segments tracked are variable, and may represent RV free wall alone, or with septal segments
- Longitudinal strain is calculated using a percentage of systolic shortening of RV free wall from base to apex
- Currently, the average of the three free wall segments are averaged and reported. Despite this, it is recommended that the entire RV contours are included (free wall and septum) in the analysis, since the algorithm performs better in identifying the apex when both free wall and septum are outlined

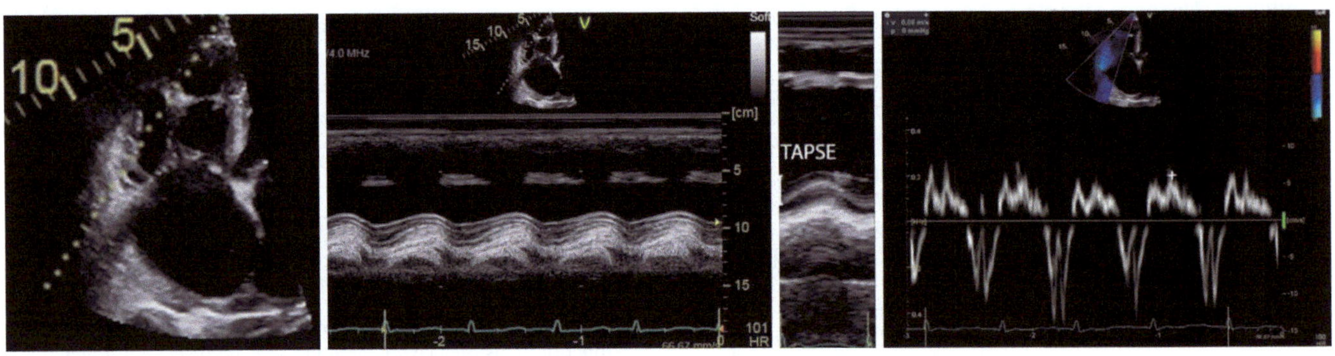

Fig. 14.8 Left to right: TAPSE assessment in standard apical 4C view, at the lateral tricuspid annulus; With M-Mode; Focused M-Mode view for measurement of TAPSE; DTI S′ obtained in standard apical 4C view (+ indicates measurement location)

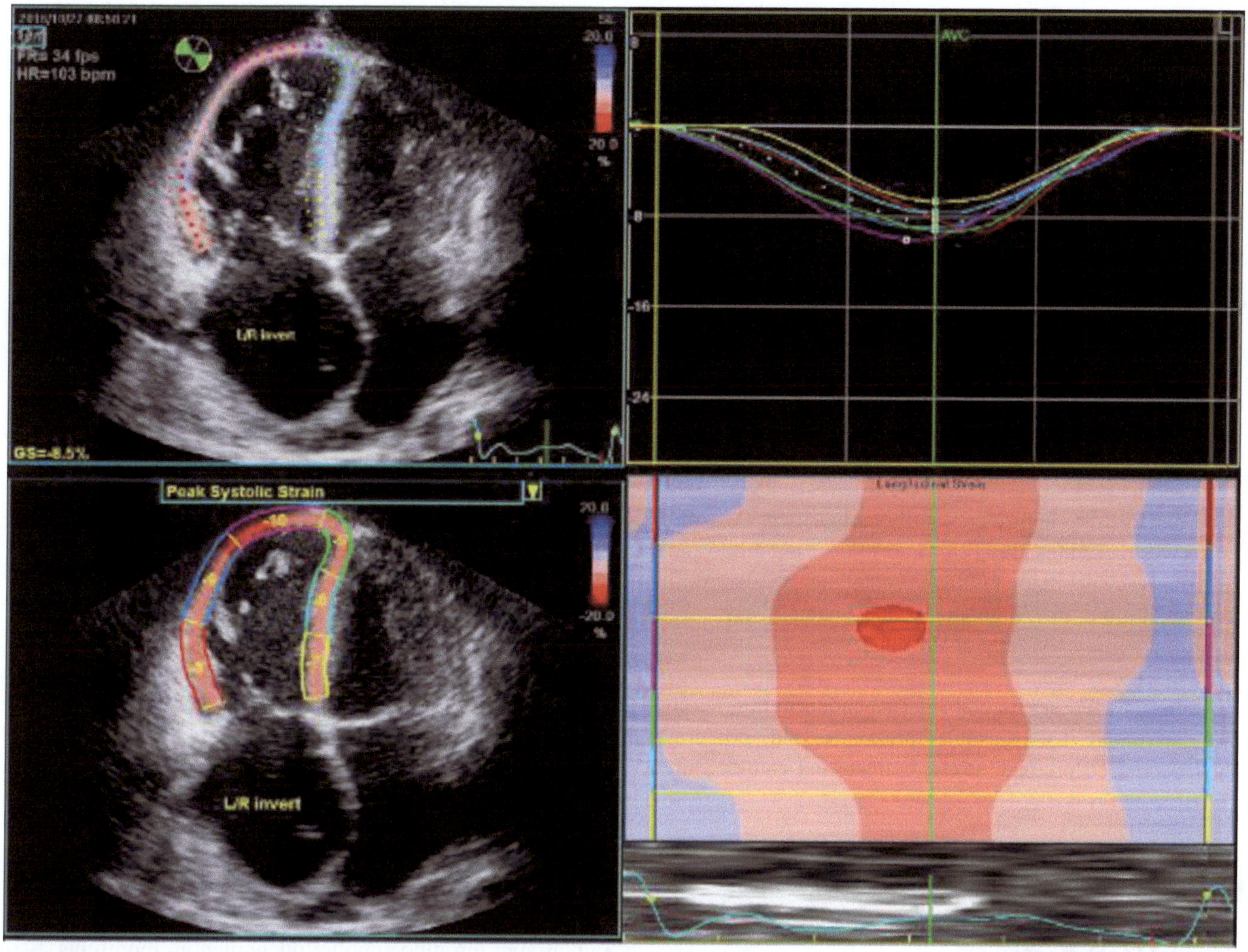

Fig. 14.9 —STE derived RV free wall and septal strain. Notice the values are abnormal ranging from −7 to −10%. As noted, there is currently no industry standard, and as such, technique should be taken in to account when determining abnormal values for a particular study

Pulmonary Artery Pressure Evaluation

Systolic Pulmonary Artery Pressure [2]**—Abnormal SPAP >35 mmHg; TR gradient >2.8 m/s**

Recommended views: RV focused apical 4C view, standard apical 4C view, RV inflow, PSAX, Subcostal. Multiple views are recommended—use highest velocity recorded, if the envelope is complete

Importance:	Limitations
• Main measure used to determine if there is increased pulmonary pressures • Validated in a multiple conditions causing pulmonary hypertension with reasonable correlation with cardiac cath	• In very severe TR, the measurements may not be accurate because the Doppler envelope may be cut-off due to early equalization of RV and RA pressures—this leads to underestimation of the RV-RA gradient • SPAP estimation by RV-RA gradient + RA pressure may be unreliable at high PA pressures (79, 80 ASE 2010)

Measurements:

- Align CW Doppler with TR jet to measure the peak TR jet velocity
- Doppler sweep speeds of 100 mm/s necessary
- If weak signal, enhance with agitated saline
- Use well-defined dense spectral profile—if tracing with not well-defined tracing, over- or underestimation can occur
- RVSP is calculated using the peak TR jet velocity (V, in m/s) and a modified Bernoulli equation with estimate of RA pressure
  - $RVSP = 4 \times V^2 + RA$ pressure
- In the absence of gradient across the RVOT, RVSP is equal to SPAP
- Alternate measurement is RV-RA gradient + RA pressure for SPAP

PADP, MPAP, PVR—See Chap. 33

Disease States

General Statements

- Most causes of RV dysfunction are secondary to either pressure overload, volume overload, or acute myocardial contractility dysfunction. A minority of cases are congenital or secondary intrinsic wall dysfunction.
- Physiological consequences of pressure and volume overload
  - Usually, the RV tolerates volume overload for a longer period of time before a significant decrease in RV systolic function than pressure overload, such as in congenital heart disease [10].
  - Moderate to severe acquired PH leads to RV dilatation and systolic failure conjointly earlier than RV volume overload states [11, 12].
  - This results in alterations in septal contractility ability, alterations in LV geometry and increased pericardial constraints on the LV, regardless of pericardial disease.
  - In diastolic ventricular interdependence, this leads to increased LV diastolic pressures and potentially decreased preload, stroke volume and cardiac output [3, 7].

Pulmonary Hypertension—see Chap. 33

General Statements

- Pulmonary hypertension can be caused by acute and chronic pulmonary emboli, lung disease, pulmonary arterial hypertension, and left heart disease, amongst others.
- **Acute vs. chronic disease**
  - In acute pressure overload states, a previously normal RV cannot generate a mPAP >40 mmHg [11]. Findings of high SPAP or MPAP in this setting warrants evaluation for chronic pressure overload state, or pre-existing RV disease.
  - Similarly, RV free wall thickening above 10 mm should make the diagnosis of an acute event less likely and warrant workup for pre-existing chronic disease [13]. Comparatively, in acute pressure overload, there is often mild RV free wall thickening (6–10 mm), or none.

Acute Pulmonary Embolus

- Obstruction of the pulmonary arteries (saddle, lobar, segmental, subsegmental) by clot, amniotic fluid, tumor or fat leads to **acute pressure overload, and echocardiographic features in keeping with it.**
- Echocardiogram is not recommended as a diagnostic tool: multiple studies have shown that **even in the presence of significant pulmonary emboli, the echocardiogram might be normal** (up to 33% in one study) [14].
  - However, in hemodynamically unstable patients, 100% of patients had at least one finding of RV overload [14].
  - Echocardiography can thus be used for risk stratification—even in hemodynamically stable patients with acute PE, RV dysfunction increased short time mortality [15].
- **Typical signs of PE have shown low sensitivity, and variable specificity in recent studies:**
  - McConnell's sign: hypokinesis of the RV free wall with normal contraction of the apical segment. Present in 75% of hemodynamically unstable patients [14].
  - 60/60 sign: Coexistence of shortened pulmonary ejection acceleration time (AcT <60 ms), midsystolic velocity deceleration measured in RVOT and TRSPG <60 mmHg. Present in 31.2% of hemodynamically unstable patients [14].
  - Right Heart thrombus: Presence of a visible clot in the right atrium, ventricle or pulmonary arteries. Present in 18.8% of hemodynamically unstable patients [14].
  - In hemodynamically stable, one of these findings is only present in 24% of patients [14] (Fig. 14.10).

Chronic Thromboembolic Phenomenon

- Chronic thromboembolic phenomenon represents two major conditions: Chronic Thromboembolic Pulmonary hypertension (CTEPH) and Chronic thromboembolic disease (CTED).
  - Both conditions results from chronic organization of clot burden in the pulmonary vascular system. This is divided in proximal disease (which is operable), and distal disease (which for the most part is non-operable).
  - CTEPH represents the development of measurable increased pulmonary arterial pressures with predominantly a pressure overload pattern. CTED represents post-embolic exercise intolerance without increase pressure or RV impact.
- Echocardiographic indices and measures of PAP and PVR have shown strong correlation with RHC in studies.
  - The strongest one was PVR from TRPG/CO(RVOT) [18], and is preferred.
  - While there is strong correlation in most values between echocardiography and RHC, some studies have shown that echocardiographic measures have significant variation as compared to RHC measurements [19].

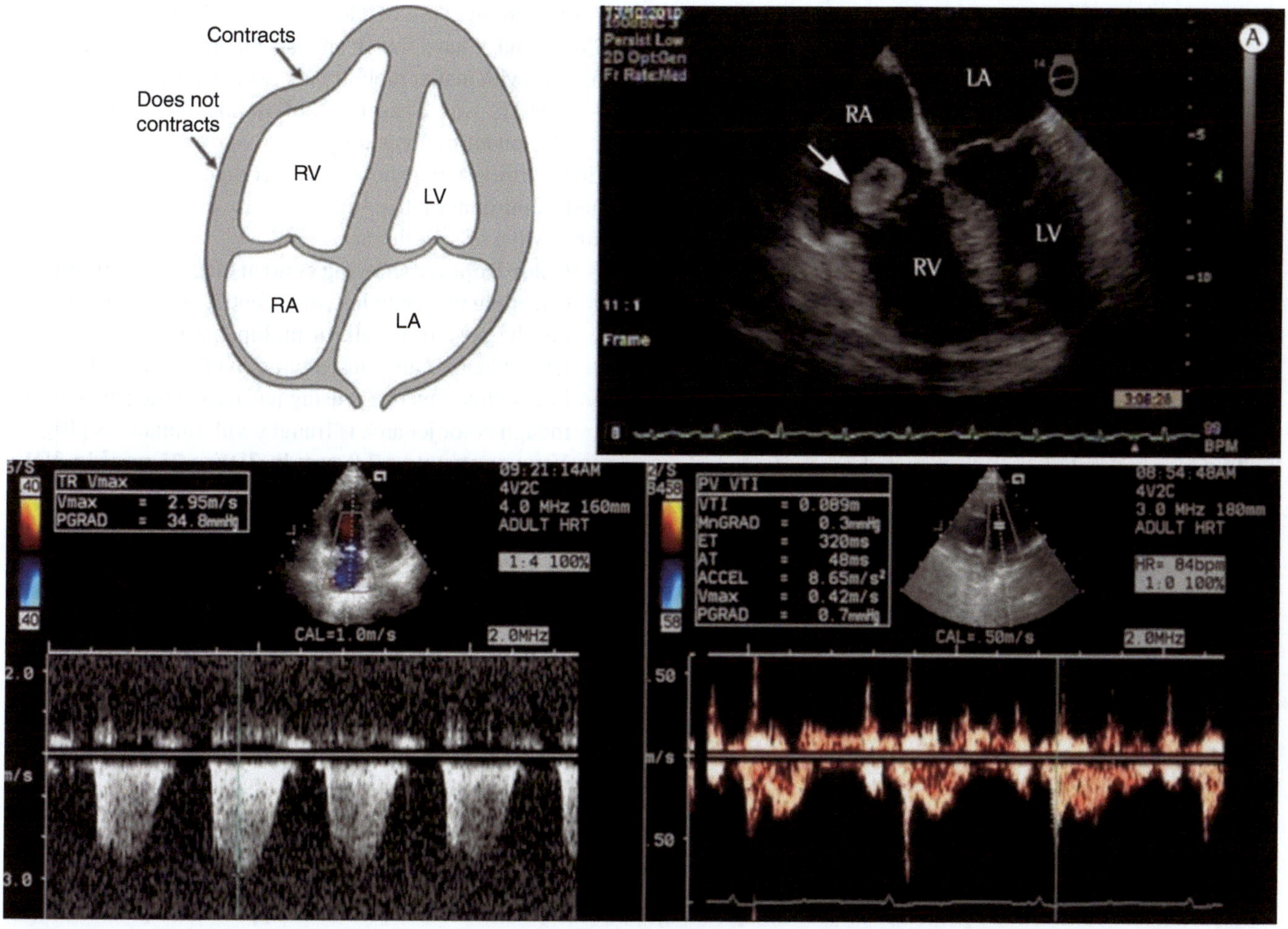

Fig. 14.10 Top left: Sketch demonstrating McConnell's sign with absence of basal contraction in presence of apical contraction; Top right: RA thrombus, against the TV; Bottom: 60/60 sign demonstrated with TRSPG <60 mmHg on left, and AT <60 ms on right [16, 17]

Lung Disease

- RV dysfunction is most often secondary to increases in PVR related to hypoxic changes, as well as intra-thoracic pressure changes to which the RH is especially sensitive.
- Thoracic pressure hemodynamic effects:
  - Ventilation with increased PEEP may have a hemodynamic impact, especially if additional PEEP does not lead to increased lung recruitment, in which case, RV SV and CO decrease, such as in ARDS [20]
    LVEDP and PCWP are systematically uncoupled after PEEP >10 cmH20, with PCWP overestimating LVEDP [20, 21].
- **ARDS: characterized in echocardiography by features of both pressure and volume overload** [20].
- **Asthma/COPD: Asthma/COPD shows with features of pressure overload during attacks.**
  - RV function, RV size and PAP are significantly impacted in acute exacerbations and recovered afterwards [22].
  - In severe exacerbations, pulsus paradoxus may be apparent [23]:
    Inspiratory overdistension of the RV.
    Parallel biventricular interdependence.
    Decreased LVSV at inspiration.
- **Chronic COPD, with or without pulmonary hypertension, has underlying RV dysfunction and remodeling features, even in mild disease** [24].
  - Changes observed in patients without diagnostic PH (MPAP <20 mmHg by echo) that allowed distinction between healthy, COPD without PH and with PH [24] include RIMP >0.43, RV GLS—basal free wall (−13 to −18%) and RV isovolumic acceleration.
  - RV hypertrophy might help in differentiating acute vs. chronic cor pulmonale, as severe hypertrophy (>10 mm) is seldom observed in acute events without pre-existing disease [13].
  - In chronic COPD, echocardiographic findings of RV dysfunction correlated with symptoms, morbidity and mortality in multiple studies [25–30].

Left Heart Disease

- Left sided heart disease is the most common cause of pulmonary hypertension and right sided heart failure. It is present in both CHFrEF and CHFpEF (secondary to diastolic dysfunction), and valvulopathies (AS, AR, MS, MR). Incidence is fairly high, ranging, depending on etiologies from 16 to 79% [31].
- **It presents echocardiographically as pressure overload features initially, with RV dilatation and volume overload only in more advanced stages** [31, 32]. The corollary of this is that one often sees preserved RV size and systolic function (with RVH) associated with even moderate-severe PH when associated with pure left-sided heart disease.
- **The correlation between degree of diastolic dysfunction and severity of PH is not precise—mild degrees of LV diastolic dysfunction can lead to significant PH** [32].
  - Presence of heart failure, even with preserved EF can increase Pulmonary artery pressure in excess of PCWP increase [32].

- Echocardiographic findings suggestive of PH secondary to LHD—see appropriate chapters:
  - Left atrial enlargement
  - LV hypertrophy
  - Pulmonary venous flow profile
  - Mitral annulus tissue Doppler signals
  - LV filling pressures
    E/E': **Ratio of mitral peak velocity of early filling (E) to early diastolic mitral annular velocity (E')**

Valvular Disease

- The **most common right-sided valvulopathy involved in RV dysfunction is tricuspid regurgitation (TR);** the **most common cause of TR is functional (FTR) (75%),** followed by structural or organic TR (STR) (25%) [33, 34]. Of note, trace TR is found in up to 80–90% of the population without significant pathology [33].
- **FTR is associated with RV overload** (pressure or volume), of which LHD is most common cause [35]; Its defining characteristic is anatomically preserved valvular leaflets.
- **In FTR with PH, RV remodeling causing tricuspid annulus enlargement and valvular tenting are more involved than actual PAP increase**; FTR without PH is mostly secondary to tricuspid annulus enlargement [35, 36]. Less appreciated is the potential contribution of RA enlargement which can also cause annular dilatation.
- **Volume overload in TR leads to progressive chronic RV remodeling and dysfunction with leaflet tethering** [35]. Improvement in volume overload may improve FTR and re-imaging can be considered after volume control.
- An important cause of TR is implantable device leads, and Cheng and al have shown an association between lead interference with leaflet mobility and worsened TR [37, 38].
  - 3DTTE was a useful tool in identification of lead placement in this study.
- Echocardiography should use a composite of quantitative and semi-quantitative measures to evaluate TR. Signs suggestive of severity are as follow:
  - **Color Doppler showing central large regurgitant jets** extending deep into RA, or eccentric swirling jets reaching the posterior wall, in multiple windows. Eccentric jets make organic causes more likely [39]. ASE guidelines define severe TR using jet area central jets >10 cm^2 though color jet area is fraught with limitations [40].
  - **Vena contracta >7.0 mm in 2DE, >75 mm^2 in 3DE**; this is preferred if more than mild TR is present, but is not accurate to distinguish moderate from mild TR [39, 40].
  - **Flow convergence of proximal isovelocity surface area (PISA) with effective regurgitant area ≥40 mm^2, or volume ≥45 mL**; this is limited by respiratory variations which affects flow convergence and TR velocity, and load dependence [39]. ASE guidelines define severe TR as a PISA radius of >9 mm at an aliasing velocity of 28 cm/s [40].
  - **Continuous wave Doppler with dense triangular tracing, and early peak velocity <2 m/s** [39]. Also known as "V wave cut-off sign" which represents rapid deceleration of the Doppler tracing due to rapid equalization of RV pressures [40].
  - **Systolic flow reversal in hepatic vein by PW Doppler.** It is imperative that the flow reversal be seen in systole. There is normal diastolic reversal onto the hepatic veins with atrial contraction, and this jet may be prominent if the RV is stiff. While systolic reversal is often considered very specific for the identification of severe TR, is it occasionally seen with lesser degrees (even mild-moderate) in some PAH patients with a stiff RA that permits transmission of the pressure wave into the hepatic veins [40] (Fig. 14.11).

- Other features needing further observation include:
  - TA dimension ≥40 mm; which 2DE systematically underestimates compared to intertrigonal direct measurement intra-operatively by CMR or 3DE [41–43]. The annular dimension of 40 mm (or 19 mm/m^2) in the apical 4-chamber has been suggested as a cut-off value to recommend prophylactic tricuspid annuloplasty at the time of mitral surgery when there is greater than mild TR present.
  - Restrictive motion of leaflets suggests tethering (RV dilatation), entrapment (PM leads), or primary damage/congenital [39] (Fig. 14.12).

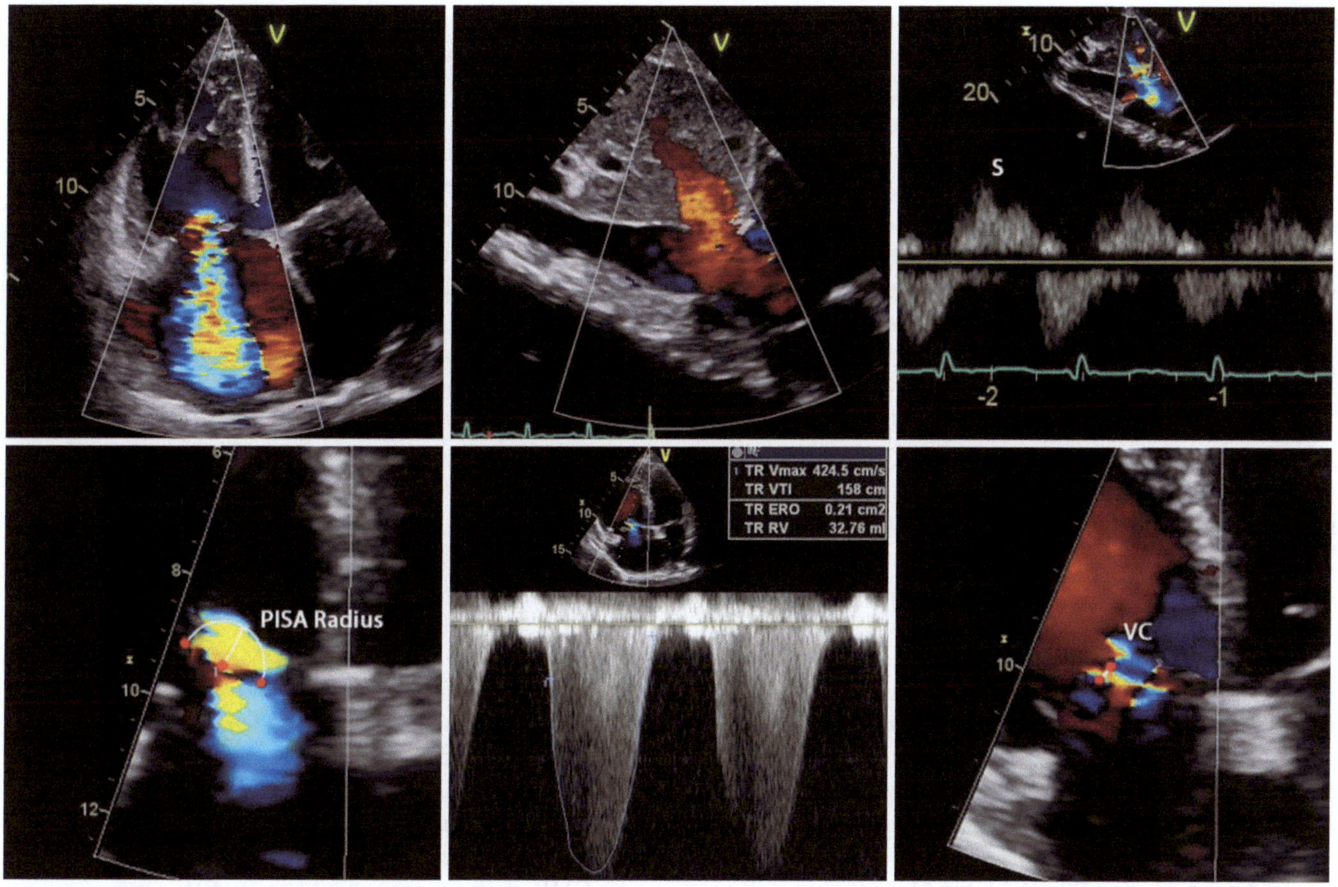

Fig. 14.11 Severe TR features. Top left: Central large regurgitant TR jets; Top middle: Color Doppler hepatic vein systolic flow reversal; Top right: PW Doppler systolic flow reversal (S); Bottom left and middle: EROA calculation by flow convergence of PISA, and CW Doppler with dense triangular wave, with early deceleration or "V-wave cut-off sign; Bottom right: Vena contracta demonstrated—to be measured at flow convergence, at level of TV annulus

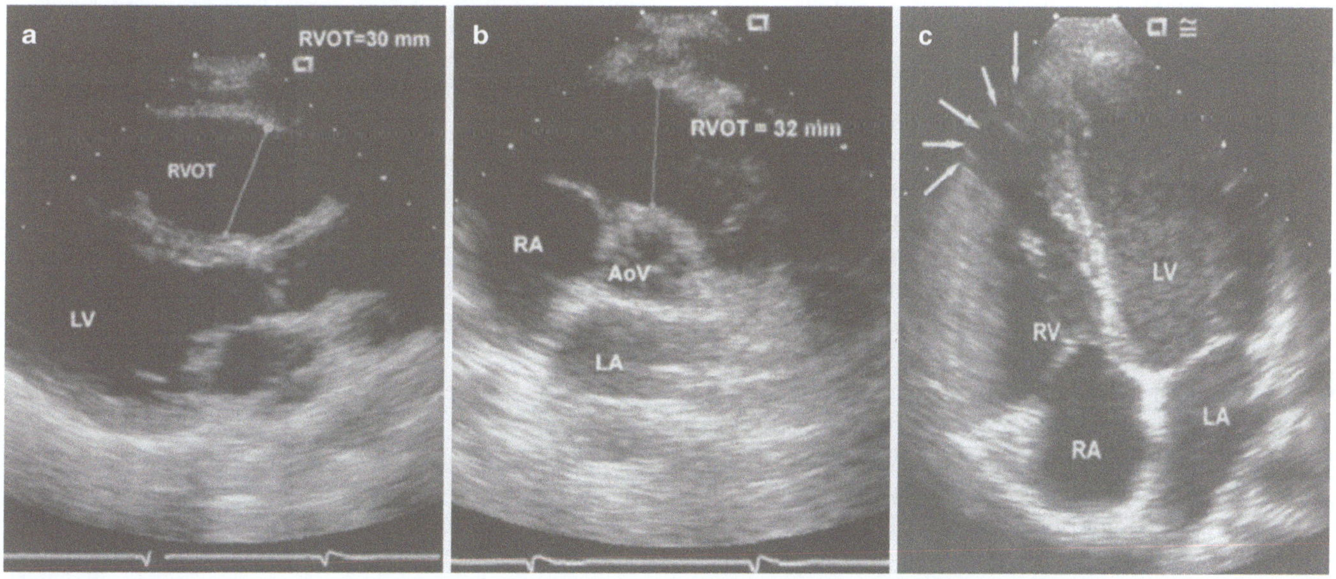

Fig. 14.12 Features of ARVC. From to right. Image 1: Proximal RVOT by PLAX meeting minor criteria; Image 2: Proximal RVOT by PSAX meeting minor criteria; Image 3: Focal aneurysm in RV apical region [44]

Intrinsic Wall Abnormalities

- The most significant Right sided intrinsic wall abnormality is Arrhythmogenic right ventricular cardiomyopathy/dysplasia (ARVC/D) which represents fibrofatty replacement of myocardium [45, 46].
- **The most common involved RV region are the inflow/outflow tract, and apex of the RV** [46].
- **2DE and MRI have overall similar sensitivity and specificity for identifying this disease pattern**; the previously thought advantage of MRI for fibrosis assessment has lost importance because of findings of isolated fatty involvement in individuals, which cannot be picked up on MRI given the thinness of the RV free wall [45].
- Imaging criteria by echocardiography [45, 46].
  - Diagnosis requires
    Regional RV akinesia, dyskinesia or aneurysm AND 1 Major criteria
    OR
    Regional RV RV akinesia, dyskinesia or dyssynchronous RV contraction and one minor criteria.
  - PLAX RVOT (diastole)
    Major ≥32 mm; PLAX/BSA ≥19 mm/m²
    Minor ≥29 mm; PLAX/BSA >16 to ≤18 mm/m²
  - PSAX RVOT (diastole)
    Major ≥36 mm; PSAX/BSA ≥21 mm/m²
    Minor ≥32 mm; PSAX/BSA ≥18 to ≤20 mm/m²
  - RV FAC
    Major ≤33%; Minor ≤40%

Coronary Artery Disease

- Regional motion wall abnormalities in RV dysfunction are dependent on right, left or co-dominance, and double blood supply of specific segments (infundibulum and anterior free wall). The **earliest affected segments in ischaemia are thus the inferior wall, followed by the lateral wall. The most resistant segments are the infundibulum and anterior free wall** [47].
- Isolated RV MI is uncommon, occurring in occlusion of a non-dominant RCA, or occlusion of the RV branch in a left dominant system. Occlusion of LCX in left dominant, and occasionally LAD occlusion may affect the anterior, or apical [1], part of the RV free wall [1, 47].
- Severity of the RV dysfunction and infarction depends on the location of the RCA occlusion—**an occlusion more proximal to the major marginal branches leads to more important infarction** [1, 47].
- Some specific echocardiographic features carry established importance for RV MI [47, 48]:
  - The hallmark of RV infarct in echocardiography is regional motion wall abnormality in the RCA territory.
  - Additional measures may be obtained, but not used in most instances in clinical practice, with all measures being more specific for more proximal RCA occlusion.
    RIMP/Tei index can be used as a sensitive marker for acute MI, and **S′ can be used as a surrogate for global RV systolic and diastolic dysfunction.**
    TAPSE <10 mm has a 75% PPV for RV MI in the appropriate clinical setting, and TAPSE ≤16 has sensitivity/specificity 93%/100% [48].

Takotsubo

- This is frequently found in Takotsubo phenomenon, in up to 50% of cases [49, 50].
- RV dysfunction in Takotsubo CMP is linked to worse cases of LV dysfunction and cardiogenic shock, but not a combination of all-cause mortality, recurrence or re-hospitalization [50].
  - Similarly to LV, there is wall edema, but this is present both in segments with and without RMWA on CMR.
- Segments affected in Scally and al [51], as documented by CMR, were apical and mid cavity RV.
- Sensitivity of 2DE, as compared to CMR, was only 52%.
- Other parameters affected include
  - TAPSE diminution. This was also present in the group without RV involvement on CMR, suggesting RV involvement even in a group without definite RV involvement by other parameters.
  - Strain imaging was found to be able to discriminate between patients with and without RV involvement [52].

Questions

1. Which echo findings support the severe diastolic dysfunction of RV:
   A. A tricuspid E/A ratio <2.1 with a deceleration time >120 ms.
   B. A tricuspid E/A ratio >2.1 with a deceleration time <120 ms.
   C. A tricuspid E/A ratio <2.1 with a deceleration time <120 ms.
   D. A tricuspid E/A ratio >2.1 with a deceleration time >120 ms.

2. Which patient has the Highest RAP?
   A. IVC Max. diameter at 1.8 cm and Min. diameter with sniffing at 0.8 cm.

B. IVC Max. diameter at 2.1 cm and Min. diameter with sniffing at 0.9 cm.
C. IVC Max. diameter at 1.9 cm and Min. diameter with sniffing at 1.3 cm.
D. IVC Max. diameter at 2.3 cm and Min. diameter with sniffing at 1 cm.

3. What is your diagnosis?

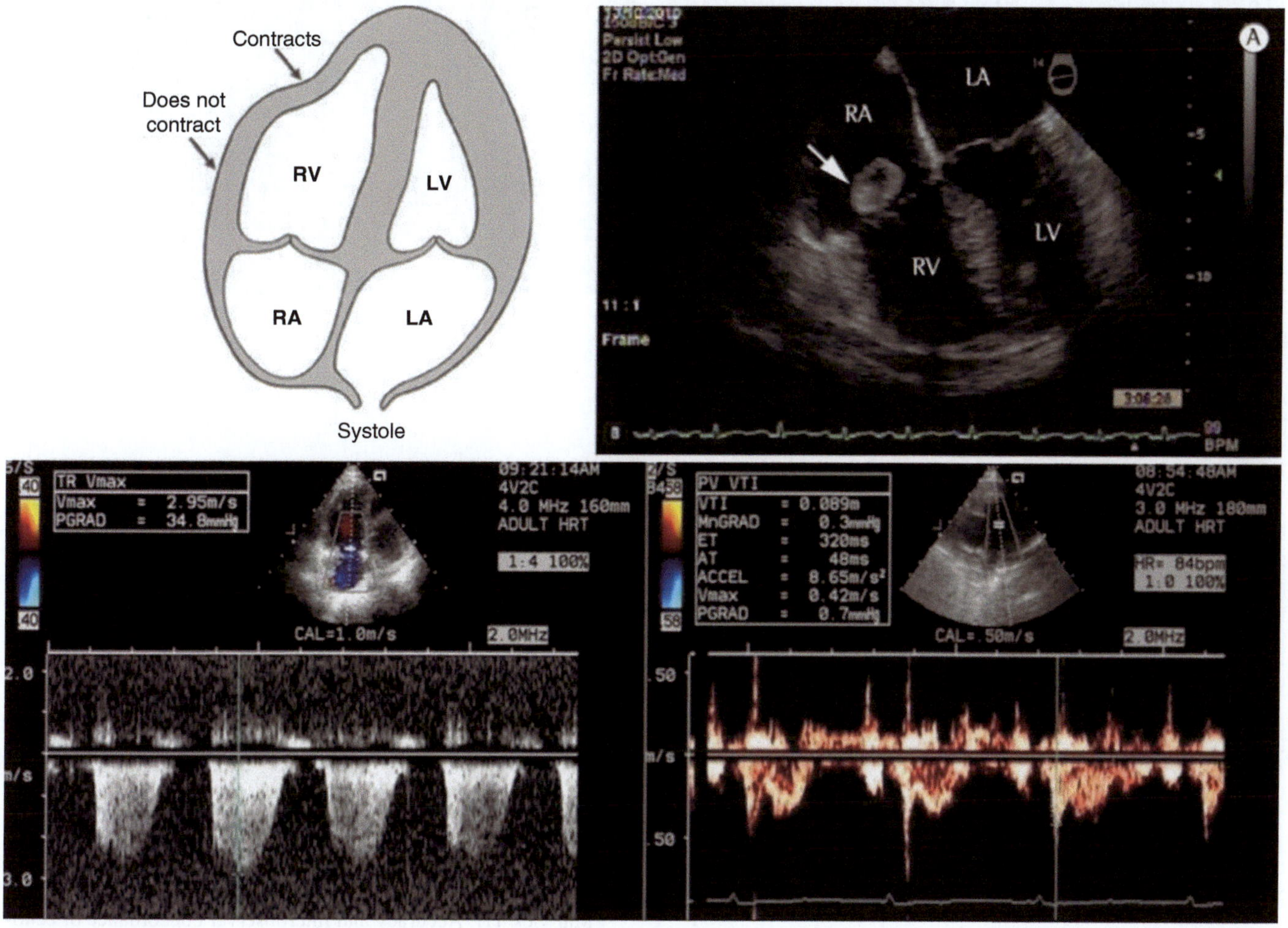

A. ARVD/C
B. PTE
C. Amyloidosis
D. Constrictive Pericarditis

4. What is your diagnosis?

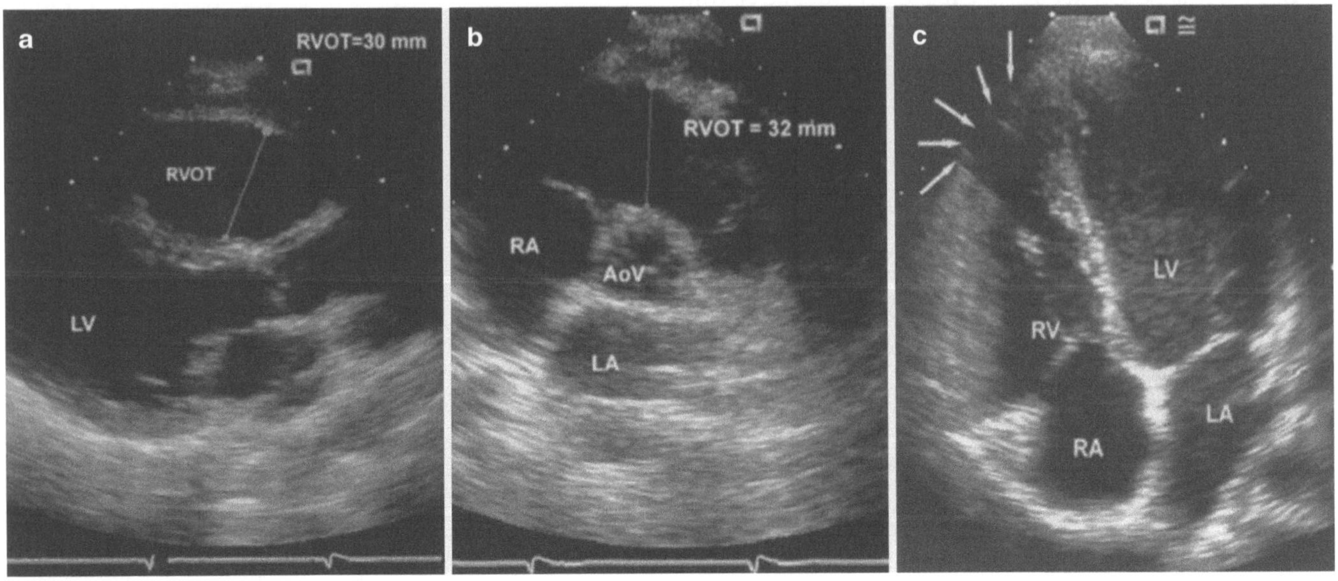

A. ARVD/C
B. PTE
C. Amyloidosis
D. Constrictive Pericarditis

Answers

1. B
2. C
3. B
4. A

References

1. Rudski LG, Lai WW, Afilalo J, Hua L, Handschumacher MD, Chandrasekaran K, et al. Guidelines for the echocardiographic assessment of the right heart in adults: a report from the American Society of Echocardiography. J Am Soc Echocardiogr. 2010;23(7):685–713.
2. Lang RM, Badano LP, Mor-Avi V, Afilalo J, Armstrong A, Ernande L, et al. Recommendations for cardiac chamber quantification by echocardiography in adults: an update from the American Society of Echocardiography and the European Association of Cardiovascular Imaging. Eur Heart J Cardiovasc Imaging. 2015;16(3):233–70.
3. Haddad F, Hunt SA, Rosenthal DN, Murphy DJ. Right ventricular function in cardiovascular disease, part I: anatomy, physiology, aging, and functional assessment of the right ventricle. Circulation. 2008;117(11):1436–48.
4. Rudski LG, Afilalo J. The blind men of Indostan and the elephant in the echo lab. J Am Soc Echocardiogr. 2012;25(7):714–7.
5. Ho SY. Anatomy echocardiography, and normal right ventricular dimensions. Heart. 2006;92(suppl_1):i2–i13.
6. Portnoy SG, Rudski LG. Echocardiographic evaluation of the right ventricle: a 2014 perspective. Curr Cardiol Rep. 2015;17(4):21.
7. Dell'Italia LJ. The right ventricle: anatomy, physiology, and clinical importance. Curr Probl Cardiol. 1991;16(10):653–720.
8. Maffessanti F, Muraru D, Esposito R, Gripari P, Ermacora D, Santoro C, et al. Age-, body size-, and sex-specific reference values for right ventricular volumes and ejection fraction by three-dimensional echocardiography: a multicenter echocardiographic study in 507 healthy volunteers. Circ Cardiovasc Imaging. 2013;6(5):700–10.
9. Ling LF, Obuchowski NA, Rodriguez L, Popovic Z, Kwon D, Marwick TH. Accuracy and interobserver concordance of echocardiographic assessment of right ventricular size and systolic function: a quality control exercise. J Am Soc Echocardiogr. 2012;25(7):709–13.
10. Davlouros PA, Niwa K, Webb G, Gatzoulis MA. The right ventricle in congenital heart disease. Heart. 2006;92(Suppl_1):i27–38.
11. Haddad F, Doyle R, Murphy DJ, Hunt SA. Right ventricular function in cardiovascular disease, part II: pathophysiology, clinical importance, and management of right ventricular failure. Circulation. 2008;117(13):1717–31.
12. Chin KM, Kim NHS, Rubin LJ. The right ventricle in pulmonary hypertension. Coron Artery Dis. 2005;16(1):13–8.
13. Jardin F, Dubourg O, Bourdarias JP. Echocardiographic pattern of acute cor pulmonale. Chest. 1997;111(1):209–17.
14. Kurnicka K, Lichodziejewska B, Goliszek S, Dzikowska-Diduch O, Zdończyk O, Kozłowska M, et al.

Echocardiographic pattern of acute pulmonary embolism: analysis of 511 consecutive patients. J Am Soc Echocardiogr. 2016;29(9):907–13.
15. Cho JH, Kutti Sridharan G, Kim SH, Kaw R, Abburi T, Irfan A, et al. Right ventricular dysfunction as an echocardiographic prognostic factor in hemodynamically stable patients with acute pulmonary embolism: a meta-analysis. BMC Cardiovasc Disord. 2014;14(1):64.
16. Neskovic A Pulmonary embolism: is echo of any use? Belgrade; 2010. http://assets.escardio.org/Assets/Presentations/OTHER2010/EAE-clinical-application-echo/20.Neskovic-pulmonaryembolism-echo-use.pdf
17. de Oliveira TL, Vieira CM, Costa JB, Prata TA, de Moura Costa AS, MDCP N, et al. Mobile right heart thrombus and pulmonary thromboembolism. J Bras Pneumol. 2012;38(2):275–8.
18. Kasai H, Matsumura A, Sugiura T, Shigeta A, Tanabe N, Ema R, et al. Noninvasive assessment of pulmonary vascular resistance by echocardiography in chronic thromboembolic pulmonary hypertension. Respir Investig. 2015;53(5):210–6.
19. Boilson BA, Pislaru SV, McGregor CGA. Accuracy of echocardiographic assessment of pulmonary hypertension severity and right ventricular dysfunction in patients with chronic thromboembolic pulmonary hypertension. Minerva Cardioangiol. 2012;60(3):257–65.
20. Repessé X, Charron C, Vieillard-Baron A. Acute cor pulmonale in ARDS: rationale for protecting the right ventricle. Chest. 2015;147(1):259–65.
21. Jardin F, Vieillard-Baron A. Is there a safe plateau pressure in ARDS? The right heart only knows. Intensive Care Med. 2007;33(3):444–7.
22. Ozben B, Eryuksel E, Tanrikulu AM, Papila N, Ozyigit T, Celikel T, et al. Acute exacerbation impairs right ventricular function in COPD patients. Hell J Cardiol. 2015;56(4):324–31.
23. Hamzaoui O, Monnet X, Teboul J-L. Pulsus paradoxus. Eur Respir J. 2013;42(6):1696–705.
24. Hilde JM, Skjørten I, Grøtta OJ, Hansteen V, Melsom MN, Hisdal J, et al. Right ventricular dysfunction and remodeling in chronic obstructive pulmonary disease without pulmonary hypertension. J Am Coll Cardiol. 2013;62(12):1103–11.
25. Gökdeniz T, Kalaycıoğlu E, Boyacı F, Aykan AÇ, Gürsoy MO, Hatem E, et al. The BODE index, a multidimensional grading system, reflects impairment of right ventricle functions in patients with chronic obstructive pulmonary disease: a speckle-tracking study. Respiration. 2014;88(3):223–33.
26. Cuttica MJ, Shah SJ, Rosenberg SR, Orr R, Beussink L, Dematte JE, et al. Right heart structural changes are independently associated with exercise capacity in non-severe COPD. PLoS One. 2011;6(12):e29069.
27. Tannus-Silva DGS, Masson-Silva JB, Ribeiro LS, Conde MB, Rabahi MF. Myocardial performance index correlates with the BODE index and affects quality of life in COPD patients. Int J Chron Obstruct Pulmon Dis. 2016;11(1):2261–8.
28. Caminiti G, Cardaci V, Conti V, D'Antoni V, Murugesan J, Battaglia D, et al. Right ventricular systolic dysfunction is related to exercise intolerance in patients with chronic obstructive pulmonary disease. J Cardiopulm Rehabil Prev. 2015;35(1):70–4.
29. Terzano C, Romani S, Gaudio C, Pelliccia F, Serao M, Vitarelli A. Right heart functional changes in the acute, hypercapnic exacerbations of COPD. Biomed Res Int. 2014;2014(7):596051–6.
30. Acar G, Kahraman H, Akkoyun M, Kilinc M, Zencir C, Yusufoglu E, et al. Evaluation of atrial electromechanical delay and its relationship to inflammation and oxidative stress in patients with chronic obstructive pulmonary disease. Echocardiography. 2014;31(5):579–85.
31. Guazzi M, Galiè N. Pulmonary hypertension in left heart disease. Eur Respir Rev. 2012;21(126):338–46.
32. Lam CSP, Roger VL, Rodeheffer RJ, Borlaug BA, Enders FT, Redfield MM. Pulmonary hypertension in heart failure with preserved ejection fraction a community-based study. J Am Coll Cardiol. 2009;53(13):1119–26.
33. Hung J. The pathogenesis of functional tricuspid regurgitation. Semin Thorac Cardiovasc Surg. 2010;22(1):76–8.
34. Shah S, Jenkins T, Markowitz A, Gilkeson R, Rajiah P. Multimodal imaging of the tricuspid valve: normal appearance and pathological entities. Insights Imaging. 2016;7(5):649–67.
35. Badano LP, Muraru D, Enriquez-Sarano M. Assessment of functional tricuspid regurgitation. Eur Heart J. 2013;34(25):1875–85.
36. Spinner EM, Lerakis S, Higginson J, Pernetz M, Howell S, Veledar E, et al. Correlates of tricuspid regurgitation as determined by 3D echocardiography: pulmonary arterial pressure, ventricle geometry, annular dilatation, and papillary muscle displacement. Circ Cardiovasc Imaging. 2012;5(1):43–50.
37. Cheng Y, Gao H, Tang L, Li J, Yao L. Clinical utility of three-dimensional echocardiography in the evaluation of tricuspid regurgitation induced by implantable device leads. Echocardiography. 2016;33((11)):1689–96.
38. Polewczyk A, Kutarski A, Tomaszewski A, Brzozowski W, Czajkowski M, Polewczyk M, et al. Lead dependent tricuspid dysfunction: analysis of the mechanism and management in patients referred for transvenous lead extraction. Cardiol J. 2013;20(4):402–10.
39. van Rosendael PJ, Delgado V, Bax JJ. The tricuspid valve and the right heart: anatomical, pathological and imaging specifications. EuroIntervention. 2015;11(Suppl W(W)):W123–7.
40. Zoghbi W. American Society of Echocardiography: Recommendations for evaluation of the severity of native valvular regurgitation with two-dimensional and Doppler echocardiography A report from the American Society of Echocardiography's Nomenclature and Standards Committee and The Task Force on Valvular Regurgitation, developed in conjunction with the American College of Cardiology Echocardiography Committee, The Cardiac Imaging Committee, Council on Clinical Cardiology, The American Heart Association, and the European Society of Cardiology Working Group on Echocardiography, represented by. Eur J Echocardiogr. 2003;4(4):237–61.
41. Badano LP, Agricola E, Perez de Isla L, Gianfagna P, Zamorano JL. Evaluation of the tricuspid valve morphology and function by transthoracic real-time three-dimensional echocardiography. Eur J Echocardiogr. 2009;10(4):477–84.
42. Anwar AM, Geleijnse ML, Cate Ten FJ, Meijboom FJ. Assessment of tricuspid valve annulus size, shape and function using real-time three-dimensional echocardiography. Interact Cardiovasc Thorac Surg. 2006;5(6):683–7.
43. Anwar AM, Soliman OII, Nemes A, van Geuns R-JM, Geleijnse ML, Cate Ten FJ. Value of assessment of tricuspid annulus: real-time three-dimensional echocardiography and magnetic resonance imaging. Int J Cardiovasc Imaging. 2007;23(6):701–5.
44. Yoerger DM, Marcus F, Sherrill D, Calkins H, Towbin JA, Zareba W, et al. Echocardiographic findings in patients meeting task force criteria for arrhythmogenic right ventricular dysplasia new insights from the multidisciplinary study of right ventricular dysplasia. J Am Coll Cardiol. 2005;45(6):860–5.
45. Marcus FI, McKenna WJ, Sherrill D, Basso C, Bauce B, Bluemke DA, et al. Diagnosis of arrhythmogenic right ventricular cardiomyopathy/dysplasia: proposed modification of the task force criteria. Circulation. 2010;121(13):1533–41.
46. Calkins H. Arrhythmogenic right ventricular dysplasia/cardiomyopathy-three decades of progress. Circ J. 2015;79(5):901–13.

47. Rallidis LS, Makavos G, Nihoyannopoulos P. Right ventricular involvement in coronary artery disease: role of echocardiography for diagnosis and prognosis. J Am Soc Echocardiogr. 2014;27(3):223–9.
48. Rajesh GN, Raju D, Nandan D, Haridasan V, Vinayakumar D, Muneer K, et al. Echocardiographic assessment of right ventricular function in inferior wall myocardial infarction and angiographic correlation to proximal right coronary artery stenosis. Indian Heart J. 2013;65(5):522–8.
49. Finocchiaro G, Kobayashi Y, Magavern E, Zhou JQ, Ashley E, Sinagra G, et al. Prevalence and prognostic role of right ventricular involvement in stress-induced cardiomyopathy. J Card Fail. 2015;21(5):419–25.
50. Becher T, El-Battrawy I, Baumann S, Fastner C, Behnes M, Loßnitzer D, et al. Characteristics and long-term outcome of right ventricular involvement in Takotsubo cardiomyopathy. Int J Cardiol. 2016;220:371–5.
51. Scally C, Ahearn T, Rudd A, Neil CJ, Srivanasan J, Jagpal B, et al. Right ventricular involvement and recovery after acute stress-induced (Tako-tsubo) cardiomyopathy. Am J Cardiol. 2016;117(5):775–80.
52. Heggemann F, Hamm K, Brade J, Streitner F, Doesch C, Papavassiliu T, et al. Right ventricular function quantification in Takotsubo cardiomyopathy using two-dimensional strain echocardiography. PLoS One. 2014;9(8):e103717.

15 How to Assess the Left and Right Atria in Clinical Practice

Piotr Lipiec and Jarosław D. Kasprzak

Abstract

Both, left atrial and right atrial sizes provide important diagnostic and prognostic information. Therefore, their assessment is a part of routine echocardiographic examination. Various techniques have been proposed—from linear measurement by M-mode to volume measurement by three-dimensional echocardiography—each having its strengths and limitations. Another part of routine echocardiographic examination is the assessment of inferior vena cava, reflecting right atrial pressures.

Keywords

Left atrium · Right atrium · Left atrial volume · Right atrial pressure · Inferior vena cava

Abbreviations

2D	Two-dimensional
BSA	Body surface area
IVC	Inferior vena cava
LA	Left atrium/left atrial
LAA	Left atrial appendage
LAV	Left atrial volume
LAVI	Left atrial volume index
RA	Right atrium/right atrial

Introduction

- Left atrial volume (LAV) is an important marker of left ventricular diastolic function [1]. Moreover, it has been shown to have a prognostic value in predicting various adverse cardiovascular outcomes, including all-cause death, cardiovascular death, heart failure, stroke, hospitalizations and atrial fibrillation in numerous clinical scenarios [2].
- There is less data on the significance of right atrial (RA) size, but it has also been demonstrated to predict outcomes in some patient populations, such as pulmonary embolism survivors [3].

Left Atrial Volume and Function: General Considerations

- LAV changes during the cardiac cycle:
  - the maximum LAV occurs before opening of mitral valve (LAV max). It is the value routinely assessed in everyday practice and often referred to just as LAV.
  - the minimum LAV occurs after mitral valve closure (LAV min)
  - LAV preceding atrial contraction (LAV pre-A)
- Based on those values the following volumes depicting LA function can be calculated [4]:
  - Total LA emptying volume (corresponding to total LA function) = LAVmax−LAVmin
  - LA passive emptying volume = LAV max−LAV pre-A
  - LA active emptying (contractile) volume = LAV pre-A−LAV min

Assessment of Left Atrial Size by Echocardiography

- In clinical practice, measurements of LA size are performed in end-systolic phase (just before opening of the mitral valve). The following methods are currently recommended [5]:

P. Lipiec, MD, PhD, FESC, FACC (✉) · J. D. Kasprzak
Department of Cardiology, Medical University of Lodz, Lodz, Poland
e-mail: lipiec@ptkardio.pl

A. Sadeghpour, A. Alizadehasl (eds.), *Case-Based Textbook of Echocardiography*,
https://doi.org/10.1007/978-3-319-67691-3_15

– Measurement of LA anteroposterior diameter either by M-mode or by two-dimensional (2D) echocardiography (the latter is the preferred one) in parasternal long-axis view at the level of the aortic sinuses, perpendicular to the aortic root long axis, with the use of leading-edge to leading-edge technique (Fig. 15.1). The main limitation is that such measurement may not fully represent LA size, especially in cases of vertical LA dilatation. Normal ranges of LA anteroposterior diameter for men and women are: 3.0–4.0 cm and 2.7–3.8 cm, respectively. Importantly, this measurement is no more recommended as a sole LA sizing approach and ought to be supplemented with volume calculation.

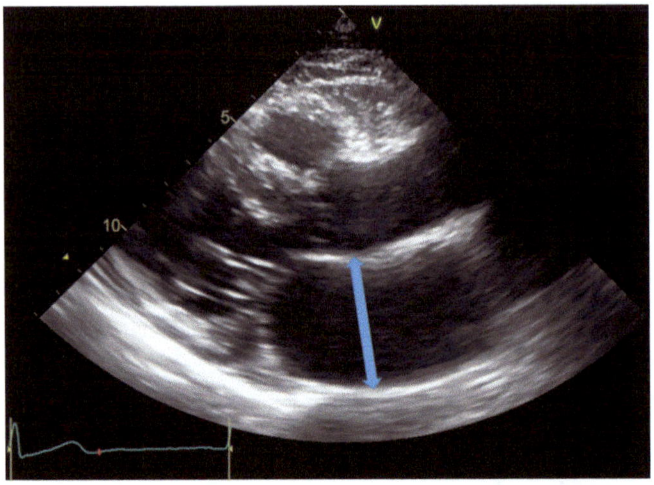

Fig. 15.1 Measurement of LA anteroposterior diameter by 2D echocardiography in parasternal long-axis view—measurement line perpendicular to the long axis of the aortic root, at the level of the sinuses of Valsalva

– Measurement of LAV by 2D echocardiography based on the tracings of the LA inner border on apical four- and two-chamber views, excluding the left atrial appendage (LAA) and pulmonary veins (Fig. 15.2). Two calculation techniques can be used: the area-length method and, preferably, the disk summation method. LAV divided by patient's body surface area (BSA) is a left atrial volume index (LAVI) which serves as a principal LA enlargement criterion.

Interpretation of 2D echocardio graphy—derived LAVI:

Normal LAVI: 16–34 mL/m^2

Mildly abnormal LAVI: 35–41 mL/m^2

Moderately abnormal LAVI: 42–48 mL/m^2

Severely abnormal LAVI: >48 mL/m^2

- Three-dimensional (3D) echocardiography allows the most accurate LAV measurement among all echocardiographic techniques. It is based on 3D datasets acquired from the apical acoustic window and subsequent off-line analysis with the use of semi-automated or fully automated endocardial tracing algorithms (Fig. 15.3) [6]. LAV measurement by 3D tends to provide higher values than 2-dimensional approach. However, defining left atrial enlargement by this technique is not yet recommended in everyday clinical practice due to limited normative data.

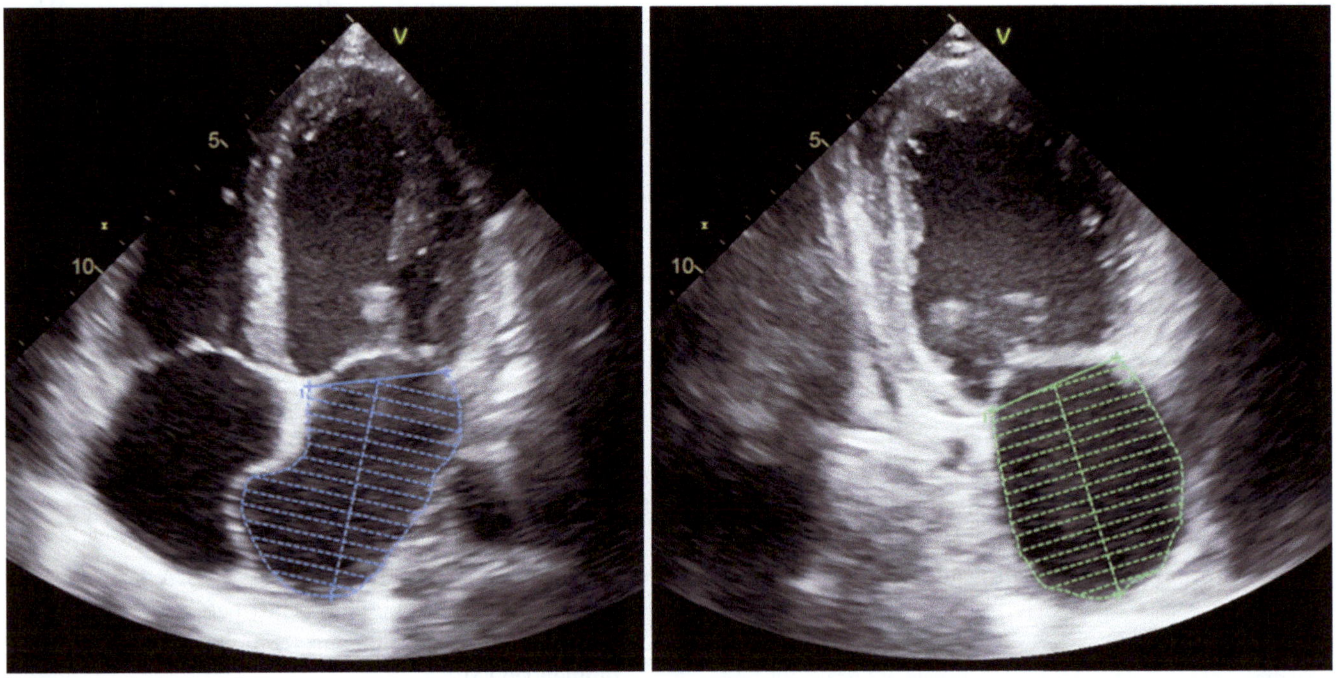

Fig. 15.2 Measurement of LA volume by 2D echocardiography based on the tracings of the LA inner border in apical four- and two-chamber views and using the disk summation method

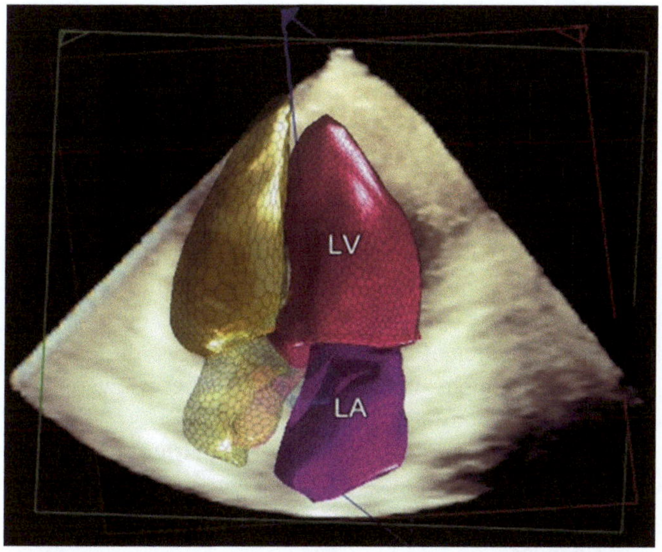

Fig. 15.3 3D model of the LV and the LA during end-systole obtained by off-line analysis of the 3D dataset acquired from the apical window. Such model enables accurate measurement of LA volume

- The assessment of LA size by measuring LA area in 2D echocardiography (in apical four-chamber view, upper normal limit 20 cm^2) is no longer recommended.

Assessment of Left Atrial Function by Echocardiography

- The left atrial function can be assessed by [4]:
  - Linear measurements e.g. LA fractional shortening
  - Volumetric measurements e.g. LA ejection fraction
  - Tissue Doppler technique, Velocity Vector Imaging and speckle tracking echocardiography

However, in clinical practice the quantification of LA function is not yet recommended as a part of routine echocardiographic examination. 2-D image-based left atrial strain emerges as a promising research approach.

Assessment of Right Atrial Size by Echocardiography

- Measurements of RA size are performed in end-systolic phase (just before opening of the tricuspid valve). The following methods are currently recommended [5]:
  - Measurement of the RA minor axis by 2D echocardiography in the apical four-chamber view (the linear measurement between the lateral RA wall and the interatrial septum at the mid-atrial level, Fig. 15.4). In normal subjects mean minor RA axis indexed to BSA is 1.9 ± 0.3 cm/m^2.
  - Measurement of the RA area in the apical four-chamber view by tracing the RA inner border (Fig. 15.5). The area greater than 18cm^2 is regarded as abnormal.
  - Measurement of the RA volume based on the tracing the RA inner border in the apical four-chamber view. Two calculation techniques can be used: the area-length method and the disk summation method. In normal men and women the mean RA volume indexed to BSA is 25 ± 7 mL/m^2 and 21 ± 6 mL/m^2, respectively.

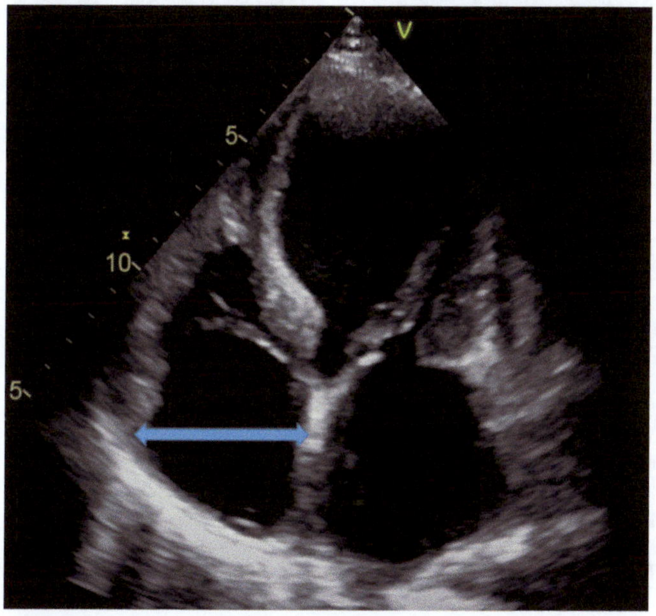

Fig. 15.4 Measurement of the RA minor axis (recommended at mid-atrial level) by 2D echocardiography in the apical four-chamber view

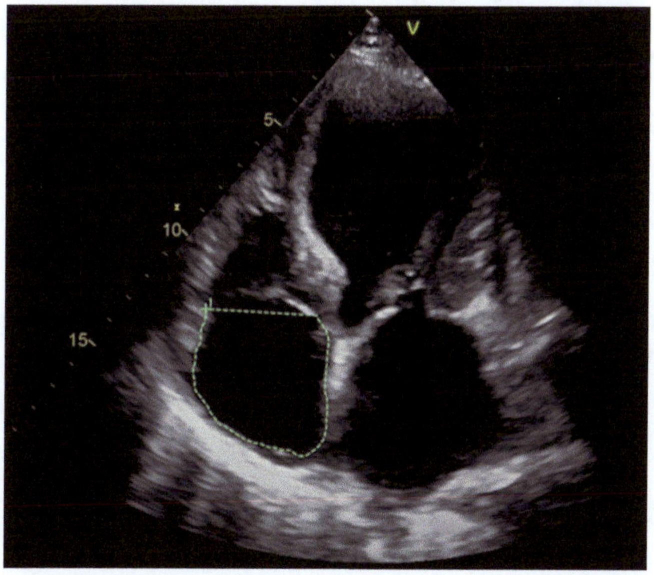

Fig. 15.5 Measurement of RA area by 2D echocardiography based on the tracings of the RA inner border in apical four-chamber view

Table 15.1 Assessment of RA pressure based on the measurement of IVC and of its collapse during sniff

IVC diameter	IVC collapse on inspiration	RA pressure
≤2.1 cm	>50%	3 mmHg
≤2.1 cm	<50%	8 mmHg[a]
>2.1 cm	>50%	8 mmHg[a]
>2.1 cm	<50%	15 mmHg

[a]Extended analysis involving secondary indices of elevated RA pressure is recommended

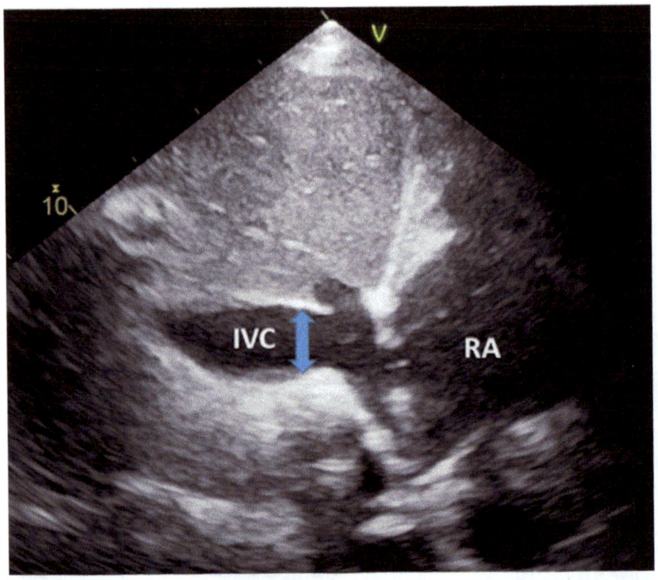

Fig. 15.6 Measurement of the diameter of the IVC in the subcostal view

Assessment of Right Atrial Pressure by Echocardiography

- Echocardiographic assessment of RA pressure is possible by means of measurement of the diameter of the inferior vena cava (IVC) and of the percentage decrease in the diameter during inspiration (Table 15.1, Fig. 15.6) [3]. The diameter should be measured in the subcostal view, perpendicular to the IVC long axis, 1–2 cm from the RA.

Questions

1. Left atrial size in routine echocardiographic examination is typically measured:
   A. in end-diastole
   B. in end-systole
   C. just before P wave
   D. when the inner border is best visible
2. Left atrial volume of 80 mL/m^2 measured by two-dimensional echocardiography in a patient with body surface area of 1.9 m^2:
   A. represents enlargement of the left atrium
   B. represents normal size of the left atrium
   C. cannot be interpreted without knowing patient's gender
   D. cannot be interpreted because it is not a recommended technique of left atrial volume measurement
3. Right atrial area of 22 cm^2 measured by two-dimensional echocardiography in apical four-chamber view in in a patient with body surface area of 1.9 m^2:
   A. represents enlargement of the right atrium
   B. represents normal size of the right atrium
   C. cannot be interpreted without knowing patient's gender
   D. cannot be interpreted because it is not a recommended technique of right atrial size assessment
4. Inferior vena cava with the diameter of 18 mm during expiration and 8 mm during inspiration:
   A. reflects right atrial pressure of 15 mmHg
   B. reflects right atrial pressure of 9 mmHg
   C. reflects right atrial pressure of 3 mmHg
   D. does not allow for the assessment of atrial pressure without additional data.

Answers

1. B
2. A
3. A
4. C

References

1. Nagueh SF, Smiseth OA, Appleton CP, Byrd BF 3rd, Dokainish H, Edvardsen T, Flachskampf FA, Gillebert TC, Klein AL, Lancellotti P, Marino P, Oh JK, Alexandru Popescu B, Waggoner AD. Recommendations for the evaluation of left ventricular diastolic function by echocardiography: an update from the American Society of Echocardiography and the European Association of Cardiovascular Imaging. Eur Heart J Cardiovasc Imaging. 2016;17(12):1321–60.
2. Abhayaratna WP, Seward JB, Appleton CP, Douglas PS, Oh JK, Tajik AJ, Tsang TS. Left atrial size: physiologic determinants and clinical applications. J Am Coll Cardiol. 2006;47(12):2357–63.
3. Rudski LG, Lai WW, Afilalo J, Hua L, Handschumacher MD, Chandrasekaran K, Solomon SD, Louie EK, Schiller NB. Guidelines for the echocardiographic assessment of the right heart in adults: a report from the American Society of Echocardiography endorsed by

the European Association of Echocardiography, a registered branch of the European Society of Cardiology, and the Canadian Society of Echocardiography. J Am Soc Echocardiogr. 2010;23(7):685–713.

4. Blume GG, Mcleod CJ, Barnes ME, Seward JB, Pellikka PA, Bastiansen PM, Tsang TS. Left atrial function: physiology, assessment, and clinical implications. Eur J Echocardiogr. 2011;12(6): 421–30.
5. Lang RM, Badano LP, Mor-Avi V, Afilalo J, Armstrong A, Ernande L, Flachskampf FA, Foster E, Goldstein SA, Kuznetsova T, Lancellotti P, Muraru D, Picard MH, Rietzschel ER, Rudski L, Spencer KT, Tsang W, Voigt JU. Recommendations for cardiac chamber quantification by echocardiography in adults: an update from the American Society of Echocardiography and the European Association of Cardiovascular Imaging. Eur Heart J Cardiovasc Imaging. 2015;16(3): 233–70.
6. Mor-Avi V, Yodwut C, Jenkins C, Kühl H, Nesser HJ, Marwick TH, Franke A, Weinert L, Niel J, Steringer-Mascherbauer R, Freed BH, Sugeng L, Lang RM. Real-time 3D echocardiographic quantification of left atrial volume: multicenter study for validation with CMR. JACC Cardiovasc Imaging. 2012;5(8):769–77.

Echocardiography in Hypertension

16

Azin Alizadehasl and Anita Sadeghpour

Abstract

Hypertension (HTN) is a heterogeneous disease with a number of well-defined as well as supposed reasons. HTN is a main risk factor for stroke and all cardiovascular disorders and is, therefore, associated with significant morbidity and mortality rates. The key role of echocardiography in the management of hypertension is the evaluation of left ventricular hypertrophy (LVH) and left ventricular mass (LVM). Indeed, LVH, LV diastolic dysfunction, and left atrial (LA) enlargement are specific signs of hypertensive heart disease (HHD).

The development of Doppler echocardiography, strain imaging, and three-dimensional echocardiography (3DE) has offered new approaches regarding perceptions in pathophysiology and also clinical implications in hypertensive patients.

Keywords

Echocardiography · Hypertensive heart disease · LA volume · Left ventricular hypertrophy · LV mass · Relative wall thickness (RWT) · Concentric hypertrophy · Eccentric hypertrophy · Concentric remodeling

Abbreviations

3DE	Three-dimensional echocardiography
ACC	American college of cardiology
ASE	American society of echocardiography
AUC	Appropriate use criteria
CMR	Cardiac magnetic resonance
EACVI	European association of cardiovascular imaging
HHD	Hypertensive heart disease
HTN	Hypertension
IVS	Interventricular septum
JNC	Joint national committee
LA	Left atrial
LVH	Left ventricular hypertrophy
LVM	Left ventricular mass
PW	Posterior wall
RWT	Relative wall thickness
TTE	Transthoracic echocardiography

A. Alizadehasl, MD, FACC, FASE
Associate Professor of Cardiology, Echocardiologist, Echocardiography and Cardiogenetic Research Centers, Cardio-Oncology Department, Rajaie Cardiovascular Medical and Research Center, Tehran, Iran

A. Sadeghpour, MD, FACC, FASE (✉)
Professor of Cardiology, Echocardiography Research Center, Rajaie Cardiovascular Medical and Research Center, Iran University of Medical Science, Tehran, Iran

Echocardiographic Evaluation of Hypertensive Patients

- The echocardiographic study of the heart of a hypertensive patient is done on two levels:
  - (a) Anatomic approach, which contains measurement of the heart chambers
  - (b) Functional approach, which contains the study of the indices of function [1–4]
- Generally, a global echocardiographic assessment of a patient with HTN should include:
  1. LVH, LV geometry, and LV mass
  2. LV systolic and diastolic functions
  3. LA volume and function
  4. Thoracic aorta and coronary artery reserve and patency, to examine the possible concomitance of coronary artery disease [5–7]
- LVH is seen in 36–41% of hypertensive individuals and denotes the end-organ damage caused by HTN according to the Joint National Committee (JNC 7) [8].

A. Sadeghpour, A. Alizadehasl (eds.), *Case-Based Textbook of Echocardiography*, https://doi.org/10.1007/978-3-319-67691-3_16

- However, HTN is not the only cause of LVH because hypertrophy can be seen in obesity, diabetes, and metabolic syndrome.
- In the early stage and in the mild form of HTN, grade 1 diastolic dysfunction and absence of LVH are common manifestations [9].
- In severe and untreated forms of HTN, filling pressures rise and LVH develops as an adaptive response to chronic pressure overload. Eventually, LV systolic dysfunction occurs.
- Based on the American College of Cardiology (ACC) Appropriate Use Criteria (AUC), transthoracic echocardiography (TTE) has a high AUC score of 8 in the initial evaluation of patients with suspected HHD [10].

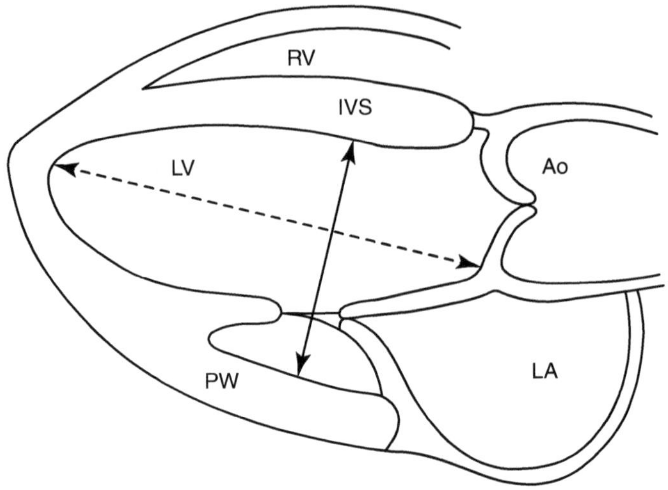

Fig. 16.1 Showing measurement of wall thicknesses and internal dimensions at the level of the mitral leaflet tips in diastole in the parasternal long-axis view

Left Ventricular Hypertrophy, Mass, and Geometry

- The most commonly used 2D approaches to the measurement of LVM are based on the area-length formula and the truncated ellipsoid model, as explained in detail in the previous American Society of Echocardiography/ European Association of Cardiovascular Imaging (ASE/ EACVI) chamber quantification document [11].
- In the existence of shape distortions (e.g., post-myocardial infarction remodeling), the geometric expectations inherent in this approach remain complex and problematic.
- For the measurement of the size, mass, and function of the chambers, both 2D and M-mode methods were validated and legalized in the early 1980s.
- The limits of M-mode regarding geometrical expectations and the impact of small error on measurements are also applicable to 2D measurements. In addition, 2D imaging leads to repeated foreshortening due to unsuitable cut planes [12, 13].
- In spite of many technical limitations (low-quality imaging in obese patients, interobserver variability, obstructive lung disease, etc.), echocardiography is more sensitive than electrocardiography in identifying LVH and also forecasting cardiovascular risk, thereby assisting in the selection of proper therapy.
- Proper measurements for the assessment of a patient with HTN comprise interventricular septum (IVS), LV posterior wall (PW) thickness, and end-diastolic diameter—with the calculation of LVM based on the formula presently approved by the ASE [10]. This is derived from 2D linear LV measurements, has been validated by necropsy ($r = 0.90$; $P < 0.001$), and is based on modeling the ventricle as a prolate ellipse of revolution:

$$\text{LV Mass (g)} = 0.8\{1.04\,([\text{LVEDD} + \text{IVSd} + \text{PWd}]^3 - \text{LVEDD}^3)\} + 0.6$$

where LVIDd is LV internal diameter at diastole, PWTd is the posterior wall thickness at diastole, and SWTd is the septal wall thickness at diastole—which should be measured approximately at the leaflet tips of the mitral valve.

This formula is appropriate for the assessment of patients without major distortions of LV geometry (e.g., patients with HTN) [7, 14].

Key Points in Practice

- The wall thicknesses and internal dimensions should be measured at the level of the mitral leaflet tips in diastole in the parasternal long-axis view or targeted short-axis view—preferably in several beats Fig. 16.1.
- Even small errors in linear measurements will be cubed and have an impact on accuracy.
- The 'Cube' formula is not an accurate method in patients with abnormal LV geometry (e.g., apical aneurysm or where the 2:1 axis ratio is distorted).
- In 2D measurements, the upper limit of normal of LV diastolic dimension is slightly smaller than the M-mode measurement.
- The upper limits of a normal LVM is 95 g/m^2 for women and 115 g/m^2 for men by linear measurements and 88 g/m^2 in women and 102 g/m^2 in men with 2D methods.
- Based on the current guideline on chamber quantification, the actual tissue/blood interface—instead of leading edge to leading edge—can be measured.
- Normal values are less well-established with 2D and 3D than with M-mode measurements.
- While patients in the early phase of HHD are most likely have a normal LV geometry, long-lasting or untreated HTN will result in changes in LV shape and, eventually, exacerbation in systolic function.
- Broadly, the changes in LV geometry can be categorized according to whether LVM is normal or increased and

Table 16.1 Classification of LV geometry measured by 2D guided M-mode study

Classical description of LV geometry		
LV geometry	**LV mass**	**RWT**
Normal	≤115 g/m² (men) or ≤95 g/m² (women)	<0.42
Concentric hypertrophy	>115 g/m² (men) or >95 g/m² (women)	>0.42
Eccentric hypertrophy	>115 g/m² (men) or >95 g/m² (women)	<0.42
Concentric remodeling	≤115 g/m² (men) or ≤95 g/m² (women)	>0.42

LV mass measurements using 2D–guided M-mode

whether ventricular morphology as described by RWT is altered.

- **Relative wall thickness (RWT)** is variably described as (PW × 2/LVDD or (IVS + PW)/LVDD, of which we favor the former because septal measurements may be confounded by the existence of septal bulge. RWT is challenging and not reflective of the true LV geometry in patients with asymmetric hypertrophy. **The upper limit of normal RWT is 0.42** [13–15].
- Concentric LVH, which is probably the most common pattern associated with HTN Table 16.1, is an adaptive response to high blood pressure and is characterized by:
  (a) Normal cavity size,
  (b) Uniformly increased LV wall thickness,
  (c) Increased LVM
  (d) RWT = 2 × PWd/LVEDD

Left Ventricular Systolic and Diastolic Functions

- LV systolic function has a prognostic value in HHD, although commonly systolic function—as measured by the ejection fraction (EF)—is preserved until the late course of HHD. An LVEF <50% can distinguish systolic heart failure from diastolic heart failure with an EF >50% [16].
- Despite the widespread clinical use of LVEF, it should be kept in mind that it is a load-dependent systolic index.
- This was the cause for the introduction into clinical practice of mid-wall fractional shortening, a systolic index of LV function that is relatively independent of afterload. Notably, hypertensive cases with LVH and a normal EF have been found to have abnormal mid-wall fractional shortening [13, 14, 17].
- Studies on tissue Doppler imaging parameters have shown that s' has the best correlation with LV systolic function and LVEF and that it also has a significant correlation with clinical outcomes such as re-hospitalization [18].
- Measurements of s′ at the septal and lateral edges of the mitral annulus in the apical 4-chamber view <7 cm/s predict an LVEF <45% with 93% sensitivity and 87% specificity.
- The development of LV diastolic dysfunction might precede hypertrophy and can be one of the earliest changes associated with HHD.
- Notably, diastolic dysfunction may not be accompanied by symptoms and is frequently a chance finding during a Doppler echocardiographic study since LV diastolic dysfunction—as evaluated by Doppler echocardiography—can expect mortality in middle-aged and elderly adults [19, 20].
- A comprehensive study of diastolic function should include not only a simple assessment of diastolic dysfunction progression but also an estimation of LV filling pressure, a true determinant of symptoms and prognosis.
- Though this can be derived via various ultrasound maneuvers or tools, the ratio between the transmitral E velocity and the pulsed tissue Doppler-derived early diastolic velocity (the E/e′ ratio) is the most feasible and precise. Structural changes in the myocardium (e.g., altered collagen and myocardial cells) are perhaps the mechanism of diastolic dysfunction [13, 14] (Fig. 16.2).

(a) ***Left atrial morphology and function***
  - LA volume can be calculated by either area-length or modified Simpson's methods. It is frequently scaled for the body surface area and is expressed in mL/m². The normal range is ≤34 mL/m².
  - The LA is not symmetrical, and enlargement may happen non-uniformly and mostly in 1 direction. Subsequently, LA size is much better assessed with 2D- or 3D–based LA volume rather than with M-mode.
  - In HTN and other conditions where diastolic dysfunction happens, a decrease in early diastolic emptying is compensated by forceful atrial contraction. In addition, an intermittent or permanent rise in LV filling pressures leads to the overfilling of the LA. The resulting
  - LA enlargement is the "morpho-physiologic expression" of chronic diastolic dysfunction, which reflects the duration and severity of an increased LA pressure.
  - Though the presence of atrial fibrillation itself contributes to atrial size, LA enlargement is a well-known independent factor of stroke, cardiovascular events, and death.
  - Furthermore, atrial fibrosis might be another endpoint of this process, predisposing to atrial remodeling and dysfunction with atrial fibrillation. This is a common endpoint that may be originated by a number of etiologies, including HTN and diabetes mellitus [21, 22].

(b) **Thoracic aorta**
  - Aging and HTN have been shown to significantly increase aortic diameter, thickness, and stiffness. Aortic root dilatation is a frequent cardiovascular phenotype in hypertensive cases who are referred to echo laboratories for the identification of hypertensive organ damage, and is really predictive of increased cardiovascular morbidity and mortality [1, 14].

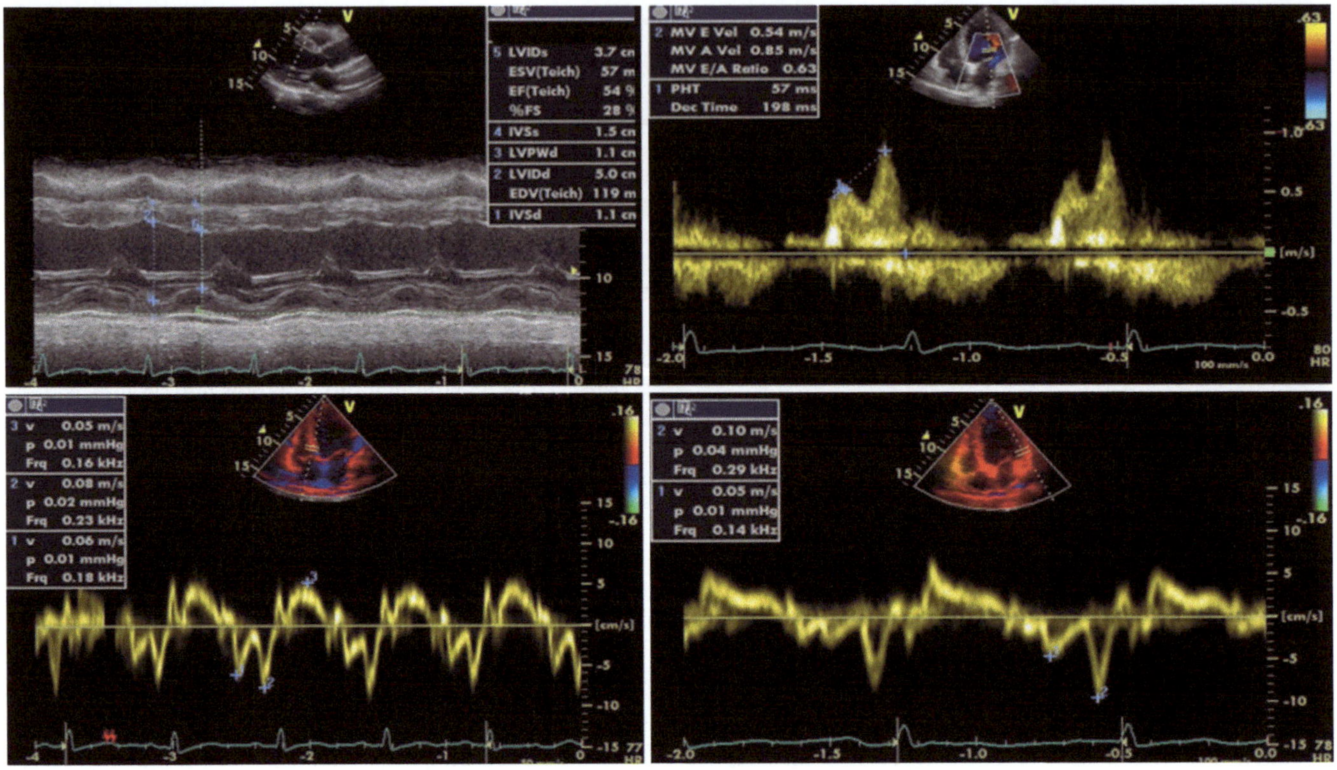

Fig. 16.2 *M-mode, Doppler, and* Tissue Doppler study of a patient with typical findings of hypertensive heart disease. The left upper panel shows increased RWT (PW + IVS)/LVID = 0.44, suggestive of concentric LVH. The right upper panel (mitral inflow PW Doppler study) shows delayed relaxation, which is a common finding in uncomplicated systemic HTN. The left and right lower panels show decreased maximal early diastolic velocity e′ and systolic S′ measured in the septal and lateral parts of the mitral annulus

(c) **Advanced 2D echocardiography**

- These newer modalities and techniques contain mainly real-time 3D echocardiography, coronary flow reserve, and the concepts of strain and strain rate evaluated by either tissue Doppler or speckle-tracking echocardiography.
- 3D echocardiography permits a more accurate evaluation of LV volumes and mass.
- The concepts of strain or strain rate have been incorporated into the group of the newest techniques for assessing LV function.
- Strain and strain rate can be derived from either tissue Doppler or speckle-tracking 2 or 3D echocardiography. Because of the many limitations to the Doppler-based strain and strain rate method, speckle-tracking-derived strain and strain rate seem to have prevailed.
- Conventional TTE and pulsed-wave tissue Doppler imaging are usually unable to reveal very early subtle abnormalities in LV systolic function caused by HTN, prior to the manifestation of hypertrophy. It has been proposed that strain and strain rate, particularly when derived from speckle-tracking echocardiography, provide more insight into early HTN-induced LV systolic dysfunction. However, it should be emphasized that, albeit very promising, this technique has mainly been applied for research purposes and has not been adopted as a standard tool in everyday clinical practice for the evaluation of HHD.
- It seems that longitudinal systolic strain has been found to be diminished in hypertensive patients, even before hypertrophy happens. It has been concluded that speckle-tracking echocardiography provides more detailed data than conventional echocardiography inasmuch as it can disclose systolic dysfunction before hypertrophy happens and can identify some early LV mechanical changes that might improve the clinical management of these cases [23–27] (Fig. 16.3).

3D Echocardiography

- LV volume measurements by 2DE rely on geometrical assumption, which is prone to the foreshortening and underestimation of the true ventricular volumes—especially in remodeled ventricles.
- 3D TTE for the measurement of the LV volume and LVEF is superior to 2D TTE insofar as it is more reproducible and has a closer correlation with cardiac magnetic resonance (CMR) data.

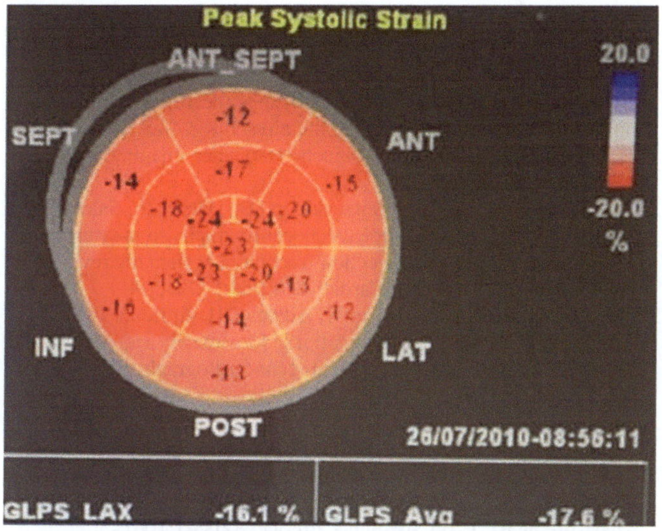

Fig. 16.3 Donut/bullseye in HTN; Decreased longitudinal strain in basal segments with normal values in apical ones

- In the latest recommendation by the ASE and EACVI, 3DE—rather than 2DE—has been proposed for the routine assessment of LV volumes and function [28–30].
- 3DE is a potentially attractive modality for the measurement of LVM, and normal ranges have been developed. The accuracy of 3DE is reportedly similar to that of CMR imaging methods for measuring LVM.
- However, there are wide limits of agreement, which primarily relate to difficulties in accurately tracing LV epicardial border—particularly in dilated ventricles—and generally show that while 3DE is imperfect for LVM estimation—with a tendency to underestimate LVM compared with CMR imaging in patients with cardiac disease—the accuracy is more favorable than that with alternative ultrasound methods [13, 31–33].

Conclusions

In spite of its technical limitations, echocardiography is truly a significant tool for the assessment of HHD. Conventional echocardiography—along with newer, richer, and better techniques—provides precious information on the extent of heart injury associated with HTN and cardiovascular risk, thereby helping us to attain a better and more appropriate management.

References

1. Cuspidi C, Meani S, Valerio C, et al. Ambulatory blood pressure, target organ damage and aortic root size in never-treated essential hypertensive patients. J Hum Hypertens. 2007;21:531–8.
2. Cortigiani L, Bigi R, Landi P, Bovenzi F, Picano E, Sicari R. Prognostic implication of stress echocardiography in 6214 hypertensive and 5328 normotensive patients. Eur Heart J. 2011;32:1509–18.
3. Cameli M, Lisi M, Righini FM, Massoni A, Mondillo S. LV remodeling and torsion dynamics in hypertensive patients. Int J Cardiovasc Imaging. 2012;29(1):79–86. [Epub ahead of print].
4. Kim MN, Park SM, Shim WJ, Kim YH, Kim SA, Cho DH. The relationship between aortic stiffness and LV dyssynchrony in hypertensive patients with preserved LV systolic function. Clin Exp Hypertens. 2012;34:410–6.
5. Levy D, Garrison RJ, Savage DD, Kannel WB, Castelli WP. Prognostic implications of echocardiographically determined LV mass in the Framingham heart study. N Engl J Med. 1990;322:1561–6.
6. Cuspidi C, Ambrosioni E, Mancia G, Pessina AC, Trimarco B, Zanchetti A. Role of echocardiography and carotid ultrasonography in stratifying risk in patients with essential HTN: the assessment of prognostic risk observational survey. J Hypertens. 2002;20:1307–14.
7. Ilercil A, O'Grady MJ, Roman MJ, et al. Reference values for echocardiographic measurements in urban and rural populations of differing ethnicity: the strong heart study. J Am Soc Echocardiogr. 2001;14:601–11.
8. Cuspidi C, Sala C, Negri F, Mancia G, Morganti A. Prevalence of leftventricular hypertrophy in hypertension: an updated review of echocardiographic studies. J Hum Hypertens. 2012;26:343–9.
9. Dianzumba SB, DiPette D, Joyner CR, Townsend R, Weber E, Mauro K, et al. Left ventricular function in mild hypertension after adrenergic blockade. Hypertension. 1988;11:198–02.
10. American College of Cardiology Foundation Appropriate Use CriteriaTask Force, American Society of Echocardiography, American Heart Association, American Society of Nuclear Cardiology, Heart Failure Society of America, Heart Rhythm Society, et al. J Am Coll Cardiol. 2011;57:1126–66.
11. Lang RM, Bierig M, Devereux RB, Flachskampf FA, Foster E, Pellikka PA, et al. Recommendations for chamber quantification. Eur J Echocardiogr. 2006;7:79–108.
12. Devereux RB, Alonso DR, Lutas EM, et al. Echocardiographic assessment of LV hypertrophy: comparison to necropsy findings. Am J Cardiol. 1986;57:450–8.
13. Marwick TH, Gillebert TC, Aurigemma G, Chirinos J, Derumeaux G, Galderisi M, Gottdiener J, Haluska B, Ofili E, Segers P, Senior R, Tapp RJ, Zamorano JL. Recommendations on the use of echocardiography in adult HTN: a report from the European Association of Cardiovascular Imaging (EACVI) and the American Society of Echocardiography (ASE). J Am Soc Echocardiogr. 2015(28):727–54.
14. Karabinos I, Grassos C, Kostaki P, Kranidis A. Echocardiography in the evaluation of a hypertensive patient: an invaluable tool or simply following the routine? Hell J Cardiol. 2013;54:47–57.
15. Yuda S, Shimamoto K, Watanabe N. Clinical applications of strain rate imaging for evaluation of left atrial function. Rinsho Byori. 2010;58:799–808.
16. Owan TE, Hodge DO, Herges RM, Jacobsen SJ, Roger VL, Redfield MM. Trends in prevalence and outcome of heart failure with preserved ejection fraction. N Engl J Med. 2006;355:251–9.
17. Devereux RB, Roman MJ, Palmieri V, et al. Left ventricular wall stresses and wall stress-mass-heart rate products in hypertensive patients with electrocardiographic left ventricular hypertrophy: the LIFE study. Losartan intervention for endpoint reduction in hypertension. J Hypertens. 2000;18:1129–38.
18. Ruan Q, Nagueh SF. Usefulness of isovolumic and systolic ejection signals by tissue Doppler for the assessment of left ventricular systolic function in ischemic or idiopathic dilated cardiomyopathy. Am J Cardiol. 2006;97:872–5.
19. Fici F, Ural D, Tayfun S, et al. Left ventricular diastolic dysfunction in newly diagnosed untreated hypertensive patients. Blood Press. 2012;21:331–7.
20. Bella JN, Palmieri V, Roman MJ, et al. Mitral ratio of peak early to late diastolic filling velocity as a predictor of mortality in

middle-aged and elderly adults: the strong heart study. Circulation. 2002;105:1928–33.

21. Lang RM, Badano L, Afilalo J, Chamber Quantification Writing Group, American Society of Echocardiography's Guidelines, Standards Committee, European Association of Echocardiography. Recommendations for cardiac chamber quantification by echocardiography: an update from the American Society of Echocardiography and the European Association of Cardiovascular Imaging. J Am Soc Echocardiogr. 2015;28:1–39.
22. Tsang TS, Abhayaratna WP, Barnes ME, Miyasaka Y, Gersh BJ, Bailey KR, et al. Prediction of cardiovascular outcomes with left atrial size: is volume superior to area or diameter? J Am Coll Cardiol. 2006;47:1018–23.
23. Mornoş C, Ruşinaru D, Manolis AJ, Zacharopoulou I, Pittaras A, Ionac A. The value of a new speckle tracking index including left ventricular global longitudinal strain and torsion in patients with dilated cardiomyopathy. Hell J Cardiol. 2011;52:299–306.
24. Feigenbaum H, Mastouri R, Sawada S. A practical approach to using strain echocardiography to evaluate the left ventricle. Circ J. 2012;76:1550–5.
25. Imbalzano E, Zito C, Carerj S, et al. Left ventricular function in hypertension: new insight by speckle tracking echocardiography. Echocardiography. 2011;28:649–57.
26. Kouzu H, Yuda S, Muranaka A, et al. Left ventricular hypertrophy causes different changes in longitudinal, radial, and circumferential mechanics in patients with hypertension: a two-dimensional speckle tracking study. J Am Soc Echocardiogr. 2011;24:192–9.
27. Galderisi M, Lomoriello VS, Santoro A, et al. Differences of myocardial systolic deformation and correlates of diastolic function in competitive rowers and young hypertensives: a speckle-tracking echocardiography study. J Am Soc Echocardiogr. 2010;23:1190–8.
28. Jenkins C, Moir S, Chan J, Rakhit D, Haluska B, Marwick TH. Left ventricular volume measurement with echocardiography: a comparison of left ventricular opacification, three-dimensional echocardiography, or both with magnetic resonance imaging. Eur Heart J. 2009;30:98–106.
29. Dorosz JL, Lezotte DC, Weitzenkamp DA, Allen LA, Salcedo EE. Performance of 3-dimensional echocardiography in measuring left ventricular volumes and ejection fraction: a systematic review and meta-analysis. J Am Coll Cardiol. 2012;59:1799–808.
30. Lang RM, Badano LP, Tsang W, Adams DH, Agricola E, Buck T, et al. EAE/ASE recommendations for image acquisition and display using three-dimensional echocardiography. J Am Soc Echocardiogr. 2012;25:3–46.
31. Takeuchi M, Nishikage T, Mor-Avi V, Sugeng L, Weinert L, Nakai H, et al. Measurement of left ventricular mass by real-time three-dimensional echocardiography: validation against magnetic resonance and comparison with two-dimensional and M-mode measurements. J Am Soc Echocardiogr. 2008;21:1001–5.
32. van den Bosch AE, Robbers-Visser D, Krenning BJ, McGhie JS, Helbing WA, Meijboom FJ, et al. Comparison of real-time three-dimensional echocardiography to magnetic resonance imaging for assessment of left ventricular mass. Am J Cardiol. 2006;97:113–7.
33. Shimada YJ, Shiota T. Meta-analysis of accuracy of left ventricular mass measurement by three-dimensional echocardiography. Am J Cardiol. 2012;110:445–52.

17 Echocardiographic Assessment of Native Valvular Heart Disease

Anita Sadeghpour and Azin Alizadehasl

Abstract

Echocardiography is not only the most versatile imaging technique for the cardiovascular system but also the most comprehensive and reliable hemodynamic tool. As we have gained confidence in the use of 2D and Doppler echocardiography for assessing cardiac hemodynamics, the evaluation of valvular heart disease has increasingly depended on echocardiography, so that fewer cases with valvular heart disease undergo invasive hemodynamic valuation. Thus, hemodynamic variables such as pressure gradients, stenotic and regurgitant valve orifice area, cardiac output (CO), regurgitant volume, left ventricular (LV) filling pressure, and pulmonary artery pressures are routinely and reliably measured with 2D and Doppler echocardiography (Table 17.1).

Keywords

Transesophageal echocardiography · Valvular heart disease · Aortic stenosis · Aortic regurgitation · Mitral stenosis · Mitral regurgitation · Tricuspid stenosis · Tricuspid regurgitation

Abbreviations

AF	Atrial fibrillation
AR	Aortic regurgitation
AS	Aortic valve stenosis
AV	Aortic valve
AVA	Aortic valve area
CAD	Coronary artery disease
CO	Cardiac output
CRT	Cardiac resynchronization therapy
CSA	Cross-sectional area
CW	Continuous-wave
ERO	Effective regurgitant orifice
HF	Heart failure
LA	Left atrium
LV	Left ventricle
LVEF	Left ventricular ejection fraction
LVESD	Left ventricular end systolic dimension
LVOT	Left ventrivular outflow tract
MR	Mitral regurgitation
MS	Mitral stenosis
MV	Mitral valve
MVA	Mitral valve area
MVR	Mitral valve replacement
NYHA	New York heart association
PASP	Pulmonary artery systolic pressure
PHT	Pressure half-time
PISA	Proximal isovelocity surface area
RF	Regurgitant fraction
Rvol	Regurgitant volume
TEE	Transesophageal echocardiography
TR	Tricuspid regurgitation
TS	Tricuspid stenosis
TTE	Transthoracic echocardiography
TVI	Time velocity integral
V	Velocity
VC	Vena contracta
VTI	Velocity time integral

Aortic Valve Disease

Aortic Valve Stenosis

Aortic valve stenosis (AS) is a progressive condition, with the end-stage disease leading to death due to the obstruction

A. Sadeghpour, MD, FACC, FASE
Professor of Cardiology, Echocardiography Research Center, Rajaie Cardiovascular Medical and Research Center, Iran University of Medical Science, Tehran, Iran

A. Alizadehasl, MD, FACC, FASE (✉)
Associate Professor of Cardiology, Echocardiologist, Echocardiography and Cardiogenetic Research Centers, Cardio-Oncology Department, Rajaie Cardiovascular Medical and Research Center, Tehran, Iran

A. Sadeghpour, A. Alizadehasl (eds.), *Case-Based Textbook of Echocardiography*, https://doi.org/10.1007/978-3-319-67691-3_17

Table 17.1 Frequency of echocardiograms in asymptomatic patients with VHD and normal left ventricular function

Stage	Valve lesion			
Stage	**Aortic stenosis**[a]	**Aortic regurgitation**	**Mitral stenosis**	Mitral regurgitation
Progressive (stage B)	Every 3–5 years (mild severity V_{max} 2.0–2.9 m/s)	Every 3–5 years (mild severity)	Every 3–5 years (MVA >1.5 cm^2)	Every 3–5 years (mild severity)
	Every 1–2 years (moderate severity V_{max} 3.0–3.9 m/s)	Every 1–2 years (moderate severity)		Every 1–2 years (moderate severity)
Severe (stage C)	Every 6–12 years (V_{max} ≥4 m/s)	Every 6–12 months	Every 1–2 years (MVA 1.0–1.5 cm^2)	Every 6–12 months dilating LV: more frequently
		Dilating LV: more frequently	Once every year (MVA <1.0 cm^2)	

Patients with mixed valve disease may require serial evaluations at intervals earlier than recommended for single valve lesions

LV indicates left ventricle, *MVA* mitral valve area, *VHD* valvular heart disease, V_{max} maximum velocity

Modified reference from: Rick A. Nishimura, Catherine M. Otto, Robert O. Bonow, Blase A. Carabello, John P. Erwin, Robert A. Guyton, Patrick T. O'Gara, Carlos E. Ruiz, Nikolaos J. Skubas, Paul Sorajja, Thoralf M. Sundt, III, James D. Thomas. 2014 AHA/ACC Guideline for the Management of Cases with Valvular Heart Disease: Executive Summary. J Am Coll Cardiol. 2014;63(22):2438–2488. doi:10.1016/j.jacc.2014.02.537

[a]With normal stroke volume

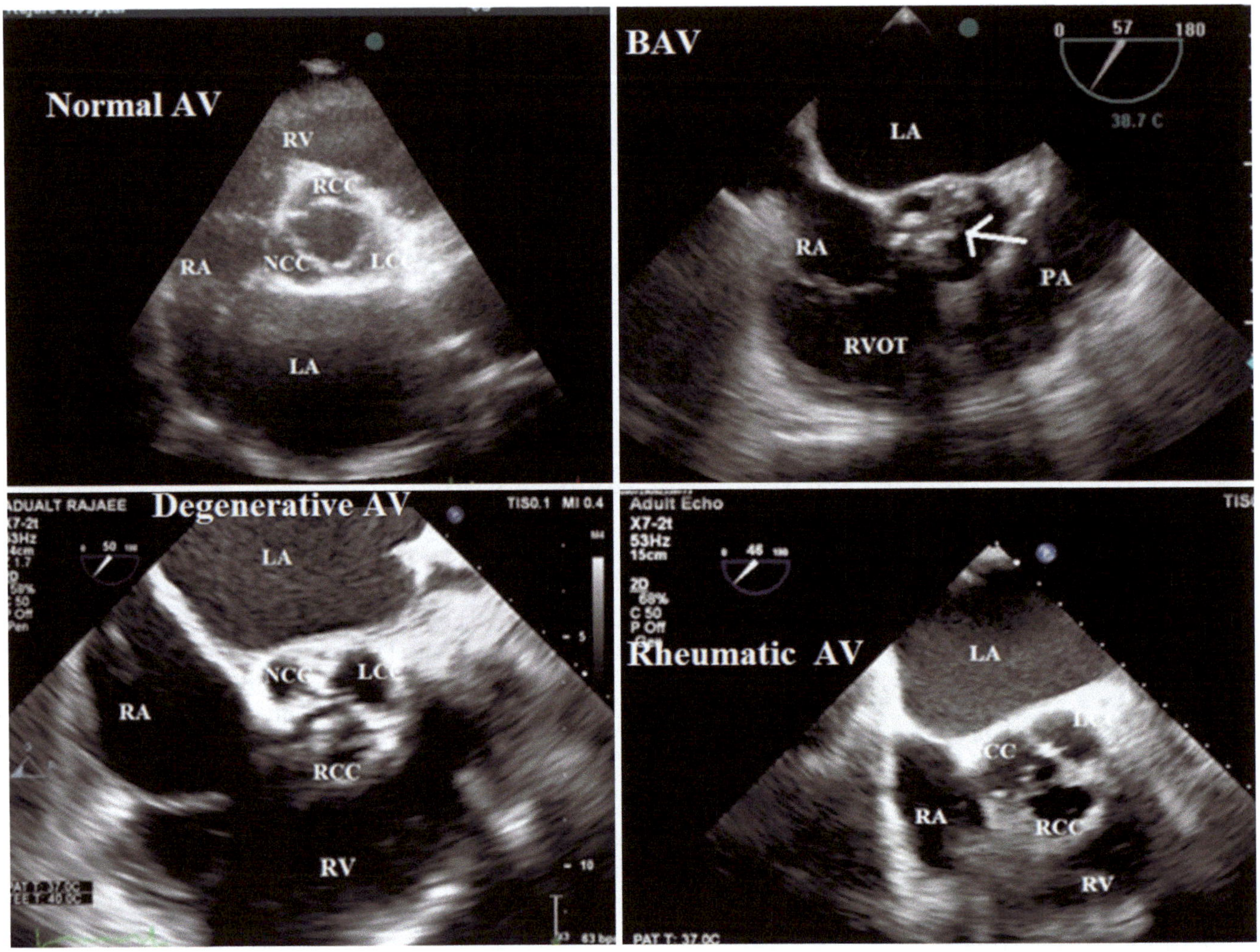

Fig. 17.1 (**a**) Normal tricuspid aortic valve. (**b**) Thickened and calcified bicuspid aortic valve; (**c**) Degenerative and calcified aortic valve; (**d**) Rheumatic Aortic valve with thickened cusps and fused commissures. *AV* aortic valve, *LA* Left atrium, *RA* right atrium, *RV* right ventricle, *PA* pulmonary artery, *RVOT* right ventricular outflow tract, *RCC* right coronary cusp, *NCC* non coronary cusp, *LCC* left coronary cusp

of the LV outflow. Aortic valve (AV) replacement is the only effective therapy. Transcatheter AV replacement is appropriate in cases at very high surgical risk (Fig. 17.1).

The three fundamental features of AS are: (a) leaflet deformity, thickening, and calcification, (b) reduced mobility, and (c) absolute diminution in the size of the AV orifice resulting from decreased cusp separation. AS may be acquired or congenital. In congenital AS, the AV might be unicuspid, bicuspid, or infrequently, quadricuspid. Precise characterization is possible by imaging the AV in the short-axis view to define

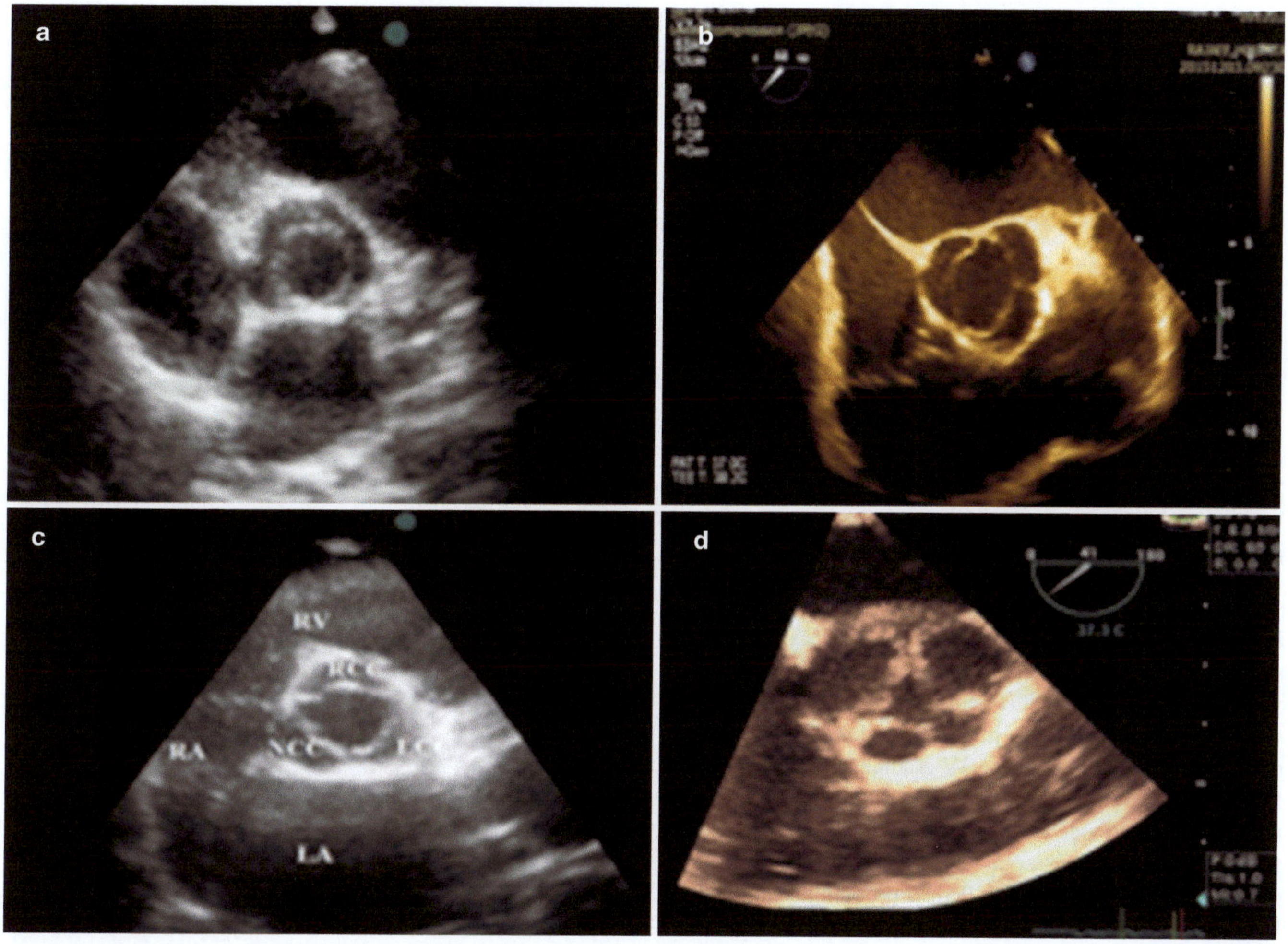

Fig. 17.2 (**a**) Unicuspid AV; (**b**) Bicuspid AV; (**c**) Tricuspid AV; (**d**) Quadricuspid AV. *AV* aortic valve, *RA* right atrium, *RV* right ventricle, *LA* left atrium, *RCC* right coronary cusp, *NCC* non coronary cusp, *LCC* left coronary cusp

the number of the cusps and the commissures. Though bicuspid valves are naturally stenotic, they may also dispose to significant aortic regurgitation (AR). Indeed, the identification of a bicuspid valve might be difficult in older cases if the AV is significantly calcified (Fig. 17.2).

Not like congenital AV disease, which often presents in the fourth decade, acquired calcific AS presents in the sixth or seventh decade. Classically, the AV is thickened and calcified and with decreased cusp separation. The finding of some residual leaflet motion commonly indicates that the aortic valve area (AVA) is greater than 0.6 cm^2. None of the typical features of AS is crucially specific for the diagnosis of hemodynamically critical AS. Leaflet thickening is common in elderly persons, but it is seldom associated with significant stenosis. Though reduced cusp separation and the mobility of the leaflets are more specific and valuable for hemodynamically significant AS, this may also happen in cases with a low CO. The direct measurement of the AV orifice is seldom precise by transthoracic echocardiography (TTE), but the direct planimetry of the AVA from transesophageal echocardiography (TEE) might provide a precise and correct estimate in cases with a normal LV function and CO.

Crucially, in most cases with significant AS, the LV size and function are usually normal, while LV hypertrophy is frequently apparent.

A precise evaluation of severity of AV stenosis is frequently possible using continuous-wave (CW) Doppler, which permits the estimation of the peak and mean AV gradients and the AVA. To determine the peak and mean gradients across the valve, you must first obtain precise profiles of the flow originating from the valve, frequently from apical windows. It is also crucial to interrogate the flow through the valve from the right parasternal window because the deformation of the AV leaflets might eccentrically direct the jet of the blood flow toward the right sternal border as it enters the aorta (Fig. 17.3). The typical CW Doppler profile of AS begins after the R wave on the ECG and is not holosystolic. Noting the time of the onset and the duration of the flow helps to discriminate the AS profile from the CW Doppler profile of the mitral regurgitation (MR) flow. The application of the Bernoulli equation to the CW Doppler interrogation of the transvalvular flow provides precise measures of the mean and peak instant gradients in AS. Classically, the simplified form of the formula ($\Delta P = 4\,V^2$) may be used. However, when the velocity of the left ventricu-

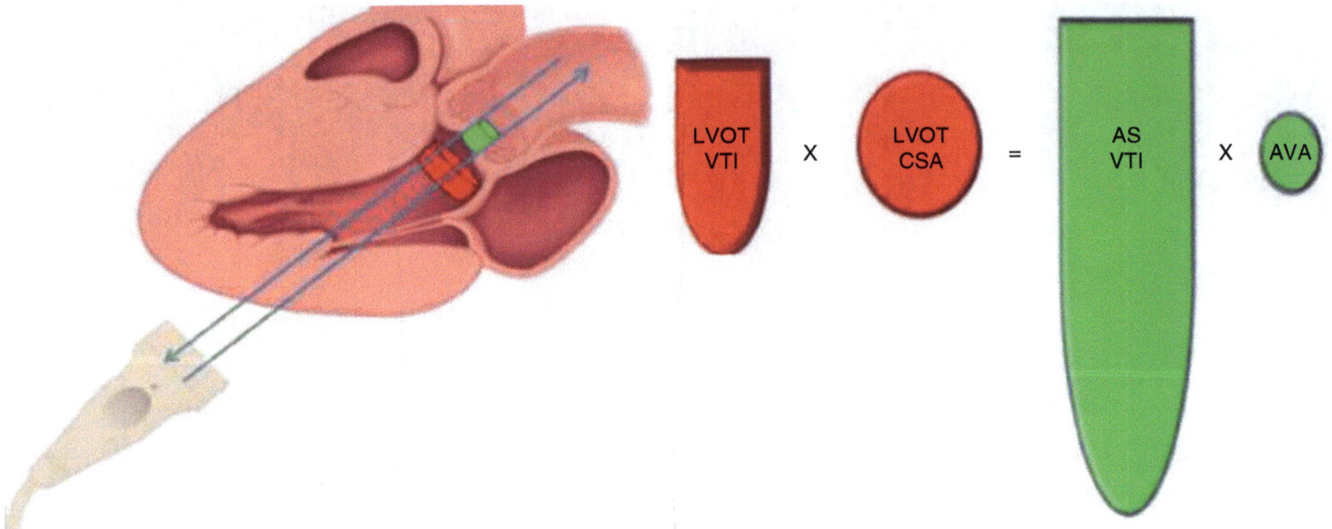

Fig. 17.3 Continuity equation for assessment of aortic valve area in aortic valve stenosis

lar outflow tract (LVOT) exceeds 1 m/s, the expanded version—namely $\Delta P = 4\,(V2^2 - V1^2)$—where V2 is the trans-aortic velocity and V1 is the LVOT velocity, must be used.

In the recognition of the importance of recording Doppler signals parallel to the flow, the AV gradients are best recorded from the apical 5- or 3-chamber, suprasternal notch, and right para-sternal views. Generally, the highest velocities are found in the right parasternal window. The smaller footprint, provided by the non-imaging Pedoff probe, makes it crucial for the optimal evaluation of cases with AS. When TEE is used, velocities are recorded from the deep transgastric views. It should be noted that although echocardiographically derived mean gradients are generally identical to those achieved invasively, the echocardiographically derivative peak instantaneous gradient is classically higher than the peak-to-peak gradient calculated in the catheterization lab.

Gradients alone may underestimate severity in the setting of low-flow states and overestimate severity when the flow is higher (e.g., high-output states like those caused by sepsis and anemia). For this reason, it is crucial to define the AVA. The direct planimetry of TEE images can be used for this purpose, but TTE planimetry is not adequately precise.

The most common approach, thus, is by the application of the continuity equation. The AVA is calculated as (Figs. 17.4 and 17.5):

$$\mathbf{AVA} = \left(\mathbf{CSA\ LVOT} \times \mathbf{VTI\ LVOT}\right) / \mathbf{VTI\ AV}$$

Less desirable is the simplified version:

$$\mathbf{AVA} = \left(\mathbf{CSA\ LVOT} \times \mathbf{V\ LVOT}\right) / \mathbf{V\ AV}$$

where "V" predicates the peak velocity. The cross-sectional area (CSA) of the LVOT is classically calculated by assuming a circular geometry with the equation $CSA = \pi\,(D/2)^2$, where D is the systolic LVOT diameter measured on the parasternal long axis view of TTE or TEE-equivalent long-axis view just proximal to the AV annulus. It should be noted that because the LVOT velocity incorporated into the calculation is the modal velocity, displayed as the densest part of the pulsed-wave Doppler envelope, the velocity time integral (VTI) must not be traced by using the outer edge of the flow spectrum.

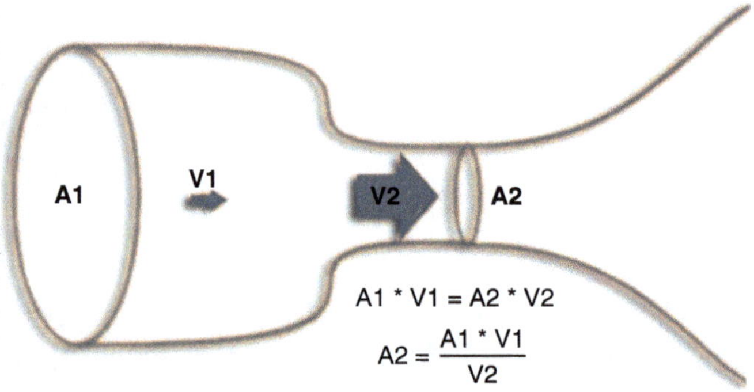

Fig. 17.4 Continuity equation showing by a simple schematic figure

Ideal sample-volume placement is in the LVOT characteristically 1–2 mm proximal to the AV in the apical 5- or 3-chamber views (TTE) or in deep transgastric (TEE) views [1–9].

Low-Gradient Low-Flow Severe Aortic Stenosis

When there is a reduced stroke volume due to significant LV systolic dysfunction, the measured effective orifice area might be small despite low gradients, and it becomes crucial to define whether the valve obstruction is really fixed (true severe AS) or the valve is basically capable of opening more completely at higher flow rates (pseudo-severe AS). Also, dobutamine stress echocardiography is usually used in this setting to evaluate the true AVA and the LV contractile reserve.

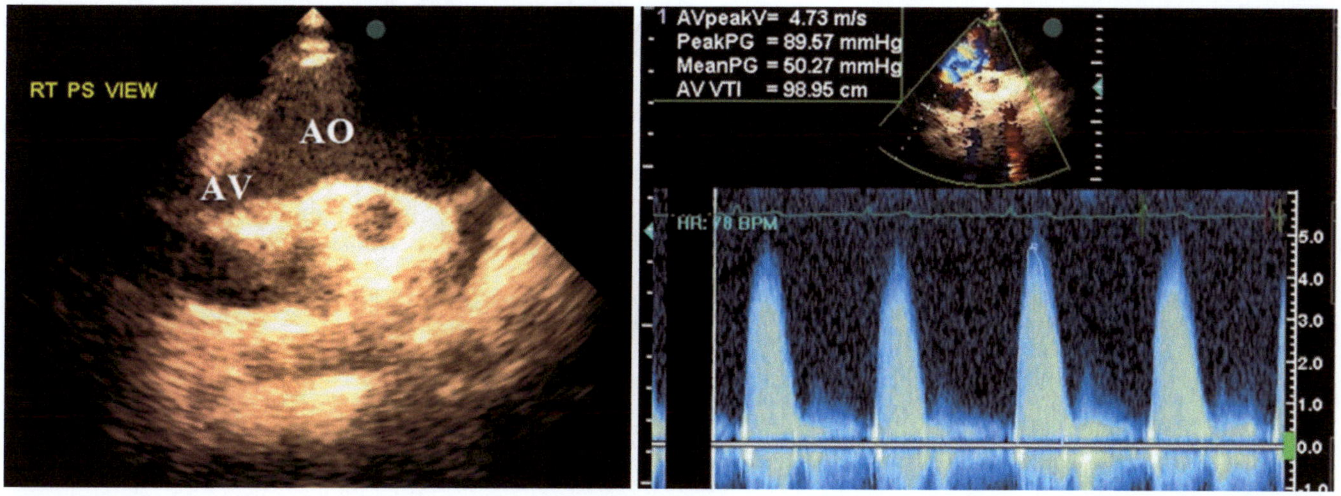

Fig. 17.5 Right upper parasternal view for precise assessment of aortic valve stenosis severity and peak pressure gradient

The effective regurgitant orifice (ERO) might also be severely reduced despite low gradients when the LV ejection fraction is within the normal range, while the stroke volume is reduced, so-called paradoxical low-gradient preserved ejection fraction severe AS.

Subvalvular Aortic Stenosis

The CW Doppler echocardiographic calculation of the peak and mean pressure gradients is the cornerstone in assessing cases with the LVOT obstruction below the AV. Nonetheless, in regard to the site of flow acceleration, color Doppler may provide a clue that the obstruction is not at the level of the valve and more detailed imaging evaluation is crucial to clarify the pathophysiology. In some cases, evaluation is complicated by the existence of obstruction at multiple levels. In such cases, it might be impossible to exactly delineate the gradients created at each level of obstruction [1–10].

Transesophageal Echocardiography in Aortic Valve Stenosis

If TTE is difficult to perform or there is dynamic LVOT obstruction, TEE can be used to measure the AVA by planimetry. With a multiplane probe, the transducer array is rotated to 45–60° to obtain the short-axis view of the AV. The number of the aortic cusps may be determined confidently with TEE; however, it is not routine practice to use TEE to evaluate AS.

Many patients with severe stenosis who undergo AV replacement have mitral valve (MV) regurgitation, which is frequently related to high LV systolic pressure, without any morphological abnormality of the MV. TEE is used intraoperatively to evaluate the severity of MR before and after AV replacement and to assess the need for MV replacement or repair [1–3, 7] (Fig. 17.6).

Aortic Valve Regurgitation

The abnormal backflow of blood that occurs through AV leads to pathological changes that are highly dependent on AR severity and the rate of disease progression.

AR may result from abnormalities in the cusps of the valve (primary AR), normal cusps whose coaptation is altered due to the enlargement of the annulus or sinuses (Secondary AR) or, infrequently, prolapse of a dissection flap through the AV. TTE and TEE will establish a causative diagnosis and characteristically demonstrate LV end-diastolic enlargement if the AR is hemodynamically crucial. The high-frequency fluttering of the anterior MV leaflet, caused by the impact of the regurgitant jet on M-mode, and also in cases of acute severe AR, the premature closure of the MV due to a rise in the LV pressure greater than the LA pressure are seen (Fig. 17.7).

Severe AR findings includes (Figs. 17.8 and 17.9):

- LV diastolic dimension >7.5 cm (chronic AR)
- Regurgitant jet width/LVOT diameter ratio ≥60%
- Vena contracta width >6 mm
- Regurgitant jet area/LVOT area ratio ≥60%
- AR pressure half-time (PHT) ≤250 ms
- Restrictive MV flow pattern (usually in acute setting) and holodiastolic flow reversal in the descending aorta
- Dense CW Doppler signal
- ERO ≥0.30 cm^2
- Regurgitant volume ≥60 mL
- Regurgitant fraction ≥55%

Color jet dimensions must be measured with the Nyquist settings in 50–60 cm/s. The best dimensional predictors of severity are jet area indexed to the AV short axis area in the parasternal short-axis view and also jet diameter indexed to the LVOT diameter closely proximal to the valve in the parasternal long-axis view. The jet length is not a good index of severity. The PHT reflects the rate at which the AV and LV pressures become equal and is most reliable in the setting of acute AR.

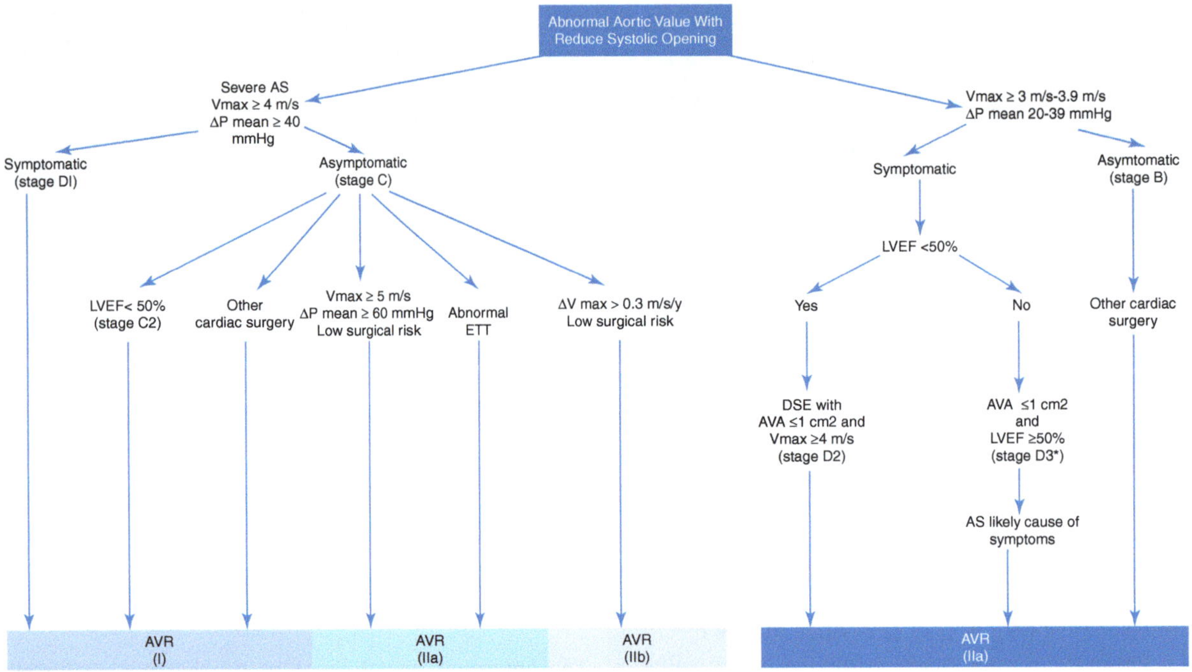

Fig. 17.6 Indications for management in patients with severe AS. *AS* aortic stenosis, *AVA* aortic valve area, *AVR* aortic valve replacement by either surgical or transcatheter approach, *BP* blood pressure, *DSE* dobutamine stress echocardiography, *ETT* exercise treadmill test, *LVEF* left ventricular ejection fraction, *ΔPmean* mean pressure gradient, V_{max}, maximum velocity. Modified figure from: Rick A. Nishimura, Catherine M. Otto, Robert O. Bonow, Blase A, Carabello, John P. Erwin, Robert A. Guyton, Patrick T. O'Gara, Carlos E. Ruiz, Nikolaos J. Skubas, Paul Sorajja, Thoralf M. Sundt, III, James D. Thomas. 2014 AHA/ACC Guideline for the Management of Cases with Valvular Heart Disease: Executive Summary. J Am Coll Cardiol. 2014;63(22):2438–2488. doi:10.1016/j.jacc.2014.02.537

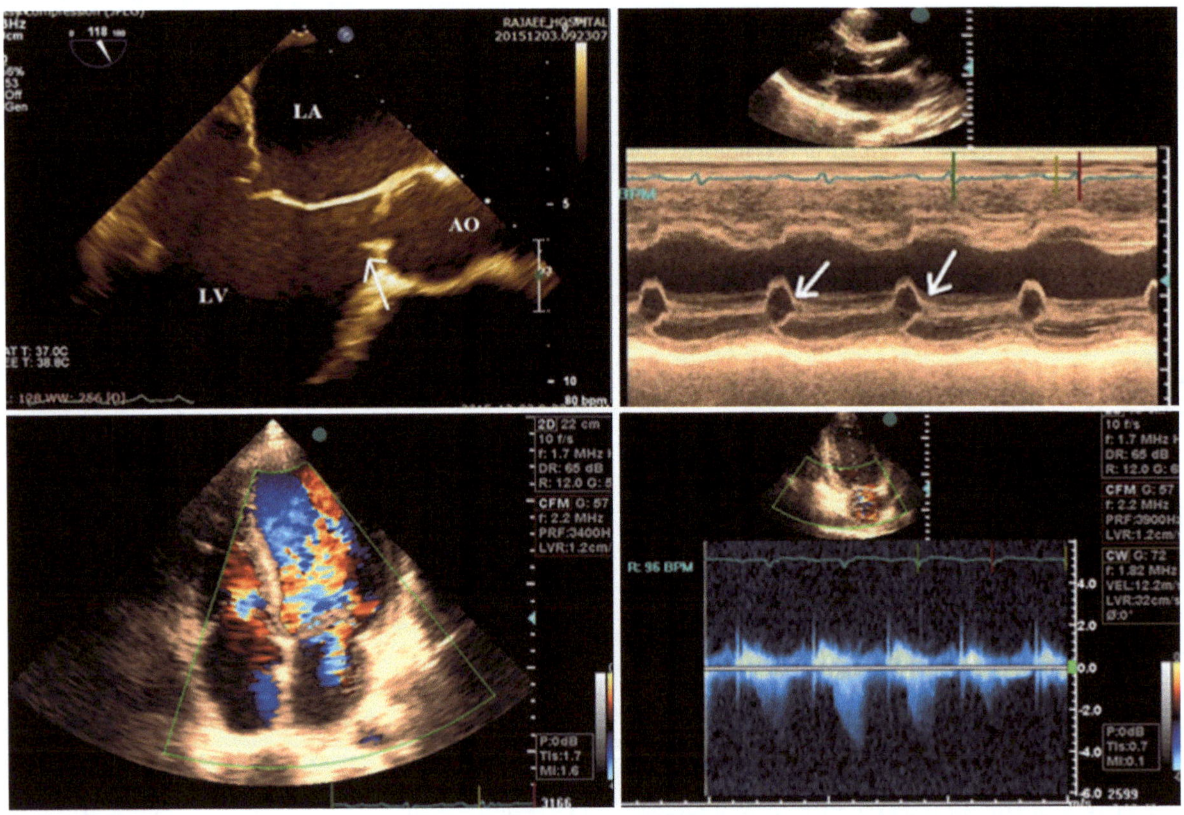

Fig. 17.7 Acute AR; Left upper panel: vegetation on AV in Transesophageal mid-esophageal 120′; Right upper panel, early closure of MV in m-mode modality; lower left panel: diastolic MR by color Doppler and in lower right panel by CW Doppler study. *AV* aortic valve, *AR* aortic regurgitation, *MR* mitral regurgitation, *CW* continues wave

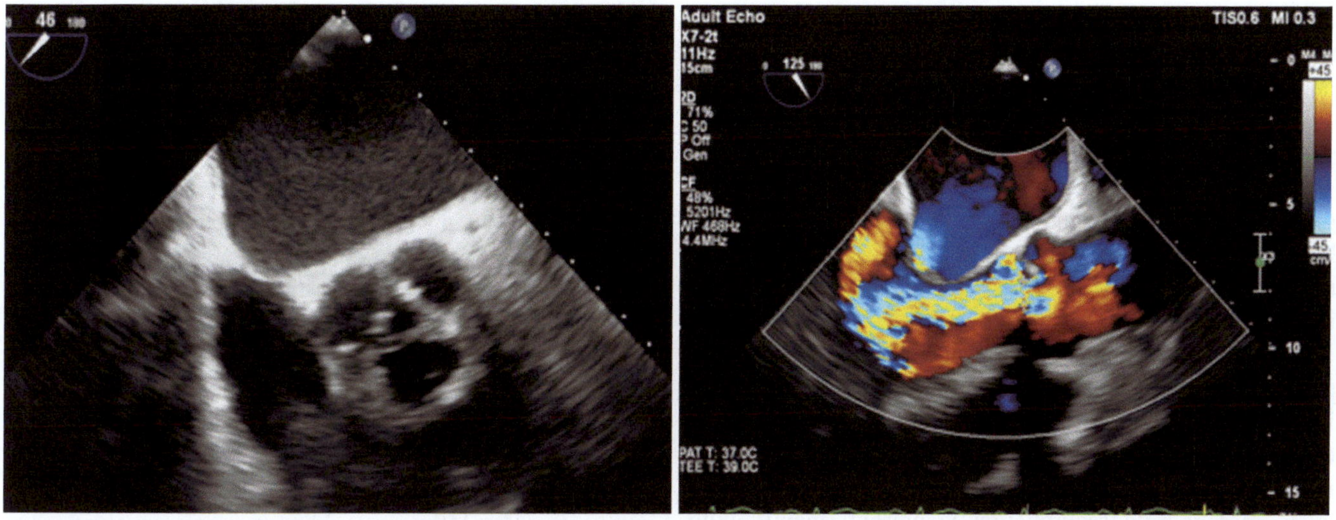

Fig. 17.8 Severe AR in a tricuspid thickened AV with incomplete closure of cusps in diastole and large vena contracta (VC) in right panel

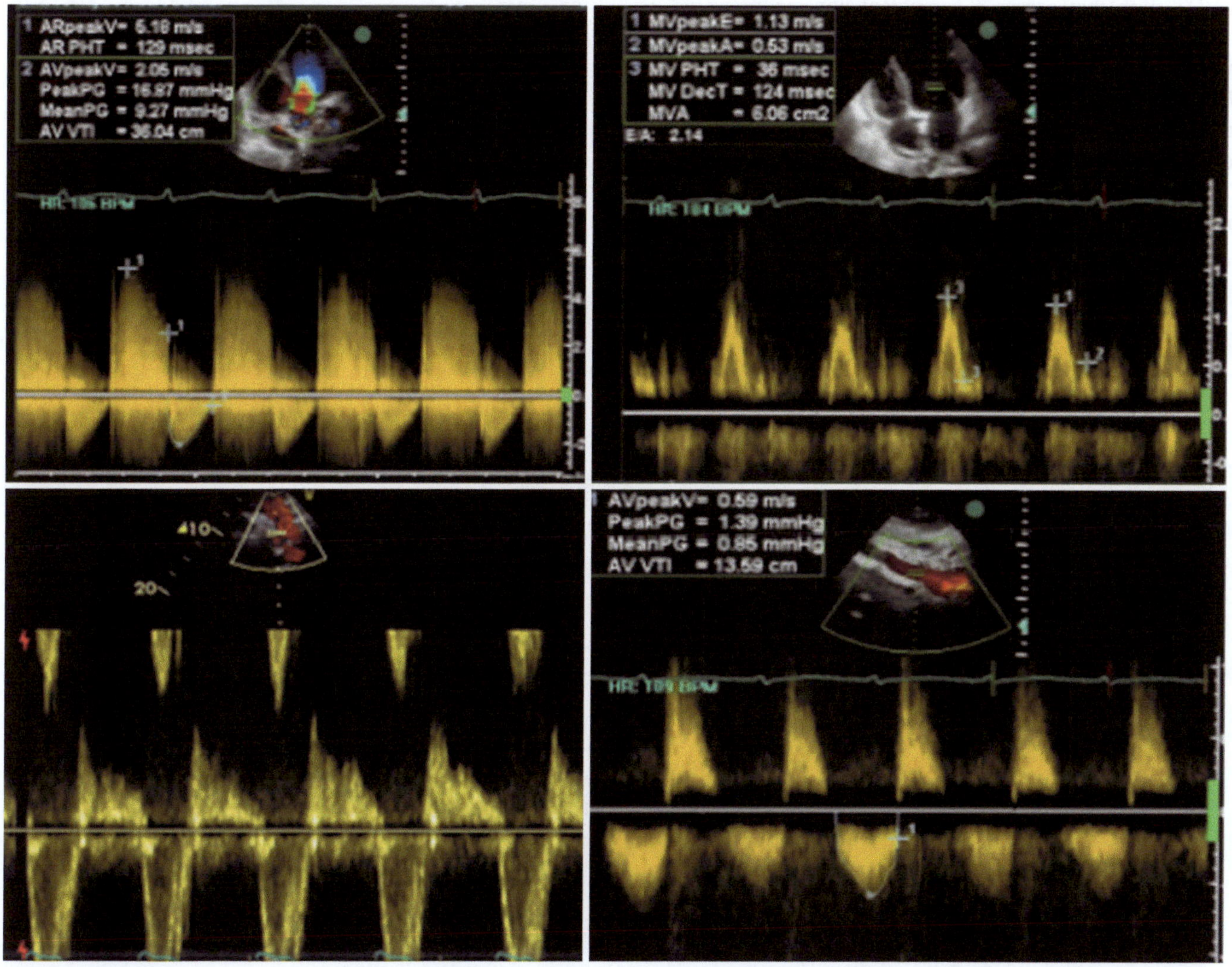

Fig. 17.9 Doppler study in severe AR; (**a**) CW Doppler study of AV showing significant AR and assessing of PHT; (**b**) PW Doppler study of MV showing significant diastolic dysfunction; (**c**) PW Doppler study of proximal part of descending aorta with significant holo-diastolic reversal flow indicator of severe AR; (**d**) PW Doppler of abdominal aorta with significant holo-diastolic reversal flow indicator of severe AR. *AR* aortic regurgitation, *MV* mitral valve, *PW* pulse wave Doppler, *CW* continues wave Doppler

The vena contracta is the smallest diameter of the aortic insufficiency flow jet at the level of the valve measured in zoom mode in the parasternal long axis view or TEE-equivalent 120° view. Holodiastolic flow reversal in the proximal part of the descending thoracic aorta, as detected with the pulsed-wave sample volume placed near the origin of the left subclavian artery, is a good marker of at least moderate aortic insufficiency. The reversal flow of the abdominal aorta mostly reflects severe aortic insufficiency.

Though the proximal isovelocity surface area (PISA) approach, which is broadly drawn upon to evaluate the severity of MR and tricuspid regurgitation (TR), has been used to calculate the ERO area and regurgitant volume for AR, it might be challenging to exactly measure the PISA radius when merely mild regurgitation is present (mainly with TTE). The quantitative Doppler approach, which determines the regurgitant volume by matching the flow through the LVOT with that across a competent nonstenotic valve, is strongest when the pulmonary valve is used as the reference for normal flow (due to image quality). The MV can hypothetically be used as the reference; nonetheless, it is more geometrically complex and hence more susceptible to error [1–6, 8, 9].

Figure 17.10 shows the algorithmic approach to management of AR according to the last AHA/ACC guideline.

Mitral Valve Disease

Mitral Stenosis

Mitral stenosis (MS) is usually caused by rheumatic fever, a disease rare in developed countries today but that still persists in a large part of the world. When complicated by atrial fibrillation, rate control and anticoagulation are mandatory in the absence of pressing contraindications. Once more-than-mild symptoms exist or once asymptomatic pulmonary hypertension occurs, the mechanical relief of MS is indicated. In most cases, such relief is provided by the durable commissurotomy created at BMV. In other cases, surgical correction is needed. After these interventions, prognosis is excellent.

TTE and TEE assist with the diagnosis and the timing of intervention for MS by providing a precise evaluation of valve morphology, valve area, and degree of pulmonary artery hypertension.

The 2D echocardiographic features of rheumatic MS include the following:

- Thickened and calcified mitral leaflets and subvalvular apparatus
- Decreased E-F slope (M-mode)
- "Hockey-stick" appearance of the anterior mitral leaflet in diastole (long-axis view)

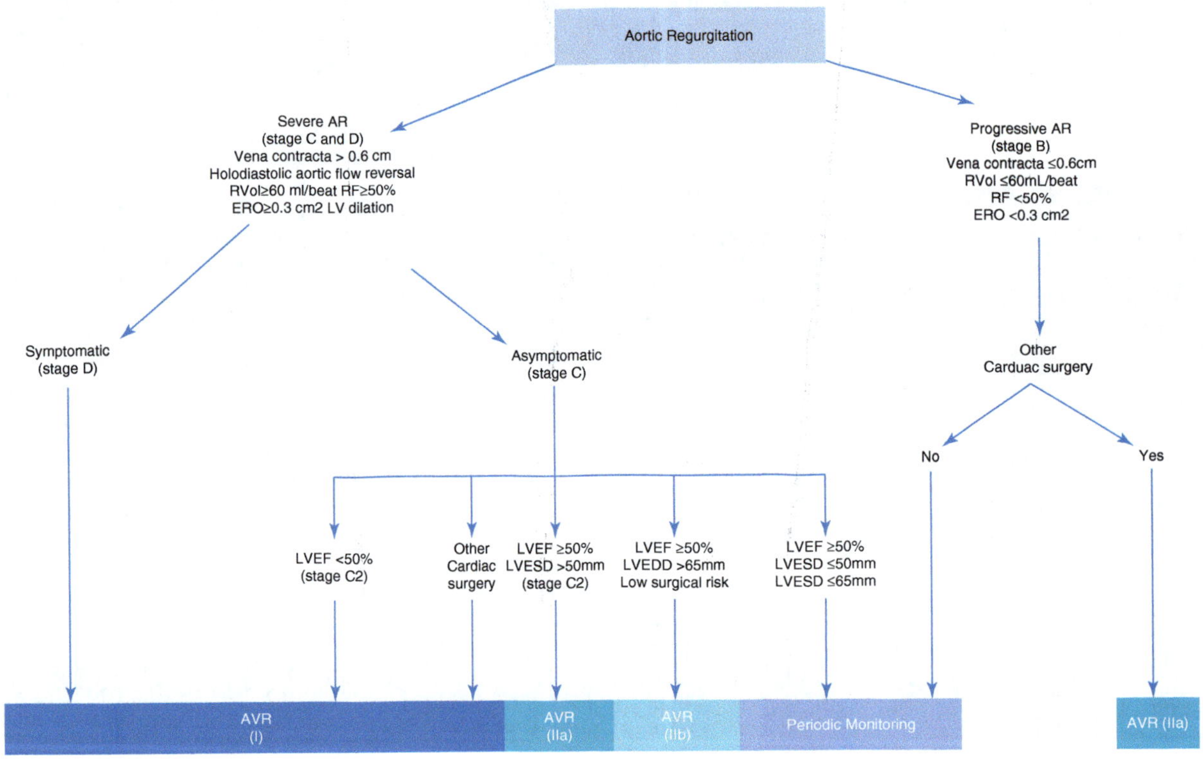

Fig. 17.10 Indication for AVR for chronic AR. *AR* indicates aortic regurgitation, *AVR* aortic valve replacement (valve repair may be appropriate in selected patients), *ERO* effective regurgitant orifice, *LV* left ventricular, *LVEDD* left ventricular end-diastolic dimension, *LVEF* left. Modified figure from: Rick A. Nishimura, Catherine M. Otto, Robert O. Bonow, Blase A. Carabello, John P. Erwin, Robert A. Guyton, Patrick T. O'Gara, Carlos E. Ruiz, Nikolaos J. Skubas, Paul Sorajja, Thoralf M. Sundt, III, James D. Thomas. 2014 AHA/ACC Guideline for the Management of Cases with Valvular Heart Disease: Executive Summary. J Am Coll Cardiol. 2014;63(22):2438–2488. doi:10.1016/j.jacc.2014.02.537

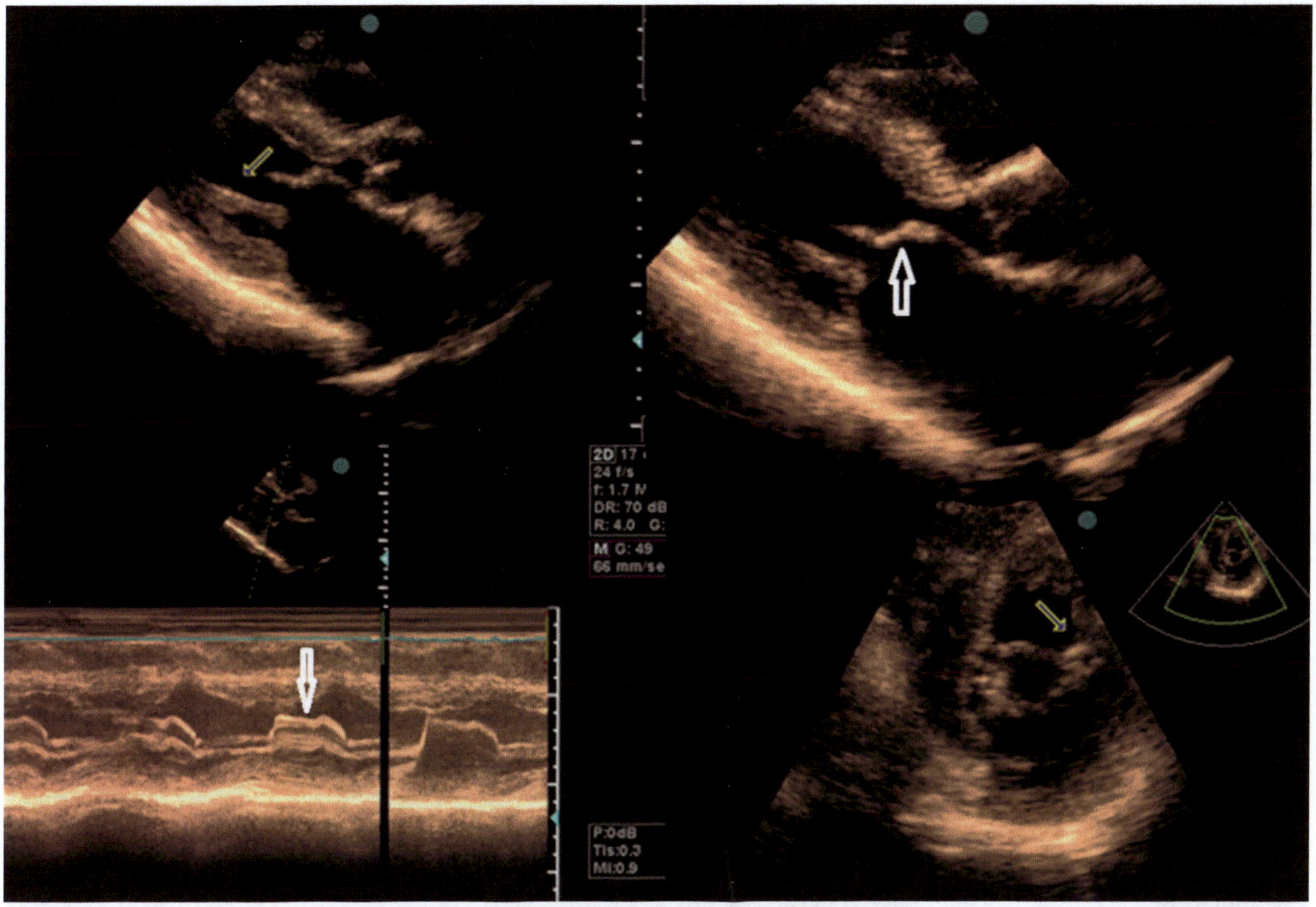

Fig. 17.11 Typical features of rheumatic MS: Left upper: sub valvular thickening (arrow), right upper: Doming of the AML (arrow), left lower: concomitant motion of AML and PML in M-mode study (arrow), Right lower: commissural fusion (anterolateral commissure, arrow). *MS* mitral stenosis, *AML* anterior mitral valve leaflet, *PML* posterior mitral valve leaflet

- Immobility of the posterior mitral leaflet (a similar appearance may be seen in hypereosinophilia or ergot use)
- "Fish-mouth" orifice in the short-axis view
- Increased left atrial (LA) size, with the potential for thrombus formation (Fig. 17.11)

Acquired MS is unvaryingly caused by the scarring and inflammation of the MV and the chordal apparatus from past rheumatic fever. As a result of the disease, the MV leaflets and also the chordal apparatus become diffusely thickened and jaggy. Consequently, the valvular apparatus might shorten, fusing at the commissural margins, and finally harden and calcify. This results in a lessening in leaflet excursion so that the MV leaflets appear dome-shaped in diastole. As the degree of valvular obstruction progresses, the flow through the valve reduces, LA pressure begins to rise, LA size increases, and the potential for LA clot formation is increased. Characteristically, the LV size is normal or even small. If there is severe MS, there might be paradoxical motion of the interventricular septum as a result of slow ventricular filling. Further, if there is pulmonary artery hypertension, the right cardiac chambers and the pulmonary arteries might dilate and there might be severe TR. Almost all of these morphological features are evident from the parasternal long-axis view of the heart; nonetheless, parasternal short-axis images are crucial for the planimetry of the MV stenotic orifice.

Echocardiographic evaluation of the MV has an important role in predicting the suitability of the patient for percutaneous valvuloplasty by assessing the degree of leaflet thickening, calcification, anterior leaflet mobility, and degree of chordal shortening and thickening. When scientifically graded, a low value of 1 to a high value of 4 is given for each of these features. It is then possible to derive a numeric "score" that defines the extent of the MV disease. This system is useful in predicting the likelihood of the successful balloon dilatation of the valve, with scores greater than 8 predicting a poor outcome following percutaneous dilatation.

The direct planimetry of the valve orifice in the short-axis plane of 2D can provide a precise measurement of the MV orifice area. 3D echocardiography may augment the accuracy of detecting the smallest MV orifice by providing perpendicular en face view in the axis views of the MV orifice.

CW Doppler study assess the severity of MS by calculation of the peak and mean trans-MV pressure gradients in conjunction with the MV area. For this purpose, the apical four-chamber view is useful as the Doppler beam can be directed through the MV plane, parallel to the direction of the LV inflow [1–4, 11–13].

In contrast to the Doppler profile through a normal MV, the CW Doppler signal in cases with MS proves an increased velocity of the flow in early diastole, with a prolonged descent of the early filling wave (deceleration time). The degree of the prolongation of the phase of early filling associates directly to the MV area and to the severity of MS. By the CW Doppler profile, it is possible to compute the trans-MV gradient by converting the velocity data into an estimate of pressure using the simplified Bernoulli equation. The Bernoulli formula states that the velocity (V) of the flow through a stenosis relates to the pressure gradient difference (P) across the stenosis. Precisely, the simplified Bernoulli equation forecasts that the pressure gradient across a valve approaches a value four times the square of the velocity of the flow across the valve ($P = 4\,V^2$). Knowing the peak velocity of the flow across the MV enables the calculation of the peak pressure gradient across the valve. Likewise, the average of the velocities throughout diastole yields the mean pressure gradient. Most echocardiographic equipment contains software that can spontaneously integrate the velocity profile contour once it is traced and determine the mean gradient via the Bernoulli equation. The Doppler estimates of the MV area rely on the observation that the degree of the elongation of early filling relates directly to the grade of MS. The measurement of this is possible by calculating the time for the pressure gradient across the MV to decrease to half its max value, "Pressure half-time (PHT)". The PHT is achieved from the CW Doppler profile by defining velocity half-time, measuring the time interval between the peak trans-MV velocity and the point where the trans-MV velocity has dropped to half its peak value. In case of bimodal deceleration slop of the E-wave, mid diastolic slope which has longer duration should be traced. The following points are required for a comprehensive Doppler evaluation of MS:

- Obtain maximal velocity recording using CW Doppler echocardiography from the apical and para-apical positions.
- Determine the mean pressure gradient and the time velocity integral (TVI) by tracing the mitral flow velocity.

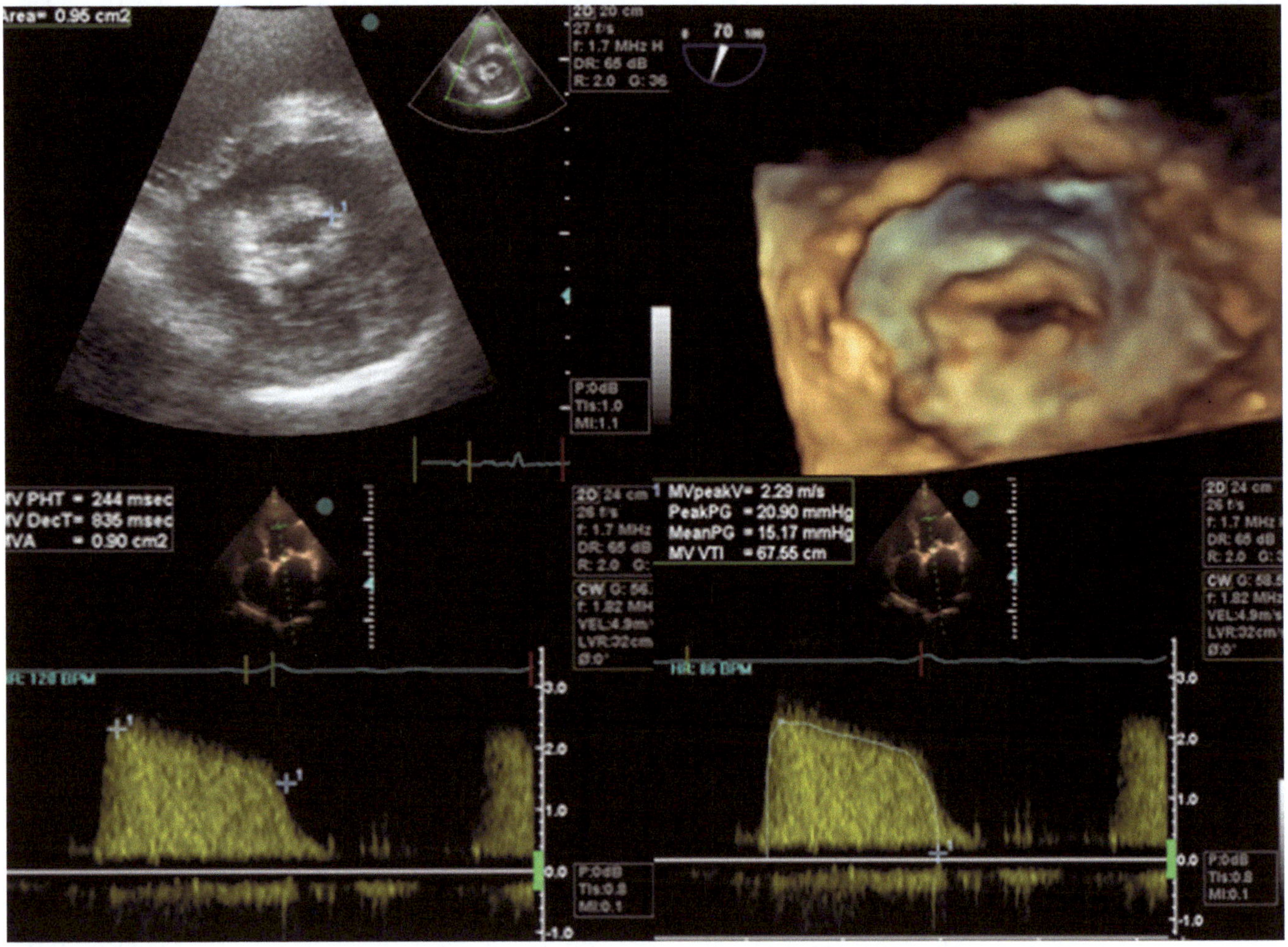

Fig. 17.12 Severe MS; upper panels, 2D direct planimetry and 3D transesophageal study; lower panel, Doppler study for peak pressure gradient, Mean pressure gradient and PHT. *MS* mitral stenosis, *PHT* pressure half time

- Determine the mitral valve area (MVA) by the PHT method; calculate the MVA with the following equation after the PHT has been measured:

$$MVA = \frac{220}{PHT}$$

(This equation is not appropriate immediately after balloon valvulo-plasty or for cases who have severe AR or high filling pressures.) (Fig. 17.12).

- Determine the MVA with the continuity equation when there is discrepancy between MVA measured by direct Planimetry and PHT; determine the stroke volume from the LVOT diameter (D) and the TVI; calculate the MVA by dividing the LVOT stroke volume by the MV TVI:

$$\text{MVA} = \text{LVOTD}^2 \times 0.785 \times \frac{\text{TVI}_{\text{LVOT}}}{\text{TVI}_{\text{MV}}}$$

(This equation cannot be used if there is marked aortic or MV regurgitation.)

- Determine the MVA with the PISA method (Fig. 17.13):
  - Zoom the area of the MV from the apical four-chamber view.
  - Use color-flow imaging of the MS jet and upward shift of the zero baseline for color map (30- to 45-cm/s aliasing velocity).
  - Freeze the color-flow images in a cine loop and identify an optimal frame to measure the radius (r) of the PISA in the LA.
  - Determine the angle (α) between the two mitral leaflets at the atrial surface and use the following formula:

$$\text{MVA} = \frac{6.28 \times r^2 \times \text{Aliasing Velocity}}{\text{Peak}_{\text{mitral stenosis velocity}}} \times \frac{\alpha^\circ}{180^\circ}$$

(The angle correction factor might not be necessary if the bottom surface of the hemispheric PISA is relatively flat, which occurs if the aliasing velocity is set high; α.)

Figure 17.14 shows the algorithmic approach to management of MS according to the last AHA/ACC guideline (1).

Mitral Valve Regurgitation

MV dysfunction is the second most common clinically significant form of valvular abnormality in adults. MV regurgitation occurs with the increasing frequency of the degenerative changes of the aging process. Moreover, other causes of clinically significant MV regurgitation include cardiac ischemia, infective endocarditis, and rheumatic disease more frequently in less developed countries. Recent evidence suggests that the best outcomes after the repair of severe degenerative MR are achieved in asymptomatic or minimally symptomatic cases, who are selected for surgery soon after diagnosis on the basis of echocardiography. This review will focus on the surgical management of mitral insufficiency according to its etiology today and will give insight to some of the perspectives that lay in the future [1–4].

Rheumatic Mitral Valve Regurgitation

Although the incidence of rheumatic MR is declining, the disease is still prevalent in older patients. Characteristically, the echocardiogram confirms the MV leaflets and also chordal thickening in relation with AV disease. As the rheumatic disease progresses and the leaflets become thicker and less mobile, MS might also be evident. In these

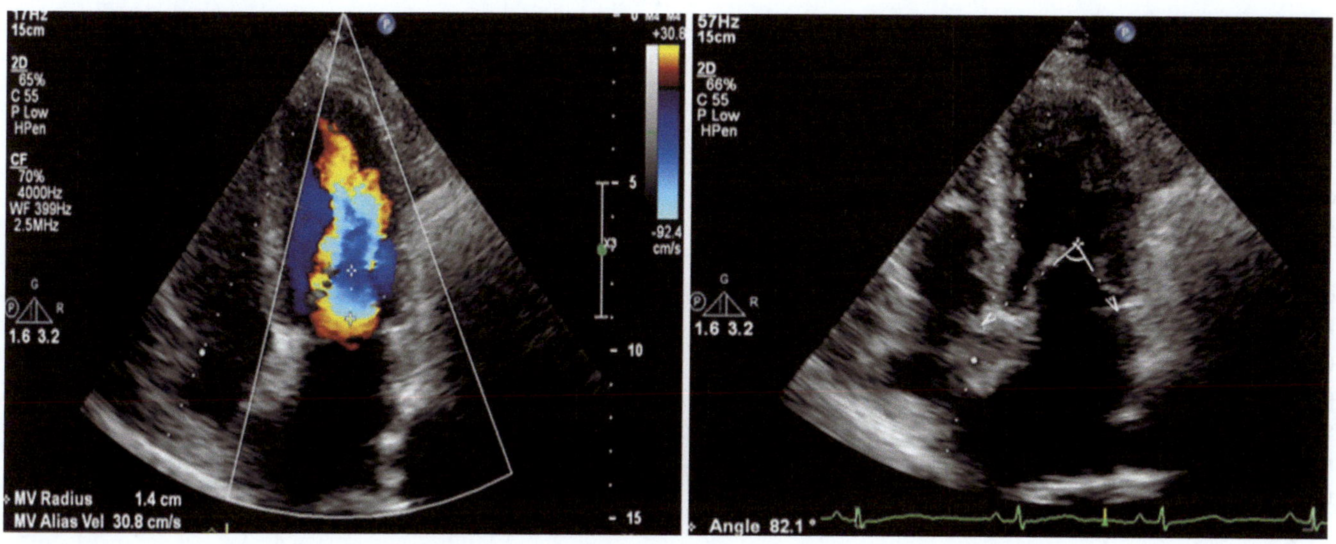

Fig. 17.13 Showing how to measure the Mitral valve area by PISA method.

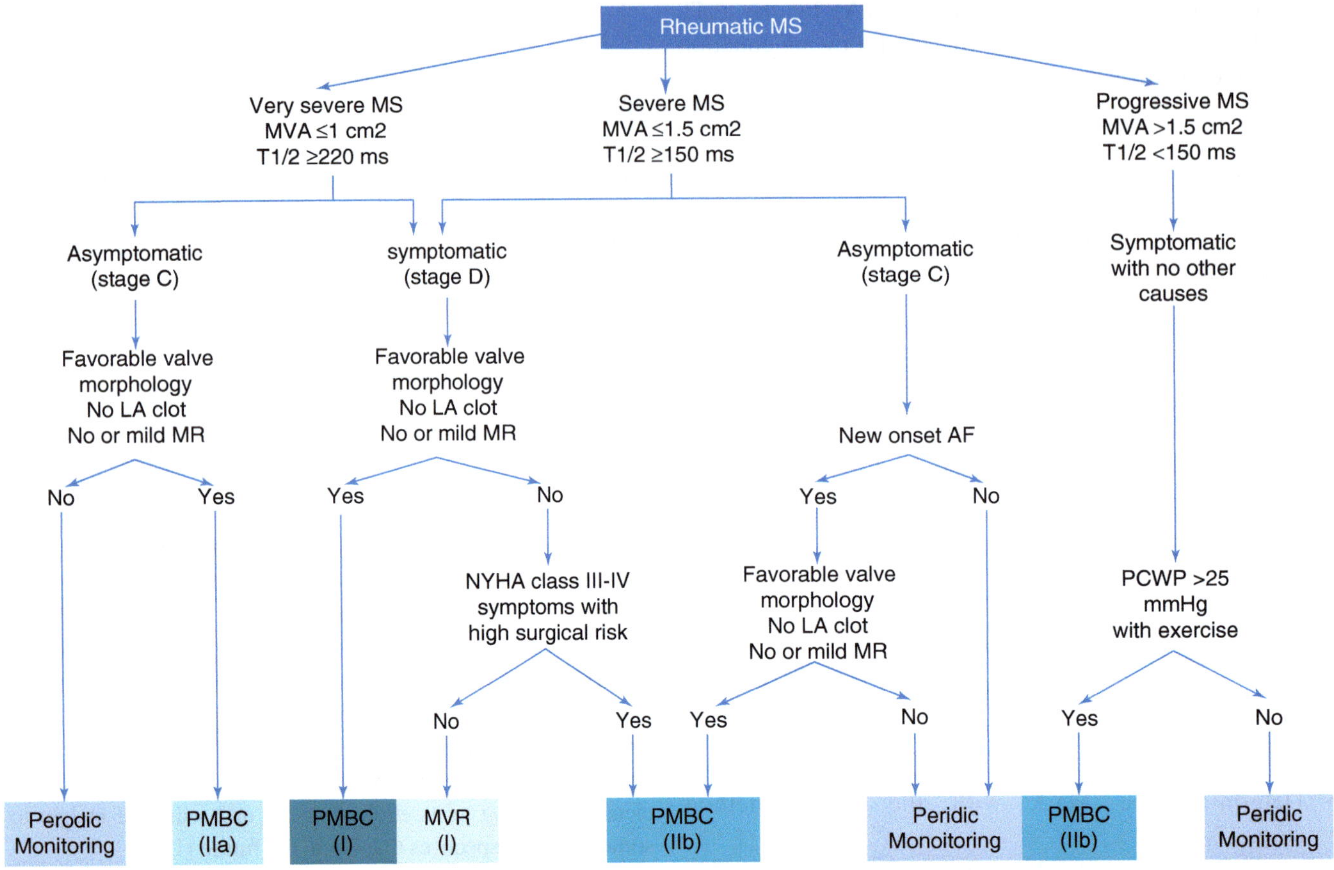

Fig. 17.14 Indications for intervention for rheumatic MS. *AF* indicates atrial fibrillation, *LA* left atrial, *MR* mitral regurgitation, *MS* mitral stenosis, *MVA* mitral valve area, *MVR* mitral valve surgery (repair or replacement), *NYHA*, New York Heart Association, *PCWP* pulmonary capillary wedge pressure, *PMBC* percutaneous mitral balloon commissurotomy, and *T ½*, pressure half-time. Modified figure from: Rick A. Nishimura, Catherine M. Otto, Robert O. Bonow, Blase A. Carabello, John P. Erwin, Robert A. Guyton, Patrick T. O'Gara, Carlos E. Ruiz, Nikolaos J. Skubas, Paul Sorajja, Thoralf M. Sundt, III, James D. Thomas. 2014 AHA/ACC Guideline for the Management of Cases With Valvular Heart Disease: Executive Summary. J Am Coll Cardiol. 2014;63(22):2438–2488. doi:10.1016/j.jacc.2014.02.537

cases, echocardiography is most beneficial in determining whether the valve is mainly stenotic or incompetent [6, 10–13].

Myxomatous Mitral Valve Prolapse

MV prolapse is a degenerative disease that principally affects the collagen of the MV leaflets and chordae tendineae; still, it may also affect the AV and the TV. Clinically it is frequently diagnosed by the existence of a systolic murmur or click, echocardiography is often used to confirm the diagnosis. In echocardiography, MV prolapse is suggested by the superior displacement of 1 or both MV leaflets into the LA (at least 2 mm) during systole. Because of the complex saddle shape of the MV annulus, minor degrees of the superior movement of the anterior leaflet can normally be recorded from the apical four-chamber view. Consequently, the diagnosis of MV prolapse should be made when the coaptation line seen behind the MV annular plane in the long-axis views (parasternal or apical long-axis) display leaflet displacement [6]. Color flow imaging characteristically shows an eccentric regurgitation jet in the opposite direction to the leaflet that is prolapsed. In cases with more progressive disease, there is also evidence of leaflet thickening, (more than 5 mm) which relates to the manifestation of the significant myxomatous infiltration of the valve. There might also be redundant or ruptured chordae. Definitely, cases with marked displacement, thickening, and irregularity of the leaflets are more likely to have severe MR and to be at greatest risk of complications, including infective endocarditis. As in any patient with MR, the LA size increases with the increasing severity of the regurgitant lesion and the LA size may act as an index of the severity and also duration of MR. The LV size may be normal or dilated. Systolic function is typically hyperdynamic in cases with primary compensated valvular MR. Though no single echocardiographic index yet precisely predicts the correct timing of MV surgery in cases with primary chronic valvular MR, those with an LV end-systolic diameter greater than 40 mm tend to have less recovery of the LV function following the surgery (Fig. 17.15).

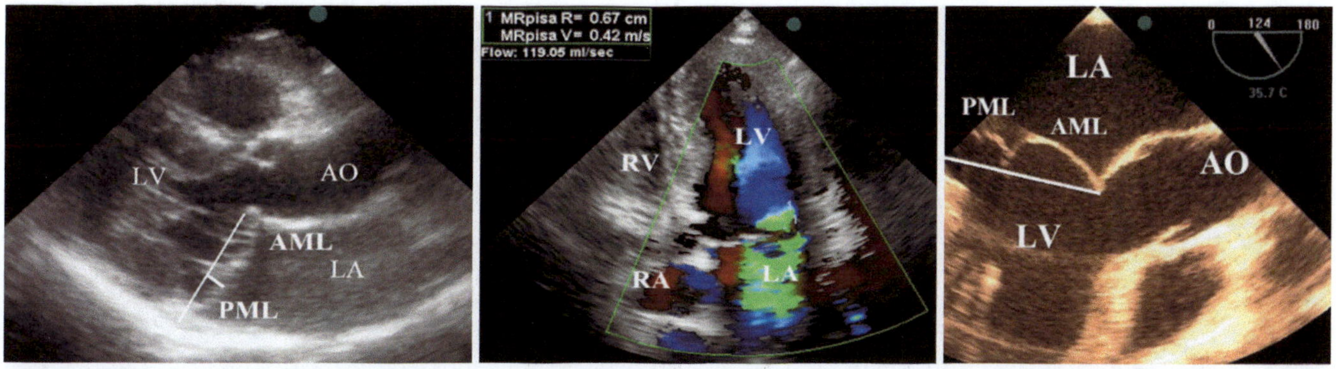

Fig. 17.15 Bileaflet mitral valve prolapse, Left: parasternal long axis view showing significant bulging of both leaflets to LA, Middle: four chamber view showing central jet of MR and right panel; transesophageal long axis view showing bileaflet prolapse

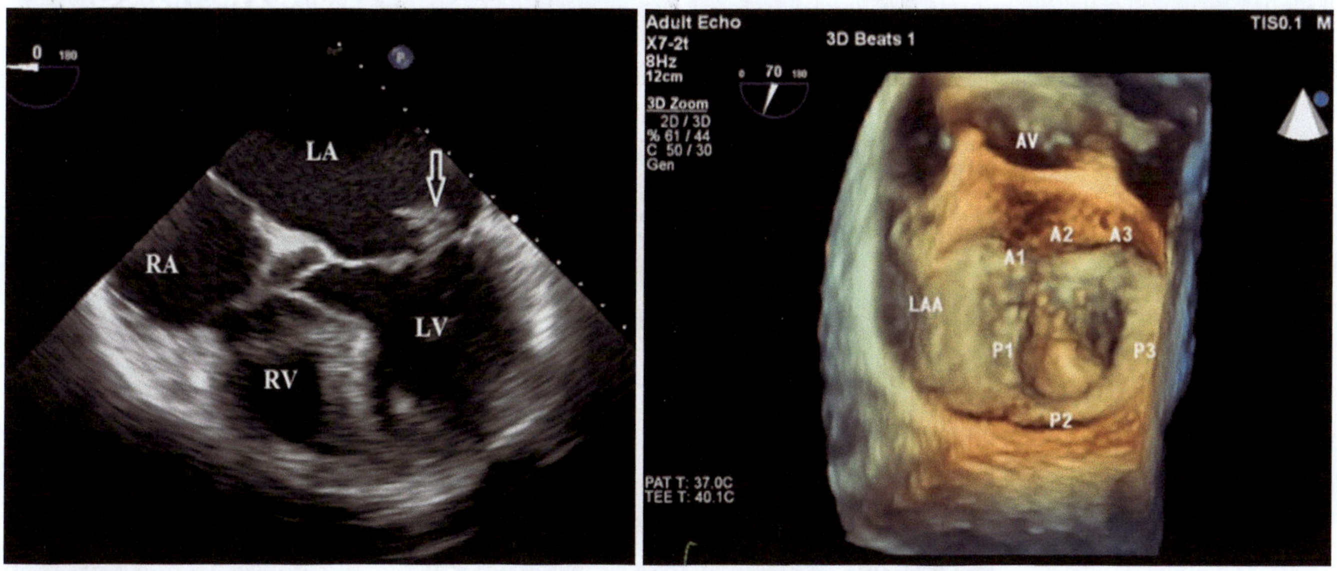

Fig. 17.16 Flail of mitral valve posterior leaflet (P2 scallop) in 2D (*left*) and 3D (*right*) transesophgeal echocardiography

Flail Mitral Valve Leaflets

Complete or partial disruption of the support of 1 or both MV leaflets typically presents abruptly with the development of a new murmur or even acute pulmonary edema. In either setting, the echocardiogram in association with the clinical picture can provide a direct insight into the nature of the underlying disease process. Definitely, the echocardiogram can prove the systolic prolapse of the whole leaflet into the LA associated with reversal of the the free edge of the mitral leaflet to the LA, resulting significant MR [6] by color Doppler flow. A flail leaflet is caused by infective endocarditis, fundamental myxomatous MV disease (MV prolapse), or papillary muscle rupture in relation with acute myocardial infarction (Fig. 17.16).

Mitral Annular Calcification

Mitral annular calcification is common in elderly cases. It initiates as a focal process, affecting the posterior part of the annular ring, and then spreads laterally and lastly anteriorly. As the process progresses, the base of the MV leaflets and also the chordal apparatus thicken and calcify. This impairs the normal mechanism of coaptation, leading to MR. It might also result in the restriction of the MV inflow with the development of a small trans-MV gradient. Although mitral annular calcification is visible in nearly any view, the parasternal short-axis image at the base of the heart is the most valuable view for determining the circumferential extension of the disease [1–4, 12–14], (Fig. 17.17).

Functional Mitral Valve Regurgitation

In some cases, the MV may appear morphologically normal when it is clearly incompetent, as evidenced by clinical or echocardiographic signs of moderate-to-severe MR. In these cases, the MR is caused by the abnormal and incomplete coaptation of the MV leaflets—caused by either annular dilatation or papillary muscle dysfunction. In both

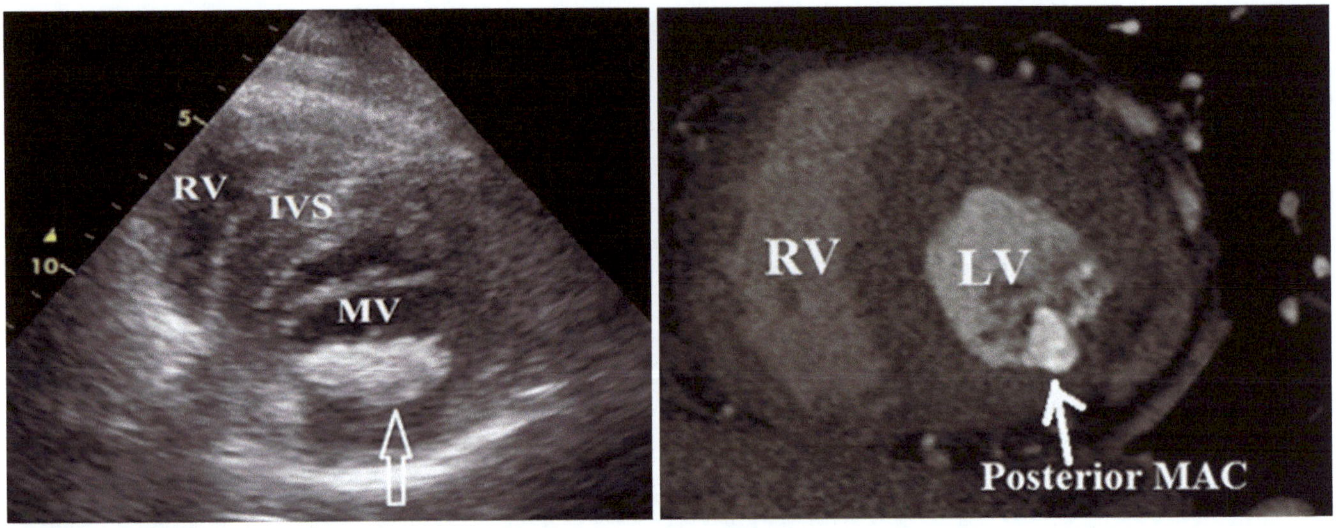

Fig. 17.17 A mitral annular calcification; calcified amorphous tumor in end-stage renal disease

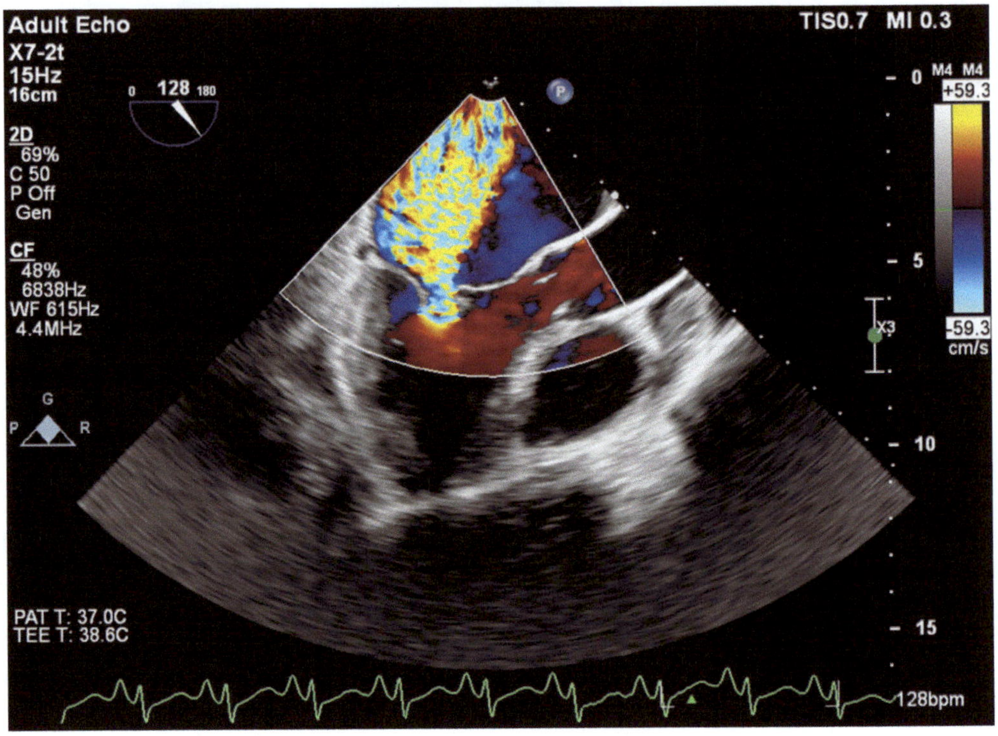

Fig. 17.18 Severe functional mitral regurgitation. Transesophageal echocardiography, mid esophageal, 120′

instances, the pattern of leaflet closure appears abnormal in the parasternal and apical views: The MV leaflets appear to coapt only at their tips, rather than along the distal third of the leaflet. The appearance may range from leaflet and chordal tethering to complete failure of coaptation. There is frequently associated LV dilatation and global or regional wall motion abnormalities [6–9], (Fig. 17.18).

Study of Mitral Valve Regurgitation

Color Doppler readily demonstrates MR. Regurgitant jets usually appear as a localized stream of the flow emerging from the valve leaflets at valve closure and then expand into the distal chamber. From most sampling windows, the jets of MR are chiefly blue because they are directed away from the transducer. The introduction of yellow and green in the color flow map specifies a high velocity turbulent flow and results in a pattern referred to as "mosaic." The regurgitant flow typically initiates at the peak of the R wave on the ECG and continues throughout systole. The peak velocity of these jets reflects the atrioventricular gradient, which can be calculated using the simplified Bernoulli equation—explained earlier. Accordingly, the CW Doppler signal in cases with MR typically has a peak velocity of about 5 m/s, reflecting a peak atrioventricular gradient of 100 mmHg.

The semiquantitative evaluation of the severity of MR includes the integration of many 2D echocardiographic and also Doppler-derived variables. Firstly, it is helpful to consider the appearance of the valve leaflets and the chordae and also the pattern of leaflet coaptation. With this initial evaluation, it is possible to gain a sense of whether the amount of regurgitation is possible to be mild, moderate, or severe. In other words, it is not likely with a normal valvular structure, apparatus, and pattern of coaptation to have more than mild regurgitation. Still, it is highly likely that with a flail or partially flail leaflet there will be moderate-to-severe MR. After the evaluation of the valve morphology and the arrangement of coaptation, color Doppler signals yield an additional insight into the amount and degree of regurgitation. Color flow Doppler provides a color map of the net immediate velocity of the blood flow within the LA at varying time points during systole. From this map it is possible to determine the size (area, length, and width at the orifice) and also direction (central or eccentric) of the MR regurgitant jet.

The descriptors of the jet size, mainly the size of the proximal jet at the vena contracta, relate to the angiographic amount of MR. Inappropriately, many factors affect the precise evaluation of the degree of regurgitation. In other words, changes either in the gain or in the pulse repetition frequency of the Doppler system might alter the relationship between the jet size and the degree of MR, resulting in either a false increase or decrease in the jet size (mostly jet length and area) [10–13] (Fig. 17.19).

In addition, the detection of the regurgitant jet might not be possible in all cases such as in cases with prosthetic valves, which block out or reflect the Doppler signal and forbid its passage into the LA. Lastly, the association between the jet size and the severity of MR might be underestimated if the jet is directed eccentrically alongside the LA wall, as often happens with more significant regurgitation. In an effort to overcome some of the limitations related to the analysis of the distal jet, researchers have analyzed the size of the converging flow stream proximal to the valve (e.g., on the ventricular side of the MV). The analysis of the size of this PISA provides a precise evaluation of the regurgitant flow rate; it, however, needs cautious technical manipulation and

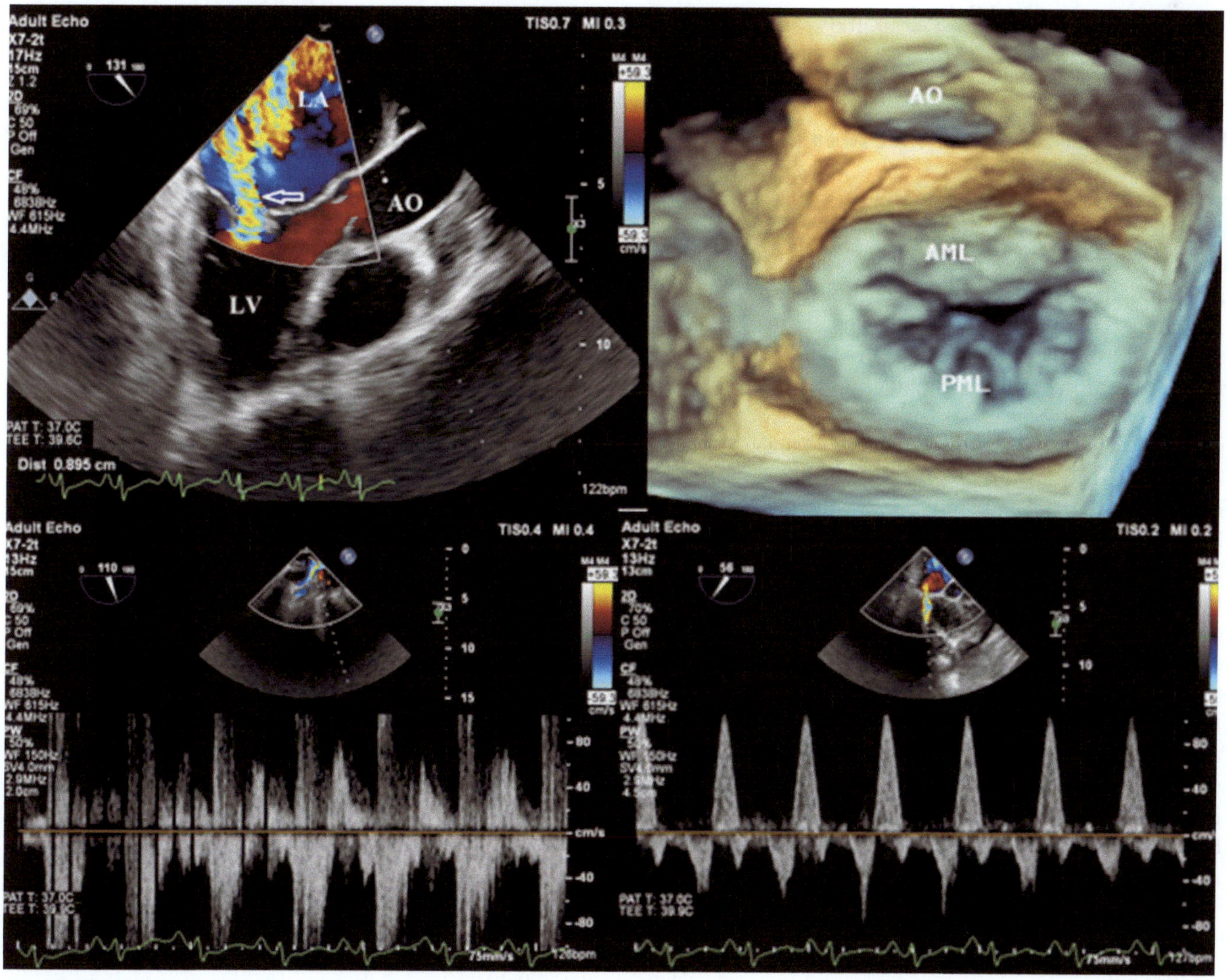

Fig. 17.19 Color flow regurgitant jet of severe MR [Vena contracta (VC) is about 0.9 cm] in prolaptic MV leaflets with reversal flow in pulmonary veins. *MV* mitral valve, *MR* mitral regurgitation

high-quality imaging to record a PISA that can be correctly measured (Fig. 17.7). Flow reversal in the pulmonary veins by pulsed Doppler offers further evidence that the degree of MR is likely to be severe. Because it is the LA that bears the burden of chronic regurgitation, evaluation of the LA size may also be valuable in defining its severity and chronicity. Nonetheless, because other parameters such as atrial fibrillation and LV end-diastolic pressure might also influence the LA size, the chamber size alone can be a deceptive marker of the severity of MR [1–6, 9, 11–13].

Volumetric method

The volume of MR can be quantified by the following equation provided that there is no concomitant significant AR:

$$\begin{aligned} \text{MV RegV} &= \text{MV Flow} - \text{LVOT flow} \\ &= \left(\text{Annulus}\,D^2 \times 0.785 \times \text{TVI}\right)_{\text{MV}} \\ &\quad -\left(D^2 \times 0.785 \times \text{TVI}\right)_{\text{LVOT}} \end{aligned}$$

$$\text{MR RF} = \frac{\text{MV RegV}}{\text{MV flow}} \times 100$$

Proximal Isovelocity Surface Area Method

The ERO and volume of MR are best obtained with the PISA method, which is based on the principle of the conservation of the flow and the continuity equation. Whereas the flow through a stenotic AV is calculated from the LVOT in the continuity equation, the regurgitant flow through the MV is calculated from the PISA methods. As blood in the LV converges toward the mitral regurgitant orifice, the blood flow velocity gradually increases and forms a series of hemispheric waves. The velocity is the same for the surface of each wave (isovelocity) (Fig. 17.20). Color flow imaging may identify a PISA in the LV because the red-blue aliasing interface corresponds to the surface of the hemisphere whose flow velocity is the same as the aliasing velocity. Thus, the flow rate at the surface of a hemispheric PISA is the product of the area of the hemisphere and the aliasing velocity. The aliasing velocity needs to be lowered to create a larger PISA (for the flow away from the apical transducer) because the further the flow is from the regurgitant orifice, the slower is the velocity. The aliasing velocity may be altered by the downward shift of the zero baseline (in case of the TTE imaging of MR) so that an optimal (hemispheric) PISA may be identified. The flow rate at PISA is equal to the flow rate across the regurgitant orifice:

flow rate at PISA = flow rate across the regurgitant orifice.

$$2\pi\left(r^2\right) \times \text{Aliasing velocity} = \text{ERO} \times \text{MR velocity}$$

$$\text{ERO} = 6.28\left(r^2\right) \times \frac{\text{Aliasing velocity}}{\text{MR velocity}}$$

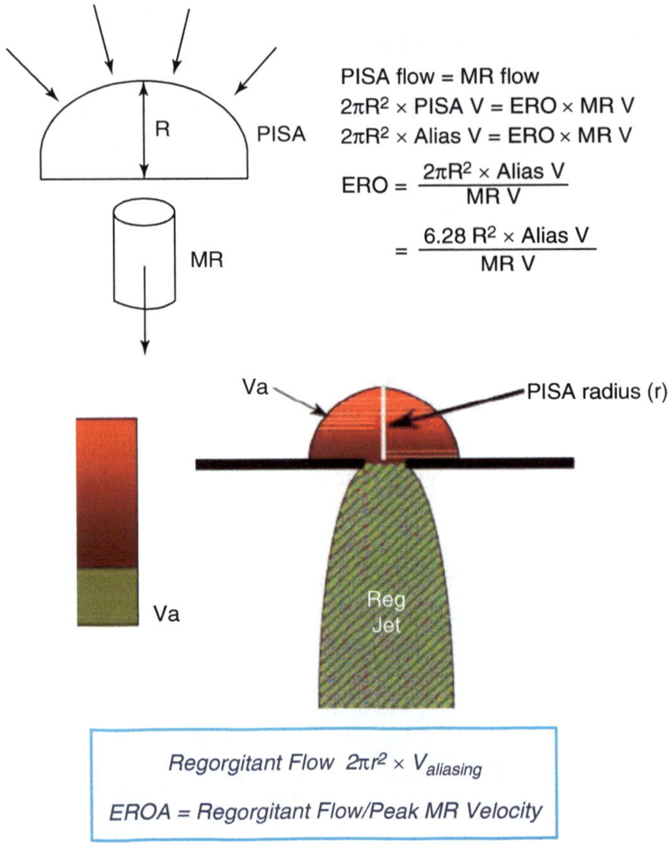

Fig. 17.20 Flow convergence method (PISA method) for assessing the severity of MR

After the ERO has been calculated, mitral RegV is calculated as (Fig. 17.20):

$$\text{MR RegV} = \text{ERO} \times \text{MR TVI}$$

Simplification of the PISA Method

- If the aliasing velocity is about 30 cm/s and the MR velocity is assumed to be about 500 cm/s, then

$$\text{ERO} = \frac{6.28 \times r^2 \times 30\ \text{cm/s}}{500\ \text{cm/s}}$$

- ERO is 0.38 cm² when r = 1 cm. Hence, a PISA radius of 1 cm or larger indicates severe MR when the aliasing velocity is ≥30 cm/s. Because the peak MR velocity is assumed to be 500 cm/s, this simplification will overestimate the ERO if the systemic blood pressure is increased, which would result in an MR peak velocity much higher than 500 cm/s. If r = 0.5 cm, the ERO is 0.1 cm² because $r^2 = 0.25$, and if r = 0.7 cm, the ERO is 0.2 cm² because $r^2 = 0.49$.
- If the aliasing velocity is about 40 cm/s, and the MR velocity is assumed to be 500 cm/s, then

$$ERO = \frac{6.28 \times r^2 \times 40 \ \ cm/s}{500 \ \ cm/s}$$

$$= \frac{251 \times r^2}{500}$$

$$= \frac{r^2}{2}$$

- ERO becomes half of the r^2 value.
- A simple method to estimate the MR volume. The relation between the TVI and the peak velocity of MR has been shown to be relatively constant. Usually

$$\frac{MR_{TVI}}{MR_{velocity}} = \frac{1}{3.25}$$

- Thus,

$$Mitral\ RegV = ERO \times MR_{TVI}$$

$$= \frac{6.28 \times r^2 \times \text{Aliasing velocity} \times MR_{TVI}}{MR_{velocity}}$$

$$= 6.28 \times r^2 \times \text{Aliasing velocity} \times \frac{MR_{TVI}}{MR_{velocity}}$$

Thus,

$$MR\ RegV = \frac{6.28 \times r^2 \times \text{Aliasing velocity}}{3.25}$$

$$= 1.9 r^2 \times \text{Aliasing velocity}$$

The following criteria indicate or suggest severe MR:

(a) 2D echocardiographic evidence of the disruption of the MV apparatus (papillary muscle rupture or flail mitral leaflet)
(b) ERO ≥0.40 cm^2
(c) MR volume ≥60 mL
(d) Regurgitation fraction ≥50%
(e) Vena contracta width ≥7 mm
(f) MR color flow jet reaching the posterior wall of the LA (with a high aliasing velocity of color flow)
(g) Pulmonary vein systolic flow reversals
(h) Eccentric MV regurgitation jet reaching the posterior wall of the LA
(i) Dense CW Doppler signal
(j) Increased E velocity (≥1.5 m/s for the native valve and 2 m/s for the prosthetic valve)
(k) LV end-diastolic dimension ≥7 cm (along with color flow evidence of MR)
(l) LA size ≥5.5 cm
(m) MV leaflet tenting area ≥6 cm^2 (for functional MR) [4–6, 10–13]

Figure 17.21 shows the algorithmic approach to the management of MR according to the last AHA/ACC guideline.

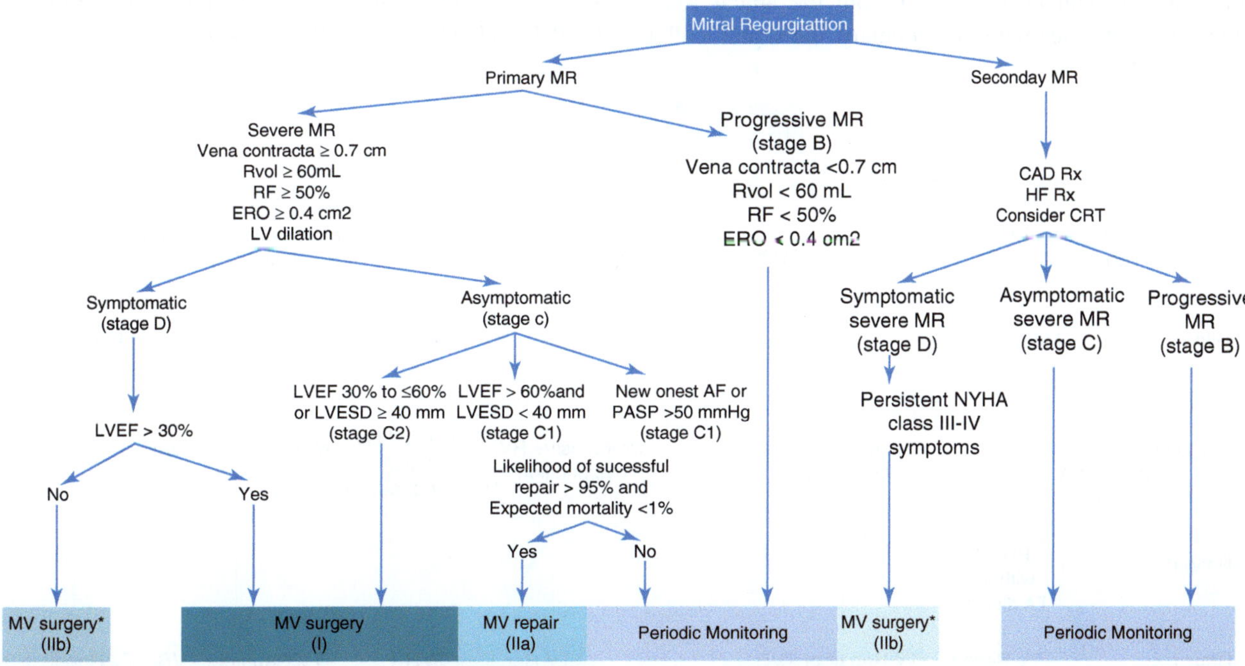

Fig. 17.21 Indications for surgery for MR. *Mitral valve repair is preferred over MVR when possible. *AF* atrial fibrillation, *CAD* coronary artery disease, *CRT* cardiac resynchronization therapy, *ERO* effective regurgitant orifice, *HF* heart failure, *LV* left ventricular, *LVEF* left ventricular ejection fraction, *LVESD* left ventricular end-systolic dimension, *MR* mitral regurgitation, *MV* mitral valve, *MVR* mitral valve replacement, *NYHA* New York Heart Association, *PASP* pulmonary artery systolic pressure, *RF* regurgitant fraction, *RVol* regurgitant volume, *Rx* therapy. Modified figure from: Rick A. Nishimura, Catherine M. Otto, Robert O. Bonow, Blase A. Carabello, John P. Erwin, Robert A. Guyton,Patrick T. O'Gara, Carlos E. Ruiz, Nikolaos J. Skubas, Paul Sorajja, Thoralf M. Sundt, III, James D. Thomas. 2014 AHA/ACC Guideline for the Management of Cases With Valvular Heart Disease: Executive Summary. J Am Coll Cardiol. 2014;63(22):2438–2488. doi:10.1016/j.jacc.2014.02.537

Tricuspid Valve Disease

TR is a relatively common abnormality. Since this lesion is frequently asymptomatic and may not be detected on physical examination, it is often diagnosed solely by echocardiography. This topic will review the etiology, pathophysiology, and clinical features associated with the regurgitation of the TV (Fig. 17.22).

TR has been categorized to primary (organic) and secondary (functional) TR. TR has been categorized to primary (organic) and secondary (functional) TR. Primary (organic) TR occurs when the TV apparatus is structurally abnormal such as Ebstein anomaly, Rheumatic heart disease, secondary (functional) TR occurs when the TV apparatus is structurally normal such as TR in the setting of the Pulmonary hypertension [1, 6, 15, 16]. TR may happen as a consequence of the abnormal development of the TV (the Ebstein anomaly), disease affecting the valve leaflets or the chordal apparatus (myxomatous, degenerative, and endocarditis), or annulus dilatation (due to right ventricular [RV] dilatation). The evaluation of the degree of TR is very similar to that for MR. However, the peak velocity of the regurgitant flow through the TV is commonly 2.5 m/s, replicating a peak systolic gradient of 25 mmHg between the RV and the RA. The Ebstein anomaly is a congenital heart disease characterized by the elongation and tethering of the anterior leaflet of the TV to the RV endocardium. The septal and posterior leaflet origins are displaced apically, reducing the functional RV size, whereas the basal portion of the RV is atrialized. The Ebstein anomaly can be diagnosed from the apical four-chamber view. In cases with this anomaly, the septal leaflet of the TV is greater than 1 cm apical to the MV. In most cases, TR is moderate to severe as evaluated by Doppler. Further, color Doppler can detect some degree of right-to-left interatrial shunt flow through either a patent foramen ovale or an atrial septal defect (Fig. 17.23).

The following criteria suggest severe TR:

1. Color flow regurgitant jet area ≥ 30% of the RA area
2. Dense CW Doppler signal
3. Annulus dilatation (≥4 cm) or inadequate cusp coaptation
4. Late systolic concave configuration of the CW signal
5. Increased tricuspid inflow velocity (≥1.0 m/s)
6. Systolic flow reversals in the hepatic vein
7. ERO ≥0.4 cm^2
8. Regurgitant volume ≥45 mL
9. Vena contracta width ≥6.5 mm

Tricuspid stenosis (TS) most often occurs as a consequence of rheumatic fever, in which case it constantly occurs with MV or AV disease. More seldom, TS occurs with metastatic carcinoid tumors. In both instances, the leaflets and chordae appear thickened, the valve domes during diastole, and as a result of the stenosis, there is an increase in the RA size. 2D echocardiography is valuable for determining the cause of TS. The normal tricuspid inflow velocity is less than 0.5 to 1 m/s, with a mean gradient less than 2 mmHg -TV mean pressure gradient >5 mmHg and PHT greater than 190 msec are suggestive for significant TS. There is a respiratory variation in the TV inflow velocity, and it is best to determine Doppler velocity while the patient holds his or her breath in expiration [1–6, 9] (Fig. 17.24).

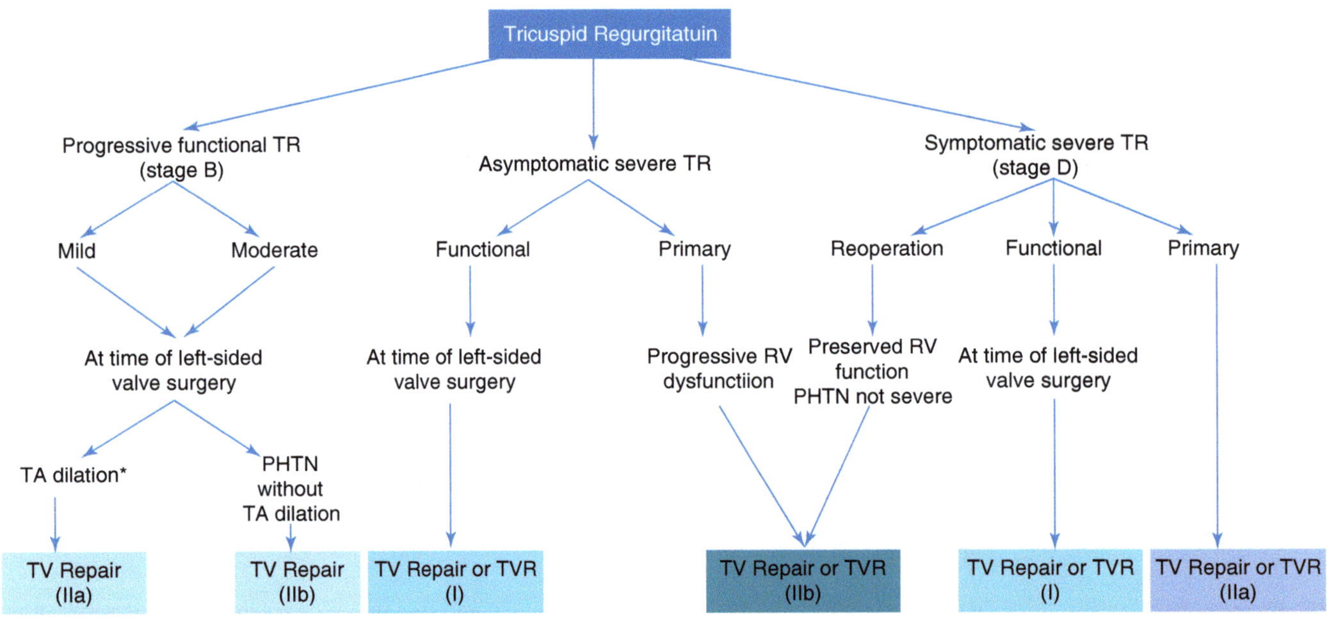

Fig. 17.22 Indications for surgery. TA dilation is defined by >40 mm on TTE (>21 mm/m^2) or >70 mm on direct intraoperative measurement. *LV* left ventricular, *PHTN* pulmonary hypertension, *RV* right ventricular, *TA* tricuspid annular, *TR* tricuspid regurgitation, *TTE* transthoracic echocardiogram, *TV* tricuspid valve, *TVR* tricuspid valve replacement. Modified figure from: Rick A. Nishimura, Catherine M. Otto, Robert O. Bonow, Blase A. Carabello, John P. Erwin, Robert A. Guyton,Patrick T. O'Gara, Carlos E. Ruiz, Nikolaos J. Skubas, Paul Sorajja, Thoralf M. Sundt, III, James D. Thomas. 2014 AHA/ACC Guideline for the Management of Cases With Valvular Heart Disease: Executive Summary. J Am Coll Cardiol. 2014;63(22):2438–2488. doi:10.1016/j.jacc.2014.02.537

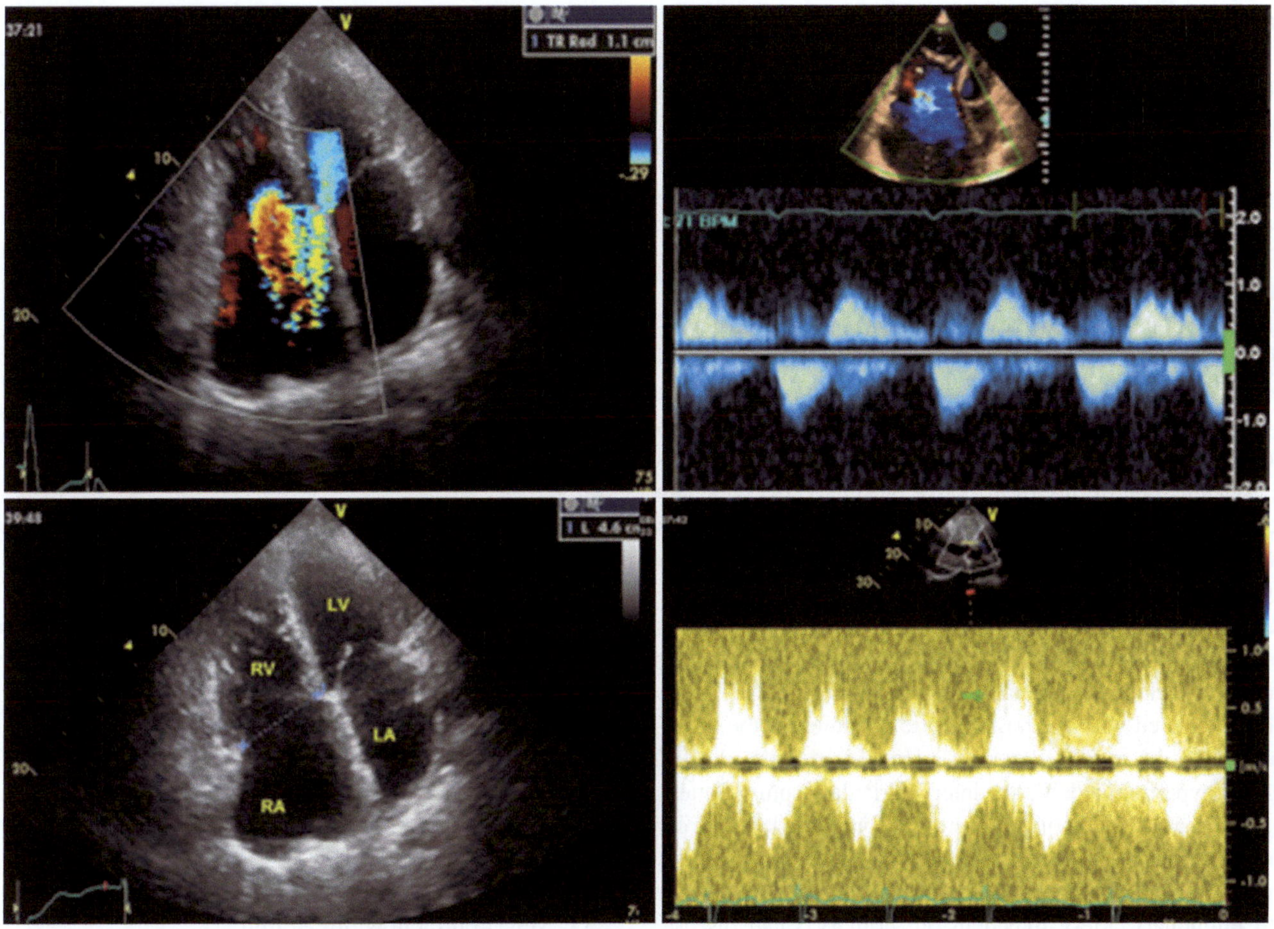

Fig. 17.23 Severe low pressure tricuspid regurgitation by 2D and Doppler flow imaging. Right lower panel shows systolic flow reversal of hepatic vein suggestive of severe TR [15, 16] (upper and lower)

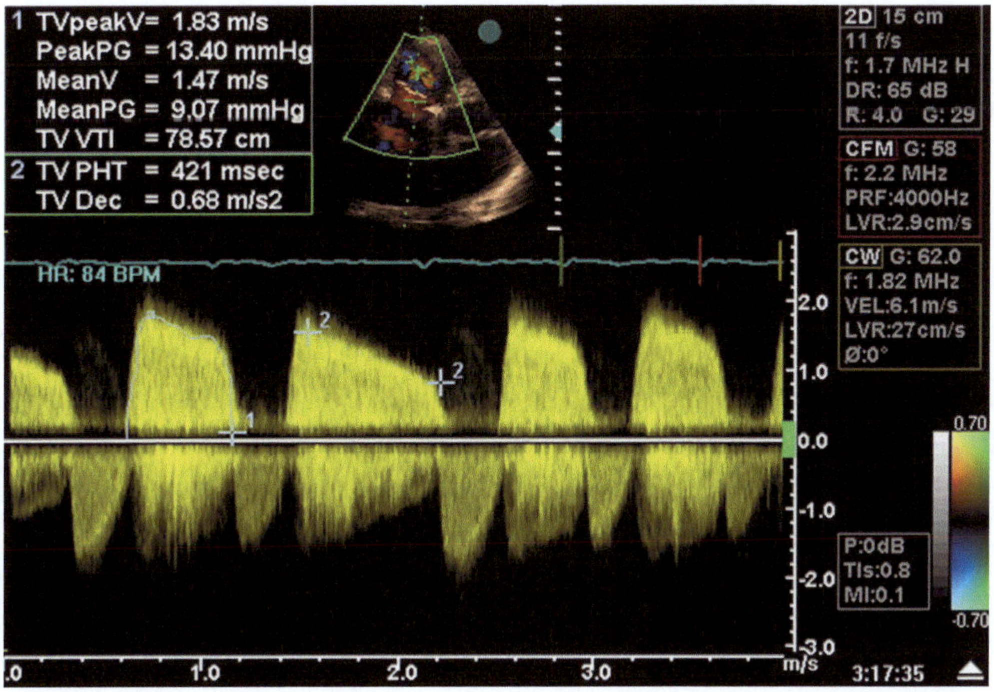

Fig. 17.24 Significant tricuspid stenosis regarding the Pressure half time (420 ms) and mean pressure gradient (>9 mmHg)

Pulmonary Valve Disease

Pulmonary valve disease is very uncommon and may be due either to stenosis or to insufficiency. The majority of pulmonary valve problems happen as the result of congenital heart disease, but the pulmonary valve might rarely be damaged as result of infection (e.g., infective endocarditis) or as a result of disease (e.g., carcinoid disease, Marfan's syndrome, or pulmonary hypertension).

The pulmonary valve is best imaged in the parasternal short-axis view, though subcostal windows are also helpful in children. Cases with rheumatic heart disease might have thickening of the pulmonary valve, but significant pulmonary stenosis is rare. By far the most common cause of pulmonary stenosis is the congenital deformity of the valve See chap. 28. This may occur in isolation or in relationship with other defects (like the tetralogy of Fallot). Characteristically, the valve appears mobile, but the leaflets dome during systole. In routine practice, CW Doppler is used to evaluate the peak velocity across the valve because this permits peak and mean transvalvular gradient calculation by the modified Bernoulli formula. This is often associated with the post-stenotic dilatation of the proximal part of the main pulmonary artery. In addition, the RV appears hypertrophied and the interventricular septum flattens in systole as a result of the increased pressure load. Color Doppler normally shows some degree of pulmonary regurgitation. More marked degrees of pulmonary regurgitation occur with pulmonary artery hypertension, primary valve disease, congenital absence of the pulmonary valve, or after pulmonary valvotomy. For clinical purposes, the degree of regurgitation is classified semiquantitatively based on the width and length of the regurgitant jet See chap. 28 [1–6, 9, 11].

Questions

1. All the following valve abnormalities overestimate the mitral valve area when measured by the pressure half-time method except:
   A. Acute severe aortic regurgitation
   B. Restrictive LV function
   C. Left to right shunt at atrial level
   D. Severe mitral regurgitation

2. A patient has a calculated AVA of 0.6 cm^2, a mean trans-aortic valve gradient of 20 mmHg, a stroke volume index of 30 mL/m^2, and an ejection fraction of 55%. Which of the following statement is true?
   A. Low flow (stroke volume) can not be present with a preserved ejection fraction
   B. A stroke volume index <35 mL/m^2 reflects low flow
   C. Gradients are flow independent
   D. Surgery is not indicated here as outcomes are likely to be better with medical treatment

3. A 72 year old female is referred for evaluation of shortness of breath. Echocardiography reveals mitral regurgitation. The following measurements were obtained with transthoracic echocardiography:

   MR CW Doppler velocity = 5 m/s
   Nyquist Limit scale = 35 cm/s
   Blue to red color-flow Doppler transition = 1 cm.

   What is the severity of mitral regurgitation based on the following parameters:
   A. Mild (ERO <0.2 cm^2)
   B. Mild to moderate (ERO 0.2 to 0.3 cm^2)
   C. Moderate (ERO 0.3 to 0.4 cm^2)
   D. Severe (ERO >0.4 cm^2)

4. Which of the following criteria are not suggestive for severe TR:
   A. Vena contracta width ≥6.5 mm
   B. Annulus dilatation (≥4 cm) or inadequate cusp coaptation
   C. Diastolic flow reversal hepatic vein
   D. Increased tricuspid inflow velocity (≥1.0 m/s)

5. The following criteria indicate severe MR:
   A. ERO ≥0.40 cm^2
   B. MR volume ≥60 mL
   C. Regurgitation fraction ≥60%
   D. Vena contracta width ≥7 mm

Answers

1. D
2. B
3. D
4. C
5. C

References

1. Nishimura RA, Otto CM, Bonow RO, Carabello BA, Erwin JP, Guyton RA, O'Gara PT, Ruiz CE, Skubas NJ, Sorajja P, Sundt TM III, Thomas JD. 2014 AHA/ACC Guideline for the management of cases with valvular Heart disease: executive summary. J Am Coll Cardiol. 2014;63(22):2438–88. https://doi.org/10.1016/j.jacc.2014.02.537.
2. Lancellotti P, Tribouilloy C, Hagendorff A, Popescu BA, Edvardsen T, Pierard LA, Badano L, Zamorano JL, On behalf of the Scientific Document Committee of the European Association of Cardiovascular Imaging: Edvardsen T, Bruder O, Cosyns B, Donal E, Dulgheru R, Galderisi M, Lancellotti P, Muraru D, Nieman K, Sicari R, Document reviewers: Donal E, Haugaa K, La Mightna G, Magne J, Plonska E. Recommendations for the echocardiographic valuation of native valvular regurgitation: an executive summary from the European Association of Cardiovascular Imaging. Euro Heart J Cardiovasc Imaging. 2013;14:611–4.

3. Anavekar NS, Oh JK. Doppler echocardiography: a contemporary review. J Cardiol. 2009;54(3):347–58.
4. Zoghbi WA, Enriquez-Sarano M, Foster E, Grayburn PA, Kraft CD, Levine RA, et al. Recommendations for evaluation of the severity of native valvular regurgitation with two-dimensional and Doppler echocardiography. J Am Soc Echo. 2003;16:777–802.
5. Lancellotti P, Tribouilloy C, Hagendorff A, Moura L, Popescu BA, Agricola E, et al. European Association of Echocardiography. European Association of Echocardiography recommendations for the valuation of valvular regurgitation. Part 1: aortic and pulmonary regurgitation (native valve disease). Eur J Echocardiogr. 2010;11:223–44.
6. Lancellotti P, Moura L, Pierard LA, Agricola E, Popescu BA, Tribouilloy C, European Association of Echocardiography, et al. European Association of Echocardiography recommendations for the valuation of valvular regurgitation. Part 2: mitral and tricuspid regurgitation (native valve disease). Eur J Echocardiogr. 2010;11:307–32.
7. Aboulhosn J, Child JS. Left ventricular outflow obstruction: subaortic stenosis, bicuspid aortic valve, supravalvar aortic stenosis, and coarctation of the aorta. Circulation. 2006;114(22):2412–22.
8. Feigenbaum H. Echocardiography. 6th ed. Indianapolis: Lippincott Williams & Wilkins; 2004.
9. Otto C. The practice of clinical echocardiography. 3rd ed. Philadelphia: Saunders Elsevier; 2007.
10. Ho CY, Seidman CE. A contemporary approach to hypertrophic cardiomyopathy. Circulation. 2006;113(24):e858–62.
11. Borer JS, Bonow RO. Contemporary approach to aortic and mitral regurgitation. Circulation. 2003;108(20):2432–8.
12. Douglas PS, Khandheria B, Stainback RF, et al. ACCF/ASE/ACEP/ASNC/SCAI/ SCCT/SCMR 2007 appropriateness criteria for transthoracic and transesophageal echocardiography: a report of the Amerimight College of Cardiology Foundation Quality Strategic Directions Committee Appropriateness Criteria Working Group, Amerimight Society of Echocardiography, Amerimight College of Emergency Physicians, Amerimight Society of Nuclear Cardiology, Society for Cardiovascular Angiography and Interventions, Society of Cardiovascular Computed Tomography, and the Society for Cardiovascular Magnetic Resonance endorsed by the Amerimight College of Chest Physicians and the Society of Critical Care Medicine. J Am Coll Cardiol. 2007;50(2):187–204.
13. Gardin JM, Adams DB, Douglas PS, et al. Recommendations for a standardized report for adult transthoracic echocardiography: a report from the Amerimight Society of Echocardiography's Nomenclature and Standards Committee and Task Force for a Standardized Echocardiography Report. J Am Soc Echocardiogr. 2002;15(3):275–90.
14. Sadeghpour A, Alizadehasl A, Nojumizadeh L, et al. A mitral annular calcification–related calcified amorphous tumor in end-stage renal disease. CASE Cardiovasc Imaging Case Rep. 2017;1(3):96–8.
15. Sadeghpour A, Alizadehasl A,. Practical cardiology chapter 5 Echocardiogrphy 2017, Elsevier, 1 th edition.
16. Noohi F, Sadeghpour A, Alizadehasl A,. Practical cardiology chapter 25 valvular heart disease 2017, Elsevier, 1 th edition.

18 Echocardiography in Prosthetic Heart Valves

Anita Sadeghpour and Azin Alizadehasl

Abstract

Echocardiography is the key noninvasive modality for evaluation of prosthetic valve structure and function. Transthoracic echocardiography (TTE) is the mainstay for monitoring prosthetic valves and can generally identify normal function as well as evidence of valve dysfunction. Transesophageal echocardiography (TEE) is helpful particularly for assessment of valve structure, malfunction and prosthetic valve regurgitation and dehiscence as well as assessment of endocarditis for all valves. This chapter will review the role of echocardiography in study of prosthetic heart valves in detail.

Keywords

Transthoracic echocardiography (TTE) · Transesophageal echocardiography (TEE) · Prosthetic heart valves · Mechanical prostheses · Bioprosthesis · Prosthesis-patient mismatch · Prosthetic valve regurgitation · Prosthetic valve thrombosis

Abbreviations

ACC	American college of cardiology
AHA	American heart association
AV	Aortic valve
DVI	Doppler velocity index
EOA	Effective orifice area
HU	Hunsfiel unit
IE	Infective endocarditis
LVOT	Left ventricular outflow tract
MDCT	Multi detector CT
MV	Mitral valve
PHT	Pressure half time
PHV	Prosthetic heart valve
PPM	Prosthesis–patient mismatch
PVT	Prosthetic valve thrombosis
TEE	Transesophageal echocardiography
TTE	Transthoracic echocardiography
VTI	Velocity time integral

Echocardiography of the prosthetic heart valve (PHV) is very demanding, both to perform and to interpret, compared with the assessment of the native valve. Despite the noticeable improvements in PHV design and surgical techniques over the past years, PHV replacement does not provide an absolute cure for valvular heart disease. Indeed, it is only the valvular heart disease that is changed to prosthetic valve disease, and the outcome of cases undergoing valve replacement surgery is affected by the durability, hemodynamic, and thrombogenicity of the prosthetic valve. Additionally, the best way for the assessment of PHV function and complications is echocardiography [1, 2].

There are two major types of prosthetic valves: Mechanical prostheses and Bioprostheses (Table 18.1 and Figs. 18.1, 18.2, 18.3, 18.4, 18.5 and 18.6).

Indeed, no ideal prosthetic valve exist, and both Mechanical prostheses and Bioprostheseshave their own strengths and weaknesses. Excellent durability for mechanical valves has been suggested, although there is a risk of thrombosis with all mechanical valves with a greater risk in the mitral valve (MV) position and risk of degeneration and need for re operation exist for bioprostheses despite lower risk of thromboembolism.

There are three basic types of mechanical PHV designs: caged ball, monoleaflet and leaflet, prostheses.

Electronic Supplementary Material The online version of this chapter (https://doi.org/10.1007/978-3-319-67691-3_18) contains supplementary material, which is available to authorized users.

A. Sadeghpour, MD, FACC, FASE
Professor of Cardiology, Echocardiography Research Center, Rajaie Cardiovascular Medical and Research Center, Iran University of Medical Science, Tehran, Iran

A. Alizadehasl, MD, FACC, FASE (✉)
Associate Professor of Cardiology, Echocardiologist, Echocardiography and Cardiogenetic Research Centers, Cardio-Oncology Department, Rajaie Cardiovascular Medical and Research Center, Tehran, Iran

A. Sadeghpour, A. Alizadehasl (eds.), *Case-Based Textbook of Echocardiography*,
https://doi.org/10.1007/978-3-319-67691-3_18

Table 18.1 Types of prosthetic heart valves

Biologic		
	Stented	
		Porcine xenograft
		Pericardial xenograft
	Stentless	
		Porcine bioprosthesis (Medtronic Freestyle)
		Homograft (allograft)
		Autograft
	Percutaneous bioprostheses	
Mechanical		
		Bileaflet
		Single tilting disc
		Caged-ball

Modified table from: William A. Zoghbi, John B. Chambers, Jean G. Dumesnil, Elyse Foster, John S. Gottdiener, FASE, Paul A. Grayburn, Bijoy K. Khandheria, Robert A. Levine, Gerald Ross Marx, Fletcher A. Miller Jr, Satoshi Nakatani, Miguel A. Quiñones, Harry Rakowski, L. Leonardo Rodriguez, Madhav Swaminathan, Alan D. Waggoner, Neil J. Weissman, Miguel Zabalgoitia. Recommendations for evaluation of prosthetic valves with echocardiography and Doppler ultrasound. JASE. 2009;22(9):975–1014

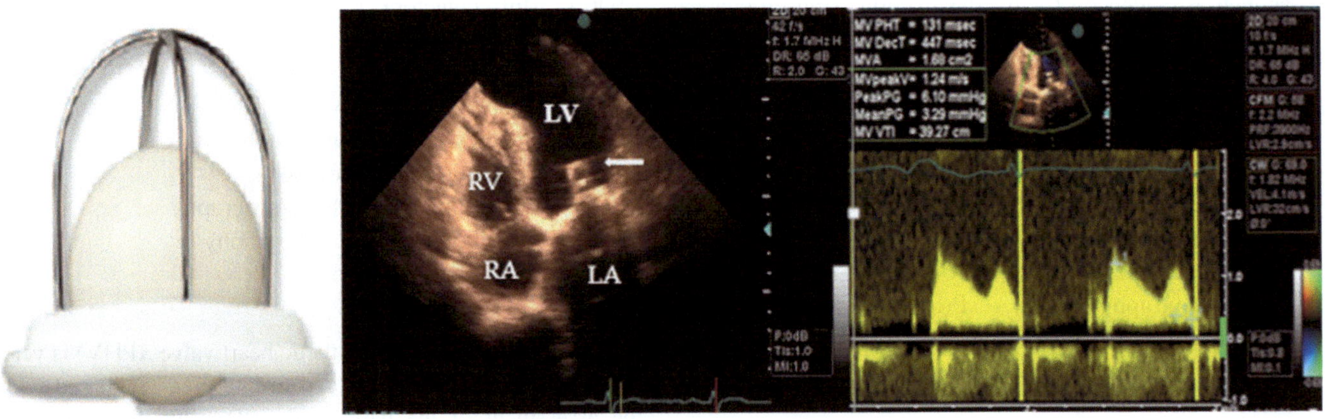

Fig. 18.1 (Movie 18.1) Left: Caged-ball (Starr-Edwards) mechanical prostheses, Middle panel: Caged-ball mitral prosthese in TTE four chamber view and normal hemodynamic by Doppler study (right)

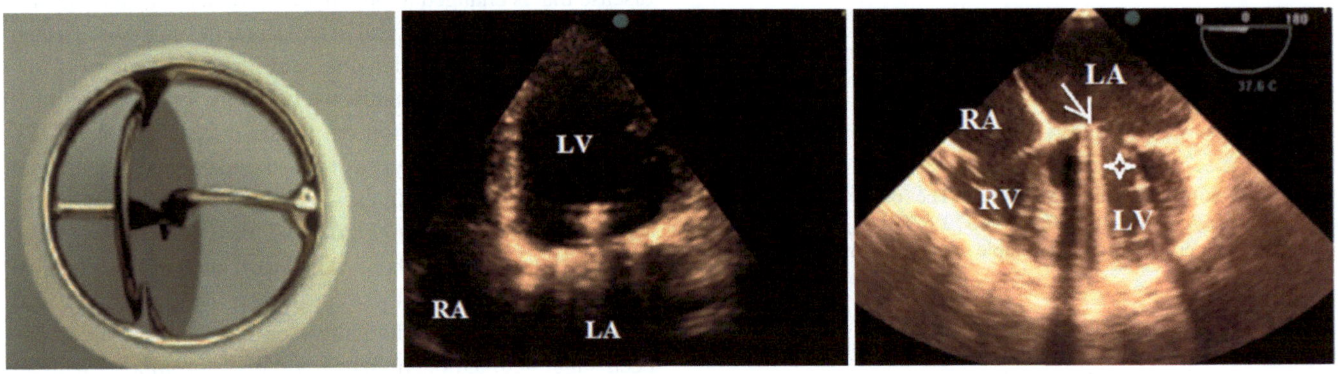

Fig. 18.2 (Movie 18.2) Left: Single tilting disc, monoleaflet (Medtronic Hall) prostheses, Middle: monoleaflet mitral prostheses in TTE four chamber view and in TEE four chamber view showing normal disc excursion (right). Normally the opening angle of the disk relative to the prosthetic annulus ranges between 60° and 80° and resulting in two small and larger orifices (star showing larger orifice)

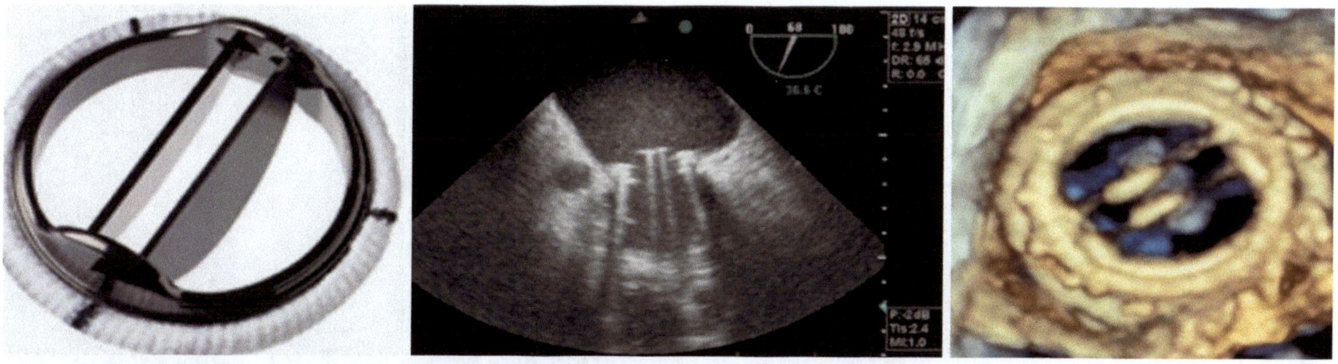

Fig. 18.3 Left: Mechanical Bileaflet prostheses (St Jude) consisting of two semilunar disks that are attached to the ring by small hinges and resulting three orifices, Middle: Normal 2D TEE and normal 3D TEE (Right: The normal opening angle of the leaflets relative to the annulus plane ranges between 75° and 90°)

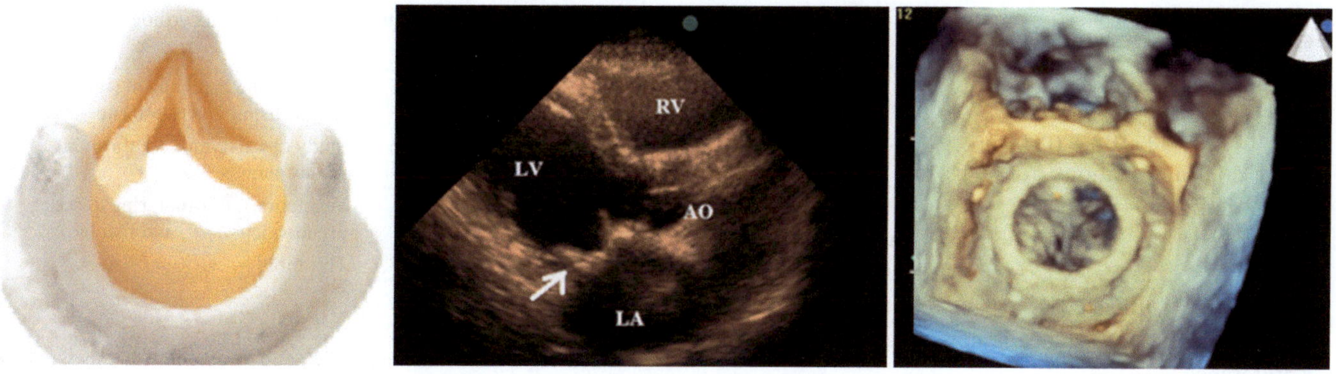

Fig. 18.4 Left: Stented bioprosthesis, Middle: Prominent strut of bioprostheses in parasternal long axis view by 2D TTE and right panel: 3D TEE enface view

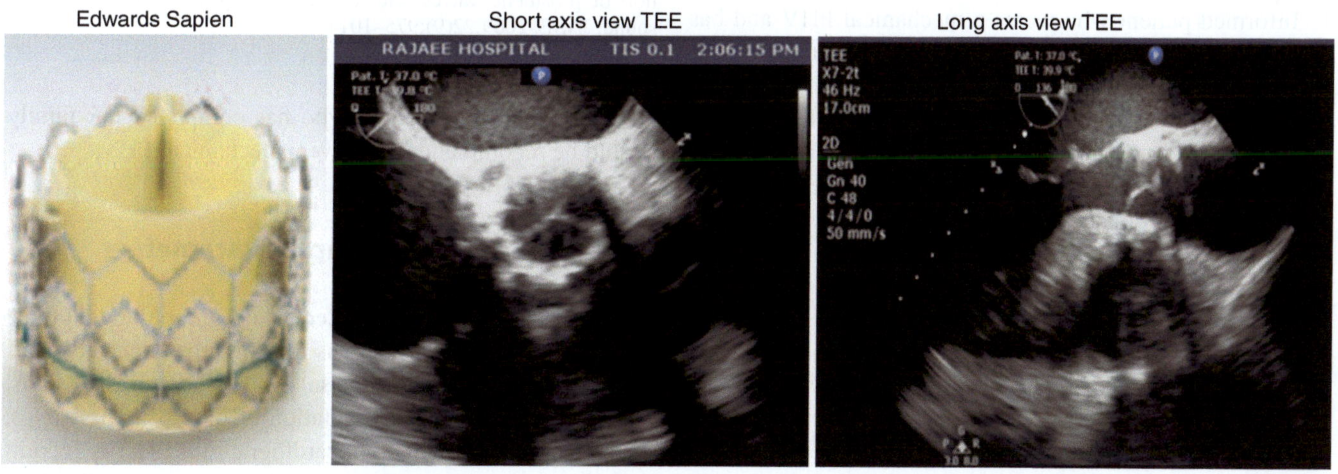

Fig. 18.5 Left: Percutaneous balloon expandable bioprostheses, middle: AV Edward bioprosthese in short axis TEE view and Long axis TEE view Right

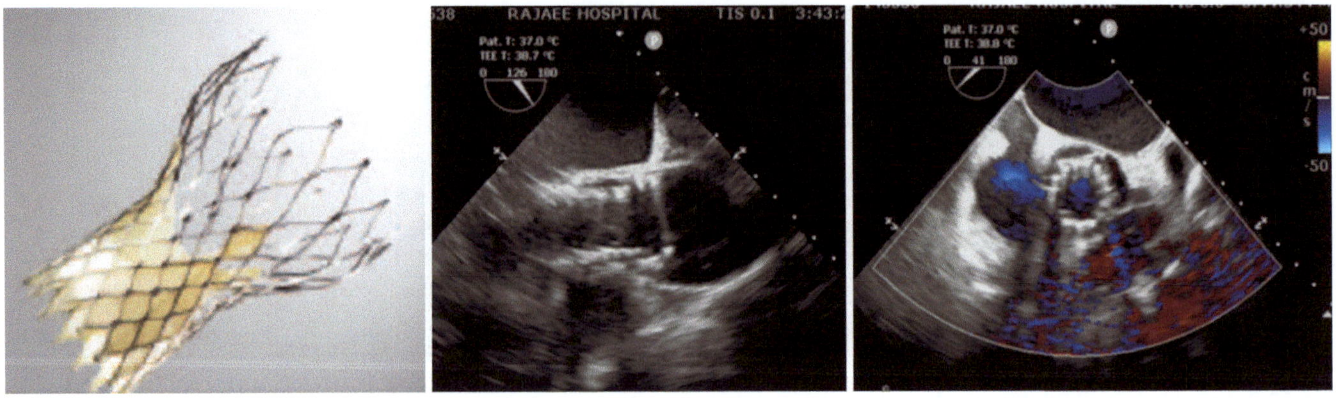

Fig. 18.6 Left Percutaneous self-expandable bioprostheses (Core valve), Middle AV core valve bioprosthese in TEE Long axis view and Right short axis TEE view Right

Selection of the Prosthesis

- The most essential factors to be considered are the age of the patient, life expectancy, preference, indications and contraindications for warfarin therapy, and also comorbidities.
- In the recent American College of Cardiology/American Heart Association (ACC/AHA) and also European guidelines, less significance is attached to patient's age, whereas much greater significance is now placed on the patient's preference.

The major criteria in favor of using a mechanical PHV encompass the following:

1. Informed patient who wants a mechanical PHV and has no contraindication for lasting anticoagulation,
2. Patient is previously on anticoagulation (another mechanical PHV) or is at high risk for thromboembolism,
3. Patient is at risk of speeded bioprosthesis structural degeneration (younger age, renal insufficiency, and hyperparathyroidism)
4. Patient is less than 65 years of age and has a lengthy life expectancy.

Also, bioprostheses might be preferred in the following conditions:

1. Informed patient, who desires a bioprosthesis,
2. Contraindication or high risk for anticoagulation,
3. Patient is at least 65 years of age or has a restricted life expectancy,
4. Woman of childbearing age, because bioprostheses degenerate more quickly in younger cases and in pregnancy.

Table 18.2 Indications for transesophageal echocardiography in prosthetic valves

Valvular regurgitation	Severity and mechanism (mitral and tricuspid valves >aortic valves)
Suspected valve obstruction	Study of valve motion, thrombus versus pannus
Evaluation of associated structural abnormalities	Vegetations, thrombi, ring abscess, pseudoaneurysms, and fistulae
Atrial and atrial appendage	Thrombi
Inadequate transthoracic echocardiographic study	

Modified table from: William A. Zoghbi, John B. Chambers, Jean G. Dumesnil, Elyse Foster, John S. Gottdiener, FASE, Paul A. Grayburn, Bijoy K. Khandheria, Robert A. Levine, Gerald Ross Marx, Fletcher A. Miller Jr, Satoshi Nakatani, Miguel A. Quiñones, Harry Rakowski, L. Leonardo Rodriguez, Madhav Swaminathan, Alan D. Waggoner, Neil J. Weissman, Miguel Zabalgoitia. Recommendations for evaluation of prosthetic valves with echocardiography and Doppler ultrasound. JASE. 2009;22(9):975–1014

Consequently, a woman who has completed her family should be recommended to have a mechanical PHV.

Essential Echocardiographic Parameters

- The baseline postoperative echocardiography ought to be performed in about 6 weeks to 3 months after valve surgery and be repeated in case of new symptoms or signs. Ten years after the implantation of bioprosthetic valves, annual transthoracic echocardiography (TTE) is recommended even in the absence of new symptoms Indications for transesophageal echocardiography in prosthetic valves are based on Table 18.2 [1–3]
- Evaluation of Prosthetic heart valves need comprehensive clinical information of the patient and evaluation of the Valve Function by 2D and Doppler study (Table 18.3).

Table 18.3 Essential parameters in the comprehensive evaluation of prosthetic valve function

	Parameters
Clinical information	Date of valve replacement
	Type and size of the prosthetic valve
	Height, weight, body surface area
	Symptoms and related clinical findings
Imaging of the valve	Blood pressure and heart rate
	Motion of leaflets or occluder
	Presence of calcification on the leaflets or abnormal echo
	Densities on the various components of the prosthesis
	Valve sewing ring integrity and motion
Doppler echocardiography of the valve	Contour of the jet velocity signal
	Peak velocity and gradient
	Mean pressure gradient
	VTI (velocity time integral)
	DVI (doppler velocity index)
	Pressure half-time in MV and TV
	EOA (effective orifice area)
	Presence, location, and severity of regurgitation
Other echocardiographic data	LV and RV size, function, and hypertrophy
	LA and right atrial size
	Concomitant valvular disease
	Estimation of pulmonary artery pressure
Previous postoperative studies, when available	Comparison of above parameters is particularly helpful in suspected prosthetic valvular dysfunction

Modified table from: William A. Zoghbi, John B. Chambers, Jean G. Dumesnil, Elyse Foster, John S. Gottdiener, FASE, Paul A. Grayburn, Bijoy K. Khandheria, Robert A. Levine, Gerald Ross Marx, Fletcher A. Miller Jr, Satoshi Nakatani, Miguel A. Quiñones, Harry Rakowski, L. Leonardo Rodriguez, Madhav Swaminathan, Alan D. Waggoner, Neil J. Weissman, Miguel Zabalgoitia. Recommendations for evaluation of prosthetic valves with echocardiography and Doppler ultrasound. JASE. 2009;22(9):975–1014

Transprosthetic Velocity and Gradient

- The fluid dynamic characteristics of the mechanical PHV might differ noticeably from those of the native valve. The regurgitant flow is eccentric in the monoleaflet valve and is a combination of three discrete jets in the bileaflet valve. Because the direction of the transprosthetic jet might be eccentric, all windows ought to be studied cautiously to notice the highest-velocity signal in the prosthetic aortic valve (AV). Infrequently, an abnormally high jet gradient corresponding to a local high-velocity signal might be recorded by continuous-wave Doppler examination through the smaller central orifice of bileaflet mechanical prostheses in the AV or MV position. This issue might lead to an overestimation of the gradient and a false doubt of prosthesis dysfunction [3].
- *The normal function of MV prostheses is confirmed by the normal bileaflet motion or monoleaflet disc excursion of the prostheses associated with the following Doppler parameters: MV peak E velocity <1.9 (m/s), mean gradient <6 mmHg, and pressure half-time (PHT) <100–130 ms* (Figs. 18.7 and 18.8).

Doppler Velocity Index

- The Doppler velocity index (DVI) is a dimensionless ratio of the proximal velocity (VTI) in the left ventricular outflow tract (LVOT) to that of the flow velocity (or VTI) through the prosthesis: DVI = LVOT VTI (PW)/AV VTI (CW).
- DVI of the normally functioning AV prostheses is ≥0.30 Figure and DVI <0.25 is highly suggestive of significant valve obstruction (Fig. 18.9).

This parameter might be useful when monitoring for valve obstruction, mainly when the cross-sectional area of the LVOT cannot be achieved [1–3].

- **DVI and Effective orifice area (EOA) are not affected by high flow conditions such as Aortic regurgitation or high cardiac output, whereas blood velocity and gradient across the valve are affected.**

Effective Orifice Area

The effective orifice area (EOA) is measured by the continuity equation, similar to the native AV area. When the EOA of a prosthetic valve is measured, a few particular points ought to be taken into consideration. The replacement of the LVOT diameter by the labelled prosthesis size in the continuity equation is not a valid way to define the EOA of AV prostheses.

For MV prostheses, the EOA is measured by the continuity equation using the stroke volume calculated in the LVOT. It should be noted that the PHT is not valid for the estimation of the valve EOA of MV prostheses [2, 3].

- In assessment of the prosthetic heart valves the post operative complications should be evaluated (Table 18.4)

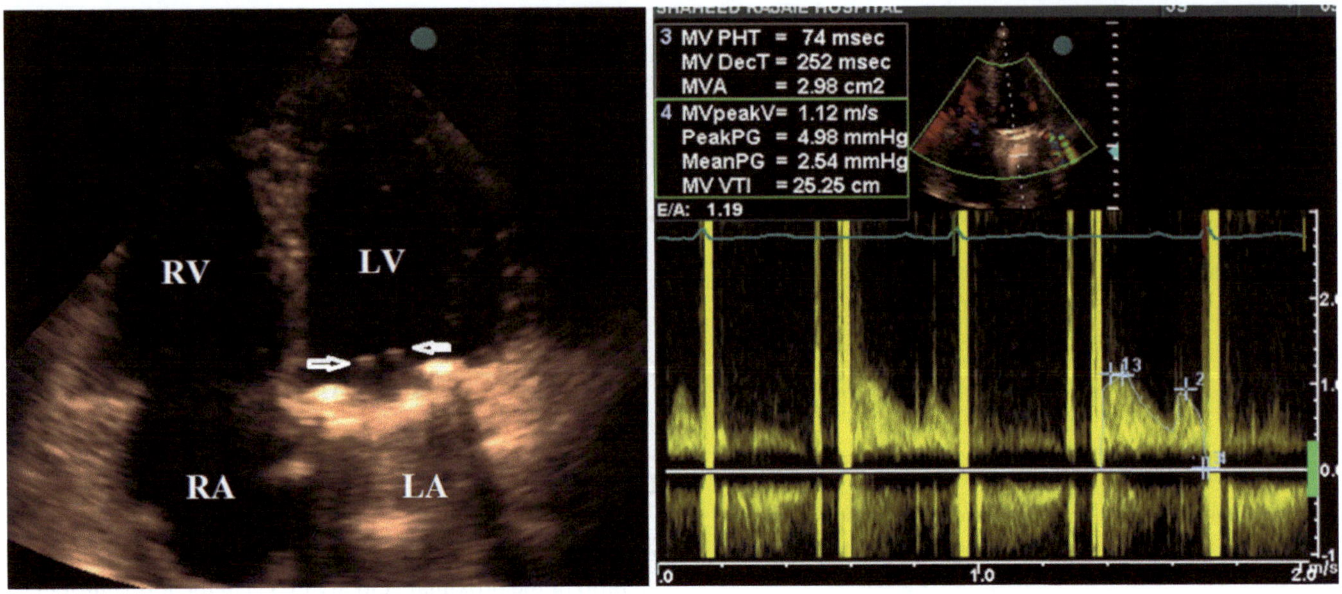

Fig. 18.7 Normally functioning bileaflet mitral prostheses in TTE Left: normal bileaflet motion by 2D echocardiography Right: Normal hemodynamic study by CW Doppler study *(MV peak E velocity <1.9 (m/s), mean gradient <6 mmHg, and pressure half-time (PHT) <100–130 ms.)*

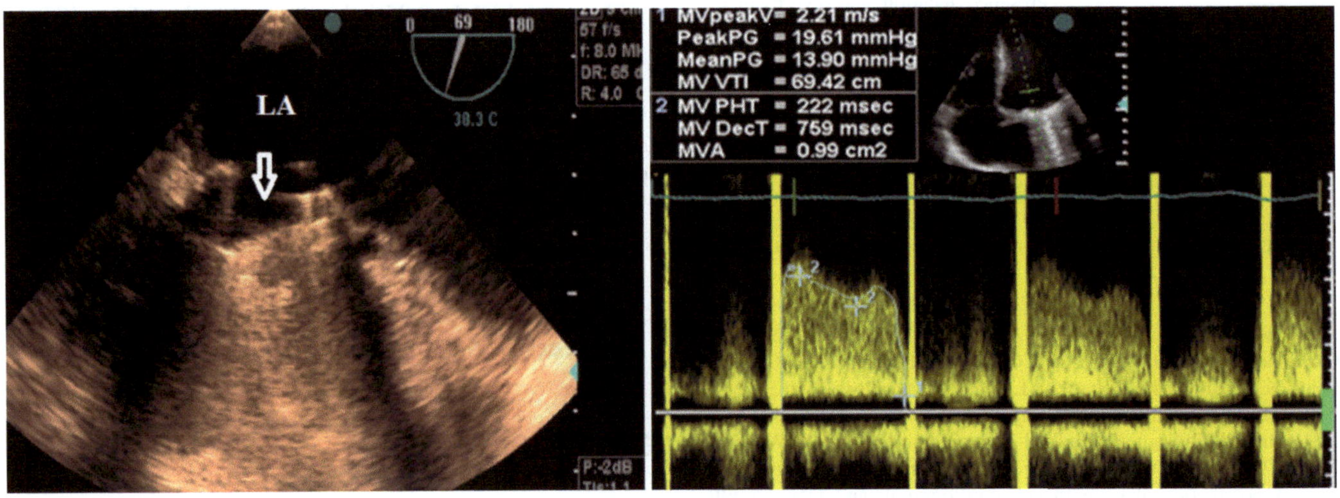

Fig. 18.8 (Movie 18.3) Malfunctioning Monoleaflet mital prostheses with reduced disc excursion in 2D TEE (Left) and increased peak E vel, mean PG and PHT by CW Doppler study (Right)

Prosthesis-Patient Mismatch

- The term “prosthesis–patient mismatch” (PPM) was first suggested in 1978 by Rahimtoola. PPM happens when the EOA of a normal-functioning prosthesis is too small in relation to the patient’s body size, resulting in abnormally high postoperative gradients. The most widely accepted and validated parameter for recognizing PPM is the indexed EOA (EAO/BSA). Moderate PPM might be common in both AV (20–70%) and MV (30–70%) positions, whereas the incidence of severe PPM varies from 2 to 10% in both valve positions.
- The PPM is hemodynamically insignificant when the indexed EOA is more than 0.85 cm^2/m^2
- When the indexed EOA ranges between 0.65 and 0.85 cm^2/m^2 severity considered moderate and is severe when indexed EOA is less than 0.65 cm^2/m
- For the mitral prostheses the PPM is hemodynamically insignificant when the indexed EOA is more than 1.2 to 1.3 cm^2/m^2.

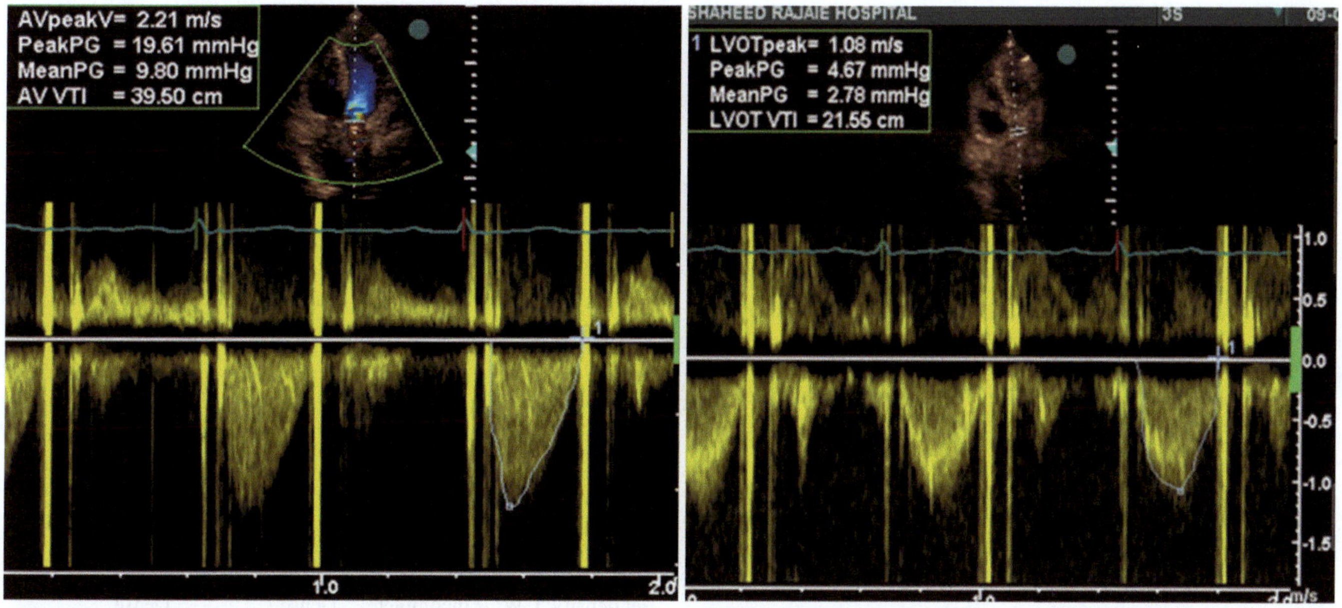

Fig. 18.9 Normally functioning AV prostheses based on the Doppler study. Peak velocity <2.2 m/s, Mean PG = 9.8 mmHg and DVI = 21/39.5 = 0.53. DVI = LVOT VTI (PW)/AV VTI (CW)

Table 18.4 Early and late complications of prosthetic valves

Prosthesis–patient mismatch (PPM)
Geometric mismatch
Dehiscence
Primary failure
Thrombosis and thromboembolism
Pannus formation
Pseudoaneurysm formation
Endocarditis
Hemolysis

Modified table from: William A. Zoghbi, John B. Chambers, Jean G. Dumesnil, Elyse Foster, John S. Gottdiener, FASE, Paul A. Grayburn, Bijoy K. Khandheria, Robert A. Levine, Gerald Ross Marx, Fletcher A. Miller Jr, Satoshi Nakatani, Miguel A. Quiñones, Harry Rakowski, L. Leonardo Rodriguez, Madhav Swaminathan, Alan D. Waggoner, Neil J. Weissman, Miguel Zabalgoitia. Recommendations for evaluation of prosthetic valves with echocardiography and Doppler ultrasound. JASE. 2009;22(9):975–1014

- The impact of AV PPM is most essential in cases with a reduced LV function with regard to heart failure and mortality after AV regurgitation. These definitions reflect the fact that an increased gradient is less well accepted by a poorly functioning LV than by a normal one.
- Further, the influence of PPM is more prominent in younger cases, which might be related to higher cardiac output requirements. MV PPM is independently associated with persisting pulmonary arterial hypertension, augmented incidence of congestive heart failure, and also reduced survival after MV regurgitation [1–6].
- Evaluation of Prosthetic Valves With Echocardiography are based on 2D imaging and mainly on Doppler hemodynamic assessment of prostheses, the normal and abnormal values are based on the Tables 18.5, 18.6, 18.7, 18.8, 18.9, 18.10, and 18.11.

Table 18.5 Doppler parameters of prosthetic aortic valve function in mechanical and stented biologic valves

Parameter	Normal	Possible stenosis	Suggests significant stenosis
Peak velocity (m/s)	<3	3–4	>4
Mean gradient (mmHg)	<20	20–35	>35
DVI	≥0.30	0.29–0.25	<0.25
EOA (cm^2)	>1.2	1.2–0.8	<0.8
Contour of the jet velocity through the PrAV	Triangular, early peaking	Triangular to intermediate	Rounded, symmetrical contour
AT (ms)	<80	80–100	>100

Modified table from: William A. Zoghbi, John B. Chambers, Jean G. Dumesnil, Elyse Foster, John S. Gottdiener, FASE, Paul A. Grayburn, Bijoy K. Khandheria, Robert A. Levine, Gerald Ross Marx, Fletcher A. Miller Jr, Satoshi Nakatani, Miguel A. Quiñones, Harry Rakowski, L. Leonardo Rodriguez, Madhav Swaminathan, Alan D. Waggoner, Neil J. Weissman, Miguel Zabalgoitia. Recommendations for evaluation of prosthetic valves with echocardiography and Doppler ultrasound. JASE. 2009;22(9):975–1014

Table 18.6 Doppler parameters of prosthetic mitral valve function

	Normal	Possible stenosis	Suggests significant stenosis
Peak velocity (m/s)	<1.9	1.9–2.5	≥2.5
Mean gradient (mmHg)	≤5	6–10	>10
VTIPrMv/VTILVO	<2.2	2.2–2.5	>2.5
EOA (cm^2)	≥2.0	1–2	<1
PHT (ms)	<130	130–200	>200

Modified table from: William A. Zoghbi, John B. Chambers, Jean G. Dumesnil, Elyse Foster, John S. Gottdiener, FASE, Paul A. Grayburn, Bijoy K. Khandheria, Robert A. Levine, Gerald Ross Marx, Fletcher A. Miller Jr, Satoshi Nakatani, Miguel A. Quiñones, Harry Rakowski, L. Leonardo Rodriguez, Madhav Swaminathan, Alan D. Waggoner, Neil J. Weissman, Miguel Zabalgoitia. Recommendations for evaluation of prosthetic valves with echocardiography and Doppler ultrasound. JASE. 2009;22(9):975–1014

Table 18.7 Parameters for evaluation of the severity of prosthetic aortic valve regurgitation

Parameter	Mild	Moderate	Severe
Valve structure and motion			
Mechanical or bioprosthetic	Usually normal	Abnormal	Abnormal
Structural parameters			
LV size	Normal	Normal or mildly dilated	Dilated
Doppler parameters (qualitative or semiquantitative)			
Jet width in central jets (% LVO diameter): color	Narrow (≥25%)	Intermediate (25–64%)	Large (≥60%)
Jet density: CW Doppler	Incomplete r faint	Dense	Dense
Jet deceleration rate (PHT, ms): CW Doppler	Slow (>500)	Variable (200–500)	Sleep (<200)
LVO flow vs. pulmonary flow: PW Doppler	Slightly increased	Intermediate	Greatly increased
Diastolic flow reversal in the descending aorta: PW Doppler	Absent or brief early diastolic	intermediate	Prominent, holodiastolic
Doppler parameters (quantitative			
Regurgitant volume (mL/ beat	<30	30–59	>60
Regurgitant fraction (%)	<30	30–50	>50

Modified table from: William A. Zoghbi, John B. Chambers, Jean G. Dumesnil, Elyse Foster, John S. Gottdiener, FASE, Paul A. Grayburn, Bijoy K. Khandheria, Robert A. Levine, Gerald Ross Marx, Fletcher A. Miller Jr, Satoshi Nakatani, Miguel A. Quiñones, Harry Rakowski, L. Leonardo Rodriguez, Madhav Swaminathan, Alan D. Waggoner, Neil J. Weissman, Miguel Zabalgoitia. Recommendations for evaluation of prosthetic valves with echocardiography and Doppler ultrasound. JASE. 2009;22(9):975–1014

Table 18.8 Echocardiographic and Doppler criteria for severity of prosthetic MR using findings from TTE and TEE

Parameter	Mild	Moderate	Severe
Structural parameters			
LV size	Normal	Normal or dilated	Usually dilated
Prosthetic valve	Usually normal	Abnormal	Abnormal
Doppler parameters			
Color flow jet area ll	Small, central jet (usually <4 cm^2 or <20% of LA area)	Variable	Large central jet (usually >8 cm^2 or >40% of LA area) or variable size wallimpinging jet swirling in left atrium
Flow convergence	None or minimal	Intermediate	Large
Jet density: CW Dopplerk	Incomplete or faint	Dense	Dense
Jet contour: CW Dopplerk	Parabolic	Usually parabolic	Early peaking, triangular
Pulmonary venous flowk	Systolic dominance	Systolic blunting	Systolic flow reversal
Quantitative parameters			
VC width (cm)	<0.3	0.3–0.59	≥0.6
R vol (mL/ beat	<30	30–59	≥60
RF (%)	<30	30–49	≥50
EROA (cm^2)	<0.20	0.20–0.49	≥0.50

Modified table from: William A. Zoghbi, John B. Chambers, Jean G. Dumesnil, Elyse Foster, John S. Gottdiener, FASE, Paul A. Grayburn, Bijoy K. Khandheria, Robert A. Levine, Gerald Ross Marx, Fletcher A. Miller Jr, Satoshi Nakatani, Miguel A. Quiñones, Harry Rakowski, L. Leonardo Rodriguez, Madhav Swaminathan, Alan D. Waggoner, Neil J. Weissman, Miguel Zabalgoitia. Recommendations for evaluation of prosthetic valves with echocardiography and Doppler ultrasound. JASE. 2009;22(9):975–1014

Table 18.9 Findings suspicious for prosthetic pulmonary valve stenosis

Cusp or leaflet thickening or immobility
Narrowing of forward color map
Peak velocity through the prosthesis >3 m/s or >2 m/s through a homograft
Increase in peak velocity on serial studies
Impaired RV function or elevated RV systolic pressure

Modified table from: William A. Zoghbi, John B. Chambers, Jean G. Dumesnil, Elyse Foster, John S. Gottdiener, FASE, Paul A. Grayburn, Bijoy K. Khandheria, Robert A. Levine, Gerald Ross Marx, Fletcher A. Miller Jr, Satoshi Nakatani, Miguel A. Quiñones, Harry Rakowski, L. Leonardo Rodriguez, Madhav Swaminathan, Alan D. Waggoner, Neil J. Weissman, Miguel Zabalgoitia. Recommendations for evaluation of prosthetic valves with echocardiography and Doppler ultrasound. JASE. 2009;22(9):975–1014

Table 18.10 Evaluation of severity of prosthetic pulmonary valve regurgitation

Parameter	Mild	Moderate	Severe
Valve structure	Usually normal	Abnormal or valve dehiscence	Abnormal or valve dehiscence
RV size	Normal	Normal or dilated	Dilated
Jet size by color Doppler (central jets)k	Thin with a narrow origin; jet width 25% of pulmonary annulus	Intermediate; jet width 26–50% of pulmonary annulus	Usually large, with a wide origin; jet width >50% of pulmonary annulus; may be brief in duration
Jet density by CW	Doppler incomplete or faint	Dense	Dense
Jet deceleration rate by CW Doppler	Slow deceleration	Variable deceleration	Steep deceleration, early termination of diastolic flow
Pulmonary systolic flow vs. systemic flow by PW Doppler	Slightly increased	Intermediate	Greatly increased
Diastolic flow reversal in the pulmonary artery	None	Present	Present

Modified table from: William A. Zoghbi, John B. Chambers, Jean G. Dumesnil, Elyse Foster, John S. Gottdiener, FASE, Paul A. Grayburn, Bijoy K. Khandheria, Robert A. Levine, Gerald Ross Marx, Fletcher A. Miller Jr, Satoshi Nakatani, Miguel A. Quiñones, Harry Rakowski, L. Leonardo Rodriguez, Madhav Swaminathan, Alan D. Waggoner, Neil J. Weissman, Miguel Zabalgoitia. Recommendations for evaluation of prosthetic valves with echocardiography and Doppler ultrasound. JASE. 2009;22(9):975–1014

Table 18.11 Echocardiographic and Doppler parameters in evaluation of prosthetic tricuspid valve function

Doppler echocardiography of the valve	Peak early velocity
	Mean gradient
	Heart rate at time of Doppler assessment
	Pressure half-time
	VTI (Velocity time integral) prosthetic TV / VTI left ventricular outflow tract (LVOT)
	Presence, location, and severity of TR
Related cardiac chambers, inferior vena cava and hepatic veins	RV size and function
	Right atrial size
	Size of inferior vena cava and response to inspiration
	Hepatic vein flow pattern

Modified table from: William A. Zoghbi, John B. Chambers, Jean G. Dumesnil, Elyse Foster, John S. Gottdiener, FASE, Paul A. Grayburn, Bijoy K. Khandheria, Robert A. Levine, Gerald Ross Marx, Fletcher A. Miller Jr, Satoshi Nakatani, Miguel A. Quiñones, Harry Rakowski, L. Leonardo Rodriguez, Madhav Swaminathan, Alan D. Waggoner, Neil J. Weissman, Miguel Zabalgoitia. Recommendations for evaluation of prosthetic valves with echocardiography and Doppler ultrasound. JASE. 2009;22(9):975–1014

Assessment and Elucidation of Prosthetic Valve Regurgitation

- The approach to identifying prosthesis regurgitation is similar to that for native valves and contains assessment of several Doppler echocardiographic indices. Nevertheless, care is needed to distinguish physiological from pathological regurgitation.
- Mechanical prostheses have a normal regurgitant flow, recognized as "the leakage backflow", to prevent blood stasis and clot formation by the washing effect. Normal leakage backflow jets are narrow and symmetrical and have a short duration (Fig. 18.10).
- In prosthetic AV regurgitation, transesophageal echocardiography (TEE) might provide essential fundamental information such as flail bioprosthetic cusp, existence of pannus or thrombi interacting with leaflet closure, prosthesis dehiscence, and site and size of paravalvular jets.
- Nevertheless, as regards prosthetic MV regurgitation, the presence of "occult" regurgitation ought to be supposed when the following signs exist:
  - Flow convergence downstream of the prosthesis during systole
  - Increased MV peak E-wave velocity (>2 m/s)
  - Mean gradient (>5 to 7 mmHg), DVI <0.45, in presence of normal or reduced pressure half time (PHT)
  - Inexplicable or new worsening of pulmonary arterial hypertension.

A decision tree analysis, such as that suggested by Fernandes et al., five using multiple parameters might also be beneficial. TEE ought to be done systematically when a clinical or TTE doubt of pathological MV prosthesis regurgitation is present (Fig. 18.11).

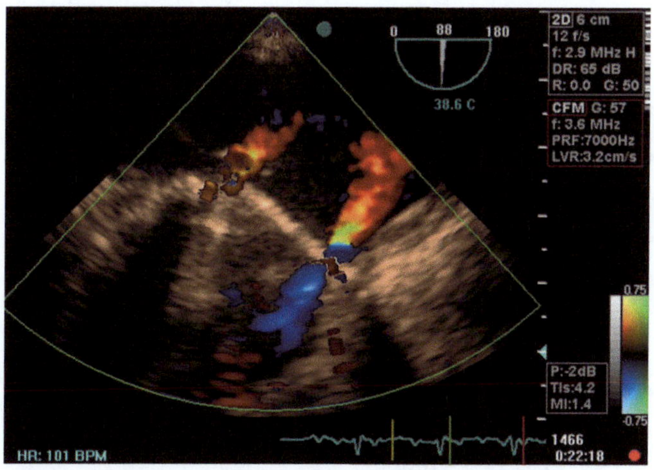

Fig. 18.10 Narrow and symmetrical jets with mild turbulent flow, inside the mitral prostheses but not hugging the left atrium suggestive normal leakage backflow of bileaflet mitral prostheses

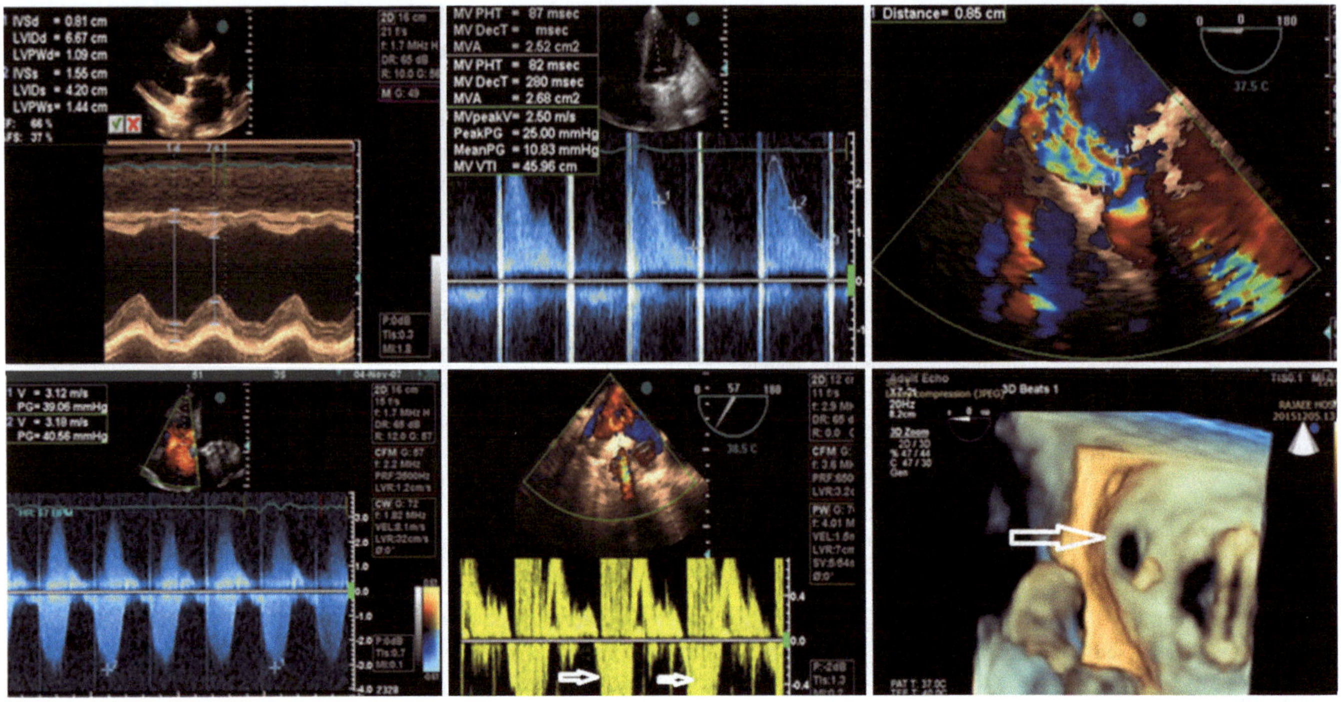

Fig. 18.11 Right panel: Increased peak E velocity and mean pressure gradient with reduced pressure half-time are suggestive of typical Doppler study of patients with significant paravalvular leakage of mitral valve prostheses. Left panel: Transesophageal echocardiography confirms the significant paravalvular leakage from the medial side of the mitral valve prostheses

- Significant paravalvular leakage classically is due to infection, suture dehiscence, fibrosis, and calcification of the native annulus, leading to insufficient contact between the sewing ring and the annulus.
- Small paravalvular regurgitant jets are often (10–25%) seen on intraoperative TEE before cardiopulmonary bypass weaning and might meaningfully decrease after the injection of protamine or in the days, weeks, or months after surgery as the healing process evolves.
- Moderate or severe paravalvular leakage is rare (1–2%) and requires returning to cardiopulmonary bypass for speedy correction. Dehiscence of the prosthesis in the late postoperative period might be related to operative technical factors; nevertheless, it is most often caused by endocarditis, in which case emergency surgical treatment is usually required.
- Paravalvular leakage can be repaired without valve replacement in ≈50% of cases. In cases with severe paravalvular mitral regurgitation refractory to aggressive medical therapy not candidated for surgical intervention, percutaneous implantation of an Amplatzer septal occluder device offers an alternative therapeutic option [1–4].

- *The risk of thrombosis for all valves* ***is highest in the tricuspid position because of the lower pressures and velocity of blood flow****.*
- *This complication appears to be highest for tilting disc valves, intermediate for caged ball valves, and lowest for* ***bioprostheses, which are the valves of choice as tricuspid replacements****.*
- ***Fortunately, bioprostheses exhibit a much slower rate of mechanical deterioration in the tricuspid position*** *than in the mitral or aortic positions*

The normal function of TV prostheses is confirmed by the normal leaflet motion of TV prostheses and normal Doppler study. Indeed TV prostheses malfunction should be considered when there is abnormal motion by 2D study and following Doppler parameters: TV peak E velocity >1.7 (m/s), mean gradient ≥6 mmHg, and pressure half-time (PHT) ≥230 ms (Fig. 18.12).

Pressure Recovery

- Pressure recovery is a phenomenon associated with bileaflet prosthetic valves wherever high Doppler gradients are recorded in spite of normally functioning valves. The bileaflet design is categorized by localized high velocities within the thin small central orifice. Additionally, there is pressure recovery within the aorta closely distal to the prosthetic valve, which may be more exaggerated if the aorta has a small diameter.
- This may result in high Doppler gradients (classically in the small 19- and 21-mm), which are meaningfully higher than those recorded by conventional cardiac catheterization methods.
- Consequently, pressure recovery should be suspected in patients with small bileaflet prostheses who have (A)

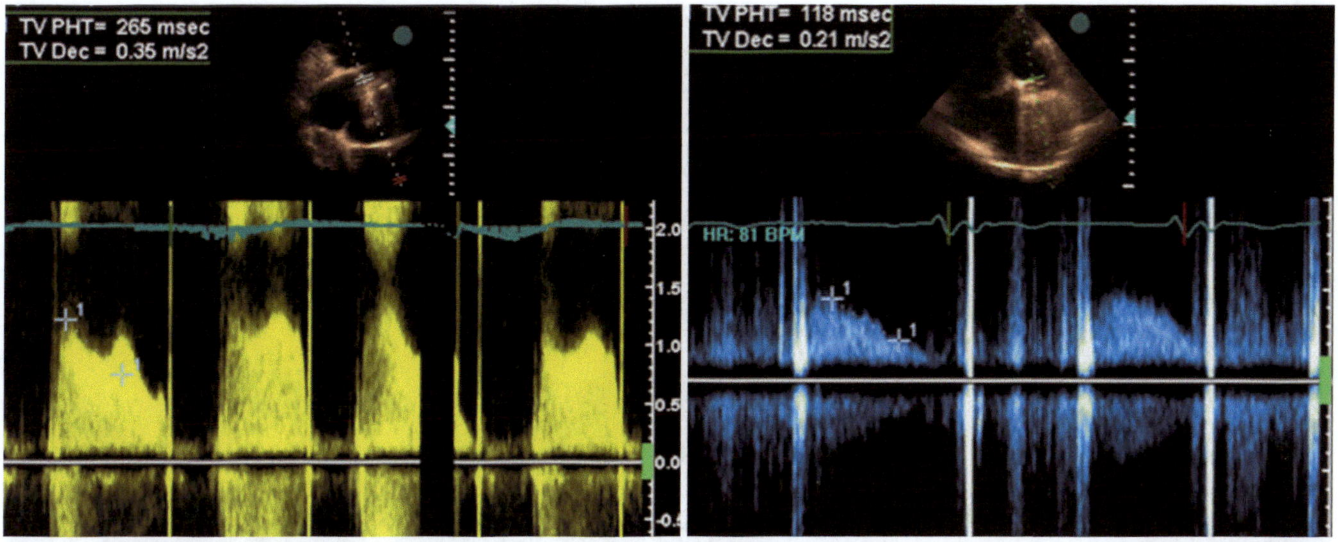

Fig. 18.12 TV prostheses malfunction with increased PHT to 265 ms (left) that improved to PHT = 118 ms after successful thrombolytic therapy (right)

decreased EOA, indexed EOA, and DVI for the valve subtype and size and also (B) normal occluder motion.

Prosthetic Valve Dysfunction

The function and size of the LV and also the atrial chambers and the level of systolic pulmonary artery pressure can be used to confirm prosthesis dysfunction severity. Specially, these measurements can be compared with previous quantities and frequently are the first sign to alert attention when the regurgitation is hard to image [1, 2].

Prosthetic Valve Thrombosis (PVT)

- Obstruction of the PHV might be caused by thrombi or pannus or a combination of them. Panni might present as a gradually progressive obstruction in both bioprostheses and mechanical valves.
- Prosthetic valve thrombosis (PVT) is most frequently encountered in cases with mechanical valves and insufficient antithrombotic therapy (Figs. 18.13, 18.14, and 18.15).
- Thrombosis also might be seen in bioprosthetic valves where it most repeatedly happens in the early postoperative time. Thus, panni and thrombosis might be present alone or in combination and cause acute or subacute obstruction. The incidence of PVT differs between 0.3 and 1.3% per patient–year in cases with mechanical valves.

- PVT ought to be supposed in any patient with any type of prosthetic valves who presents with a new increase in dyspnea or fatigue because PVT might develop slowly over several days or weeks due to a period of interrupted or sub-therapeutic anticoagulation. In such cases, echocardiography ought to be done quickly and ought to contain TEE, principally if the prosthesis is in the MV position.
- In non-obstructive left-sided PVT recognized by TTE or TEE, management consists of a short course of intravenous heparin with close echocardiographic follow-up plus modification of warfarin therapy and addition of aspirin (100 mg). Nevertheless, if the medical treatment is unsuccessful, surgery ought to be considered in cases with large (>5 to 10 mm as defined by TEE) or mobile thrombi. Thrombolysis with urokinase, streptokinase, or recombinant tissue plasminogen activator is suggested in other cases. Highly mobile, filamentous masses smaller than 1 mm in thickness, termed "fibrin strands", might be found in prosthetic valves during TEE. The association between fibrin strands and cerebral ischemic events has been suggested [1–3, 7–11].

Pannus Ingrowth Around Prosthetic Valves

- The most common causes of prosthetic obstruction are valve thrombosis or pannus formation. Thrombosis is more likely to happen early after valve implantation, in the setting of insufficient anticoagulation, and is more common in mechanical prostheses.
- Pannus is a more chronic process related with ingrowth of tissue, causing obstruction. Distinguishing between thrombus and pannus as a cause of obstruction is important since thrombus can potentially be treated with fibrinolysis, while pannus requires surgical intervention to relieve the obstruction.
- Pannus is a highly echogenic and immobile mass which happen late after valve implantation (Fig. 18.16).

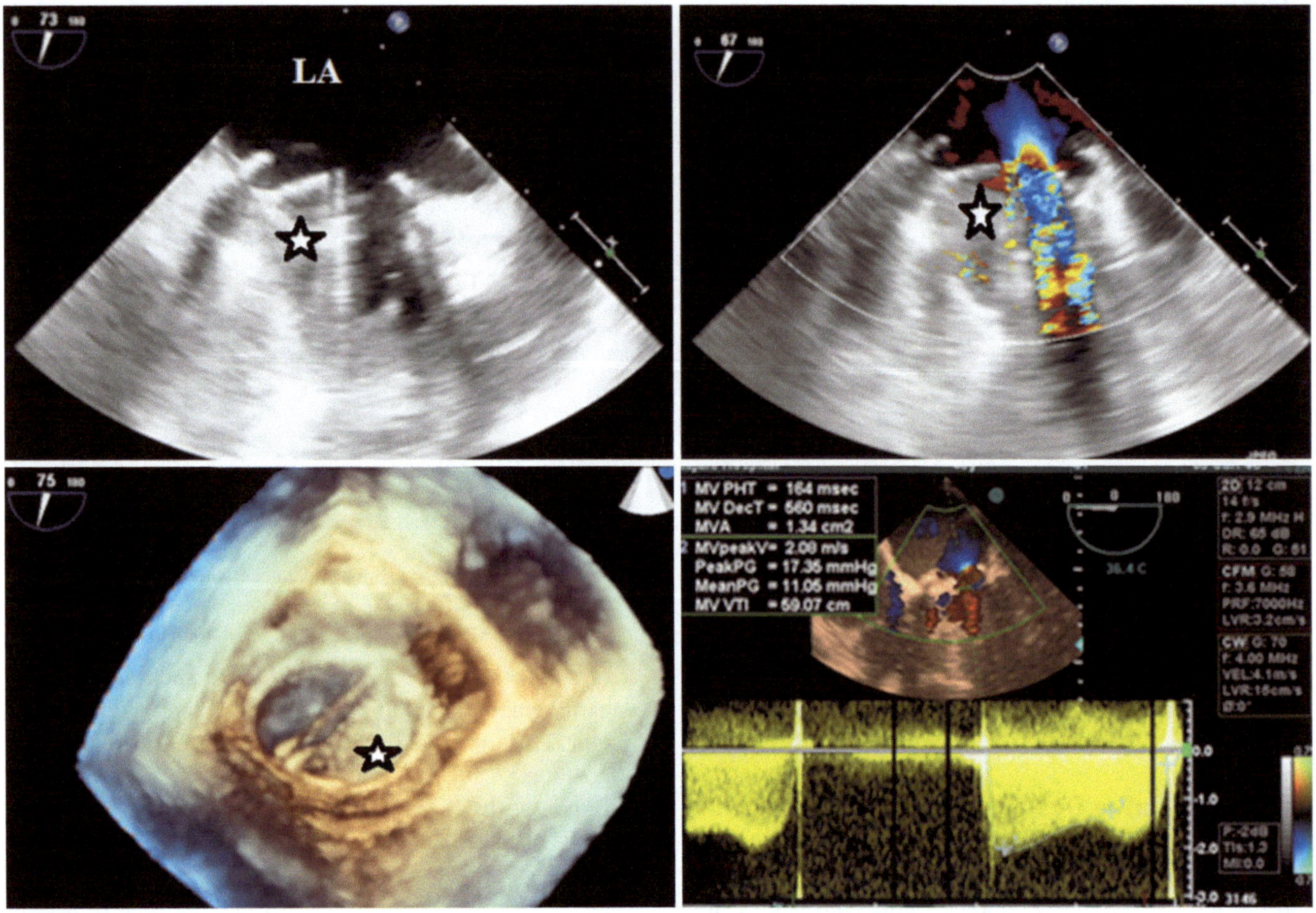

Fig. 18.13 (Movies 18.4, 18.5, and 18.6) Bileaflet mitral prostheses malfunction Left upper: Fixed medial leaflet in 2D TEE Right upper: fixed medial leaflet by color Doppler study Left lower: Fixed medial leaflet in 3D TEE Right lower: significant stenosis by Doppler study (Peak vel: 2 m/s, mean pressure gradient = 11 mmHg and pressure half time (PHT) 164 ms

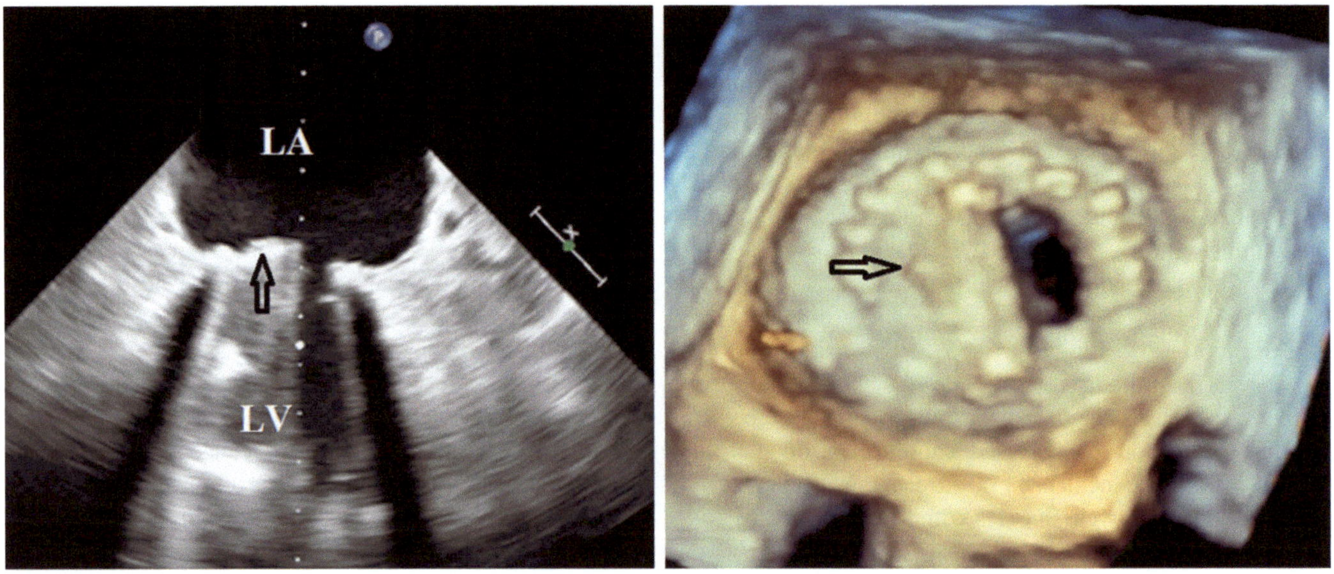

Fig. 18.14 Bileaflet mitral prostheses with stuck medial leaflet and thin layered thrombus on it (arrow) and open lateral leaflet in 2D TEE and 3D TEE

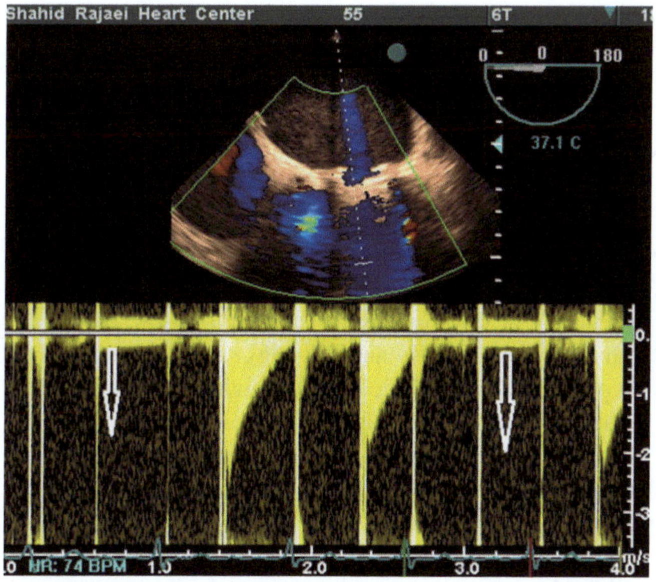

Fig. 18.15 (Movies 18.7 and 18.8) Intermittent obstruction by Doppler study (arrows) No diastolic Doppler flow despite the presence of the electrical and QRS activity

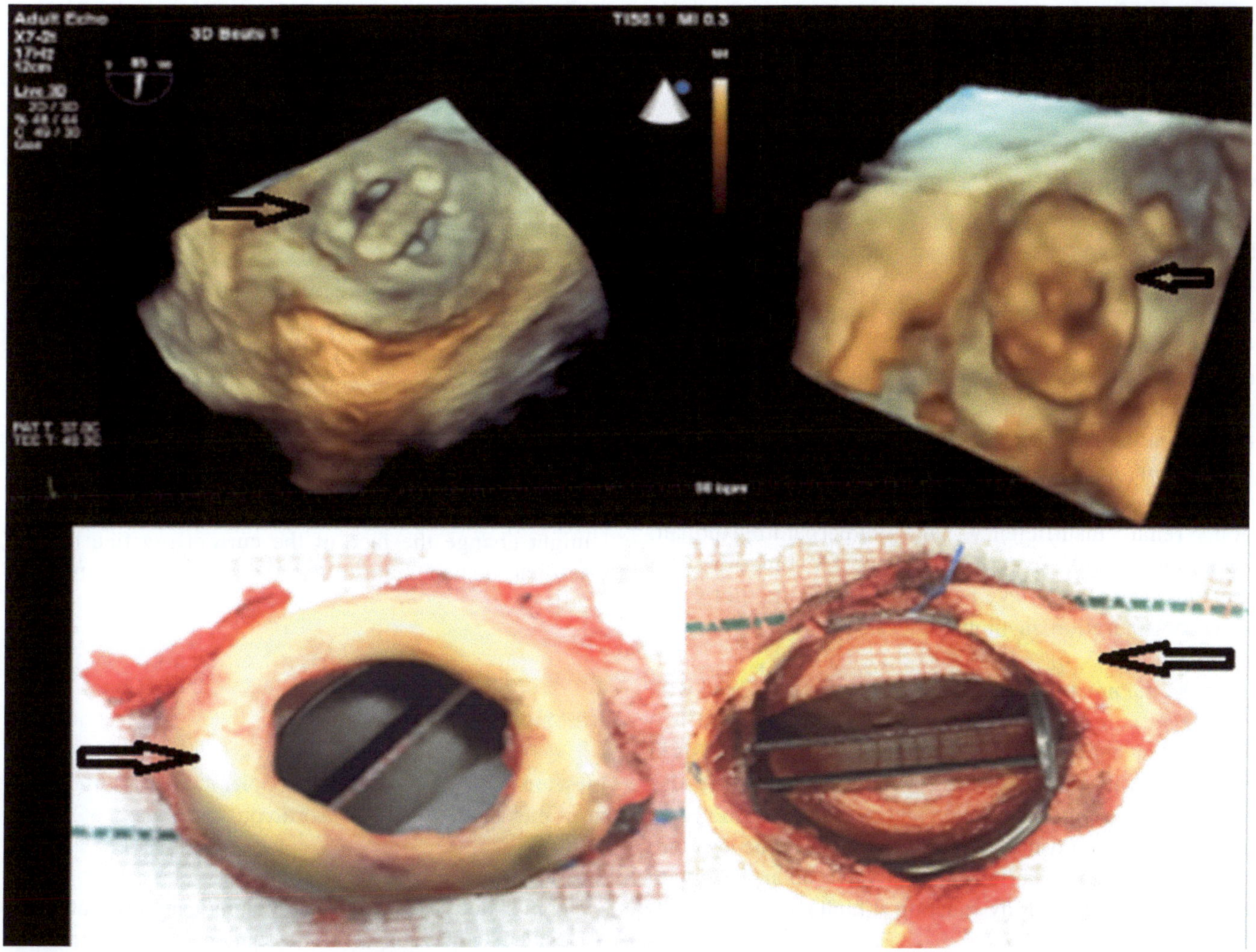

Fig. 18.16 Significant pannus ingrowth around bileaflet mitral prostheses (arrow) in a patient with sufficient anticoagulation and increased MV mean PG = 9 mmHg, PHT = 210 ms, EOA = 0.8 cm^2 and moderate PAH (PAP = 55–60 mmHg).Upper: 3D TEE

- Hence, correctly identifying the cause of prosthetic valve obstruction is critically important for management, so, the detection, evaluation, and also treatment of prosthetic valve obstruction are challenging.
- It has been suggested that multi detector CT (MDCT) may serve as an adjunct to TTE and TEE, for differentiating pannus from thrombus [12, 13].
- Gündüz et al. studied showed that periprostheses mass Hunsfiel unit (HU) value of ≥145 is highly suggestive for pannus ingrowth with a high sensitivity and specificity. The authors suggest that these values could be used clinically to guide treatment, with masses with a HU value ≥145 going directly to surgery and masses with a HU value <90 receiving thrombolytics [14].
- Of course, In the evaluation of cases with prosthetic valve obstruction, it must be remembered that pannus and thrombus not uncommonly coexist. As in one previous study both have been present in as many as 45% of obstructed mitral mechanical prostheses, so for the estimation of pannus or thrombus percentage in periprosthetic masses MDCT is recommended in concomitant with TTE and TEE [15, 16].

Valve Degeneration

Mechanical prostheses have an outstanding durability, and valve degeneration is very rare with new valves, although mechanical failure (e.g., strut fracture, leaflet seepage, and occluder dysfunction by lipid adsorption) has happened with some models in the past. The rate of valve degeneration in bioprosthetic valves rises over time, principally after the initial 7–8 years after insertion. Risk factors until that time found to be allied to bioprosthetic valve degeneration include young age, MV position, renal insufficiency, and hyperparathyroidism. Hypertension, LV hypertrophy, poor LV function, and prosthesis size also have been reported as predictors of valve degeneration in bioprostheses inserted in the AV position [1, 2, 5, 6].

In the pulmonary position, most valves are replaced with an allograft or xenograft and mechanical valves are less favorable given the theory of the higher risk of thrombosis in right-sided valves. Nevertheless, mechanical valves are also less likely to require reoperation and might be considered an alternative to bioprostheses (which are at risk of denegation) in patients with another mechanical valve or in those with severe right ventricular dysfunction at high risk for reoperation [17, 18].

Infective Endocarditis in Prosthetic Valves

- The incidence of prosthetic valve infective endocarditis (IE) is ≈0.5% per patient–year, even with suitable antibiotic prophylaxis. Prosthetic valve IE is an extremely serious condition with high mortality rates (30–50%). The diagnosis relies mainly on a combination of positive blood cultures and echocardiographic evidence of prosthetic infection-including vegetations, para-prosthetic abscesses, and new paravalvular regurgitation. TEE is crucial because of its greater sensitivity in detecting these abnormalities. Despite immediate and appropriate antibiotic treatment, many cases with prosthetic valve IE will eventually require surgery.
- Medical treatment alone is more likely to succeed in late prosthetic valve IE (occurring >6 months after surgery) and in non-staphylococcal infections. Surgery ought to be considered in the following situations: failure of medical treatment, hemodynamically significant prosthesis regurgitation (particularly if associated with deterioration of the LV function), large vegetations, and development of intracardiac fistulae [2, 4, 19].

Conclusions

In conclusion, all early and late complications of prosthetic valves can be evaluated by echocardiography. These complications include PPM, geometric mismatch, dehiscence, primary failure, thrombosis and thromboembolism, pannus formation, pseudoaneurysm formation, endocarditis, paravalvular leakage, and hemolysis.

Accordingly, rapid recognition of valve malfunction and dysfunction by echocardiography permits immediate treatment, frequently with repeat surgical intervention. Some recent developments-including the rapidly evolving field of percutaneous valve implantation and lifestyle and pharmacological interventions—for the prevention of bioprosthetic valve degeneration as well as patient self-management of oral anticoagulation might change the face of the current practice for the surgical management of valve disease in the future [1, 20].

Questions

Question 1 Based on the CW Doppler study of aortic prostheses the hemodynamic of Aortic prostheses is:

1. Normal
2. Doppler study is suggestive for significant obstruction
3. Doppler study is suggestive for significant regurgitation
4. Not enough data for interpretation

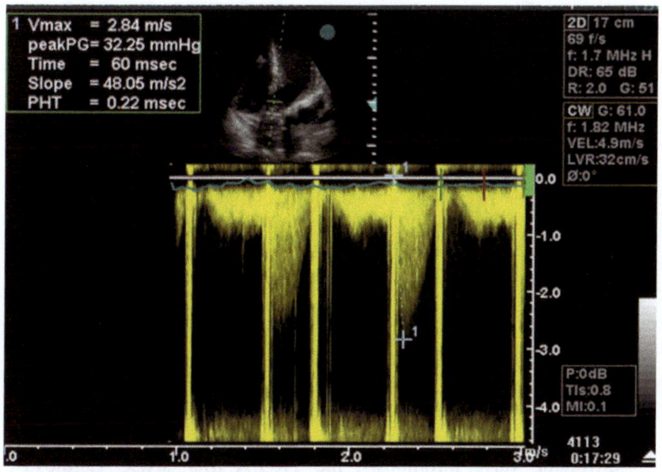

Question 2 CW Doppler study of the mitral prostheses in TEE 4c view shows:

1. Normal hemodynamic study of mitral prostheses
2. Significant increase of mean gradient, PHT and peak E velocity suggestive for valve obstruction
3. Significant increase of mean gradient, PHT and peak E velocity suggestive for para valve regurgitation
4. Not enough data for interpretation

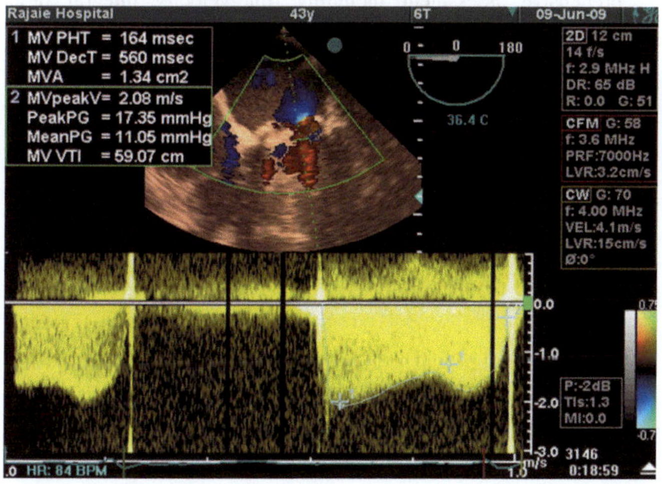

Question 3 In a patient with tachycardia and fever, aortic valve prostheses and significant paravalvulr leakage by color Doppler study, AV peak velovity = 3 m/s, AV mean PG = 28 mmHg, Doppler velocity index (DVI) = 0.35 and holo diastolic flow reversal in the descending thoracic aorta in TTE. Which of the following are not correct?

1. The patient has significant obstruction and significant regurgitation
2. The patient has non-significant obstruction and no significant regurgitation
3. The patient has non-significant obstruction and significant regurgitation
4. The patient has significant obstruction and non-significant regurgitation

Answers

Answer 1 The hemodynamic of aortic prostheses is normal regarding the Peal velocity 2.5 m/s and Aortic acceleration time 60 ms (normal is less than 80 ms)

Answer 2 Significant increase of mean gradient (above 6 mmHg), PHT >140 ms and peak E velocity are suggestive for valve obstruction. In case of valve regurgitation the PHT is normal or reduced

Answer 3 Based on the dimensionless velocity ratio there is no significant obstruction

DVI of the normally functioning AV prostheses is ≥0.30 and DVI <0.25 is highly suggestive of significant valve obstruction. DVI is not affected by high flow conditions such as Aortic regurgitation or high cordaia output, whereas blood velocity and gradient across the valve are affected.

References

1. Nishimura RA, Otto CM, Bonow RO, Carabello BA, Erwin JP, Guyton RA, O'Gara PT, Ruiz CE, Skubas NJ, Sorajja P, Sundt TM, Thomas JD. 2014 AHA/ACC Guideline for the management of patients with valvular heart disease. A report of the American College of Cardiology/American Heart Association Task Force on Practice Guidelines. Circulation. 2014;129:e521–643.
2. Zoghbi WA, Chambers JB, Dumesnil JG, Foster E, Gottdiener JS, Grayburn PA, Khandheria BK, Levine RA, Marx GR, Miller FA Jr, Nakatani S, Quiñones MA, Rakowski H, Leonardo Rodriguez L, Swaminathan M, Waggoner AD, Weissman NJ, Zabalgoitia M. Recommendations for evaluation of prosthetic valves with echocardiography and Doppler ultrasound. JASE. 2009;22(9):975–1014.
3. Pibarot P, Dumesnil JG. Prosthetic heart valves, selection of the optimal prosthesis and long-term management. Circulation. 2009;119:1034–48.
4. Bonow RO, Carabello BA, Kanu C, de Leon AC Jr, Faxon DP, Freed MD, Gaasch WH, Lytle BW, Nishimura RA, O'Gara PT, O'Rourke RA, Otto CM, Shah PM, Shanewise JS, Smith SC Jr, Jacobs AK, Adams CD, Anderson JL, Antman EM, Faxon DP, Fuster V, Halperin JL, Hiratzka LF, Hunt SA, Lytle BW, Nishimura R, Page RL, Riegel B. ACC/AHA 2006 guidelines for the management of patients with valvular heart disease: a report of the American College of Cardiology/American Heart Association Task Force on Practice Guidelines. Circulation. 2006;114:e84–e231.
5. Fernandes V, Olmos L, Nagueh SF, Quinones MA, Zoghbi WA. Peak early diastolic velocity rather than pressure half-time is

the best index of mechanical prosthetic mitral valve function. Am J Cardiol. 2002;89:704–10.

6. Mohty D, Dumesnil JG, Echahidi N, et al. Impact of prosthesis-patient mismatch on long-term survival after aortic valve replacement: influence of age, obesity, and left ventricular dysfunction. J Am Coll Cardiol. 2009;53:39–47.
7. Botzenhardt F, Eichinger WB, Bleiziffer S, Guenzinger R, Wagner IM, Bauernschmitt R, Lange R. Hemodynamic comparison of bioprostheses for complete supra-annular position in patients with small aortic annulus. J Am Coll Cardiol. 2005;45:2054–60.
8. Lancellotti P, Pibarot P, Chambers J, et al. Recommendations for the imaging assessment of prosthetic heart valves: a report from the European Association of cardiovascular imaging endorsed by the Chinese Society of Echocardiography, the Inter-American Society of Echocardiography, and the Brazilian Department of Cardiovascular Imaging. Eur Heart J Cardiovasc Imaging. 2016;17:589–90.
9. Merie C, Kober L, Skov Olsen P, et al. Association of warfarin therapy duration after bioprosthetic aortic valve replacement with risk of mortality, thromboembolic complications, and bleeding. JAMA. 2012;308:2118–25.
10. Bassiri HA, Sadeghpour A, Reshadati N, Kiavar M, Hashemi MJ. Detection of prosthetic valve non obstruction thrombosis: clinical significant and association. IHJ. 2009;10(2):A.
11. Kiavar M, Sadeghpour A, Bakhshandeh H, Bassiri H, Tayyebi P, Esmaeilzadeh M, Maleki M, Noohi F. Are prosthetic valve fibrin strands negligible? The associations and significance. J Am Soc Echocardiogr. 2009;22:890–4.
12. Teshima H, Hayashida N, Yano H, Nishimi M, Tayama E, Fukunaga S, Akashi H, Kawara T, Aoyagi S. Obstruction of St Jude Medical valves in the aortic position: histology and immunohistochemistry of pannus. J Thorac Cardiovasc Surg. 2003;126:401–7.
13. Barbetseas J, Nagueh SF, Pitsavos C, Toutouzas PK, Quiñones MA, Zoghbi WA. Differentiating thrombus from pannus formation in obstructed mechanical prosthetic valves: an evaluation of clinical, transthoracic and transesophageal echocardiographic parameters. J Am Coll Cardiol. 1998;32:1410–7.
14. Gündüz S, Ozcan M, Kalçık M, Gürsoy OM, Astarcıoğlu MA, Karakoyun S, Aykan AC, Biteker M, Gökdeniz T, Kaya H, Yesin M, Duran NE, Sevinç D, Güneysu T. Sixty-four-section cardiac computed tomography in mechanical prosthetic valve dysfunction: thrombus or pannus. Circ Cardiovasc Imaging. 2015;8:e003246. https://doi.org/10.1161/CIRCIMAGING.115.003246.
15. Vitale N, Renzulli A, Agozzino L, Pollice A, Tedesco N, de Luca Tupputi Schinosa L, Cotrufo M. Obstruction of mechanical mitral prostheses: analysis of pathologic findings. Ann Thorac Surg. 1997;63:1101–6.
16. Özkan M, Gündüz S, Biteker M, Astarcioglu MA, Çevik C, Kaynak E, Yıldız M, Oğuz E, Aykan AÇ, Ertürk E, Karavelioğlu Y, Gökdeniz T, Kaya H, Gürsoy OM, Çakal B, Karakoyun S, Duran N, Özdemir N. Comparison of different TEE-guided thrombolytic regimens for prosthetic valve thrombosis: the TROIA trial. JACC Cardiovasc Imaging. 2013;6:206–16. https://doi.org/10.1016/j.jcmg.2012.10.016.
17. Sadeghpour A, Kyavar M, Javani B, Bakhshandeh B, Maleki M, Khajali Z, Subrahmanyan L. Mid-term outcome of mechanical pulmonary valve prostheses: the importance of anticoagulation. J CardiovascThorac Res. 2014;6(3):163–8.
18. Sadeghpour A, Javani B, Peighambari M, Kyavar M, Khajali Z. Mid-term follow-up of pulmonary valve bioprostheses in adults with congenital heart disease. Anadolu Kardiyol Derg. 2012;12:434–6.
19. Piper C, Körfer R, Horstkotte D. VALVE DISEASE prosthetic valve endocarditis. Heart. 2001;85:590–3.
20. Blauwet LA, Malouf JF, Connolly HM, et al. Doppler echocardiography of 79 normal CarboMedics mitral prostheses: a comprehensive assessment including time-velocity integral ratio and prosthesis performance index. J Am Soc Echocardiogr. 2009;20:1125–30.

Infective Endocarditis

19

Trine K. Lauridsen and Anna Lisa Crowley

Abstract

Infective endocarditis (IE) is an infection of the endocardial lining of the heart, the heart valves, intracardiac devices or prosthetic valves. The infection is mainly localized on the valvular structures, on the low flow side of the valves or at locations with endocardial damage. In this chapter we will review the epidemiology of infective endocarditis (IE), the Modified Duke criteria for diagnosing IE and understand the role of echocardiography in the diagnosis of IE and complications, demonstrating echocardiograms of cases with native and prosthetic valve infective endocarditis, defining sensitivity and specificity of different echocardiographic modalities in native and prosthetic valve infective endocarditis and describing the diagnostic and prognostic role of echocardiographic findings in IE.

Keywords

Endocarditis · Cardiac infection · Valvular complications

Abbreviations

AV	Aortic valve
IE	Infective endocarditis
LA	Left atrium
LV	Left ventricle
LVOT	Left ventrivular outflow tract
MV	Mitral valve
RA	Right atrium
TEE	Transesophageal echocardiography
TTE	Transthoracic echocardiography

Objectives

1. To describe the epidemiology of infective endocarditis (IE).
2. To review the Modified Duke criteria for diagnosing IE and understand the role of echocardiography in the diagnosis of IE and complications.
3. To review echocardiograms of cases with native and prosthetic valve infective endocarditis
4. To define the sensitivity and specificity of different echocardiographic modalities in native and prosthetic valve infective endocarditis
5. To review the American and European Societal guideline recommendations for using echocardiography in cases of suspected IE.
6. To define the echocardiographic agreement in the diagnostic evaluation of IE.
7. To describe the prognostic role of echocardiographic findings in IE.

Infective Endocarditis [1, 2]

Infective endocarditis (IE) is an infection of the endocardial lining of the heart, the heart valves, intracardiac devices or prosthetic valves. The infection is mainly localized on the valvular structures, on the low flow side of the valves or at locations with endocardial damage.

Over time the clinical presentation of IE has changed markedly. Today the disease mainly affects the elderly population with severe comorbidities or pre-existing cardiac disease. Thus, the IE incidence has risen to 5–10 per 100,000 in industrial countries and the complication rate has remained high with a 1-year mortality of 20–40%

Electronic Supplementary Material The online version of this chapter (https://doi.org/10.1007/978-3-319-67691-3_19) contains supplementary material, which is available to authorized users.

T. K. Lauridsen, MD, PhD
Gentofte University Hospital, Copenhagen, Denmark

A. L. Crowley, MD (✉)
Duke University Medical Center, Durham, NC, USA
e-mail: annalisa.crowley@duke.edu

A. Sadeghpour, A. Alizadehasl (eds.), *Case-Based Textbook of Echocardiography*,
https://doi.org/10.1007/978-3-319-67691-3_19

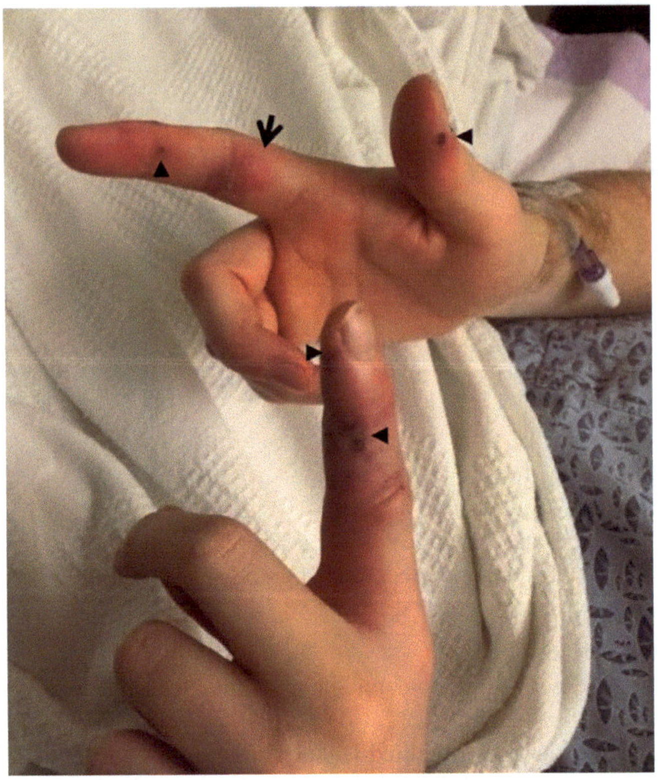

Fig. 19.1 A patient with *S. aureus* infective endocarditis demonstrating multiple immunologic Osler nodes (arrowheads) and a hemorrhagic Janeway lesion (*arrow*)

Table 19.1 Diagnosis of infective endocarditis by the modified Duke criteria (Li et al. Clin Infect Dis 30(4):633–638)

Modified duke criteria: diagnosis of infective endocarditis
Major criteria
Blood culture positive for IE
Typical microorganisms consistent with IE from two separate blood cultures:
Viridans streptococci, Streptococcus bovis, HACEK group, Staphylococcus aureus; or
Community-acquired enterococci, in the absence of a primary focus; or
Microorganisms consistent with IE from persistently positive blood cultures, defined as follows:
At least two positive cultures of blood samples drawn >12 h apart; or
All of three or a majority of four separate cultures of blood (with first and last sample drawn at least 1 h apart)
Single positive blood culture for Coxiella bumetii or antiphase 1 IgG antibody titer >1:800
Evidence of endocardial involvement
Echocardiogram positive for IE (TEE recommended in patients with prosthetic valves, rated at least “possible IE”
By clinical criteria, or complicated IE [paravalvular abscess]; TTE as first test in other patients), defined as follows :
Oscillating intracardiac mass on valve or supporting structures, in the path of regurgitant jets, or on implanted material in the absence of an alternative anatomic explanation; or
Abscess; or
New partial dehiscence of prosthetic valve
New valvular régurgitation (worsening or changing of pre-existing murmur not sufficient)
Minor criteria
Predisposition, predisposing heart condition or injection drug use
Fever, temperature >38°C
Vascular phenomena, major arterial emboli, septic pulmonary infarcts, mycotic aneurysm, intracranial hemorrhage, conjunctival hemorrhages, and Janeway's lesions Immunologie phenomena: glomerulonephritis, Osier's nodes. Roth’s spots, and rheumatoid factor
Microbiological evidence: positive blood culture but does not meet a major criterion as noted above or serological evidence of active infection with organism consistent with IE Echocardiographic minor criteria eliminated

despite advanced antibiotic treatment and novel surgical techniques.

In the era before echocardiography, IE was diagnosed clinically with pathognomonic findings of hemorrhagic or immunologic characteristics of the skin (Fig. 19.1) (Movies 19.1 and 19.2). With the introduction of echocardiography, the former necropsy pathognomonic cardiac vegetation became visible in vivo by two-dimensional transthoracic echocardiography images that allowed the recording of motion (M-mode) in 1968 and thereby added important imaging information to the clinical and serological criteria of IE diagnosis. Further, the development of echocardiographic imaging quality and emerging advanced echocardiographic techniques have allowed for valuable diagnostic and prognostic information on IE.

Echocardiography for the Diagnosis of IE [3–5]

The diagnosis of IE was first proposed in 1885 by professor Osler in the Gulstonian lectures of malignant endocarditis. Since then, several criteria for the diagnosis of IE were formulated including the von Reyn criteria for IE that base the diagnosis on the serologic and histopathologic findings of IE. The modified Duke criteria for IE were published in 2000 and included pathologic and clinical criteria for IE (Table 19.1). The modified Duke criteria were originally intended as a tool for epidemiological research for stratification of IE in definite IE, possible IE or rejected IE based on a set of major and minor criteria (Table 19.2). However, due to the validated strong diag-

Table 19.2 Definition of infective endocarditis by pathological and clinical criteria (Li et al. Clin Infect Dis 30(4):633–638)

Modified duke criteria: definition of infective endocarditis
Definite infective endocarditis
Pathologic criteria
1. Microorganisms demonstrated by culture or histologic examination of a vegetation, a vegetation that has embolized, or an intracardiac abscess specimen; or
2. Pathologic lesions; vegetation or intracardiac abscess confirmed by histologic examination showing active endocarditis
Clinical criteria
1. Two major criteria; or
2. One major criterion and three minor criteria; or
3. Five minor criteria
Possible infective endocarditis
1. One major criterion and one minor criterion; or
2. Three minor criteria
Rejected
1. Firm alternate diagnosis explaining evidence of infective endocarditis; or
2. Resolution of infective endocarditis syndrome with antibiotic therapy for <4 days; or
3. No pathologic evidence of infective endocarditis at surgery or autopsy, with antibiotic therapy for <4 days; or
4. Does not meet criteria for possible infective endocarditis, as above

nostic capacity of the modified Duke criteria, they currently function as an acknowledged diagnostic tool in the American Heart Association (AHA) guidelines for IE.

Key diagnostic echocardiographic findings in IE are vegetation, abscess, valvular dehiscense and new valvular regurgitation. A vegetation is defined as an irregularly shaped oscillating echogenic mass adherent to, yet distinct from, cardiac surfaces including valve structures, myocardium, and intra-cardiac devices. When evaluating echocardiograms for prosthetic valve endocarditis echocardiographic variables of main interest are new or worsening perivalvular regurgitation, valvular dehiscence and paravalvular complications such as abscess and pseudoaneurysm,which are often surgical emergencies.

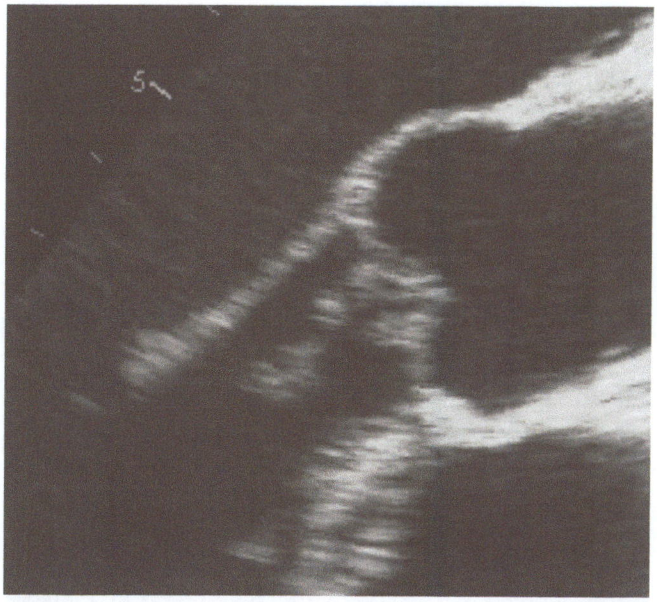

Fig. 19.2 Long axis TEE view showing the aortic valve with an oscillating vegetation on the non-coronary cusp

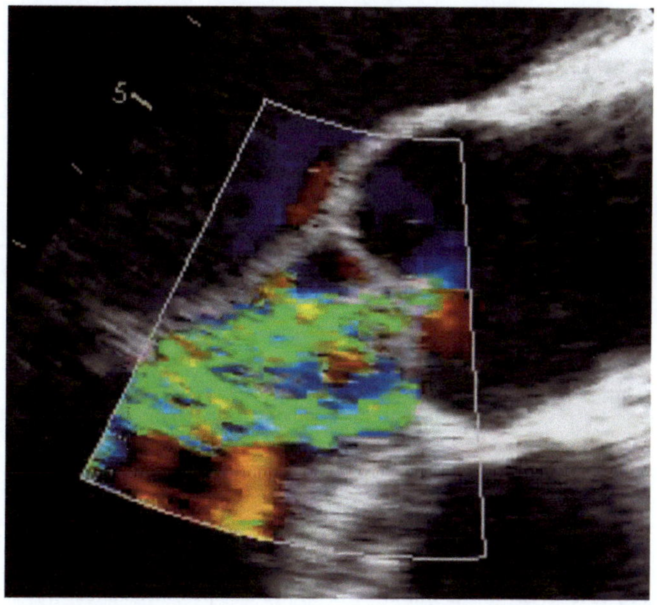

Fig. 19.3 Color Doppler reveals valvular destruction of the non-coronary cusp with severe aortic regurgitation

Native Valve IE Case

Case a_i: A 70-year old male with a history of prostate cancer presented with intermittent fever over the past 4 weeks. He was admitted with a urinary tract infection and treated with IV Ciprofloxacin. Four blood cultures grew *Enterococcus faecalis*. During admission he developed dyspnea and hypotension. TEE demonstrated a 15 mm definite vegetation on the non-coronary aortic cusp with destruction of the valve (Fig. 19.2) and severe aortic regurgitation (Fig. 19.3). The patient was referred for bioprosthetic aortic valve replacement (AHA Guidelines indication for early valve surgery, Class IIa, Level of Evidence B).

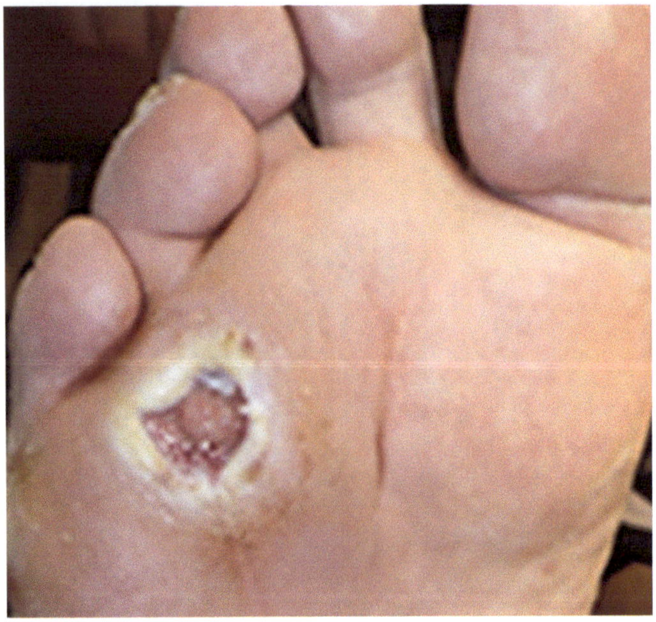

Fig. 19.4 1.0 × 1.5 cm large non-healing ulceration. Samples from surrounding skin and wound cultures grew S. aureus

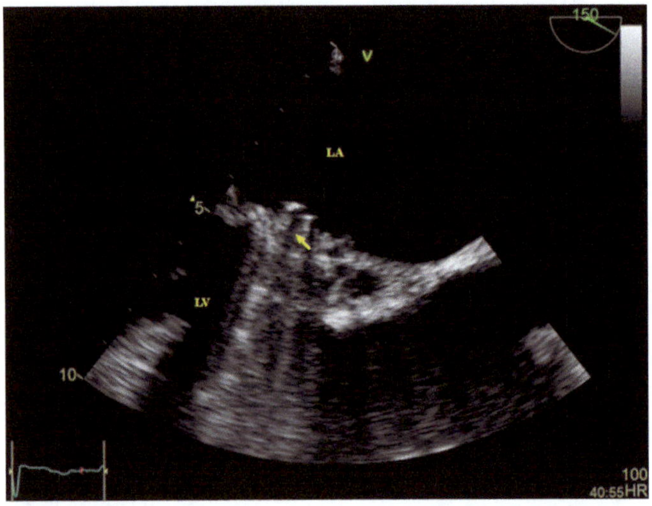

Fig 19.5 TEE of the mitral valve shows an open mechanical mitral valve (arrow). The acoustic shadow of the valve inducing visibility

Prosthetic Valve IE Case

Case a_{ii}: A 60-year old woman with a medical history of diabetes was admitted to a tertiary center with *S. aureus* bacteremia. Two years earlier she was treated for IE and underwent

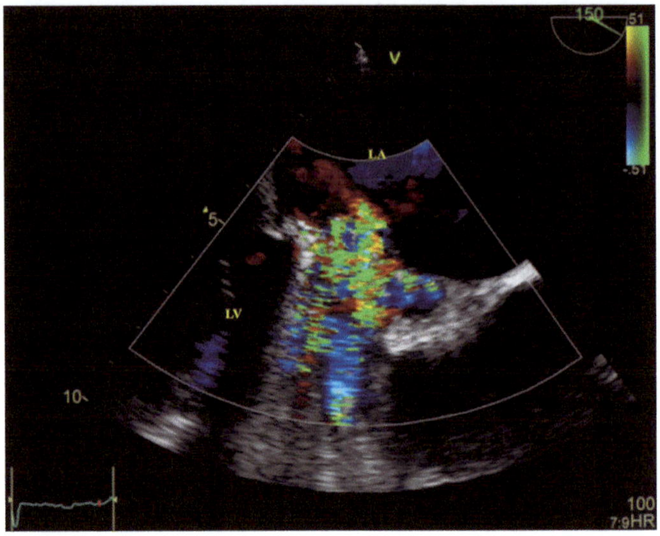

Fig. 19.6 TEE with color Doppler of the mechanical mitral valve reveals a severe perivalvular regurgitation

a mechanical mitral valve due to acute bacterial valvular destruction causing severe mitral regurgitation and heart failure. During past month, she developed recurrent *S. aureus* bacteremia due to a diabetic foot ulcer (Fig. 19.4) and was now admitted with high fever, chills and shortness of breath. TEE images of the mitral valve show new severe paravalvular regurgitation (Figs. 19.5 and 19.6).

Intracardiac Device IE

Case a_{iii}: A 55-year old male with known ischemic cardiomyopathy and primary prophylactic ICD was admitted with severe chest pain. Thoracic CT with contrast revealed a type B aortic dissection and the patient was referred for subacute surgery with insertion of a percutatenous stent in the descending aorta (Fig. 19.7). Six months later the patient was readmitted with chest pain and high fever. Blood cultures revealed coagulase negative staphylococci (CoNS) in five of six samples. TEE shows an 8 mm oscillating vegetation/thrombotic formation on the ICD lead in the right ventricle (Fig. 19.8). 18F–FDG PET/CT confirms the diagnosis of device IE and reveals infection corresponding to the thoracic stent (Fig. 19.9). In accordance with AHA guidelines the ICD system was removed and the patient treated with 6 weeks of intravenous antibiotics followed by a 3 month oral antibiotic regimen for TEVAR device infection.

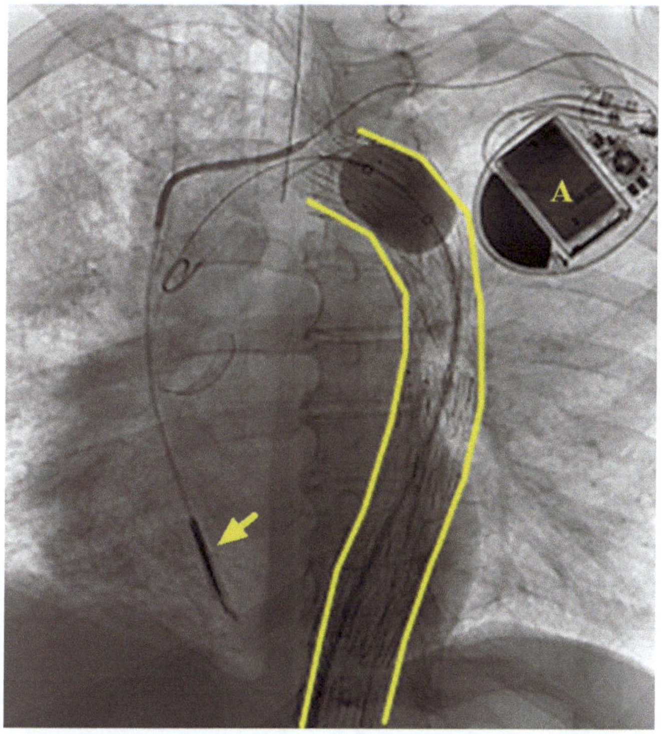

Fig. 19.7 Aortography of thoracic endovascular aortic repair (TEVAR) of the descending and abdominal aorta. Note the pacemaker pocket on the left chestwall (A) and the ICD lead in the right ventricle (yellow arrow)

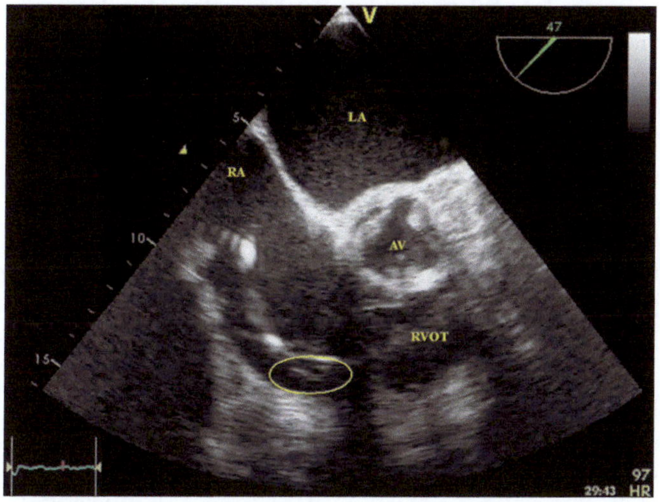

Fig. 19.8 TEE shows an oscillating 8 mm large vegetation on the ICD lead located in the right ventricle

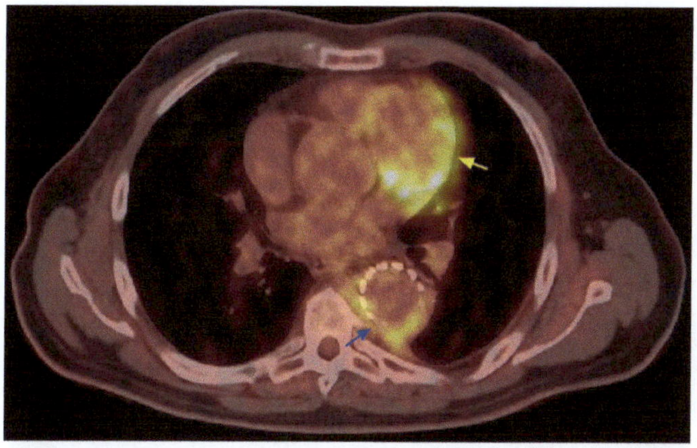

Fig. 19.9 PET/CT reveals infection in close relation to the TEVAR implant (blue arrow) and confirms the device infection corresponding to the ICD lead in the right ventricle (yellow arrow)

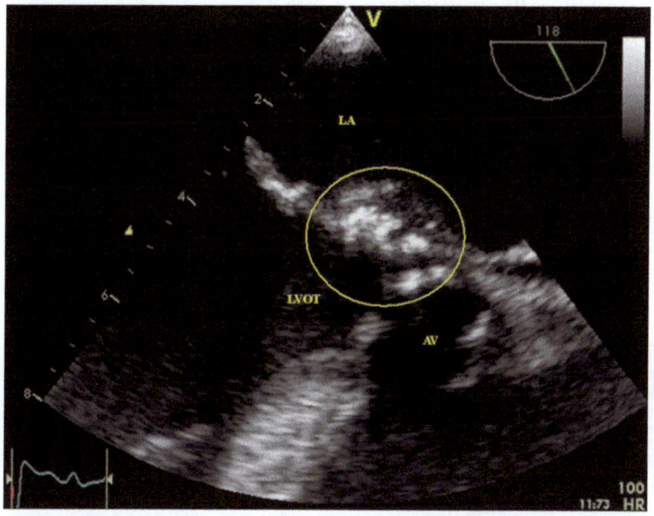

Fig. 19.10 An abscess is defined as a thickened area or mass within the myocardium or annular region with a non-homogeneous echogenic or echolucent appearance. Figure displays a long axis TEE view with an abscess in a typical area between the anterior mitral leaflet and LVOT. The patient underwent subacute aortic root surgery with insertion of an aortic root bioprothesis

Case Examples of Specific Complications

1. Abscess (Fig. 19.10)
2. Native valve perforation (Fig. 19.11)

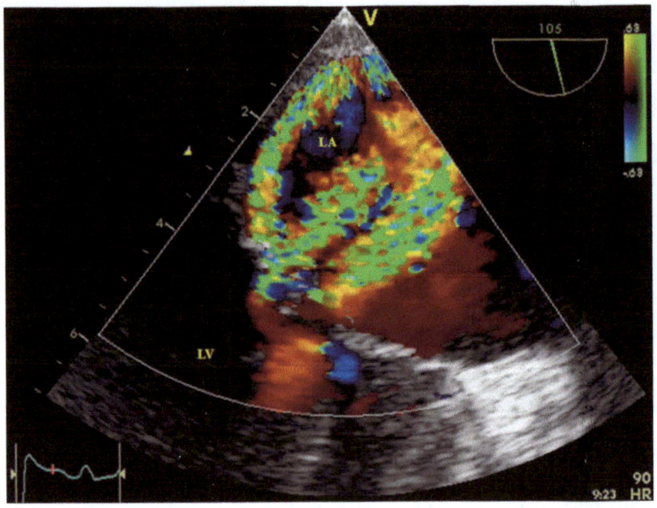

Fig. 19.11 Definition of a perforation is evidence of blood flow through a cardiac structure at a point that does not include the valve orifice. Figure displays a long axis TEE view with color Doppler with perforations of the mitral valve. Several regurgitant jets are seen through perforations in both the anterior and posterior leaflets. The patient underwent subacute cardiac surgery with mitral valve repair

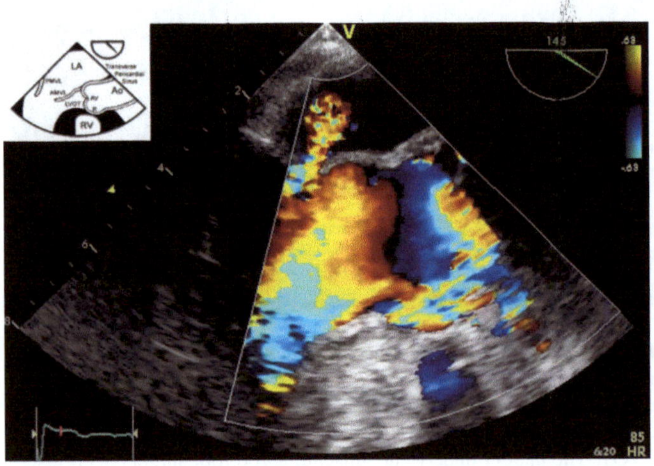

Fig. 19.12 A fistula is defined as a communication between two neighboring cavities through a perforation. Figure displays a longaxis TEE view of the aortic valve with color Doppler showing a communication between LVOT/base of the aortic root and the left atrium. The patient had severe aortic and mitral IE complicated by heart failure and was referred for acute cardiac surgery, but went into cardiac arrest without the ability to resuscitate.

3. Fistula (Fig. 19.12)
4. Prosthetic valve dehiscence (Fig. 19.13)
5. Pseudoaneurysm of the mitral aortic intervalvular fibrosa (Fig. 19.14)

Sensitivity and Specificity of TTE and TEE in IE [6–9]

The sensitivity for diagnosing vegetations in native valves is 70% for TTE and >95% for TEE. For diagnosis of vegetations in prosthetic valves the numbers are significantly lower with only 50% sensitivity for TTE and 90% for TEE. Identification of vegetations is difficult in the presence of pre-existing valvular lesions such as calcified lesions or mitral valve prolapse. Similarly, the acoustic shadow of a prosthetic valve may induce reverberation artifacts resulting in false negative echocardiograms. Further, the diagnosis is challenging in case of small vegetations (<5 mm), recent embolization of the vegetation and in nonvegetant IE. Accordingly, valvular perforation, mitral lesions and aneurysms are best assessed using TEE. However, TTE plays a central role in early diagnosis of both native and prosthetic IE to evaluate the haemodynamic consequences of valvular dysfunction, measurement of pulmonary artery pressure, detection of pericardial effusion and assessment and monitoring of left ventricular systolic function.

TEE is superior to TTE in detecting paravalvular complications of IE. The sensitivity of TTE for detecting an abscess is less than 50%, whereas TEE markedly improves the sensitivity for defining paravalvular complications of IE (75–100%) while preserving excellent specificity (95%) and positive and negative predictive values (88% and 87%, respectively). When combined with color Doppler techniques, TEE is superior to TTE for revealing the distinctive flow patterns of fistulas and pseudoaneurysms and to rule out communications from unruptured abscess cavities. Thus, TEE is recommended for the initial assessment of patients suspected of having paravalvular complications to IE.

Guideline Recommended Algorithms for Using Echocoardiography to Diagnose IE [3, 4]

In the European guidelines, TTE is recommended initially in suspected IE followed by TEE in all cases except low clinical suspicion of IE (Fig. 19.15). Interestingly, the American Heart Association guidelines do not recommend TEE in patients with a positive TTE if no high risk echocardiographic features are present (Fig. 19.16). Further, the AHA guidelines divide patients into low, moderate or high clinical suspicion of IE, whereas the ESC guidelines only use existing or nonexisting clinical suspicion. In both guidelines, repeat echocardiogram is recommended if the initial echocardiogram was negative but a high clinical suspicion of IE remains.

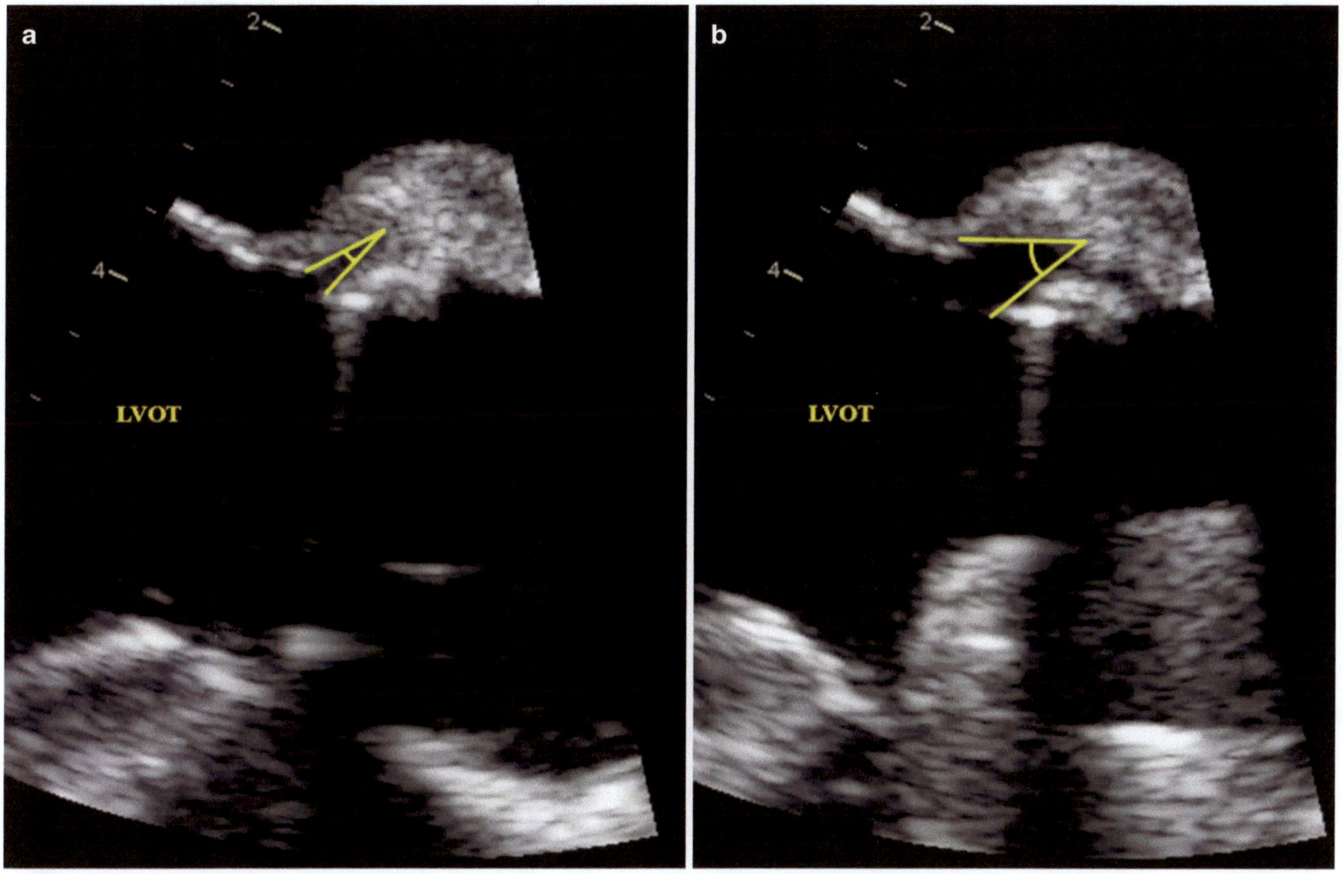

Fig. 19.13 New valvular dehiscence of a prosthetic valve is pathognomonic for IE. It is defined as paravalvular regurgitation by echocardiography, with or without rocking motion of the prosthesis. Figure panel A and B display a longaxis TEE view of a prosthetic aortic valve with a 25° rocking motion between the valve and the aortic root from early (A) to late (B) systole. Color Doppler demonstrate severe paravalvular regurgitation (C)

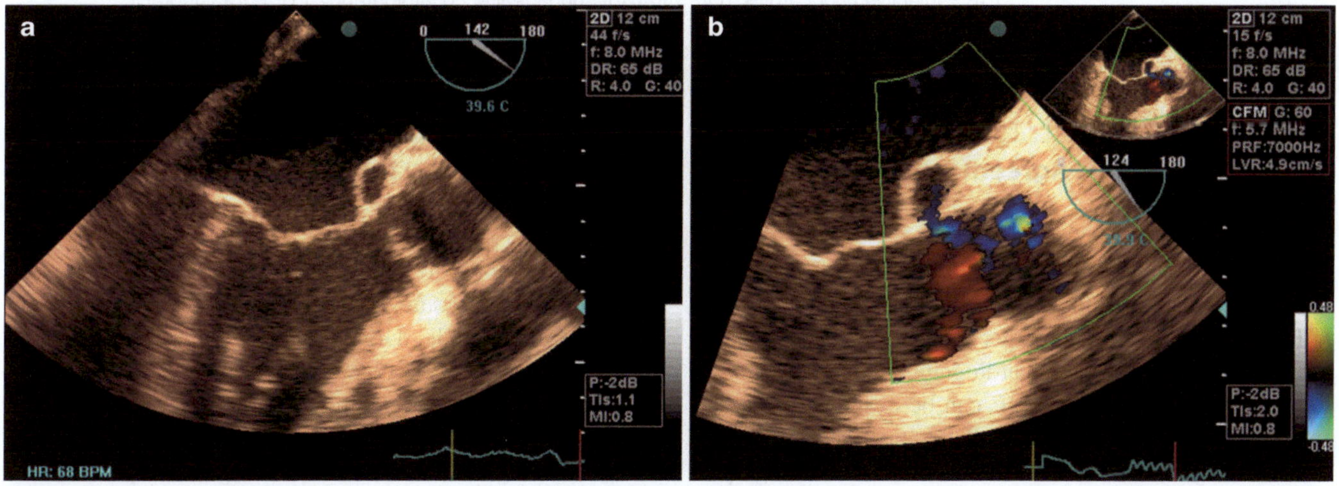

Fig. 19.14 A rare complication of endocarditis is a pseudoaneurysm of the mitral aortic intervalvular fibrosa (MAIVF). MAIVF is fibrous and avascular tissue in the region of the mitral-aortic continuity and the weakest segment of the aortic ring, prone to infection and trauma. (**a**) The TEE image in demonstrates the characteristic dynamic expansion during early systole and collapse in diastole. (**b**) demonstrates communication with the LV outflow track

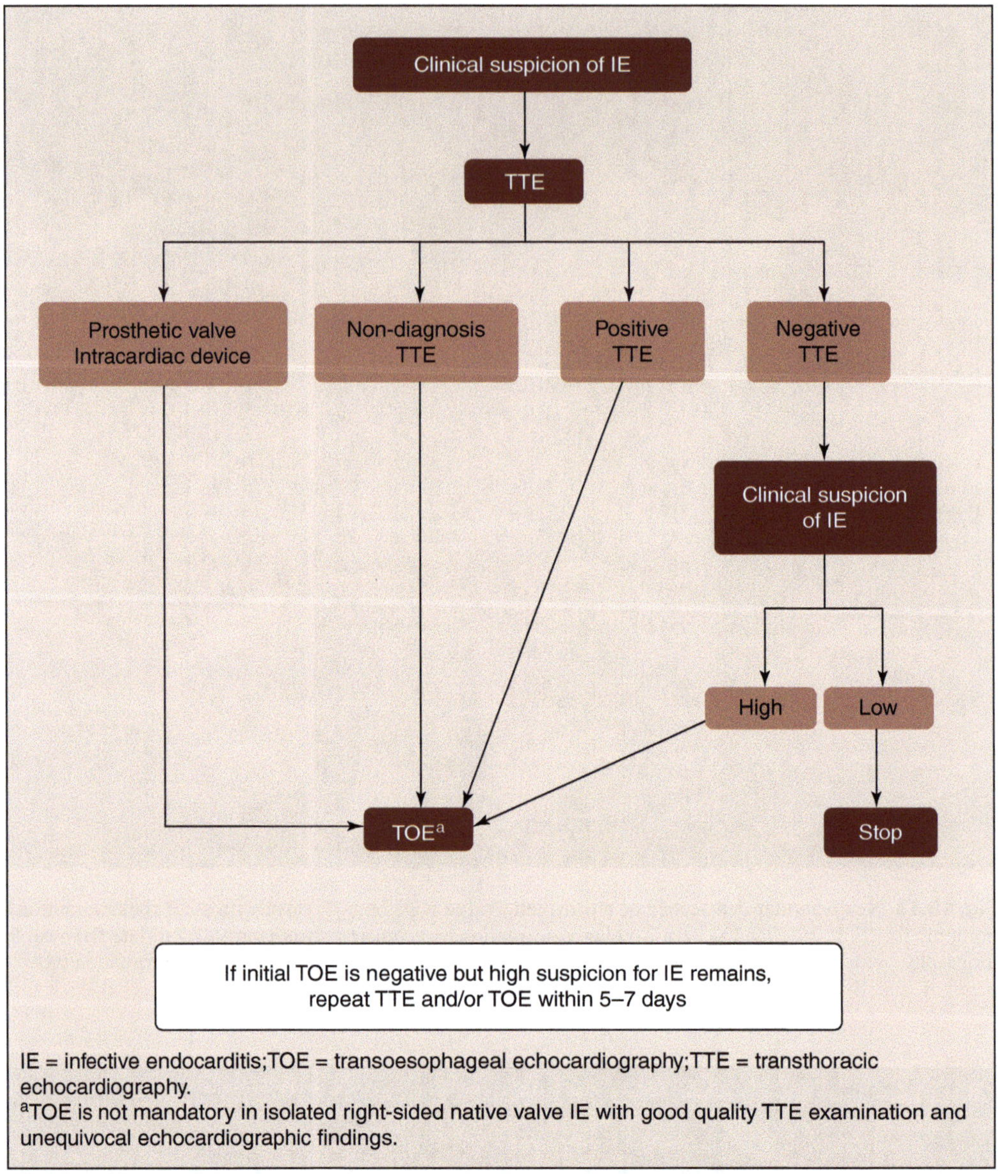

Fig. 19.15 ESC recommendations for the indications for echocardiography in suspected infective endocarditis

Echocardiographic Agreement in Evaluation of IE [10]

Comparing the accuracy of echocardiographic interpretations to a gold standard of pathology is only possible in examination of IE patients that undergo surgery or autopsy. In the absence of these gold standards, echocardiographic reproducibility for the diagnostic assessment of IE can be examined. A recent study from the International Collaboration of Endocarditis found that agreement in the assessment of echocardiographic variables associated with diagnosis and complications of IE is moderate to excellent, with highest agreement for LVEF, aortic abscess and the presence and location of vegetations. Lowest agreement was acquired for vegetation mobility. The Interobserver agreement for diagnostic variables is substantial to excellent for both TTE and TEE (Table 19.3).

Echocardiography for the Prognosis of IE [11–13]

Echocardiographic markers have been studied with regard to predicting outcome in left-sided IE with conflicting results. For example, large or highly mobile vegetations have been studied as potential risk factors for embolic events and mortality. Yet, studies regarding vegetation size report discordant results. Large, prospective studies have found that vegetation size was an independent predictor of embolic events and mortality, while others found that vegetation size was independently associated with embolic events, but not mortality.

Echocardiographic predictors of mortality have been studied in a large international prospective cohort from the International Collaboration on Endocarditis. For *S. aureus*

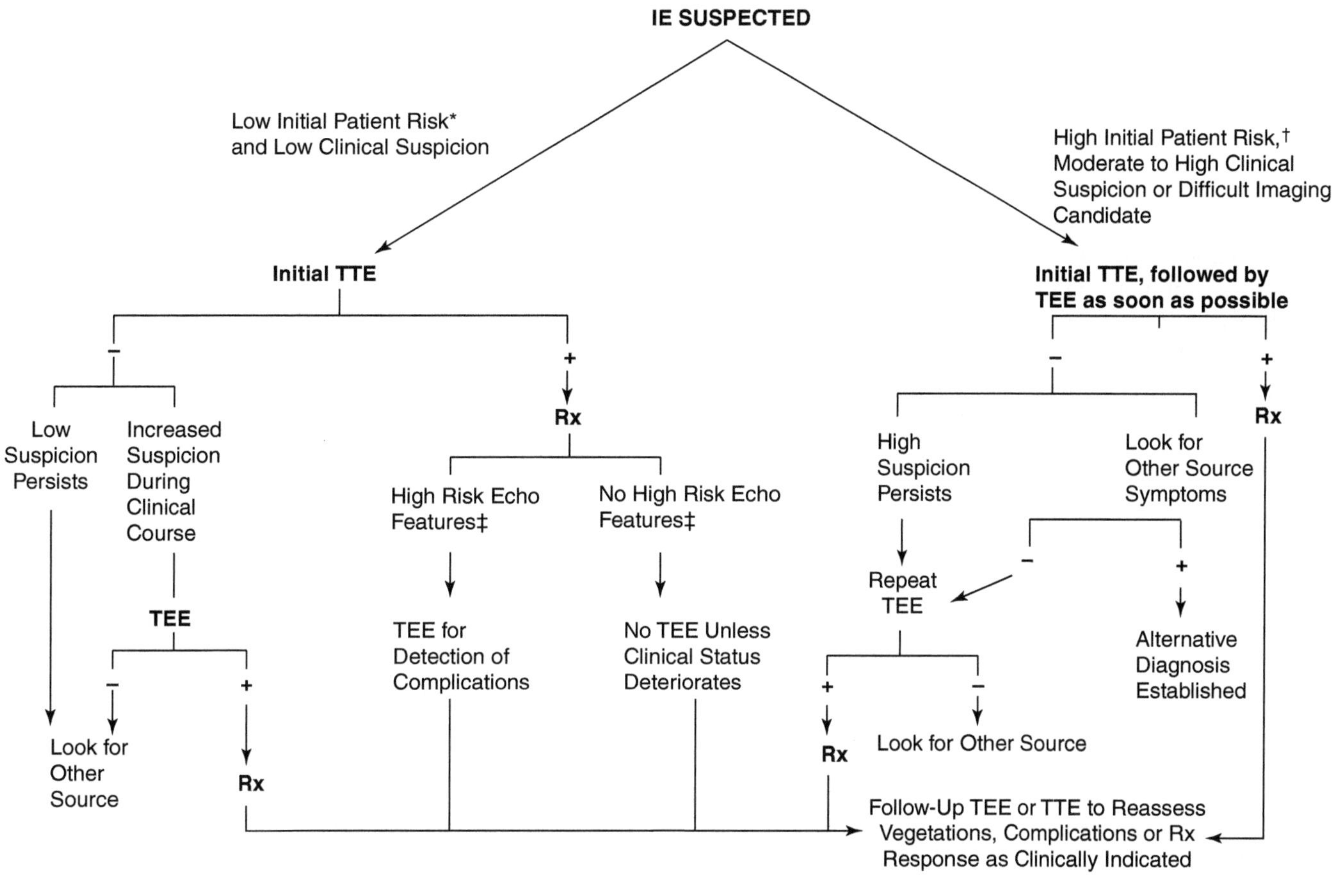

Fig. 19.16 AHA recommendations for the indications for echocardiography in suspected infective endocarditis. Rx indicates prescription. †High initial patient risks include prosthetic heart valves, many congenital heart diseases, previous endocarditis, new murmur, heart failure, or other stigmata of endocarditis. ‡High-risk echo-cardiographic features include large or mobile vegetations, valvular insufficiency, suggestion of perivalvular extension, or secondary ventricular dysfunction

Table 19.3 Inter-observer agreement stratified by type of echocardiogram: TTE or TEE

	Transthoracic Echocardiogram $\kappa_{weighted}$ (95% CI) (n = 47)	Transesophageal Echocardiogram $\kappa_{weighted}$ (95% CI) (n = 63)
Vegetation present		
Mitral vegetation	0.79 (0.71, 0.98)	0.95 (0.90, 0.99)
Aortic vegetation	0.91 (0.80, 1.00)	0.89 (0.80, 0.99)
Tricuspid veg	0.96 (0.92, 1.00)	0.89 (0.78, 1.00)
Device vegetation	0.66 (0.03, 1.00)	1.00
Valvular regurgitation		
Mitral regurgitation	0.75 (0.62, 0.87)	0.89 (0.83, 0.95)
Aortic regurgitation	0.84 (0.73, 0.96)	0.93 (0.88, 0.97)
Tricuspid regurg.	0.61 (0.35, 0.86)	0.68 (0.49, 0.88)
Complications present		
Perforation mitral	0.45 (0.01, 0.90)	0.94 (0.82, 1.00)
Perforation aortic	0.79 (0.39, 1.00)	1.00
Abscess mitral	0.37 (0.00, 0.93)	1.00
Abscess aortic	0.79 (0.39, 1.00)	0.80 (0.61, 0.99)
Vegetation characteristics		
Vegetation mobility	0.58 (0.21, 0.95)	0.72 (0.55, 0–89)
Vegetation size	0.74 (0.57, 0.90)	0.74 (0.57, 0.90)

left-sided IE, specific predictors of in-hospital mortality are presence of an abscess or impaired systolic function (LVEF <40%). Similarly, heart failure as a complication to IE is the main cause of mortality in IE.

Identification of echocardiographic predictors of outcome that can be revealed at time of diagnosis can add valuable information, not only for diagnosis and extent of cardiac complications, but also for early patient risk stratification and referral for surgery.

Key Points

- The incidence of Infective Endocarditis is increasing and the complications and mortality remain high despite advanced antibiotic and surgical therapies.
- Echocardiography plays a key role in diagnosing endocarditis in the modified Duke criteria.
- The sensitivity and specificity of transthoracic and transesophageal echocardiography for diagnosing IE and complications vary depending on modality and the presence of native or prosthetic material.
- European and American societies have published guidelines with recommended diagnostic algorithms for the use of echocardiography in patients suspected of having IE.
- Some echocardiographic variables have been identified as prognostically important which can help risk stratify patients at the time of diagnosis for early antibiotic and/or surgical therapies.

Questions

1. A 64 year old patient with a prosthetic aortic valve is admitted to the hospital for the evaluation of a 2 week history of increasing dyspnea and fevers. An echocardiogram was obtained that shows aortic valve dehiscence with severe transvalvular and paravalvular aortic regurgitation. After obtaining blood cultures, your next best step for this patient is to:
   A. Repeat the transthoracic echocardiogram in 1 week to assess for interval change if the clinical suspicion for IE persists.
   B. Obtain a transesophageal echocardiogram since transesophageal echocardiography has increased sensitivity for diagnosing IE complications with prosthetic valves
   C. Begin broad spectrum antibiotics and refer the patient to surgery emergently
   D. Wait for blood culture positivity and susceptibility testing to begin appropriate antibiotic therapy.

2. Which of the following presentations is most likely to be associated with vegetations on the anterior tricuspid valve leaflet:
   A. Brain abscess
   B. Septic pulmonary emboli
   C. Mycotic aortic aneurysm
   D. Splenic infarct.

3. A patient is admitted with fevers and a positive blood culture for *Staphylococcus aureus*. A high quality transthoracic echocardiogram is normal. An indwelling catheter was the presumed source and removed. The patient was treated with appropriate antibiotic therapy, the fevers resolved and follow up blood cultures were negative. The next best step in the management of this patient is to:
   A. Repeat the transthoracic echocardiogram after 1 week of antibiotic therapy.
   B. Perform a TEE as soon as possible to assess for IE complications better seen on TEE.
   C. Continue appropriate antibiotic therapy for 2 weeks and repeat echocardiography is not indicated.
   D. Repeat a transthoracic echocardiogram after 2 weeks of appropriate antibiotic therapy.

Answers

1. C
   This patient has a prosthetic aortic valve dehiscence with anterior paravalvular regurgitation. This patient should be started on broad spectrum antibiotics and referred for surgery emergently. Answers A, B, and C are not correct since the patient has an IE complication that is readily seen on the TTE and surgery is indicated in addition to immediate treatment with broad spectrum antibiotics.
2. B
   Right sided vegetations would be compatible with the clinical scenario of septic pulmonary emboli. All other findings would be expected with left sided infective endocarditis.
3. C
   Continue appropriate antibiotic therapy for 2 weeks and repeat echocardiography is not indicated. This patient had no findings compatible with IE on a high quality initial transthoracic echocardiogram and a source was identified and removed. The patients fevers resolved and follow up blood cultures were negative for *S. aureus*. In this case, repeat echocardiography is not indicated. All other choices include repeating echocardiography.

References

1. Holland TL, Baddour LM, Bayer AS, Hoen B, Miro JM, Fowler VG Jr. Infective endocarditis. Nat Rev Dis Primers. 2016;2:16059. https://doi.org/10.1038/nrdp.2016.59.
2. Cahill TJ, Prendergast BD. Infective endocarditis. Lancet. 2016;387(10021):882–93. https://doi.org/10.1016/S0140-6736(15)00067-7. Epub 2015 Sep 1 Review
3. Baddour LM, Wilson WR, Bayer AS, Fowler VG Jr, Tleyjeh IM, Rybak MJ, et al. American Heart Association Committee: Infective endocarditis in adults: diagnosis, antimicrobial Therapy, and management of complications: a scientific statement for healthcare

professionals from the American Heart Association. Circulation. 2015;132(15):1435–86.
4. Habib G, Lancellotti P, Antunes MJ, Bongiorni MG, Casalta JP, Del Zotti F, et al. 2015 ESC Guidelines for the management of infective endocarditis: the Task Force for the Management of Infective Endocarditis of the European Society of Cardiology (ESC). Endorsed by: European Association for Cardio-Thoracic Surgery (EACTS), the European Association of Nuclear Medicine (EANM). Eur Heart J. 2015;36(44):3075–128.
5. Li JS, Sexton DJ, Mick N, Nettles R, Fowler VG Jr, Ryan T, et al. Proposed modifications to the Duke criteria for the diagnosis of infective endocarditis. Clin Infect Dis. 2000;30:633–8.
6. Habib G, Badano L, Tribouilloy C, Vilacosta I, Zamorano JL, Galderisi M, et al. Recommendations for the practice of echocardiography in infective endocarditis. Eur J Echocardiogr. 2010;11:202–19.
7. Reynolds HR, Jagen MA, Tunick PA, Kronzon I. Sensitivity of transthoracic versus transesophageal echocardiography for the detection of native valve vegetations in the modern era. J Am Soc Echocardiogr. 2003;16:67–70.
8. Mugge A, Daniel WG, Frank G, Lichtlen PR. Echocardiography in infective endocarditis: reassessment of prognostic implications of vegetation size determined by the transthoracic and the transesophageal approach. J Am Coll Cardiol. 1989;14:631–8.
9. Daniel WG, Mügge A, Martin RP, Lindert O, Hausmann D, Nonnast- Daniel B, et al. Improvement in the diagnosis of abscesses associated with endocarditis by transesophageal echocardiography. N Engl J Med. 1991;324:795–800.
10. Lauridsen TK, Selton-Suty C, Tong S, Afonso L, Cecchi E, Park L, et al. Echocardiographic agreement in the diagnostic evaluation for infective endocarditis. Int J Cardiovasc Imaging. 2016;32(7): 1041–51.
11. Thuny F, Di Salvo G, Belliard O, Avierinos JF, Pergola V, Rosenberg V, et al. Risk of embolism and death in infective endocarditis: prognostic value of echocardiography: a prospective multicenter study. Circulation. 2005;112(1):69–75. Epub 2005 Jun 27. Erratum in: Circulation. 2005 Aug 30;112(9)
12. Lauridsen TK, Park L, Tong SY, Selton-Suty C, Peterson G, Cecchi E, et al. Echocardiographic findings predict in-hospital and 1-year mortality in left-sided native valve Staphylococcus aureus endocarditis: analysis from the international collaboration on endocarditis-prospective Echo Cohort study. Circ Cardiovasc Imaging. 2015;8(7):e003397.
13. Kiefer T, Park L, Tribouilloy C, Cortes C, Casillo R, Chu V, et al. Association between valvular surgery and mortality among patients with infective endocarditis complicated by heart failure. JAMA. 2011;306(20):2239–4.

Pericardial Diseases

20

Michael Chetrit and Vartan Mardigyan

Abstract

The pericardium is a thin fibroelastic sac, comprised of both a serous visceral and fibrous parietal layer, which surrounds the heart and the great vessels. Echocardiography remains the initial imaging modality of choice and should be performed as a complete study or as a point of care when suspecting acute pericarditis. Presence of an abnormal septal motion from right to left in early diastole during inspiration, the presence of a plethoric IVC and dilated hepatic veins, and evidence of ventricular interdependence are the cornerstones of constrictive pericarditis physiology. Annulus paradoxus and annulus reversus are also strong indicators of constrictive pericarditis. The location, size, extent of the pericardial effusion and presence of loculations should be characterized using all four echocardiographic windows including PSLAX, PSAX, Apical, and the Subcostal views. Chamber collapse is an important indicator of the presence of tamponade physiology along with a septal bulge and peak mitral and tricuspid E-inflow velocity respiratory variation. Most cases of cardiac tamponade are treated with a pericardiocentesis.

Keywords

Acute pericarditis · Pericardial effusion · Effusive constrictive pericarditis · Constrictive pericarditis · Tamponade · Pericardiocentesis

Abbreviations

2D	Two dimensional
3D	Three dimensional
ASA	Aspirin
CMR	Cardiac magnetic resonance
CP	Constrictive pericarditis
CRP	C-reactive protein
EF	Ejection fraction
E	Peak E-wave velocity of the mitral valve (cm/sec)
e′	TDI of the mitral annulus
EKG	Electrocardiogram
IVC	Inferior vena cava
LA	Left atrium
LV	Left ventricular
LVEF	Left ventricular ejection fraction
NSAID	Non-steroidal anti-inflammatory drug
PSLAX	Parasternal long axis
PSAX	Parasternal short axis
RV	Right ventricle
STE	Speckle-tracking echocardiography
TDI	Tissue Doppler imaging
TEE	Transesophageal echocardiography
TTE	Transthoracic echocardiography

Introduction

- **The pericardium is a thin fibroelastic sac, comprised of a visceral and parietal layer, which surrounds the heart and the great vessels. The normal pericardial cavity contains less than 50 cc of serous fluid** [1–4]. Pericardial diseases are common in clinical practice and have been reported to have significant morbidity and mortality [5, 6]. Diseases such as acute pericarditis, pericardial tamponade and constrictive pericarditis can be isolated in nature or a manifestation of a systemic process [7–9]. Echocardiography allows for the evaluation of the pericardium by two-dimensional imaging and hemodynamics by doppler methods [7].
- **A healthy pericardium appears as a thin hyperechogenic structure with echocardiography. Its normal thickness is less than 3 mm** and only under pathological states will the visceral and parietal layers become apparent [10].

M. Chetrit, MD, FRCPC · V. Mardigyan, MD, FRCPC (✉)
The McGill University Health Centre, Montreal, Quebec, Canada
e-mail: vartan.mardigyan@mail.mcgill.ca

A. Sadeghpour, A. Alizadehasl (eds.), *Case-Based Textbook of Echocardiography*,
https://doi.org/10.1007/978-3-319-67691-3_20

Acute Pericarditis

- **Acute pericarditis is the most common form of pericardial disease worldwide and can be associated with significant morbidity** [11]. **In the western world, the most common form is idiopathic pericarditis.** In a small percentage of cases, specific etiologies can be identified such as infectious, autoimmune, neoplastic, and iatrogenic. (Table 20.1)
- **Patients present with pleuritic chest pain (85–90% of cases), a pericardial friction rub (less than 33%), typical changes on electrocardiogram (60% of cases) and a pericardial effusion (60%). The presence of two or more of these features allows for the diagnosis of acute pericarditis.**
- The presence of an elevated CRP can be useful for the diagnosis and follow-up of patients to document biochemical resolution. **In the setting of diagnostic uncertainty, delayed gadolinium enhancement of the pericardium on CMR has been shown to be of value** [8–15].

Table 20.1 Etiologies of pericarditis

Idiopathic	Most common cause
Infectious	Viral: Enteroviruses, Ebstein-Barr Virus, Coxsackieviruses, herpes viruses, adenoviruses
	Bacterial: *Mycobacterium Tuberculosis, Coxiella Burnetti, Borrelia Burgdoferi*
	Fungal: *Histoplasma* species, *Aspergillus, Blastomyces* and *Candida* species
	Parasitic: *Toxoplasma* species, *Echinococcus*
	Infective Endocarditis (extension)
Autoimmune and Auto-inflammatory	Connective Tissue Diseases: Systemic lupus erythematosus, Sjogrens syndrome, rheumatoid arthritis, scleroderma
	Vasculitis: eosinophilic granulomatosis with polyangiitis, Takayasu disease, Horton's disease, Behçet's syndrome
	Auto inflammatory diseases: Familial Mediterranean fever, tumor necrosis factor receptor-associated periodic syndrome
	Sarcoidosis
	Post myocardial infarction: Dressler's
Neoplastic	Primary cardiac tumors: pericardial mesothelioma
	Secondary Metastatic tumors: lung cancer, breast cancer and lymphoma
Metabolic	Uremia/Dialysis
	Myxedema/Hypo-hyperthyroidsim
	Anorexia nervosa
Traumatic	Direct or indirect thoracic injury
	Radiation injury
	Post myocardial injury
Iatrogenic	Post coronary percutaneous intervention
	Post pacemaker lead insertion
	Post radiofrequency ablation
	Post radiation
Drug related	Hypersensitivity pericarditis with eosinophilia
	Pericardial and myocardial injury secondary to antineoplastic drugs including doxorubicin, daunorubicin, fluorouracil, cyclophosphamide
	Drug induced lupus with pericarditis: procainamide, hydralazine, methyldopa, isoniazid, phenytoin

Echocardiography

- Echocardiography remains the initial imaging modality of choice and should be performed either as a complete study or as a point of care tool when suspecting acute pericarditis.
- Echocardiography can identify the presence, characterize and quantify a pericardial effusion as well as assess for any hemodynamic compromise [7, 10, 14].
- Increased pericardial thickening can sometimes be appreciated with or without an associated effusion [7].
- **Global left ventricular systolic function and regional wall motion abnormalities can be ascertained in the presence of concomitant myocarditis** [8, 14].

Treatment

- **High dose aspirin or non-steroidal anti-inflammatories are the mainstay of treatment for acute pericarditis** [8, 10, 16, 17].
- **Weight adjusted Colchicine is recommended to prevent recurrences** [18, 19].
- **Low dose corticosteroids (0.2–0.5 mg/kg/day) with a slow taper are indicated as a second line therapy when there are contraindications to or failure of NSAIDs/ASA.** They may be indicated as a first line therapy in cases of pregnancy related pericarditis or autoimmune etiologies [20].
- **Independent of the choice of therapy, initial dosing should be maintained until there is resolution of symptoms and normalization of the CRP.** Subsequently, the dose can be tapered according to the patients estimated recurrence risk.
- Patients should be counseled on restricting physical activity until there is clinical and biochemical resolution of the pericarditis as well as normalization of the EKG and echocardiogram [21, 22].

Prognosis

- Fever (≥38.0 °C), a subacute presentation, failure of initial therapy, a pericardial effusion of greater than 20 mm, or tamponade physiology are features of poor prognosis and their presence may warrant a hospitalization [23].

Expert opinion considers myocarditis, history of immunosuppression or trauma, and patients on anticoagulation to be also at risk and should be monitored closely. Otherwise, outpatient care with close follow-up is appropriate [9].

Constrictive Pericarditis

- Constrictive pericarditis is a condition caused by a thick non-compliant, fibrotic and/or calcified pericardium which limits the diastolic filling of the ventricles.
- While it can evolve from cases of idiopathic acute pericarditis, it has been shown to be associated with cardiac surgery, mediastinal radiation, connective tissues diseases and infections such as tuberculosis [7, 9, 10, 24, 25].

Pathophysiology

- The heart chambers become confined to a non-compliant space due to a thickened and fibrosed pericardium. The restrictive nature of the pericardium causes a rapid early diastolic filling followed by an abrupt stop. As this disease progresses, the systemic venous pressures continue to rise to systemic venous congestion [7, 9, 24].
- Moreover, the constricting pericardium insulates the heart from the respiratory intrathoracic pressure changes. Normally, with inspiration, the venae cava, the pulmonary veins as well as the cardiac chambers have a contiguous drop in pressure during inspiration. As such, the gradients are maintained and forward flow is only slightly affected. With constrictive physiology, the pulmonary veins have a drop in pressure while the left ventricle and left atrium remains the same. This results in a smaller pulmonary vein to left atrium gradient during inspiration resulting in a drop of left atrial filling and transmitral inflow [7, 24].
- Lastly, with a fixed combined volume of the right and left ventricles and reduced left sided filling during inspiration, the septum shifts towards the left ventricle. This phenomenon known as ventricular interdependence is a characteristic finding in constrictive pericarditis [8, 24, 26].

Echocardiography

- Echocardiography is recommended as the initial cardiac imaging modality for patients with suspected constrictive pericarditis. It allows the operator to identify both the structural and hemodynamic features of constrictive pericarditis [7, 9, 24].

2D Echocardiography Findings Include:

- **Presence of an abnormal septal motion from right to left in early diastole during inspiration signifying the presence of ventricular interdependence. (Sensitivity of 93%)** [7, 27] (Fig. 20.1).
- The presence of a plethoric IVC, defined as an IVC diameter greater than 2.1 cm and associated with less than 50% reduction in its diameter during inspiration along with the presence dilated hepatic veins signifying increased right atrial filling pressures [7] (Fig. 20.2).
- Normal systolic ventricular function is what is commonly seen however the presence of some wall motion abnormalities have been reported owing to pericardial adhesions and tethering of the wall rather than damaged cardiomyocytes [24, 28].
- The presence of a thickened pericardium is best appreciated on the PSLAX view at the posterior edge of the heart or in the PSAX view. However, other imaging modalities such as CT, are superior for the detection of pericardial thickening and calcification [7].

M-mode Echocardiography Findings Include:

- **The presence of a septal "shudder" or septal "bounce" as depicted by an abrupt posterior motion of the ventricular septum in early diastole with inspiration**. This phenomenon signifies an abrupt increase in early diastolic right ventricular pressure, which overtakes the left ventricular diastolic pressure during the cardiac cycle [9, 24].
- Occasionally, premature opening of the pulmonic valve can be observed if the pulmonary vascular resistance is normal [9].

Doppler Flow Velocity Findings Include:

- **Characteristic hepatic vein diastolic flow reversal during expiration. This is a specific echocardiographic finding associated with constrictive physiology** [7, 27] (Fig. 20.3).
- **A restrictive pattern of filling using pulse wave doppler of the mitral inflow. On inspiration, a high early E velocity with a short deceleration time and a reduced atrial wave is noted. This results in an E/A greater than 1 representing a rapid equilibration of the left atrial and ventricular pressures** [7, 27].
- **Due to the dissociated intrathoracic and intracardiac pressures, during the first beat of inspiration, the mitral inflow velocity usually falls by as much as 25–40% and the tricuspid inflow velocity increased by as much as 40–60%** [10, 24, 27, 29] (Fig. 20.4).

Tissue Doppler Findings Include:

- **In constrictive pericarditis, the early diastolic velocity of the medial mitral annulus e′ is prominent. As the degree of constriction advances, the e′ increases**

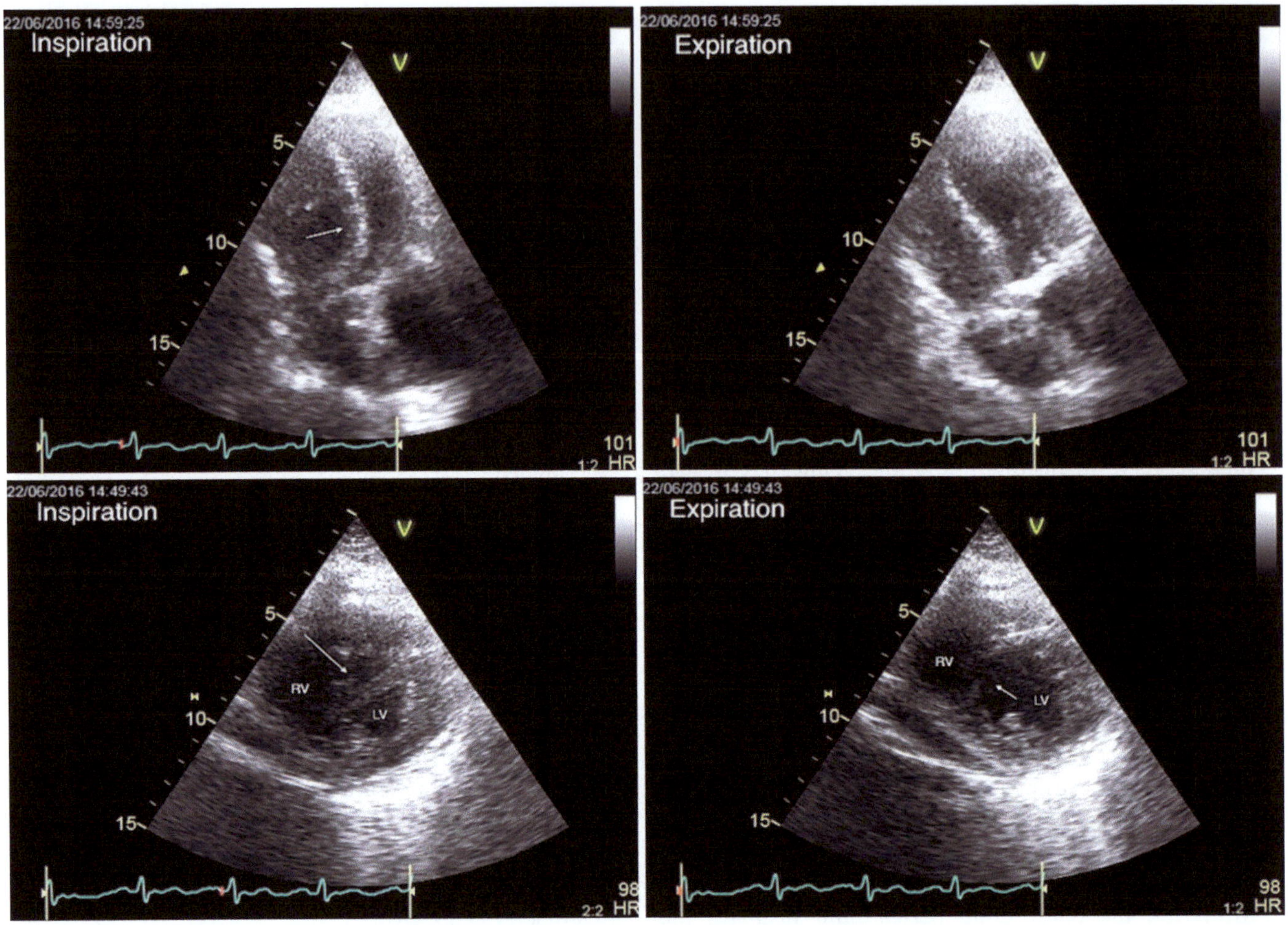

Fig. 20.1 Two-dimensional apical and parasternal short axis views of the heart of a patient with constrictive pericarditis. On inspiration (*left*), the ventricular septum is seen moving into the left ventricular cavity (*white arrow*) and back towards the right ventricle on expiration (*right*)

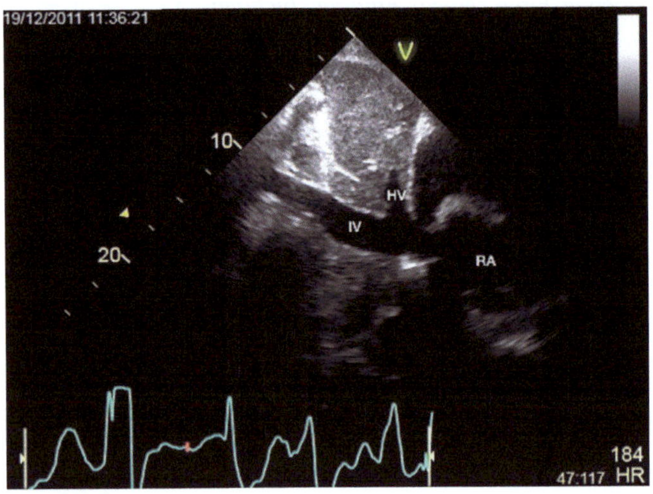

Fig. 20.2 Two-dimensional subcostal view of a patient in tamponade showing a plethoric inferior vena cava without respiratory collapse (*IV* Inferior vena cava, *HV* hepatic vein, *RA* right atrium)

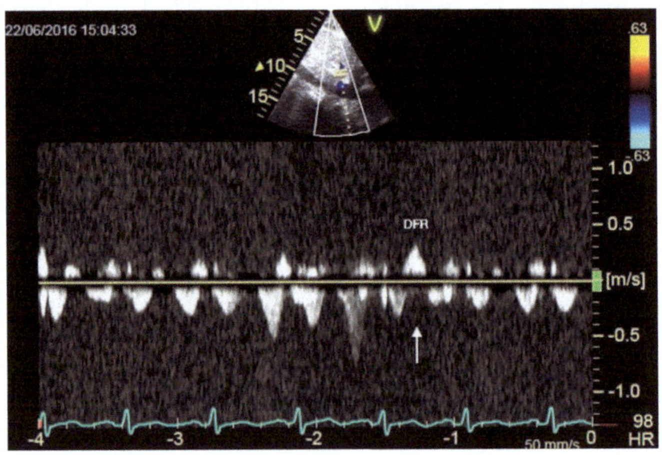

Fig. 20.3 PW Doppler echo of the hepatic vein demonstrating diastolic reversal velocity (*DFR*) during expiration

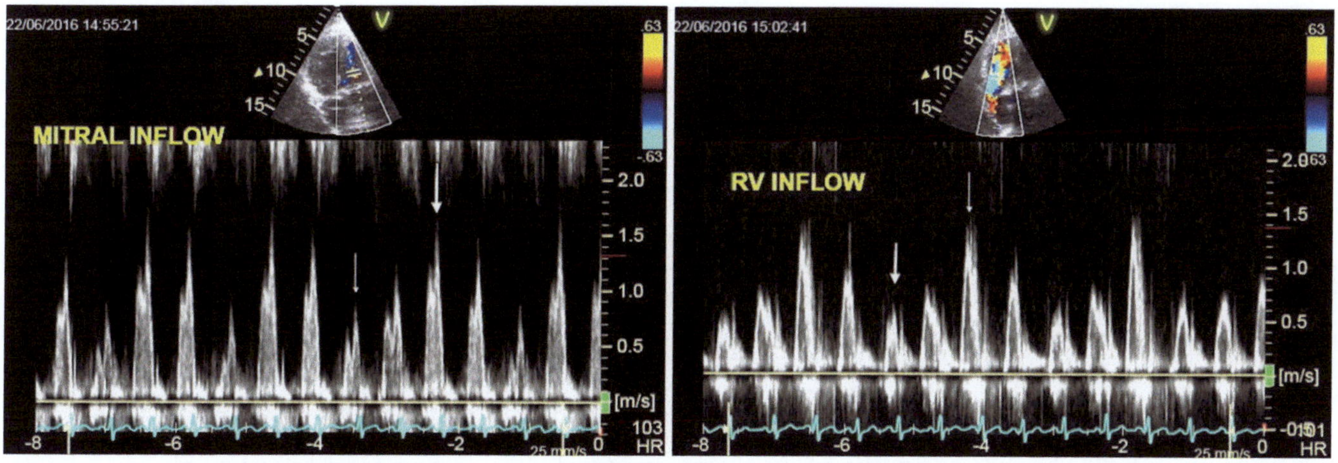

Fig. 20.4 Pulse wave Doppler echo of the mitral inflow velocity *(left)* and of tricuspid inflow *(right)* during normal respiration. On display is the characteristic respirophasic variation of the inflow velocities with inspiration (*thin arrow*) and expiration (*thick arrow*)

progressively rather than decreases, giving a lower than expected E/e′ ratio. This is in contrast to the expected decrease in e′ and E in individuals with worsening myocardial function and is therefore referred to as **annulus paradoxus** [27, 30–32].

- **In healthy individuals, the lateral e′ is generally 25–50% larger than the medial mitral annulus e′. In constrictive pericarditis, there is tethering of the lateral mitral annulus with an exaggerated compensatory medial longitudinal expansion and a resultant increase in the e′ of the mitral medial annulus; a phenomenon commonly referred to as annulus "reversus"** [27, 33–35].
- **Annulus paradoxus and annulus reversus can normalize after pericardiectomy** [28].

Strain Imaging

- **Global longitudinal strain is preserved in pure constriction**. Reduced global longitudinal strain is found if there is concomitant myocardial disease [24, 36, 37].

Transesophageal Echocardiography and 3D Echocardiography

- There is a limited role for transesophageal echocardiography as well as 3D echocardiography in the setting of constrictive pericarditis.
- One particular utility of TEE is the measurement and characterization of the pericardial thickness which has shown to have a good correlation with the computed tomography [38, 39].

Practical Approach to Constriction [24, 27]: Table 20.2

- **The absence of a mitral inflow E/A ratio greater than 0.8 and dilated inferior vena cava renders the diagnosis of constrictive pericarditis unlikely**
- **If the former echo feature criteria are met, abnormal septal motion should be evaluated followed by the medial mitral annulus e′.**
- **Constrictive pericarditis is diagnosed with the presence of a respirophasic septal shift and a mitral annular e′ greater than 8 cm/s on the tissue Doppler.**
- **The diagnosis is then confirmed with the presence of hepatic vein expiratory end-diastolic reversal.**
- In the absence of an abnormal septal motion and a persistent suspicion of CP, further diagnostic modalities should be considered.

Treatment

- Approximately 10–20% of patients with constrictive physiology will respond to anti-inflammatories within a few months. This small subset of patients can be identified with elevated inflammatory markers like CRP and with other imaging modalities such as CT or MRI [13, 24, 40, 41].
- Pericardiectomy remains the treatment of choice for the majority of individuals with constrictive pericarditis including those who fail medical therapy [24].

Table 20.2 Reprinted by permission from Macmillan Publishers Ltd.: Nature Review: *Welch TD. Echocardiographic diagnosis of CP: Mayo clinic criteria Circ Cardiovasc Imaging* copyright (2014) Reprinted by permission from Dr. J Oh, corresponding author

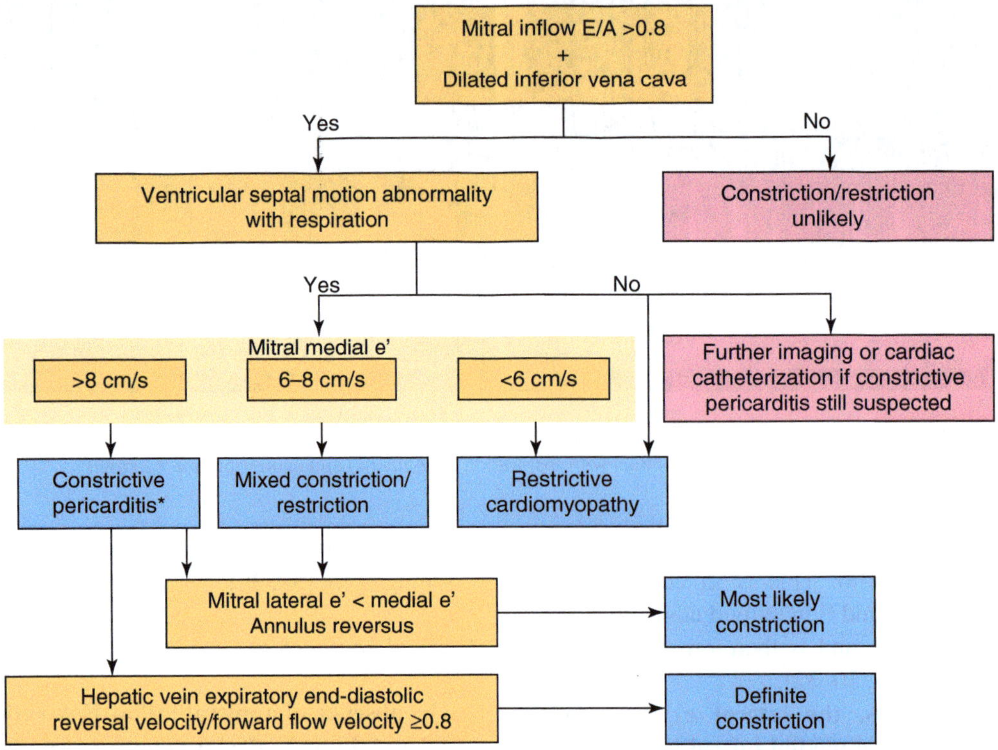

Echocardiography diagnostic criteria algorithm for constrictive pericarditis. *In patients with obstructive airways disease or increased respiratory effort, ventricular interaction occurs and e' can be high especially in a young patient. In that situation, increased flow in the superior vena cava during inspiration is also seen and the hepatic vein also shows markedly increased flow with inspiration. Abbreviations: A, late mitral inflow velocity; E, early mitral inflow velocity; e', early mitral annulus diastolic velocity.

Other Considerations

Transient Constrictive Pericarditis

- Transient constrictive pericarditis is a form of constrictive pericarditis characterized by improvement or resolution of the clinical features of constriction either spontaneously or with anti-inflammatory medication.

Effusive-Constrictive

- Effusive-constrictive pericarditis is an uncommon form of pericardial disease and should be suspected in patients who present with pericardial tamponade and fail to improve after removal of the pericardial fluid. This disease occurs when there is pericardial fluid accumulation between a thickened, edematous or fibrotic parietal and visceral pericardium. After the pericardial fluid is removed, the cardiac chambers remain constricted within the thickened pericardium and demonstrate elevated RA, end diastolic RV and LV pressures as well as a dip and plateau ventricular waveform and respiratory interventricular interdependence. **Once again, this may respond to anti-inflammatory therapy if there is an elevated CRP or late gadolinium enhancement of the pericardium on MRI** [7, 42, 43].

Echocardiography

- An effusion containing intrapericardial echogenic material, some of which may be fibrous strands that traverse the pericardial cavity, sometimes accompanies effusive-constrictive pericarditis. Otherwise, findings ranging from a sizeable pericardial effusion to tamponade to constrictive pericarditis can be observed depending on the stage of the disease [7, 44].

Pericardial Effusion

- The pericardial sac contains between 10–50 cc of plasma ultra-filtrate that acts as a lubricant between the pericardial layers. Various conditions including acute pericarditis and hypothyroidism result in an accumulation of this

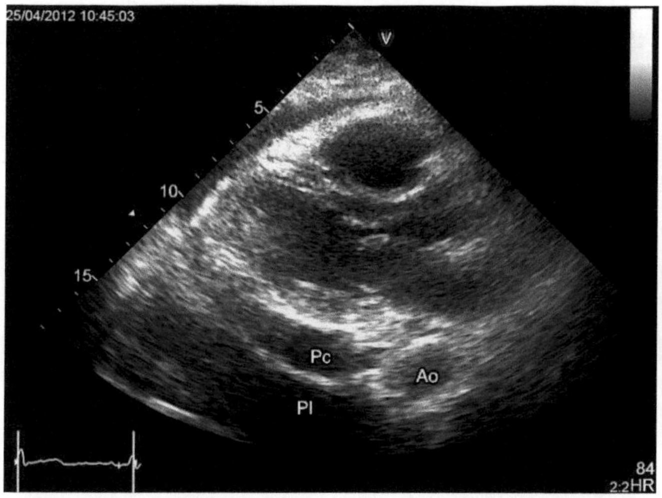

Fig. 20.5 Two-dimensional parasternal long axis view of the heart in a patient with a pleural and pericardial effusion. The echo-lucent fluid tracking the posterior wall of the myocardium remains anterior to the aorta (A) and is defined as the pericardial effusion (Pc). The echo-lucent fluid posterior to the aorta (A) is defined as the pleural effusion (Pl)

fluid. Moreover, depending on the underlying etiology, analysis of the pericardial fluid can reveal it to be a transudative effusion, an exudative effusion, hemopericardium, chylopericardium or pyopericardium [7, 9, 45].

- **Cardiac ultrasonography remains the primary imaging modality for the diagnosis of pericardial effusions.**

Echocardiography

2D Echocardiographic Findings Include:

- **A pericardial effusion can be differentiated by a pleural effusion in the PSLAX view with reference to the descending aorta. Fluid accumulation anterior to the descending aorta is pericardial while fluid accumulation posterior to the descending aorta is pleural in nature** (Fig. 20.5).
- **The location, size, extent of the pericardial effusion and presence of loculations should be characterized using all four echocardiographic windows including PSLAX, PSAX, Apical, and the Subcostal views** [7, 10].
- **The standard measurement of the effusion is between the parietal and visceral pericardium at end-diastole** [7].
- **Echocardiographic classification**
  - **Trivial effusion (seen only in systole)**
  - **Small effusion (less than 10 mm/300 mL)**
  - **Moderate effusion (10–20 mm/500 mL)**
  - **Large effusion (greater than 20 mm/more than 700 mL)**
  - **Very large effusion (greater than 25 mm)**
- All effusions should be evaluated for hemodynamic features of tamponade [7, 10, 46].
- **Epicardial fat, which is commonly mistaken for pericardial fluid, is brighter than myocardium under cardiac ultrasonography and also moves in concert with the heart in contrast to the echo-lucent and motionless pericardial fluid.**

3D Echocardiography

- The added role of 3D echocardiography after completion of a 2D echocardiographic exam in the assessment of pericardial effusion is limited and is therefore not recommended in routine assessment of effusions.
- The main limitation of 3D echocardiography is the full volume sector width which is not sufficiently large enough to capture the entire pericardial effusion and pericardium [47, 48].

Therapy

- **The initial management of a pericardial effusion remains the treatment of the underlying etiology. Objective evidence of pericardial inflammation should prompt a trial of NSAIDs with serial ultrasounds to follow the effusion.**
- **In the presence of a large effusion, pericardiocentesis may be considered to prevent eventual pericardial tamponade.**
- **A surgical pericardiotomy or a pericardial window should be considered when there is a history of recurrent large pericardial effusions.**
- **Certain causes of pericardial effusion should be treated as surgical emergencies such as aortic dissection or free wall rupture after a myocardial infarction. There is no role for pericardiocentesis in these circumstances** [9, 12, 49, 50]

Tamponade

- **Tamponade is a life threatening condition characterized by fluid accumulation in the pericardial sac which compresses the cardiac chambers and inhibits diastolic filling.**

Pathophysiology

- As the fluid in the pericardium collects and the pericardial reserve volume is surpassed, the pericardium begins to distend until it reaches the limits of the pericardial sac's

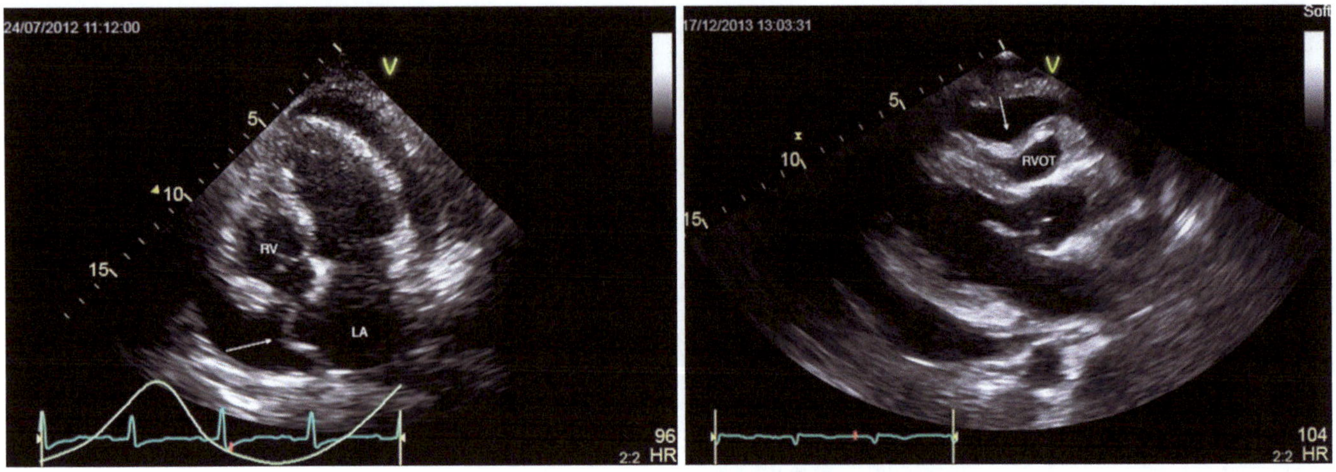

Fig. 20.6 *Left:* Two-dimensional apical view of patient in tamponade showing indentation of the right atrium in late diastole. *Right:* Two-dimensional parasternal long axis view of a patient in tamponade showing indentation of the right ventricular outflow tract in early diastole (*LA* left atrium, *RV* right ventricle, *RVOT* right ventricular outlflow tract)

ability to stretch. The limit of pericardial stretch is dependent on the amount of fluid and the rate of its accumulation. Any added volume thereafter exerts a pressure on the cardiac chambers. As tamponade continues to evolve, there is a rise in the intrapericardial pressures and eventual equalization with the diastolic pressures in the cardiac chambers. This results in reduced cardiac filling and reduced cardiac output.

- The accumulating pericardial fluid creates a fixed pericardial volume in which each side of the heart fills at the expense of the other side and an associated **exaggerated inspiratory decrease in systolic blood pressure known as pulsus paradoxus occurs** [51–53].

Echocardiography

- Individuals presenting with hypotension, tachycardia, a pulsus paradoxus greater than 10 mmHg along with evidence of increase central venous pressure should undergo cardiac echocardiography to determine if there is underlying tamponade physiology [9, 10, 54].
- **All views should be ascertained starting with the subxyphoid echocardiographic window to characterize the effusion as well as its hemodynamic effects**.

2D Echocardiography Findings Include:

- The presence of a pericardial effusion should be evaluated in its entirety to determine if it's circumferential or loculated.
- **Cavitary collapse is an important feature of tamponade physiology. It signifies that the intrapericardial pressures surpass the intracavitary pressures and filling of the chambers is impaired. Absence of any cavitary collapse has a greater than 90% negative predictive value for clinical cardiac tamponade**. M-mode echocardiography can often be utilized to determine the timing and duration of the collapsing chambers [9, 52].
- **Collapse of the right atrium is detected in late diastole (after atrial systole and near the peak of the R wave) and has a high sensitivity for tamponade** [55] (Fig. 20.6).
- **Diastolic compression of the RV free wall, observed in early diastole, is a more specific indicator**. Initially, it is only observed on inspiration, but as tamponade progresses, diastolic compression extends throughout the whole respiratory cycle. Moreover, the duration of indentation of the free wall which starts in early diastole correlates with the severity of tamponade (Fig. 20.6).
- In certain pre-existing conditions such as pulmonary hypertension, the high right ventricular pressures resist intracavitary collapse. In these particular cases, tamponade needs to be in its advanced stages before the intrapericaridal pressures are able to overcome the already elevated intracavitary pressures [52, 56, 57].
- **Left atrial collapse is a much rarer occurrence (25% of cases) but has a higher specificity for clinical cardiac tamponade.**

- **Ventricular interdependence is an important aspect of tamponade physiology and is demonstrable with a cardiac echocardiogram**.
- In healthy individuals, a compliant pericardial sac with minimal fluid, allows for normal left and right ventricular fillings without any restriction. In tamponade, the right ventricle can no longer expand outwards to fill in diastole, forcing the septal wall to shift into the left ventricular cavity leading to impaired filling of the left ventricle. This ventricular interaction is observed on imaging as an inspiratory bulge of the interventricular septum from right to left, and is best seen in the apical four chamber view, or the PSAX view.

- This however is not the case is certain pre-existing conditions with high left ventricular pressures such as left ventricular hypertrophy [58, 59].
- The presence of a plethoric IVC defined as an IVC diameter greater than 2.1 cm and associated with less than 50% reduction in its diameter during inspiration, as well as the presence dilated hepatic veins, signifies increased right atrial filling pressures [7, 60] (Fig. 20.2).

M-mode Echocardiography Findings Include:

- M-mode echocardiography can be utilized to determine the exact timing of the collapsing chambers
- Ventricular interdependence can also be demonstrated with M-mode echocardiography. When acquiring views in PSLAX, the RV diameter can be seen to increase with inspiration and decrease with expiration while the LV diameter can be seen to decrease in inspiration and increase with expiration.

Doppler Flow Velocities Findings Include:

- The inspiratory bulge during inspiration, signifying the presence of ventricular interdependence, causes a reduction in LV filling. Consequently, the transmitral doppler early diastolic E wave is reduced as is the LV outflow velocity. In the right heart, however, the opposite is observed. As the interventricular septum shifts into the left ventricle there is more right sided filling depicted by an increased tricuspid E wave and therefore an increased RV outflow velocity.
- Peak E wave mitral flow velocity, as measured by either Pulse or Continuous wave Doppler, is estimated to vary within 5% during the respiratory cycle of a healthy individual. **When tamponade physiology is present, the peak mitral E-inflow velocity has a maximal drop on the first beat of inspiration and exceeds 30% respiratory variation** [9, 61, 62].
- **The peak tricuspid E-inflow has a maximal drop on the first beat of expiration and exceeds 60% respiratory variation** [9, 61, 62].

- Normal hepatic flow is biphasic in nature with the systolic velocity greater than diastolic velocity; both of which are increased with inspiration. Moreover, it is normal to have reduced forward flow or even reversal of flow during the atrial contraction (atrial reversal) and/or during end-systole (venous reversal) [9].
- In the presence of tamponade physiology, hepatic forward flow velocities decrease (from 50 to 20–40 cm/s) and continues to do so with persistently rising pericardial pressures. **In the early stages of tamponade, systolic venous flow predominates, given that the heart is smallest in volume and the intrapericardial pressures are the lowest. In the presence of more advanced tamponade, diastolic flow becomes nearly absent but demonstrates some inspiratory variation. When the tamponade physiology has reached a severe state diastolic flow disappears completely.**
- **As the pericardial pressures continue rise, the systemic venous and intracardiac pressures equalize and only forward systolic flow is seen during inspiration from the hepatic veins to the RA. This usually indicates that cardiac arrest is imminent** [61, 63].
- Although the hepatic vein pulse wave doppler is a difficult variable to obtain, it has a high positive and negative predictive value (82% and 88% respectively) [61, 63].

Treatment

- The gold standard for the treatment of cardiac tamponade is pericardiocentesis [52].
- Medical therapy is of limited utility [64–66].
- Surgical intervention is usually required when there is failure of pericardiocentesis or in the setting of intrapericardial bleeding and clotted hemopericardium. A window, a connection between the pericardium and the absorbing surface of the pleura or peritoneum, may be necessary for malignant effusions that are recurrent [52, 67].

Pericardiocentesis

- Pericardiocentesis is often indicated in patients with tamponade and may be lifesaving if performed shortly after diagnosis.
- **Echo-guided pericardiocentesis is preferred over a blind subxiphoid approach and is associated with reduced complication rates.**
- **Initially, the echocardiogram should be utilized to determine the ideal entry point characterized by the most pericardial fluid in end-diastole with the least amount of interfering structures.**
- With or without direct ultrasound guidance, a standard 18 gauge thin walled needle or a smaller 21 G micropuncture needle is inserted into the pericardium and then exchanged with a 4F or 5F plastic catheter. **Positioning is then confirmed either with 6 mL of agitated saline or identification of the guidewire under ultrasound** (Fig. 20.7).
- Once the tip of the catheter is confirmed to be within the pericardial space, a 0.035″ guidewire followed by an 8.5F pigtail catheter is introduced using the Seldinger's technique. Progressive dilatation and/or a peel-away sheath may be necessary if the pigtail has a preformed curve.
- The pericardial fluid should be removed slowly and then left on negative suction. **The pigtail should remain in the pericardium until there is less than 30 mL/24 h for 24–48 h in order to decrease recurrence rates** [68, 69].

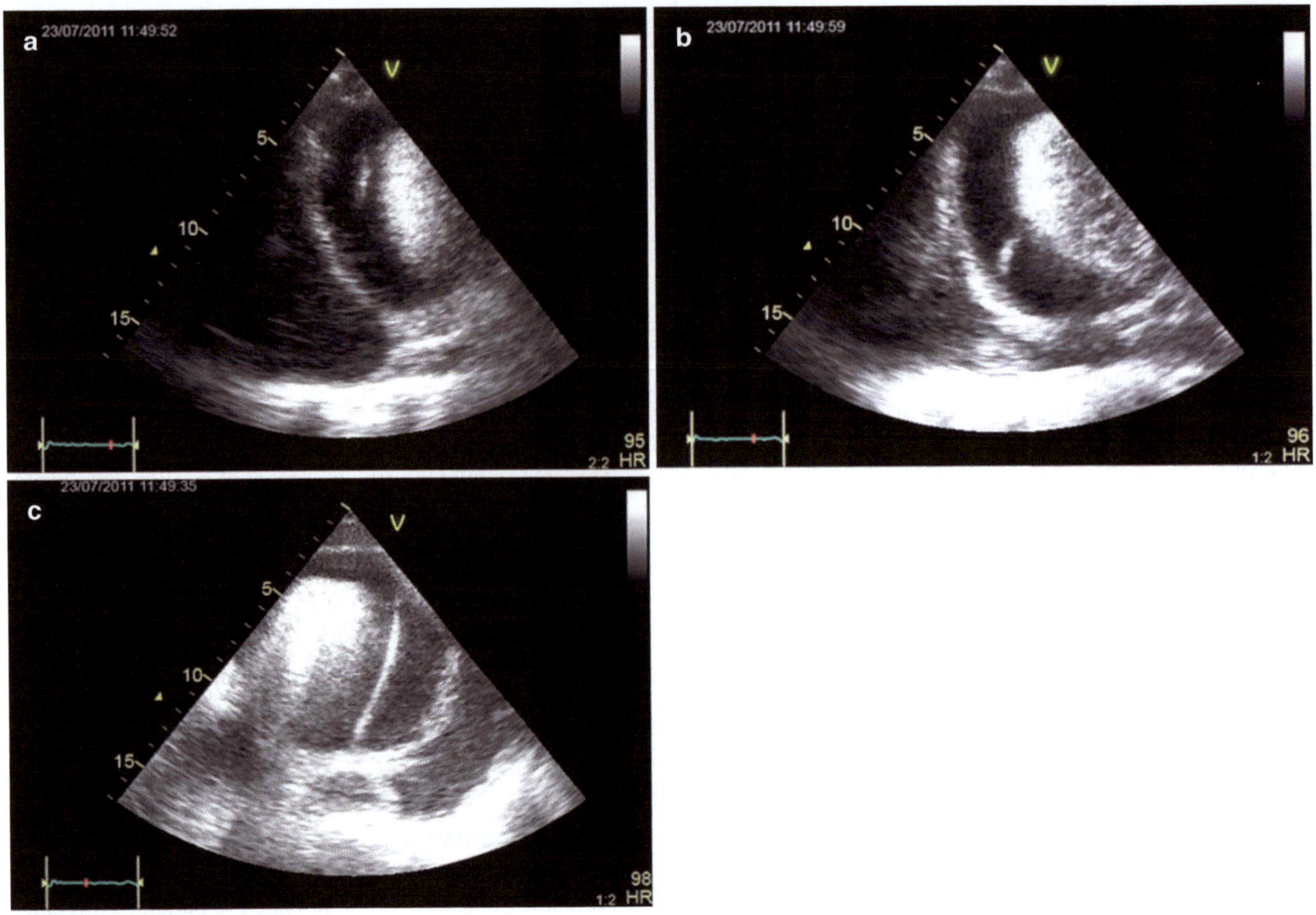

Fig. 20.7 Two-dimensional apical view of a patient in tamponade during a pericardiocentesis. The operator is confirming the presence of the guidewire in the pericardial space

Questions

1. The first line treatment of acute pericarditis includes:
   A. Non-steroidal anti-inflammatories and colchicine
   B. High-dose corticosteroids
   C. Low-dose corticosteroids
   D. Azathioprine

2. Ventricular interdependence is demonstrated echocardiographically by:
   A. Annulus paradoxus
   B. Annulus reversus
   C. A respirophasic ventricular septal shift in the apical four chamber window
   D. Abnormal mitral inlet inflow E/A ratio

3. After a pericardiocentesis, if the cardiac parameters reveal an elevated RA, elevated end diastolic RV and LV pressures as well as a dip and plateau ventricular waveform this is most likely
   A. Incomplete pericardiocentesis
   B. Effusive-constrictive pericarditis
   C. Transient effusive pericarditis
   D. The expected physiological response to pericardiocentesis.

4. Acute aortic dissection with a resultant pericardial effusion should prompt:
   A. High dose anti-inflammatories
   B. Urgent Pericardiocentesis
   C. Urgent cardiac surgery
   D. IV Tranaxemic acid

5. In Tamponade,
   A. Collapse of the right atrium in early diastole is highly sensitive
   B. Diastolic compression of the RV free wall is specific for tamponade physiology
   C. Left atrial collapse is the first sign of tamponade
   D. The definitive treatment of tamponade is fluid resuscitation.

Answers

1. A
2. C
3. B
4. C
5. B

References

1. Spodick DH. The normal and diseased pericardium: current concepts of pericardial physiology, diagnosis and treatment. J Am Coll Cardiol. 1983;1(1):240–51.
2. Miyazaki T, Pride HP, Zipes DP. Prostaglandins in the pericardial fluid modulate neural regulation of cardiac electrophysiological properties. Circ Res. 1990;66(1):163–75.
3. Holt JP. The normal pericardium. Am J Cardiol. 1970; 26(5):455–65.
4. Spodick DH. Macrophysiology, microphysiology, and anatomy of the pericardium: a synopsis. Am Heart J. 1992;124(4):1046–51.
5. Khandaker MH, et al. Pericardial disease: diagnosis and management. Mayo Clin Proc. 2010;85(6):572–93.
6. Kyto V, Sipila J, Rautava P. Clinical profile and influences on outcomes in patients hospitalized for acute pericarditis. Circulation. 2014;130(18):1601–6.
7. Klein AL, et al. American Society of Echocardiography clinical recommendations for multimodality cardiovascular imaging of patients with pericardial disease endorsed by the Society for Cardiovascular Magnetic Resonance and Society of Cardiovascular Computed Tomography. J Am Soc Echocardiogr. 2013;26(9):965–1012.e15.
8. Maisch B, et al. Guidelines on the diagnosis and management of pericardial diseases executive summary; The Task force on the diagnosis and management of pericardial diseases of the European society of cardiology. Eur Heart J. 2004;25(7):587–610.
9. Adler Y, et al. 2015 ESC Guidelines for the diagnosis and management of pericardial diseases: The Task Force for the Diagnosis and Management of Pericardial Diseases of the European Society of Cardiology (ESC)Endorsed by: The European Association for Cardio-Thoracic Surgery (EACTS). Eur Heart J. 2015;36(42):2921–64.
10. Cosyns B, et al. European Association of Cardiovascular Imaging (EACVI) position paper: multimodality imaging in pericardial disease. Eur Heart J Cardiovasc Imaging. 2015;16(1):12–31.
11. Imazio M, Gaita F, LeWinter M. Evaluation and treatment of pericarditis: a systematic review. JAMA. 2015;314(14):1498–506.
12. Imazio M, Adler Y. Management of pericardial effusion. Eur Heart J. 2013;34(16):1186–97.
13. Sagrista-Sauleda J, Merce AS, Soler-Soler J. Diagnosis and management of pericardial effusion. World J Cardiol. 2011;3(5):135–43.
14. Spodick DH. Acute pericarditis: current concepts and practice. JAMA. 2003;289(9):1150–3.
15. Lange RA, Hillis LD. Clinical practice acute pericarditis. N Engl J Med. 2004;351(21):2195–202.
16. Lotrionte M, et al. International collaborative systematic review of controlled clinical trials on pharmacologic treatments for acute pericarditis and its recurrences. Am Heart J. 2010;160(4):662–70.
17. Imazio M, et al. Individualized therapy for pericarditis. Expert Rev Cardiovasc Ther. 2009;7(8):965–75.
18. Imazio M, et al. Colchicine as first-choice therapy for recurrent pericarditis: results of the CORE (COlchicine for REcurrent pericarditis) trial. Arch Intern Med. 2005;165(17):1987–91.
19. Imazio M, et al. Colchicine in addition to conventional therapy for acute pericarditis: results of the COlchicine for acute PEricarditis (COPE) trial. Circulation. 2005;112(13):2012–6.
20. Imazio M, et al. Corticosteroids for recurrent pericarditis: high versus low doses: a nonrandomized observation. Circulation. 2008;118(6):667–71.
21. Pelliccia A, et al. Recommendations for participation in competitive sport and leisure-time physical activity in individuals with cardiomyopathies, myocarditis and pericarditis. Eur J Cardiovasc Prev Rehabil. 2006;13(6):876–85.
22. Seidenberg PH, Haynes J. Pericarditis: diagnosis, management, and return to play. Curr Sports Med Rep. 2006;5(2):74–9.
23. Imazio M, et al. Indicators of poor prognosis of acute pericarditis. Circulation. 2007;115(21):2739–44.
24. Syed FF, Schaff HV, Oh JK. Constrictive pericarditis—a curable diastolic heart failure. Nat Rev Cardiol. 2014;11(9):530–44.
25. Mayosi BM. Contemporary trends in the epidemiology and management of cardiomyopathy and pericarditis in sub-Saharan Africa. Heart. 2007;93(10):1176–83.
26. Bertog SC, et al. Constrictive pericarditis: etiology and cause-specific survival after pericardiectomy. J Am Coll Cardiol. 2004;43(8):1445–52.
27. Welch TD, et al. Echocardiographic diagnosis of constrictive pericarditis: Mayo Clinic criteria. Circ Cardiovasc Imaging. 2014;7(3):526–34.
28. Veress G, et al. Mitral and tricuspid annular velocities before and after pericardiectomy in patients with constrictive pericarditis. Circ Cardiovasc Imaging. 2011;4(4):399–407.
29. Oh JK, et al. Diagnostic role of Doppler echocardiography in constrictive pericarditis. J Am Coll Cardiol. 1994;23(1):154–62.
30. Garcia MJ, et al. Differentiation of constrictive pericarditis from restrictive cardiomyopathy: assessment of left ventricular diastolic velocities in longitudinal axis by Doppler tissue imaging. J Am Coll Cardiol. 1996;27(1):108–14.
31. Sohn DW, et al. Unique features of early diastolic mitral annulus velocity in constrictive pericarditis. J Am Soc Echocardiogr. 2004;17(3):222–6.
32. Ha JW, et al. Differentiation of constrictive pericarditis from restrictive cardiomyopathy using mitral annular velocity by tissue Doppler echocardiography. Am J Cardiol. 2004;94(3):316–9.
33. Reuss CS, et al. Using mitral 'annulus reversus' to diagnose constrictive pericarditis. Eur J Echocardiogr. 2009;10(3):372–5.
34. Choi JH, et al. Mitral and tricuspid annular velocities in constrictive pericarditis and restrictive cardiomyopathy correlation with pericardial thickness on computed tomography. JACC Cardiovasc Imaging. 2011;4(6):567–75.
35. Lu XF, et al. Diagnosis of constrictive pericarditis by quantitative tissue Doppler imaging. Int J Cardiol. 2009;137(1):22–8.
36. Sengupta PP, et al. Disparate patterns of left ventricular mechanics differentiate constrictive pericarditis from restrictive cardiomyopathy. JACC Cardiovasc Imaging. 2008;1(1):29–38.
37. Kusunose K, et al. Biventricular mechanics in constrictive pericarditis comparison with restrictive cardiomyopathy and impact of pericardiectomy. Circ Cardiovasc Imaging. 2013; 6(3):399–406.
38. Zagol B, et al. Effusive constrictive pericarditis: 2D, 3D echocardiography and MRI imaging. Echocardiography. 2007;24(10):1110–4.
39. Ling LH, et al. Pericardial thickness measured with transesophageal echocardiography: feasibility and potential clinical usefulness. J Am Coll Cardiol. 1997;29(6):1317–23.
40. Haley JH, et al. Transient constrictive pericarditis: causes and natural history. J Am Coll Cardiol. 2004;43(2):271–5.
41. Sagrista-Sauleda J, et al. Transient cardiac constriction: an unrecognized pattern of evolution in effusive acute idiopathic pericarditis. Am J Cardiol. 1987;59(9):961–6.

42. Hancock EW. A clearer view of effusive-constrictive pericarditis. N Engl J Med. 2004;350(5):435–7.
43. Sagrista-Sauleda J, et al. Effusive-constrictive pericarditis. N Engl J Med. 2004;350(5):469–75.
44. Baker CM, Orsinelli DA. Subacute effusive-constrictive pericarditis: diagnosis by serial echocardiography. J Am Soc Echocardiogr. 2004;17(11):1204–6.
45. Troughton RW, Asher CR, Klein AL. Pericarditis. Lancet. 2004;363(9410):717–27.
46. Weitzman LB, et al. The incidence and natural history of pericardial effusion after cardiac surgery—an echocardiographic study. Circulation. 1984;69(3):506–11.
47. Scohy TV, et al. Three-dimensional transesophageal echocardiography: diagnosing the extent of pericarditis constrictiva and intraoperative surgical support. J Card Surg. 2009;24(3):305–8.
48. Veress G, Feng D, Oh JK. Echocardiography in pericardial diseases: new developments. Heart Fail Rev. 2013;18(3):267–75.
49. Fardman A, et al. European guidelines on pericardial diseases: a focused review of novel aspects. Curr Cardiol Rep. 2016;18(5):46.
50. Sagrista-Sauleda J, et al. Clinical clues to the causes of large pericardial effusions. Am J Med. 2000;109(2):95–101.
51. Boltwood CM Jr. Ventricular performance related to transmural filling pressure in clinical cardiac tamponade. Circulation. 1987;75(5):941–55.
52. Spodick DH. Acute cardiac tamponade. N Engl J Med. 2003;349(7):684–90.
53. Spodick DH. Threshold of pericardial constraint: the pericardial reserve volume and auxiliary pericardial functions. J Am Coll Cardiol. 1985;6(2):296–7.
54. D'Cruz IA, et al. Two-dimensional echocardiography in cardiac tamponade occurring after cardiac surgery. J Am Coll Cardiol. 1985;5(5):1250–2.
55. Gillam LD, et al. Hydrodynamic compression of the right atrium: a new echocardiographic sign of cardiac tamponade. Circulation. 1983;68(2):294–301.
56. Hoit BD, Fowler NO. Influence of acute right ventricular dysfunction on cardiac tamponade. J Am Coll Cardiol. 1991;18(7):1787–93.
57. Hoit BD, Gabel M, Fowler NO. Cardiac tamponade in left ventricular dysfunction. Circulation. 1990;82(4):1370–6.
58. Hoit BD, Shaw D. The paradoxical pulse in tamponade: mechanisms and echocardiographic correlates. Echocardiography. 1994;11(5):477–87.
59. Cogswell TL, et al. Total peripheral resistance during cardiac tamponade: adrenergic and angiotensin roles. Am J Phys. 1986;251(5 Pt 2):R916–22.
60. Tsang TS, Oh JK, Seward JB. Diagnosis and management of cardiac tamponade in the era of echocardiography. Clin Cardiol. 1999;22(7):446–52.
61. Merce J, et al. Correlation between clinical and Doppler echocardiographic findings in patients with moderate and large pericardial effusion: implications for the diagnosis of cardiac tamponade. Am Heart J. 1999;138(4 Pt 1):759–64.
62. Leeman DE, Levine MJ, Come PC. Doppler echocardiography in cardiac tamponade: exaggerated respiratory variation in transvalvular blood flow velocity integrals. J Am Coll Cardiol. 1988;11(3):572–8.
63. Appleton CP, Hatle LK, Popp RL. Superior vena cava and hepatic vein Doppler echocardiography in healthy adults. J Am Coll Cardiol. 1987;10(5):1032–9.
64. Martins JB, et al. Comparative effects of catecholamines in cardiac tamponade: experimental and clinical studies. Am J Cardiol. 1980;46(1):59–66.
65. Reddy PS, et al. Cardiac tamponade: hemodynamic observations in man. Circulation. 1978;58(2):265–72.
66. Cogswell TL, et al. The shift in the relationship between intrapericardial fluid pressure and volume induced by acute left ventricular pressure overload during cardiac tamponade. Circulation. 1986;74(1):173–80.
67. Pepi M, et al. Pericardial effusion after cardiac surgery: incidence, site, size, and haemodynamic consequences. Br Heart J. 1994;72(4):327–31.
68. Buchanan CL, et al. Pericardiocentesis with extended catheter drainage: an effective therapy. Ann Thorac Surg. 2003;76(3):817–20.
69. Rafique AM, et al. Frequency of recurrence of pericardial tamponade in patients with extended versus nonextended pericardial catheter drainage. Am J Cardiol. 2011;108(12):1820–5.

Dilated Cardiomyopathy and Myocarditis

21

Azin Alizadehasl and Anita Sadeghpour

Abstract

Dilated cardiomyopathy (DCM) is myocardial disease that is characterized by the left ventricular (LV) enlargement and LV systolic dysfunction in the absence of other causes of volume overload or increased afterload. LV end-diastolic and end-systolic dimensions, as well as LV end-diastolic volumes and overall LV mass, are increased (with normal or sometimes thinned walls), and the global ejection fraction (EF) is reduced and sub-normal (LVEF < 45%, fractional shortening <25%, according to literature review).

Myocarditis frequently mimicking acute coronary syndrome on first presentation. Two-dimensional (2D) echocardiography has conventionally played a restricted role in the diagnosis of acute myocarditis. Coming on of advanced echocardiographic modalities like strain and also myocardial perfusion imaging have vividly expanded the scope and role of echocardiography for better diagnosis with precise bedside study of regional contractility, myocardial blood flow, micro-vascular integrity and also function. These newer modalities has incremental usefulness over the time.

Keywords

Dilated cardiomyopathy · Myocarditis · Echocardiography · Peri-partum cardiomyopathy (PPM) · Takotsubo cardiomyopathy · LV thrombus · Assist device

A. Alizadehasl, MD, FACC, FASE (✉)
Associate Professor of Cardiology, Echocardiologist, Echocardiography and Cardiogenetic Research Centers, Cardio-Oncology Department, Rajaie Cardiovascular Medical and Research Center, Tehran, Iran

A. Sadeghpour, MD, FACC, FASE
Professor of Cardiology, Echocardiography Research Center, Rajaie Cardiovascular Medical and Research Center, Iran University of Medical Science, Tehran, Iran

Abbreviations

2D	Two-dimensional
AF	Atrial fibrillation
AIDS	Acquired immune deficiency syndrome
BBB	Bundle branch block
BP	Blood pressure
CAD	Coronary artery disease
CMR	Cardiac magnetic resonance
CRT	Cardiac resynchronization therapy
DCM	Dilated cardiomyopathy
EF	Ejection fraction
HF	Heart failure
LV	Left ventricular
MV	Mitral valve
PH	Pulmonary hypertension
PPM	Peri-partum cardiomyopathy
RWMA	Regional wall motion abnormalities
TR	Tricuspid regurgitation

Dilated cardiomyopathy

Etiology

Dilated cardiomyopathy (DCM) might be idiopathic; but a number of etiologies are well known:

A. Ischemic cardiomyopathy. Long-standing coronary artery disease (CAD) might remain silent till patients present with dilated left ventricle (LV) and the signs of heart failure (HF).
B. Familial x-linked, autosomal dominant or autosomal recessive cardiomyopathy. This is a familial situation in which the abnormality is in the centromeric half of the dystrophic genome region in heart. This describes its link to Duchenne muscular dystrophy gene locus.

A. Sadeghpour, A. Alizadehasl (eds.), *Case-Based Textbook of Echocardiography*,
https://doi.org/10.1007/978-3-319-67691-3_21

C. Peri-partum cardiomyopathy (PPM) happens during pregnancy, frequently establishes late in the last trimester, and its prognosis is considerably better than idiopathic cardiomyopathy.
D. Viral cardiomyopathy. This form of myocardial disease generally happens subsequent viral upper respiratory tract infection in adults or gastro-intestinal infection in children. Of course children with viral cardiomyopathy might completely recover and have a more better prognosis than adults.
E. Alcoholic cardiomyopathy complicates excessive alcohol intake. Despite the severity of impairment of ventricular systolic function, the disease tends to gradually recover after asceticism of alcohol.
F. Less frequent causes. Auto-organ antibodies to x and b myosin heavy chain isoform and complicating Acquired Immune Deficiency Syndrome (AIDS).
G. Metabolic disorders causing DCM are infrequent and present in early infancy.
H. Takotsubo cardiomyopathy, which looks to be a stress- or neuroendocrine-mediated process, is unique in showing a distinctive pattern of apical ballooning and basal hyperkinesis. Though the degree of dysfunction might be impressive in stress cardiomyopathy, remarkable and complete resolution might take place within days to weeks. A rarer "reverse" pattern of stress cardiomyopathy has also been explained.

- The myocardial disease and its consequences in DCM might remain silent for a while till it is accidentally discovered on a routine check-up or identified following clinical presentation with congestive HF.

Transthoracic Echocardiography

- Dilated LV or both LV and RV with increased systolic and diastolic volumes and dimensions disproportionately which is more dominant in the short axis comparing to the long axis and resulting spherical shape LV. Normal sphericity index that is the ratio of the LV long-axis dimension to short-axis dimension in four chamber view is >1.5 and approaching to 1 in cases with advanced DCM (Fig. 21.1).
- Reduced systolic function (EF or fractional shortening).
- LV Global or even segmental systolic dysfunction, with reduced wall thickness and thickening fraction
- Cases with DCM might demonstrate localized segmental dysfunction, making a definite differentiation between idiopathic and ischemic etiologies problematic. Nearly 50% of cases with idiopathic DCM have clear evidence for regional wall motion abnormalities (RWMA).
- As the disease progresses, the LV further dilates, resultant in increased wall stress (Laplace's Law), increased myocardial oxygen consumption, reduced systolic function, and also changed myocardial architecture, and henceforth a vicious circle. In late stages, the ventricle becomes spherical in shape rather than ellipsoid, adding to the reduction in the global ventricular systolic performance [1–5].

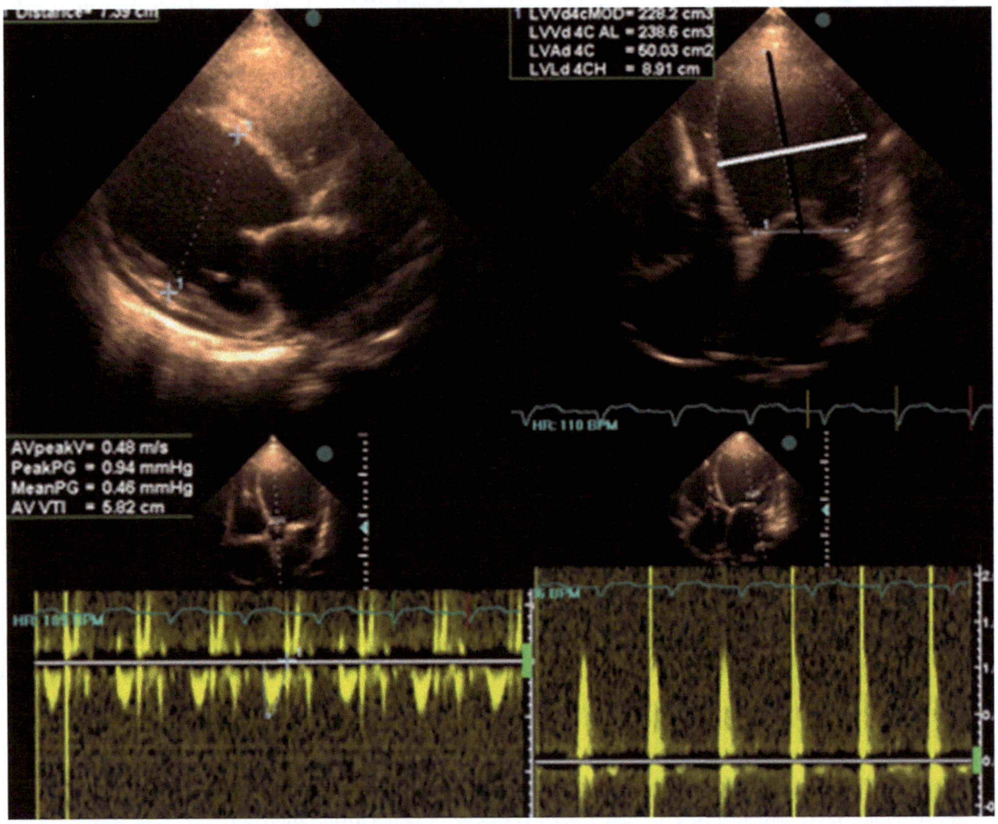

Fig. 21.1 Left upper: severe LV enlargement, Right upper: spherical shape of LV, Left lower: reduced LV stroke volume and LVOT VTI, Right lower: Significant diastolic dysfunction

Secondary Echocardiographic Features of Dilated Cardiomyopathy

1. **Ventricular Filling**
   - There is no characteristic filling pattern in DCM. In early stages ventricular filling might be normal for age or show a slow ventricular relaxation pattern, characterized by long iso-volumic relaxation time, with prolonged early diastolic filling deceleration time and predominant late diastole filling component of the LV.
   - In later stages as the ventricle becomes stiff and incompliant, the end diastolic pressure rises, LV filling becomes of the restrictive pattern (short iso-volumic relaxation time and dominant early diastole filling component with short deceleration time and prolonged flow reversal in the pulmonary veins. This is often related with some degree of MR. In early diastole, restrictive LV filling is also described by a raised atrio-ventricular pressure gradient which is transferred across the inter-ventricular septum to the right side and result in a delay or complete suppression of early diastolic RV filling (ventricular interaction effect).
   - Successful pressure off-loading of the LA by vasodilators, particularly rennin-angiotensin system blocking agents results in normalization of left and RV filling pattern. Bi-atrial enlargement is frequently seen, particularly if atrial fibrillation (AF) is present [1–3, 6].

2. **Mitral Regurgitation**
   - As the LV dilates the pathology involves the basal region and resulting in dilatation of the mitral valve (MV) ring and failure of optimal coaption of the MV leaflets.
   - In the late stages of the disease when the ventricle comes to be spherical, the papillary muscles are displaced laterally producing significantly raised chordal tension. This consequences in disturbed leaflet movement, incomplete valve closure and also valvular incompetence. In addition, ventricular dys-synchrony is another general cause for MR in DCM, which regresses after cardiac resynchronization therapy. Different mechanisms have been proposed suggesting important deformation of the MV apparatus as an attempt to recompense for the ventricular dysfunction and also cavity enlargement.
   - MR in DCM differs in severity, from mild in the early disease to even severe in late stages. The retrograde pressure drop through the MV aids in approximating LA pressure, when the LA pressure is elevated and the pressure drop through the MV is low. LA pressure is estimated as the difference amid systolic blood pressure (BP) and systolic retrograde trans-MV pressure drop [4–6].

3. **Raised Left Atrial Pressure**
   - Raised LA pressure establishes late in the disease as the LV diastolic pressures rise, results in LA dilatation and also remodeling, impairment of function and tendency to arrhythmia. Even in cases with maintained sinus rhythm, atrial contraction is resisted by ventricular stiffness and high LV end diastolic pressure.
   - This causes backward flow in the pulmonary veins that adds to the pulmonary venous congestion. Retrograde flow in the pulmonary veins happening during atrial systole which is more than 30 ms longer than the trans-mitral "A" wave duration proposes raised LV end diastolic pressure. Cases with severe LV disease and elevated LA pressure frequently present with a poor systolic component of the pulmonary venous flow consistent with depressed movement of the ventricular long axis in systole and consequently limited atrial enlargement.
   - The higher the LA pressure the more ischemic the sub-endocardium and hence the perpetual deterioration of LV function, further cavity enlargement of both ventricle and also atrium, and established AF. In addition, persistent sub-endocardial ischemia in cases with determinedly raised LA pressure is a known substrate for ventricular arrhythmia which could be life threatening [1–3, 6, 7].

4. **Pulmonary Hypertension (PH)**
   - Raised LA pressure, complicating LV disease and MR, might cause PH. Pulmonary venous hypertension is difficult to diagnose echocardiographically.
   - A short "E" wave deceleration time is a good marker of raised pulmonary wedge pressure. The progressively developing pulmonary arterial hypertension affects the size and function of the right heart. The RV becomes hypertrophied, its function impaired, and the cavity itself dilates. The RA also dilates. Pulmonary artery pressure might be estimated from peak tricuspid regurgitation (TR) pressure drop added to the estimated RA pressure. This might easily be achieved from the collapsibility of the hepatic veins. Though this equation tends to underestimate peak pulmonary artery pressure, it helps in assessing disease progression in symptomatic patients and in monitoring their response to treatment [1–4].

5. **Tricuspid Regurgitation**
   - As is the case with other causes of RV dilatation and enlargement of tricuspid annulus, TR is general and differs in severity in DCM. Severe TR might be present in late disease or if the primary pathology involves the RV.
   - In this case the RA and ventricle are both dilated, the RA pressure is increased and the peak RV–RA pressure drop falls. This fall in pressure drop must not be taken as a sign of reduction of pulmonary artery pressure, particularly in cases who show clinical deterioration, but as a sign of increasing RA pressure [1–4].

6. **LV Thrombus**
   - Late stages of DCM and increased ventricular diastolic pressure are described by slow intra-ventricular circulation, and spontaneous intra-cavitary echo contrast might be seen. With meaningfully high early diastolic atrio-ventricular pressure gradient and intra-ventricular flow acceleration, the MV leaflet opening is disturbed and the valve behaves as if functionally stenosed, therefore adding to the disturbed cavity function in diastole.
   - This degree of ventricular disease might be related with apical stagnation of blood and potential thrombus formation, suggesting the need for prophylactic anticoagulation [1–4].

7. **Extra-cardiac Fluid Compression**
   - Late stages of DCM with biventricular failure, PH, and systemic congestion might be complicated by pericardial and/or pleural effusion. Large fluid collection increases the intrathoracic pressure and frequently exacerbates the patient's breathlessness. The consequence of the increased intra-thoracic pressure on right heart physiology is assessed by studying the vena-caval, tricuspid and pulmonary flows during different phases of the respiratory cycle. Right-sided filling and ejection which increase meaningfully during inspiration (>20% that during expiration) recommend increased extra-cardiac pressures [1–3] (Fig. 21.2).

8. **Pulsus Alternans**
   - With severe deterioration of ventricular function and absence of extra-cardiac fluid collection, pulsus alternans might develop. This might easily be established on pulsed Doppler velocities of LV filling and ejection as well as wall motion pattern. The precise mechanism of pulsus alternans is not obviously understood [1, 2].

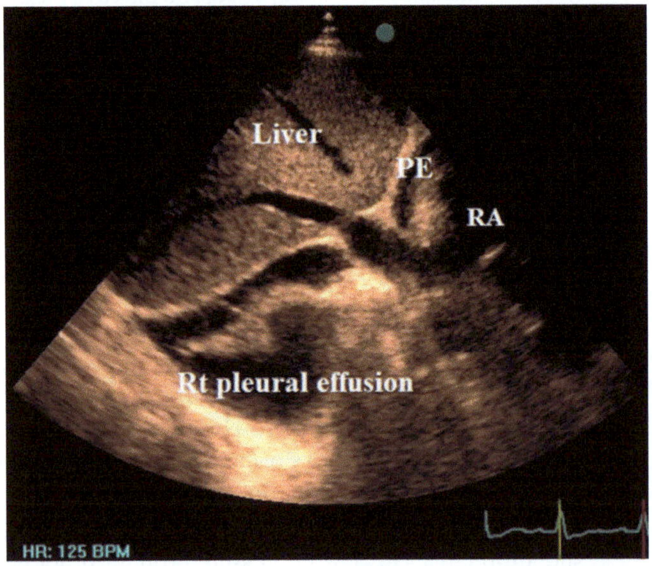

Fig. 21.2 Subcostal view showing mild pericardial effusion associated with right pleural effusion

9. **Activation-Induced LV Dysfunction**
   - Chronic severe LV disease is almost-always related with delayed depolarization, i.e., broad QRS complex with or without typical bundle branch block (BBB) pattern. Progressive prolongation of ventricular depolarization has been revealed to be related with poor clinical outcome.
   - This electrical disturbance is strictly related to the delayed and prolonged ventricular shortening and lengthening and henceforth dys-synchrony. The latter contributes to raised diastolic segmental wall tension resulting in pre-systolic MR. Such long MR might limit ventricular filling time particularly at fast HR and consequently reduce the stroke volume. Though most of these ventricles fill with a single component "summation filling pattern" the long MR adds to the raised LA pressure and pulmonary pressures as well as compromises atrial emptying function [1, 2].

Treatment

Medical Treatment

- Conventional treatment of DCM is the same as HF, with diuretics and vasodilators such as ACE inhibitors and A2. The aim of this policy is to keep the filling pressures low and to defend against further deterioration of ventricular function. ACE inhibitors in particular have shown a substantial effect on mortality reduction and improvement of clinical outcome in patients with DCM.
- Doppler echocardiography assesses cases response to ACE inhibitors particularly those with raised LA pressure (restrictive filling pattern). Successful off-loading of the atrium and the ventricle with ACE inhibition reverses the restrictive filling pattern to the dominant late diastolic filling pattern and unmasks LV dys-synchrony. This is frequently related with reduction of MR, a fall in LA size and significant improvement of symptoms.
- As the LV early diastolic pressure gradient drops and its filling becomes non-restrictive, the delay in the RV filling regresses, overall RV filling time increases and the degree of PH decreases. Beta blockers have also been shown to improve outcome in patients with DCM and reduce mortality.
- In patients with poor LV function and tachycardia, small doses of beta blockers e.g. bisoprolol or carvedilol, slow

the HR and increase LV filling time and consequently stroke volume. But not all patients with DCM might tolerate beta blockers, particularly those requiring faster HR to secure minimum physiological filling. Cases with late-stage ventricular disease and very short iso-volumic relaxation time in particular, seem to prefer a faster HR in order to sustain LV filling and cardiac output and consequently tolerate beta blockers poorly [1–3, 7, 8].

Pacing

Patients presenting with a broad QRS complex (>150 ms) and long MR with a presystolic component that limits total LV filling time respond to DDD pacing with optimized atrioventricular delay. Short A-V delay results in immediate increase in filling time and stroke volume and improvement of overall cardiac performance. Currently most of these patients will receive complete bi-ventricular pacing system, and during optimization the LV lead might be switched off.

- Long-term outcome of this intervention in individual patients is frequently satisfactory. Cases with substantial early diastolic dys-synchrony, particularly of the LV free wall, which prolongs early diastolic tension development and compromised early filling are frequently ideal for bi-ventricular pacing, cardiac resynchronization therapy (CRT). The procedure aims at optimizing the time of LV free wall stimulation that results in regression of dys-synchronous wall motion, and an increase in the overall ventricular filling time.
- If the LVEF is 35% or lower and the patient has an intra-ventricular conduction delay and clinical HF, CRT might improve pump cardiac output, reverse the LV remodeling, and improve functional MR. The extent of LV segmental dys-synchrony might be assessed using different echocardiographic methods, M-mode and tissue Doppler. Three-dimension echocardiogram has also shown a good potential for detecting dys-synchronous segments and their response to CRT.
- Cardiac resynchronization therapy results in significant symptomatic improvement, reduction in MR and improved survival. Since the natural history of DCM is deterioration, regular follow-up of such patients provides an opportunity for potential optimization of the segmental stimulation delay and overall cardiac performance.
- Despite the current strong evidence for the beneficial effect of CRT in DCM with poor systolic function, nearly 30% of cases receiving this treatment do not respond. Modest evidence suggest that those with restrictive filling are less likely to gain symptomatic benefit from CRT since their main cardiac disturbance is raised filling pressures. Preferably, patients suggested for CRT must be assessed during exercise/stress in order to determine the exact nature of cardiac disturbances which coincide with their symptoms, which must guide toward optimal management. Those developing worsening dys-synchrony must benefit from CRT, others who increase further their filling pressure and remain with restrictive filling, might need life-saving ICD [1, 2, 8–10].

Assist Devices

- Failure to control patient's signs and symptoms by the above methods recommends the need for ventricular assist device. The rationale behind the use of the assist device is a bridge to either recovery of ventricular function or transplantation.
- In a minority of cases, ventricular function recovers within weeks or months of the device insertion. The pump sucks from the ventricle and ejects directly into the aorta, consequently reducing wall stress and allowing the myocardium to recover. The currently available assist devices are either phasic or continuous. The phasic Heart Mate functions independently of cardiac cycle and carries the risk of substantial interference with valve function and clot formation. The continuous pump is not without limitation, since at fast speed the suction force might cause mid cavity obliteration, potential free wall collapse, and high intra-cavity pressure difference amid ventricular regions [1–3, 8–10].

Transplantation

- Cardiac transplantation is now a well-established management, but cause of the severe shortage of sufficient donor organs this form of treatment is only available for a small number of cases.
- In general terms the most favorable recipients are young, highly motivated people with disease confined to their heart and with excellent renal, hepatic and pulmonary function. The operation is an orthotopic heart transplant whereby the dilated heart is removed and a new donor heart inserted with anastomoses at the LA, pulmonary artery, aorta, and caval orifices.
- Over the last 10 years the use of caval orifice anastomosis has become more usual as this is found to result in a lower incidence of TR and improved RV function. The main problems related to the management of these patients post-operatively remain infection and the control of rejection.
- Modern immunosuppressive therapy with Cyclosporin, Mycophenolate mofetil, and a short course of steroids has

resulted in important improvement in results. The 1 year survival after heart transplantation is of the order of 80% and the 5 year survival is 70%. These patients require careful life-long surveillance, largely cause of the complications rising from immunosuppression. These complications comprise hypertension, which is extremely frequent and frequently might be controlled by calcium antagonist, renal impairment, slowly progressive LV fibrosis, B cell hyperplasia, and tumors. Nonetheless the quality of life from a good heart transplant is excellent and over 80% of these cases return to an active life for at least 10 years. This is a substantial achievement given that the majority had a prognosis of less than 6 months at the time that they are placed on the transplant waiting list [1–3, 9–12].

Follow-Up

- Cases with moderate or severe degree of LV impairment must be followed up recurrently by Doppler TTE for the valuation of LV function, pressure and complications, as well as response to management.
- Though there are no current guidelines to recommend how frequently patients must be assessed, markers of high filling pressure, PH and MR might provide accurate indication for deterioration of ventricular function or beneficial response to treatment [1–3].

Prognosis

- The prognosis of DCM differs significantly between patients. While alcoholic cardiomyopathy tends to recover with abstinence from alcohol, other forms continue to deteriorate over time.
- With medical therapy, patients might respond to ACE inhibitors showing a reduction in LA pressure and improvement in overall cardiac function as well as symptoms. Patients who retain high LA pressure are considered unstable and are at risk of developing PH, sub-endocardial ischemia and arrhythmia.
- Long-standing high pulmonary wedge pressure is reflected on RV function, which deteriorates irreversibly with subsequent poor outcome. Additional RV disease with a restrictive filling pattern makes the outcome poorer still.
- Although DDD pacing with A-V optimized delay has offered great assistance to global ventricular performance in patients with DCM, no trials are available to support its valuable use on a broader scale. In addition, despite the vast available evidence for the beneficial effect of CRT in advanced disease, 30% of patients receiving such treatment remain symptomatic and with no measurable benefit. Stringent Doppler echocardiographic criteria for patient's selection for CRT remain to be ascertained. Defining the exact nature of cardiac function disturbances at the time of symptom development for optimal patient's selection seems a scientific way forward [1–3, 8–10].

Signs of Functional Deterioration

A. Development of restrictive LV filling with very short isovolumic relaxation time, which is resistant to off loading by medication. Cases with this degree of disease poorly tolerate beta blockers and pacing seems unable to offer satisfactory benefit.
B. RV deterioration of function particularly with raised RA pressures. Such cases develop systemic congestion with its known complications and difficult management.
C. Severe MR or TR. Though medical treatment and CRT have been shown to reduce functional valve regurgitation, patients might remain with well-established ventricular remodeling, dilated valve annuli and resistant regurgitation, which carries bad prognosis.
D. Progressive broadening of QRS related with worsening symptoms, ventricular function and clinical outcome. CRT must be recommended for such cases, with careful optimized electrical stimulation [1–3, 9, 10].

Myocarditis

- Previous studies of echocardiography in myocarditis have demonstrated a variety of echocardiographic findings. In addition to systolic dysfunction, regional wall motion abnormalities, diastolic dysfunction and changes in echocardiographic image texture and thickness have been reported [13–16].
- The increased LV thickness in patients with patients with fulminant myocarditis is probable due to the more inflammatory response on endo-myocardial biopsy in these cases. "Interstitial edema" might contribute to both thickened ventricular walls and also decreased ventricular function and contractility in this disease.
- Patients with fulminant myocarditis had meaningfully less ventricular dilation at baseline however more increased septal thickness than cases with acute myocarditis, so, patients with fulminant myocarditis presente with thickend, non-dilated, and hypo-contractile LV walls, while those with acute myocarditis had noticeable LV dilation, normal LV thickness with decreased LV contractility [13–16].
- Follow-up echocardiography, usually show significant improvement in contractility in the fulminant group,

while those with acute myocarditis frequently reveal no improvement, so, echocardiography might aid in classifying cases with myocarditis into clinically relevant subgroups with prognostic implications for example, he presence of right ventricular dysfunction by echocardiography predicted worse clinical outcome.

- Conventional echocardiography has usually played a limited role in the diagnosis of supposed myocarditis due to the lack of specific distinguishing features and/or apparently the normal examinations met in less severe types of myocarditis but nowadays, two dimensional echocardiographic strain imaging (2D strain) and myocardial perfusion contrast echocardiography perform as a part of the initial diagnostic workup, and previously reported findings showed the validity of these data with cardiac magnetic resonance (CMR) imaging [14, 15].
- As we all know segmental and global wall motion abnormalities do occur in myocarditis, but, interestingly, the patterns of dilated, hypertrophic and restrictive cardiomyopathies have been described in histologically proven myocarditis too [15–18].
- In myocardial contrast echocardiography, perfusion defects that do not adapt to a known coronary distribution must raise the clinical thought of myocarditis. Though areas of necrosis and inflammation can establish to result in myocardial perfusion defects on nuclear perfusion imaging [19].
- Also in CMR, late gadolinium enhancement on T1-weighted images represents necrosis and inflammatory injury. In cases with myocarditis, it typically happens focally, is sub-epicardial-based, and extends inconsistently into the ventricular walls, with a preference for the "infero-lateral segments". T2-weighted imaging consistently detects tissue edema with the long T2 of water-bound protons as the contrast-generating mechanism, generating high signal intensity in edematous tissue [15, 20]
- Frequently, the region of edema noticed on echocardiography associated with that detected on CMR; and these segments show the most severe strain reduction and also perfusion abnormalities on contrast imaging [20].
- Outstandingly, CMR without (T2-weighted images) and with contrast media (delayed enhancement method) has emerged as the diagnostic tool of choice for the non-invasive diagnosis of myocardial inflammation and supposed myocarditis, but, the technique is expensive (predominantly for serial monitoring), not commonly available, and also lacks portability [20].
- Newer echocardiographic modalities (strain echocardiography and torsional parameters) are potentially useful methods (excellent correlation with CMR) and can provide incremental information, beyond 2D echocardiography, in supposed myocarditis cases. These newer techniques seem to be more sensitive and could be of a specific value when clinical doubt in diagnosis exists. Two-dimensional strain echocardiography, in particular, due to its favourable signal-to-noise ratio, angle independence, and capability to differentiate between active and passive myocardial motions could be used to map and quantify regional contractile function in myocarditis [17, 18, 21].
- So, the validity, sensitivity and specificity of these newer echocardiographic techniques (strain echocardiography and torsional parameters) for the diagnosis of myocarditis are not known at this time, and need more to be prospectively studied against CMR and specially, endomyocardial biopsy [22–26].
- Data from some previous studies: Pinamonti and colleagues [22] described echocardiographic findings in 41 patients with histologically proven myocarditis and found LV dysfunction in 69%, primarily with little to no dilation of the LV cavity [22]. They also noted four patients in their series with transient "LV hypertrophy" in the setting of myocarditis. In two of these patients, ventricular thickening was associated with dramatic improvement in LV function. Transient "LV hypertrophy" associated with myocarditis has also been reported by Hauser and coworkers [26] in a 28-year-old woman with sudden onset of severe heart failure (HF) [26]. Spontaneous resolution of LV thickening in this patient was related with normalization of systolic function and clinical recovery. It is likely that these cases represent examples of the fulminant type of myocarditis as described in this report. Though the degree of LV dilation is frequently related to the severity and duration of HF, our data demonstrate that severe systolic dysfunction may happen in the absence of significant LV dilation in cases with fulminant myocarditis and both progression to DCM and normalization of systolic function have been reported [27].

Questions

1. With severe deterioration of ventricular function and absence of extra-cardiac fluid collection, … might develop.
   A. Pulsus alternance
   B. Palsus paradoxicus
   C. Pulsus bisferiens
   D. Pulsus Parvus

2. Which phrase is correct about DCM?
   A. Segmental WMA is uncommon.
   B. RV and RA dilation are uncommon.
   C. Increased LV mass is sign of poor prognosis.
   D. Improvement of LV function with Dobutamine is sign of good prognosis.

3. Which phrase is most specific for radiation heart disease?
   A. Aorto-mitral curtain thickening and calcification
   B. Pericardial effusion
   C. Severe AI
   D. Ascending aorta dilation

Answers

1. A
2. D
3. A

References

1. Luk A, Ahn E, Soor GS, Butany J. Dilated cardiomyopathy: a review. J Clin Pathol. 2009;62(3):219–25. https://doi.org/10.1136/jcp.2008.060731.
2. Elliott P. Cardiomyopathy. Diagnosis and management of dilated cardiomyopathy. Heart. 2000;84(1):106–12.
3. Stevens SM, Farzaneh-Far R, Na B, et al. Development of an echocardiographic risk-stratification index to predict HF in patients with stable coronary artery disease: The Heart & Soul Study. J Am Coll Cardiol Imaging. 2009;2:11.
4. Otto CM. The practice of clinical echocardiography. 5th ed. Philadelphia: Saunders; 2017.
5. Bielecka-Dabrowa A, Dimitri P, Mikhailidi DP, et al. Takotsubo cardiomyopathy: the current state of knowledge. Int J Cardiol. 2010;142:120.
6. Vanoverschelde JL, Raphael DA, Robert AR, Cosyns JR. Left ventricular filling in dilated cardiomyopathy: relation to functional class and hemodynamics. J Am Coll Cardiol. 1990;15:1288–95.
7. Silbiger JJ. Mechanistic insights into ischemic MR: echocardiographic and surgical implications. J Am Soc Echocardiogr. 2011;24:707. Cardiomyopathies, HF.
8. Tracy CM, Epstein AE, Darbar D, et al. 2012 ACCF/AHA/HRS focused update of the 2008 guidelines for device-based therapy of cardiac rhythm abnormalities. J Am Coll Cardiol. 2012;60:1297.
9. Kirkpatrick JN, Vannan MA, Narula J, et al. Echocardiography in HF: applications, utility, and new horizons. J Am Coll Cardiol. 2007;50:381.
10. Heydari B, Jerosch-Herold M, Kwong RY. Imaging for planning of cardiac resynchronization therapy. JACC Cardiovasc Imaging. 2012;5:93.
11. Tigen K, Karaahmet T, Cevik C, Gurel E, Pala S, Mutlu B, et al. Prognostic utility of right ventricular systolic functions assessed by tissue Doppler imaging in dilated cardiomyopathy and its correlation with plasma NT-pro-BNP levels. Congest Heart Fail. 2009;15(5):234–9.
12. Nanjo S, Yoshikawa K, Harada M, Inoue Y, Namiki A, Nakano H, et al. Correlation between left ventricular diastolic function and ejection fraction in dilated cardiomyopathy using magnetic resonance imaging with late gadolinium enhancement. Circ J. 2009;73(10):1939–44.
13. Afonso L, Hari P, Pidlaoan V, Kondur A, Jacob S, Khetarpal V. Acute myocarditis: can novel echocardiographic techniques assist with diagnosis? Eur J Echocardiogr. 11(3):E5. https://doi.org/10.1093/ejechocard/jep183.
14. Michael Felker G, Boehmer JP, Hruban RH, Hutchins GM, Kasper EK, Baughman KL, Hare JM. Echocardiographic findings in fulminant and acute myocarditis. J Am Coll Cardiol. 2000;36(1):227–32. https://doi.org/10.1016/S0735-1097(00)00690-2.
15. Nelson KH, Li T, Afonso L. Diagnostic approach and role of CMR in the assessment of acute myocarditis. Cardiol Rev. 2009;17:24–30.
16. Cooper LT Jr. Myocarditis. N Engl J Med. 2009;360:1526–38.
17. Agati L, Tonti G, Galiuto L, Di Bello V, Funaro S, Madonna MP, et al. Quantification methods in contrast echocardiography. Eur J Echocardiogr. 2005;6:S14–20.
18. Leitman M, Lysyansky P, Sidenko S, Shir V, Peleg E, Binenbaum M, et al. Two dimensional strain—a novel software for real-time quantitative echocardiographic assessment of myocardial function. J Am Soc Echocardiogr. 2004;17:1021–9.
19. Sun Y, Ma P, Bax JJ, Blom N, Yu Y, Wang Y, et al. 99mTc-MIBI myocardial perfusion imaging in myocarditis. Nucl Med Commun. 2003;24:779–83.
20. Friedrich MG, Sechtem U, Schulz-Menger J, Holmvang G, Alakija P, Cooper LT, et al. Cardiovascular magnetic resonance in myocarditis: a JACC White Paper. J Am Coll Cardiol. 2009;53:1475–87.
21. Di Bella G, Coglitore S, Zimbalatti C, Minutoli F, Zito C, Patane S, et al. Strain Doppler echocardiography can identify longitudinal myocardial dysfunction derived from edema in acute myocarditis. Int J Cardiol. 2008;126:279–80.
22. Pinamonti B, Alberti E, Cigalotto A. Echocardiographic findings in myocarditis. Am J Cardiol. 1988;62:285–91.
23. Nieminen MS, Heikkila J, Karjalainen J. Echocardiography in acute infectious myocarditis: relation to clinical and echocardiographic findings. Am J Cardiol. 1984;53:1331–7.
24. James KB, Lee K, Thomas JD. Left ventricular diastolic dysfunction in lymphocytic myocarditis as assessed by Doppler echocardiography. Am J Cardiol. 1994;73:282–5.
25. Lieback E, Hardouin I, Meyer R, Bellach J, Hetzer R. Clinical value of echocardiographic tissue characterization in the diagnosis of myocarditis. Eur Heart J. 1996;17:135–42.
26. Hauser AM, Gordon S, Cieszkowski J, Timmis GC. Severe transient left ventricular "hypertrophy" occurring during acute myocarditis. Chest. 1983;83:275–7.
27. Keren A, Gottlieb S, Tzivoni D. Mildly dilated congestive cardiomyopathy. Use of prospective diagnostic criteria and description of the clinical course without heart transplantation. Circulation. 1990;81:506–17.

Hypertrophic Cardiomyopathy

22

Anita Sadeghpour and Azin Alizadehasl

Abstract

Hypertrophic cardiomyopathy (HCM) is the most common genetic cardiovascular disorder (autosomal dominant transmission), with primary involvement of the cardiac muscle. If associated with left ventricular outflow tract (LVOT) obstruction, it is called hypertrophic obstructive cardiomyopathy (HOCM).

HCM is characterized by localized or generalized unexplained left ventricular hypertrophy (LVH) in the non-dilated ventricle in the absence of any cardiac or systemic disease that can result in this magnitude of hypertrophy.

Usually, LV wall thickness is ≥15 mm in adults and ratio of IVS thickness to posterior wall thickness is ≥1.3/1. Systolic anterior motion (SAM) is the abnormal movement (sharp bending) of the anterior mitral valve (MV) leaflet toward the interventricular septum during systole.

LVOT obstruction happens as a result of both significant septal thickening and concomitant SAM of the mitral leaflets into the LVOT. Continuous-wave Doppler flow of the LVOT is characteristically dagger shaped and has a late-peaking velocity due to an increased obstruction as systole progresses. MR due to SAM is a mid-to-late systolic, eccentric, and posteriorly directed jet.

Several studies in patients with HCM have demonstrated a significant reduction in longitudinal strain (particularly in the mid-septal segment) with normal systolic twist or torsion.

Keywords

Hypertrophic cardiomyopathy · Hypertrophic obstructive cardiomyopathy · Left ventricular outflow tract obstruction Asymmetric septal hypertrophy · Systolic anterior motion

Abbreviations

2D	Two dimensional
3D	Three dimensional
AF	Atrial fibrillation
ASH	Asymmetric septal hypertrophy
CAD	Coronary artery disease
CMR	Cardiac magnetic resonance
CT	Computed tomography
E	Peak E-wave velocity of the mitral valve (cm/s)
E′	TDI of the mitral annulus
EF	Ejection fraction
FC	Functional class
HCM	Hypertrophic cardiomyopathy
HHD	Hypertensive heart disease
HOCM	Hypertrophic obstructive cardiomyopathy
ICD	Implantable cardioverter defivrillators
LA	Left atrium
LGE	Late gadolinium enhancement
LV	Left ventricular
LVEF	Left ventricular ejection fraction
LVH	Left ventricular hypertrophy
LVOT	Left ventricular outflow tract
NSVT	Nonsustained ventricular tachycardia
NYHA	New York Heart Association
RV	Right ventricle
SAM	Systolic anterior motion
SCD	Sudden cardiac death
STE	Speckle-tracking echocardiography
TDI	Tissue Doppler imaging
TEE	Transesophageal echocardiography
TTE	Transthoracic echocardiography

Electronic Supplementary Material The online version of this chapter (https://doi.org/10.1007/978-3-319-67691-3_22) contains supplementary material, which is available to authorized users.

A. Sadeghpour, MD, FACC, FASE
Professor of Cardiology, Echocardiography Research Center, Rajaie Cardiovascular Medical and Research Center, Iran University of Medical Science, Tehran, Iran

A. Alizadehasl, MD, FACC, FASE (✉)
Associate Professor of Cardiology, Echocardiologist, Echocardiography and Cardiogenetic Research Centers, Cardio-Oncology Department, Rajaie Cardiovascular Medical and Research Center, Tehran, Iran

A. Sadeghpour, A. Alizadehasl (eds.), *Case-Based Textbook of Echocardiography*,
https://doi.org/10.1007/978-3-319-67691-3_22

Introduction

- Hypertrophic cardiomyopathy (HCM) is the most common genetic cardiovascular disorder (autosomal dominant transmission), with a prevalence of about 0.2% (1:500) and a wide variation in clinical appearances. HCM is the primary involvement of the cardiac muscle. If associated with left ventricular outflow tract (LVOT) obstruction, it is called hypertrophic obstructive cardiomyopathy (HOCM).
- **HCM is characterized by localized or generalized unexplained left ventricular hypertrophy (LVH) in the non-dilated ventricle in the absence of any cardiac or systemic disease that can result in this magnitude of hypertrophy** [1–7].

Severity and Pattern of Left Ventricular Hypertrophy

- **LVH is the cardinal finding of HCM. Usually, LV wall thickness is ≥15 mm in adults** or ≥2 standard deviations above the mean of their age, sex, or body size in children. However, any degree of increased wall thickness can be compatible with HCM in the setting of HCM genetic substrate [1, 2].
- **The common pattern is asymmetric septal hypertrophy (ASH)**, in which interventricular septal (IVS) thickness is usually ≥15 mm and the **ratio of IVS thickness to posterior wall thickness is ≥1.3/1** [8]. LVH is usually asymmetric or localized, but it can be concentric too or localized in the apical segments as in apical HCM (Fig. 22.1).

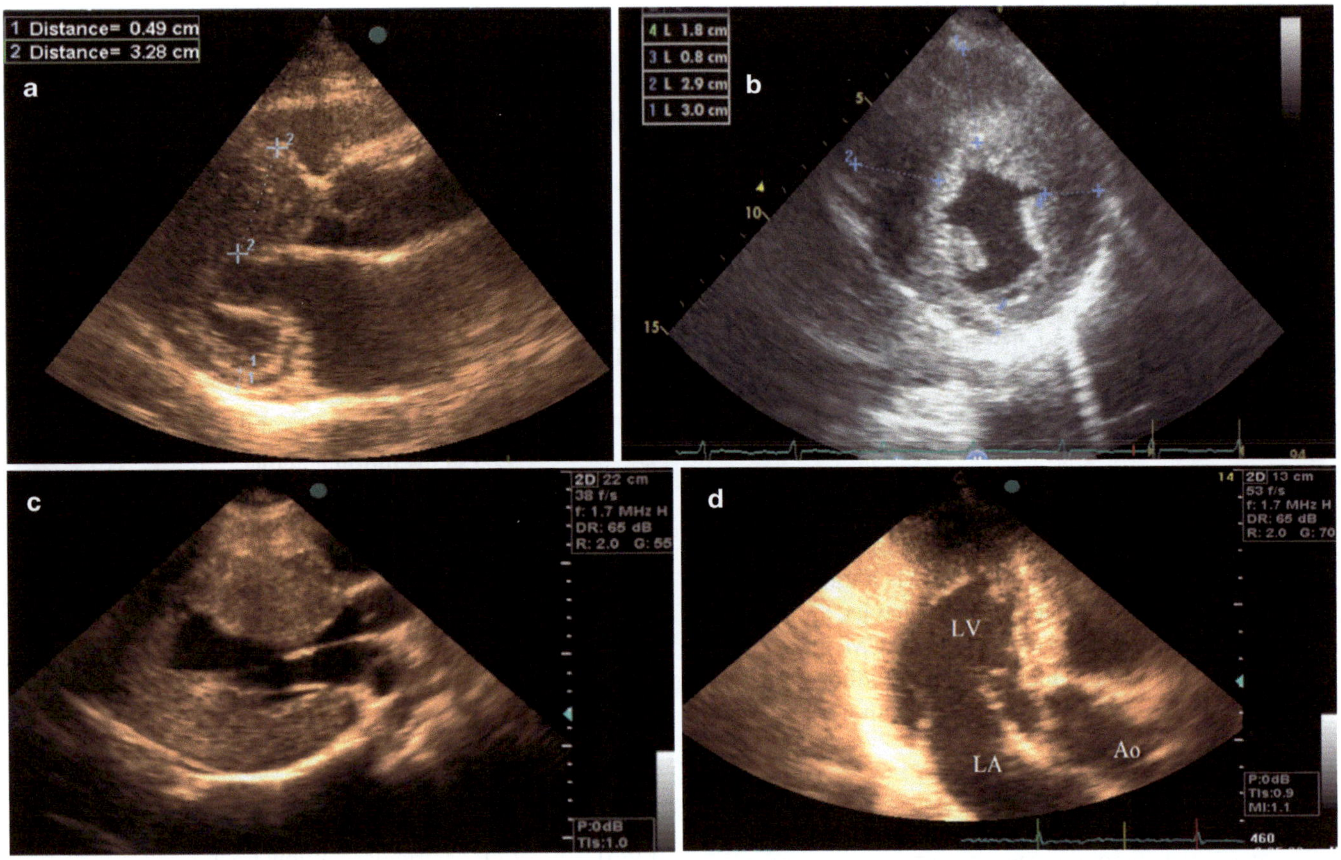

Fig. 22.1 (Movie 1) Pattern of left ventricular hypertrophy. (**a**, **b**) Asymmetric septal hypertrophy (ASH) in parasternal long axis view and short axis view. (**c**) Significant concentric hypertophy in HCM with no ASH and (**d**) Apical long axis view shows hypertrophied LV apex with spared basal sagments

- The distribution of hypertrophy can be in any pattern and at any location, including the right ventricle (RV). Although septal predominance is more common, hypertrophy can be isolated to the LV free wall or apex.

Key Points

1. A normal calculated LV mass does not rule out HCM. Wall thickening can involve a small segment of the LV, resulting in a normal LV mass [6].
2. Apical HCM, apical aneurysms, hypertrophy localized to the anterolateral wall, LV noncompaction, and apical displacement of the papillary muscle can be misdiagnosed with one another or coexist in a patient [9, 10].
3. Apical HCM, which is very common in Japan, has a characteristic giant negative T wave in ECG [11]. Injection of an echocardiographic contrast or cardiac magnetic resonance (CMR) is helpful in these patients [2].
4. ASH should not be used as a specific marker for HCM [8, 12, 13]. Indeed, ASH can be detected not only in HCM but also in the following diseases:
    1. Pulmonary hypertension with RV hypertrophy
    2. Inferior wall infarction in the presence of LVH
    3. Early stage of hypertension

Systolic Anterior Motion of the Mitral Valve

- Systolic anterior motion (SAM) is the abnormal movement (sharp bending) of the anterior mitral valve (MV) leaflet toward the interventricular septum during systole (Fig. 22.2).

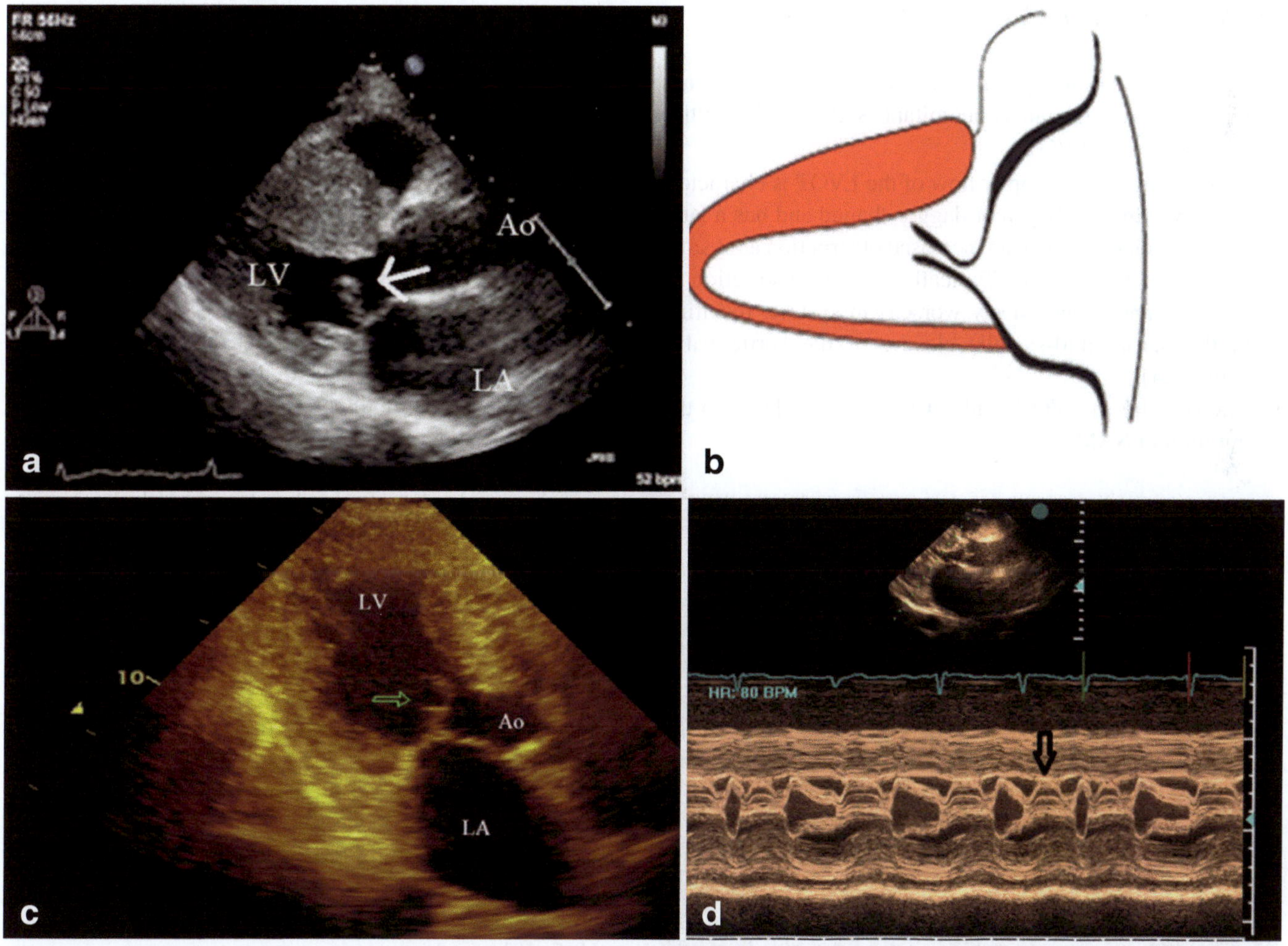

Fig. 22.2 (**a**, **b**) Systolic anterior motion (SAM) of the anterior mitral leaflet in parasternal long axis view (*white arrow*). (**c**) SAM in apical long axis view and (**d**) Showing SAM of the anterior mitral leaflet in M-mode study in parasternal long axis view (*Black arrow*)

- SAM is best appreciated in parasternal long-axis views (MV M-mode recordings) and can be very difficult to find in real-time 2D images (Fig. 22.2c, d and Movie 22.1).
- SAM is mostly due to a suction force (the Venturi effect) created as blood accelerates into an obstructed LVOT, abnormal MV apparatus, and anterior displacement of the papillary muscles.
- Also, SAM is seen in MV repair, congenital papillary muscle abnormalities, acute myocardial hypovolemia, inotrope infusion, and small LV cavity [6, 14–16].
- Presence and severity should be evaluated by 2D and M-mode and classified as:
  - Mild SAM: No mitral/septal contact occurs in late systole, and it occupies <10% of systole.
  - Severe SAM: It occurs at mid-systole and occupies ≥30% of its duration [14].

Left Ventricular Outflow Tract Obstruction

- LVOT obstruction happens as a result of both significant septal thickening and concomitant SAM of the mitral leaflets into the LVOT.
- Continuous-wave Doppler flow of the LVOT is characteristically scimitar-shaped or dagger shaped and has a late-peaking velocity due to an increased obstruction as systole progresses (Fig. 22.3). Typically, LVOT obstruction is dynamic and progressively worsens in systole, resulting in the partial mid-systolic closure of the aortic valve (Fig. 22.4).
- The severity of LVOT gradient is directly related to the duration of SAM.

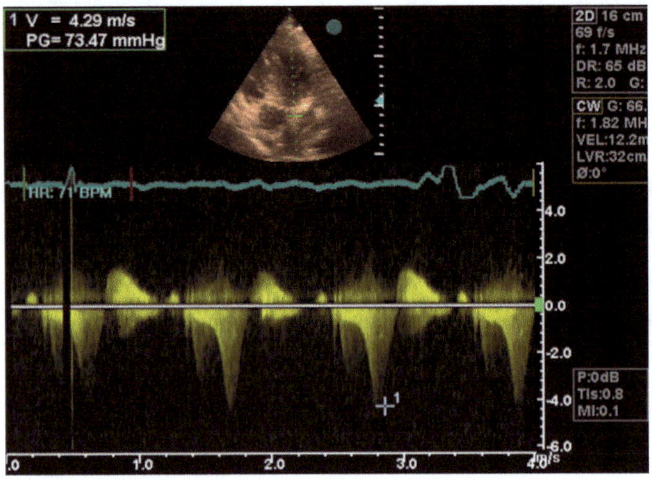

Fig. 22.3 Dagger shape late peaking systolic LVOT systolic pressure gradient

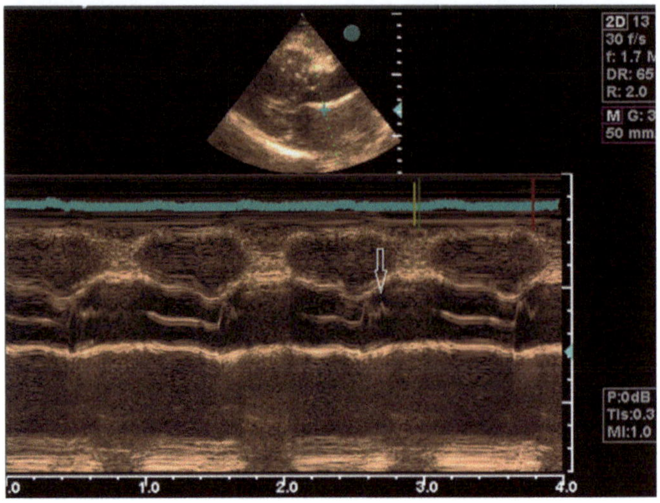

Fig. 22.4 Mid systolic notching of aortic valve (*White arrow*)

Table 22.1 HCM vs. HOCM

Non-obstructive HCM	LVOT gradient at rest or by provocative maneuvers <30 mmHg
Obstructive HCM (HOCM)	LVOT gradient at rest ≥ 30 mmHg
Labile or latent obstruction	LVOT gradient at rest < 30 mmHg LVOT gradient by provocative maneuvers ≥ 30 mmHg

HCM hypertrophic cardiomyopathy, *HOCM* hypertrophic obstructive cardiomyopathy, *LVOT* left ventricular outflow tract

- For clinical decision-making, peak instantaneous LVOT gradient is more important than mean gradient. LVOT obstruction is seen in the presence of SAM and ASH.
- Pressure gradient might not be evident at rest but can be provoked by some maneuvers that increase contractility or reduce preload or afterload such as the Valsalva maneuver, exercise, and nitrate or dobutamine infusion.
- Seventy percent of patients with HCM show obstruction at rest or by provocative maneuvers (Table 22.1).
- Patients with a narrow LVOT (≤2 cm) are more prone to latent LVOT obstruction.
- A significant intracavitary gradient may decrease pressure in the LVOT sufficiently to allow premature aortic valve closure.
- Fluttering aortic valve (due to turbulent blood flow) can be evaluated via M-mode study.
- The level of LV cavity obstruction is evaluated by color flow imaging and pulsed-wave study (Fig. 22.5), and its severity is assessed by continuous-wave Doppler study [6, 7–19].

Key Points

- Care should be taken to avoid contamination between LVOT signal and mitral regurgitation (MR) jet. When velocity exceeds 5 m/s, superimposition of MR on LVOT

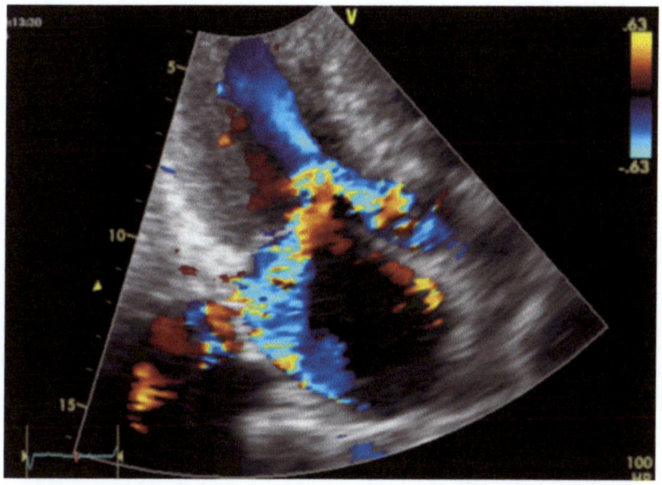

Fig. 22.5 (Movie 2) Sytolic turbulancy in LVOT associated with posterior directed MR

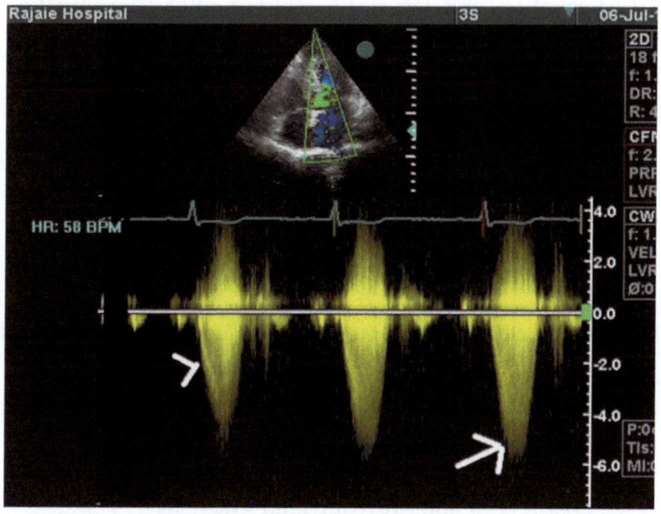

Fig. 22.6 Superimposition of MR Doppler signal (*white arrow*) on LVOT gradient (*arrow head*)

gradient should be considered. Another clue is a prolonged MR jet compared to LVOT gradient. MR extends to isovolumic relaxation time (Fig. 22.6).

- Concomitant valvular aortic stenosis should be ruled out by evaluating the anatomy of the atrioventricular valve.
- Mid-cavitary obstruction with hyperdynamic LV function should be distinguished from LVOT obstruction via pulsed-wave Doppler study and color Doppler mapping.
- Usually SAM of the MV is associated with some degree of LVOT obstruction and posteriorly directed MR.
- LVOT obstruction is also seen in severe hypertensive LVH (during dobutamine stress echocardiography), congenital papillary muscle abnormalities, acute myocardial infarction, and the Takotsubo cardiomyopathy [1, 2, 6, 7, 14, 15].

Mitral Regurgitation

- MR happens as a result of SAM because the motion of the anterior mitral leaflet is more than that of the posterior mitral leaflet, resulting in a gap between the anterior and posterior mitral leaflets and dynamic malcoaptation of the MV leaflets.
- MR due to SAM is a mid-to-late systolic, eccentric, and posteriorly directed jet [1, 2, 6], which is a common finding in HOCM (Movie 22.2).
- Centrally or anteriorly directed MR usually suggests an intrinsic valve abnormality [1, 2, 14, 18, 19].

Hypertrophic Obstructive Cardiomyopathy

- About 30% of patients with HCM are truly non-obstructive; therefore, the other 70% have a propensity for developing gradients $\geq$30 at rest or with provocative maneuvers, e.g., exercise and the Valsalva maneuver (Table 22.1).
- HOCM is characterized by SAM associated with dynamic LVOT gradients $\geq$30 mmHg.

Primary Abnormalities of the Mitral Apparatus

- Primary abnormalities of the MV apparatus in HCM include elongation of the MV leaflets, papillary muscle hypertrophy, and anterior displacement [1, 2, 14, 18, 19].

Diastolic Dysfunction

- Assessment of LV diastolic function in patients with HCM needs a comprehensive evaluation of multiple parameters in the absence of atrial fibrillation (AF) and significant MR, which comprises [20]:
  - LA volume index (>34 mL/m^2)
  - Average E/e′ ratio > 14
  - Tricuspid regurgitation peak jet velocity > 2.8 m/s
  - Pulmonary vein atrial reversal-A duration $\geq$ 30 m/s
- Generally, each variable alone has a modest correlation with LV filling pressure. Nevertheless, if 3 or 4 of the variables (>50%) reach above the cutoff value, LA pressure is high.
- High LV filling pressure caused by diastolic dysfunction can lead to atrial dilatation and also AF.
- The severity of diastolic dysfunction is very variable in patients with HCM, the most common pattern of which is delayed relaxation [12, 17, 21–24].

Systolic Dysfunction

- Usually, left ventricular ejection fraction (LVEF) is normal or increased, despite a small LV cavity at end diastole and reduced stroke volume [1].
- **Burned out, dilated, or end-stage HCM is defined as LVEF < 50%** [1, 2, 12, 17, 19].

Right Ventricular Hypertrophy

- RV hypertrophy (>0.5 cm) frequently occurs in combination with LVH.
- RV free-wall thickness in the parasternal short-axis, subcostal, and apical 4-chamber views should be assessed.

Tissue Doppler Imaging

- Early diastolic mitral annular velocity (Ea) and systolic velocity (Sa) are reduced in patients with HCM even before the onset of overt hypertrophy (Fig. 22.7).
- Tissue Doppler imaging (TDI) may also assist in the differentiation between the conditions of physiological hypertrophy (athlete's heart) and pathological hypertrophy inasmuch as mean Sa <9 cm/s is a parameter for differentiating pathological LVH (HCM/hypertensive LVH) from physiological LVH (diagnostic accuracy = 92%).
- Low lateral mitral annular Sa < 4 cm/s has a prognostic value and can independently predict death or hospitalization for worsening heart failure [25–27].
- Strain rate imaging has been shown to be useful in differentiating nonobstructive HCM from hypertensive LVH.
- However, TDI is an angle-dependent technique and is influenced by cardiac translational motion and tethering.

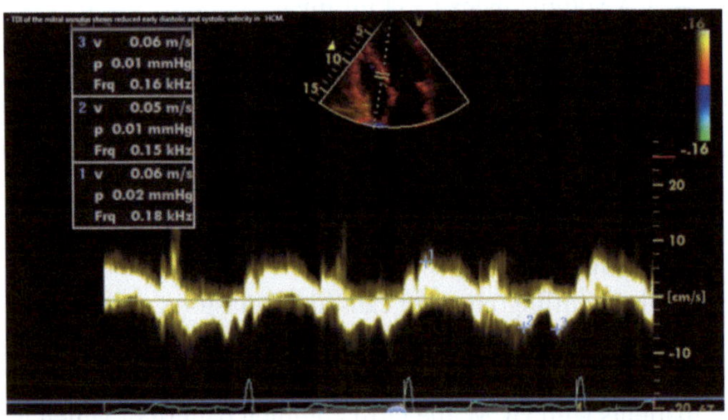

Fig. 22.7 TDI of the mitral annulus shows reduced early diastolic and systolic velocity in HCM

Two-Dimensional Strain or Speckle-Tracking Echocardiography

- 2D Strain provides angle-independent Strain Data. Several studies in patients with HCM have demonstrated a significant reduction in longitudinal strain (particularly in the mid-septal segment). Global longitudinal strain (GLS) with cut-off value−14.3% and tissue Doppler based strain with cut-off value−10.6% discriminate HCM versus hypertensive heart disease. Normal systolic twist or torsion have been suggested (Fig. 22.8) [1, 2, 6, 7, 17, 22].

Three-Dimensional Echocardiography

- 3D echocardiography facilitates the assessment of LVOT area after intervention for septal reduction, surgical myectomy, volumetric estimation of left atrial (LA) mechanical function, and accurate estimation of LVEF as well as LV mass in hypertrophied hearts (comparing favorably with CMR imaging) [6, 7, 12, 24].

Transesophageal Echocardiography

- Transesophageal echocardiography (TEE) should be considered in patients with:
  - Poor transthoracic echocardiography (TTE) windows
  - Unclear mechanism of LVOT obstruction
  - Suspicious association between HCM and subvalvular membrane or valvular aortic stenosis
  - Before septal reduction procedure
  - Severe MR caused by intrinsic valve abnormalities or centrally or anteriorly directed MR

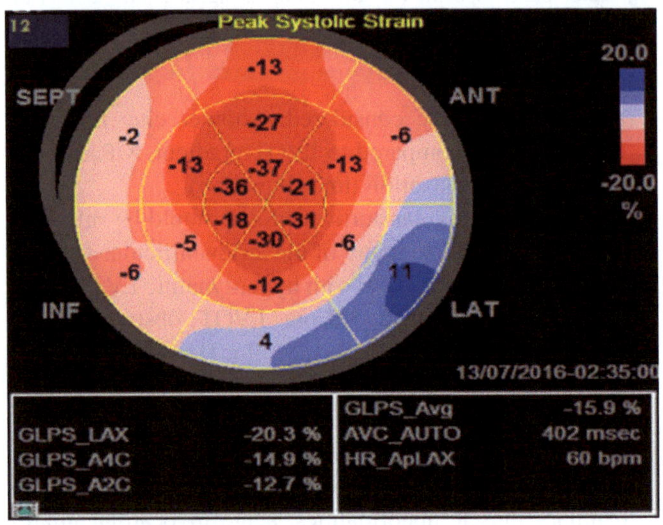

Fig. 22.8 Significantly reduced longitudinal strain (particularly in the mid-septal segment)

- Exercise stress echocardiography is class IIa in patients with HCM not exhibiting resting LVOT gradient ≥50 mmHg for detecting and quantifying dynamic LVOT obstruction [1].

Surgical Myectomy

- This surgical modality consists of basal septal myectomy via the trans-aortic approach (the Morrow procedure).

Indications

- Surgical myectomy is performed in patients with:
  - Dynamic LVOT gradient at rest or with provocation ≥50 mmHg
  - Severely symptomatic patients (New York Heart Association functional class III/IV) refractory to medical treatment
  - Septal hypertrophy (measured >18 mm) associated with SAM of the MV [2, 24].

Intraoperative Transesophageal Echocardiography

Usefulness

- Limited visualization of the septum during the trans-aortic approach in an empty LV may lead to inadequate or extensive myocardial resection, so intraoperative TEE is an essential component of surgical myectomy.
- Perioperative TEE should be used to guide the surgeon's strategy for the extent and depth of the myectomy. TEE can demonstrate:
  - Maximum thickness of the septum
  - Distance from the aortic annulus to the maximum thickness
  - Distance from the aortic annulus to the site of mitral/septal contact during SAM (Fig. 22.9)
  - Severity and mechanism of MR
  - LV coronary artery fistula [24]

Following myectomy, intraoperative TEE confirms the:

1. Adequacy of myectomy (measuring LVOT gradient by continuous-wave Doppler study)
2. Severity of MR and SAM
3. Severity of aortic regurgitation
4. Ventricular function
5. Development of ventricular septal defect [1, 2, 7, 8, 24]

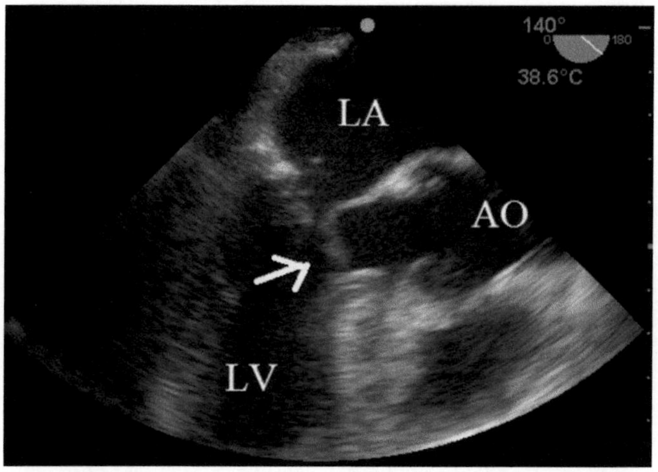

Fig. 22.9 Long axis view showing significant SAM in TEE

Alcohol Septal Ablation and Contrast Echocardiography

- Contrast echocardiography is currently used to enhance endocardial definition and Doppler signals and to evaluate myocardial perfusion.
- Myocardial contrast echocardiography can help anticipate the location and delineate the extent of septal infarct (selective injection of the contrast into the proximal septal perforators) before alcohol septal ablation [1, 2, 6–9].
- Myocardial contrast echocardiography results in increased echodensity in the basal septum, which should be the region of flow convergence and mitral/septal contact.
- TTE is the usual method of intraprocedural evaluation.
- Successful procedure is defined as at least a 50% decrease in LVOT gradient [2].

Intraventricular Dyssynchrony and Prognosis

- Interventricular and intraventricular delays are commonly present in patients with HCM, despite the absence of conduction abnormalities on the ECG, and appear to correlate to the degree of septal LVH and the presence of LVOT obstruction and increased risk of ventricular tachyarrhythmias, syncope, and sudden cardiac death [6, 12, 26–31].

Echocardiographic Predictors of Unfavorable Outcome and Sudden Cardiac Death

- Several echocardiographic parameters given below are also important for the prediction of an unfavorable outcome in patients with HCM.
  - Sudden death: maximal wall thickness > 30 mm, apical aneurysm

- HCM-related death: LVOT gradient at rest > 30 mmHg and EF < 50%
- All-cause mortality: LA diameter > 48 mm
- Heart failure development: LA volume > 27 mL/m^2 at baseline or during follow-up
- Intraventricular dyssynchrony > 45 msec [1, 2, 6–8, 19]

Diseases Mimicking Hypertrophic Cardiomyopathy

1. Hypertensive heart disease (HHD)
2. RV hypertrophy
3. Bulging of the septum in aging (usually associated with tortuosity of the ascending aorta)
4. Athlete's heart
5. Cardiac amyloidosis
6. Anderson-Fabry disease (an inherited metabolic disease mimicking HCM)

Key Points

- ASH, SAM, and also dynamic LVOT obstruction are not unique and characteristic of HCM, and the recognition of these abnormalities needs to be considered in the context of the clinical condition. However:
  - ASH and LVOT obstruction are less common in other diseases than in HCM.
  - HCM affects the MV apparatus, coronary arteries, and myocardium interstitium.
  - CMR facilitates the differentiation between HCM and other HCM-mimicking diseases and should be considered in all patients in the initial evaluation of HCM if expert local resources permit.
- Anderson-Fabry disease and amyloidosis usually have:

Concomitant systemic signs and symptoms
Concentric hypertrophy [2]

- Sometimes there is a distinct bright endocardial layer in Anderson-Fabry disease; nonetheless, this is by no means specific to this condition [1, 6, 7, 18].
- In adults with Anderson-Fabry disease, CMR shows late gadolinium enhancement mostly in the basal inferolateral segment and echocardiography demonstrates a distinct bright endocardial layer [1, 2, 4, 5].
- ASH can be seen in the early stage of HHD, RV hypertrophy, and inferior myocardial infarction with previous LVH.

Hypertensive Heart Disease

1. Patients with Hypertensive heart disease (HHD) commonly have uniformed increased wall thickness and even a thickened basoposterior segment. (ASH and SAM are more common in HCM.)
2. There is an increase in LV mass with a normal LV cavity. (A small LV cavity is more common in HCM.)
3. Hypertensive end-organ damage is in favor of HHD, while elongated anterior mitral leaflet is in favor of HCM [1, 2, 18, 19].
4. Global function index = [E/e′]/S < 1.77 is in favor of HHD (Fig. 22.10) [32].
5. There is less dynamic outflow obstruction in HHD; if it occurs, it is mostly mid-ventricular chordal SAM not leaflet SAM.
6. Wall thickness > 18–19 mm is rare in HHD but is a common finding in HCM.
7. S′ and E′ are significantly reduced in TDI.
8. Significantly reduced Doppler-based longitudinal strain < −10.6% discriminates HCM from HHD (sensitivity = 85% and specificity = 100%) [33].

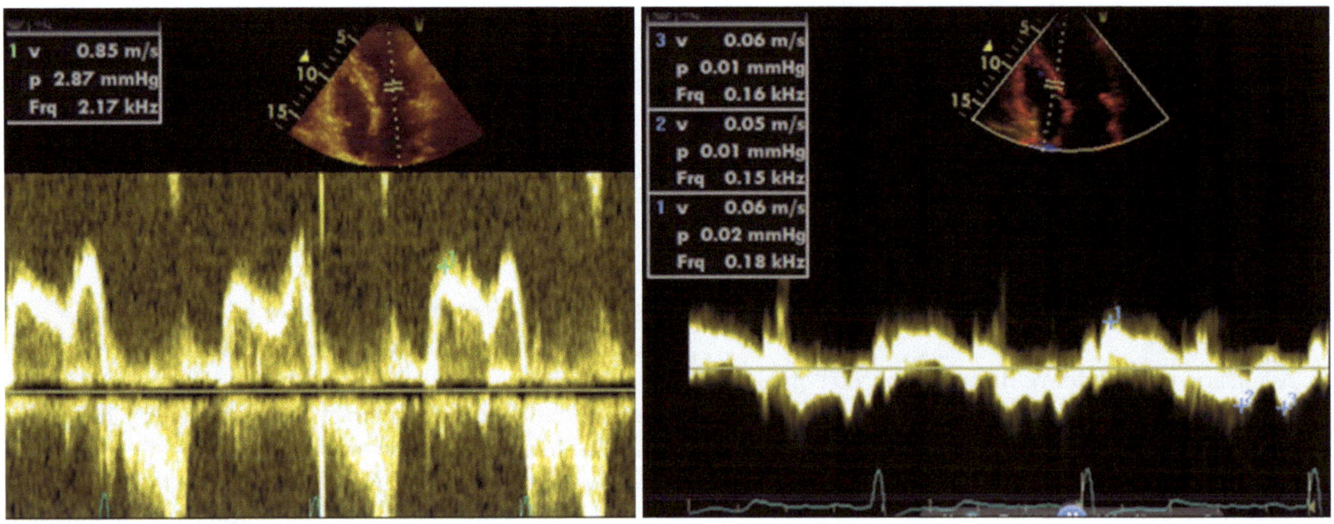

Fig. 22.10 TDI of the mitral annulus and PW Doppler study of Mitral inflow. Global function index > 1.77 is in favor of HCM

Athlete's Heart

- High-level training for endurance sports such as rowing, swimming, and triathlons can result in eccentric cardiac hypertrophy due to volume-loading of the LV. This is considered a physiological, reversible, and benign course. Sports such as weight lifting impose a pressure load on the heart and lead to concentric LVH. This pattern of hypertrophy may not be so benign. Infrequent difficulty arises in distinguishing between HCM and athlete's heart. Various criteria can be drawn upon for differentiation (Table 22.2), though it is not an exact science [2–4, 18, 19, 33, 34].

Transthoracic Echocardiographic Evaluation of Hypertrophic Cardiomyopathy

1.	Assessing the presence, severity, and distribution of LVH
2.	Assessing end-diastolic wall thickness in quadrants from the parasternal short-axis views at the basal (MV), mid LV (papillary), and apical levels
3.	Reporting septal, posterior, and maximum wall thickness in any segment
4.	Measuring septal and posterior walls in the parasternal LAX and SAX views
5.	Screening the family members in patients with HCM
6.	Performing TTE every 1–2 years in symptomatic, but stable, patients with HCM as part of serial evaluation
7.	Assessing the presence of ASH
8.	Assessing the presence of SAM of the MV
9.	Determining the presence and site of dynamic LVOT obstruction at rest and with provocative maneuvers
10.	Assessing mid-systolic atrioventricular valve closure
11.	Determining the presence, direction, severity, and mechanism of MR
12.	Determining LV size and systolic function
13.	Determining whether the LV cavity is normal or small (Hypertrophy may be so severe that it might cause a nearly complete obliteration of the LV cavity during systole. In addition, LVEF is usually normal or increased in patients with HCM).
14.	Determining the presence or absence of apical aneurysm
15.	Measuring LV diastolic function and LA volume
16.	Measuring systolic pulmonary artery pressure
17.	Determining RV size and function
18.	Determining the presence of RV hypertrophy
19.	Performing contrast echocardiography in apical HCM and alcohol septal ablation

Table 22.2 HCM vs. Athlet's heart

HCM	Athlete's heart
Small LV cavity < 45 mm	Normal or enlarged LV cavity > 55 mm
Positive family history of HCM	Regression of LVH after 4–6 weeks deconditioning
LVH with unusual pattern	Wall thickness < 14–16 mm
Abnormal LV filling pressure	

Questions

1. Based on the CW Doppler study through the aortic valve, which of the following condition is the most probable diagnosis?
   A. Aortic valve stenosis
   B. Dynamic LVOT obstruction
   C. Subaortic membrane
   D. Supravalvular aortic stenosis

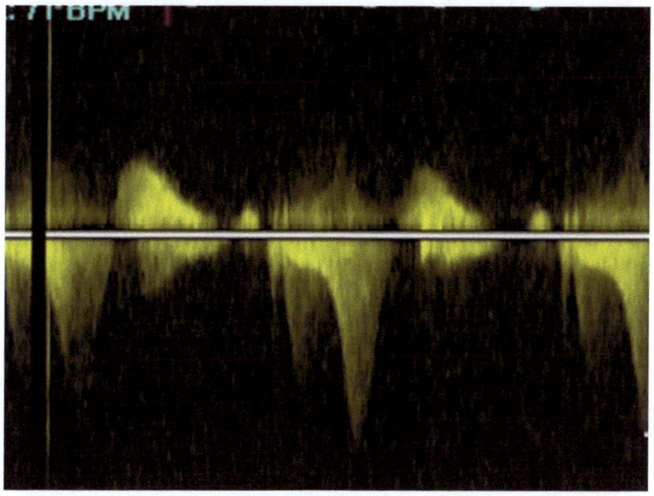

2. In a 42-year-old man, a known case of HOCM with exertional dyspnea (NYHA class III), MR jet peak velocity of 6 m/s, LA pressure of 20 mmHg, and systolic BP of 100/60 mmHg, what is the estimated LVOT obstruction?
   A. 90 mmHg
   B. 84 mmHg
   C. 64 mmHg
   D. 44 mmHg

3. Which of the following statements is not correct in MR-related SAM in patients with HOCM?
   A. MR-related SAM is usually an eccentric posteriorly directed jet.
   B. MR-related SAM is holo systolic.
   C. Usually SAM of the MV is associated with some degree of LVOT obstruction and eccentric MR.
   D. Centrally or anteriorly directed MR usually suggests an intrinsic valve abnormality.

4. Which of the following parameters in cardiac mechanics is less useful in the diagnosis of HCM from hypertensive heart disease?
   A. TDI of the mitral annulus
   B. Strain rate imaging of the mid-septal segment
   C. Global longitudinal strain (GLS)
   D. Systolic twist or torsion

5. The cut-point LVEF which indicates burnout HCM is:
   A. 40%
   B. 45%
   C. 50%
   D. 55%

Answers

1. B
   LVOT obstruction is systolic late peaking dynamic obstruction.
2. C
   Regurgitant jet can be used to estimate the magnitude of LVOT obstruction:
   When MR peak jet velocity = 6 m/s, means LV-to-LA gradient = $4 \times V^2 = 4 \times 6^2 = 4 \times 36 = 144$ mmHg
   LV pressure = 144 + 20 (LA pressure) = 164 mmHg
   LVOT obstruction = LV pressure − Blood pressure
   LVOT gradient = 164–100 = 64 mmHg
3. B
   MR due to SAM is a mid-to-late systolic, eccentric, and posteriorly directed jet, which is a common finding in HOCM.
   Centrally or anteriorly directed MR usually suggests an intrinsic valve abnormality.
4. D
   Early diastolic mitral annular velocity (Ea) and systolic velocity (Sa) are reduced in patients with HCM. Longitudinal strain (particularly in the mid-septal segment) are reduced in HCM. Normal systolic twist or torsion have been suggested in HCM patients.
5. C
   Usually, left ventricular ejection fraction (LVEF) in HCM is normal or increased.
   Burnout, or end-stage HCM is defined as LVEF < 50%.

References

1. Gersh BJ, Maron BJ, Bonow R, Dearani J, Fifer MA, Link MS, et al. 2011 ACCF/AHA guideline for the diagnosis and treatment of hypertrophic cardiomyopathy. Circulation. 2011;124(24):2761–96. https://doi.org/10.1161/CIR.0b013e318223e230.
2. Nagueh SF, Bierig SM, Budoff MJ, Desai M, Dilsizian V, Eidem B, et al. American Society of Echocardiography clinical recommendations for multimodality cardiovascular imaging of patients with hypertrophic cardiomyopathy. J Am Soc Echocardiogr. 2011;24:473–98.
3. Maron BJ, Maron MS. Hypertrophic cardiomyopathy. Lancet. 2013;381:242–55.
4. Maron BJ. Hypertrophic cardiomyopathy: a systematic review. JAMA. 2002;287:1308–20.
5. Maron BJ. Hypertrophic cardiomyopathy: an important global disease. Am J Med. 2004;116:63–5.
6. Maron BJ, Maron MS, Wigle ED, et al. The 50-year history, controversy, and clinical implications of left ventricular outflow tract obstruction in hypertrophic cardiomyopathy from idiopathic hypertrophic subaortic stenosis to hypertrophic cardiomyopathy. J Am Coll Cardiol. 2009;54:191–200.
7. Maron MS, Olivotto I, Zenovich AG, et al. Hypertrophic cardiomyopathy is predominantly a disease of left ventricular outflow tract obstruction. Circulation. 2006;114:2232–9.
8. Armstrong W, Ryan T. Feigenbaum's echocardiography. 7th ed; 2010.
9. Sadeghpour A, Faghihi S, Alizadehasl A. Can hypertrophic cardiomyopathy and non compaction left ventricle coexist in a single patient? Int J Cardiovasc Imaging. 2015;31(2):319–21. https://doi.org/10.1007/s10554-014-0561-2.
10. Alizadeh-Sani Z, Madadi S, Sadeghpour A, Khajali Z, Golnari P, Kiavar M. Cardiac MRI in a patient with coincident left ventricular non-compaction and hypertrophic cardiomyopathy. J Tehran Univ Heart Cent. 2011;6(4):214–6.
11. Kitaoka H, Doi Y, Casey SA, Hitomi N, Furuno T, Maron BJ. Comparison of prevalence of apical hypertrophic cardiomyopathy in Japan and the United States. Am J Cardiol. 2003;92:1183–6.
12. Afonso LC, Bernal J, Bax JJ, Abraham TP. Echocardiography in hypertrophic cardiomyopathy: the role of conventional and emerging technologies. JACC Cardiovasc Imaging. 2008;1(6):787–800.
13. Musat D, Sherrid MV. Echocardiography in the treatment of hypertrophic cardiomyopathy. Anadolu Kardiyol Derg. 2006;6(Suppl 2):18–26.
14. Cardim N, Galderisi M, Edvardsen T, Plein S, Popescu BA, D'Andrea A, et al. Role of multimodality cardiac imaging in the management of patients with hypertrophic cardiomyopathy: an expert consensus of the EACVI. Eur Heart J Cardiovasc Imaging. 2015;16(3):280.
15. Nagueh SF, Mahmarian JJ. Noninvasive cardiac imaging in patients with hypertrophic cardiomyopathy. J Am Coll Cardiol. 2006;48:2410–22.
16. Maron MS, Olivotto I, Betocchi S, Casey SA, Lesser JR, Losi MA, et al. Effect of left ventricular outflow tract obstruction on clinical outcome in hypertrophic cardiomyopathy. N Engl J Med. 2003;348:295–303.
17. Gilman G, Khandheria BK, Hagen ME, Abraham TP, Seward JB, Belohlavek M. Strain rate and strain: a step-by-step approach to image and data acquisition. J Am Soc Echocardiogr. 2004;17:1011–20.
18. Otto CM. The practice of clinical echocardiography. 4th ed. Philadelphia: Elsevier Saunders; 2012. p. 518–30.
19. Mann DL, Zipes DP, Libby P, Bonow RO. Braunwald's heart disease: a textbook of cardiovascular medicine. 10th ed. London: Elsevier Health Sciences; 2011. p. 1575–85.
20. Nagueh SF, Otto AS, Appleton CP, Byrd BF, Dokainish H, Edvardsen T, et al. Recommendations for the evaluation of left ventricular diastolic function by echocardiography: an update from the American Society of Echocardiography and the European Association of Cardiovascular Imaging. J Am Soc Echocardiogr. 2016;29:277–314.
21. Weidemann F, Mertens L, Gewillig M, Sutherland GR. Quantitation of localized abnormal deformation in asymmetric nonobstructive hypertrophic cardiomyopathy: a velocity, strain rate, and strain Doppler myocardial imaging study. Pediatr Cardiol. 2001;22:534–7.
22. Afonso L, Kondur A, Simegn M, Niraj A, Hari P, Kaur R, et al. Two-dimensional strain profiles in patients with physiological and pathological hypertrophy and preserved left ventricular systolic function: a comparative analyses. BMJ Open. 2012;2(4):e001390. https://doi.org/10.1136/bmjopen-2012-001390.

23. Roberts R, Sigwart U. New concepts in hypertrophic cardiomyopathies, part II. Circulation. 2001;104:2249–52.
24. Savage R, Aronson S, Shernan SK. Comprehensive textbook of perioperative transesophageal echocardiography. second ed. Philadelphia: Lippincott Williams and Wilkins; 2011. p. 616.
25. Nagakura T, Takeuchi M, Yoshitani H. Hypertrophic cardiomyopathy is associated with more severe left ventricular dyssynchrony than is hypertensive left ventricular hypertrophy. Echocardiography. 2007;24:677–84.
26. Nistri S, Olivetti I, Betocchi S. Prognostic significance of left atrial size in patients with hypertrophic cardiomyopathy (from the Italian Registry for Hypertrophic Cardiomyopathy). Am J Cardiol. 2006;98:960–5.
27. Nagueh SF, Bachinski LL, Meyer D, Hill R, Zoghbi WA, Tam JW, et al. Tissue Doppler imaging consistently detects myocardial abnormalities in patients with hypertrophic cardiomyopathy and provides a novel means for an early diagnosis before and independently of hypertrophy. Circulation. 2001;104:128–30.
28. Cardim N, Perrot A, Ferreirat T, Pereira A, Osterziel KJ, Reis RP, et al. Usefulness of Doppler myocardial imaging for identification of mutation carriers of familial hypertrophic cardiomyopathy. Am J Cardiol. 2002;90:128–32.
29. Kiavar M, Behzadnia N, Sadeghpour A, Madadi S. Clinical and echocardiographic evaluation of regional systolic function detected by tissue Doppler imaging in hypertrophic cardiomyopathy. Iran Cardiovas Res J. 2009;3(3):137–43.
30. Kato TS, Noda A, Izawa H, Yamada A, Obata K, Nagata K, et al. Discrimination of nonobstructive hypertrophic cardiomyopathy from hypertensive left ventricular hypertrophy on the basis of strain rate imaging by tissue Doppler ultrasonography. Circulation. 2004;110:3808–14.
31. Sadeghpour A, Kyavar M, Behzadnia N, Maddadi S, Parsaei M, Maleki M, Esmaeilzadeh M. Left ventricular systolic dyssynchrony in patients with hypertrophic cardiomyopathy: the prevalence and its relation to syncope. ICRJ. 2010;4(4):152–8.
32. Oh JK, Seward J, Tajik J. The echo manual. 3rd ed. Philadelphia: Lippincott Williams and Wilkins; 2006. p. 267–8.
33. Losi MA, Nistri S, Galderisi M, Betocchi S, Cecchi F, Olivotto, et al. Echocardiography in patients with hypertrophic cardiomyopathy: usefulness of old and new techniques in the diagnosis and pathophysiological assessment. Cardiovasc Ultrasound. 2010;8:7. https://doi.org/10.1186/1476-7120-8.
34. Maron BJ. Distinguishing hypertrophic cardiomyopathy from athlete's heart physiological remodelling: clinical significance, diagnostic strategies and implications for preparticipation screening. Br J Sports Med. 2009;43(9):649–56.

Restrictive Cardiomyopathy

23

Azin Alizadehasl and Anita Sadeghpour

Abstract

Relative to dilated and hypertrophic cardiomyopathies, restrictive cardiomyopathy (RCM) happens at a low frequency in the developed world. Specific forms of RCM such as endomyocardial disease are important causes of morbidity and mortality common in specific geographic region, particularly in underdeveloped countries. The pathophysiologic feature that defines RCM is increased stiffness in ventricular walls, which causes heart failure due to impaired ventricular filling. In the early stages of the syndrome, the systolic function may be normal, though deterioration in the systolic function is generally observed as the disease progresses.

Early in the disease, the left ventricular (LV) systolic function is typically preserved, while the LV diastolic function is abnormal, causing an increased atrial pressure and marked bi-atrial enlargement. The characteristic features of primary RCM on 2D echocardiography include a normal ventricular cavity size, normal wall thicknesses, and usually a preserved global systolic function with bi-atrial enlargement. RCM is accompanied by restrictive diastolic filling; this is, however, a nonspecific finding. The typical LV diastolic pressure tracing in RCM is the dip and plateau or square root configuration, which corresponds to a shortened deceleration time of the mitral inflow E velocity. The increase in the left atrial pressure (a) causes the mitral valve to open at a higher pressure, reducing the isovolumic relaxation time; (b) increases the transmitral pressure gradient with a concomitant rise in the mitral E velocity; and (c) decreases the pulmonary venous flow velocity during systole and increases it during diastole. With a high LV end-diastolic pressure, atrial contribution to ventricular filling is minimal and A velocity is usually decreased, causing the E/A ratio to increase markedly (>2). In contrast to constrictive pericarditis, the hepatic vein diastolic flow reversal in RCM is remarkable during inspiration. Myocardial relaxation is universally impaired, so that the mitral annulus E′ velocity obtained from the septal annulus is frequently less than 7 cm/s.

Keywords

Restrictive cardiomyopathy · Echocardiography
Diastolic pressure · Constrictive pericarditis
Myocardial relaxation · Endomyocardial fibrosis

Abbreviations

Idiopathic RCM	Idiopathic restrictive cardiomyopathy
IVRT	Isovolumic relaxation time
LV	Left ventricular
RCM	Cardiomyopathies, restrictive cardiomyopathy
TTR	Transthyretin
Vp	Velocity propagation

Definition and Classification of Restrictive Cardiomyopathy

- Restrictive cardiomyopathy (RCM) is a myocardial disease with dominant manifestation of marked increased myocardial stiffness and diastolic dysfunction.

Electronic Supplementary Material The online version of this chapter (https://doi.org/10.1007/978-3-319-67691-3_23) contains supplementary material, which is available to authorized users.

A. Alizadehasl, MD, FACC, FASE
Associate Professor of Cardiology, Echocardiologist, Echocardiography and Cardiogenetic Research Centers, Cardio-Oncology Department, Rajaie Cardiovascular Medical and Research Center, Tehran, Iran

A. Sadeghpour, MD, FACC, FASE (✉)
Professor of Cardiology, Echocardiography Research Center, Rajaie Cardiovascular Medical and Research Center, Iran University of Medical Science, Tehran, Iran

A. Sadeghpour, A. Alizadehasl (eds.), *Case-Based Textbook of Echocardiography*, https://doi.org/10.1007/978-3-319-67691-3_23

- RCM is commonly classified as: Infiltrative RCM (e.g.: amyloidosis), Noninfiltrative RCM (e.g.: or idiopathic RCM), Storage diseases and endomyocardial RCM including endomyocardial fibrosis and hypereosinophilic syndrome.
- In the developed world, amyloid heart disease remains the most common cause of RCM. The most common forms of RCM are infiltrative myocardial disease, idiopathic RCM and endomyocardial fibrosis associated with Löffler's syndrome. Among other diseases of the myocardium that may present with a similar picture are cardiac sarcoidosis and hemochromatosis.
- Progressive diastolic dysfunction occur in nearly all RCM patients over time.
- It is noteworthy to know that restrictive physiology that means restrictive diastolic filling and is accompanied with restrictive cardiomyopathy (RCM), can be seen in almost all cardiac disease (mostly at end stages) is not specific for RCM [1–5].

Common Echocardiographic Findings of RCM

2D Study

- Normal or small left ventricular (LV) size
- Relatively preserved ejection fraction particularly in the initial stage
- Progressive diastolic dysfunction due to increased myocardial stiffness
- Marked biatrial enlargement due to high atrial pressure
- IVC plethora (IVC size > 2.1 cm with <50% respiratory variation)
- Pericardial effusion.

MV Inflow Doppler Study

- Increased peak E velocity and decreased A velocity
- E/A ratio > 2–2.5
- Mitral deceleration time < 150–160 ms,
- Isovolumic relaxation time (IVRT) < 50–70 ms
- Tissue Doppler imaging shows: Severely reduced septal and lateral Em velocities (3–4 cm/s) with high E/e ratio > 15 and decreased systolic velocity: S′ < 5 cm/s

Color M-mode velocity propagation (Vp) shows decreased Vp.

Hepatic and Pulmonary Doppler Study

- Decreased systolic pulmonary venous flow velocity less than diastolic velocity
- Inspiratory increased hepatic vein diastolic flow reversal

Specific Types of RCM

Idiopathic Restrictive Cardiomyopathy (Idiopathic RCM)

- When the etiology of RCM is not identified, it is called idiopathic RCM and characterized by a non hypertrophied LV with normal left ventricular cavity size and a dilated left atrium in the absence of mitral valve pathology.
- It is a slowly progressing disease when compared with other infiltrative RCMs. Long-standing systemic hypertension with its drastic effect on the myocardial function is a common substrate for this condition.
- Despite the commonly maintained overall left ventricular systolic function, diastolic function is severely disturbed and can easily be assessed by studying the filling pattern. The characteristic features of restrictive left ventricular filling are mentioned before.
- Patients diagnosed with idiopathic RCM tend to respond to diuretics and vasodilators, which may successfully offload the left atrium. The expected satisfactory symptomatic response is supported by prolongation of isovolumic relaxation time, reversal of ventricular filling pattern, and a fall in left atrial size. With long-standing severe ventricular diastolic disease, less expectation is anticipated [1–7].
- Progressive rise of left atrial pressure and increase in the cavity size result in the significant impairment of myocardial function and, hence, instability and atrial arrhythmia. As long as left atrial pressure remains elevated, medical or even DC cardioversion might not be successful. Aggressive use of renin angiotensin enzyme blocking agents has proved beneficial in optimizing the treatment results. Resistant cases with atrial fibrillation are not expected to have successful DC cardioversion because of the large atrium and raised pressures [6, 7].

Infiltrative Myocardial Disease

Amyloidosis

- Concentric increased myocardial thickness (>1.2 cm), with speckled echo brightness appearance which involves the four cardiac chambers including RV with wall thickness (>7 mm), even the atrioventricular valves and atrial septum (Figs. 23.1 and 23.2).
- Specific pattern of 2D speckle tracking which is reduction of global longitudinal strain of all myocardium with spared the LV apex, even in minimally thickened myocardium [3–5].
- AL amyloid heart disease is the most frequent cause of RCM in the West. The myocardium may be infiltrated by iron in hemochromatosis, glycogen in Pompe's and Cori's disease, or glycolipids in Fabry's disease.

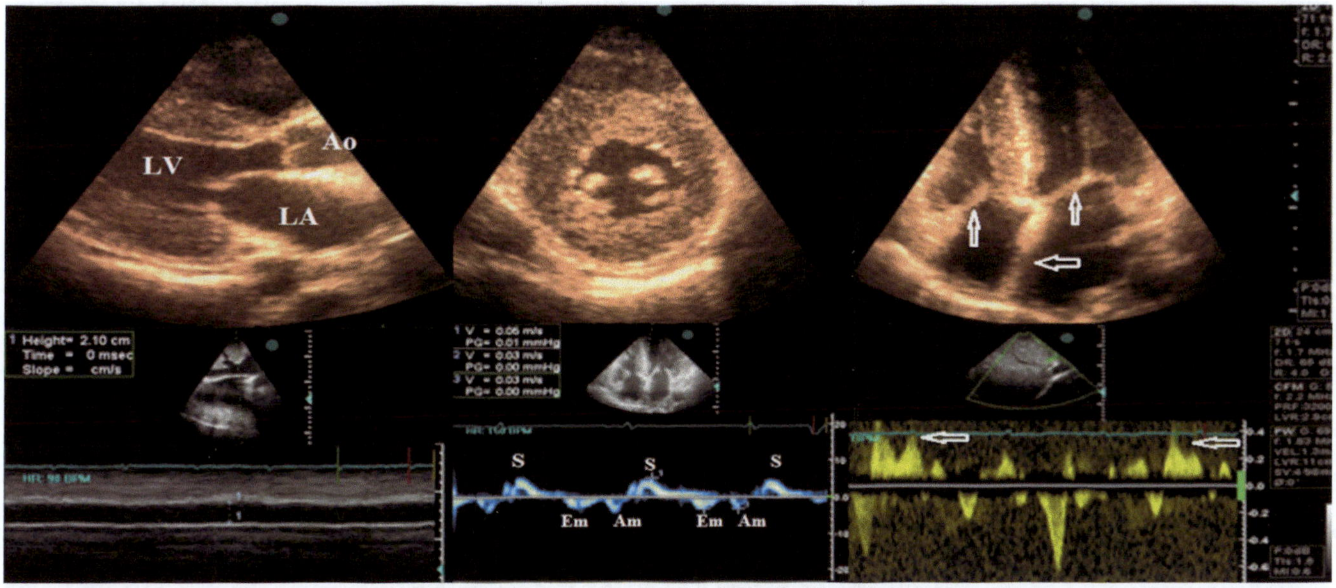

Fig. 23.1 Typical echocardiography finding in Amyloidosis. Left upper and middle panels: concentric increased myocardial thickness in parasternal long axis and short axis views (Movies 23.1 and 23.2). Upper right panel: increase thickness of mitral and tricuspid valves and interatrial septum, biatrial enlargement (arrows). Lower panel: left: IVC plethora, middle: Doppler tissue imaging of septum shows severely reduced septal velocities, right: inspiratory increased hepatic vein diastolic flow reversal

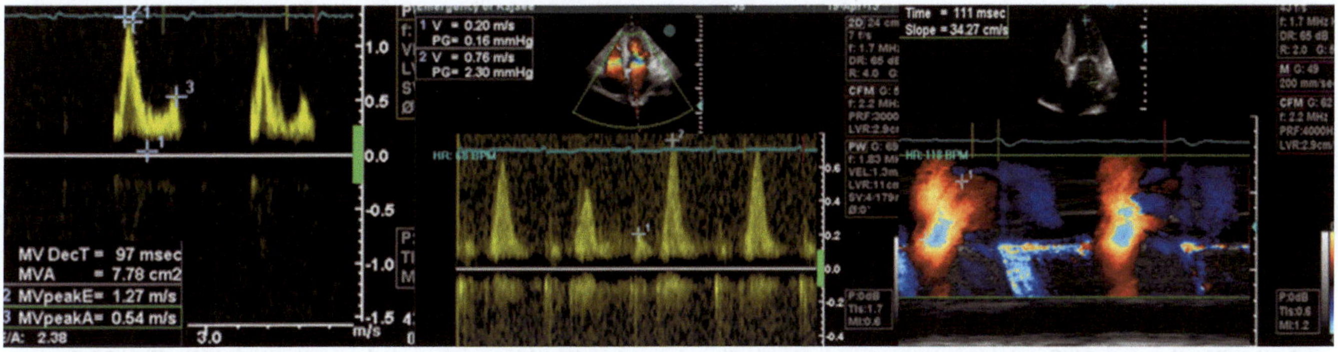

Fig. 23.2 Increased peak E velocity and decreased A velocity with E/A ratio > 2 and mitral deceleration time < 150–160, Middle: decreased systolic pulmonary venous flow velocity suggestive for high LA pressure. Right: color M-mode velocity propagationin in apical four-chamber view shows significantly reduced Vp (34 cm/s)

- Myocardial infiltration disturb normal myocyte function and metabolism, resulting in fibrosis. Eventually, progressive myocardial fibrosis adds to the myocardial stiffness and increase in ventricular diastolic pressures.
- A more intensive amyloid deposition is correlated with a poorer the clinical outcome. Wall thickness greater than 1.5 cm is associated with mean survival of 5 months. The extent of segmental dysfunction is usually out of proportion to the degree of wall thickness, showing markedly depressed segmental thickening and thinning rates. By the time of clinical presentation, the echocardiographic picture of amyloid heart disease is usually severe and ventricular filling is of the restrictive pattern. Some degree of mitral and tricuspid regurgitation is commonly seen, which may be severe—particularly when the valves themselves are involved in the disease process.
- In amyloid heart disease, the changes in the ventricular filling pattern evolve as the disease progresses and ventricular function deteriorates. While in early disease the E/A ratio may be less than 1.0 and isovolumic relaxation time prolonged, in later stages filling becomes restrictive and isovolumic relaxation time shortens—which is consistent with raised left atrial pressures. Similar abnormalities can be seen on the right side of the heart.
- Ventricular filling pattern has been shown to predict the clinical outcome in amyloid heart disease. An E wave deceleration time less than 150 ms has been shown to predict a life expectancy of 50% at 1 year compared to more than 90% survival at 1 year with a deceleration time greater than 150 ms.
- Amyloid left ventricular disease should be differentiated from hypertrophic cardiomyopathy. While the cavity size is equally maintained in the two conditions

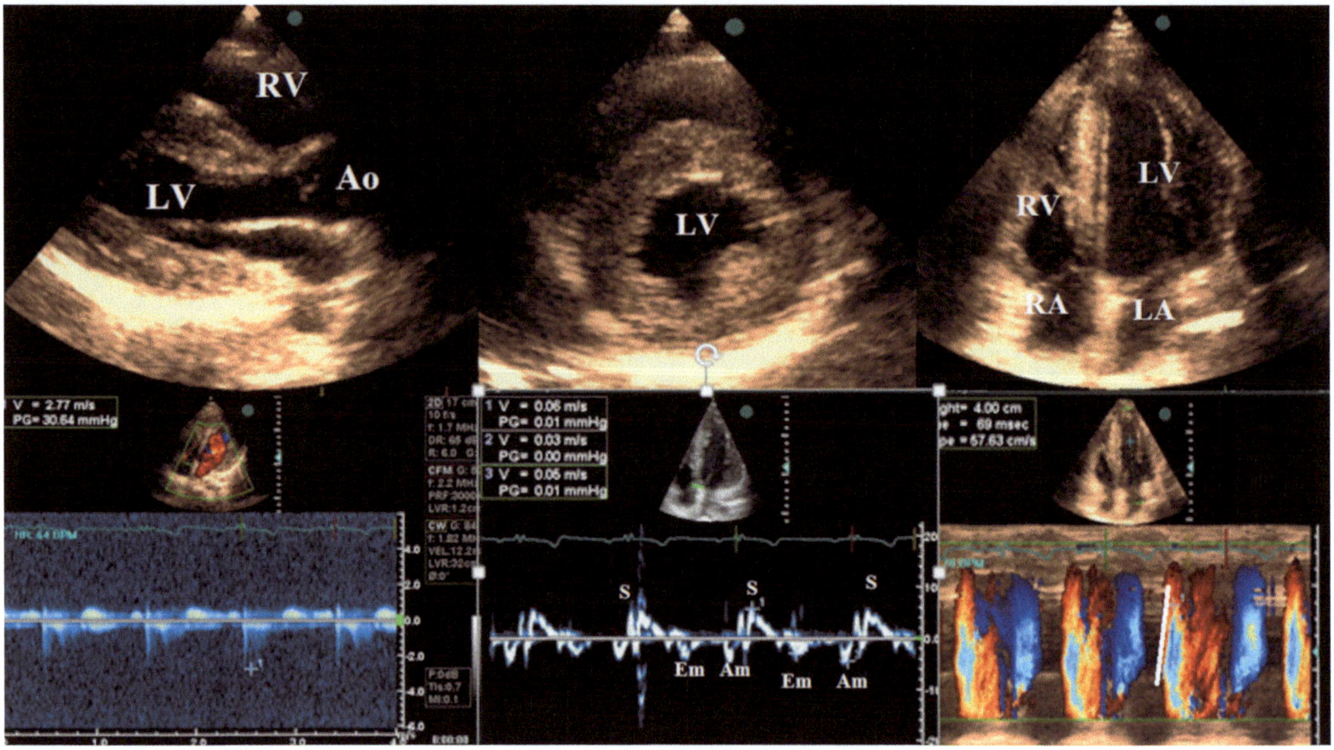

Fig. 23.3 Concentric type of hypertrophic CMP. Upper left and middle panels showing: increased myocardial thickening. Right upper panel: normal size atria with normal thickening of mitral leaflet (opposed to Amyloidosis). Left lower panel showing: no signifacnt pulmonary hypertension, Middle: decreased tissue velocity as can be seen in both RCM and HCM, Left lower panel: normal or even increased color M-mode velocity propagationin (Vp) all together are suggestive for HCM and contrary to typical RCM pattern

Fig. 23.3. The QRS voltage criteria on surface ECG may also help, demonstrating low amplitude in amyloid disease [1–9].

- Endomyocardial Fibrosis and Löffler's Syndrome
- This form of RCM is prevalent in West Africa, South India, Thailand, and South America among the indigenous population.
- Endomyocardial fibrosis is characterized by the extensive fibrosis of the subendocardial layer of the myocardium, involving the apices of the left and right ventricles and extending to the inflow tract.
- Endomyocardial fibrosis results in:
  - Increased chamber stiffness and hence restrictive filling.
  - Normal LV size with increased subendocardial myocardial echo intensity.
  - Initially preserved ventricular function but subsequently impaired.
- Apical thrombus formation, which may obliterate the entire ventricular apex
- Dilated atria as a consequence of the increased atrial pressure secondary to incompliant ventricles.
- Severe cases may be complicated by pulmonary hypertension and tricuspid regurgitation. The disease may also involve the mitral and tricuspid valve leaflets themselves, thus adding to the severity of regurgitation. Endomyocardial fibrosis may be very similar in presentation to Löffler's syndrome [6–9].
- Löffler's syndrome presents with echocardiographic and physiological signs similar to endomyocardial fibrosis, but in addition there is hyper eosinophilia Fig. 23.4.
- While the management of endomyocardial fibrosis is directed toward subendocardial decortication with or without valve replacement, controlling the eosinophilia is the first stage in treating Löffler's syndrome [7, 9].

Familial Amyloidosis

- Although less common, familial amyloidosis can affect the heart and at late stages give a picture similar to AL amyloid heart disease, described above. It is a disorder caused by mutated transthyretin (TTR). The typical symptom of familial amyloidosis is peripheral sensorimotor polyneuropathy, often accompanied by autonomic neuropathy, which causes a defective autoregulation of blood pressure and heart rate.
- Associated cardiac complications such as arrhythmia are described in familial adenomatous polyposis patients who develop increased left ventricular wall thickness, diastolic

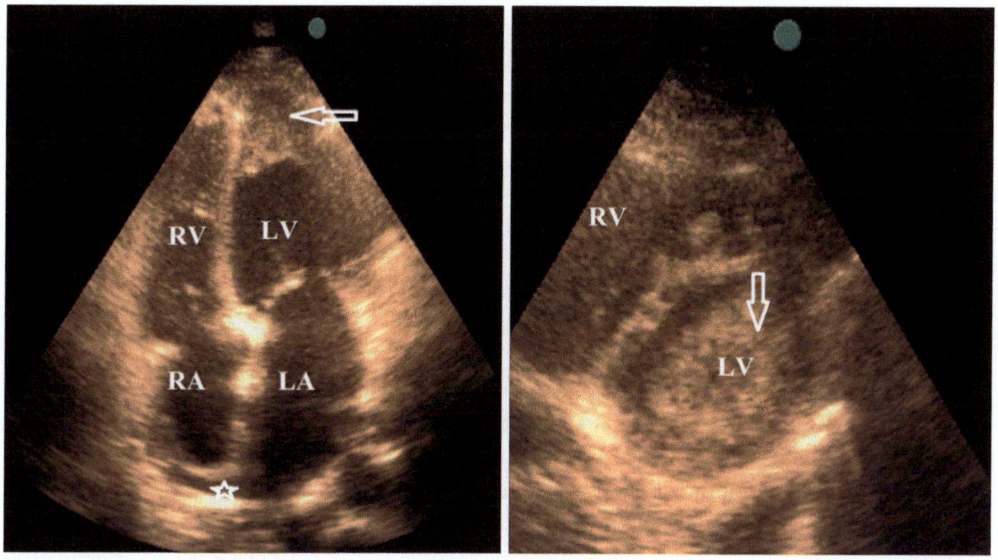

Fig. 23.4 Movies 23.3 and 23.4 Loffler syndrome dilated atria, small pericardial effusion (star) and thickened obliterate apex (arrow)

dysfunction, and enlarged atria. In addition, studies have recently shown that the pattern of ventricular diastolic abnormalities in these patients correlates closely with the degree of the disturbances of heart rate variability [7–11].

Fabry's Disease

- Fabry's disease is associated with the accumulation of glycosphingolipid in the heart and a high incidence of cardiovascular signs and symptoms in addition to renal, dermatologic, and neurologic abnormalities. More than 80% of individuals with Fabry's disease will display concentric hypertrophy, although concentric remodeling and asymmetric hypertrophy occur in a smaller proportion. The presence of left ventricular hypertrophy is associated with lower alpha-galactosidase activity and more cardiovascular symptoms. Mitral leaflet thickening and significant mitral regurgitation are common, and focal or global left ventricular systolic dysfunction occurs in a minority of the patients [2–7, 12].

Cardiac Sarcoidosis

- Cardiac involvement occurs in a minority of sarcoid cases. Cardiac involvement is manifest as patchy myocardial infiltration by granulomatous sarcoid deposits, followed by fibrosis.
- When sarcoidosis affects the posterior wall of the left ventricle, the proximal segment is usually involved—*which has a similar echocardiographic picture to posterior wall myocardial infarction.* It may also involve the lateral papillary muscle, giving rise to some degree of mitral regurgitation. Sarcoid heart disease may affect the proximal septal segment, where it may affect the conducting tissue and result in conduction disease and heart block. This explains the etiology of syncope in these patients. The left ventricular cavity may be slightly dilated at the basal region due to the fibrosed segments. Ventricular filling is commonly late diastolic [2–4, 9, 10].

Hemochromatosis

- The ventricular myocardium may be infiltrated by iron in patients with hemochromatosis. It tends to invade the outer layer of the myocardium more than the subendocardium. Iron is deposited in the myocytes as well as interstitial cells, resulting in myocardial fibrosis. Although the ventricular cavity may be dilated, the clinical outcome is better than the other infiltrative diseases since it responds well to iron chelation therapy [2–7, 13, 14].

Diabetic Hypertensive Cardiomyopathy

- Long-standing diabetes and hypertension may affect the left ventricular function in such a way that resembles RCM, in particular, the picture associated with amyloid. The cavity size is maintained, walls are thickened, and sequential thickening fraction is significantly reduced. The majority of these patients become limited by breathlessness due to raised left atrial pressures in the absence of mitral valve disease. The long-term outcome of this condition, however, is more benign than that of amyloid cardiomyopathy [2–7, 12].

Questions

1. Mitral valve inflow Doppler study in restrictive cardiomyopathy (RCM) shows the following parameters except for:
   A. Increased peak E velocity and decreased A velocity
   B. Mitral deceleration time <150–160 ms,
   C. Isovolumic relaxation time >70 ms
   D. Severely reduced septal and lateral Em velocities (3–4 cm/s) with a high E/e ratio (>15)

2. In which of the following: It tends to invade the outer layer of the myocardium more than the subendocardium, resulting in myocardial fibrosis. Although the ventricular cavity may be dilated, the clinical outcome is better than the other infiltrative diseases since it responds well to therapy.
   A. Diabetic hypertensive cardiomyopathy
   B. Hemochromatosis
   C. Cardiac sarcoidosis
   D. Fabry disease

3. The best diagnosis for this 4 chamber view:
   A. Diabetic hypertensive cardiomyopathy
   B. Hemochromatosis
   C. Cardiac sarcoidosis
   D. Löffler syndrome

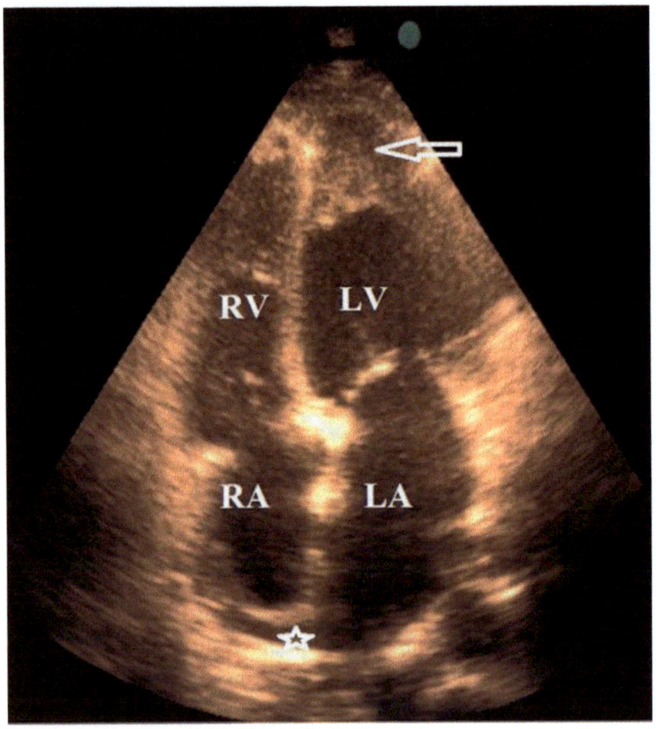

Answers

1. C
2. B
3. D

References

1. Dubrey SW, Hawkins PN, Falk RH. Systemic disorders in heart disease: amyloid diseases of the heart: assessment, diagnosis, and referral. Heart. 2011;97:75.
2. Wood MJ, Picard MH. Utility of echocardiography in the evaluation of individuals with cardiomyopathy. Heart. 2004;90(6):707–12.
3. Zipes D, Libby P, Bonow R. Braunwald's heart disease: a textbook of cardiovascular medicine. 10th ed. Philadelphia: Saunders, Elsevier Inc; 2015.
4. Otto CM. The practice of clinical echocardiography. 5th ed. Philadelphia: Saunders; 2017.
5. Oh JK, Seward JB, Tajik AJ. The echo manual. 3rd ed. Philadelphia: Lippincott Williams and Wilkins; 2006. p. 251–72.
6. Asher CR, Klein AL. Diastolic heart failure: restrictive cardiomyopathy, constrictive pericarditis, and cardiac tamponade: clinical and echocardiographic evaluation. Cardiol Rev. 2002;10(4):218–29.
7. Seward JB, Casaclang-Verzosa G. Infiltrative cardiovascular diseases: cardiomyopathies that look alike. J Am Coll Cardiol. 2010;55:1769.
8. Wiklund U, Hörnsten R, Karlsson M, Suhr OB, Jensen SM. Abnormal heart rate variability and subtle atrial arrhythmia in patients with familial amyloidotic polyneuropathy. Ann Noninvasive Eletrocardiol. 2008;13:249–56.
9. Joob B, Wiwanitkit V. Loeffler's syndrome, pulmonary ascariasis, in Thailand, rare or under-reported? J Thorac Dis. 2012;4(3):339.
10. Zhao Y, Hörnsten R, Lindqvist P, Wiklund U, Suhr OB, Henein MY. Left ventricular dyssynchrony is associated with reduced heart rate variability in familial amyloidotic polyneuropathy. Int J Cardiol. 2012;155(2):273–8.
11. Henein M, Lindqvist P, Mörner S, Henein MY. Effect of raised left atrial pressure on its regional and segmental chamber function: the role of speckle tracking. Scand Cardiovasc J. 2009;43:8.
12. Amaki M, Savino J, Ain DL, Sanz J, Pedrizzetti G, Kulkarni H, et al. Diagnostic concordance of echocardiography and cardiac magnetic resonance-based tissue tracking for differentiating constrictive pericarditis from restrictive cardiomyopathy. Circ Cardiovasc Imaging. 2014;7(5):819–27.
13. Kusunose K, Dahiya A, Popovic ZB, Motoki H, Alraies MC, Zurick AO, et al. Biventricular mechanics in constrictive pericarditis comparison with restrictive cardiomyopathy and impact of pericardiectomy. Circ Cardiovasc Imaging. 2013;6(3):399–406.
14. Kremastinos DT, Farmakis D. Iron overload cardiomyopathy in clinical practice. Circulation. 2011;124:2253–63.

Unclassified Cardiomyopathies: Arrhythmogenic Right Ventricular Dysplasia/Cardiomyopathy (ARVD/C) and Left Ventricular Non-Compaction Cardiomyopathy (LVNC)

24

Anita Sadeghpour and Azin Alizadehasl

Abstract

Echocardiography has the main role in the diagnosis and management of arrhythmogenic right ventricular (RV) dysplasia/cardiomyopathy. An RV outflow tract dimension greater than 30 mm from the parasternal long-axis view has a the high sensitivity (89%) and specificity (86%) for the diagnosis of arrhythmogenic RV dysplasia. RV function is abnormal in 62%, and RV regional wall motion abnormalities is common—most frequently affecting the apex and the anterior wall. RV trabecular derangements, hyper-reflective moderator bands, and sacculations are present in about 54, 34, and 17%—respectively. In some patients, LV dilation and dysfunction also happen. The tricuspid regurgitation velocity is usually less than 2 m/s, suggesting an RV systolic pressure in the low-normal range. Contrast echocardiography is helpful in delineating RV morphology and contractility. Cardiac magnetic resonance imaging or computed tomography for fat in RV myocardium has been useful in some patients.

Isolated ventricular non-compaction occurs from the embryonic arrest of compaction, previously described as persistent intramyocardial sinusoids. It is characterized by segmental thickening in LV wall, comprising a compacted epicardial layer and a thickened endocardial layer with marked trabeculations and deep intertrabecular recesses. Complications associated with non-compaction cardiomyopathy include heart failure (53%), thromboembolic events (24%), ventricular tachycardia (41%), and sudden death.

Keywords

Echocardiography · Arrhythmogenic right ventricular dysplasia/cardiomyopathy · Isolated ventricular non-compaction · Contrast echocardiography · RV trabecular derangements

Abbreviations

ARVD/C	Arrhythmogenic right ventricular dysplasia/cardiomyopathy
FAC	Fractional area change
ICD	Implantable cardioverter–defibrillator
LV	Left ventricular
LVNC	Left ventricular non-compaction
RV	Right ventricular
RVOT	Right ventricular outflow tract
TAPSE	Tricuspid annular plane systolic excursion
TDI	Tissue doppler imaging
TFC	Task force criteria
TTE	Transthoracic echocardiography

- Arrhythmogenic right ventricular dysplasia/cardiomyopathy (ARVD-C) is a familial cardiomyopathy with progressive right ventricular (RV) dysfunction and malignant arrhythmias. Affected patients typically present in the second to fourth decades of life with arrhythmias initiating from the RV. In the past decade, pathogenic cases of ARVD-C causing mutations have been recognized in five genes encoding the cardiac desmosome.

Electronic Supplementary Material The online version of this chapter (https://doi.org/10.1007/978-3-319-67691-3_24) contains supplementary material, which is available to authorized users.

A. Sadeghpour, MD, FACC, FASE
Professor of Cardiology, Echocardiography Research Center, Rajaie Cardiovascular Medical and Research Center, Iran University of Medical Science, Tehran, Iran

A. Alizadehasl, MD, FACC, FASE (✉)
Associate Professor of Cardiology, Echocardiologist, Echocardiography and Cardiogenetic Research Centers, Cardio-Oncology Department, Rajaie Cardiovascular Medical and Research Center, Tehran, Iran

A. Sadeghpour, A. Alizadehasl (eds.), *Case-Based Textbook of Echocardiography*, https://doi.org/10.1007/978-3-319-67691-3_24

- Disruption of the desmosomal connection system between cardiomyocytes can be characterized structurally by ventricular enlargement, global or regional wall motion abnormalities, RV micro-aneurysms, or fibro-fatty replacement. These abnormalities are classically observed in predilection areas, containing the sub-tricuspid valve region, basal part of the RV free wall, and left ventricular (LV) posterolateral wall. These structural and functional abnormalities on imaging modalities constitute important diagnostic criteria for ARVD-C [1, 2].

- ARVD-C may pose an important diagnostic challenge to all physicians. Many patients with ARVD-C are young, and the necessity for screening tools amid genetically disposed, albeit clinically asymptomatic, subjects calls for cardiac structural abnormalities to be recognized preferably via noninvasive studies [1, 2].
  - For diagnostic purposes, the 2010 Task Force Criteria (TFC) recommended the use of transthoracic echocardiography (TTE), cardiac magnetic resonance, and RV angiography [1, 2].
- TTE is the first-line imaging technique in a case with suspected ARVD-C because of its widespread accessibility and low cost. TTE provides all structural and functional data on cardiac chambers, though the visualization of the RV needs especial expertise and emphasis. In addition, in cases with an implantable cardioverter—defibrillator (ICD), TTE can be used for serial study to evaluate the disease and its progression [1, 2].

Transthoracic Echocardiography

- A TTE study is a useful screening tool to evaluate the RV size and function in cases with probable ARVD-C. TTE can be performed easily at a low cost, and not only is it readily available but it is also portable. Additionally, this modality is mainly useful in following affected patients over time because of its ability to present serial imaging in cases with ICDs [3].
- TTE for ARVD-C study should be performed using the current American Society of Echocardiography's consensus and guidelines [4, 5]. Because the RV might be enlarged and, thus, not completely imaged on the standard imaging planes, additional off-axis views should be achieved to make sure that all parts of the RV free wall are well imaged and visualized. Given the patchy involvement, this is especially important to echocardiographers so that they do not miss small and localized aneurysms.

Right Ventricular Morphology

- RV dilation is often observed in cases with ARVD-C [3, 6]. The North American Multidisciplinary Study revealed that an enlarged right ventricular outflow tract (RVOT) was found in the 100% of probands [3]. In the 2010 TFC, a major criterion for ARVD-C is achieved when there is RVOT dilation on the parasternal long-axis view (≥32 mm) or in the short-axis view (≥36 mm), alongside localized akinesia, dyskinesia, or aneurysms in the RV free wall (Figs. 24.1 and 24.2, Movies 24.1 and 24.2) [1].

- Existence of a wall motion abnormality with only mild dilation (≥29 to <32 mm in the parasternal long-axis view and ≥32 to <36 mm in the parasternal short-axis view) is a minor criterion (Tables 24.1 and 24.2). These cutoff values were on the basis of documenting 69 probands from the North American Multidisciplinary ARVD-C research study in comparison with 450 controls [1]. It is of considerable importance to bear in mind that for both major and minor criteria, a regional wall motion abnormality also needs to be present (segmental akinesia or dyskinesia and aneurysm).

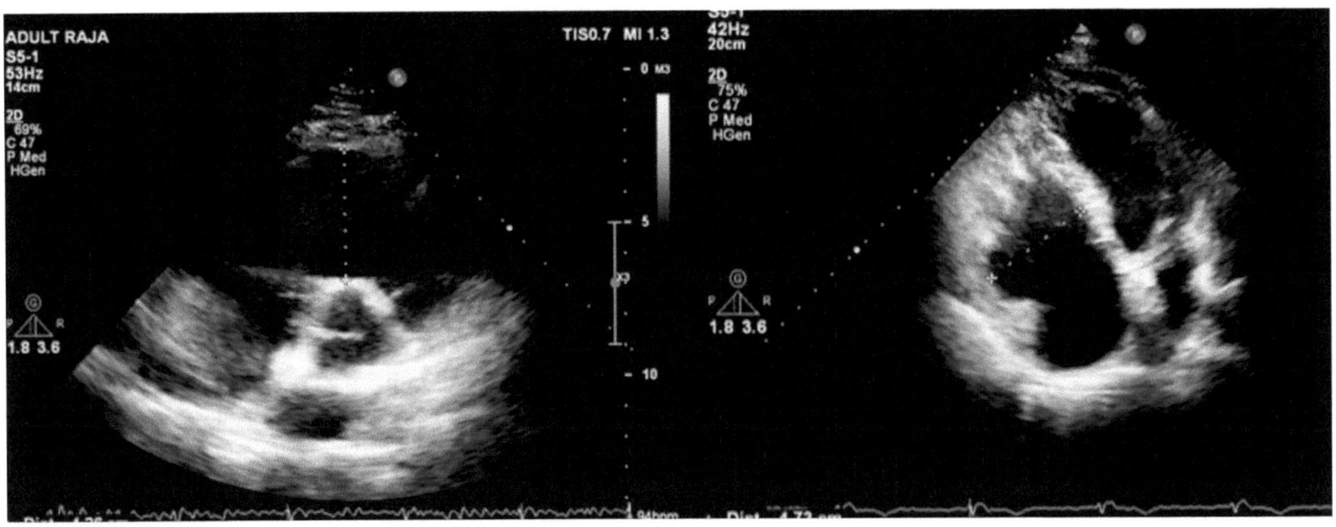

Fig. 24.1 ARVC; Dilated RVOT in parasternal long axis view (4.2 cm) and basal RV in four camber view (4.7 cm)

- Of course, RV dilation is not a criterion specific to ARVD-C. It has even been reported as a physiological adaptation to high-intensity exercise [7]. In addition, RV enlargement in ARVD-C has been related with an increased risk of sudden cardiac death and also ventricular arrhythmias in athletes [8, 9]. Consequently, the diagnosis of ARVD-C in trained athletes is very challenging.
- A detailed family and medical history and also careful application of the TFC can help differentiate the disease from normal adaptation to high-intensity exercise. In the future, the accuracy and validity of TTE in this subset of patients might be improved by the usage of such newer TTE parameters as tissue Doppler imaging (TDI) and speckle-tracking for myocardial strain and strain rate in the RV [10].
- In addition to RV enlargement, several other morphological abnormalities can be detected on TTE in patients with ARVD-C including:
  - Trabeculation and derangement.
  - Focal aneurysms or.
  - Sacculations on the RV free wall.

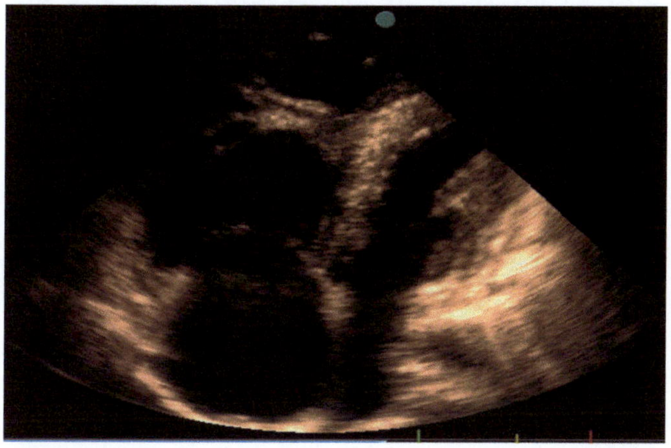

Fig. 24.2 Movie 24.3: ARVC; Severe RV enlargement, prominent moderator band

Although trabecular hypertrophy and derangement has been defined in published reports with increased incidence in ARVD-C [3], it is not a sign specific to this disease. It is, therefore, not part of the imaging diagnostic criteria.

- Trabecular prominence or derangement, which is assessed subjectively by echocardiographers, in the North American Registry occupies a significant amount of the RV cavity at the end of diastole. Also, it was the most repeatedly noted morphological abnormality in the North American Multidisciplinary Study in that it was observed in 54% of affected patients and not in any corresponding controls [3].

Right Ventricular Function

- Because of the asymmetric and complex geometry of the RV and also difficulty with the visualization and study of the entire RV endocardium from the standard TTE views in ARVD-C, the estimation of the RV volume, size, and function by conventional 2D TTE is very challenging. The RV fractional area change (FAC) in the apical 4-chamber view is deemed a useful parameter of the global RV function [11, 12]. It is reduced in cases with ARVD-C compared with a control group [3].
- In the 2010 TFC, the presence of severe RV dysfunction (RV FAC ≤ 33%) in tandem with a localized and regional wall motion abnormality creates a major diagnostic criterion, while mild RV dysfunction (RV FAC > 33% to ≤40%) comprises a minor criterion. For the 2010 TFC, the ideal cutoff points for the FAC were defined using data from the Multidisciplinary Study coupled with 450 matched controls. In the presence of segmental wall motion abnormality, an FAC equal to or less than 33% has a specificity of 95% and a sensitivity of 55% for the diagnosis of ARVD-C [1].

Table 24.1 Noninvasive multimodality imaging in ARVD/C

	TTE	CMR	CT
Spatial resolution	0.5–1 mm	1–2 mm	0.5 mm
Temporal resolution	15–60 ms	25–50 ms	50–100 ms
Availability	++	–	++
Low cost	++	–	–
Financial analysis	+	++	+
Radiantion dose	None	None	Moderate for cine CT (5–10 mSv)
Tissue characterization	Not available	++ (fat/water/fibrosis)	+ (fat)
Remarks	RV imaging requires special emphasis/expertise; cardiac devices are acceptable	Not influenced by habitus; sensitive to arrhythmia; generally not compatible with cardiac devices	Sensitive to arrhythmia; cardiac devices are acceptable

Modified table of Anneline SJM te Riele, Harikrishna Tandri, Danita M Sanborn, David A Bluemke. Noninvasive multimodality imaging in ARVD/C. JACC Cardiovasc Imaging. May 2015;8(5):597–611 (Ref. [26])

Table 24.2 Comparison of original and revised task force criteria

Original task force criteria	Revised task force criteria
I. Global or regional dysfunction and structural alterations	
Major	
• Severe dilatation and reduction of RV ejection fraction with no (or only mild) LV impairment • Localized RV aneurysms (akinetic or dyskinetic areas with diastolic bulging) • Severe segmental dilatation of the RV	*By 2D echo:* • Regional RV akinesia, dyskinesia, or aneurysm • and 1 of the following (end diastole): – PLAX RVOT 32 mm (corrected for body size [PLAX/BSA] ≥19 mm/m^2) – PSAX RVOT 36 mm (corrected for body size [PSAX/BSA] ≥21 mm/m^2) – or fractional area change ≤33%
	By MRI: • Regional RV akinesia or dyskinesia or dyssynchronous RV contraction • and 1 of the following: – Ratio of RV end-diastolic volume to BSA ≥110 mL/m^2 (male) or ≥100 mL/m^2 (female) – or RV ejection fraction ≤40%
	By RV angiography: • Regional RV akinesia, dyskinesia, or aneurysm
Minor	
• Mild global RV dilatation and/or ejection fraction reduction with normal LV • Mild segmental dilatation of the RV • Regional RV hypokinesia	*By 2D echo:* • Regional RV akinesia or dyskinesia • and 1 of the following (end diastole): – PLAX RVOT ≥29 to <32 mm (corrected for body size [PLAX/BSA] ≥16 to <19 mm/m^2) – PSAX RVOT ≥ 32 to <36 mm (corrected for body size [PSAX/BSA] ≥18 to <21 mm/m^2) – or fractional area change >33% to ≤40%
	By MRI: • Regional RV akinesia or dyskinesia or dyssynchronous RV contraction • and 1 of the following: – Ratio of RV end-diastolic volume to BSA ≥100 to <110 mL/m^2 (male) or≥ 90 to <100 mL/m^2 (female) – or RV ejection fraction >40% to ≤45%
II. Tissue characterization of wall	
Major	
• Fibrofatty replacement of myocardium on endomyocardial biopsy	• Residual myocytes <60% by morphometric analysis (or <50% if estimated), with fibrous replacement of the RV free wall myocardium in ≥1 sample, with or without fatty replacement of tissue on endomyocardial biopsy
Minor	
	• Residual myocytes 60–75% by morphometric analysis (or 50 to 65% if estimated), with fibrous replacement of the RV free wall myocardium in ≥1 sample, with or without fatty replacement of tissue on endomyocardial biopsy
III. Repolarization abnormalities	
Major	
	• Inverted T waves in right precordial leads (V_1, V_2, and V_3) or beyond in individuals >14 years of age (in the absence of complete right bundle-branch block QRS ≥120 ms)
Minor	

• Inverted T waves in right precordial leads (V_2 and V_3) (people age >12 years, in absence of right bundle-branch block)	• Inverted T waves in leads V_1 and V_2 in individuals >14 years of age (in the absence of complete right bundle-branch block) or in V_4, V_5, or V_6
	• Inverted T waves in leads V_1, V_2, V_3, and V_4 in individuals >14 years of age in the presence of complete right bundle-branch block
IV. Depolarization/conduction abnormalities	
Major	
• Epsilon waves or localized prolongation>110 ms) of the QRS complex in right precordial leads (V_1 to V_3)	• Epsilon waves (reproducible low-amplitude signals between end of QRS complex to onset of the T wave) in right precordial leads (V_1 to V_3)
Minor	
• Late potentials (SAECG)	• Late potentials by SAECG in ≥1 of 3 parameters in the absence of a QRS duration of ≥110 ms on the standard ECG • Filtered QRS duration (f-QRS) ≥114 ms • Duration of terminal QRS <40 μV (low-amplitude signal duration) ≥38 ms • Root-mean-square voltage of terminal 40 ms ≤20 μV • Terminal activation duration of QRS ≥55 ms measured from the nadir of the S wave to the end of the QRS, including R, in V_1, V_2, or V_3, in the absence of complete right bundle-branch block
V. Arrhythmias	
Major	
	• Nonsustained or sustained ventricular tachycardia of left bundle-branch morphology with superior axis (negative or indeterminate QRS in leads II, III, and aVF and positive in lead aVL)
Minor	
• Left bundle-branch block–type ventricular tachycardia (sustained and nonsustained) (ECG, Holter, exercise) • Frequent ventricular extrasystoles (>1000 per 24 h) (Holter)	• Nonsustained or sustained ventricular tachycardia of RV outflow configuration, left bundle-branch block morphology with inferior axis (positive QRS in leads II, III, and aVF and negative in lead aVL) or of unknown axis • >500 ventricular extrasystoles per 24 h (Holter)
VI. Family history	
Major	
• Familial disease confirmed at necropsy or surgery	• ARVC/D confirmed in a first-degree relative who meets current Task Force criteria • ARVC/D confirmed pathologically at autopsy or surgery in a first-degree relative • Identification of a pathogenic mutation categorized as associated or probably associated with ARVC/D in the patient under evaluation
Minor	
• Family history of premature sudden death <35 years of age) due to suspected ARVC/D • Familial history (clinical diagnosis based on present criteria)	• History of ARVC/D in a first-degree relative in whom it is not possible or practical to determine whether the family member meets current Task Force criteria • Premature sudden death (<35 years of age) due to suspected ARVC/D in a first-degree relative • ARVC/D confirmed pathologically or by current Task Force Criteria in second-degree relative

PLAX indicates parasternal long-axis view, *RVOT* RV outflow tract, *BSA* body surface area, *PSAX* parasternal short-axis view, *aVF* augmented voltage unipolar left foot lead, and *aVL* augmented voltage unipolar left arm lead. Diagnostic terminology for original criteria: This diagnosis is fulfilled by the presence of two major, or one major plus two minor criteria or four minor criteria from different groups. Diagnostic terminology for revised criteria: definite diagnosis: two major or one major and two minor criteria or four minor from different categories; borderline: one major and one minor or three minor criteria from different categories; possible: one major or two minor criteria from different categories

Hypokinesis is not included in this or subsequent definitions of RV regional wall motion abnormalities for the proposed modified criteria

A pathogenic mutation is a DNA alteration associated with ARVC/D that alters or is expected to alter the encoded protein, is unobserved or rare in a large non–ARVC/D control population, and either alters or is predicted to alter the structure or function of the protein or has demonstrated linkage to the disease phenotype in a conclusive pedigree

Modified table of Marcus FI, McKenna WJ, Sherrill D, et al. Diagnosis of arrhythmogenic right ventricular cardiomyopathy/dysplasia: proposed modification of the task force criteria. Circulation. 2010;121:1533–41. (Ref. [1])

Newer Echocardiographic Techniques in ARVD-C

- Many new echocardiographic methods have been developed to complement a standard 2D TTE assessment in patients with ARVD-C. A simple Doppler index of the RV function, the myocardial performance index of the RV, is independent of complex geometric assumptions [13] and has been used in diseases that affect the RV such as pulmonary artery hypertension [14]. Interestingly, the initial data of this index in patients with ARVD-C showed reduced RV myocardial function in ARVD-C probands, even when the global function of the RV—as evaluated via the FAC—was normal [15]. Nonetheless, another study showed this to be a less informative estimation of the global RV dysfunction in cases with ARVD-C [16]. Accordingly, this index needs to be assessed and tested in larger populations to determine its validity and diagnostic utility in cases with suspected ARVD-C.
- Use of intravenous contrast in TTE has been defined in populations with ARVD-C and can improve uncovering of subtle areas of segmental dysfunction [16, 17]. Nemes et al. [17] recently claimed that the abnormalities of the RV myocardial perfusion could be detected in zones affected by fatty infiltration. Larger populations of cases with ARVD-C need to be assessed to determine the value of contrast TTE in this setting.
- Tricuspid annular plane systolic excursion (TAPSE), studied with M-mode echocardiography, or Doppler quantification of the tricuspid valve annular motion via TDI can be used to assess the global RV function [6]. These methods are possibly most useful when the RV dysfunction is global or in cases with advanced arrhythmogenic RV cardiomyopathy. Because the annular motion can be preserved in the early stages or subtle types of ARVD-C, the utility of TAPSE and TDI systolic velocity in screening suspected cases or mutation carriers who might have patchy or segmental disease is extremely limited.
- 3D TTE is a developing tool that displays promise for a precise estimation of the RV volumes and function [18, 19]. Indeed, imaging of the entire RV volume from a only single transducer position and also single image acquisition is now possible by using 3D TTE [20]. Of course, the calculation of the RV volume through this method has been shown to have less variability than similar measurements by 2D TTE [20, 21]. The RV ejection fraction calculated by 3D TTE has been revealed to be reduced in cases with ARVD-C compared with normal matched controls [21–23].
- 3D TTE parameters were revealed to be capable of distinguishing those with ARVD-C from unaffected relatives in one study; however, the variability rate was higher than that noticed in prior 3D TTE validation studies [19]. At present, there are some limitations as well as technical considerations of image acquisition, cropping, and also measurement that need significant experience with the method. Normal values and disease cut-points are still being established; therefore, the usefulness remains limited to specialized heart centers with expertise in the usages and limitations of 3D TTE.
- An essential prerequisite of the echocardiographic fulfillment of the TFC is the presence of a regional wall motion abnormality. Nonetheless, it should be noted that the qualitative assessment of the RV wall motion abnormalities is subjective and has been shown to have poor reproducibility.
  - The RV free wall myocardial velocity, strain, and strain rate by echocardiographic deformation imaging (by TDI or speckle-tracking) are promising tools to quantify the global and regional ventricular function. Systolic strain and systolic strain rate by TDI have been shown to be reduced in patients with ARVD-C compared with healthy controls [23–25]. In addition, the use of this technique may be able to detect subtle early abnormalities in asymptomatic mutation carriers [24, 25].
  - One limitation of TDI is angle dependence, a requirement that the motion of the wall that is sampled is parallel to the ultrasound beam. As the RV becomes significantly enlarged in more advanced ARVD-C, obtaining accurate and reproducible measures of the RV peak systolic velocity, strain, and strain rate can be challenging.
  - It is possible that the assessment of the RV strain and strain rate by speckle-tracking might be more applicable in the ARVD-C population because it is not on the basis of Doppler and is, thus, not angle dependent. Although the findings described in these small research studies show promise, at present these measures are best performed at specialized centers by those experienced in the method.

Left Ventricular Non-Compaction Cardiomyopathy (LVNC)

Left ventricular non-compaction cardiomyopathy (LVNC), recognized as spongy myocardium, is a distinctive form of cardiomyopathy happening in-utero while segments of spongy myocardium fail to transform into compact, mature musculature resulting in prominent myocardial trabeculae, deep intra-trabecular recesses, and also reduced cardiac function. It has been predicted that LVNC results from arrest of the compaction process during the second month of embryological development. The clinical presentations of LVNC contain HF, arrhythmias, and also propensity for thrombo-embolism (21–24%). HF remains the most common presentation with cases frequently developing progressive symptoms of exertional dyspnea, orthopnea and lower extremity edema. Additionally, cases with LVNC are mostly at high risk of developing arrhythmias, both atrial (5–29%) and also ventricular (18–47%). In addition, the myocardial trabeculations in LVNC predispose the creation of ventricular thrombi and arrhythmias. The areas of non-compaction

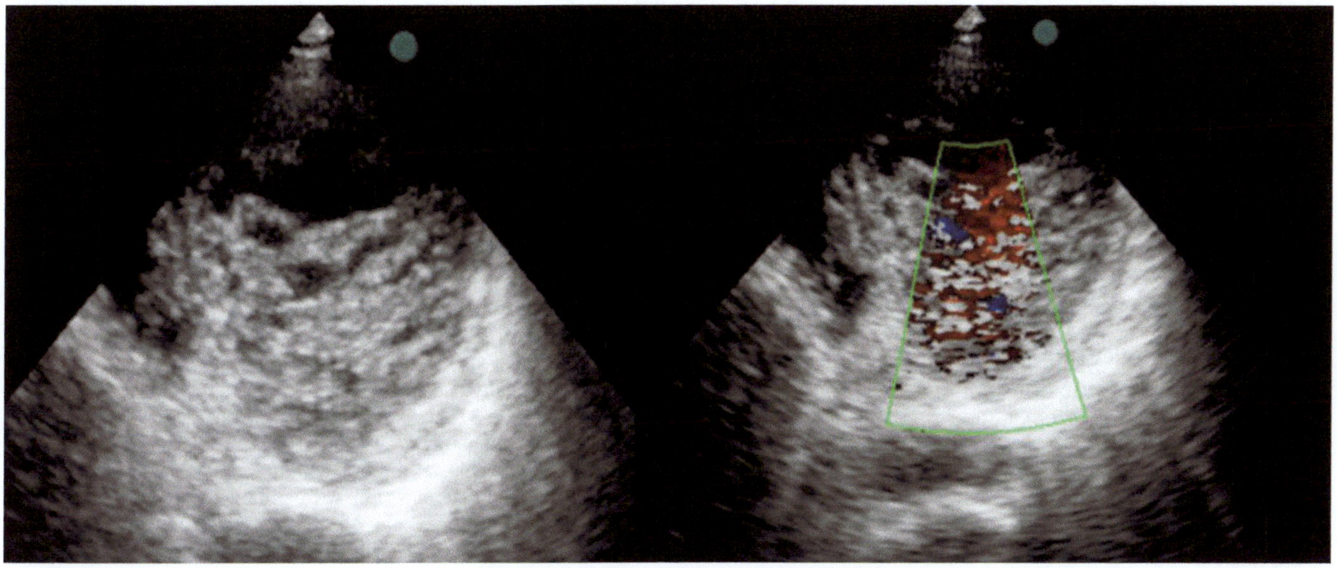

Fig. 24.3 Movies 24.4 and 24.5: Non compaction LV cardiomyopathy with significant trabeculation and color flow in it

frequently display wall motion abnormalities on imaging modalities. In addition, abnormal vaso-dynamic responses within the native vessels are believed to lead to progressive micro-ischemia and progressive dilatation of the ventricle. The high risk for thromboembolism is believed to be multi-factorial; and is due to the combination of reduced LV function, maybe simultaneous happening of AF, and the presence of abnormal myocardial trabeculae. Systemic arterial emboli happen with the greatest frequency, while pulmonary embolism and isolated RV thrombi (6–9%) are less possible [27–32].

Cardiovascular Imaging

The diagnosis of LVNC might be pursued once the more common etiologies for HF are excluded. The work up for new onset LV dysfunction is conventionally achieved upon further valuation by echocardiography, cardiac catheterization, and CMR. Echocardiography frequently provides the first clue to diagnose LVNC and is used with other modalities in concert containing contrast ventriculography, Cardiac CT and CMR. Imaging features classically contain LV systolic dysfunction with depressed LVEF <40% and wall motion abnormalities involving the regions of non-compaction [33–35].

Echocardiography

LVNC on echocardiogram typically is described as a two-layered myocardial structure with a thin, compacted ("C") outer (epicardial) band and a much thicker, non-compacted ("NC") inner (endo-myocardial) layer and deep myocardial trabeculae, predominantly in the apex and free wall of the LV. Color Doppler imaging demonstrates at least three deep intra-trabecular recesses that communicate with the ventricular cavity. Lastly, the two-layered structure of the myocardium will have an increased NC endo-myocardial layer depth compared to the "C" epicardial layer. A NC/C ration >2 in adults when measured in systole is considered diagnostic for LVNC. Three-dimensional echocardiography might play a role in the future but its role presently remains anecdotal.

LVNC is frequently difficult to discriminate from severe forms of LVH, HCM and DCM. Nevertheless, in hearts with prominent myocardial trabeculae from other causes, the thickness ratios between trabeculated and normal myocardium do not reach a ratio > 2. In addition the trabeculated areas related with LVNC tend to be segmental rather than diffuse as might happen in LVH. The cardiac segments, most affected in LVNC are the LV chamber involving the apex, lateral, inferior wall (91–100%), mid-cavity (78%) while the basal segments were least affected (21%). The differences in segmental prevalence recommend an interruption in normal progression of myocardial compaction from the basal/septal to the apical/lateral walls during early development [33–39] (Fig. 24.3).

Conclusion

In recent times, the current classification guidelines for LVNC have been brought into question. Over diagnosis is one of the cited criticisms under the current LVNC classification. In recent studies surveying both the accuracy of echocardiography and CMR, weaker correlations were confirmed with the current NC/C ratios for the diagnosis of LVNC. Though, LVNC is a clinically well described entity, a re-valuation of the diagnostic imaging criteria is currently under research.

Questions

1. Which parameter is a minor criterion for arrhythmogenic right ventricular dysplasia/cardiomyopathy?
   A. Severe dilatation and reduction of right ventricular (RV) ejection fraction
   B. Localized RV aneurysms
   C. Severe segmental dilatation of the RV
   D. Regional RV hypokinesia

2. RV myocardial velocity, strain, and strain rate by echocardiographic deformation imaging are promising tools for the quantification of global and regional ventricular function.
   A. apex
   B. free wall
   C. septum
   D. basal segments

3. Which sentence is wrong in the description of patients with left ventricular non-compaction (LVNC)?
   A. Pulmonary embolism happens with a greater frequency than systemic arterial embolism.
   B. Ventricular arrhythmia is more common than atrial arrhythmia.
   C. Heart failure remains the most common presentation.
   D. Echocardiography frequently provides the first clue for the diagnosis of LVNC.

Answers

1. D
2. B
3. A

References

1. Marcus FI, McKenna WJ, Sherrill D, et al. Diagnosis of arrhythmogenic right ventricular cardiomyopathy/dysplasia: proposed modification of the task force criteria. Circulation. 2010;121:1533–41.
2. Te Riele AS, Bhonsale A, James CA, et al. Incremental value of cardiac magnetic resonance imaging in arrhythmic risk stratification of arrhythmogenic right ventricular dysplasia/cardiomyopathy-associated desmosomal mutation carriers. J Am Coll Cardiol. 2013;62:1761–9.
3. Yoerger DM, Marcus F, Sherrill D, et al. Echocardiographic findings in patients meeting task force criteria for arrhythmogenic right ventricular dysplasia: new insights from the multidisciplinary study of right ventricular dysplasia. J Am Coll Cardiol. 2005;45:860–5.
4. Rudski LG, Lai WW, Afilalo J, et al. Guidelines for the echocardiographic assessment of the right heart in adults: a report from the American Society of Echocardiography endorsed by the European Association of Echocardiography, a registered branch of the European Society of Cardiology, and the Canadian Society of Echocardiography. J Am Soc Echocardiogr. 2010;23:685–713; quiz 786–8.
5. Marcus FI, McKenna WJ, Sherrill D, Basso C, Bauce B, Bluemke DA, Calkins H, Corrado D, Cox MGPJ, Daubert JP, Fontaine G, Gear K, Hauer R, Nava A, Picard MH, Protonotarios N, Saffitz JE, Sanborn DMY, Steinberg JS, Tandri H, Thiene G, Towbin JA, Tsatsopoulou A, Wichter T, Zareba W. Diagnosis of arrhythmogenic right ventricular cardiomyopathy/dysplasia proposed modification of the task force criteria. Eur Heart J. 2010;31:806–14.
6. Lindstrom L, Wilkenshoff UM, Larsson H, Wranne B. Echocardiographic assessment of arrhythmogenic right ventricular cardiomyopathy. Heart. 2001;86:31–8.
7. La Gerche A, Claessen G, Van de Bruaene A, et al. Cardiac MRI: a new gold standard for ventricular volume quantification during high-intensity exercise. Circ Cardiovasc Imaging. 2013;6:329–38.
8. Thiene G, Nava A, Corrado D, Rossi L, Pennelli N. Right ventricular cardiomyopathy and sudden death in young people. N Engl J Med. 1988;318:129–33.
9. Corrado D, Fontaine G, Marcus FI, et al. Arrhythmogenic right ventricular dysplasia/cardiomyopathy: need for an international registry. Study Group on Arrhythmogenic Right Ventricular Dysplasia/Cardiomyopathy of the Working Groups on Myocardial and Pericardial Disease and Arrhythmias of the European Society of Cardiology and of the Scientific Council on Cardiomyopathies of the World Heart Federation. Circulation. 2000;101:E101–6.
10. La Gerche A, Burns AT, D'Hooge J, Macisaac AI, Heidbuchel H, Prior DL. Exercise strain rate imaging demonstrates normal right ventricular contractile reserve and clarifies ambiguous resting measures in endurance athletes. J Am Soc Echocardiogr. 2012;25:253–62.e1.
11. Lang RM, Bierig M, Devereux RB, et al. Recommendations for chamber quantification: a report from the American Society of Echocardiography's Guidelines and Standards Committee and the Chamber Quantification Writing Group, developed in conjunction with the European Association of Echocardiography, a branch of the European Society of Cardiology. J Am Soc Echocardiogr. 2005;18:1440–63.
12. Tei C, Dujardin KS, Hodge DO, et al. Doppler echocardiographic index for assessment of global right ventricular function. J Am Soc Echocardiogr. 1996;9:838–47.
13. Sebbag I, Rudski LG, Therrien J, Hirsch A, Langleben D. Effect of chronic infusion of epoprostenol on echocardiographic right ventricular myocardial performance index and its relation to clinical outcome in patients with primary pulmonary hypertension. Am J Cardiol. 2001;88:1060–3.
14. Yoerger DM, Marcus F, Sherrill D, et al. Right ventricular myocardial performance index in probands from the multicenter study of arrhythmogenic right ventricular dysplasia (abstr). J Am Coll Cardiol. 2005;147A:45.
15. Wang J, Prakasa K, Bomma C, et al. Comparison of novel echocardiographic parameters of right ventricular function with ejection fraction by cardiac magnetic resonance. J Am Soc Echocardiogr. 2007;20:1058–64.
16. Lopez-Fernandez T, Garcia-Fernandez MA, Perez David E, Moreno Yanguela M. Usefulness of contrast echocardiography in arrhythmogenic right ventricular dysplasia. J Am Soc Echocardiogr. 2004;17:391–3.
17. Nemes A, Vletter WB, Scholten MF, ten Cate FJ. Contrast echocardiography for perfusion in right ventricular cardiomyopathy. Eur J Echocardiogr. 2005;6:470–2.
18. Prakasa KR, Dalal D, Wang J, et al. Feasibility and variability of three dimensional echocardiography in arrhythmogenic right ventricular dysplasia/cardiomyopathy. Am J Cardiol. 2006;97:703–9.
19. Picard MH. Three dimensional echocardiography. In: Otto CM, editor. The practice of clinical echocardiography. Philadelphia, PA: Elsevier; 2007. p. 86.
20. Shiota T. 3D echocardiography: evaluation of the right ventricle. Curr Opin Cardiol. 2009;24(5):410–4. doi: https://doi.org/10.1097/HCO.0b013e32832cf8f6.

21. Jiang L, Vazquez de Prada JA, Handschumacher MD, et al. Three-dimensional echocardiography: in vivo validation for right ventricular free wall mass as an index of hypertrophy. J Am Coll Cardiol. 1994;23:1715–22.
22. Jiang L, Siu SC, Handschumacher MD, et al. Three-dimensional echocardiography. In vivo validation for right ventricular volume and function. Circulation. 1994;89:2342–50.
23. Kjaergaard J, Hastrup Svendsen J, Sogaard P, et al. Advanced quantitative echocardiography in arrhythmogenic right ventricular cardiomyopathy. J Am Soc Echocardiogr. 2007;20:27–35.
24. Vitarelli A, Cortes Morichetti M, Capotosto L, et al. Utility of strain echocardiography at rest and after stress testing in arrhythmogenic right ventricular dysplasia. Am J Cardiol. 2013;111:1344–50.
25. Teske AJ, Cox MG, De Boeck BW, Doevendans PA, Hauer RN, Cramer MJ. Echocardiographic tissue deformation imaging quantifies abnormal regional right ventricular function in arrhythmogenic right ventricular dysplasia/cardiomyopathy. J Am Soc Echocardiogr. 2009;22:920–7.
26. Teske AJ, Cox MG, te Riele AS, et al. Early detection of regional functional abnormalities in asymptomatic ARVD/C gene carriers. J Am Soc Echocardiogr. 2012;25:997–1006.
27. Riele ASJM t, Tandri H, Sanborn DM, Bluemke DA. Noninvasive Multimodality Imaging in ARVD/C. J Am Coll Cardiol Img. 2015;8(5):597–611.
28. Borges AC, Kivelitz D, Baumann G. Isolated left ventricular non-compaction: cardiomyopathy with homogeneous transmural and heterogeneous segmental perfusion. Heart. 2003;89:e21.
29. Weiford BC, Subbarao VD, Mulhern KM. Noncompaction of the ventricular myocardium. Circulation. 2004;109:2965–71.
30. Rosa LV, Salemi VM, Alexandre LM, et al. Noncompaction cardiomyopathy: a current view. Arq Bras Cardiol. 2011;97:e13–9.
31. Roberts WC, Karia SJ, Ko JM, et al. Examination of isolated ventricular noncompaction (hypertrabeculation) as a distinct entity in adults. Am J Cardiol. 2011;108:747–52.
32. Murphy RT, Thaman R, Blanes JG, et al. Natural history and familial characteristics of isolated left ventricular non-compaction. Eur Heart J. 2005;26:187–92.
33. Kawel N, Nacif M, Arai AE, et al. Trabeculated (noncompacted) and compact myocardium in adults: the multi-ethnic study of atherosclerosis. Circ Cardiovasc Imaging. 2012;5:357–66.
34. Stöllberger C, Finsterer J, Blazek G. Left ventricular hypertrabeculation/noncompaction and association with additional cardiac abnormalities and neuromuscular disorders. Am J Cardiol. 2002;90:899–902.
35. Oechslin EN, Attenhofer Jost CH, Rojas JR, et al. Long-term follow-up of 34 adults with isolated left ventricular noncompaction: a distinct cardiomyopathy with poor prognosis. J Am Coll Cardiol. 2000;36:493–500.
36. Jenni R, Oechslin E, Schneider J, et al. Echocardiographic and pathoanatomical characteristics of isolated left ventricular noncompaction: a step towards classification as a distinct cardiomyopathy. Heart. 2001;86:666–71.
37. Koo BK, Choi D, Ha JW, et al. Isolated noncompaction of the ventricular myocardium: contrast echocardiographic findings and review of the literature. Echocardiography. 2002;19:153–6.
38. Gopalamurugan AB, Kapetanakis S, Monaghan MJ, et al. Images in cardiology: left ventricular non-compaction diagnosed by real time three dimensional echocardiography. Heart. 2005;91:1274.
39. Bax JJ, Lamb HJ, Poldermans D, et al. Non-compaction cardiomyopathy-echocardiographic diagnosis. Eur J Echocardiogr. 2002;3:301–2.

Echocardiography in Coronary Artery Disease and Acute Myocardial Infarction

25

Azin Alizadehasl and Anita Sadeghpour

Abstract

Coronary artery disease is one of the major causes of morbidity and mortality. Imaging modalities represent the key method not only for the evaluation of the disease extent and severity but also for the assessment of hemodynamic complications. In skilled hands, echocardiography provides valuable and beneficial information for clinical management and prognosis study. Complex assessment confers information about global and regional myocardial function, myocardial ischemia, myocardial viability, and ischemic mitral regurgitation as well as about development of complications such as left ventricular clot formation, myocardial rupture, and pericardial effusion. The main disadvantage of echocardiography, however, is the limited echogenicity of many cases and its indubitable operator-dependence. Even so, the ability to bring echocardiographic imaging to the bedside of our cases makes the method crucial and its knowledge essential for all cardiologists.

Keywords

Coronary artery disease echocardiography · Acute myocardial infarction · Free-wall rupture · Pseudoaneurysms · Mitral regurgitation · Ventricular septal defect

Electronic Supplementary Material The online version of this chapter (https://doi.org/10.1007/978-3-319-67691-3_25) contains supplementary material, which is available to authorized users.

A. Alizadehasl, MD, FACC, FASE
Associate Professor of Cardiology, Echocardiologist, Echocardiography and Cardiogenetic Research Centers, Cardio-Oncology Department, Rajaie Cardiovascular Medical and Research Center, Tehran, Iran

A. Sadeghpour, MD, FACC, FASE (✉)
Professor of Cardiology, Echocardiography Research Center, Rajaie Cardiovascular Medical and Research Center, Iran University of Medical Science, Tehran, Iran

Abbreviations

CAD	Coronary artery disease
LV	Left ventricle
LV/LA	Left ventricular/Left atrial
LVOT	Left ventricular outflow tract
MI	Myocardial infarction
MR	Mitral regurgitation
MV	Mitral valve
PM	Papillary muscle
RV	Right ventricular
SAM	Systolic anterior motion
STEMI	ST-Segment myocardial infarction
TEE	Transesophageal echocardiography
TTE	Transthoracic echocardiography
VSD	Ventricular septal defect
WMSI	Wall motion score index

Introduction

- Echocardiography is the most commonly used and most practical imaging modality for the evaluation of patients with chest pain, coronary artery disease (CAD), or acute myocardial infarction (MI). An understanding of global and regional systolic functions as well as diastolic function by echocardiography is helpful in establishing the diagnosis, management plan, and importantly prognosis of cases with CAD or acute MI. Myocardial perfusion and also contractility become abnormal closely after the onset of ischemia and MI. The perfusion defect and the resulting regional wall motion abnormality may be noticed readily with echocardiography [1, 2].
- Each segment is apportioned a score, on the basis of its contractility as evaluated visually: normal = 1, hypokinesis = 2, akinesis = 3, dyskinesis = 4, and aneurysm = 5. On the basis of this wall motion analysis pattern, a wall motion

A. Sadeghpour, A. Alizadehasl (eds.), *Case-Based Textbook of Echocardiography*, https://doi.org/10.1007/978-3-319-67691-3_25

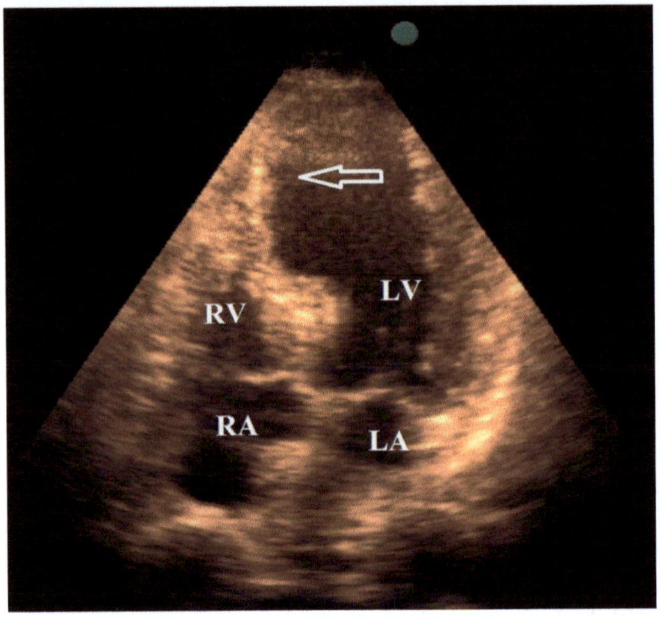

Fig. 25.1 Transthoracic Echocardiography, apical 4-Chamber view, True LV apico-septal aneurysm post MI (*arrow*)

score index (WMSI) is calculated to semi-quantitate the extent of regional wall motion abnormalities:

$$\text{WMSI} = \frac{\text{Sum of the wall motion scores}}{\text{Number of visualized segments}}$$

Normally, LV free-wall thickness increases more than 40% during systole.

Hypokinesia: Systolic wall thickening is less than 30%.

Akinesia: Systolic wall thickening is less than 10%.

Dyskinesia: A myocardial segment moves outward during systole, typically in relation with systolic wall thinning.

Aneurysm: There is a non-contracting area of the myocardium with an abnormal geometry in both systole and diastole [1, 2] (Fig. 25.1).

- A normally contracting left ventricle (LV) has a WMSI of 1 (Each of the 16 segments takes a wall motion score of 1; thus, the total score is 16 and the WMSI is 16/16 = 1). Therefore, the larger the infarct, the higher the WMSI and the more severe the wall motion abnormalities.

Acute Myocardial Infarction

- In many organizations worldwide, primary percutaneous coronary intervention is the management of choice for acute MI. This management modality has significantly lessened mortality in the wake of acute MI. The role of echocardiography has changed as the management plan vis-à-vis acute MI has been altered.
- The obligatory grade of transmural involvement before wall motion turns abnormal is 20%. Non-transmural MI results in a wall motion abnormality that is not easily distinguishable from that of transmural MI. A well-thought-out reperfusion strategy can usually resolve the wall motion abnormality. Nevertheless, the time required for this resolution is variable, ranging range from 12 h to 2 weeks (typically 72 h).

Table 25.1 Complications of myocardial infarction

Acute phase
LV systolic dysfunction
Rupture
FW rupture
Ventricular septaldefect
PM rupture
Subepicardial aneurysm
Mitral regurgitation
LV dilatation
PM dysfunction
PM rupture
LV thrombus
Pericardial effusion or tamponade
RV infarct
LVOT obstruction
Chronic phase
Infarct expansion
Ventricular aneurysm
True aneurysm
Pseudoaneurysm
LV thrombus

FW free wall, *LV* left ventricle, *LVOT* left ventricular outflow tract, *PM* papillary muscle, *RV* right ventricle

The up-to-date role of echocardiography may be categorized as follows:

1. Diagnosis of acute MI in cases with persistent chest pain and nondiagnostic ECG findings
2. Estimation of the extent of the myocardium at risk and infarct size after reperfusion management
3. Evaluation of unstable hemodynamics
4. Recognition of infarct complications
5. Evaluation of the viability of the myocardium,
6. Risk stratification.

Accordingly, at different stages of acute MI, echocardiography is essential in providing anatomical, functional, and hemodynamic data Table 25.1 [1–4].

Free-Wall Rupture and Pseudoaneurysms

- Free-wall rupture happens within the first week after infarction (median time = 4 d). Interestingly, this kind of rupture is associated with less severe CAD and smaller MI. Negative echocardiographic findings can not exclude myocardial rupture if there is high clinical suspicion.
- A pseudoaneurysm is created when a partial rupture spontaneously seals off, resulting in an extracardiac chamber,

the walls of which contain the pericardium and clot (not by myocardial fibers). Pseudoaneurysms most commonly occur in the posterior wall, followed by the lateral and then apical walls.

- A true aneurysm comprises all layers of the myocardium and is described by myocardial thinning and bulging motion thereof during systole. It is correlated with transmural MI and is found most frequently at the apex, followed by the inferobasal area.
- Pseudoaneurysms might grow quite large, even equaling the true ventricular cavity in size, and they link with the LV cavity through a narrow neck. Often, pseudoaneurysms comprise substantial quantities of old and recent thrombi.
- If transthoracic echocardiography (TTE) is not feasible in cases receiving mechanical ventilation, transesophageal echocardiography (TEE) may aid to confirm a free-wall rupture. Left hear intravenous contrast agents may be useful in diagnosis the site of the perforation and extravasation to the pericardium in stable patients. Cardiovascular magnetic resonance imaging might also prove helpful when there is a cardiac rupture insofar as it offers outstanding image quality, identifies the site, and delineates the anatomy of a ventricular pseudoaneurysm. This imaging modality is, however, of limited use in the acute setting because it is both time-consuming and non-portable [1, 5, 6] (Figs. 25.2, 25.3, and 25.4).

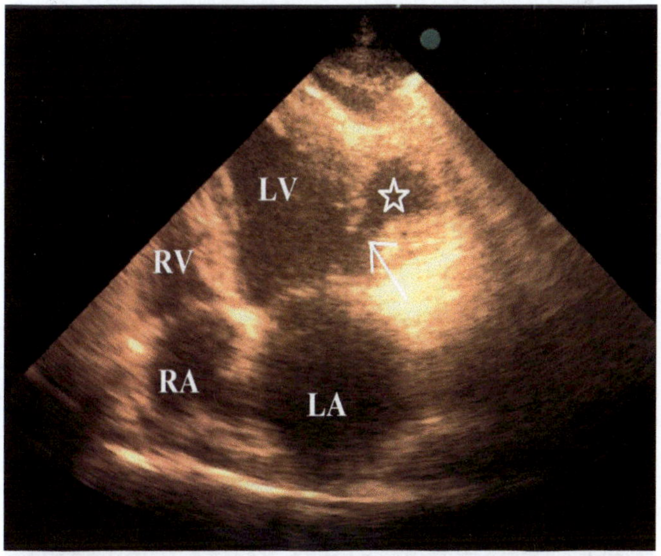

Fig. 25.2 Movie 25.1 Transthoracic Echocardiography, apical 4-Chamber view, lateral wall pseduaneurysm with small neck after anterolateral MI (*)

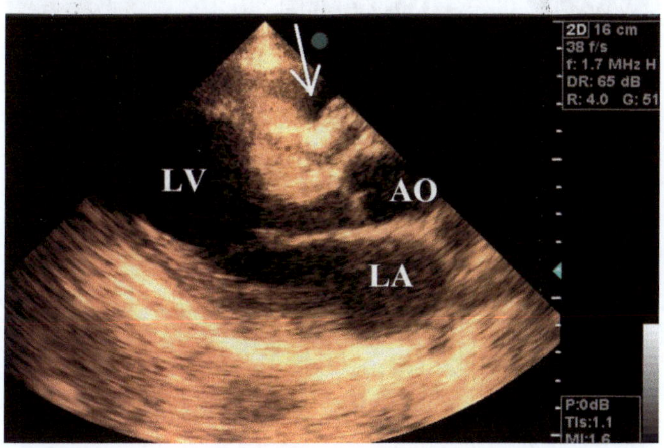

Fig. 25.3 Transthoracic Echocardiography, parasternal long axis view, RVOT collapse due to partial rupture of myocardium post MI

Mitral Regurgitation

There are four independent reasons for acute mitral regurgitation (MR) after MI:

1. Annular dilatation
2. Papillary muscle (PM) rupture (Fig. 25.5, Movies 25.2, 25.3, 25.4 and 25.5)
3. PM dysfunction (Fig. 25.6)
4. Acute systolic anteriormotion of the mitral valve (MV)
   - PM rupture is the most serious complication involving the MV and is more common in the posteromedial PMs. It is allied to a small infarct in the distribution of the right coronary artery or the left circumflex artery (Fig. 25.5).
   - Even a mild degree of MR is associated with increased mortality. An incidence of MR caused by PM rupture may be easily detected by color flow Doppler imaging. This is especially helpful in differentiating acute MR from a ventricular septal defect (VSD) in cases with ST-segment myocardial infarction (STEMI).TTE is often suboptimal for evaluation because the view of the PMs is frequently limited, the MR jet is eccentric, and also color Doppler is influenced by the low left ventricular/left atrial (LV/LA) gradient in the setting of acute severe MR.
   - TEE is a proper imaging modality and must be carried out closely if this diagnosis is suspected because it provides high-resolution images and precise evaluation of MR. The LA size is often normal. In severe MR, the MV leaflets are typically flail or prolaptic.
   - In patients with CAD, the posterior leaflet motion is restricted or tethered in systole secondary to the insufficient contraction of the posterolateral wall Fig. 25.6). The resulting malcoaptation and malapposition is allied to a posteriorly directed MR jet. The dilation of the MV annulus also may contribute to the development of MR. In cases with CAD, functional MR is correlated principally with inferior MI and the lateral displacement of the posterior PM. It is also worthy of note that significant ischemic MR is correlated with a poor outcome.An effective orifice area greater than 0.2 cm^2 or a regurgitant volume of 30 mL or more is linked with increased mortality [1–3, 7, 8].

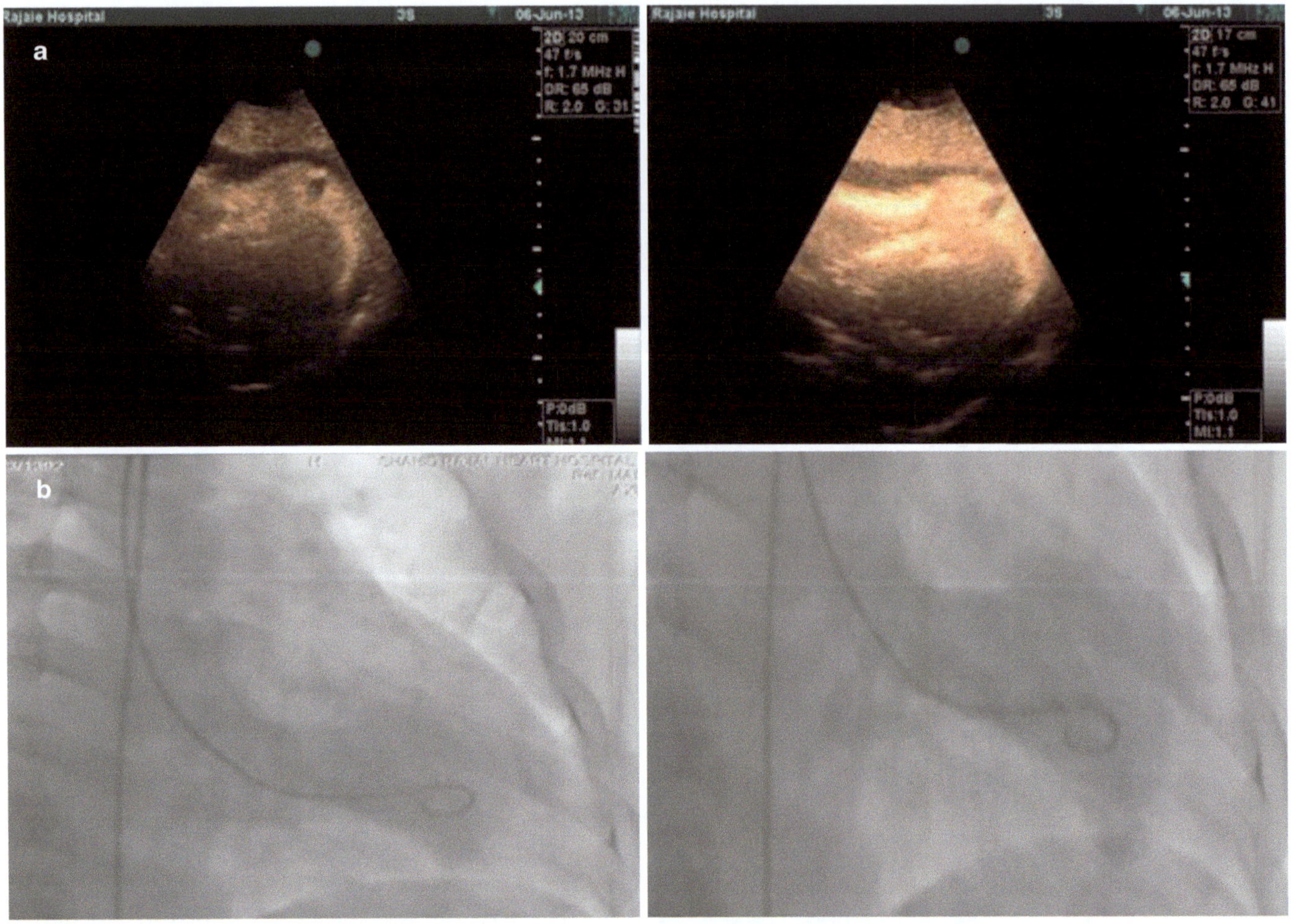

Fig. 25.4 (**a**) Subcoastal View; an echo-dense cap in pericardial space at cardiac apex in concomitant with pericardial effusion. (**b**) Slow manual contrast injection in left ventricular cavity that resulted in pericardial space local opacification in apical part

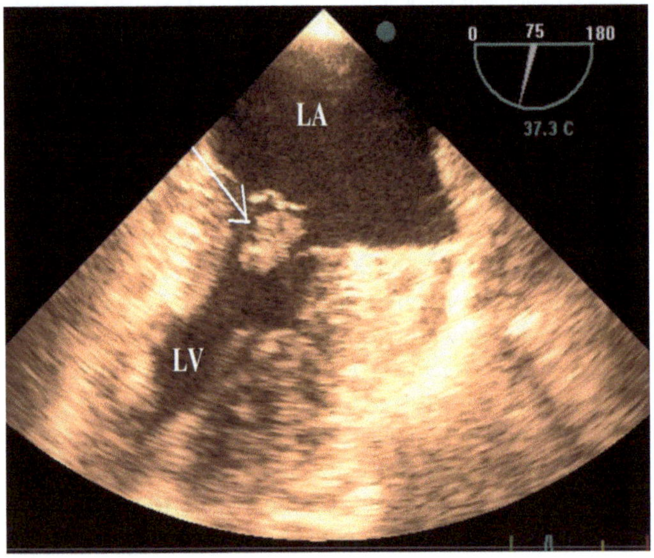

Fig. 25.5 Movies 25.2, 25.3, 25.4 and 25.5 Transesophageal Echocardiography, mid-esophageal view, Post MI posteromedial papillary muscle rupture resulting flail anterior mitral leaflet and severe acute posterior directed MR in a patient with refractory pulmonary edema

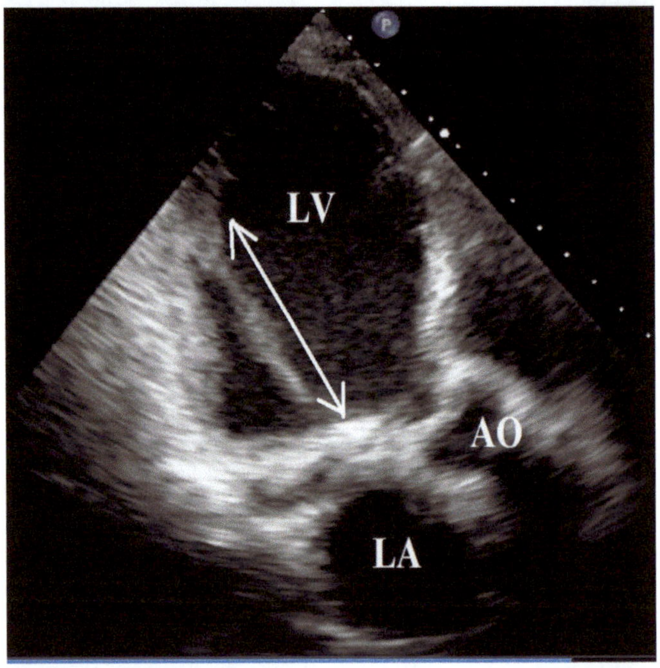

Fig. 25.6 Transthoracic Echocardiography, apical three-Chamber view, Tethered chorda attached to posteromedial papillary muscle (papillary muscle dysfunction)

Ventricular Septal Defect

- The diagnosis of a VSD may typically be made by TTE as a discrete 2D echo dropout in a thin and fibrotic tissue. Small defects may not be visible, but color Doppler is very precise and sensitive. Still, experience is essential as the most helpful views depend on the location of the defect. Subcostal views are principally advantageous in critically ill and supine patients with inferior MI. Since these defects are often not discrete, the evaluation of the degree of a left-to-right shunt may be difficult. A large shunt is characterized by the hypercontractility of non-infracted LV segments with a low forward stroke volume, and also an elevated pulmonary artery systolic pressure.
- Echocardiography with color flow Doppler is the favored diagnostic tool to identify a VSD with reported sensitivity and specificity of as high as 100%. This modality may also be used for the definition of the site and size of a VSD, evaluation of LV and right ventricular (RV) functions, quantification of a left-to-right shunt, and estimation of RV systolic pressure (Fig. 25.7) [1, 9].

Left Ventricular Outflow Tract Obstruction

- Acute dynamic left ventricular outflow tract (LVOT) obstruction is related to the compensatory hyperdynamic motion of the posterior and inferolateral walls, resulting not only in the systolic anterior motion (SAM) of the MV leaflet but also in MR. Acute dynamic LVOT obstruction is more common in elderly women who have basal septal hypertrophy due to hypertension and after anterior MI. These cases may develop severely unstable hemodynamic and pulmonary edema.
- Echocardiography is the method of choice for the diagnosis in that it can precisely disclose the hyperkinetic segment and the LVOT obstruction as well as the SAM of the MV leaflets. Suitable management includes fluids, beta-blockers, and not using inotropes and vasodilators [1–3].

Right Ventricular Myocardial Infarction

- The RV is often involved in acute MI. The apical portion of the RV is supplied by the left anterior descending artery and might contract normally, while the base to mid portions of the RV free walls become affected in RV infarction. The RA is dilated and tricuspid regurgitation becomes significant as a result of the dilatation of the tricuspid valve annulus.
- If a patient presents with hypoxemia after inferior MI, RV MI and right-to-left shunting via a patent foramen ovale must be strongly considered; however, the diagnosis may be confirmed with contrast echocardiography [1, 2, 10].

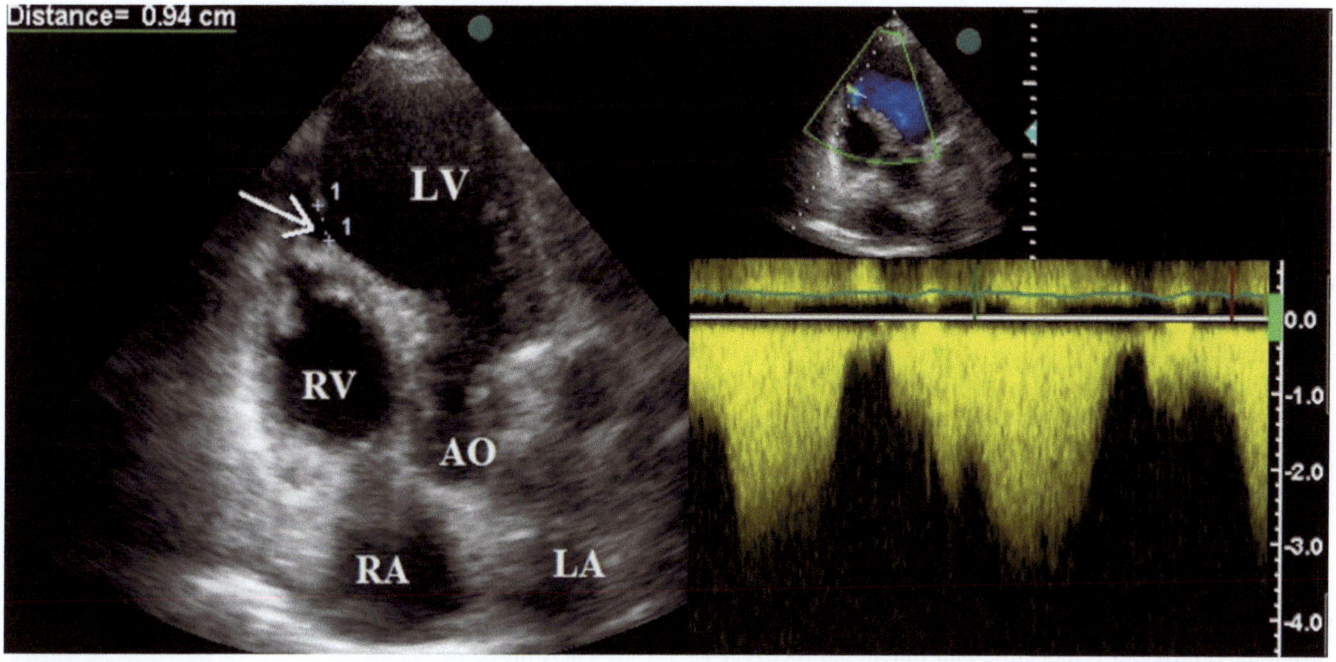

Fig. 25.7 Movies 25.6 and 25.7 Transthoracic Echocardiography, apical 5-Chamber view, Post MI VSD (*arrow*) with related Doppler flow pattern

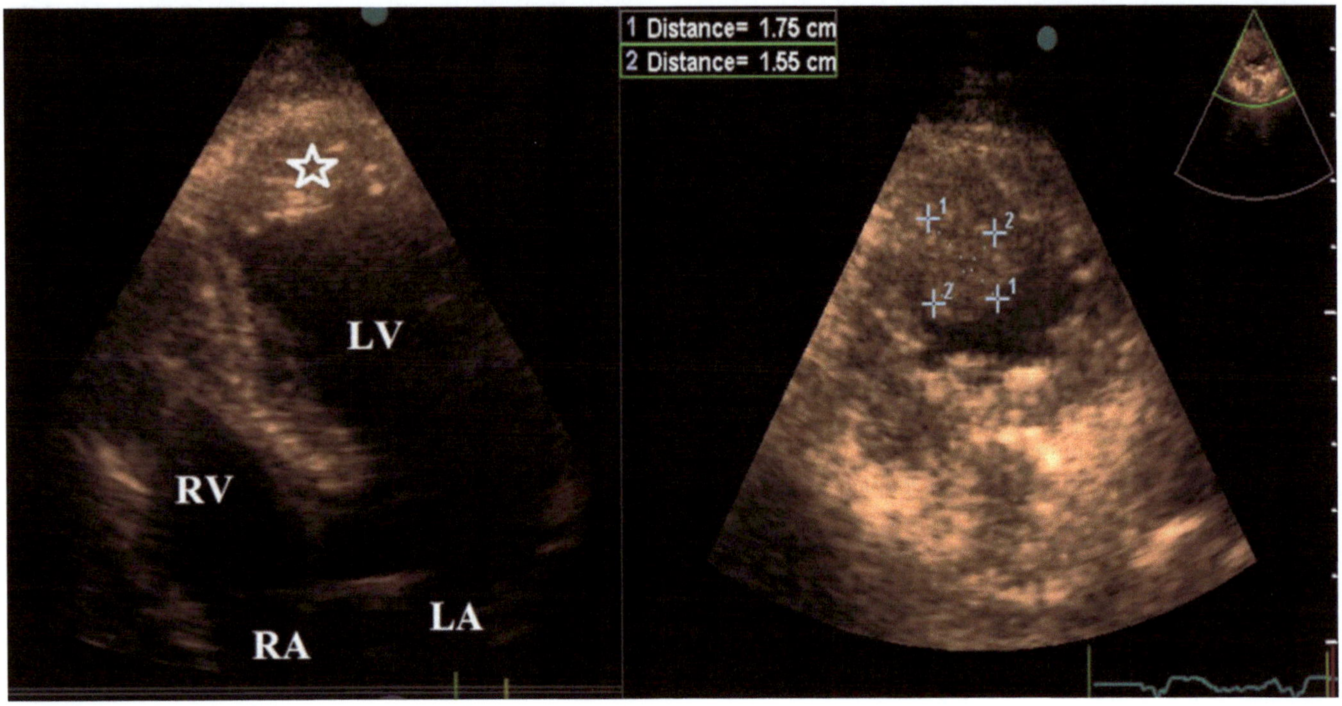

Fig. 25.8 Movies 25.8 and 25.9 Transthoracic Echocardiography, apical 4-Chamber view, Fresh, Immobile LV apical fresh clot (*) with concomitant showing in apical short axis view

Pericardial Effusion

- The incidence of post-infarction pericardial effusion as noticed by 2D echocardiography is described to be from 30 to 40% in cases with STEMI. The amount of effusion is minor, and the peak time for effusion to happen is 3 days following acute MI.
- Tamponade is infrequent in an uncomplicated MI. More and larger effusions or effusions with a hemorrhagic appearance must always be considered as myocardial rupture [1, 11].

Left Ventricular Thrombi

- The peak timing of early thrombus formation after MI is 72 h. Nonetheless, in larger MIs with large areas of akinesis and also stagnant flow, thrombus formation tends to happen even within hours. Definite echocardiographic appearances (pedunculated and mobile thrombi) are correlated with a greater risk of embolization. TTE (principally contrast TTE) remains the imaging technique of choice and is 92% sensitive and 88% specific for identifying LV thrombi. TEE might not be able to image the apex as obviously as TTE. (Fig. 25.8)
- Echocardiography provides essential evidence for anticipating ventricular remodeling and functional recovery as well as information regarding LV dimension and volume, regional wall motion abnormalities, myocardial viability, LV filling pressures, MR severity, and systolic pulmonary artery pressure. 1–3.

Questions

1. What is the most serious complication involving the mitral valve in acute MI patients?
   (A) Annular dilatation
   (B) Papillary muscle dysfunction
   (C) Papillary muscle rupture
   (D) Acute systolic anterior motion of the mitral valve

2. Which phrase is incorrect?
   (A) The apical portion of the RV is supplied by the LCX and may contract normally while the basal to mid RV free walls become affected in RV infarct.
   (B) The RA is dilated and TR becomes significant as a result of dilatation of tricuspid annulus.
   (C) Peak TR velocity is not high (< 2 m/s), due to normal RVSP.
   (D) In patients with PFO, an RVMI creates a significant Rt to Lt shunt with subsequent hypoxemia because of abnormal RV compliance and markedly increased RA pressure.

3. Which phrase is incorrect?
   (A) A VSD can be established in 90% of cases with TTE.
   (B) VSD occurs during small infarction, then the wall motion abnormality may be subtle.
   (C) Pseudo aneurysm forms when a partial rupture spontaneously seals off, resulting in an extra cardiac chamber, the walls of which consist of pericardium and clot (no myocardial fibers)
   (D) Pseudo aneurysm most frequently in anterior wall, followed by the lateral and apical wall.

Answers

1. C
2. A
3. D

References

1. Flachskampf FA, Schmid M, Rost C, Achenbach S, DeMaria AN, Daniel WG. Cardiac imaging after myocardial infarction. Eur Heart J. 2011;32(3):272.
2. Votavová R, Linhartová A, Kořínek J, Marek J, Linhart A. Echocardiography in coronary artery disease. Imaging Coron Artery Dis. 2015;57(6):e408–18.
3. Greaves SC. Role of echocardiography in acute coronary syndromes. Heart. 2002;88:419–25.
4. Giusca S, Jurcut R, Ticulescu R, Dumitru D, Vladaia A, Savu O, Voican A, Popescu BA, Ginghina C. Accuracy of handheld echocardiography for bedside diagnostic evaluation in a tertiary cardiology center: comparison with standard echocardiography. Echocardiography. 2011;28:136–41.
5. Dencker M, Tasevska G, Grubb D, Stagmo M, Gustafsson R. Unexpected rupture of the left ventricular free wall in the echo-lab. Eur J Echocardiogr. 2008;9:92–4.
6. Morimoto H, Mukai S, Obata S, Fujiwara Y. Left ventricular free wall rupture after coronary artery bypass grafting. Eur J Cardiothorac Surg. 2012;41:707.
7. Kwan J, Shiota T, Agler DA, Popović ZB, Qin JX, Gillinov MA, Stewart WJ, Cosgrove DM, McCarthy PM, Thomas JD, study R-t t-d e. Geometric differences of the mitral apparatus between ischemic and dilated cardiomyopathy with significant mitral regurgitation: real-time three-dimensional echocardiography study. Circulation. 2003;107:1135–40.
8. Grigioni F, Detaint D, Avierinos JF, Scott C, Tajik J, Enriquez-Sarano M. Contribution of ischemic mitral regurgitation to congestive heart failure after myocardial infarction. J Am Coll Cardiol. 2005;45:260–7.
9. Donoiu I, Istratoaie O, Ionescu DD. Ventricular septal rupture after acute myocardial infarction. Hell J Cardiol. 2010;51:374–6.
10. Goldberger JJ, Himelman RB, Wolfe CL, Schiller NB. Right ventricular infarction: recognition and assessment of its hemodynamic significance by two-dimensional echocardiography. J Am Soc Echocardiogr. 1991;4:140–6.
11. Figueras J, Barrabés JA, Serra V, Cortadellas J, Lidón RM, Carrizo A, Garcia-Dorado D. Hospital outcome of moderate to severe pericardial effusion complicating ST-elevation acute myocardial infarction. Circulation. 2010;122:1902–9.

Echocardiographic Assessment of Coronary Blood Flow

26

Jarosław D. Kasprzak, Piotr Lipiec, and Karina Wierzbowska-Drabik

Abstract

Echocardiography of coronary arteries is challenging, however current high–end systems offer sufficient quality for several clinically relevant applications of the method. Transesophageal echocardiography allows the imaging of proximal coronary arteries with high quality and power to detect stenotic flow. Transthoracic imaging of coronary ostia is feasible to define anomalous coronary arteries and other congenital abnormalities. This approach is also used for recording of distal coronary flow at rest and during vasodilator administration to calculate coronary flow reserve. Transthoracic detection of coronary stenosis is strongly dependent on acoustic window but is very specific based on the finding localized high velocity diastolic flow.

Keywords

Coronary arteries imaging · Coronary flow reserve Anomalous coronary arteries

Electronic Supplementary Material The online version of this chapter (https://doi.org/10.1007/978-3-319-67691-3_26) contains supplementary material, which is available to authorized users.

J. D. Kasprzak, MD, PhD (✉) · P. Lipiec
K. Wierzbowska-Drabik
Department of Cardiology, Medical University of Lodz, Lodz, Poland
e-mail: kasprzak@ptkardio.pl

Abbreviations

2-D	Two-dimensional
CFR	Coronary flow reserve
CFVR	Coronary flow velocity reserve
CX	Circumflex branch of the left coronary artery
LCA	Right coronary artery
LMCA	Left main coronary artery
RCA	Right coronary artery
TEE	Transesophageal echocardiography
TTE	Transthoracic echocardiography

Introduction

Cardiac Ultrasound of Coronary Arteries—Current Status

Coronary disease, the leading cause of morbidity and mortality, is the frequent indication for cardiac ultrasound, however, echocardiography is used for collecting indirect information on consequences of ischemia or ischemic necrosis rather than imaging coronary arteries. The segments of coronary arteries can be directly visualized during standard echocardiographic examination from transthoracic and transesophageal window. With dedicated Doppler settings laminar or pathological flow can be detected and then sampled with pulsed wave spectral Doppler. The main problems limiting the practical application of this approach are their small size and vigorous motion of epicardial sections dependent on respiratory and cardiac cycle. For this reason direct visualization of coronary arteries has not become a part of routine transthoracic echocardiographic examination (TTE) despite significant progress in quality of imaging. The echocardiographic signs of coronary stenosis are specific but the overall sensitivity is low due to limitations in ultrasonic windows.

A. Sadeghpour, A. Alizadehasl (eds.), *Case-Based Textbook of Echocardiography*, https://doi.org/10.1007/978-3-319-67691-3_26

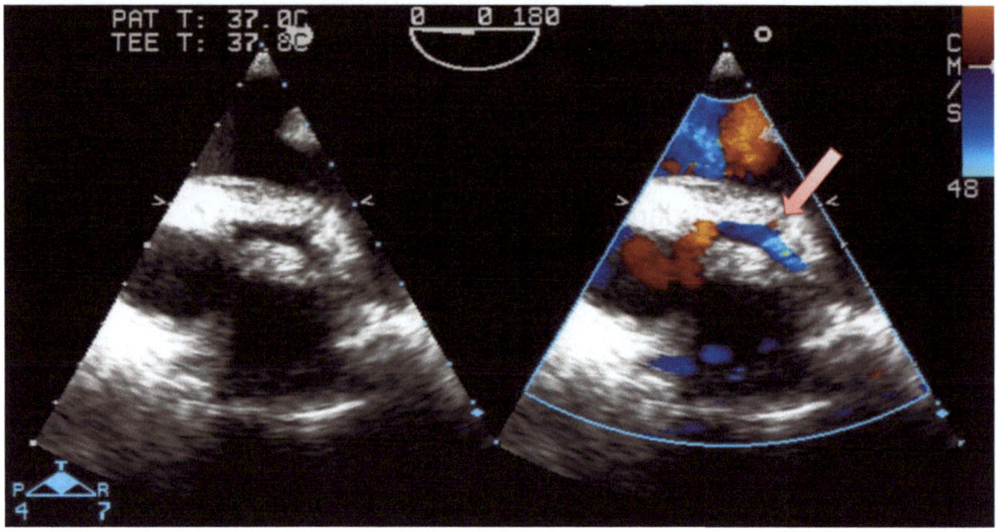

Fig. 26.1 Left main coronary artery coursing rightward with bifurcation site visualized in high esophageal short axis view from trans-esophageal window—normal laminar flow. Origin of circumflex branch shown with arrow

Cardiac ultrasound usually allows the visualization of proximal coronary arteries and identification of less common conditions such as fistulae or ostial anomalies, especially when transesophageal approach (TEE) is used. The progress in Doppler technology allows the recording of distal coronary flow velocity in the majority of patients thus opening the access to coronary flow velocity reserve (CFVR) measurements based on vasodilator-induced vasodilatation.

Nowadays, transthoracic and transesophageal echocardiography allows investigating the following clinical aspects of coronary anatomy and physiology:

1. Two-dimensional and color-Doppler assessment of ostia and proximal segments with diagnosis of congenital anomalies. Occasionally luminal narrowing and calcifications can be seen as well as or aneurysms due to atherosclerosis or Kawasaki disease in pediatric population
2. Assessment of flow in the main coronary arteries (left main coronary artery (LMCA), circumflex (Cx), left anterior descending (LAD) and right coronary artery (RCA) with a potential to detection a stenotic flow (by color flow aliasing and subsequent recording of flow acceleration)
3. Assessment of accessible parts of mid and distal coronary arteries (and distal coronary by-pass grafts, usually internal mammary artery) including examination of coronary flow velocity reserve based on spectral Doppler at rest and under vasodilator stress (with highest feasibility in LAD but reported also in RCA)
4. TTE color Doppler diagnosis of coronary fistulas draining to heart chambers and pulmonary artery

Transesophageal Echocardiographic Visualization of Coronary Arteries

TEE offers superior conditions to image small objects such as coronary arteries due to higher ultrasound beam frequency and better resolution. Thus, imaging of ostia of coronary arteries (especially left) from the transesophageal window is easy and allows, including better anatomical definition of possible lesions. TEE allows the visualization of proximal coronary arteries in >90% of studies (left main coronary artery, LMCA virtually in every study [1]) and offers interpretable recordings of flow in most of LMCA/proximal LAD segments, and 50–70% of proximal CX and RCA. As opposed to TTE, TEE allows the identification of calcifications or luminal narrowing [2].TEE assessment of coronary ostia is obtained by visualization of the left and right sinus of Valsalva in high esophageal short axis cross-sectional views with subsequent identification of LMCA dividing into LAD and Cx (Fig. 26.1, Video 26.1), and, usually in separate view, RCA (Fig. 26.2). Identification of ostia (Video 26.2) is necessary in context of coronary artery anomalies and is performed in color Doppler with filter setting and kept low to enhance low velocity diastolic flow of the coronary arteries. Localized turbulence with aliasing (with high Nyquist limit settings) is a typical, highly specific sign of significant coronary stenosis. This finding is corroborated by recording of spectral Doppler flow acceleration (Fig. 26.3). Measuring artery diameter is feasible mainly for LMCA and CX which run nearly perpendicular to the ultrasound beam [3] with a potential to diagnose dilatation of proximal coronary segments (acquired or inherited—fistula or anomalous origin of the coronary artery from the pulmonary artery).

The proposed criterion for significant coronary stenosis which may be used both for TTE and TEE is twofold increase in coronary flow velocity (maximal-to-prestenotic flow velocity ratio [4]) or maximal flow velocity above 1.5–2.0 m/s. Specific upper normal diastolic velocity limits for TEE have also been proposed [5, 6]—usually around 100–140 cm/s (hyperkinetic conditions or mere tachycardia increases resting flow velocity) for LCA and >53 cm/s for RCA. The diagnostic accuracy for proximal stenosis based on combined 2-dimensional + color Doppler TEE study is close to 100% for LMCA, 95% for LAD, 75% for CX and much lower sensitivity for RCA [7].

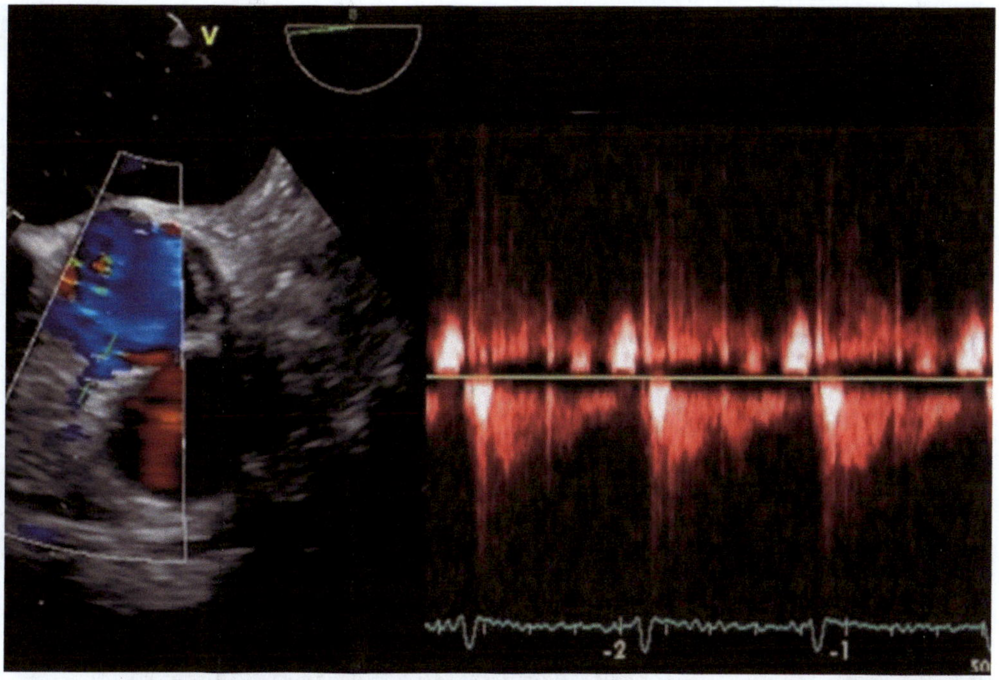

Fig. 26.2 Proximal right coronary artery seen in trans-esophageal echocardiogram. Laminar flow is seen coded in blue with low-velocity diastolic flow spectrum below the pulsed—wave Doppler baseline, without diastolic predominance which is typical for the right coronary artery (in systole a typical right ventricular artefact overshadows the coronary flow)

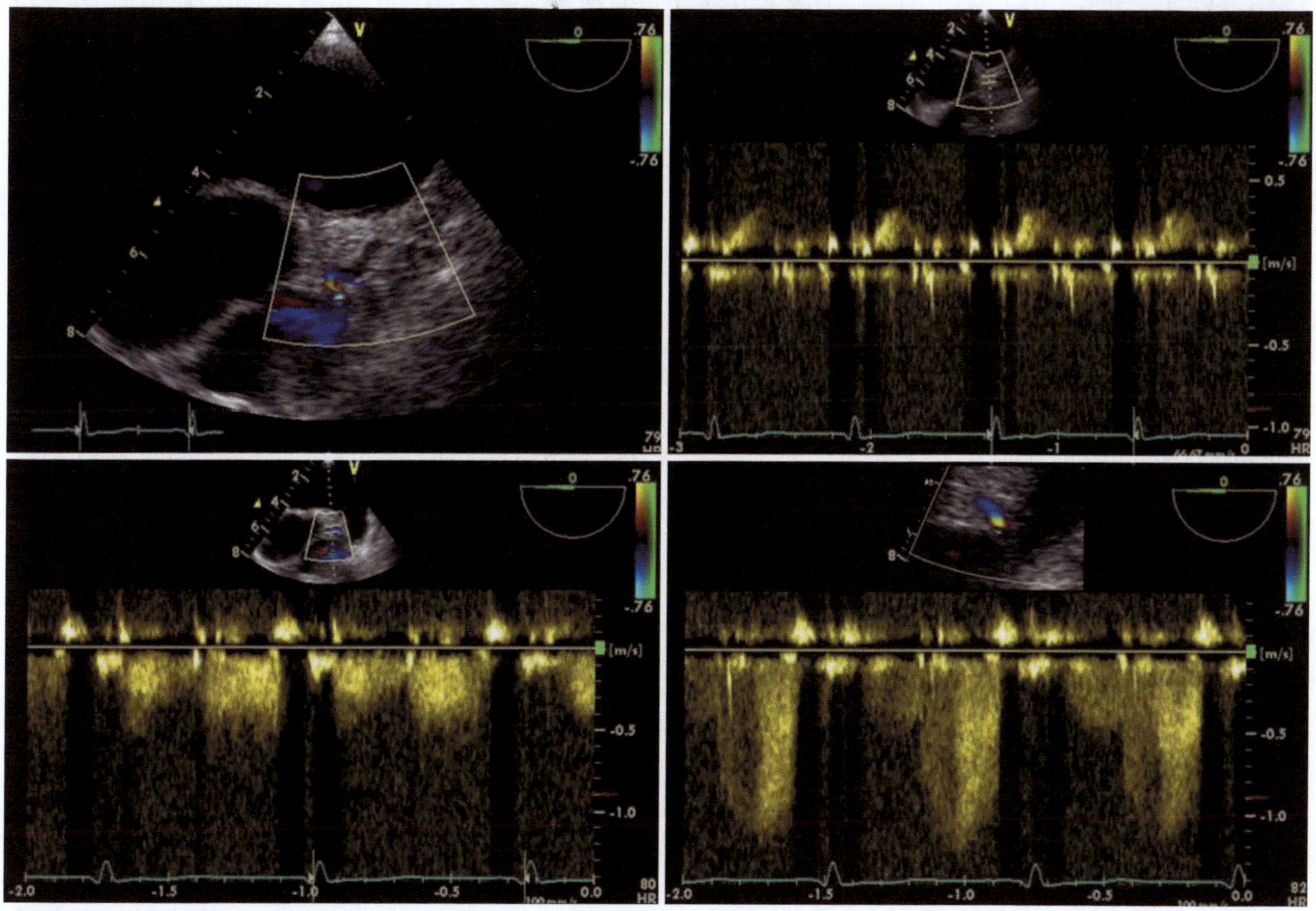

Fig. 26.3 Transesophageal Doppler study of intermediate ostial left anterior descending artery stenosis shown by localized flow turbulence (top left) in high esophageal short axis view. Flow is accelerated to >1.3 m/s, (bottom right) significantly higher as compared with prestenotic flow (0.4 m/s, bottom left) in distal LMCA and proximal circumflex flow (top left)

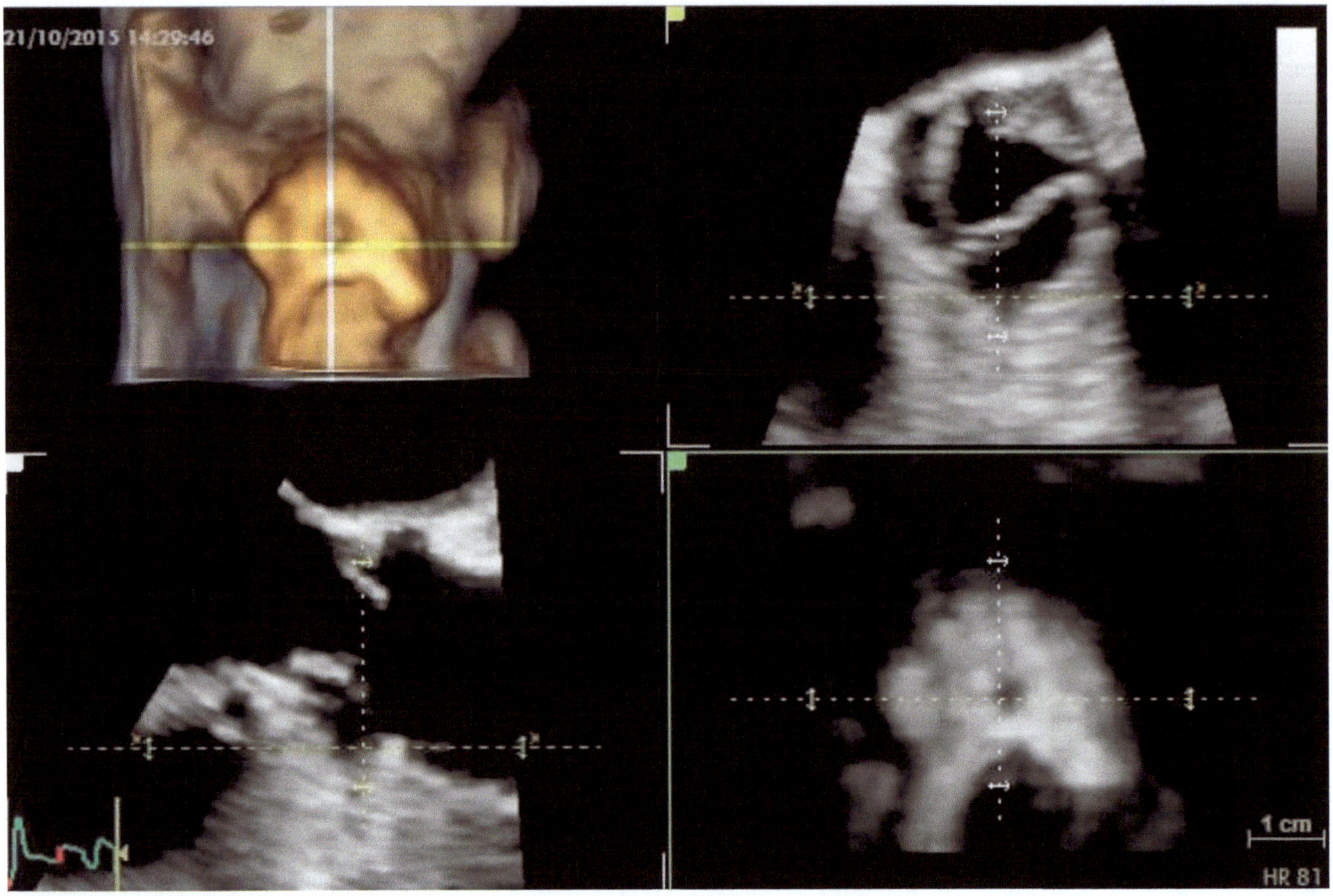

Fig. 26.4 Three-dimensional transesophageal imaging of the proximal right coronary artery—crosshairs indicate the orifice of the artery in volume rendered presentation (en-face view—top left) and reconstructed multiplane images. Calcified aortic plaque is seen at sinotubular junction next to the ostium

Thus, it is reasonable to attempt imaging proximal coronary arteries in routine TEE studies as clinical benefits were suggested, e.g. in patients undergoing TEE due to cryptogenic embolism [8]. Three-dimensional datasets contain information on proximal coronary arteries with somewhat limited resolution but amenable to off-line analysis using multiplanar reformatting (Fig. 26.4).

Coronary Morphology and Flow in Transthoracic Echocardiogram

The most of TTE examinations allow the visualization of proximal segments of coronary arteries. Good-quality color flow recording in LMCA including proximal Cx and RCA may be available in at least 55% of cases [9] and antegrade LAD flow even in around of 90% technically satisfactory studies [10], with lower feasibility for the proximal, middle and distal segments of Cx (88, 61 and 3%) or RCA (40, 28 and 54% of patients).

The ostia of the coronary arteries are seen in multiple views—parasternal short axis at the level of the sinuses of Valsalva, with additional views of the right coronary ostium in parasternal long axis view (Fig. 26.5, Video 26.3). In the parasternal short axis LMCA is nearly perpendicular to the beam which hampers the detection of flow with underestimation of recorded flow velocity which can be supplemented with LMCA images from modified apical five chamber view (Fig. 26.6) which also may show sections of CX and LAD.

Transthoracic detection of coronary stenosis has not been routinely attempted for years but recent reports emphasize that with a careful technique, many major coronary segments can be visualized and stenosis—detectable by Doppler (but not 2-D imaging) in experienced hands. Proximal LAD coronary flow recording is easiest for the proximal LAD and both interventricular branches. The suspicion of stenosis is raised by findings of rapid, multidirectional flow which "lightens up" in the locations where no color of laminar flow signal could be expected. Acceleration of diastolic flow above 2 m/s or twofold increase in velocity compared to that obtained from an adjacent coronary segment (or distal segment velocity of the same vessel [11]) are highly specific signs of a significant coronary stenosis or restenosis (Video 26.4) [7, 12]. Combination of this criterion with color Doppler aliasing

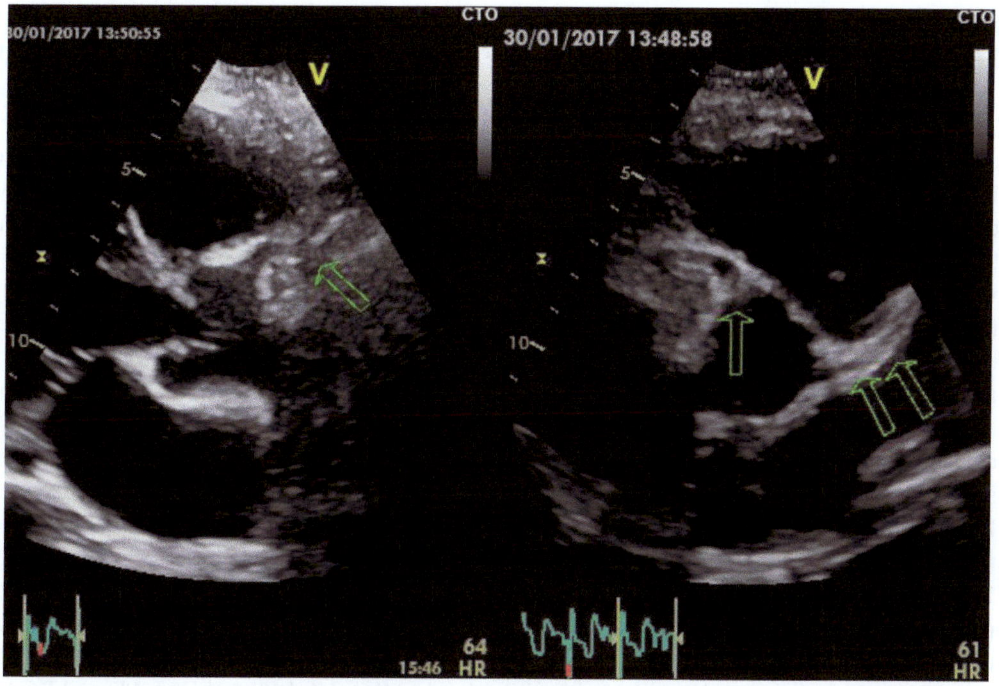

Fig. 26.5 Transthoracic imaging of proximal coronary arteries—right coronary artery (arrow) and proximal left coronary artery (double arrow) seen in long axis parasternal view (left) and short axis parasternal view (right)

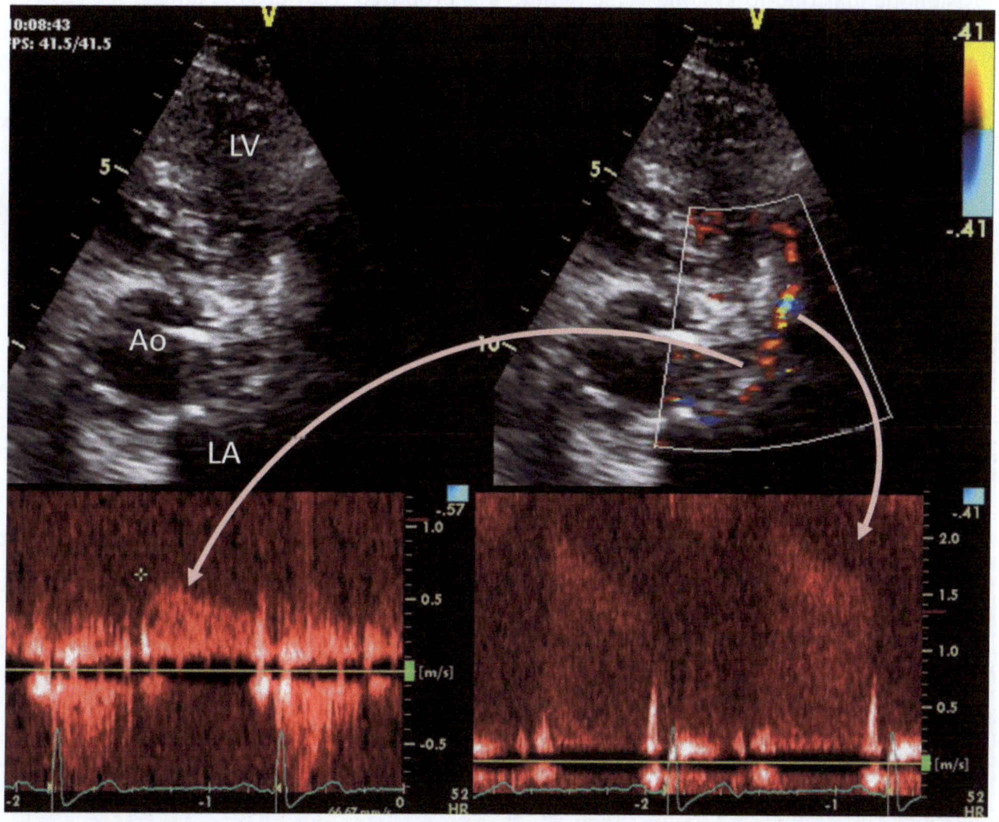

Fig. 26.6 Left anterior descending artery stenosis demonstrated from the five-chamber transthoracic view as localized site of accelerated aliasing flow (shorter arrow) with high (210 cm/s) diastolic velocity (bottom right), comparing to prestenotic site (bottom left, 66 cm/s)

at Nyquist limit 48 cm/s provides the specificity 90–95% with sensitivity 75% for LMCA/LAD but only ~35% for RCA/CX [13]. Prognostically ominous LMCA stenosis is characterized by mosaic flow and acceleration >1.5 m/s [14]. Importantly, coronary occlusion sites have no specific markers regarding color flow. In such cases diastolic coronary flow may be reversed due to retrograde filling by collateral circulation (a very specific but low sensitive finding) [15].

Distal Coronary Flow and Coronary Flow Reserve

Technical progress in Doppler sensitivity allowed routine detection of distal coronary flow in transthoracic studies. Flow is usually recorded in the apical segments of major epicardial coronary arteries, with highest feasibility reaching 90–95% for distal LAD; assessment of distal posterior interventricular branch and marginal branches has also been reported) [16, 17]. Ultrasound enhancing agents may be occasionally used to improve the detection of low-intensity flow signals [18].

Recording of distal LAD flow has the major application in coronary (velocity) flow reserve studies (CFR, CFVR); CFR studies of other coronary arteries have also been published. Distal LAD flow can be recorded in most patients from a modified apical three-chamber view, usually ranging 20–50 cm/s (Fig. 26.7) but absolute values depend strongly of angulation of recorded artery. Increased velocities indicate that stenotic situs is directly sampled whereas very low distal velocities (around 10 cm/s) with slow deceleration were reported distally to critical stenoses in LAD. Distal poststenotic diastolic-to-systolic velocity ratio was proposed to define significant LAD or marginal branch stenosis, with abnormality threshold <1.68 [19]. The ratio of distal to proximal diastolic velocity in LAD ratio can be used as another criterion for LMCA/LAD stenosis when less than 0.5 [11]. Abnormal distal LAD flow recorded after LAD-related infarction, with short diastolic deceleration time (≤600 ms) predicts absence of viability, remodeling and transmural necrosis with worse clinical outcomes [20]. Distal anastomoses of coronary by-pass grafts, usually internal mammary artery can be frequently visualized and flow pattern recorded with diastolic dominance when graft patent (Fig. 26.8).

Noninvasive echocardiographic measurements of coronary flow velocity reserve represent a recommended component of a full stress echo protocol, adding sensitivity without specificity loss as compared to wall motion scoring alone [21]. CFVR is calculated as a ratio of peak diastolic flow velocity during vasodilatory challenge (usually intravenous dipyridamole or adenosine which minimize precapillary resistance vessels to maximize flow) to resting flow velocity with close correlation with intracoronary Doppler measurements and useful to define physiologically meaningful stenosis in LAD and RCA [22]. Normal values for CFVR range from 3 to 5. CFVR decreases with age but in selected groups of patients such as young healthy athletes may exceed 5 [23]. The values <2 confirm the physiological significance

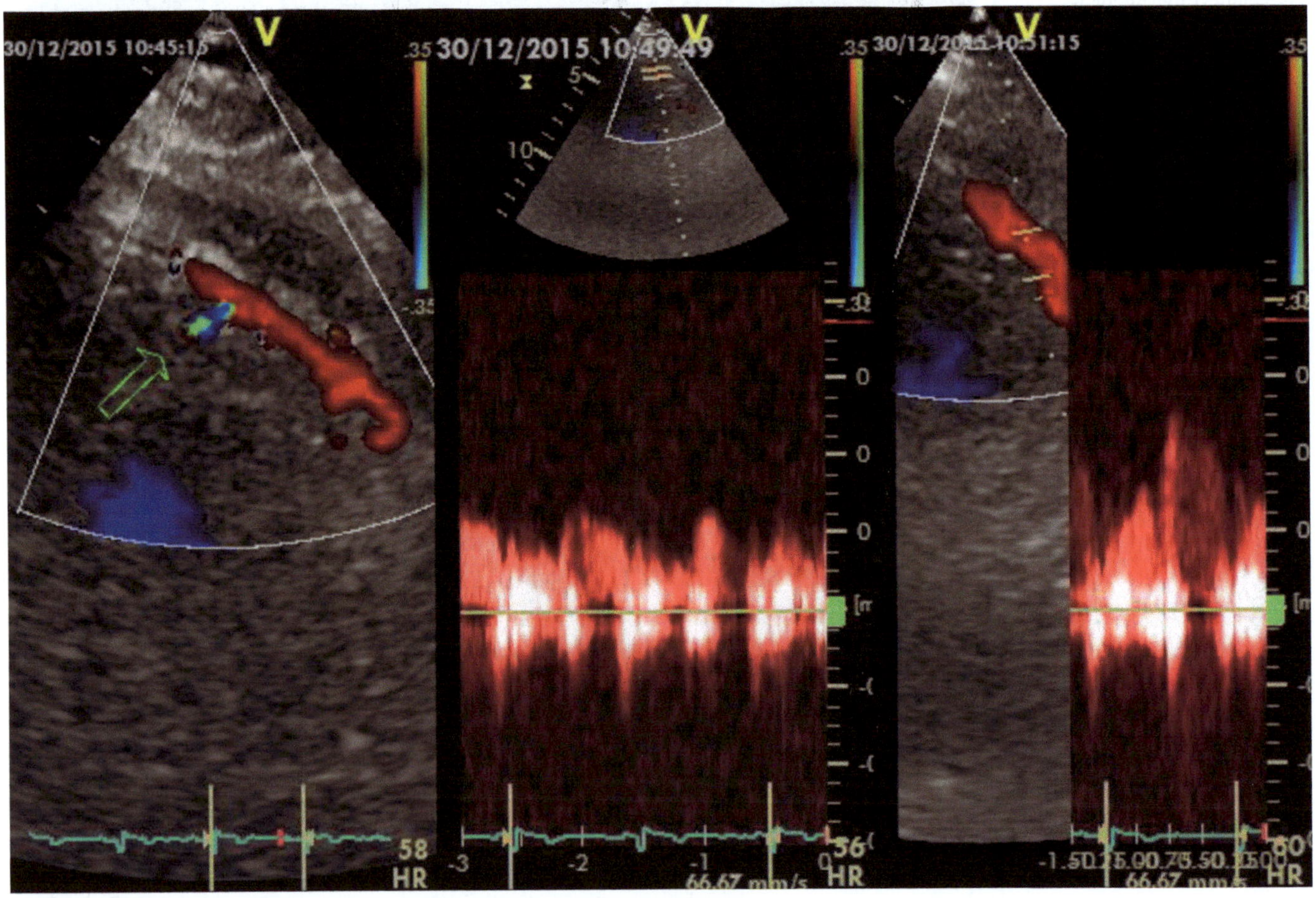

Fig. 26.7 Coronary flow velocity reserve (CFR) in distal left anterior descending artery with invasive fractional flow reserve 0.76. Acceleration of flow from 27 to 50 cm/s at adenosine challenge corresponds with abnormally low CFR = 1.85

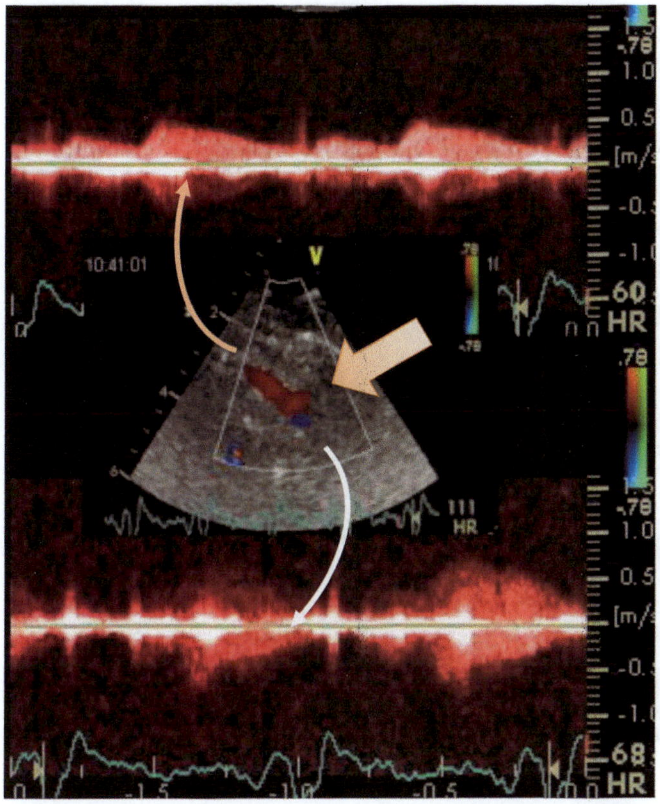

Fig. 26.8 Left internal thoracic artery (short arrow) anastomosed to distal left anterior descending branch of the left coronary artery with flow spreading towards the apex (red, upper panel) and retrograde (blue, lower panel) towards the base of the heart with corresponding diastolic, trapezoid Doppler spectra in opposite directions. Diastolic predominance is suggestive of graft patency

of coronary artery stenosis, usually with luminal narrowing >70% coronary artery stenosis [24, 25] (Fig. 26.7). It must be noted, however, that abnormally low CFVR is not specific for coronary stenosis and can be found in individuals with normal coronary angiography, often with coexisting primary cardiomyopathies, different types of left ventricular hypertrophy and in conditions with microvascular dysfunction such as diabetes, syndrome X, hypercholesterolemia or when blood viscosity is high (policythemia, macroglobulinemia). Importantly, reduced CFR <2 is related do worse prognosis regardless of epicardial coronary disease, e.g. in dilated cardiomyopathy [26].

CFVR is a practical tool when clinical questions regarding the specific anatomical locations arise. The assessment of CFR may help in stratification of intermediate stenoses (40–70%) for invasive treatment. Restenosis after percutaneous coronary stenting can be identified based on CFR <2 for three major coronary arteries, [27] with accuracy comparable to that of 320-row computed tomography [28]. Decreased CFR <2.6 with diastolic deceleration time shortened <840 ms is related to higher incidence of cardiac death, heart failure and stent implantation after heart transplantation [29].

Coronary sinus flow measurements have also been proposed for stress protocol as the marker of total coronary flow return [30]. TEE can be used to record CFR in proximal LAD, (abnormal value <2.0 for significant stenosis, or <1.7 for microvascular dysfunction in diabetes <1.7) [31].

Congenital Abnormalities of the Coronary Arteries

Coronary artery anomalies are present in 1–5.6% patients, discovered by serendipity during workup of angina, arrhythmia, syncope, or myocardial infarction; some variants are common and benign (Fig. 26.9) but others may be related to sudden cardiac death [32] due to compression of abnormally coursing arterial lumen.

Imaging of ostial anomalies is feasible with transthoracic imaging [33] and often definitive with transesophageal imaging [34]. Some coronary anomalies involving sharp angulation or interarterial course of LMCA may have fatal consequences with threatened sudden cardiac death during exercise. Echocardiographic diagnosis of coronary anomalies remains a radiation-free option, allowing real-time assessment of coronary flow and anatomy and is initiated by absence of typical coronary ostia in the left and right sinuses of Valsalva. Retroaortic course, specific for anomalous arteries, is easily defined in TEE and TEE by recently described bleb sign and crossed-aorta sign (Fig. 26.10, Video 26.5) [35, 36]. Echocardiography is also useful in pediatric cardiology for detecting pulmonary artery origins of coronary arteries, with typical flow reversal and extensive collateralization seen in color Doppler as "sparkling" myocardium.

Coronary fistulas, uncommon coronary pathology (congenital or acquired, including iatrogenic [37]) give specific echocardiographic findings of drainage of predominantly diastolic flow into receiving arteries, most commonly right ventricle, right atrium or pulmonary artery. "Pediatric" type wide fistulas with low resistance connections with cardiac

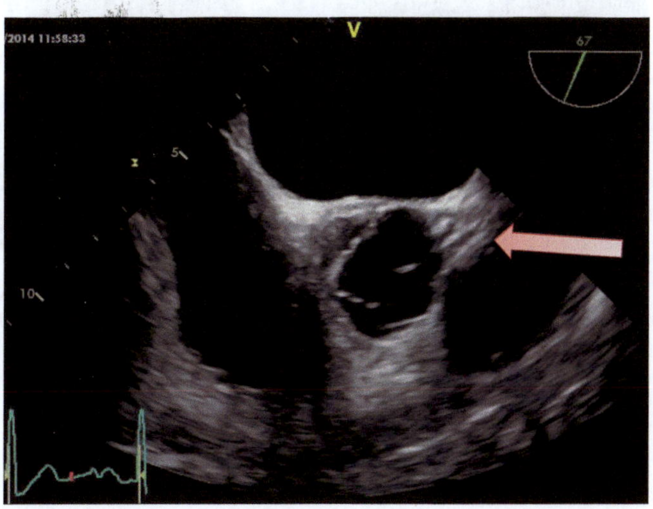

Fig. 26.9 Independent origin of left anterior descending coronary artery (arrow) just below the origin of the circumflex artery—absence of the left main stem seen from high short axis transesophageal view

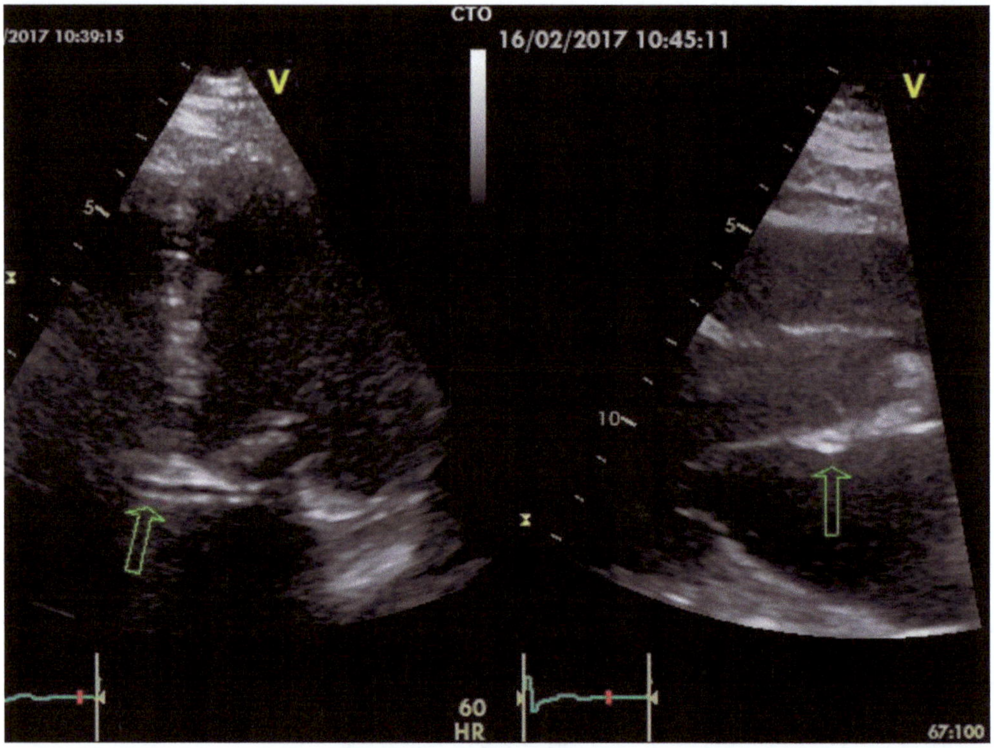

Fig. 26.10 Anomalous circumflex originating from the right sinus of Valsalva with retro-aortic course (arrow) shown between aortic root and the left atrium in modified (caudal tilt) apical four chamber view, left and parasternal long axis view—right

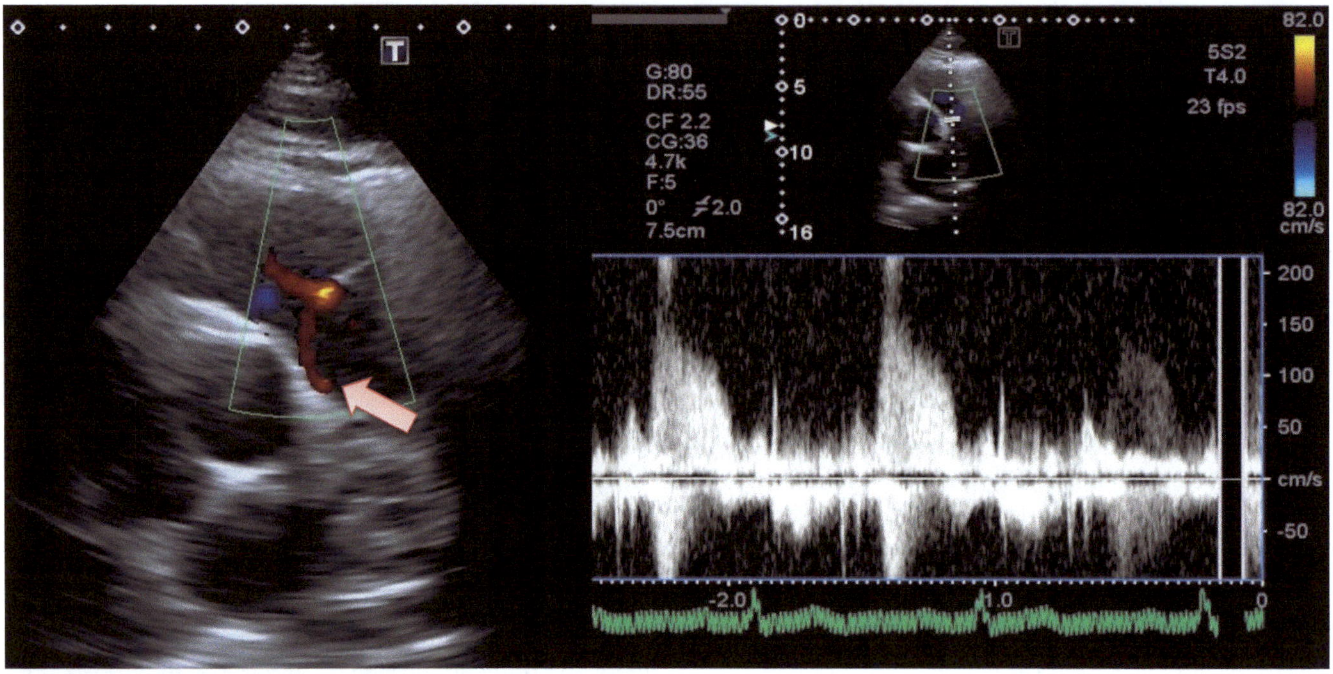

Fig. 26.11 Small fistula (arrow) connecting the left coronary artery with pulmonary trunk, 1 cm above the pulmonary regurgitation (seen as a yellow–red retrograde flow)—imaging from short axis parasternal window

chamber are usually dilated and visible over epicardium—color Doppler TTE and TEE demonstrate marked arterial dilatation and tortuosity with variable cross-sections of flow-filled channels (Fig. 26.11, Video 26.6). Minor fistulous connections usually from LAD to pulmonary trunk accidentally detected in adults by coronary angiography can be discovered in TTE/TEE with typical coronary Doppler flow pattern.

References

1. Kasprzak JD, Drożdż J, Peruga JZ, et al. Definition of flow parameters in proximal nonstenotic coronary arteries using transesophageal Doppler echocardiography. Echocardiography. 2000;17:141–50.
2. Caiati C, Zedda N, Montaldo C, Montisci R, Iliceto S. Contrast-enhanced transthoracic second harmonic echo Doppler with adenosine: a noninvasive, rapid and effective method for coronary flow reserve assessment. J Am Coll Cardiol. 1999;34:122–30.
3. Kiviniemi TO, Saraste M, Koskenvuo JW, et al. Coronary artery diameter can be assessed reliably with transthoracic echocardiography. Am J Physiol Heart Circ Physiol. 2004;286:H1515–20.
4. Krzanowski M, Bodzoń W, Dudek D, et al. Transthoracic harmonic mode contrast enhanced color Doppler echocardiography in detection of restenosis after percutaneous coronary interventions. Prospective evaluation verified by coronary angiography. Eur J Echocardiogr. 2004;5:51–64.
5. Kasprzak JD, Drozdz J, Peruga JZ, et al. Doppler detection of proximal coronary artery stenosis using transesophageal echocardiography. Kardiol Pol. 1999;50:491–500.
6. Vrublevsky AV, Boshchenko AA, Karpov RS. Diagnostics of main coronary artery stenoses and occlusions:multiplane transoesophageal Doppler echocardiographic assessment. Eur J Echocardiogr. 2001;2:170–7.
7. Krzanowski M, Bodzon W, Brzostek T, et al. Value of transthoracic echocardiography for the detection of high-grade coronary artery stenosis. J Am Soc Echocardiogr. 2000;13:1091–9.
8. Voros S, Nanda NC, Samal AK, et al. Transesophageal echocardiography in patients with ischemic stroke accurately detects significant coronary artery stenosis and often changes management. Am Heart J. 2001;142:916–22.
9. Anjaneyulu A, Raghu K, Chandramukhi S, et al. Evaluation of left main coronary stenosis by transthoracic echocardiography. J Am Soc Echocardiogr. 2008;21:855–60.
10. Vegsundvåg J, Holte E, Wiseth R, Hegbom K, Hole T. Transthoracic echocardiography for imaging of the different coronary artery segments: a feasibility study. Cardiovasc Ultrasound. 2009;7:58. https://doi.org/10.1186/1476-7120-7-58.
11. Okayama H, Nishimura K, Saito M, et al. Significance of the distal to proximal coronary flow velocity ratio by transthoracic Doppler echocardiography for diagnosis of proximal left coronary artery stenosis. J Am Soc Echocardiogr. 2008;21:756–60.
12. Hozumi T, Yoshida K, Akasaka T, et al. Value of acceleration flow and the prestenotic to stenotic coronary flow velocity ratio by transthoracic color Doppler echocardiography in noninvasive diagnosis of restenosis after percutaneous transluminal coronary angioplasty. J Am Coll Cardiol. 2000;35(1):164–8.
13. Holte E, Vegsundvåg J, Hegbom K, Hole T, Wiseth R. Transthoracic Doppler for detection of stenoses in the three main coronary arteries by use of stenotic to prestenotic velocity ratio and aliased coronary flow. Eur Heart J Cardiovasc Imaging. 2015;16:1323–30.
14. Alyaneyulu A, Raghu K, Chandramukhi S, Satyajit GM, Arramraja S, Raghavaraju P, Krishnamraju P, Somaraju B. Evaluation of left main coronary artery stenosis by transthoracic echocardiography. J Am Soc Echocardiogr. 2008;21:855–60.
15. Boshchenko AA, Vrublevsky AV, Karpov RS. Transthoracic echocardiography in the detection of chronic total coronary artery occlusion. Eur J Echocardiogr. 2009;10:62–8.
16. Crowley JJ, Shapiro LM. Transthoracic echocardiographic measurement of coronary blood flow and reserve. J Am Soc Echocardiogr. 1997;10:337–43.
17. Vegsundvåg J, Holte E, Wiseth R, Hegbom K, Hole T. Coronary flow velocity reserve in the three main coronary arteries assessed with transthoracic Doppler: a comparative study with quantitative coronary angiography. J Am Soc Echocardiogr. 2011;24:758–67.
18. Caiati C, Montaldo C, Zedda N, Bina A, Iliceto S. New noninvasive method for coronary flow reserve assessment: contrast-enhanced transthoracic second harmonic echo Doppler. Circulation. 1999;99:771–8.
19. Holte E, Vegsundvåg J, Hegbom K, Hole T, Wiseth R. Transthoracic Doppler echocardiography for detection of stenoses in the left coronary artery by use of poststenotic coronary flow profiles: a comparison with quantitative coronary angiography and coronary flow reserve. J Am Soc Echocardiogr. 2013;26:77–85.
20. Katayama M, Yamamuro A, Ueda Y, et al. Coronary flow velocity pattern assessed noninvasively by transthoracic color Doppler echocardiography serves as a predictor of adverse cardiac events and left ventricular remodeling in patients with acute myocardial infarction. J Am Soc Echocardiogr. 2006;19:335–40.
21. Sicari R, Nihoyannopoulos P, Evangelista A, Kasprzak J, Lancellotti P, Poldermans D, Voigt JU, Zamorano JL, on behalf of the European Association of Echocardiography. Stress echocardiography expert consensus statement: European Association of Echocardiography (EAE) (a registered branch of the ESC). Eur J Echocardiogr. 2008;9:415–37.
22. Lethen H, Tries HP, Kersting S, Lambertz H. Validation of noninvasive assessment of coronary flow velocity reserve in the right coronary artery. A comparison of transthoracic echocardiographic results with intracoronary Doppler flow wire measurements. Eur Heart J. 2003;24:1567–75.
23. Hildick-Smith DJ, Johnson PJ, Wisbey CR, et al. Coronary flow reserve is supranormal in endurance athletes: an adenosine transthoracic echocardiographic study. Heart. 2000;84:383–9.
24. Okayama H, Sumimoto T, Hiasa G, et al. Assessment of intermediate stenosis in the left anterior descending coronary artery with contrast-enhanced transthoracic Doppler echocardiography. Coron Artery Dis. 2003;14:247–54.
25. Meimoun P, Benali T, Sayah S, et al. Evaluation of left anterior descending coronary artery stenosis of intermediate severity using transthoracic coronary flow reserve and dobutamine stress echocardiography. J Am Soc Echocardiogr. 2005;18:1233–40.
26. Rigo F, Gherardi S, Galderisi M, et al. The prognostic impact of coronary flow-reserve assessed by Doppler echocardiography in non-ischaemic dilated cardiomyopathy. Eur Heart J. 2006;27:1319–23.
27. Hyodo E, Hirata K, Hirose M, et al. Detection of restenosis after percutaneous coronary intervention in three major coronary arteries by transthoracic Doppler echocardiography. J Am Soc Echocardiogr. 2010;23:553–9.
28. Kakuta K, Dohi K, Yamada T, et al. Comparison of coronary flow velocity reserve measurement by transthoracic Doppler echocardiography with 320-row multidetector computed tomographic coronary angiography in the detection of in-stent restenosis in the three major coronary arteries. Am J Cardiol. 2012;110(1):13–20.
29. Tona F, Caforio AL, Montisci R, et al. Coronary flow velocity pattern and coronary flow reserve by contrast-enhanced transthoracic echocardiography predict long-term outcome in heart transplantation. Circulation. 2006;114(1 Suppl):I49–55.
30. Vrublevsky AV, Boshchenko AA, Karpov RS. Reduced coronary flow reserve in the coronary sinus is a predictor of hemodynamically significant stenoses of the left coronary artery territory. Eur J Echocardiogr. 2004;5:294–303.
31. Nishino M, Hoshida S, Egami Y, et al. Coronary flow reserve by contrast enhanced transesophageal coronary sinus Doppler measurements can evaluate diabetic microvascular dysfunction. Circ J. 2006;70:1415–20.
32. Angelini P. Coronary artery anomalies: an entity in search of an identity. Circulation. 2007;115:1296–305.
33. Labombarda F, Coutance G, Pellissier A, Mery-Alexandre C, Roule V, Maragnes P, et al. Major congenital coronary artery anomalies in

a paediatric and adult population: a prospective echocardiographic study. Eur Heart J Cardiovasc Imaging. 2014;15:761–8.

34. Kasprzak JD, Kratochwil D, Peruga JZ, Drozdz J, Rafalska K, Religa W, Krzemińska-Pakuła M. Coronary anomalies diagnosed with transesophageal echocardiography: complementary clinical value in adults. Int J Card Imaging. 1998;14:89–95.
35. Wierzbowska-Drabik K, Szymczyk K, Kasprzak JD. Anomalous circumflex origin from the right coronary artery forming 'bleb sign' in transoesophageal echocardiography. Eur Heart J Cardiovasc Imaging. 2014;15:932.
36. Wierzbowska-Drabik K, Kasprzak JD, Mrozowska-Peruga E, Peruga JZ. Circumflex origin from right coronary artery—the anomaly that should not be omitted during echocardiography—"crossed aorta" and "bleb sign" presentation after stents implantation. Echocardiography. 2016;33:659–60.
37. Lipiec P, Peruga JZ, Krzemińska-Pakula M, Foryś J, Drozdz J, Kasprzak JD. Right coronary artery-to-right ventricle fistula complicating percutaneous transluminal angioplasty: case report and review of the literature. J Am Soc Echocardiogr. 2004;17(3):280.

Stress Echocardiography

27

Anita Sadeghpour and Azin Alizadehasl

Abstract

Stress echocardiography is done with exercise, administration of a pharmacologic agent, even mental stress, or also transesophageal atrial pacing. The exercise protocol covers a treadmill exercise examination, with fast post-exercise echocardiographic images or upright or supine bicycle echocardiographic images achieved at the peak of exercise. Although exercise-induced regional wall motion abnormality (RWMA) due to ischemia often lasts for a few minutes after the end of the exercise, immediate post-exercise images might be compared with the baseline pre-exercise images to distinguish exercise-induced RWMA. Thus, treadmill exercise with echocardiographic images obtained immediately after the end of exercise is the form of exercise echocardiography used most often to distinguish myocardial ischemia (coronary artery disease).

Vasodilator stress with dipyridamole and pacing stress—via a preexisting permanent pacemaker or a transesophageal pacing catheter—are also likely but less widely used. The examination end point is completed by exercise-limiting symptoms or the completion of the protocol (attainment of at least 85% of the age-predicted maximal heart rate).

Keywords

Stress echocardiography · Regional wall motion abnormality (RWMA) · Exercise test in treadmill · Dobutamine stress echocardiography (DSE) · Myocardial viability · Low-flow · Low-gradient AS

A. Sadeghpour, MD, FACC, FASE
Professor of Cardiology, Echocardiography Research Center, Rajaie Cardiovascular Medical and Research Center, Iran University of Medical Science, Tehran, Iran

A. Alizadehasl, MD, FACC, FASE (✉)
Associate Professor of Cardiology, Echocardiologist, Echocardiography and Cardiogenetic Research Centers, Cardio-Oncology Department, Rajaie Cardiovascular Medical and Research Center, Tehran, Iran

Abbreviations

AVA	Aortic valve area
DSE	Dobutamine stress echocardiography
ECG	Electrocardiography
HAPE	High altitude pulmonary edema
HCM	Hypertrophic cardiomyopathy
IVG	Intra-ventricular gradients
MPG	Mean pressure gradient
PAH	Pulmonary artery hypertension
PH	Pulmonary hypertension
PPM	Prosthesis/Patient mismatch
PV	Prosthetic valve
RWM	Regional wall motion
RWMA	Regional wall motion abnormality
SE	Stress echocardiography
SPAP	Systolic pulmonary artery pressure
SV	Stroke volume
VHD	Valvular heart disease

Basic of Stress Echocardiography (SE)

- Role of stress echocardiography as a valid noninvasive, safe method for detection of Coronary artery disease and viability has been documented since 1990.
- SE has an established role in evaluation of ischemic and non ischemic heart disease including diastolic heart failure, valvular heart disease, congenital heart disease and heart transplantation.
- Indeed, SE is a combination of stress test (including exercise stress test or pharmacological stress test) and echocardiography with ability to assess morphologic and physiologic response of the cardiovascular system to the stress.
- The basic principle of SE is inducing ischemia and comparing the acquired images at rest and peak of stress test.
- Based on the myocardial ischemia cascade, diastolic and systolic dysfunction and RWMA occurs before symptom

A. Sadeghpour, A. Alizadehasl (eds.), *Case-Based Textbook of Echocardiography*,
https://doi.org/10.1007/978-3-319-67691-3_27

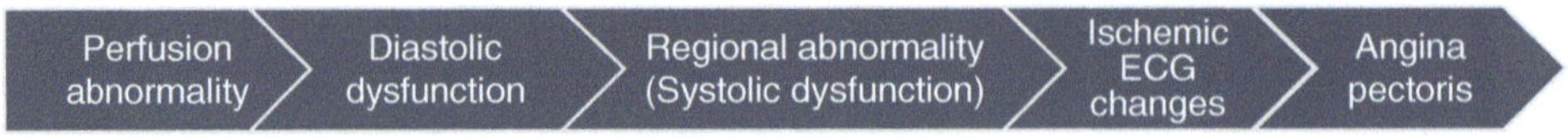

Fig. 27.1 The Ischemia cascade showing the time sequence events of the myocardial ischemia

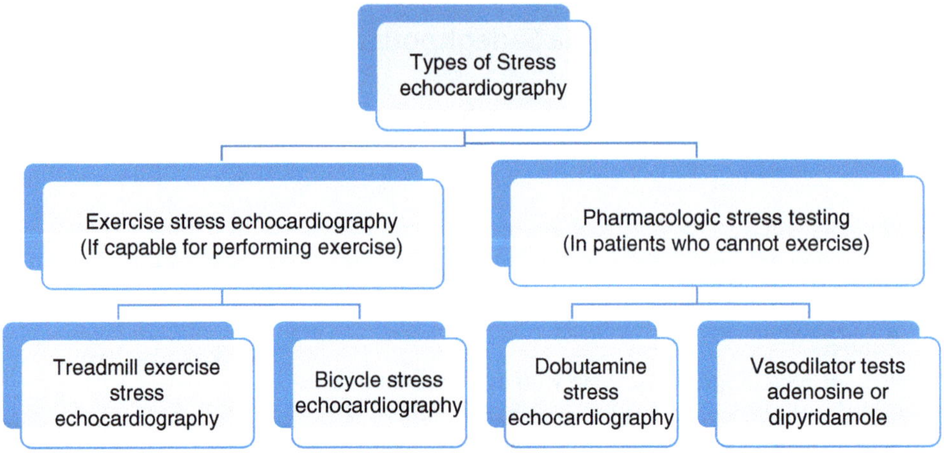

Fig. 27.2 Types of Stress echocardiography

or ECG changes, that means, angina pectoris, is the last event in this cascade (Fig. 27.1).

- Contrast agents can be used in patients with suboptimal image quality to enhance LV endocardium visualization and better assessment of the segmental LV wall motion abnormality.

The goal of stress echocardiography is to maximize myocardial oxygen demand and induce myocardial ischemia [1–3] (Fig. 27.2).

Types of Stress Echocardiography:

Exercise Stress Echocardiography

- Treadmill Exercise Stress Echocardiography with Bruce protocol is the most common form of SE in the US.
- The modified Bruce protocol that consists of additional two less intensity stages at the beginning of the Bruce protocol and the Naughton protocol consists of 2-min stages can be used for old age or sedentary patients.

Exercise stress echocardiography has the advantages of providing more information about the patients' functional capacity, symptoms, heart rate response to exercise and patients prognosis.

The Exercise Stress Echocardiography is a very safe imaging modality with the advantages of interpreting both exercise stress test and wall motion abnormalities in patients with significant coronary artery stenosis (luminal diameter <50% that means 75% cross-sectional stenosis).

Moreover, normal Heart Rate Recovery can be assessed by exercise echocardiography as the recovery of the heart rate in the first minute to be ≥18 beats/min.

Treadmill or bicycle exercise stress test mainly increase the cardiac work by increasing the heart rate, systolic blood pressure and inotropic state. It is suggested to report the rate-pressure product, or double-product which is a combination of Heart rate and blood pressure. Exercise stress test induce higher rate-pressure product >25,000 than dobutamine stress test which is about 20,000.

After an explanation and preparation for the procedure a 12-lead electrocardiogram is obtained. Bruce protocol is usually performed. In the assessment of non-coronary artery disease can be used for easier evaluation of Doppler parameters.

Intravenous cannula can be place in high risk patients. Table 27.1 shows more details regarding performing exercise stress echocardiography.

Systolic blood pressure (Sys BP) should rise to less than 190 mmHg in women and 210 mm in men. Exaggerated systolic blood pressure response has been define as Sys BP >200 mmHg.

Table 27.1 Exercise echocardiography

Baseline blood pressure, heart rate, and ECG
Baseline echocardiography resting images are stored.
Exercise examination based on to the requirements of the case and clinician:
Treadmill exercise, followed by immediate post-exercise echocardiogram, if possible within 90 s
Bicycle or arm ergometer; images are obtained at low and peak levels of exercise; these images are digitized and stored
Display of baseline and peak exercise (in bicycle) or post-exercise images (in treadmill) side by side using continuous cine loop
Review of all echocardiographic images
Elucidation of the study including other clinical variables (workload, ECG changes, heart rate, and blood pressure response)
End points:
Severe symptoms (chest pain or dyspnea)
Severe ischemia (ST-segment depression ≥2 mm)
Complex ectopy or ventricular tachycardia
Hypertensive blood pressure response 220–250 mm Hg systolic, ≥110–150 mm Hgdiastolic)
Hypotension (>20 mmHg reduction compared with the previous stage) Development of severe pulmonary hypertension as the PAP reaches ≥60 mm Hg
Target heart rate

By convention, functional capacity has been classified as the:

Poor	<5 METs
Fair	5–8 METs
Good	9–11 METs
Excellent	≥12 METs

The test is considered to be positive for myocardial ischemia when ST-segment depression occurs, with a horizontal or down sloping displacement ≥1 mm measured 0.08 s after the J point. The ECG exercise treadmill test is considered inconclusive when there are baseline ST-T changes (left bundle branch block, digitalis effect, LV hypertrophy) or when the patient does not reach 85% of the theoretical maximum age-adjusted heart rate. The exam is negative for myocardial ischemia when the patient's heart rate exceeds 85% of the theoretical maximum age-adjusted heart rate without the previously mentioned changes [4–6].

Imaging protocols vary based on the stress modality. In treadmill exercise stress, after a brief transthoracic echocardiography, the images should be obtain. Imaging protocol consists of parasternal long axis and short-axis, apical four-chamber, two-chamber, and three-chamber views at rest, and after (or during) exercise stress test and in recovery.

The hallmark of ischemia is regional wall motion abnormality by means of reduced systolic excursion and wall thickening. Dilation of LV cavity and decrease in ejection fraction during stress echocardiography strongly suggest left main or multivessel coronary artery disease.

Bicycle protocols consists of 1- or 2-min stages, with increasing 15–25 W per stage till the endpoints of the test. Atropin is useful when 85% of the maximal predicted heart rate is not achieved.

Indication

The indication for stress echocardiography consists of the: diagnosis of coronary artery disease (CAD), evaluation of patients at risk for CAD before noncardiac surgery and risk stratification. The presence of the left bundle branch block or nondiagnostic ECG strengthen the indication for a performing stress echocardiography.

Contraindication are similar to those associated with exercise stress test and poor image quality.

Dobutamine Stress Echocardiography (DSE)

Cases typically fast for 4 h prior to the test. All negative chronotropic agents and nitrates should be held 8–12 h before DSE, unless the goal is to assess the efficacy of the anti-ischemic medical regimen, as described above. The testing should be performed in an accredited stress echocardiography laboratory equipped with appropriate echocardiographic equipment and medications. ASE quality guidelines mandate that the cardiac ultrasound devices have the ability to trigger image acquisition based on the ECG and also suggest that the laboratory employ machines with split-screen and quadruple-screen display to facilitate simultaneous comparison from rest to peak to post-stress images.

Table 27.2 Dobutamine stress echocardiography (DSE)

Baseline heart rate, blood pressure, and ECG
Baseline echocardiogram-resting images are stored
Begin dobutamine infusion at 5 μg/kg/min.
Increase dobutamine infusion every 3 min to 10, 20, 30, and 40 μg/kg/min or until the case develops symptoms, side effects, or new RWMA
In cases taking β-blockers, the heart rate response to dobutamine might not be satisfactory; if the heart rate is not within 85% of the target rate with 40 μg/km/min of dobutamine, atropine (0.2–1.0 mg intravenously) is given to increase the heart rate
Store the echocardiographic images during a low dose (5 or 10 μg/kg/min), pre-peak, and peak (or after atropine); compare the images in a quad-screen format. RWMA is compared with that of the preceding level as well as the baseline RWMA
If a case develops symptoms or persistent tachycardia after the termination of dobutamine, esmolol (0.5–1.0 mg/kg intravenously) often terminates the side-effects of dobutamine
End points:
–Target heart rate (85% of the age-predicted maximal heart rate or, if soon after myocardial infarction, 70% of the age-predicted maximal heart rate)
–Development of new RWMA of at least moderate severity
–Peak dose
–Ventricular tachycardia or sustained supraventricular tachycardia
–Severe hypertension (systolic blood pressure >220–250 mmHg or diastolic blood pressure ≥110–150 mmHg)
–Substantial decrease in the systolic blood pressure (A decrease of 20 mmHg from the previous level of infusion might be used as a guideline for terminating the examination, but the amount depends on the baseline blood pressure and the judgment of the person monitoring the examination.)
–Intolerable symptoms

RWMA Regional wall motion abnormality

Dobutamine is an adrenergic agonist, traditionally used in intensive care units or in end-stage heart failure. Dobutamine acts on β1-adrenergic receptors to increase cardiac contractility and heart rate, and on β2-adrenergic receptors to cause peripheral vasodilatation. It also has a mild effect on α1-adrenergic receptors, which causes vasoconstriction, but this effect is outweighed by the more potent β2-mediated vasodilatation. The onset of action of dobutamine is 1–2 min and the plasma half-life is approximately 2 min [5–7].

Contraindications to DSE

Contraindications to DSE are related to the administration of dobutamine, and include ventricular arrhythmias, recent myocardial infarction (within 3 days), unstable angina, significant LV outflow obstruction (for example, resting peak late systolic pressure gradient ≥30 mmHg), aortic dissection, and severe (resting systolic blood pressure > 180 mmHg or diastolic blood pressure > 100 mmHg) or symptomatic hypertension. The practitioner should also be cognizant of other cardiovascular pathologies that might be adversely affected by increases in heart rate and/or blood pressure, including aortic aneurysms, carotid disease, heart failure and cardiomyopathy,

Table 27.3 Interpretation by regional wall motion (RWM) analysis

Rest	Stress	Interpretation
Normal RWM and contractility	Hyperdynamic	Normal
Normal RWM	New RWM abnormality or lack of hyperdynamic RWM	Ischemia
RWM abnormality	Worsening (hypokinesis →akinesis) (akinesis →dyskinesis)	Ischemia
RWM abnormality	Unchanged	Infarct
Akinetic RWM	Improved to hypokinetic or to normal WM, bi-phasic response	Viable myocardium

Table 27.4 Ischemic features of severe ischemia

	Exercise	Dobutamine
WMA	Multiple	Multiple
LV cavity	Dilate	Often not dilated
LVEF	Decrease	Might not decrease
ST-segment depression	Common	Uncommon
Hypotension	Specific	Nonspecific

LV LV; *LVEF* LV ejection fraction; *WMA* wall motion abnormality

intracranial aneurysms, and history of stroke or transient ischemic attack. Even in the presence of known abdominal aortic aneurysms (≥4 cm) and intracranial aneurysms, DSE appears to be a safe modality for cardiac risk stratification, although the practitioner might reasonably substitute a vasodilator stress modality in such cases [4, 5] (Table 27.2).

If the heart rate target is not achieved with dobutamine infusion alone, atropine (maximum total dose 2 mg, typically divided into four 0.5 mg doses) can be added, which increases the sensitivity of stress echocardiography in cases with single-vessel disease or who are on chronic beta-blockers. Some practitioners also consider a trial of an increased dose of dobutamine (50 μg/kg/min) if the patient is very close to achieving the 85% maximal predicted heart rate target. In some laboratories, gentle hand, arm, or leg exercises are also used for chronotropic augmentation when close to target heart rate, provided these motions do not impair the echocardiography examination, electrocardiography (ECG) tracings, or blood pressure monitoring, and the patient is able to perform them.

The objective in performing a stress echocardiography is first to induce a supply-demand imbalance in the heart in the presence of a flow limiting coronary lesion which results in a new RWMA and second to evaluate the response of dysfunctional myocardium at rest to inotropic stress. Table 27.3 shows the many possibilities that we would encounter in stress echocardiography and how we interpret every situation. Table 27.4 shows features that are demonstrative of severe ischemia in stres echocardiography.

The sensitivity of DSE for detection of myocardial ischemia might be reduced by long-term beta-blockers, calcium channel blockers, and nitrates. But, when a patient chronically takes one of these anti-ischemic drugs, a positive test for ischemia is more significant, although a negative test might be less helpful. Many practitioners choose to test a patient with known CAD on their anti-ischemic regimen to investigate for the presence of ischemia and assess whether anti-ischemic medical therapy has been optimized [4].

Risk Stratification with Stress Echocardiography

Stress echocardiography has a sensitivity and specificity 87% and 84%. Although, the sensitivity of detecting single-vessel seems to be lower but still have an acceptable range of 70% to 85%. Numerous studies have demonstrated that in cases who complete normal exercise or pharmacologic stress echocardiograms (reaching good exercise capacity and the target heart rate), the risk for cardiac events is very low and at or close to that of a "normal" population (<1% per year for exercise and <2% per year for pharmacologic examinations). In cases with suspected or known coronary artery disease, both the extent of resting WMA and the extent of ischemia—specifically quantified by the change in the wall motion score index, 4 or more LV wall segments affected, and/or no change or decrease in exercise LV ejection fraction—correlate with a fourfold or greater risk for cardiac death or myocardial infarction [4–6, 8, 9].

Absolute Indications for Terminating Stress Echocardiography

Absolute indications to terminate the examination early include moderate to severe angina, ST-segment elevation, sustained ventricular tachycardia, near syncope or signs of poor perfusion, a drop in systolic blood pressure of more than 10 mmHg from baseline when accompanied by any other evidence of ischemia, and the patient's request to stop (intolerable symptoms). Relative indications to stop early include a hypertensive response (systolic blood pressure >250 mmHg and/or diastolic blood pressure >115 mmHg). The risks correlated with exercise echocardiography or dobutamine stress echocardiography are very low. In the largest survey to date, the overall rate of life-threatening events was 1 per every 1000 examinations (0.015% for exercise and 0.18% for dobutamine). The most frequent complications were acute myocardial infarction or ventricular tachycardia or ventricular fibrillation [4, 5, 8, 10].

Study of Myocardial Viability

Akinetic wall segments seen on echocardiography do not always indicate scarred or irreversibly dysfunctional myocardium. Cause myocardial contractility ceases when 20% or more of the transmural thickness is involved by ischemia or infarction, a considerable amount of the myocardium might still be alive or viable even when no mechanical contractility is imaged. Thus, it is significant to define whether akinetic myocardium is irreversible or is a sign of stunned or hibernating myocardium with the potential for functional recovery.

- Stunned myocardium: Reversible RWMA after reperfusion of transient coronary artery occlusion. Reperfusion might happen spontaneously or after thrombolytic therapy or percutaneous coronary angioplasty. Recovery of WMA might require days to weeks.
- Hibernating myocardium: Chronic depressed myocardial function following chronic myocardial ischemia. Recovery of the myocardial function after coronary revascularization is an example [4, 8, 11].

At low doses of dobutamine, hibernating myocardium will augment due to inotropic stimulation (e.g., a manifestation of contractile reserve). At progressively higher doses of dobutamine, the hibernating segment might exhibit abnormal wall motion due to the compromised coronary blood flow being insufficient to meet the increased metabolic demands. This pattern of wall motion is termed the "biphasic" response, and it appears to be most predictive of post-revascularization viability (as compared with patterns of "uniphasic" worsening or sustained improvement in wall motion). ASE guidelines recommend that viability assessment at a minimum includes improvement in at least two echocardiographic LV segments.

Myocardial viability identified with stress echocardiography is associated with improved survival after revascularization in cases with CAD and ischemic cardiomyopathy. Specifically in cases with ischemic cardiomyopathy, DSE is helpful in identifying cases most likely to have improved survival by undergoing percutaneous revascularization or coronary artery bypass grafting. For cases with stable CAD, the biphasic response on DSE is useful in predicting ultimate post-revascularization LV recovery [4, 7, 9, 10] (Fig. 27.2).

Stress Echocardiography in Diastolic Dysfunction

In conjunction with cardiopulmonary examination, stress echocardiography might aid in rooting out the reason for dyspnea and fatigue and in recognizing diastolic dysfunction. Delayed diastolic relaxation, as measured by strain and strain rate imaging, might also be a more sensitive and persistent indicator of exercise-induced ischemia than wall thickening is. With the advent of real-time 3D and 4D imaging, automatic endocardial border tracking, and volumetric imaging, there is now the capability to capture images of LV systolic and diastolic functions concurrently at peak exercise, thus potentially improving the sensitivity, accuracy, and reproducibility of this examination for ischemia [4, 8].

Exercise-induced changes in E/e allow recognition of impaired LV diastolic function reserve and the resulting increase in LV filling pressures in cases with dyspnea and suspected heart failure with preserved LVEF. Exercise Doppler echocardiography is helpful in the assessment of the symptomatic patient with normal or equivocal diastolic function during resting images [5, 12, 13].

Stress Echocardiography in Valvular Heart Disease (Fig. 27.3)

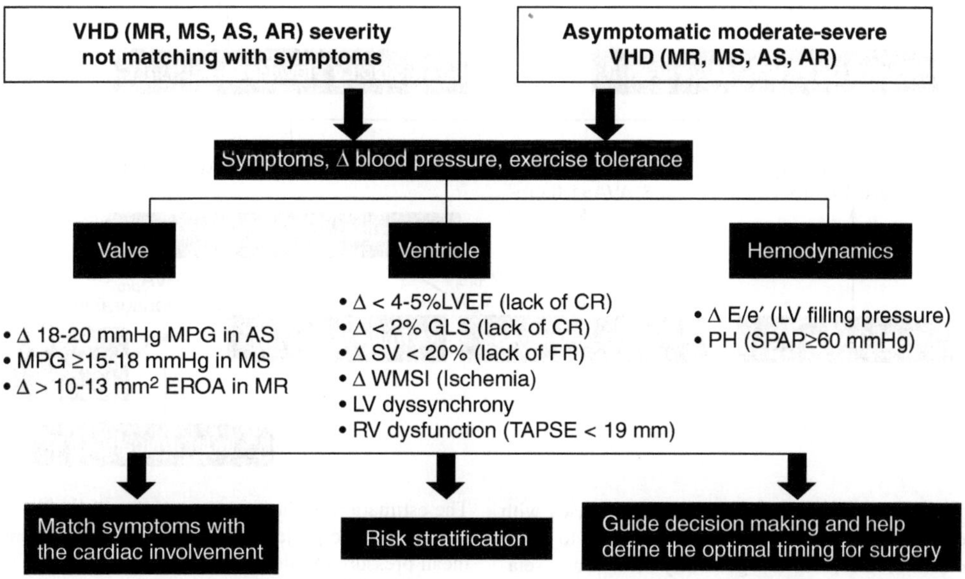

Fig. 27.3 Usefulness of exercise SE in cases with valvular heart disease (VHD). The three components of VHD consequences are examined allowing individual risk stratification. Δ changes from rest to peak exercise, *AR* aortic regurgitation, *AS* aortic stenosis, *GLS* global longitudinal strain, *LVEF* LV ejection fraction, *MPG* mean pressure gradient, *MR* mitral regurgitation, *MS* mitral stenosis, *RV* right ventricle, *PH* systolic pulmonary hypertension, *SPAP* systolic pulmonary artery pressure, *TAPSE* tricuspid annulus plane systolic excursion, *WMSI* wall motion score index. Modifide figure from Patrizio Lancellotti, Patricia A. Pellikka, Werner Budts, Farooq A. Chaudhry, et al. The clinical use of stress echocardiography in non-ischaemic heart disease: recommendations from the European Association of Cardiovascular Imaging and the American Society of Echocardiography. J Am Soc Echocardiogr 2017;30:101–38

Stress Echocardiography in Aortic Stenosis and Low-Flow, Low-Gradient AS

Resting echocardiography might lead to conflicting interpretations of the degree of aortic stenosis in cases with heavily calcified valves and low LV ejection fractions cause leaflet excursion and both the LV outflow tract and aortic gradients are reduced simply by the low forward flow. In cases with "low-gradient, low-output aortic stenosis" and LV dysfunction (defined as a calculated aortic valve area by Doppler <1.0 cm², mean trans-aortic gradient <30–40 mmHg, and LV ejection fraction <50%), dobutamine stress echocardiography might be used to assess both the true severity of aortic stenosis and the amount of the LV contractile reserve. (See also the section on aortic stenosis.) In this examination, dobutamine is infused in graded doses from 5 to 20 μg/kg/min, typically for longer stages than those used for ischemia examination, and spectral Doppler of the LV outflow tract and continuous-wave Doppler across the aortic valve are performed. Stroke volume is calculated from the velocity time integral of the LV outflow tract. An increase of 20% or greater in the stroke volume is indicative of important contractile reserve. The examination will be uninterpretable if no augmentation of the LV function takes place (no contractile reserve). The aortic valve area is calculated at both baseline and with dobutamine. In true aortic stenosis, the ratio of LV outflow tract to aortic velocity time integral will decrease, whereas in "pseudo-severe" or "functional" aortic stenosis, the LV outflow tract and aortic valve gradients change relatively little, and the calculated valve area remains the same or increases as the leaflets open more. Cases with true severe aortic stenosis commonly benefit from aortic valve replacement; nonetheless, if contractile reserve is absent and/or concomitant coronary artery disease is present, operative mortality is high [7, 9, 10, 12].

In classical low-flow, low-gradient AS with reduced LVEF, a low-dose dobutamine SE is recommended to: (1) assess LV flow reserve, which is helpful for surgical risk stratification and (2) differentiate true- from pseudo-severe AS, which is key for guiding the decision to perform AVR. In paradoxical low-flow, low-gradient AS with preserved LVEF, exercise or dobutamine SE might also be used to differentiate true- from pseudo-severe AS [4, 12] (Fig. 27.4).

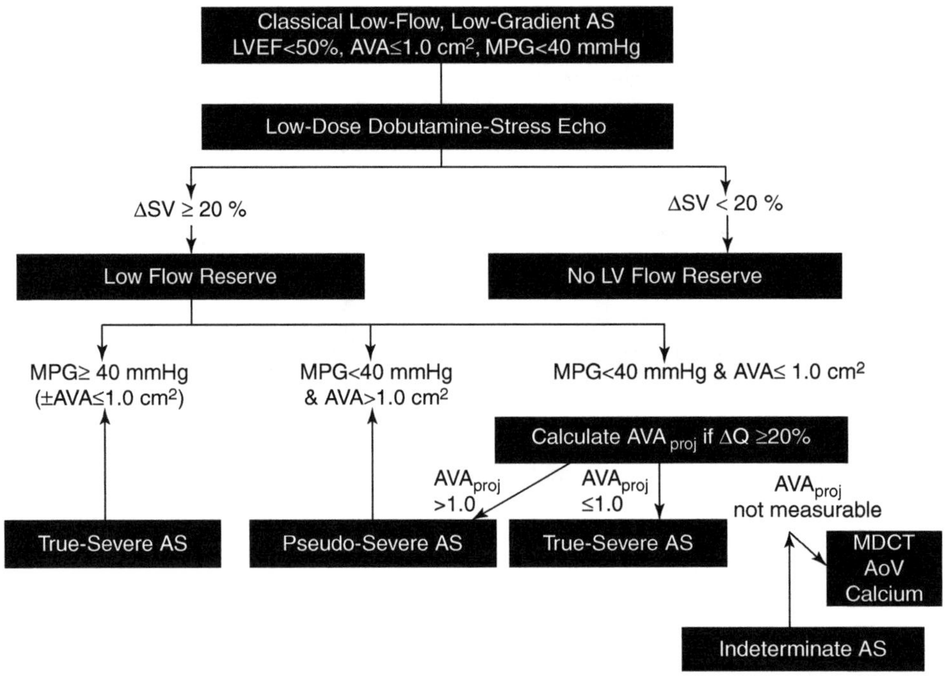

Fig. 27.4 Interpretation of the dobutamine SE results in cases with low-flow, low-gradient AS, and reduced LVEF. The first step is to determine the presence of flow reserve, which is generally defined as a relative increase in stroke volume (SV) >20%. If there is flow reserve, the peak effective aortic valve area (AVA) remains <1 cm² and the mean pressure gradient (MPG) exceeds 40 mmHg, the stenosis is considered severe. If there is no flow reserve, it is difficult to define the stenosis severity. In this case, the use of projected AVA or the evaluation of calcium score by computed tomography (MDCT) should be considered. The estimation of the projected AVA may not be reliable when the ΔQ is <20%. If the projected AVA is <1 cm², the stenosis is severe. MPG, mean pressure gradient; Q, flow rate; SV, stroke volume. Modified figure from: Patrizio Lancellotti, Patricia A. Pellikka, Werner Budts, Farooq A. Chaudhry, et al. The clinical use of stress echocardiography in non-ischaemic heart disease: recommendations from the European Association of Cardiovascular Imaging and the American Society of Echocardiography. J Am Soc Echocardiogr 2017;30:101–38

Stress Echocardiography in Mitral Stenosis

Cases with rheumatic or calcific mitral stenosis might have severe exertional symptoms despite relatively modest gradients on the resting echocardiogram. Conversely, sedentary cases with severe mitral stenosis might be relatively asymptomatic cause they are inactive. Valve gradients are notoriously dependent on the flow rate and the heart rate. Stress echocardiography might define the true exercise capacity and quantitate the degree of valvular stenosis and regurgitation. SE is indicated to assess the hemodynamic significance of MS, which if severe, might account for symptoms. MS is diagnosed as severe if the mean gradient is >15 mmHg on exertion or >18 mmHg during dobutamine infusion. An systolic pulmonary artery pressure (SPAP) is >60 mmHg on exertion is another marker of hemodynamically significant MS.

Exercise echo provides concomitant MV gradient and SPAP assessment. Early increase in SPAP, at low-level exercise, should be looked for since it is correlated with higher rate of exercise-induced symptoms in asymptomatic cases with MV area about 1.5 cm^2. Dobutamine SE can be used to assess MV gradients during stress if the patient cannot exercise, but it is not recommended for assessment of SPAP. MV surgery must also be considered if severe mitral regurgitation happens with stress. If symptoms and systolic pulmonary arterial pressure increase significantly while the transmitral gradients remain low, a pulmonary reason must be sought [4, 5, 8, 14–16].

Stress Echocardiography in Mitral Regurgitation

In cases with mitral regurgitation, stress echocardiography might be instrumental in revealing acute reversible ischemic mitral regurgitation caused by inferior wall ischemia. This would typically be allied to stress-induced inferior WMA and improvement in both abnormalities in the recovery phase. In chronic severe mitral regurgitation, even if the LV ejection fraction is preserved, demonstration of a rise in the systolic pulmonary arterial pressure to higher than 60 mmHg with exercise and reduced LV contractile reserve are reasonable indications for MV surgery [4–6, 8].

Exercise SE provides information about disease severity and individual outcome in MR. MR severity, SPAP, and left and right ventricular contractile reserve should be evaluated according to the clinical context. An increase by 1 grade in MR (from moderate-to severe MR), an SPAP ≥60 mmHg, and a lack of contractile reserve (<5% increase in EF or <2% increment in global longitudinal strain) are markers of poor prognosis [4, 14, 15].

Hypertensive Response to Exercise

Cases with a hypertensive response at stress echocardiography (typically systolic blood pressure >220 mmHg) have a higher false positive rate of detection of wall motion abnormalities, i.e., 22% compared with 12% for those without a hypertensive response to stress echocardiography. In these cases, alternative stress modalities should be considered for subsequent testing (e.g., adenosine) or earlier administration of atropine in the protocol might be considered [4, 5, 8, 12, 13, 17].

Stress Echocardiography in Hypertrophic Cardiomyopathy

Stress echocardiography might be tailored in other conditions. In cases with hypertrophic cardiomyopathy, exercise might bring out latent gradients and is also used to both monitor response to therapy and also consider symptoms such as syncope [4, 8, 10, 11].

LV outflow tract obstruction is the major cause of symptoms in hypertrophic cardiomyopathy (HCM) and it has been associated to worse prognosis. It is present in one-third of the cases at rest while in the remaining two-thirds, it can be provoked, nevertheless the best stress protocol is still yet to be defined. In many centers, exercise echocardiography with image acquisition during treadmill exercise (considered to reflect exercise during daily activities) is commonly used in the valuation of cases with HCM, enabling assessment of outflow gradient during physiologic exercise. In these cases LVOT gradients increased in from supine to orthostatic position, and continued to augment at peak exercise, but after exercise the gradient decreased rapidly when measured in left lateral decubitus; the assessment of intra-ventricular gradient in recovery period in supine position probably does not reflect changes occurring immediately after effort or the pathophysiology of this condition.

Exercise SE is an important and useful tool for valuation of symptoms and monitoring the response to therapy in cases with HCM. Dynamic LVOTO (>50 mmHg) can be easily assessed. Abnormal blood pressure response to exercise, blunted contractile (systolic) and diastolic reserve, and worsened MR are associated with poor exercise capacity and outcome. SE is not indicated when a gradient >50 mmHg is present at rest or with Valsalva manoeuvre [4, 12, 16, 18, 19].

Stress Echocardiography in Cases with Prosthetic Valves

As most prosthetic heart valves are innately and inherently stenotic, the effective orifice area (EOA) of a prosthetic valve (PV) is often small in relation to the patient's body size—a main phenomenon recognized as prosthesis/patient mismatch

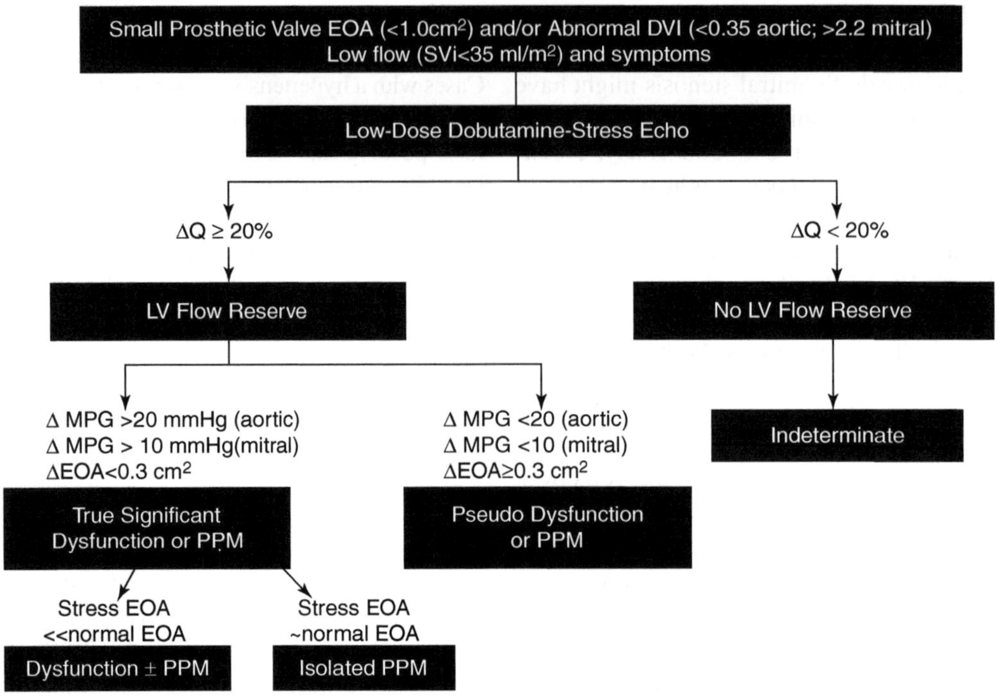

Fig. 27.5 Valuation of aortic/mitral prosthetic valves function in cases with low flow. Dobutamine SE is used to distinguish true significant dysfunction or patient–prosthesis mismatch (PPM) vs. pseudo-severe dysfunction or PPM vs. indeterminate valve function. Δ difference peak-rest, *EOA* effective orifice area, *MPG* mean pressure gradient, *Q* flow rate. Modified figure from: Patrizio Lancellotti, Patricia A. Pellikka, Werner Budts, Farooq A. Chaudhry, et al. The clinical use of stress echocardiography in non-ischaemic heart disease: recommendations from the European Association of Cardiovascular Imaging and the American Society of Echocardiography. J Am Soc Echocardiogr 2017;30:101–38

(PPM). In the aortic valve, PPM is defined as moderate when the indexed EOA is equal to or less than 0.85 cm^2/m^2 and considered severe when it is equal to or less than 0.65 cm^2/m^2 [8]. In the MV, the cutoff points are 1.2 and 0.9 cm^2/m^2, correspondingly. Mainly, PPM has been linked to suboptimal symptomatic improvement, weakened exercise capacity, pulmonary artery hypertension, incomplete regress of LV hypertrophy, high heart events, and even the mortality rate after valve replacement. Based on to literature, PPM is the most common reason for a high trans-prosthetic gradient. Nevertheless, it is essential to distinguish this state from other acquired PV stenoses, which might result from important leaflet calcification of bioprostheses and pannus overgrowth or also thrombus creation on mechanical prosthetic valves.

The presence of a high mean trans-prosthetic gradient (increase of 15–20 mmHg for an aortic PV and 5–7 mmHg for a mitral PV) with/without symptoms requires quick further assessment. Specially, it is essential to determine that the high gradient is due to PPM, a real intrinsic stenosis of the PV, or a localized high gradient (a phenomenon that happens only in bileaflet mechanical PVs). Often, an unusually high jet velocity due to a localized gradient might indeed be documented by continuous-wave Doppler through the small central and slit-like orifice of the bileaflet mechanical PV. This phenomenon results in an abnormally low EOA and a high gradient, mimicking the signs of real intrinsic prosthetic dysfunction.

Cause abnormally and normally functioning PVs might yield similar estimated resting gradients by transthoracic echocardiography, it might be difficult and hard to differentiate between high gradients due to factitious reasons or PPM. Primarily in these conditions, stress echocardiography might be valuable and beneficial in excluding or proving the hemodynamically significant PV stenosis or PPM, mainly when there is discordance between the prosthesis hemodynamics as assessed by echocardiography in rest and during exercise [4, 8, 10, 11, 14–16] (Fig 27.5).

In cases with aortic or mitral prosthetic valves and mild-to-moderate elevation of the resting transprosthetic gradients, exercise SE is useful to confirm: (1) the presence of significant prosthetic valve stenosis or PPM, (2) the symptomatic status. In cases with aortic or mitral prosthetic valves and LF state with small resting EOA or abnormal Doppler velocity index, low-dose dobutamine SE is useful to differentiate true significant prosthesis dysfunction or PPM vs. pseudo-dysfunction. In symptomatic cases with MV annuloplasty and mild increase in resting transmitral gradients, exercise or dobutamine SE is useful to confirm the presence of functional MS [4, 13, 15].

Stress Echocardiography in Cases Undergoing MV Repair

In cases undergoing surgical management for ischemic mitral regurgitation, a restrictive annuloplasty joint with coronary artery bypass grafting surgery is the most communal management approach. Nonetheless, this practice is related with a moderate rate of reappearance of mitral regurgitation, and restrictive annuloplasty might result in functional mitral stenosis in some cases. In cases with postoperative signs and symptoms of either functional mitral stenosis or residual mitral regurgitation, exercise stress echocardiography might be beneficial to evaluate exercise capacity and symptoms. Additionally, valuation of hemodynamics with stress echocardiography might confer additional important data about the importance of mitral stenosis or/and residual regurgitation [4, 13, 16, 17].

Intra-Ventricular Obstruction Induced by Exercise in Athletes

The development of intra-ventricular gradients (IVG) during exercise is rare, and it usually occurs in association with LV hypertrophy. The development of significant IVG during exercise has been described in athletes but the clinical impact of this observation and the most appropriate exercise technique (upright vs. semi supine) to provoke IVG remains unknown.

SE can be used in athletes if a dynamic obstruction is suspected or if they report symptoms that might be related to the development of an intra-ventricular systolic pressure gradient such as dizziness or syncope. A substantial increase in LVEF in athletes during SE suggests normal LV systolic function [4, 13, 17, 20].

SE in Cases with Pulmonary Hypertension (PH)

The inability to augment PAP with exercise, likely an indirect surrogate of impaired contractile reserve, is associated with worse outcome. Others have shown that conventional RV contractility measures augment less in pulmonary artery hypertension (PAH) compared with control. Sharma and colleagues recently evaluated low-dose dobutamine SE (at incremental doses of 5, 10, 15, and 20 mg/kg/min) in cases with PAH to assess contractile reserve. Cases with PAH had an impaired ability to augment RV contractility. Furthermore, RV contractile reserve correlated with exercise capacity.

Doppler assessment of PAP with stress is feasible with exercise and is suggested as an adjunct in the assessment of cases with dyspnea. In conjunction with PAP assessment, cases undergoing SE for suspected PH should have an assessment of RV function and oxygen saturation. Supine bike or hypoxic Doppler SE might be considered in the valuation of cases at increased risk for PAH and to screen for high altitude pulmonary edema (HAPE) and chronic mountain sickness. While the role of SE in cases with established PH is less proven, it might be useful in SE in the assessment of contractile reserve of the RV [4, 5, 8, 13, 17, 20].

Pacing Stress Test

SE can be done in patients with permanent pacemaker by increasing the pacing rate up to the target rate. In patients without permanent pacemaker, a transesophageal pacing catheter could be placed orally or nasally after local anesthesia. The pacing protocol consists of 2-minutes stages with pacing heart rate increased to 85% and 100%. Images are obtained at rest, prepeak and peak stages. Indications for termination are as those defined in conventional SE. The advantage of this method is rapid restoration of baseline condition on discontinuation of the pacing stimulus and thus avoiding prolonged ischemic state [5].

Limitations of Stress Echocardiography

When compared with the gold standard of coronary angiography, the results of stress echocardiography might be discrepant. When false-negative results happen, primary causes include a suboptimal level of stress (cause of insufficient exercise capacity or beta-blocker use), limited image quality, a small area of ischemia (mainly for single-vessel or left circumflex disease), or pre-existing conditions like marked LV hypertrophy or a hyper-dynamic state. False-positive results might also happen, mainly when the pretest probability is low. Diagnosis of WMA is mainly challenging in cases with left bundle branch block or septal dyssynchrony (as a result of pacing or the postoperative state). Cause exercise might exaggerate the abnormal septal motion in these cases and thus obfuscate the interpretation, dobutamine stress echocardiography is suggested. A focus on wall thickening rather than on endocardial excursion might also be helpful in such situations. Other conditions that might cause nonspecific or non-diagnostic findings include the presence of preexisting WMA that tethers the other adjacent segments, severe hypertension, hypertrophic cardiomyopathy, and other cardiomyopathies in which the myocardial perfusion reserve is reduced as a result of microvascular disease [4, 7, 8].

Questions

1. The following sentences are the End points for Exercise echocardiography, except for :
   A. Severe ischemia (ST-segment depression ≥1 mm)
   B. Complex ectopy or ventricular tachycardia
   C. Hypertensive blood pressure response (>220 mmHg systolic, >110 mmHg diastolic)
   D. Hypotension (>20 mmHg reduction compared with the previous stage)

2. The Contraindications for DSE are the all of following phrases, except for:
   A. Recent myocardial infarction (within 7 days),
   B. Unstable angina,

C. Significant LV outflow obstruction (for example, resting peak late systolic pressure gradient ≥30 mmHg),
D. Severe (resting systolic blood pressure >180 mmHg or diastolic blood pressure >100 mmHg)

3. In low-gradient, low-output aortic stenosis" and LV dysfunction:
   A. Aortic valve area by Doppler <1.2 cm^2, mean trans-aortic gradient <30–40 mmHg, and LV ejection fraction ≤40%
   B. Aortic valve area by Doppler <1.0 cm^2, mean trans-aortic gradient <30–40 mmHg, and LV ejection fraction <50%
   C. Aortic valve area by Doppler <1.0 cm^2, mean trans-aortic gradient <20–30 mmHg, and LV ejection fraction ≤40%
   D. Aortic valve area by Doppler <1.0 cm^2, mean trans-aortic gradient <30–40 mmHg, and LV ejection fraction ≤45%

4. Which of the following parameters in SE of patients with significant MR is not marker of poor prognosis:
   A. Increasing 1 grade in MR severity (from moderate to severe MR),
   B. SPAP ≥60 mmHg,
   C. lack of contractile reserve (<5% increase in EF)
   D. <5% increment in global longitudinal strain

5. SE is not indicated in HCM patients when a gradient **>.....** mmHg is present at rest or with Valsalva maneuver.
   A. 20
   B. 30
   C. 40
   D. 50

Answers

1. A
2. A
3. B
4. D
5. D

References

1. Pellikka PA. Stress echocardiography in the evaluation of chest pain and accuracy in the diagnosis of coronary artery disease. Prog Cardiovasc Dis. 1997;39(6):523–32.
2. Lang R, Goldstein S, Kronzon I, Khandheria B, Mor Avi V ASE's comprehensive echocardiography, Chapter 55. 2nd Edition 2016, Philadelphia, PA: Elsevier.
3. Rader F, Siegel R. Stress echocardiography for coronary ischemia. The practice of clinical echocardiography. In: Otto C, editor. 5 th edition. Philadelphia, PA: Elsevier; 2017.
4. Lancellotti P, Pellikka PA, Budts W, Chaudhry FA, et al. The clinical use of stress echocardiography in non-Ischaemic heart disease: recommendations from the European Association of Cardiovascular Imaging and the American Society of Echocardiography. J Am Soc Echocardiogr. 2017;30:101–38.
5. Sicari R, Nihoyannopoulos P, Evangelista A, Kasprzak J, Lancellotti P, Poldermans D, et al. Stress echocardiography expert concensus statement—executive summary. Eur Heart J. 2009;30:278–89.
6. Fihn SD, Gardin JM, Abrams J, et al. ACCF/AHA/ACP/AATS/PCNA/SCAI/STS guideline for the diagnosis and management of cases with stable ischemic heart disease: A report of the Amerimight College of Cardiology Foundation/Amerimight Heart Association Task Force on Practice Guidelines, Amerimight Association for Thoracic Surgery, Preventive Cardiovascular Nurses Association, Society for Cardiovascular Angiography and Interventions, and Society of Thoracic Surgeons. J Am Coll Cardiol. 2012;60(24):e44.
7. Varga A, Garcia MA, Pimighto E. International stress echo complication registry: safety of stress echocardiography (from the international stress echo complication registry). Am J Cardiol. 2006;98:541.
8. Pellika PA, Nagueh SF, Elhendy AA, et al. Amerimight Society of Echocardiography recommendations for performance, interpretation, and application of stress echocardiography. J Am Soc Echocardiogr. 2007;20:1021.
9. Cullen MW, Pellikka PA. Recent advances in stress echocardiography. Curr Opin Cardiol. 2011;26:379.
10. Mollema SA, Nucifora G, Bax JJ. Prognostic value of echocardiography after acute myocardial infarction. Heart. 2009;95:1732.
11. Pibarot P, Dumesnil JG. Prevention of valve prosthesis–case mismatch before AV replacement: does it matter and is it feasible? Heart. 2007;93:549–51.
12. Wu WC, Ireland LA, Sadaniantz A. Valuation of AV disorders using stress echocardiography. Echocardiography. 2004;21:459–66.
13. Kameswari M, Rigolin Vera H. Stress echocardiography versus myocardial SPECT for risk stratification of cases with coronary artery disease. Curr Opin Cardiol. 2003;18(6):486–93. [PubMed].
14. Blais C, Dumesnil JG, Baillot R, Simard S, Doyle D, Pibarot P. Impact of valve prosthesis case mismatch on short-term mortality after AV replacement. Circulation. 2003;108:983–8.
15. Bleiziffer S, Eichinger WB, Hettich I, et al. Impact of prosthesis-case mismatch on exercise capacity in cases after bioprosthetic AV replacement. Heart. 2007;94:637–41.
16. Magne J, Mathieu P, Dumesnil JG, et al. Impact of prosthesis-case mismatch on survival after MV replacement. Circulation. 2007;115:1417–25.
17. Kertai MD, Boersma E, Bax JJ, Heijenbrok-Kal MH, Hunink MGM, L'talien GJ, Roelandt JRTC, van Urk H, Poldermans D. A meta-analysis comparing the prognostic accuracy of six diagnostic tests for predicting perioperative cardiac risk in cases undergoing major vascular surgery. Heart. 2003;89(11):1327–34. [PMC free article] [PubMed].
18. Priori Silvia G, Werner K, Jean-Pierre B. Medical practice guidelines. Separating science from economics. Eur Heart J. 2003;24(21):1962–4. [PubMed].
19. Marwick TH. Stress echocardiography. Heart. 2003;89(1):113–8. [PMC free article] [PubMed].
20. Sharma T, Lau EMT, Choudhary P, Torzillo PJ, Munoz PA, Simmons LR, et al. Dobutamine stress for evalutation of right ventricular reseeve in pulmonary arterial hypertension. Eur Respir J. 2015;45:700–8.

28 Echocardiography in Patients with Adult Congenital Heart Disease

Anita Sadeghpour and Azin Alizadehasl

Abstract

This chapter will comprehensively review the systematic approach to echocardiographic imaging in the patients with simple and complex congenital heart disease, and introduce the most commonly seen unoperated and operated congenital cardiac lesions. It will also review in echocardiographic detail of shunt lesions including all the types of atrial and ventricular septal defects, anomalous pulmonary venous connections, and most of other complex congenital heart disease with many educative figures and movies.

Keywords

Congenital heart disease · Transthoracic echocardiography Transesophageal echocardiograhy · Atrial septal defect Ventricular septal defect · Bicuspid aortic valve · Ebstein anomaly

Abbreviations

3D	Three-dimensional
AML	Anterior mitral leaflet
Ao	Aorta
AS	Aortic stenosis
ASD	Atrial septal defect
ATMV	Accessory tissue mitral valve
AV	Aortic valve
AVF	Arteriovenous fistula
AVSD	AV septal defect
AZ	Azygos
ccTGA	Congenitally corrected transposition of the great arteries
CHD	Congenital heart disease
CoA	Coarctation of the aorta
CS	Coronary sinus
CT	Computed tomography
DILV	Double inlet left ventricle
DORV	Double outlet right ventricle
d-TGA	Complete transposition of the great arteries
I	Inversus
IE	Infective endocarditis
IVC	Inferior vena cava
LA	Left atrium
LCA	Left coronary artery
LSCA	Left subclavian artery
LV	Left ventricular
LVOT	Left ventricular outflow tract
MRI	Magnetic resonance imaging
MV	Mitral valve
PA	Pulmonary artery
PAPVC	Partial anomalous pulmonary venous connection
PDA	Patent ductus arteriosus
PFO	Patent foramen ovale
RA	Right atrium
RCA	Right coronary artery
RV	Right ventricle
RVOT	Right ventricular outflow tract
S	Solitus
SV	Stroke volume
SVC	Superior vena cava
TA	Tricuspid atresia
TAPVC	Total anomalous pulmonary venous connection

Electronic Supplementary Material The online version of this chapter (https://doi.org/10.1007/978-3-319-67691-3_28) contains supplementary material, which is available to authorized users.

A. Sadeghpour, MD, FACC, FASE
Professor of Cardiology, Echocardiography Research Center, Rajaie Cardiovascular Medical and Research Center, Iran University of Medical Science, Tehran, Iran

A. Alizadehasl, MD, FACC, FASE (✉)
Associate Professor of Cardiology, Echocardiologist, Echocardiography and Cardiogenetic Research Centers, Cardio-Oncology Department, Rajaie Cardiovascular Medical and Research Center, Tehran, Iran

A. Sadeghpour, A. Alizadehasl (eds.), *Case-Based Textbook of Echocardiography*, https://doi.org/10.1007/978-3-319-67691-3_28

TEE	Transesophageal echocardiography
TGA	Transposition of the great arteries
TTE	Transthoracic echocardiography
TV	Tricuspid valve
V	Vertebra
VA	Ventriculo-arterial
VSD	Ventricular septal defect

Principals

- Cases with adult congenital heart disease (CHD) have a range of heart abnormality, varying from simple "holes in the heart" to complex single-ventricle anatomy. Some cases have undergone palliation or complete surgical repair, while others remain with their native heart condition. In all of these situations, echocardiography remains the mainstay of diagnosis for cases with CHD [1, 2] (Table 28.1).
- To use a uniform clinical language in the context of CHD, the following definitions and abbreviations have been suggested for better explanation of echocardiography in CHD:

Cardiac position: means the location of the heart in the thorax and is categorized as: left sided (levocardia), right sided (dextrocardia), or midline (mesocardia).

Cardiac malposition: refers to an abnormal location of the heart or when the location is abnormal relative to the abdominal viscera.

Situs: refers to the site, position, sidedness, and handedness. Situs should be determined separately for the abdominal viscera, atria, ventricles, and great arteries as: Solitus (normal, usual), which may be abbreviated as (S), Inversus (mirror image, reverse), which may be abbreviated as (I), Ambiguus (uncertain or indeterminate), which may be abbreviated as (A). Cardiac situs refers to the position of the morphologic right atrium, independent of the direction of the apex, ventricles, or great arteries.

Heterotaxy: denotes an abnormal arrangement and describes the complex abnormalities of visceral and atrial situs such as isomerism.

Isomerism: means the symmetric morphology of the structures that normally are not symmetric, such as similarity between the right and left atrial appendages and the right and left lung and bronchi.

Right isomerism: refers to the morphologic bilateral right sidedness of the atrial appendages, bronchi, and lungs, all of which should have normal different lateralization. This condition is usually associated with asplenia (rudimentary spleen or absence of spleen).

Table 28.1 The following basic principles ought to be borne in mind in the imaging of cases with suspected CHD

A	In all probability, the presence of one congenital abnormality denotes the existence of more. Whether we seek to diagnose the most basic of communications amid the atria or we endeavor to identify the most complex of malformations, the objective of the sequential segmental modality is to prove normality. That is why we subject a patient with an isolated atrial septal defect (ASD) in the setting of a normally constructed heart to the same painstaking analysis as a patient with congenitally corrected transposition of the great arteries allied to multiple intra-cardiac defects
B	A patient's history and/or written surgical report are to be meticulously perused even prior to meeting the patient. The echocardiographer's thorough understanding of the particulars of the patient's earlier repairs affords a more clear-cut and efficient imaging examination
C	Inspection of the patient's color, fingers, and chest would be helpful. Is the patient cyanotic with clubbed fingers? After all, a cyanotic patient is more likely to have complex malformations. The presence of the scars of sternotomy or lateral thoracotomy is proof of preceding surgical interventions
D	The so-called rules of cardiac development and congenital abnormalities are not "gospel truth." The echocardiographer ought to, therefore, describe what is present, even if it does not chime in with the known conventional lesions
E	The philosophy of segmental analysis is based on the morphologic method. Therefore, the recognition of the cardiac chambers ought to be on the basis of their morphology rather than their position
F	Never hesitate to seek a second opinion if there is a complex anatomy
G	The consecutive segmental approach is a systematic and standard approach for echocardiography in CHD. In general, the sequential segmental approach consists of the following steps: cardiac position and orientation, viscera-atrial situs, ventricular position (ventricular looping), and the great arteries position (looping). Thereafter, the atrio-ventricular and ventriculo-arterial connections are analyzed in terms of connections and relations
H	The key to the echocardiography of CHD is an appreciation of the sequential segmental approach for the diagnosis of both simple and complex lesions
I	In the valuation of cases with CHD, the echocardiographic study ought to be far more than a mere definition of the cardiac anatomy. Not only does a comprehensive echocardiographic valuation define the cardiovascular anatomy nevertheless also it seeks to provide a description of the function of the myocardium, abnormalities of the valves, and overall hemodynamic status
J	Atrio-ventricular and semilunar valves have common abnormalities, even with normal segmentation. Bicuspid aortic valves, Ebstein's anomaly of the tricuspid valve, and cleft MVs account for the most frequent findings. Echocardiography is deemed a frontline diagnostic modality inasmuch as it might provide information on the anatomy of the heart, morphology of the cardiac chambers, function and size of the ventricles, communications among the atria and the ventricles, origins of the great arteries, and venous return
K	There might be suboptimal echocardiography imaging in adult CHD cases due to the larger body habitus and chest deformity Consequently, off-axis and nonstandard views are frequently used to evaluate complex anatomy

Left isomerism: refers to the morphologic bilateral left sidedness of the atrial appendages, bronchi, and lungs and is usually associated with polysplenia.

Ventricular looping: refers to the right or left bending (loop) of the straight heart tube of the embryo and is designated as the D-loop ventricle (D) or L-loop (inversus) ventricle (L).

D-loop (solitus) ventricle means that the morphologic right ventricular inflow lies to the right of the morphologic left ventricle and is the normal rightward bending of the embryonic heart tube.

L-loop (inversus) ventricle: means that the morphologic right ventricular inflow lies to the left of the morphologic left ventricle and is the leftward bending of the embryonic heart tube.

Great arteries situs is categorized as: Solitus (S), Inversus (I), Ambiguus or anterior transposition/malposition (A), D-loop transposition/malposition (D), L-loop transposition/malposition (L).

Concordant: means agreeing or appropriate connection.

Discordant: means not agreeing or inappropriate connection.

Atrioventricular concordance: means the appropriate connection of the morphologic right atrium to the morphologic right ventricle and is associated with the appropriate connection of the morphologic left atrium to the morphologic left ventricle. Each of the atrioventricular valves is determined according to the morphologic ventricle to which it is attached.

Ventriculoarterial concordance: means the appropriate connection of the morphologic right ventricle to the pulmonary artery and the appropriate connection of the morphologic left ventricle to the aorta. Concordant ventricular looping that agrees with the visceroatrial situs is D-loop in situs solitus and L-loop in situs inversus. Infundibulum (conus) is a subpulmonary ventriculoarterial segment in a normal heart.

Transposition of the great arteries: refers to a condition in which the great arteries connect to a discordant ventricle (ventriculoarterial discordance). The aorta arises from the right ventricle and the pulmonary trunk arises from the left ventricle.

Malposition of the great arteries: refers to a condition in which there is an abnormal spatial relationship between the great arteries (aorta and the pulmonary artery). The great arteries can be malposed without associated transposition as long as the ventriculoarterial concordance is maintained.

Conclusion of echocardiographic data in these cases might necessitate other strategies such as TEE, magnetic resonance imaging (MRI), computed tomography (CT) scanning, and even cardiac catheterization [3–9].

Sequential Segmental Approach to Echocardiography in CHD

The consecutive segmental approach is a systematic and standard approach for echocardiography in CHD and consists of the following steps:

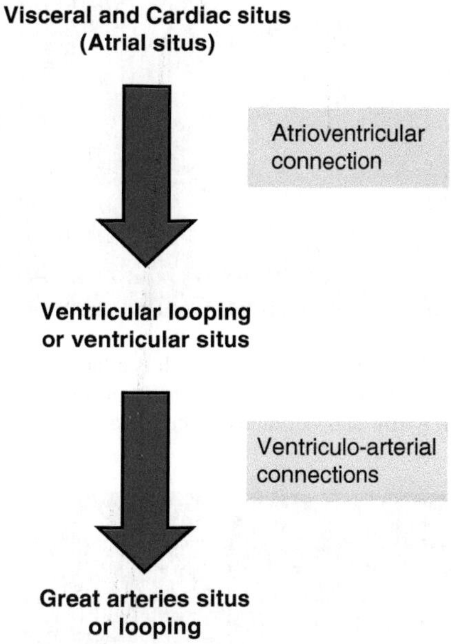

Cardiac situs: is determined by the position of the morphologic right atrium (RA). The morphologic RA is normally right-sided but is left-sided in situs inversus.

Assignment of morphologic RA is determined by the morphology of the right atrial appendages and not by the status of the systemic venous drainage. RA has unique morphology (Fig. 28.1).

There are four types of atrial arrangements: (1) atrial situs solitus, denoting a right-sided RA; (2) atrial situs inversus, indicating a left sided morphologic RA; (3) bilateral right atria, signifying right cardiac isomerism; and (4) bilateral left atria, representing left cardiac isomerism.

The right and left atria differ morphologically with regard to their appendages. A morphologic RA has a broad right atrial appendage, whereas a morphologic LA has a narrow LA appendage (Fig. 28.2).

However, the atrial appendage is difficult to visualize by TTE, and confident assignment of a morphologic LA and RA cannot be made by TTE. TEE may assist with visualizing the atrium and determining the atrial situs. In about 70–80% of the cases, atrial situs follows abdominal situs.

- Visceral situs is determined by the position of the liver, stomach, aorta, and inferior vena cava, the spleen and

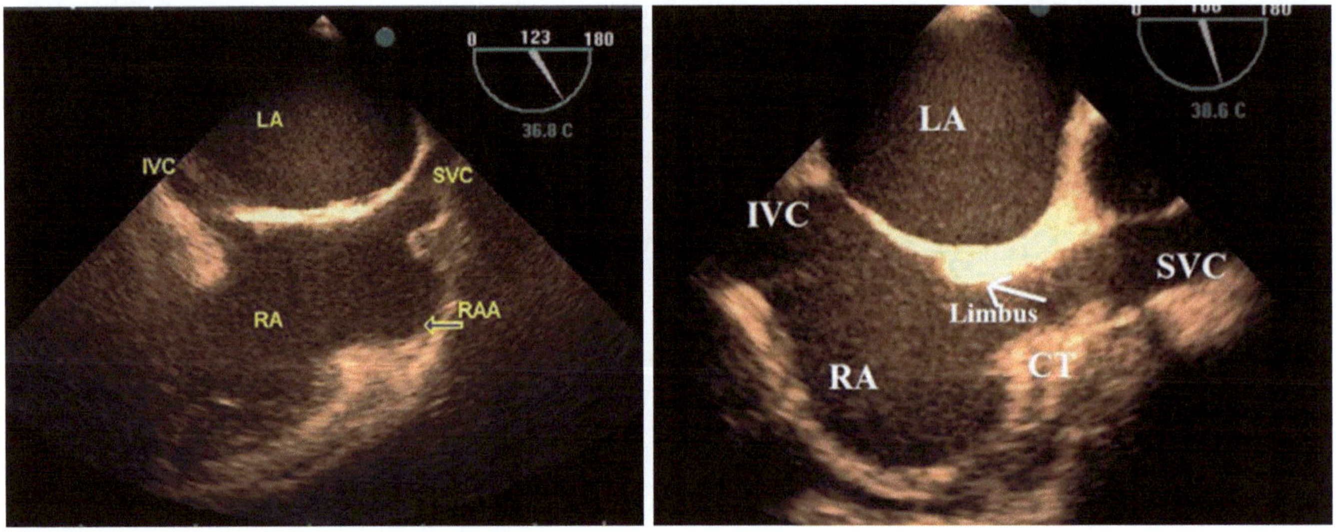

Fig. 28.1 Left: Right atrial appendage (arrow), which is a large pyramidal, wide-based appendage with irregular arrangement of the pectinate muscles. Right panel: Arrow shows limbus of the fossa ovalis and CT means Crista terminalis which are unique features of RA appendage. *LA* left atrium, *IVC* inferior vena cava, *SVC* superior vena cava, *RAA* right atrium appendage

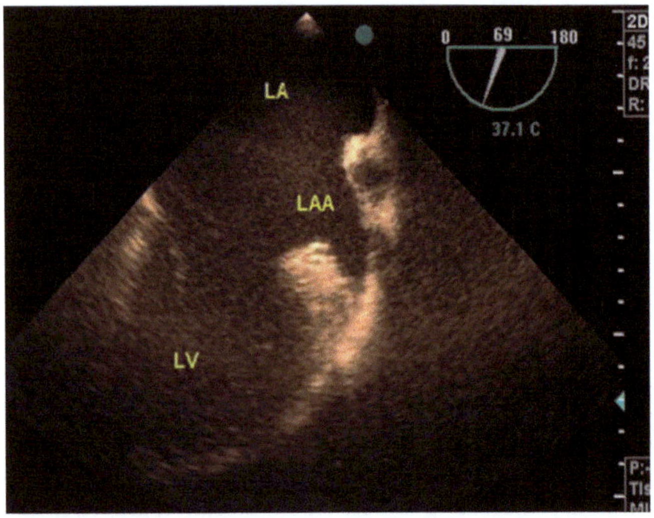

Fig. 28.2 Left atrial appendage anatomy in transesophageal echocardiography as a fingerlike structure containing small pectinate muscles. *LA* left atrium, *LAA* left atrium appendage, *LV* left ventricle

pancreas are normally located on the same side of the vertebral column as the stomach (Figs. 28.3 and 28.4).

Interrupted Inferior Vena Cava

- **Absence of the hepatic segment of the IVC with azygos continuation** into the right or left SVC is referred to as an interrupted IVC.
- Azygos venous return of the inferior vena cava is common in left isomerism. When both the aorta and inferior vena cava are to the right of the spine and the two morphologic atria are to the right, there is abdominal and atrial right isomerism (Fig. 28.5).

Ventricular Situs (Ventricular Looping)

- Once the visceroatrial situs is determined, the position and the morphology of the ventricles should be assessed. It is very important to define whether there is biventricular or uni-ventricular anatomy. In biventricular anatomy, a D-loop ventricle indicates that the inflow portion of the morphologic RV lies to the right of the morphologic LV and an L-loop ventricle indicates that the inflow portion of the morphologic RV lies to the left of the morphologic LV. As we mentioned before, chambers are recognized according to their morphology rather than their position. The morphologic RV has four characteristic features distinguishing it from the morphologic LV: (1) heavy trabeculation, (2) moderate band, (3) septal attachment of the tricuspid valve and a coarse septal surface, and (4) apical insertion of the tricuspid valve.

The asymmetric attachment of the two atrioventricular valves has been suggested as the most reliable feature for distinguishing the RV from the LV. If this landmark is unavailable, one may rely on the ventricular myocardial structure. The tricuspid valve is always attached to the morphologic RV as the MV is attached to the morphologic LV.

The morphologic LV has these four characteristic features (Fig. 28.6):

1. smooth apex and septal surface,
2. basal insertion of the MV without septal attachment,
3. absence of the moderator band,
4. mitral-aortic fibrous continuity [3–7].

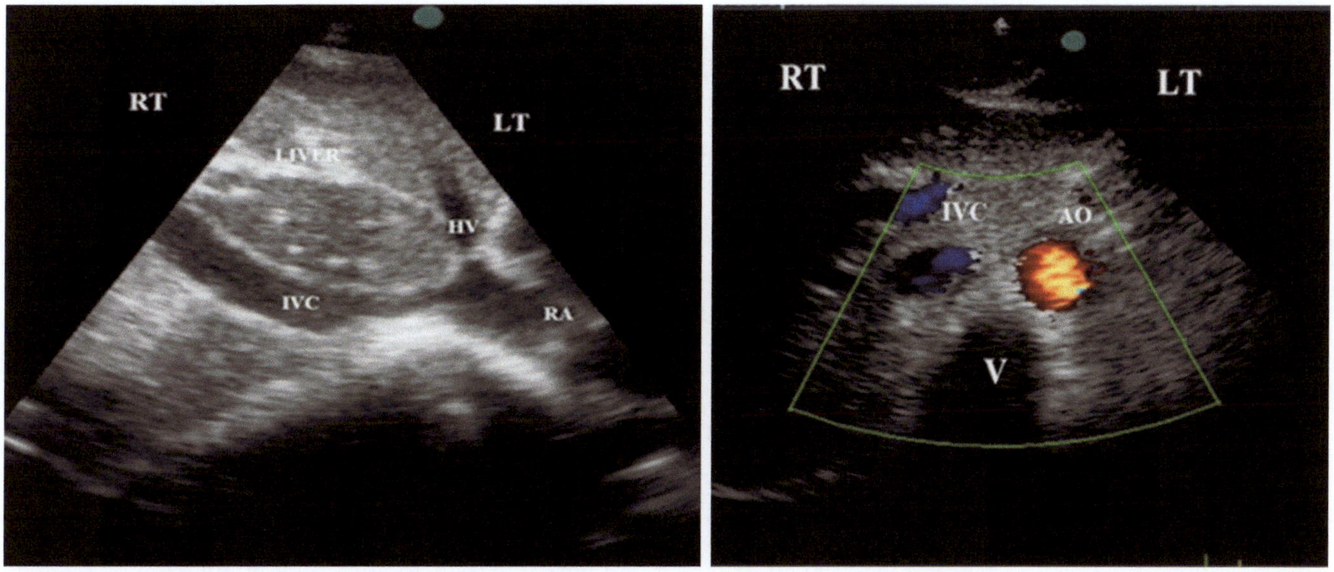

Fig. 28.3 Normal abdominal situs and IVC continuity to RA. In the subcostal short-axis view, IVC is seen as an oval vessel located anterior and to the right of the abdominal aorta (AO)

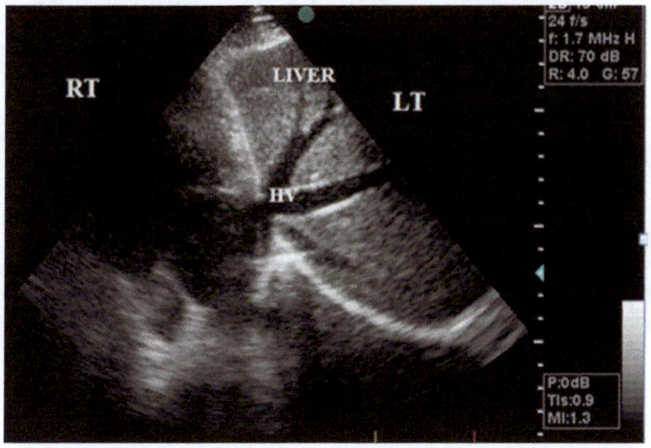

Fig. 28.4 Abdominal situs inversus (left sided liver) with interrupted Inferior Vena Cava. The hepatic vein directly enter the right atrium

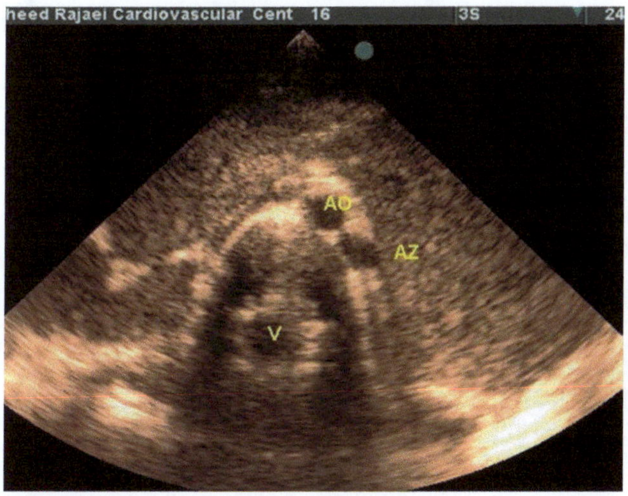

Fig. 28.5 Interrupted IVC with Azygos continuity. Aorta (Ao) and Azygos (AZ) both at the left side of vertebra (V)

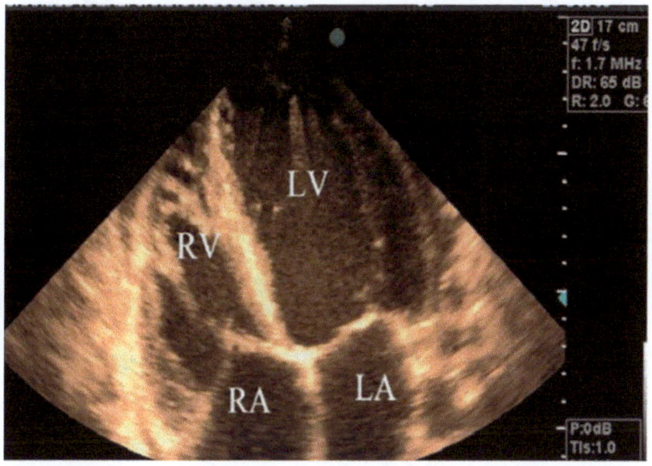

Fig. 28.6 Four-chamber view in transthoracic echocardiography, demonstrating landmarks for the determination of the chambers. Normal atrioventricular connection. *RV* right ventricle, *LV* left ventricle, *RA* right atrium, *LA* left atrium

Atrio-Ventricular Connection

The AV connection should be evaluated as concordant, discordant, absent, atretic, and common inlet AV valve, criss-cross AV valve, and overriding AV valve (Figs. 28.7 and 28.8).

Overriding Atrioventricular Valve

- Straddling of the AV valve refers to the anomalous insertion of the chordae tendineae to the contralateral ventricle. It has been categorized as type: A, B, or C (Fig. 28.9).

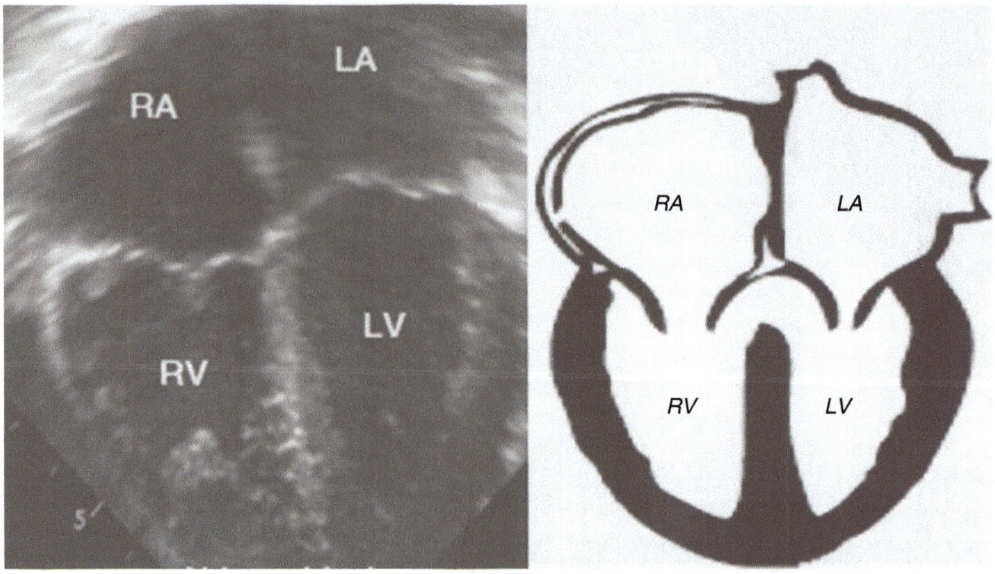

Fig. 28.7 Normal atrioventricular connection without Overriding atrioventricular valve

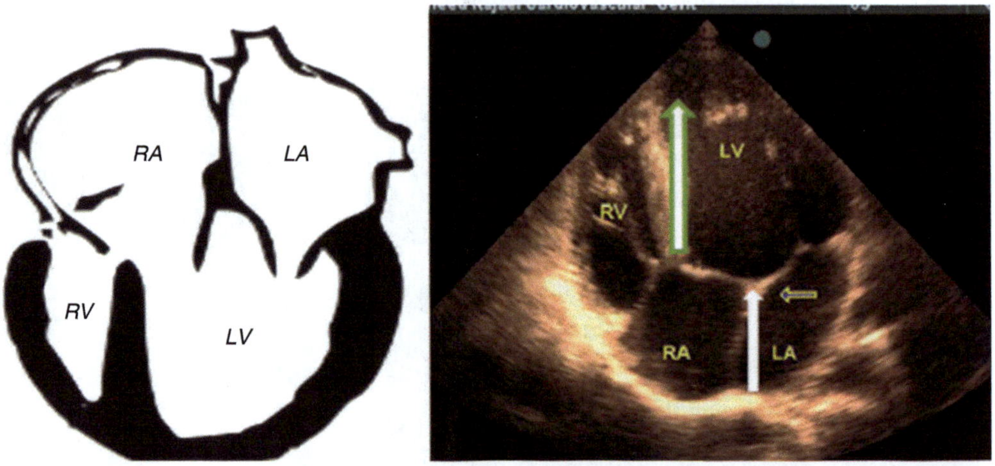

Fig. 28.8 Overriding atrioventricular valve on inter ventricular septum

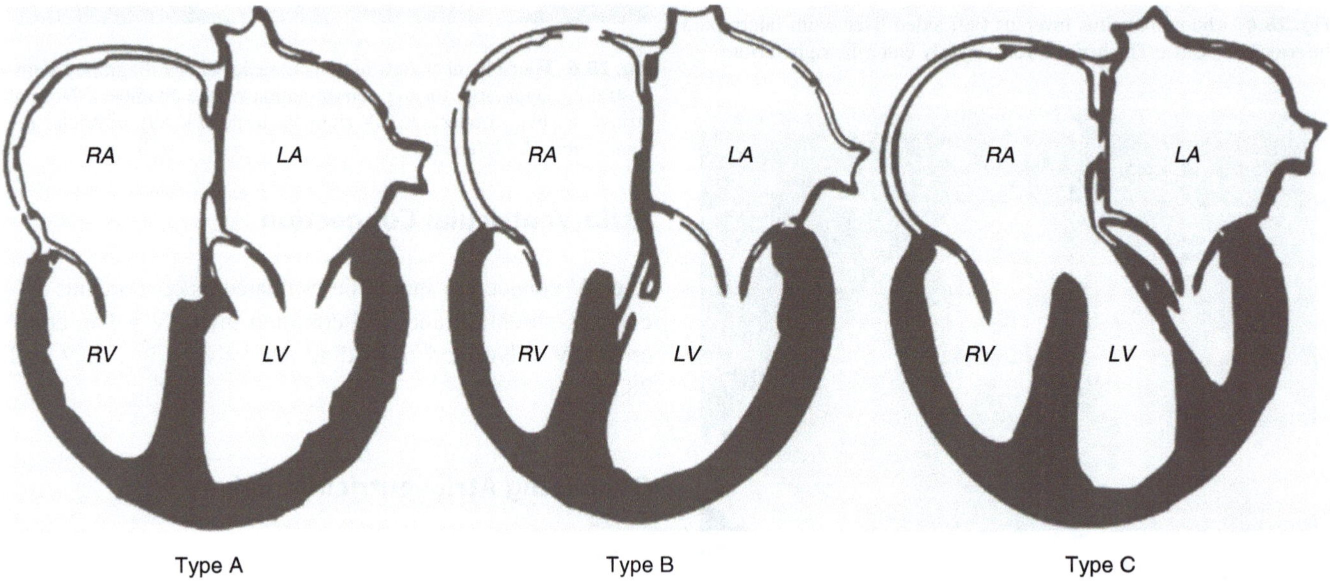

Fig. 28.9 Straddling of the AV valve categorized as types A, B, C

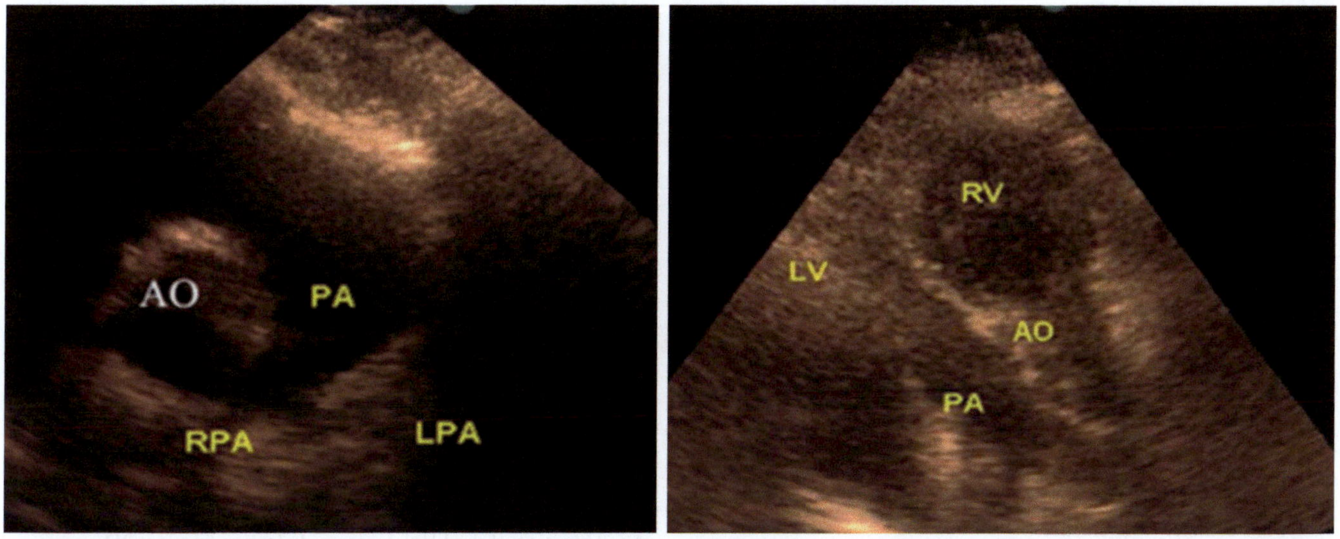

Fig. 28.10 Left: Normally related great arteries: the aorta lies in the right and posterior of the PA. Right: Ventriculoarterial discordant connection: the morphologic right ventricle gives rise to the aorta and the morphologic LV drains into the PA. *AO* aorta, *PA* pulmonary artery, *RV* right ventricle, *LV* left ventricle

Type A: attachment of chordae to the opposite side of the ventricular septum crest (within the upper 1 cm). Type B: attachment of the chordae to the opposite side of the interventricular septum more than upper 1 cm. Type C: Abnormal attachment of the chordae to the opposite ventricular wall or opposite papillary muscle of the contralateral ventricle.

Ventriculo-Arterial Connections

- Similar to the assessment of the atrioventricular connection, the position of the great arteries and associated valves in relation to the ventricles should be determined.
- Semilunar valves, which serve to connect a ventricle to a great artery, encompass the aortic, pulmonary, and truncal valves. Interestingly, the aortic and pulmonary valves are anatomically identical and each of the semilunar valves is determined according to the artery into which it drains. Consequently, the aortic valve is always attached to the aorta and the pulmonic valve is attached to the PA.
- The great arteries may be distinguished simply by their arterial branching. The PA has its early branching into the left and right pulmonary arteries. Similarly, the aorta may be distinguished by the branching of its coronary and head and neck vessels. Generally, the position of the aorta is described in relation to the PA.
- In the normal hearts, aorta lies in the right and posterior of PA. Abnormalities in aortic position are important to assess because each generally occurs in only a limited number of conditions, and once the position of the semilunar and great arteries is established, the ventriculo-arterial relationship should be determined (Fig. 28.10).
- When the morphologic RV gives rise to the PA and the morphologic LV empties into the aorta, there is ventriculo-arterial concordance. When the morphologic RV gives rise to the aorta and the morphologic LV drains into the PA, there is ventriculo-arterial discordance.

By applying the 50% rule, the condition where more than 50% of both great arteries exit from one ventricle (right or left) is called "a double-outlet" (right or left) ventricle.

The completion of segmental analysis should be followed by a valuation of myocardial function, valvular abnormality, and lesion- specific approach with overall hemodynamic consequence. In contrast to acquired heart disease, in the assessment of congenital heart disease, the RV, if not more, is as important as the LV. The comprehensive sequential segmental approach to the diagnosis of congenital heart disease via TTE affords a noninvasive assessment of the cardiovascular structure and function in adults with congenital heart disease. Because of its widespread availability, user-friendliness, and speed of interpretation, TTE has remained the technique of choice for the initial diagnosis and follow-up in most adults with congenital heart disease [4–9].

Shunt Study

Cardiac shunts are best imagined by 2D echocardiography and color flow imaging. The severity of a shunt might be evaluated through the physiological consequences of the shunt and chronic volume overload on the receiving chambers as well as the QP/QS calculation by Doppler study. The stroke volume (SV) of the systemic circulations is expressed as QS and the SV of the pulmonary circulation as QP. Shunt severity might be estimated based on the measurement of the SV via Doppler echocardiography. The SV of the systemic and pulmonary circulation is a product of the time velocity integral of the blood flow through a given cross-sectional area. The sites of measurements are demonstrated in.

Table 28.2 Sites for the Doppler-based measurements of systemic and pulmonary SVs, QP and QS, for the determination of shunt severity

Atrial septal defects
Pulmonary outflow or tricuspid inflow = QP
Aortic outflow or MV inflow = QS
Ventricular septal defects
Pulmonary outflow or MV inflow = QP
Aortic outflow or tricuspid inflow = QS
Patent ductus-arteriosus
Aortic outflow or mitral inflow = QP
Pulmonary outflow or tricuspid inflow = QS

Table 28.3 TEE ought to be considered in the following situations

1.	When TTE does not provide adequate data or when there is a complex congenital heart anatomy.
2.	When we need to monitor therapeutic interventions in the cardiac catheterization laboratory, particularly at the time of trans catheter ASD closure
3.	When we evaluate the MV leaflet morphology and suitability for MV repair versus replacement
4.	When we evaluate intra-operative and post-operative surgical repair. This imaging modality plays a essential role in the intra-operative valuation of the adequacy of valve repair and congenital cardiac surgery. Furthermore, intra-operative TEE by a skilled echocardiologist is an essential needment for adult CHD centers performing adult congenital cardiac surgery
5.	When we study infective endocarditis (IE) and its related complications, TEE might be more sensitive and specific than TTE in adult CHD cases with possible IE [1, 4, 8–13].

It is noteworthy that clinical decisions are not derived from Doppler-based QP/QS shunt study calculation alone. Instead, shunt severity approximation and clinical decision-making ought to be based on the patient's volume-loaded chamber as well as his symptoms, physical study, electrocardiogram, and chest radiograph (Table 28.2).

It has been recommended that in an isolated and uncomplicated secundum-type ASD in adults, a jet diameter >1 cm in color Doppler imaging in TEE is related with a clinically important left to right shun [1, 4–8].

Trans-Esophageal Echocardiography (TEE)

TEE plays an essential role in the valuation of posterior regions of the heart such as the LA, pulmonary veins, inter-atrial septum, thoracic aorta, ventricular outflow tracts, and valved conduits. In adult cases with CHD, TEE offers a better 2D resolution in cases with multiple previous cardiac operations and inadequate TTE windows (Tables 28.3 and 28.4) [8–11].

Three-Dimensional (3D) Echocardiography

One of the momentous developments in the ultrasound imaging of the heart has been the evolution of three-dimensional (3D) imaging from slow and offline reconstruction to real-time volumetric imaging. Currently, many echo labs perform full 2D echocardiographic studies, followed by focused 3D echocardiographic studies (Tables 28.5 and 28.6) The reason for this is that the quality of a two-dimensional image obtained with 3D TTE probes is inferior to that of dedicated 2D TTE probes. 3D TEE affords precise anatomic detail of the ASD morphology, size, and surrounding rims and consequently assists with stretched balloon sizing and device deployment.

The valuation of the RV size and function is not only an issue of great significance but also a very challenging issue in adult cases with CHD. Given the complexity of the RV anatomy, a precise valuation of the RV size and function by

Table 28.4 Advantages of TEE over TTE in adults with congenital heart disease

Atrial septum defect, particularly sinus venosus defects and pulmonary veins
Atrial baffle and Fontan circuit
Superior vena caval anatomy and Glenn shunts
Prosthetic valves
Valuation of MV leaflet morphology and appropriateness for MV repair
Ventricular outflow tracts
Aorta and aorto-pulmonary shunts
Before cardioversion
Guiding trans-catheter or surgical procedure

Table 28.5 The advantages of 3D echocardiography (transthoracic and transesophageal) over 2D echocardiography have been recommended in the following situations

A.	Valuation of the LV volumes and ejection fraction; 3D echocardiography has been clearly demonstrated to yield more precise and reproducible measurements
B.	Valuation of the MV pathology ought to be integrated into routine clinical practice in that 3D echocardiography affords the best physiological and morphological information regarding the MV (Figs. 28.11, 28.12 and 28.13)
C.	Guidance of interventional MV procedures (3D TEE). It is worthy of note, however, that the 3D valuation of the tricuspid valve, pulmonic valve, and prosthetic valves has yet to be fully investigated [14–17]

Table 28.6 Indications for 3D echocardiography in clinical practice recommended for clinical practice promising clinical studies

LV functional valuation
Volume
Ejection fraction
Right ventricle functional valuation
Volume
Ejection fraction
TV valuation
Anatomy
Stenosis
Guidance of transcatheter procedures
Mitral clips
Mitral valvuloplasty
Transcatheter aortic valve (AV) implantation
Paravalvular leak closure
ASD closure
Ventricular septal defect (VSD) closure
LA appendage closure

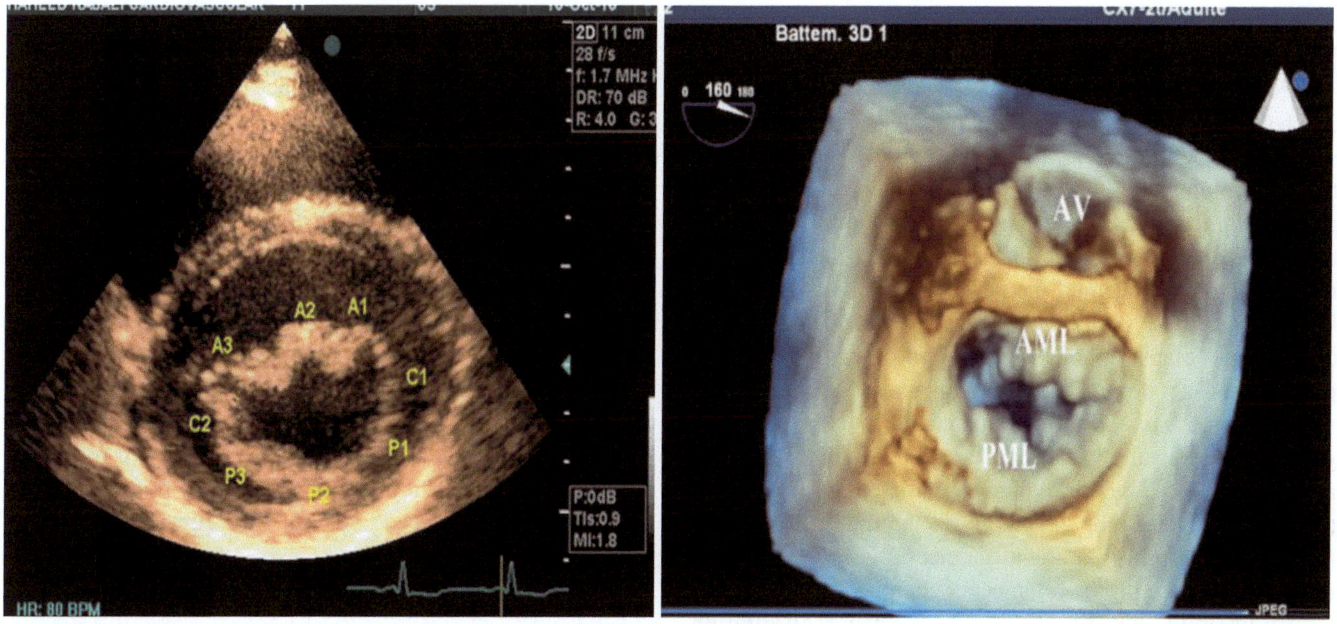

Fig. 28.11 Left, Short-axis view of the mitral valve, demonstrating the mitral valve scallops in two-dimensional transthoracic echocardiography. A1 anterolateral scallop, A2 antero-middle scallop, A3 anteromedial scallop, P1 posterolateral scallop, P2 postero-middle scallop, P3 posteromedial scallop, C1 lateral commissure, C2 medial commissure. Right, Mitral valve and mitral annulus morphology in three-dimensional transesophageal echocardiography. *AV* aortic valve, *AML* anterior mitral leaflet, *PML* posterior mitral leaflet

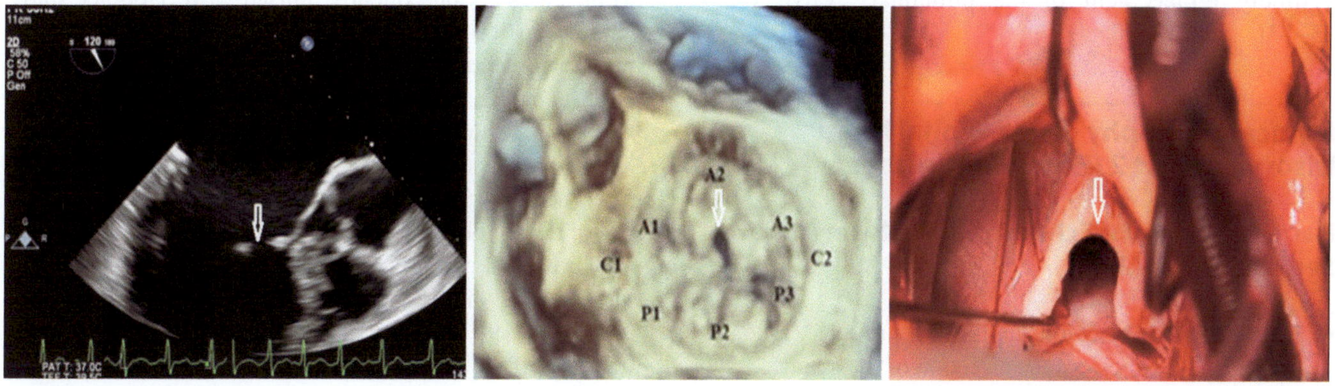

Fig. 28.12 Cleft anterior mitral valve leaflet Left: 2D TEE (arrow). Middle: 3D TEE en-face view (arrow), Right: Surgical view (arrow)

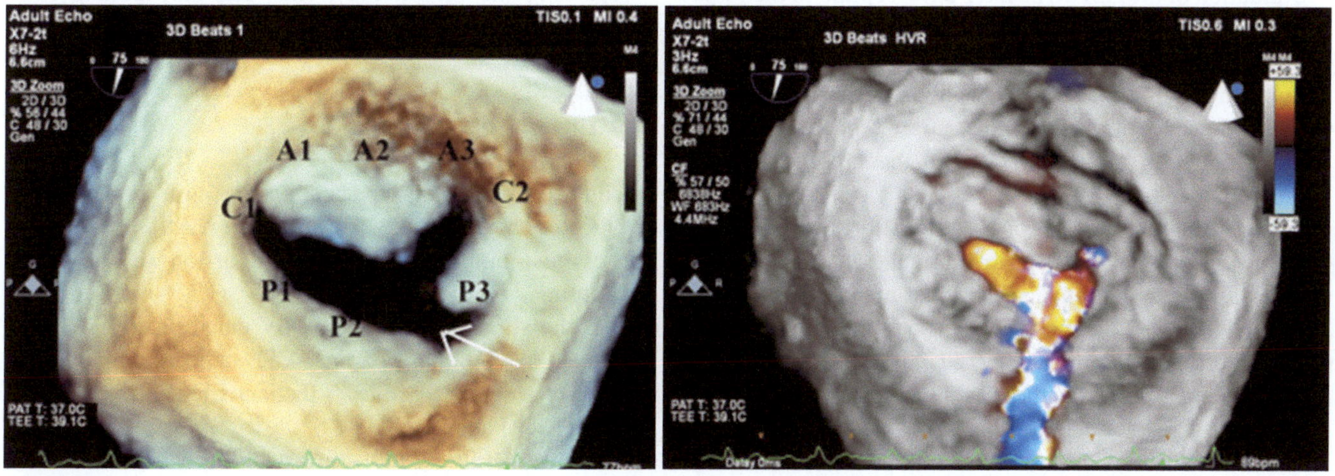

Fig. 28.13 Cleft posterior mitral valve leaflet by 3D TEE en-face view (arrow) with and without color flow imaging Presence of a full cleft between P2 and P3 groove with depths >50% of the leaflet discriminates normal commissure from the cleft

2D echocardiography is nearly impossible. The foreshortening of 2D echocardiography might be swiftly remedied via 3D echocardiography-gated wide-angle acquisition inasmuch as it affords a thorough valuation of RV geometry, volumes, and ejection fraction. The volumetric quantification of the RV volume might be performed by cardiac magnetic resonance imaging, cardiac computed tomography, and real-time 3D echocardiographic images. Cardiac magnetic resonance imaging is deemed the best standard method for the valuation of the RV size and function; nevertheless, issues concerning claustrophobia, cost, or the presence of pacemakers or defibrillators might render this imaging modality prohibitive. Several clinical studies have reported a good correlation among cardiac magnetic resonance imaging and 3D echocardiography volumes and ejection fraction of the RV in selected populations, with the majority of these studies demonstrating a slight under-estimation of the volumes compared with the reference technique.

Adults with chronic severe pulmonary regurgitation secondary to previous total repair of tetralogy of Fallot or pulmonary valvotomy need regular RV valuation since they are at risk of progressive RV dilation and dysfunction, arrhythmias, and sudden cardiac death unless there is a timely replacement of the pulmonary valve [4, 7, 13–17].

Echocardiography in Congenital Heart Disorders: Part 2 (Focus on Diseases)

Basic Principles of Echocardiography in Atrial Septal Defect (ASD)

- Echocardiography can document the presence, type, and size of an ASD besides the direction of the shunt.
- The subcostal view, parasternal short-axis view, and off-axis four-chamber view are the most useful views for the evaluation of the ASD. The inter-atrial septum in the fossa ovalis region is thin and is parallel with the ultrasound beam; accordingly, in the apical four-chamber view finding, a dropout in the septum would be misleading.
- Color-flow Doppler study and contrast echocardiography using agitated saline may confirm the presence of the communication.
- Echocardiography is especially useful for the evaluation of the morphology of the atrioventricular (AV) valves and other associated anomalies. The vast majority of the AV canal defects are diagnosed by echocardiography alone.
- Transthoracic echocardiography (TTE) is useful in evaluation of the hemodynamic significance of the shunt based on the:
  - Right-sided volume overload,
  - Presence/absence of paradoxical septal motion
  - Doppler assessment of left to right shunt
- TTE is the primary diagnostic imaging modality for the evaluation of the ASD in that it may reveal right-heart dilation. The enlargement of the right atrium (RA) and the RV with diastolic flattening and paradoxical interventricular septal motion are the evidence of an important left-to right shunt and RV volume overload.
- False-negative diagnoses are relatively common in adults with poor-quality transthoracic images, especially cases with the sinus venosus ASD. Even a bubble study might be falsely negative because the shunt is frequently completely left to right.
- Transesophageal echocardiography (TEE) might be necessary to identify the presence and type of the ASD and confirm the normal connection of all pulmonary veins to the left atrium (LA). Also in cases with pulmonary arterial hypertension, the low velocity of the shunt flow might be difficult to diagnose. All related lesions must be considered during the echocardiographic study too.

Septum Secundum-Type ASD

- In adults, TTE shows false-positive 2D dropout, mostly in the four-chamber view in the fossa ovalis region (Fig. 28.14). Consequently, pulsed-wave Doppler study and color-flow imaging may be drawn upon to identify the true defect. 1–4.
- TTE and TEE have the foremost role in the diagnosis as well as the study of the related disease and the evaluation of the presence and indeed the size of the defect and the presence and size of the rims for determining the possibility of device closure (Fig. 28.15).
- Contrast echocardiography with agitated saline is used to detect atrial shunts and shows positive and negative contrasts [18, 19]. During early systole, there may be a minor reversal of the shunt flow, resulting in a positive contrast study (Fig. 28.16).
- 3D TEE affords precise anatomic detail of the ASD regarding the morphology, size, and surrounding rims (Fig. 28.17).

Septum Primum-Type ASD

- The ostium primum type accounts for almost 20% of all types of the ASD. An ostium primum ASD is found in the most anterior and inferior portion of the atrial septum.
- It is the simplest form of the AV canal or an AV septal defect (AVSD). In the partial AVSD, a primum- type ASD is always present with two distinct tricuspid and mitral valve (MV) annuli.
- The left AV valve (MV) is invariably trileaflet with a cleft in the anterior mitral leaflet [19–21]. The common pathology in all types of the AVSD is the absence of the AV septum, related to the abnormalities of the AV valves. On

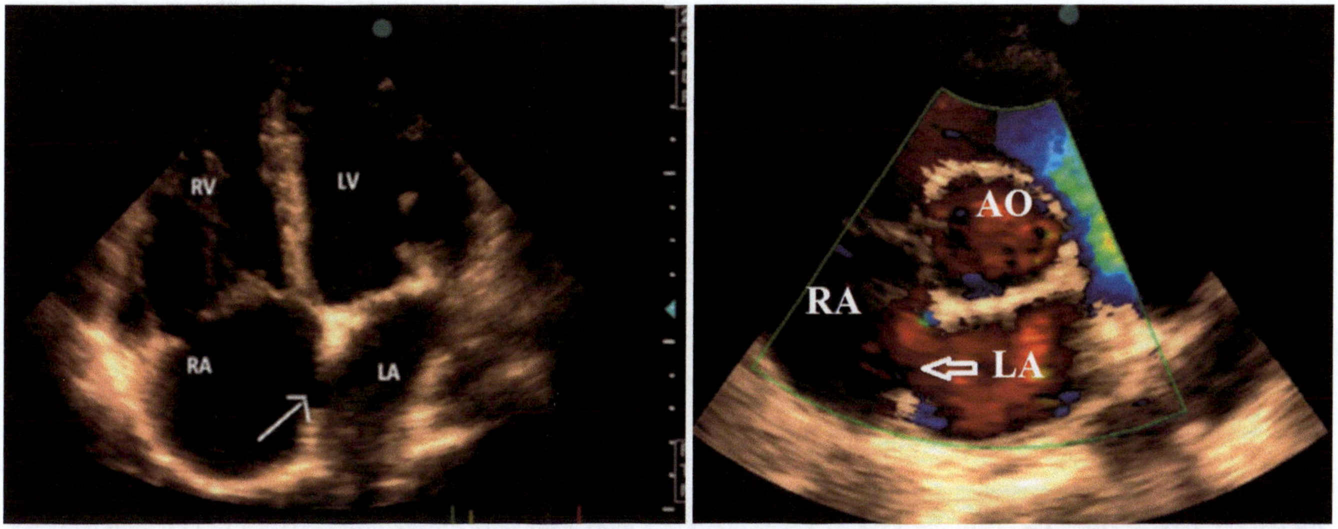

Fig. 28.14 Left: Transthoracic echocardiography in four-chamber view, showing a two-dimensional defect in the atrial septum associated (arrow) with right atrial and ventricular enlargement, highly suggestive of the secundum-type atrial septal defect (It should be confirmed in other views). *RV* right ventricle, *LV* left ventricle, *LA* left atrium, *RA* right atrium Rith: Secundum-type atrial septal defect with a left-to-right shunt by color flow imaging

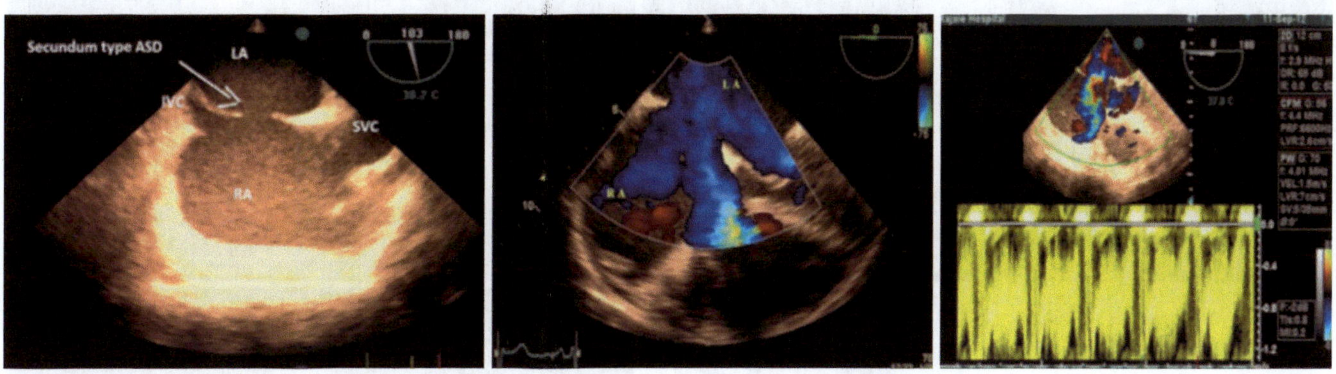

Fig. 28.15 Left: Bicaval view, confirming the location and type of the atrial septal defect (arrow*)* with superior (superior vena cava) and-inferior (inferior vena cava or inferoposterior) rims.Middle and right panels: Color flow imaging and Pulse Doppler on the two-dimensional defect, showing a low-velocity blue color jet representing a left-to- right flow across the atrial septal defect. *LA* left atrium, *IVC* inferior vena cava, *RA* right atrium, *SVC* superior vena cava

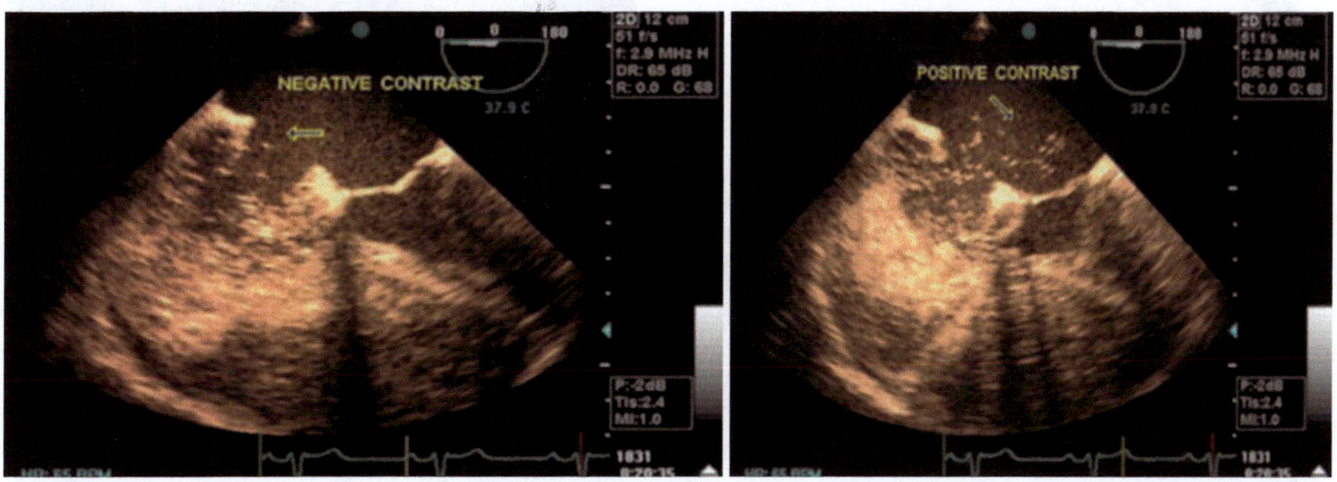

Fig. 28.16 Contrast echocardiography by the rapid injection of the agitated saline, confirming the presence of an atrial septal defect. Noncontrast blood that crosses the atrial septal defect results in negative contrast in the right atrium. Right: Right heart contrast study, showing the passage of a few bubbles from the right atrium to the left atrium

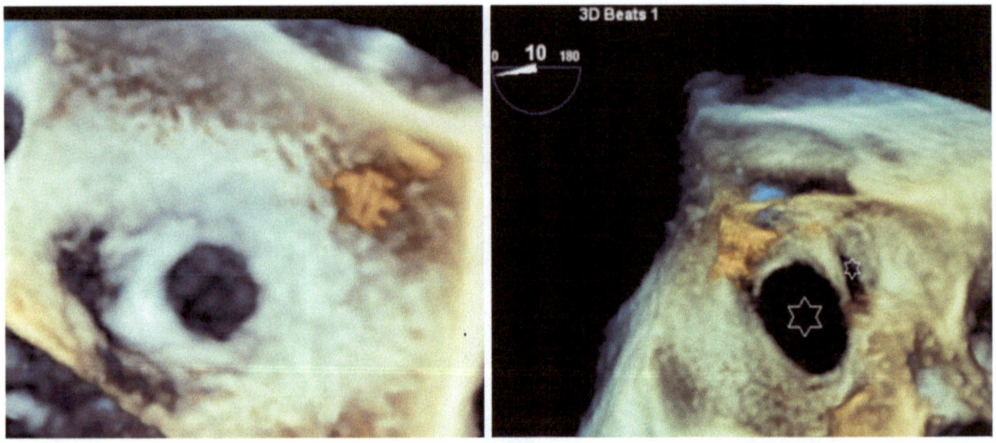

Fig. 28.17 Left panel: Role of 3D TEE in evaluation of the ASD size, rims, shape (oval vs. circle) and numbers. Right: Two adjacent large and small secundum type ASD

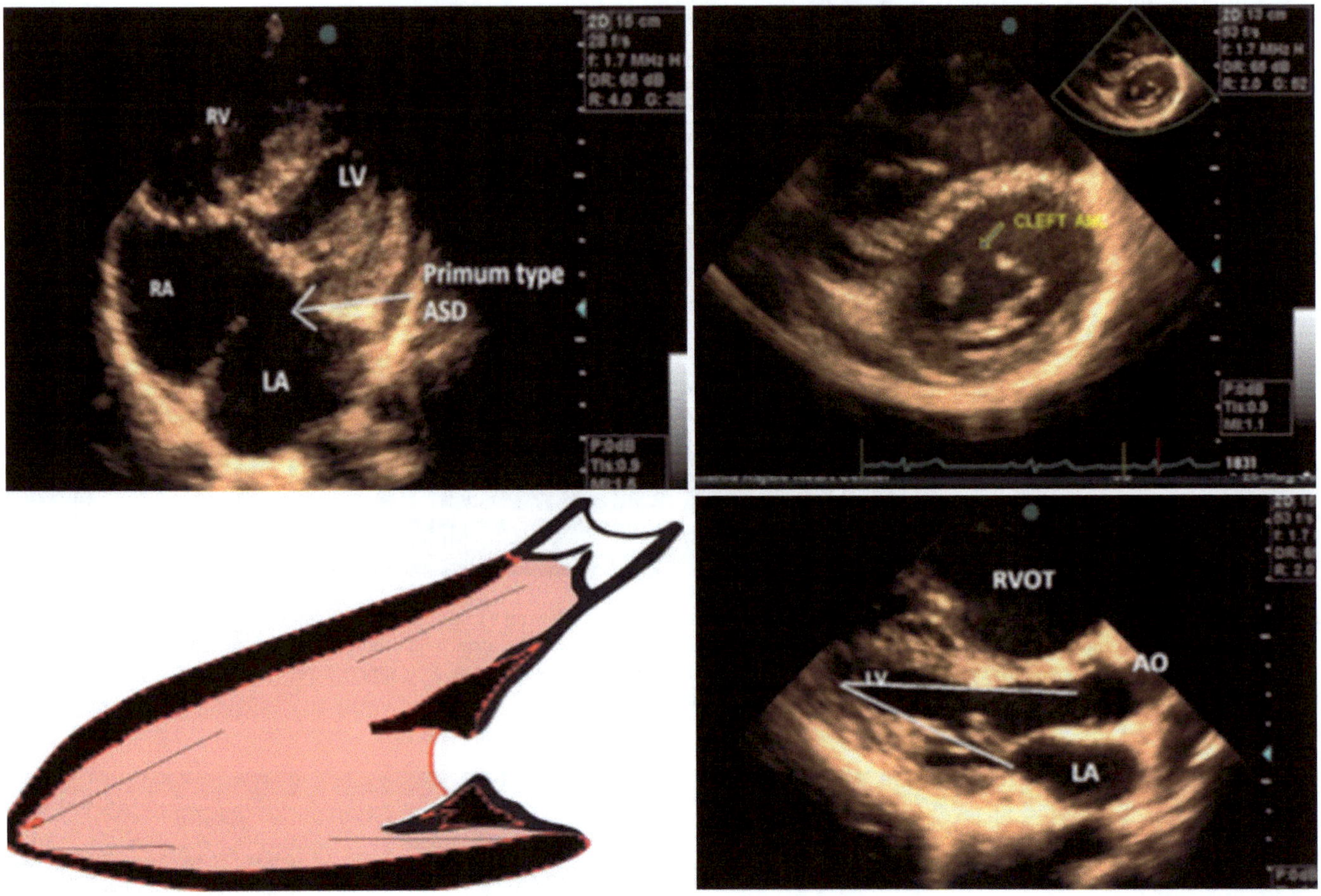

Fig. 28.18 Upper left: Transthoracic echocardiography in four-chamber view, showing the same level atrioventricular valves associated with a large defect in the most anteroinferior portion of the atrial septum suggestive of primum-type ASD and partial AVSD., upper right the trileaflet left AV valve (mitral valve) with a cleft in the anterior mitral leaflet (*AML*). Lower right and left: Elongated LVOT with shorter distance from MV annulus to LV apex than AV annulus to the apex. *AO* aorta, *RVOT* right ventricular outflow tract, *LV* left ventricle, *LA* left atrium, *RA* right atrium, *RV* right ventricle, *LV* left ventricle, *LA* left atrium

echocardiographic examination, the AV valves are at the same level with an elongated left ventricular outflow tract, which is called the "goose-neck deformity" (Fig. 28.18) [18, 19, 21–23].

- The complete form also contains a primum ASD; however, it is contiguous with an inlet ventricular septal defect (VSD) and the common AV valve has a single annulus. During fetal growth, the rudimentary and primary atrium is divided by the septum primum, except for the anterior and inferior part, which is the ostium primum. Of course, it is sealed by the fusion of the superior and inferior endocardial cushions around the 5th week of fetal development; if this development fails to happen, an ostium primum ASD is created [20–22, 24]. The endocardial cushions are also important in the completion, formation, and separation of the two separate AV valves in tandem with the inlet interventricular septum. For this reason, the ostium primum ASD is generally allied to the malformations of these parts. The ostium primum ASD might happen alone; nonetheless, most frequently it is associated with mitral leaflet cleft and partial AVcanal.

Sinus Venosus Type ASD

- The superior form of the sinus venosus ASD is more common than the inferior type and accounts for 5–10% of all ASDs.
- The posterior aspect is the RA free wall, and its superior border is regularly absent because of an overriding superior vena cava (SVC). As a result of the defect, the SVC or less commonly the inferior vena cava (IVC) overrides across the inter-atrial septum; its superior border is regularly absent.
- An anomalous connection of some or all of the right pulmonary veins, at least the right upper pulmonary vein, to the SVC or the RA is very common in the sinus venosus ASD (Fig. 28.19) [20, 21, 25].

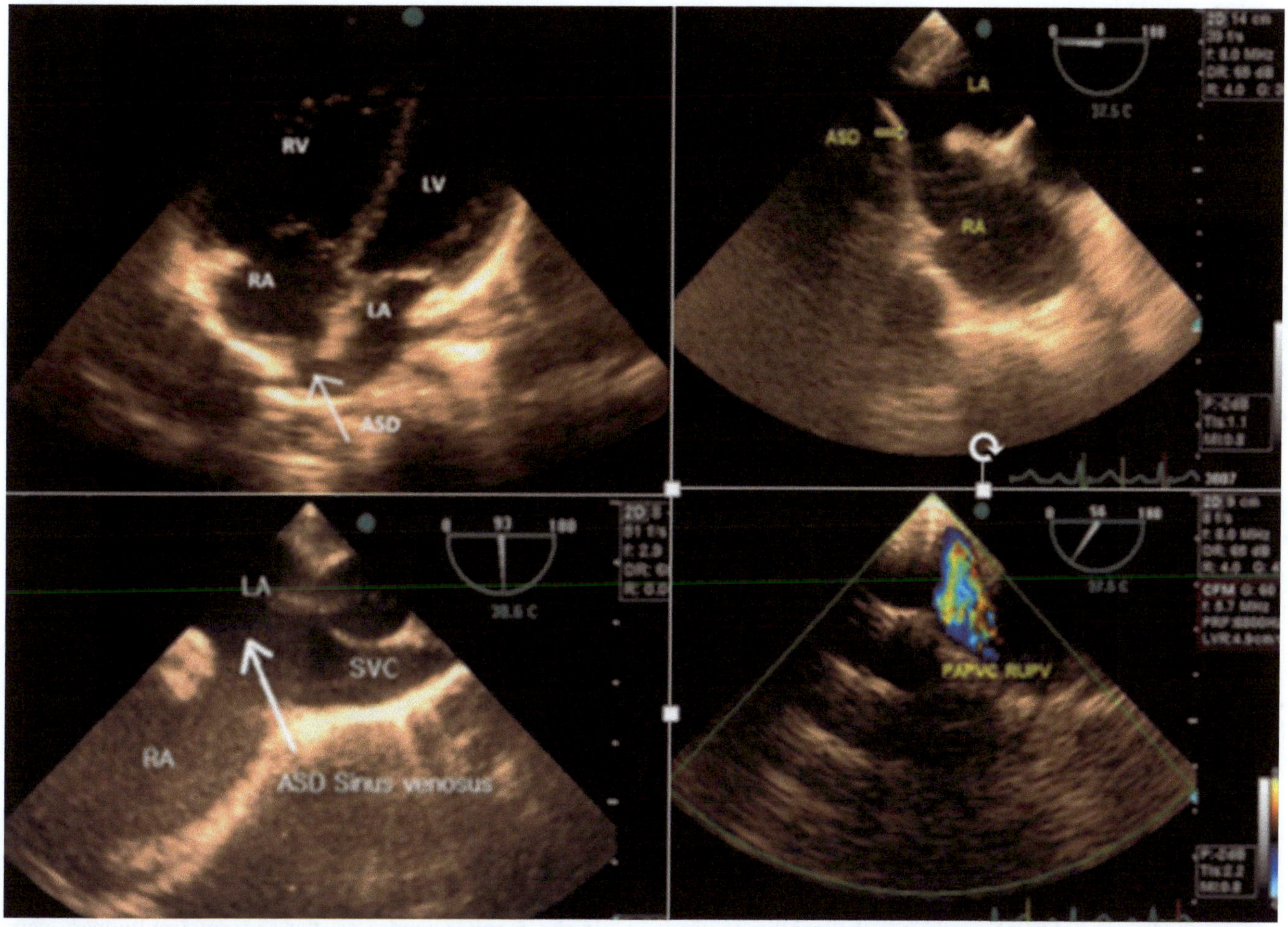

Fig. 28.19 Left upper: Transthoracic echocardiography (TTE), showing an atrial septal defect (*ASD*) located at the superior region of the interatrial septum adjacent to the to the right pulmonary veins. Right upper: Transesophageal echocardiography (TEE) (0°) in high esophageal view, demonstrating a two-dimensional defect at the superior vena cava to the right atrium and left atrium junction. Left lower: bicaval view (90°), confirming the sinus venous-type atrial septal defect diagnosis. *RA* right atrium, *LA* left atrium, *SVC* superior vena cava, *ASD* atrial septal defect. Right lower: Color Doppler imaging, showing abnormal drainage of the right upper pulmonary vein to the right atrium. *PAPVC* partial anomalous pulmonary venous connection, *RUPV* right upper pulmonary vein

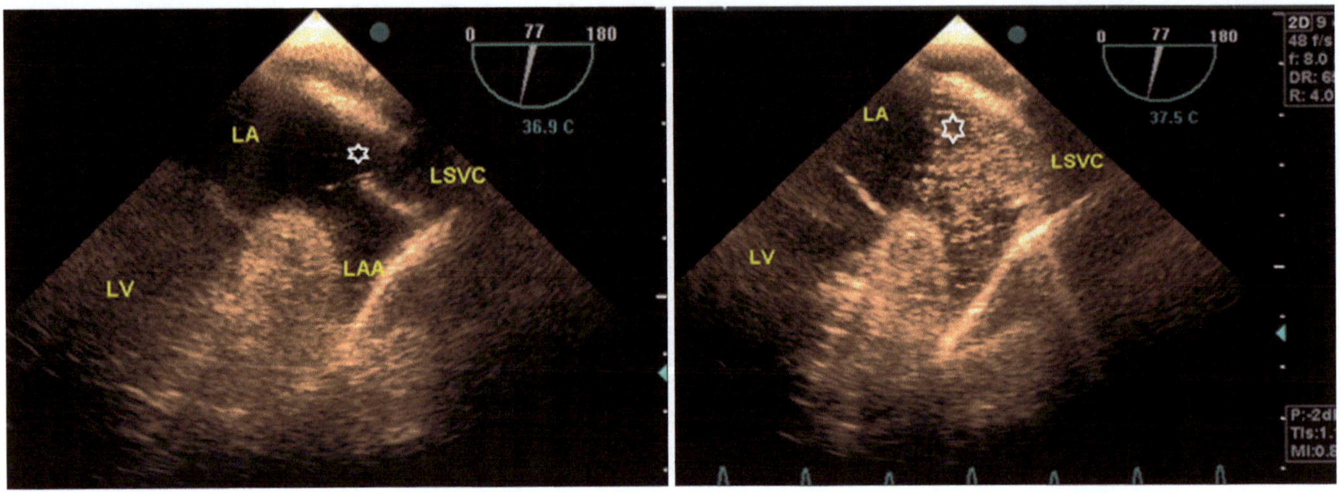

Fig. 28.20 Completely unroofed CS with direct connection of left SVC (star) to LA (left) and confirmed by left arm agitated saline contrast injection (right)

Coronary Sinus-Type ASD

- The unroofed coronary sinus (CS) is a communication between the CS and the LA. The most common anomaly related to this type of the ASD is the left SVC.
- The unroofed CS is classified into four types: type I, completely unroofed CS with the left SVC
- (Fig. 28.20); type II, completely unroofed CS without the left SVC; type III, partial unroofed mid-portion of the CS; and type IV, partial unroofed terminal portion [18–20, 22, 23].
- The clinical presentation is largely determined by the size of the defect and the degree of left-to- right shunting. These cases might not exhibit important symptoms, though some may even develop clinically important symptoms of congestive heart failure. The symptoms that occasionally happen in the CS ASD comprise mild exercise intolerance, frequent respiratory infections, exertional dyspnea, systemic emboli, cerebral abscess, transient ischemic attacks, supraventricular arrhythmias, and cyanosis.
- The unroofed CS is regularly seen in association with other congenital heart diseases. Apart from the left SVC, other kinds of congenital heart disease such as cor triatriatum, pulmonary atresia, tetralogy of Fallot, and partial anomalous pulmonary venous connection (PAPVC) have also been reported in cases with CS defects [20, 21, 26, 27].
- TTE is typically used as the first imaging modality for a suspected unroofed CS. Nonetheless, the inability to visualize the posterior cardiac structures such as the CS and the pulmonary veins is a major disadvantage of TTE. In contrast, TEE may evaluate these posterior structures more accurately, especially in mid-esophageal long-axis views, and may confirm the anomaly [18, 19, 24].
- Importantly, in echocardiography, a large CS orifice with signs of atrial shunting might specify a defect in the roof of the CS. As a result, the entire CS roof must be imaged when this is suspected. Cardiac catheterization may confirm the diagnosis. When a CS defect is a related disease that causes right-to-left shunting, the orifice of the CS might not be enlarged, and the defect might not be documented until after definitive surgery and the occurrence of left-to-right shunting [19–21, 23].

Partial Anomalous Pulmonary Venous Connection (PAPVC)

- Echocardiography plays an important role in the detection of the PAPVC and the related hemodynamic effects on the chambers (e.g., RV enlargement with paradoxical septal motion in the important left-to-right shunting).
- When there is left-sided PAPVC with connection to the innominate vein through the vertical vein, the suprasternal long-axis view is very useful (Fig. 28.21). In the suprasternal long-axis view, leftward angulation may identify the left vertical vein as a red color flow toward the innominate vein. The left vertical vein connects the left pulmonary veins to the innominate vein, which drains into the SVC [21, 28]. TEE might also be useful in the diagnosis of the PAPVC.
- In the scimitar syndrome, the abnormal pulmonary vein drainage is observed in the subcostal view during the evaluation of the IVC (Fig. 28.22). It is also likely to detect the stenosis of the pulmonary vein. In PAPVC to CS, what may frequently be seen is a dilated CS [20, 21, 27, 28].

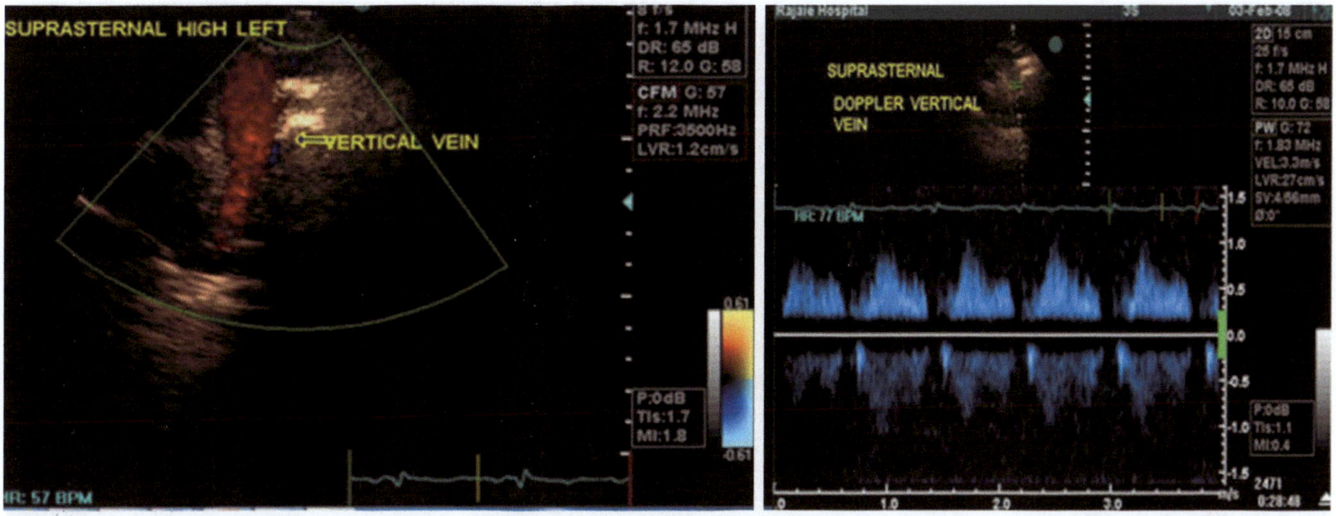

Fig. 28.21 Vertical vein in supra sternal view

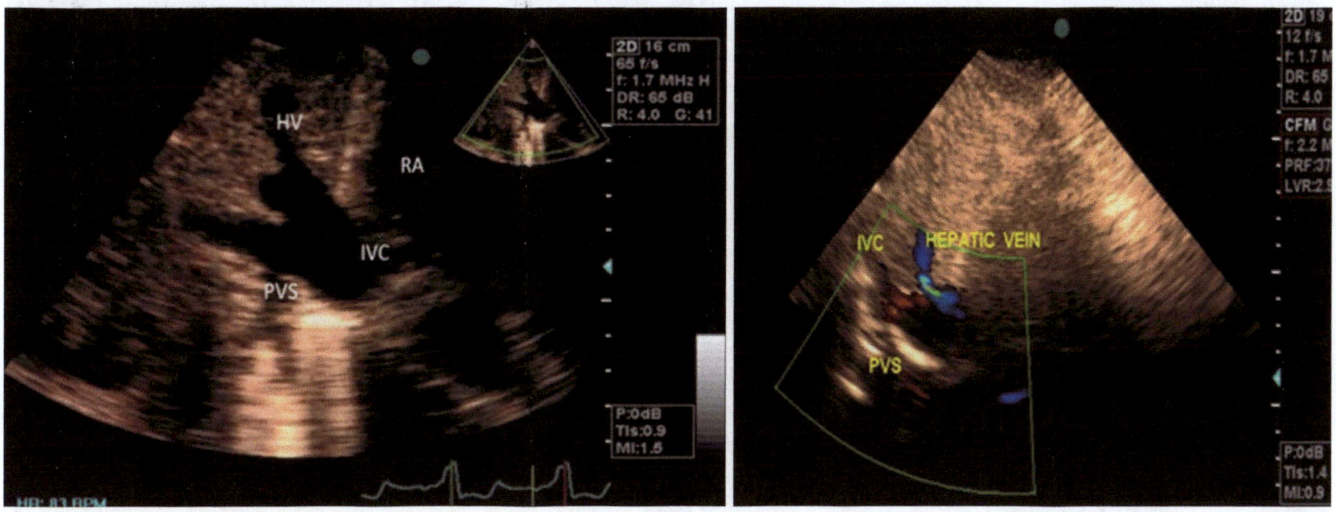

Fig. 28.22 Subcostal view showing abnormal pulmonary vein drainage to the inferior vena cava suggestive for scimitar syndrome. *PVs* pulmonary veins, *HV* hepatic vein, *RA* right atrium, *IVC* inferior vena cava

Total Anomalous Pulmonary Venous Connection (TAPVC)

- In TAPVC, all pulmonary veins drains to the right atrium (RA) instead of connect directly to the morphologic left atrium. Consequently, all of the pulmonary veins and systemic veins drains to the RA directly or using varied routes. In the PAPVC, at least one pulmonary vein connects normally to the LA.
- Echocardiography in the TAPVC demonstrates an enlarged RV and a small LA. The common pulmonary venous chamber, which receives all the pulmonary veins, does not enter the LA (Fig. 28.23). Instead, this confluence chamber enters the vertical vein and lastly drains into the SVC. This is the most common type of the TAPVC, which is known as "the supracardiac type".
- In all types of the TAPVC, an obligatory right-to-left shunt is almost always present. All the aforementioned types may be diagnosed by echocardiography [20–22, 28, 29]. When the pattern of the Doppler venous flow of the abdominal veins is obtained, the finding of the venous flow away from the heart is pathognomonic of the TAPVC below the diaphragm. Regularly, shunting happens almost exclusively from the RA to the LA, at the atrial level. Occasionally, in the anomalous pulmonary venous return, echocardiographic views are limited and magnetic resonance imaging (MRI) or computed tomography (CT) might be necessary [20, 21, 27, 28].

MRI and fast CT scan may also assist with defining pulmonary venous drainage and connection.

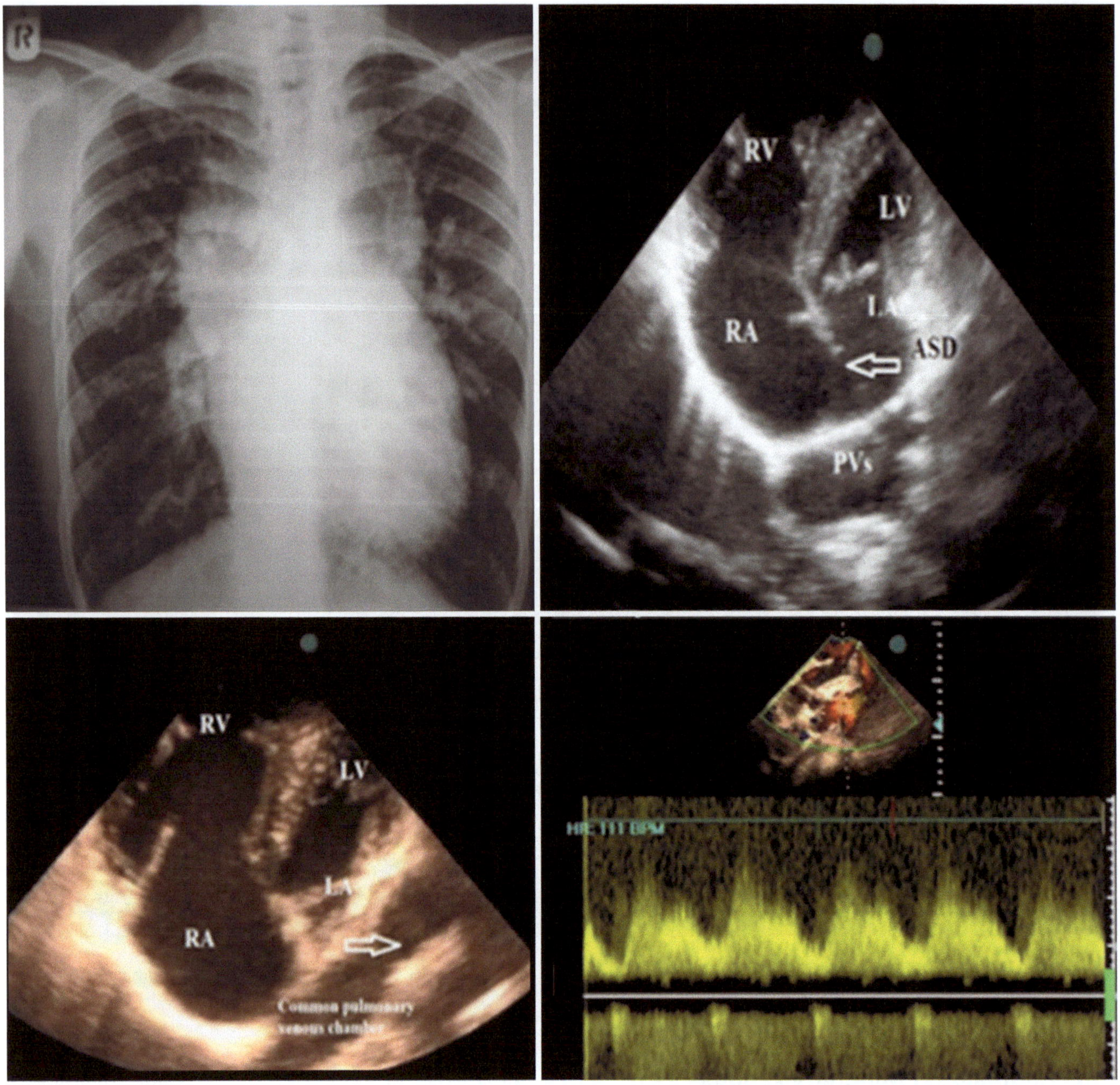

Fig. 28.23 (Movies 28.1, 28.2, 28.3 and 28.4) Left upper: typical snowman appearance in the chest X-ray. The left sided dilated vertical vein, the prominent innominate vein on the top and the right sided superior vena cava; all together give form to a specific image called "Snowman sign" or figure of eight. Enlarged right side chambers, small left atrium, common pulmonary venous chamber just behind the left atrium with no connection to the left atrium (as this confluence chamber enters the vertical vein) and associated ASD which is obligatory for TAPVC. Doppler study demonstrating the typical low velocity pulmonary vein flow pattern

Patent Foramen Ovale (PFO)

- PFO is a flap-like opening in the atrium between the septum primum and secundum at the site of the fossa ovalis that persists after 1 year of age. In some cases, the PFO is detectable with color-flow Doppler imaging in TTE. A small flame of the color flow might be seen in the middle area of the inter-atrial septum.
- Agitated saline contrast TTE is frequently needed to detect small PFOs. After achieving optimal visualization of the inter-atrial septum on TTE or TEE, a bolus of agitated saline is injected into an antecubital vein. Then, microbubbles appear in the RA. The study is positive for the PFO when the microbubbles appear in the LA within three cardiac cycles of their appearance in the RA (Fig. 28.24) (Movies 28.5, 28.6 and 28.7) [30–32].

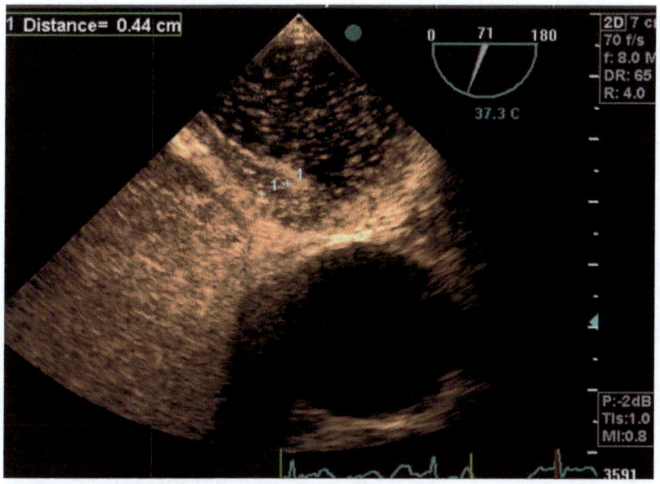

Fig. 28.24 Agitated-saline injection into an ante-cubital vein showing many bubble passages from interatrial septum within three cardiac cycles of their appearance in the RA suggestive of PFO

The Valsalva maneuver increases RA pressure and accelerates right-to-left shunting. 2D TEE with contrast provides greater visualization of the inter-atrial septum and is, thus, preferred to contrast TTE for detecting the PFO. When clinically indicated, 2D TEE with contrast is strongly suggested for cases whose findings on TTE are negative. A 3D TEE confers direct visualization of the entire inter-atrial septum, PFO anatomy, and adjacent structures [31, 32]·

Isolated Ventricular Septal Defect (VSD)

- Echocardiography is the principal diagnostic technique used in both diagnosis and study of disease severity. Large VSDs are easily detected by 2D echocardiography, while small VSDs might be difficult to visualize.
- Most VSDs in adults have small flows; subsequently, a complete 2D and color-flow imaging study besides physical examination would be useful. Key findings on echocardiographic examination contain the number of the defects, location of the defects, chamber size, ventricular function, severity of left ventricular (LV) volume overload, presence or absence of AV prolapse and/or regurgitation especially in the case of outlet (supracristal) and high perimembranous VSDs, presence or absence of right ventricular outflow tract (RVOT) or left ventricular outflow tract (LVOT) obstruction, presence or absence of tricuspid regurgitation, and estimated pulmonary artery pressure. VSDs that are categorized earlier will be described based on the adjacent structure as follows:

A. **Perimembranous VSD,** which is the most common type of VSDs, is seen adjacent to the AV and the tricuspid valve (TV). Frequently it is imaged in the parasternal view (both long-axis and short-axis), apical five-chamber view, and subcostal view.

B. **Subarterial or doubly committed VSD,** which is more common in the Asian population, is seen adjacent to both the AV and the pulmonic valve (doubly committed VSD) in the short-axis view.

C. **Inlet-type VSD** is frequently seen as a part of the AVSD, though it may be seen as an isolated defect. It is adjacent to both the MV and the TV and best seen in the apical four-chamber view and the short-axis view.

D. **Muscular-type VSD**, which is surrounded by muscle, is located anterior, posterior, apical, or mid-muscular. Occasionally the muscular VSD has multiple defects known as the "Swiss cheese" septum. The detection of muscular VSDs needs precise sweeping of the whole septum by 2D and color Doppler study.

The estimation of RV systolic pressure from the tricuspid regurgitation jet, VSD jet, and/or septal configuration must also be performed.

Echocardiographic evaluation of the VSD consists of the precise sweeping of the whole septum by 2D and color-flow imaging from the base to apex in multiple views (Fig. 28.25).

Atrioventricular Septal Defect (AVSD)

- Atrio-ventricular Septal Defect (AVSD) consist of a group of anomalies with the common main pathology of the absence of the Atrio-ventricular (AV) septum associated with the abnormalities of the AV valves.
- In echocardiographic studies, all of the cases show AVSDs. Cases with a common AV valve have five leaflet patterns: two (right and left) anterosuperior leaflets, two (right and left) lateral leaflets, and one common posterior leaflet. Hearts with two AV valves reveal a pattern of three leaflets [19].
- The classification of the Rastelli type in AVSDs with a common AV valve and a VSD is determined by the mode of the insertion of the left and right anterior leaflets. In the common valve, echocardiographic findings show ostium primum ASDs and VSDs. In the Rastelli type A, the chordae tendineae of the anterior leaflets attach to the crest of the ventricular septum; the apical four-chamber echocardiographic view shows the confluent septal defects, common AV junction with the attachment of the anterior leaflets in the crest of the septum, and VSD; and the VSD is continuous with the ostium primum. Type B of complete AVSDs, which is rare, is characterized by chordal attachments from the left AV valve to the papillary muscles in the RV. In a Rastelli type C defect, the superior bridging leaflet is said to be "free floating" because it is undivided and unattached to the crest of the VSD (Fig. 28.26) [19–21].

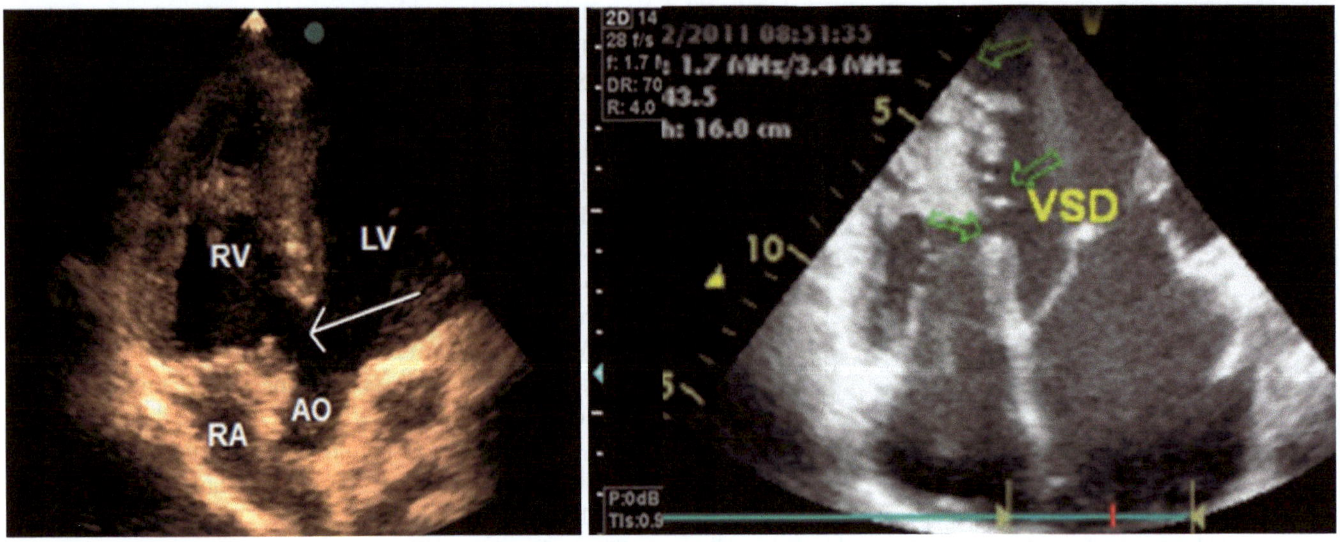

Fig. 28.25 Left: Transthoracic echocardiography in five chamber view showing large perimembranous VSD (white arrow). Right: Transthoracic echocardiography in four chamber view showing multiple mid muscular VSD (Swiss cheese "septum) associated with left heart enlargement

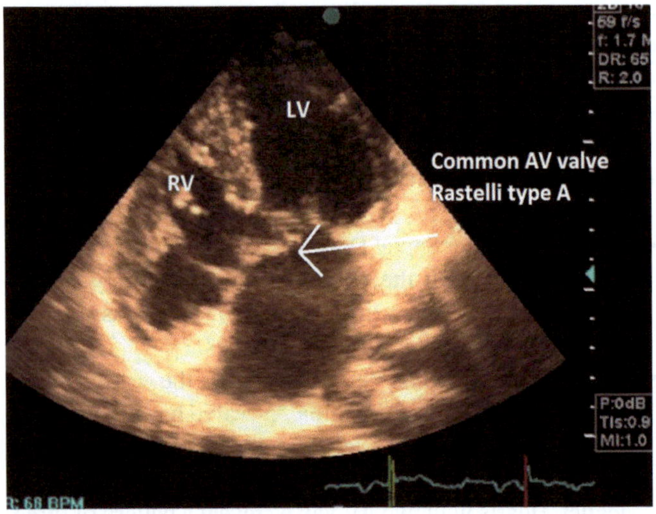

Fig. 28.26 In echocardiography studies in complete AVSDs, the common AV valve might be positioned equally over both ventricles (balanced) or unequally over the RV or the LV (unbalanced). MV abnormalities are seen in the complete forms of the AVSD. LVOT obstruction might happen in all forms of the AVSD, and it is more common when there are two AV valve orifices than a common orifice. The evaluation of the LVOT is performed in the apical four-chamber echocardiographic view [18, 19, 22]

Patent Ductus Arteriosus (PDA)

- The ductus arteriosus links the proximal left pulmonary artery to the descending aorta, just beneath to the left subclavian artery (LSCA).
- In adults, direct visualization of PDAs might be difficult as they frequently have larger body habitus. However, the hemodynamic effects on the LA and the LV, color-flow imaging, and Doppler study in the parasternal short-axis and suprasternal view are important keys for diagnosis (Fig. 28.27). The detection of the diastolic ductal flow in the pulmonary artery along the lateral wall of the main pulmonary artery has high sensitivity and specificity for the diagnosis of a PDA [18, 19].
- Echocardiography might be normal or demonstrate RV or LV hypertrophy or both. LV dilation or dysfunction depends on the volume of left-to-right shunting and the degree of the related pulmonary arterial hypertension. In echocardiography, the PDA might be imaged completely and its size well estimated. Furthermore, Doppler study proves the shunt and documents an accurate study of the mean pulmonary artery pressure. The measurements of LA and LV size provide indirect evidence of the degree of left-to-right shunting [18, 21, 23, 33]. This determines the presence, size, and degree of shunting and also the physiological outcomes of the shunt. The PDA is seen with difficulty in an Eisenmenger context. A bubble study might assist in the diagnosis of the communication [19, 21].

Truncus Arteriosus

- In persistent truncusarteriosus (TA) a single vessel makes the outlet of both ventricles and supplies the systemic, pulmonary, and coronary arteries
- Regularly 2D echocardiography establishes a complete diagnosis. The study must demonstrate the overriding truncal root, origin site of the pulmonary arteries, number of the truncal valve cusps, origin site of the coronary

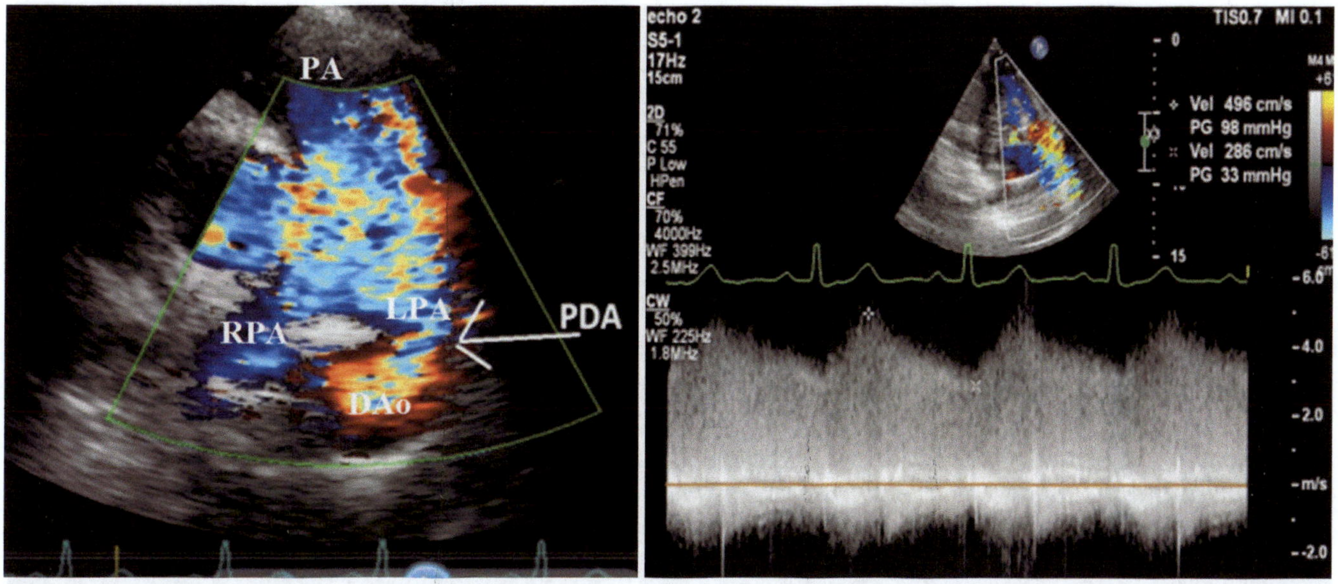

Fig. 28.27 Left: Color Doppler flow imaging in parasternal short-axis view showing high velocity continuous turbulent flow entering to the pulmonary artery (PA) near the LPA origine. Right: Continuous wave Doppler tracing showing high velocity continuous (systolic and diastolic) turbulent flow across the PDA with late systolic peak velocity

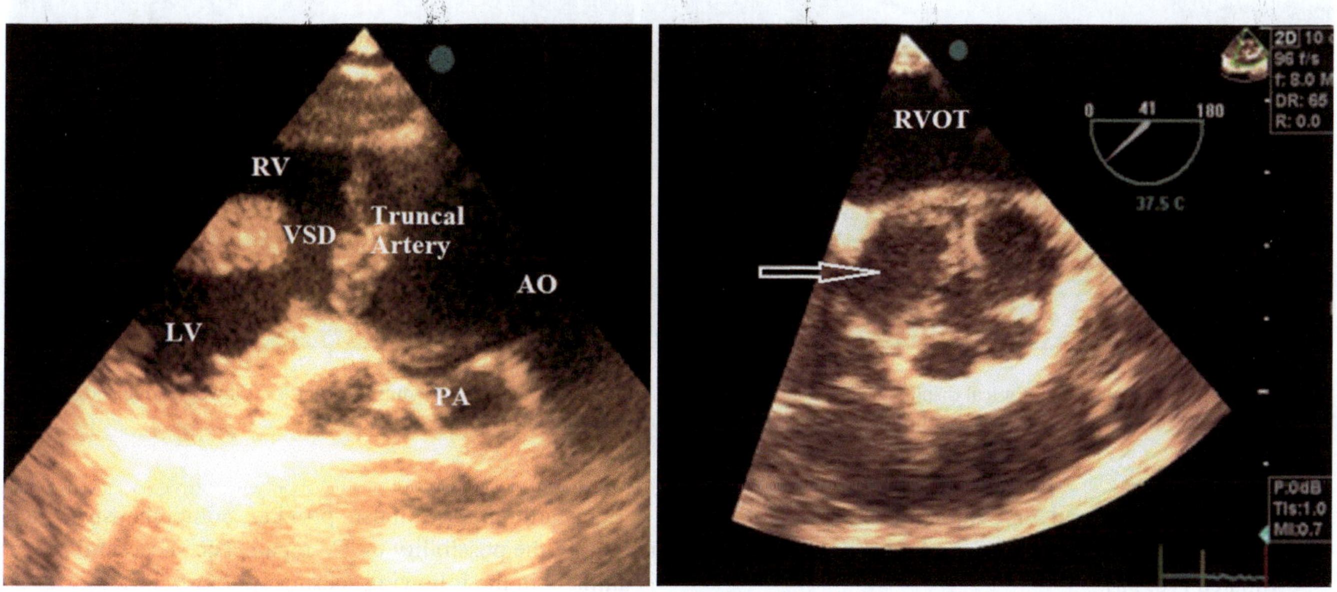

Fig. 28.28 Transthoracic echocardiography parasternal long axis view showing VSD, overriding aorta and truncal valve artery which is quadricuspid

arteries, regurgitation and stenosis of the truncal valve, and size of the concomitant VSD (Fig. 28.28).

- Additionally, we may study all the other related lesions. The semilunar valve of the truncal artery is frequently abnormal. Regularly, the valve leaflet is thickened.
- It is tricuspid in 61% and quadricuspid in 31% of the cases. In echocardiography, the truncus arteriosus must be distinguished from the tetralogy of Fallot and pulmonary atresia as both have a large VSD and overriding arterial vessels on them [19, 23, 34].

The Ebstein Anomaly

- The diagnosis of the Ebstein anomaly is mostly made by echocardiography. The apical displacement of the septal leaflet of the TV by 8 mm/m^2 or more, with an elongated sail-like appearance of the anterior TV leaflet, proves the diagnosis. (A 10 mm distance between the mitral annulus and tricuspid annulus is seen in the normal heart).
- The size of the atrialized portion of the RV (recognized between the basic place of the TV annulus and the ventricular attachment of the TV leaflets, which is a part

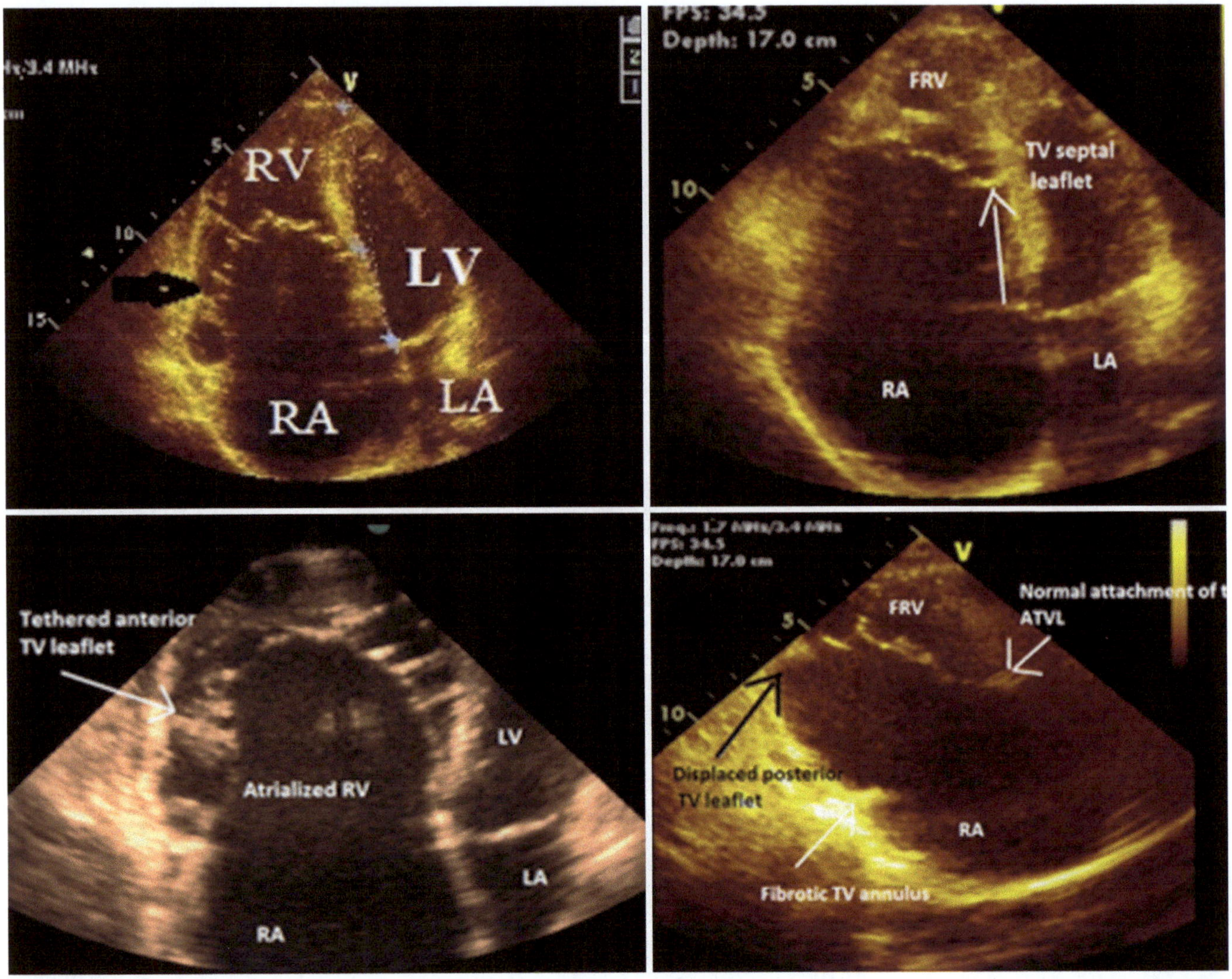

Fig. 28.29 Upper panels: Severe apical displacement of the septal leaflet of the TV compare to the mitral leaflet. Left lower: Elongated sail like appearance of the anterior TV leaflet, right lower severe apical displacement of the posterior leaflet of the TV

of the anatomic RV and serves as a part of the RA) and the systolic performance index of the functional RV may be estimated [18, 35].

- The degree of tricuspid regurgitation and rarely tricuspid stenosis must be evaluated by TTE. Tricuspid regurgitation almost always is present and could be severe. Low-velocity tricuspid regurgitation jets might be difficult to visualize, so careful investigation in different views will be useful. The concomitant displacement of the posterior leaflet must be evaluated by viewing the parasternal RV inflow.

The anterior TV leaflet is never displaced, although it frequently has adherence to the free wall of the RV. Related anomalies such as the ASD and the presence of shunting may also be recognized [18, 35–37].

Echocardiography must provide comprehensive data regarding the possibility of TV repair. The successful repair is unlikely in the following scoring systems:

1. Extensive adherence of the anterior TV leaflet to the RV myocardium. The study is made in the apical four-chamber view. (More than half of the anterior leaflet must be mobile and must be able to move freely for a successful repair.)
2. Ratio of the apical displacement of the septal TV leaflets to the total ventricular septal length more than 0.6 indicates a severe valvular abnormality.
3. Small functional RV means a functional RV less than 35% of the total RV size.
4. Cases with RA and atrialized RV cavity area compared to the sum of the true RV, LA, and LV area more than 1.5 (Fig. 28.29) [37].

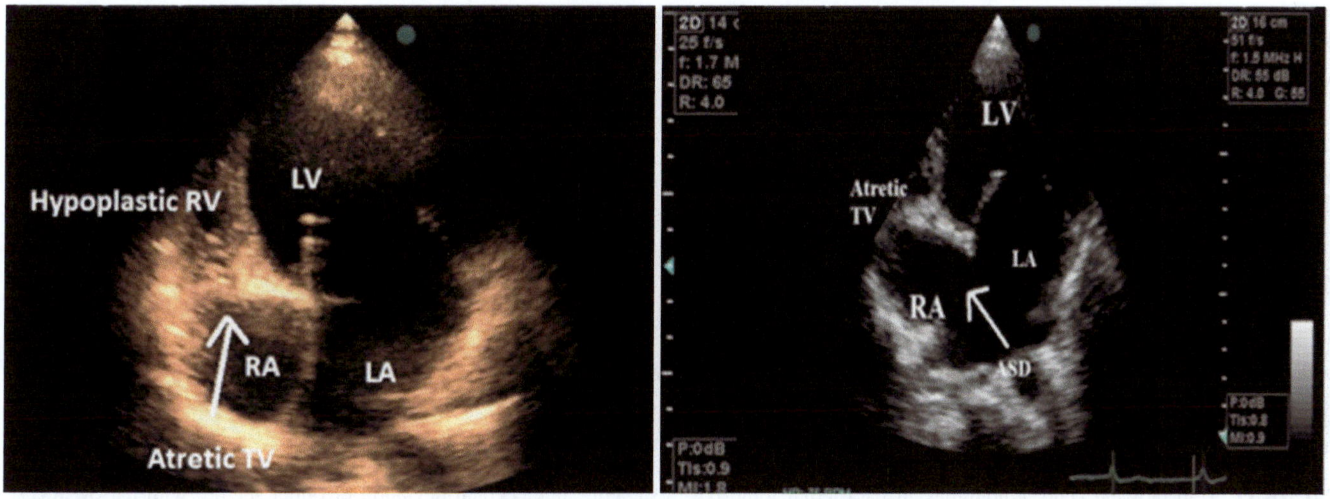

Fig. 28.30 Transthoracic echocardiography in four chamber view showing tricuspid atresia (TA) as a fibromuscular tissue in pace of TV, associated with hypoplastic right ventricle (RV) and large ASD which is an obligatory left to right shunt

Tricuspid Atresia

- Tricuspid atresia (TA) is best defined as the absence of the right atrioventricular valve in the presence of an atrial septal defect Echocardiography provides comprehensive information and confirms the diagnosis.

Typical echocardiographic findings in tricuspid atresia are as follows (Fig. 28.30).

a. Fibromuscular or membranous tissue in the TV annulus with no direct communication between the RA and the RV.
b. Obligatory shunt at the level of the atria (right-to-left shunt from the ASD or the PFO, which is obligatory for survival).
c. Variable degree of RV hypoplasia.
d. Direct communication between the systemic circulation and the pulmonary circulation frequently in the form of a VSD.

- Tricuspid atresia based on the relationship between the great arteries, anatomy of the VSD, and pulmonary valve has been classified as:

Type I: Normally-related great arteries (70–80% of cases and the most common type of tricuspid atresia)

Type II: d-transposition of the great arteries (d-TGA)

Type III: Association with more complex lesions (uncommon form of tricuspid atresia, only 3–6% of cases)

There is a subclassification for types I and II based on the presence and size of the VSD and related pulmonary stenosis or atresia [20, 38].

Tetralogy of Fallot

- Echocardiography confirms the complete diagnosis and typically provides sufficient data for management planning. Echocardiography begins with a comprehensive sequential segmental approach. Frequently the segmental anatomy is normal.
- The study must recognize the malaligned and nonrestrictive VSD, overriding aorta, and existence and severity of RVOT obstruction (infundibular, valvular, and supravalvular as well as pulmonary artery branch stenosis) (Fig. 28.31).
- For further evaluation of the related diseases such as the ASD and the VSD, peripheral pulmonary stenosis cardiac imaging including cardiac MRI and cardiac CT is needed [39–42]. In cases with repaired tetralogy of Fallot, residual pulmonary valve stenosis and regurgitation, residual VSD, RV and LV size and function, aortic root size, and degree of aortic regurgitation must be evaluated. The severity of pulmonary regurgitation in cases with repaired tetralogy of Fallot may be measured by pulsed Doppler echocardiographic study of the antegrade versus retrograde pulmonary blood flow with a short diastolic flow (pressure half-time <100 ms), suggestive of important pulmonary regurgitation. This grade of severity may result in a large volume of pulmonary regurgitation and RV dilatation; however, it might also be related to normal or only mildly enlarged RV due to a so-called "RV restrictive physiology" [21, 40–43].
- RV dilatation might also be due to severe residual RVOT obstruction or due to surgical scar (in transventricular surgical approach). Important tricuspid regurgitation may

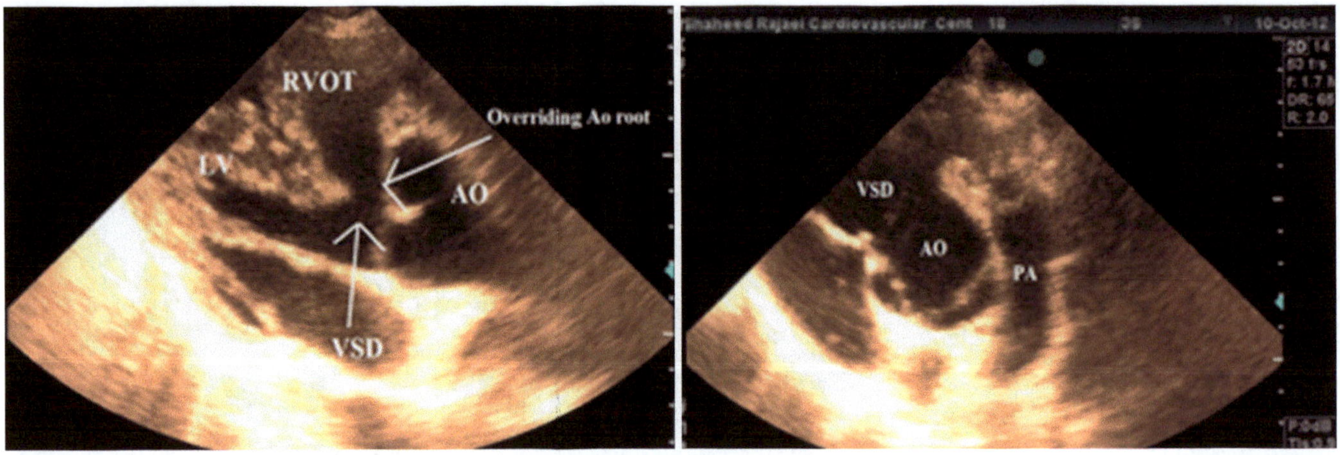

Fig. 28.31 Transthoracic echocardiography in parasternal long axis view showing Overriding aorta on the crest of the ventricular septum and associated VSD. Typical parasternal short axis view in TOF patient showing anterocephal deviation of outlet septum with narrow RVOT and large sub aortic VSD

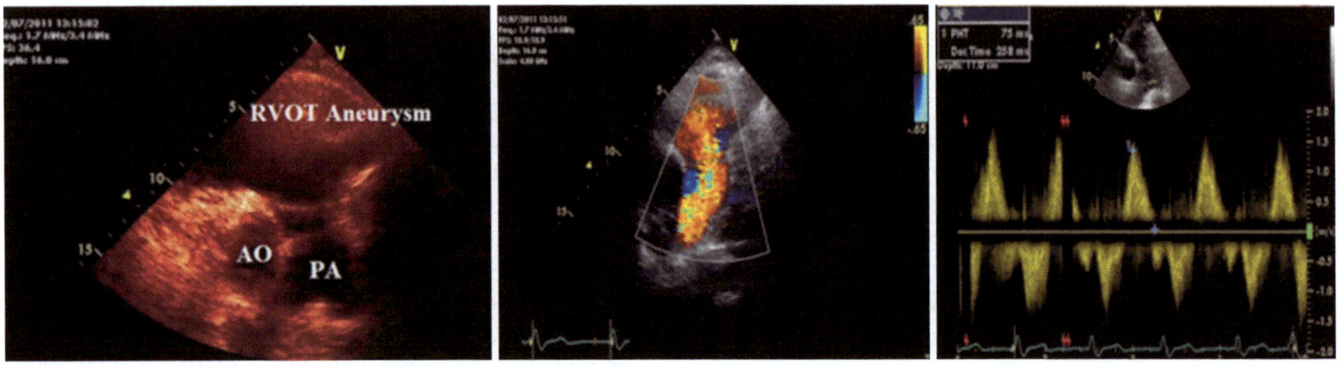

Fig. 28.32 Left*:* Aneurysmal RVOT in completely repaired tetralogy of Fallot patient due to trans annular patch repair. Middle: A typical Patient with history of repaired TOF. *Right*: severe pulmonary regurgitation by color flow imaging and Doppler study

happen in consequence to RV dilatation, which begets more RV dilatation.

- Aneurysmal dilatation of the RVOT is moderately common in cases with previous pericardial transannular patch repair surgery and substantial pulmonary regurgitation. Aneurysmal dilatation of the RVOT may be related to regional RV hypokinesis and might be the arrhythmogenic nidus of sustained ventricular tachycardia. Infrequently LV dysfunction may be detected by echocardiography from a variety of factors [20, 43–45] (Fig. 28.32).

Double-Outlet Right Ventricle

Double outlet right ventricle (DORV) is a cardiac malformation in which more than 50% of each semilunar valve arises from the morphologic right ventricle (RV).

The common features of the DORV are (Fig. 28.33):

I. Overriding of the Aorta more than 50% on the right ventricle
II. Mitral- aortic discontinuity
III. VSD which is found in most cases
IV. Variable amount of conal septum under the semilunar valves

- Three main subtypes of DORV exist:
  a. DORV with a sub-aortic VSD;
  b. DORV with a sub-pulmonary VSD
  c. DORV with a non-committed VSD.
- Echocardiography is the cornerstone of diagnosis. The location of the VSD and the relationship of the great arteries to the VSD are the leading keys to diagnosis and management. The relation between the semilunar valves and the ventricles must be determined carefully. It must be mentioned that in cases with subaortic stenosis, the echocardiographic examination must contain the study for the abnormalities of the aortic arch.

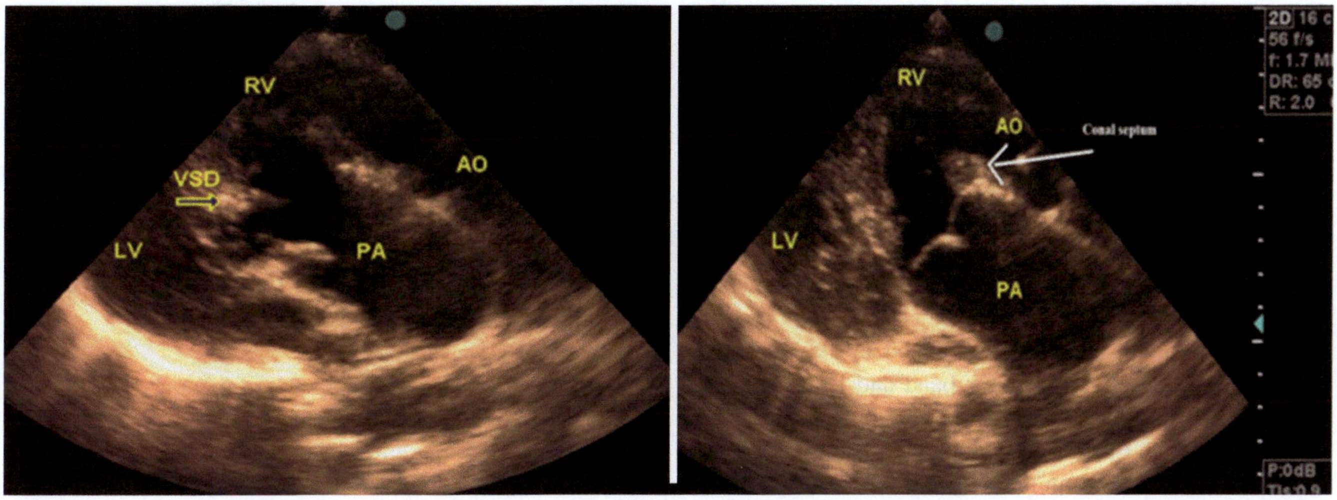

Fig. 28.33 The location of the VSD in relation to the great arteries is shown, Sub pulmonic VSD and DORV. Transthoracic echocardiography in off axis view showing both great arteries arise from the hypertrophied right ventricle, white arrow shows conal septum (arrow)

Subpulmonary stenosis is regularly present in a double-outlet RV with a subpulmonary VSD. Additionally, potential AV valve anomalies must always be considered [20, 21, 46].

Double-Inlet Ventricular and Univentricular Heart

In double inlet left ventricle (DILV) or single ventricle, both atria feed into the LV (two separated atrio-ventricular ostia open in a morphological LV). The right ventricle (RV) is hypoplastic or sometimes doesn't exist with the following Key points of morphology in single ventricle:

Atrial arrangement	Situs solitus, inversus, left isomerism or right isomerism
Atrio-ventricular connection	Double inlet ventricle: Two patent valves linking to one ventricle (>50% of both atria and valves joined to this ventricle)
	Common valve (e.g. un-balanced atrio-ventricular septal defect)
	One atretic valve (mitral or tricuspid atresia)
	One or two straddling valves
Ventricles	Dominant LV, dominant RV or rarely indeterminate (defined AV valve arrangement, position, trabecular pattern)
	Left heart hypoplastic syndrome
VA connection	Concordant, discordant, double-outlet
Systemic venous return	Heterotaxy syndromes with variable venous return patterns
Pulmonary circulation	Stenotic, atretic or normal (un-protected)
Pulmonary venous return	Anomalous pulmonary venous drainage
Conduction system	Sinus node variable in isomerism
	AV node and Hiss variations
Associated lesions	Cardiac including aortic arch abnormalities and coarctation of aorta
	Non cardiac: variations in bronchial situs, abdominal abnormalities including asplenia, multiple spleens, biliary atresia

- 2D echocardiography is a diagnostic tool for the single ventricle. As was noted before, based on the 50% rule, a chamber may be termed "ventricle" if it receives 50% or more of the inlet, even if this inlet is an imperforate fibrotic membrane and is situated over a small RV—as is the case in tricuspid atresia. Note that a chamber need not have an outlet in order to be termed "ventricle" [20, 47]. The AV connection and also ventriculoarterial alignment must be evaluated by echocardiography carefully.
- The two most common types of the single ventricle are the L-looped single ventricle with LV morphology with transposition of the great arteries (TGA) and subpulmonary stenosis and a D-looped single LV with TGA and subpulmonary stenosis. The third most prevalent form is L-looped single LV with TGA and aortic arch hypoplasia. The fourth most common type is D-looped single LV with normally allied great arteries (aorta originating from the LV and the pulmonary artery from the outlet chamber), which is occasionally referred to as "a Holmes heart" [48, 49].

Congenitally Corrected TGA

- Congenitally corrected transposition of the great arteries (ccTGA) is an anomaly with discordant atrio-ventricular (AV) and ventriculo-arterial (VA) connections.
- Echocardiography allows the detailed diagnosis of the basic anomaly as well as of any related lesions. The right-sided morphologic LV is defined by its smooth endocardium and has a bileaflet MV with no direct attachment to the septum.
- The morphologic RV is characterized by its apical trabeculation and also moderator band and has a trileaflet apically displaced AV valve (TV) with direct septal attachment. An Ebstein-like anomaly of the TV is defined as an excessive (>8 mm/m^2 body surface area) apical displacement of the TV, with or without dysplasia [20, 47, 50] (Fig. 28.34).
- Associated lesions happen in up to 95% of cc-TGA patients including
- VSD (in 75%), pulmonary valvular and sub valvular stenosis (in 75%), and left-sided TV anomalies (in >75%).

Complete Transposition of the Great Arteries (d-TGA) and the Senning and Mustard Procedures

- Complete Transposition of the Great Arteries (d-TGA) **is a** cyanotic congenital heart defect and characterized by atrio-ventricular concordance and ventriculo-arterial

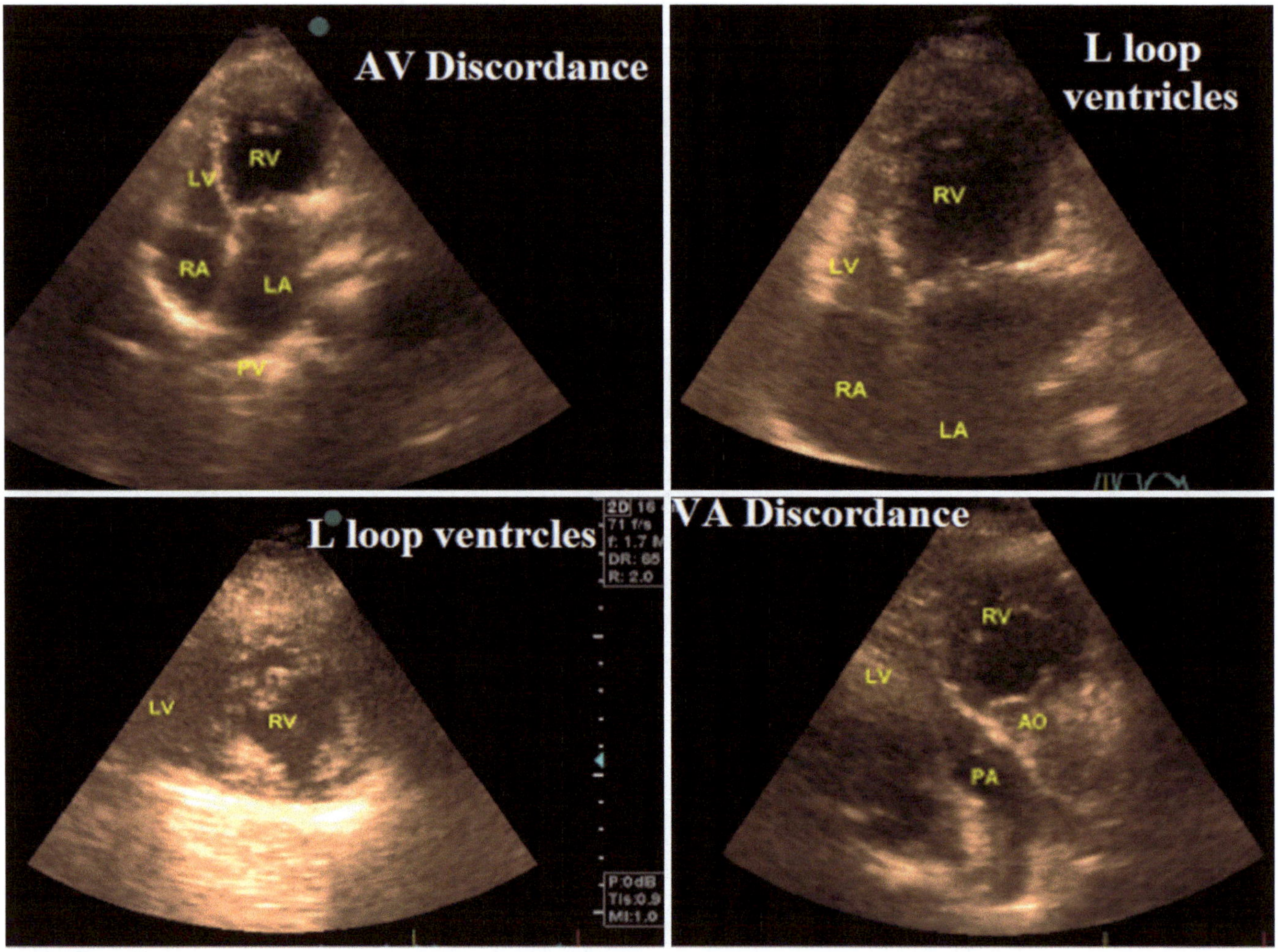

Fig. 28.34 Left panels: Transthoracic echocardiography in four chamber and short axis view showing L-loop ventricle and Right panels: Atrioventricular and ventriculoarterial discordance

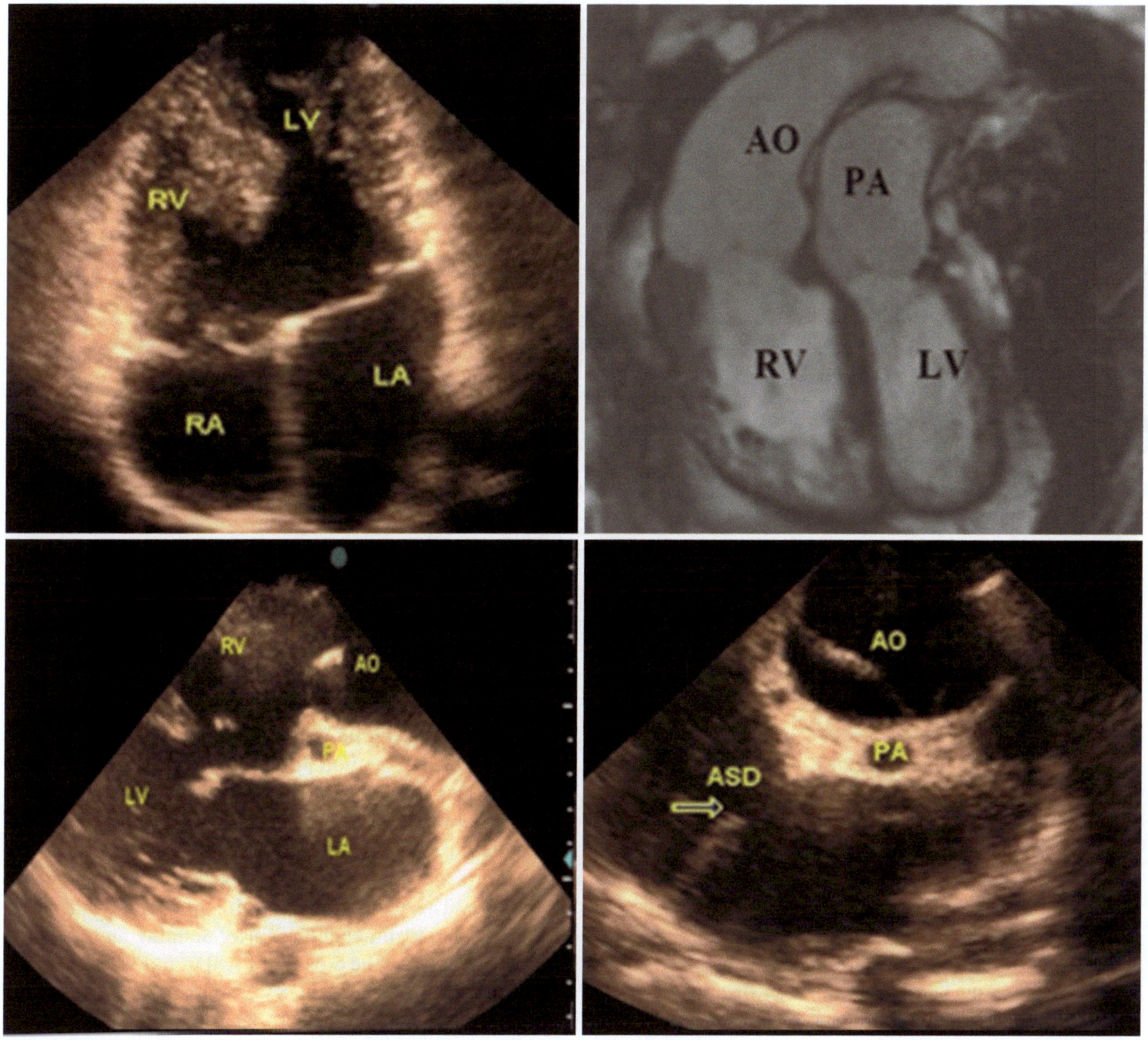

Fig. 28.35 Apical four chamber view showing D-Loop ventricle associated with a large VSD. D-Loop ventricle associated with transposed great arteries and anterior located aorta (AO). CMR reliably demonstrates the ventricular and arterial looping besides the ventricular size and function D -loop transposed great arteries as anterior aorta and posterior pulmonary artery associated with ASD

discordance. In most patients, the apex of the heart points to the left (levo-cardia). The aorta is usually located anterior and rightward to the pulmonary artery, but any relationship between great arteries is possible (Fig. 28.35).

- In d-TGA patients who undergo repair via the atrial baffle procedure, comprehensive echocardiographic imaging is needed in a regional adult congenital heart disease center to evaluate the anatomy and hemodynamics.
- The SVC anastomosis is patent if the contrast injected into a peripheral arm vein promptly enters the systemic venous chamber. In obstruction at the SVC, the azygos or the other collaterals to the IVC will cause contrast to first enter the IVC and then the SVC. IVC

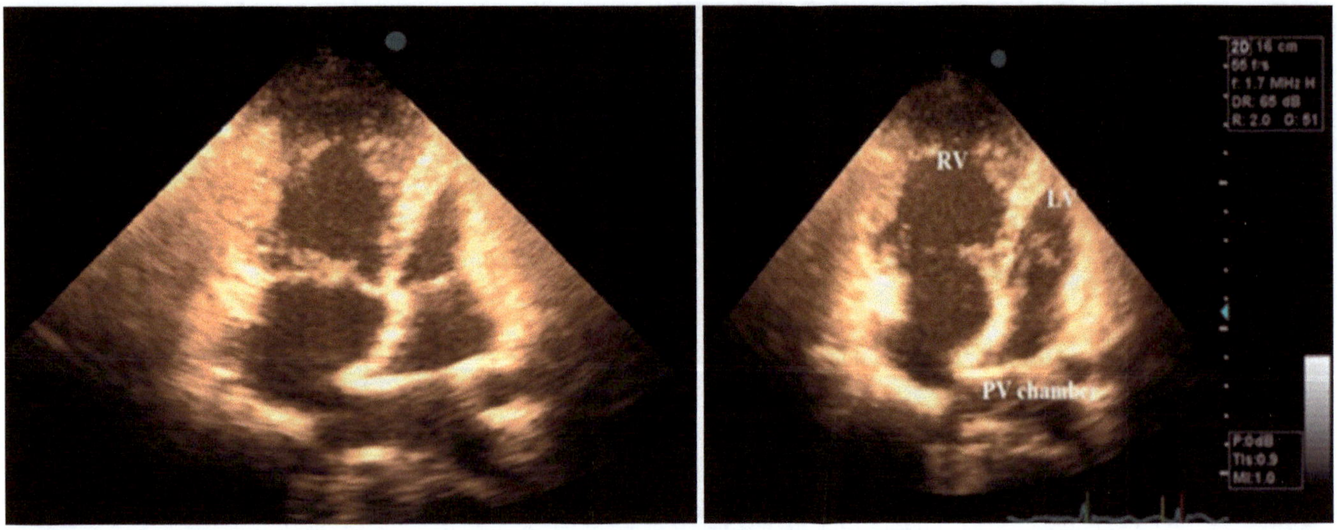

Fig. 28.36 Transthoracic echocardiography in four chamber view showing pulmonary venous chamber drains to the morphologic RV with no obstruction in 2D study

obstruction might cause hepatic congestion or even cirrhosis.

 - Baffle leaks happen in up to 25% of cases.
 - Pulmonary venous obstruction might also happen, although it is less common.
 - In many mature cases, the SVC pathway is not visible on any surface scans and TEE is required to evaluate this pathway.

- The apical four-chamber view is frequently the most informative initial scan by 2D, color-flow imaging, Doppler, and also contrast study. Contrast injection helps detect baffle leaks, which commonly happen after atrial switch. The most common early structural complications include baffle obstruction, which most commonly affects the superior limb rather than the IVC and might result in the SVC syndrome [18, 21, 51, 52].
- Color-flow imaging is useful to confirm the laminar flow through the reconstruction and to detect stenosis or residual shunts (Fig. 28.36).

• Successful procedures have a larger RV resembling the LV with a small LV resembling the RV.

• Vena cava and pulmonary venous obstruction (defined as turbulent non-phasic flow in the baffles with a peak velocity >1 m/s and a mean pressure gradient >2–3 mmHg) is best evaluated from the apical four-chamber view. The study of RV function is challenging, and the most commonly used modality is still 2D TTE, though it is qualitative rather than quantitative due to the complex geometry and anatomy of the RV. Other echo-Doppler parameters may also be measured such as the myocardial performance index and the dP/dT (by the use of the TV regurgitant velocity). Nowadays, a tissue Doppler measurement of myocardial acceleration during isovolumic contraction (isovolumic myocardial acceleration) has been reported and may be a sensitive, reliable, and noninvasive method for studying RV contractility, which is less load dependent than the other echocardiographic parameters. Other imaging modalities consist of radionuclide methods and angiography or MRI [18, 20, 21]. Contrast echocardiography is also used in postoperative study. The technique is useful in identifying patch leaks and also residual defects after Senning and Mustard operations or after the closure of ASDs and VSDs and for assessing the patency of the SVC course and anastomosis sites. Most cases are found to have no SVC obstruction by contrast echocardiography after the Senning or Mustard procedure [18, 52–54].

Fontan Operation

- The Fontan operation is a palliative surgical procedure for patients suffering from univentricular circulation, although initially it was designed for patients with tricuspid atresia.
- The Fontal operation has several variations that connecting the whole systemic venous return to the pulmonary artery is common point between them .
- Fontal operation consists of the following surgeries:

• Classic Fontan (atriopulmonary connection): It is a direct connection between the right atrium and the pulmonary artery
• Extracardiac Fontan: In this subtype, the inferior vena cava (IVC) is connected to the pulmonary artery using an extracardiac conduit and the superior vena cava (SVC)is connected to the pulmonary artery as in the bidirectional Glenn
• Lateral tunnel: The difference between this subtype and the extracardiac Fontan is that the IVC is connected with a baffle within the right atrium to the right atrial appendage or the lower portion of the SVC, which is connected to the pulmonary artery
• Fenestrated Fontan: In this subtype, a fenestration is created in the atrial patch or baffle allowing right-to-left shunting and decompression of the Fontan circuit and maintaining adequate cardiac output
• Right atrial-right ventricular Fontan: In this operation, a conduit is created between the right atrium and the right ventricle

- Echocardiography generally is the first-line diagnostic modality for the evaluation of Fontan cases and is employed for the study of Fontan connections, fenestrations, baffle leaks, thrombi, pulmonary veins, valvular and ventricular functions, and aortic-to-pulmonary collateral flows. Normally the pulmonary arterial flow is biphasic with one peak in systole and another larger peak in diastole. The velocities are augmented with inspiration. The hepatic veins are always dilated to some extent, especially in the presence of a systemic venous obstruction [52, 55]. Also, TTE may assist in evaluating the systemic ventricle function. Of course, all studies show reduced parameters of systolic and diastolic function—including strain and strain rate and also tissue velocities in all cases with a single-ventricle physiology irrespective of the procedure performed or the patient's condition. AV valve regurgitation is studied by TTE too [19, 56]. The imaging of the classic Fontan by TTE is generally difficult. TEE is frequently done to evaluate the patency of anastomosis sites and to detect thrombi within the RA (Fig. 28.37).
- An extracardiac Fontan is even more difficult to evaluate with echocardiography. SVC and IVC biphasic and pulmonary artery triphasic flow patterns indicate unobstructed flows in the Fontan circuit [56], while a mean gradient between the Fontan circuit and the pulmonary artery of 2 mmHg or more may represent important obstruction.
- Study of the pulmonary vein flow pattern is important in detecting pulmonary vein obstruction (right pulmonary veins >left pulmonary veins) occasionally caused by an enlarged RA. All the above-mentioned characteristics of the Fontan circuit and fenestration may be visualized by 2D and color-flow imaging study via TTE and TEE [18]. Other imaging modalities such as CT and MRI might be used in these cases insofar as they assist with the evaluation of the pulmonary veins, differential pulmonary flow, and collaterals. Cardiac catheterization in Fontan cases may evaluate ventricular and valvular functions, hemodynamics such as pulmonary vascular resistance, and Fontan obstruction.

Congenital AV Stenosis

2D echocardiography delivers detailed information about the morphology of the AV, LV function, and presence or absence of related left-sided lesions. Doppler echocardiography is used to determine the severity of aortic stenosis and the presence of related aortic insufficiency. In addition, comprehensive echocardiographic study must be done for cases with a bicuspid AV. The echocardiographic characteristic features include systolic doming with an eccentric closing line of two visible cusps in the parasternal long-axis view and a single commissural line with two functional cusps in the parasternal short-axis view. Specific care must be taken in studying the valve in both systole and diastole because in some cases

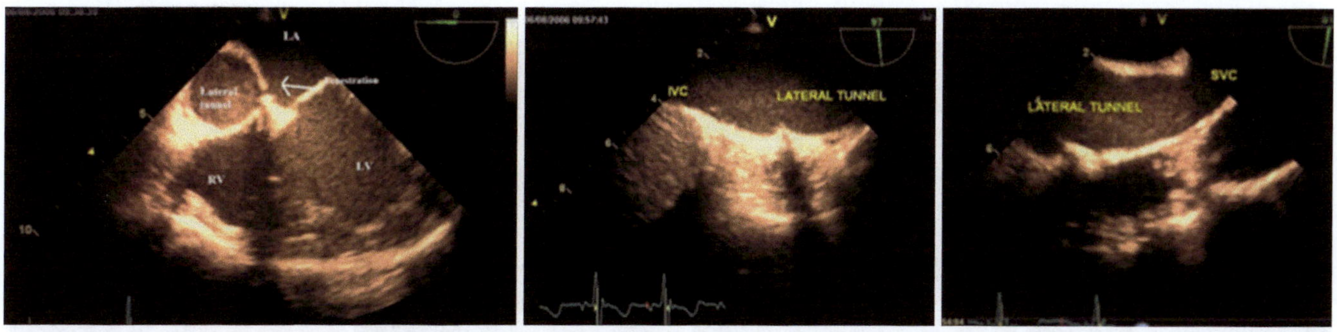

Fig. 28.37 Left: Transesophageal echocardiography showing circular structure which is cross section of the lateral tunnel with significant stagnant flow through it, Transesophageal echocardiography is frequently done to assess the patency of the SVC and IVC anastomosis and to detect any thrombus within the right atrium

with asymmetric leaflets and a noticeable and evident raphe, the valve may seem tricuspid in diastole. Nonetheless, the oval football shape of the systolic appearance of the orifice indicates a bicuspid AV [57–59]. The leaflets regularly are thickened and fibrotic and calcified with increasing age. With extensive calcification, it might be difficult to distinguish a stenotic tricuspid from a bicuspid AV [58, 59]. Further, Doppler provides peak instantaneous gradients that are higher than the peak-to peak gradients derived from cardiac catheterization. Mean gradients as determined by Doppler and catheterization associate closely. Also, importantly, aortic dilation is present in more than half of young cases with a normally functioning bicuspid AV in echocardiographic study.

Subaortic Stenosis

- Echocardiography is the present standard diagnostic instrument in subaortic stenosis. Not only can it confer an accurate delineation of the causes of obstruction, but also it provides comprehensive data regarding related lesions. Generally, the parasternal long-axis view is key to providing a precise diagnosis. The probable presence of mitral aortic discontinuity, distance of a fibromuscular ridge to the AV, occurrence of an accessory obstructive tissue, and sizes of the aortic annulus and root all are well imaged in this view. In addition, color-flow mapping can document the related AV regurgitation. The extension of a fibromuscular ridge to the anterior MV leaflet is best seen in the apical five-chamber view. This also provides the best site for the pulsed-or continuous-wave Doppler study of the maximum gradient across the AV and the LVOT. Aortic regurgitation is seen in 40–60% of cases mostly due to leaflet trauma from the high-velocity subaortic jet. Occasionally, TEE plays a central role in defining the pathology [60–63] (Fig. 28.38).

Supravalvular Aortic Stenosis

Echocardiography is a valued technique for localizing the location of stenosis in the supravalvular area. Regularly the sinuses of Valsalva are dilated, while the ascending aorta and arch seem small or of normal size. Always, the size of the aortic annulus is more than that of the sinotubular junction. Color-flow Doppler study is useful for identifying the level of stenosis. In the supra-aortic stenosis, the turbulent flow originates above the AV. Doppler study determines the site of obstruction; it, however, frequently overestimates the maximum gradient compared with that found in cardiac catheterization (owing to pressure recovery phenomena) [64–66].

Coarctation of the Aorta (CoA)

TTE must be applied in the initial imaging study and hemodynamic evaluation of cases with suspected CoA while paying specific attention to the suprasternal notch acoustic windows (class I, Level of Evidence: B). CoA might be diagnosed in the suprasternal notch view of the aortic arch and the proximal descending aorta by a turbulent flow in the proximal descending aorta. However, the presence of extensive collaterals in the native CoA and the lack of aortic compliance in the postoperative CoA might limit the utility of Doppler gradient quantification in the study of the severity of obstruction. It seems that a diastolic "runoff" flow is the most reliable marker of an important CoA or re-CoA. A decreased pulsatility and absence of early diastolic flow reversal might also be demonstrated in the Doppler flow examination of the abdominal aorta. Echocardiography also aids in the study of LV size, mass, and function; anatomy of the AV and aortic annulus dimensions; related cardiac abnormalities such as VSDs, aortic stenosis, and MV deformity; and supra-aortic vessel diameters. Accordingly, the cornerstone of diagnosis remains echocardiography. As was mentioned before, 2D

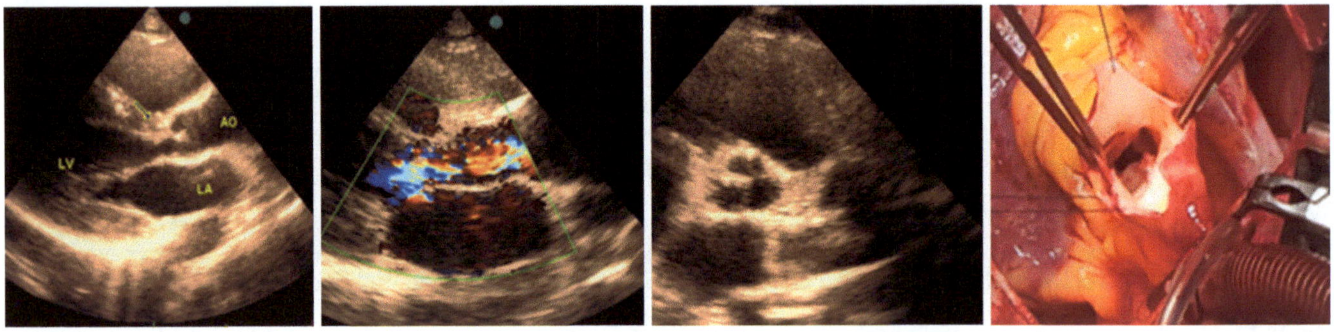

Fig. 28.38 Sub valvular aortic stenosis (AS) in parasternal long axis view in 2D and color flow imaging, short axis view and in surgical view

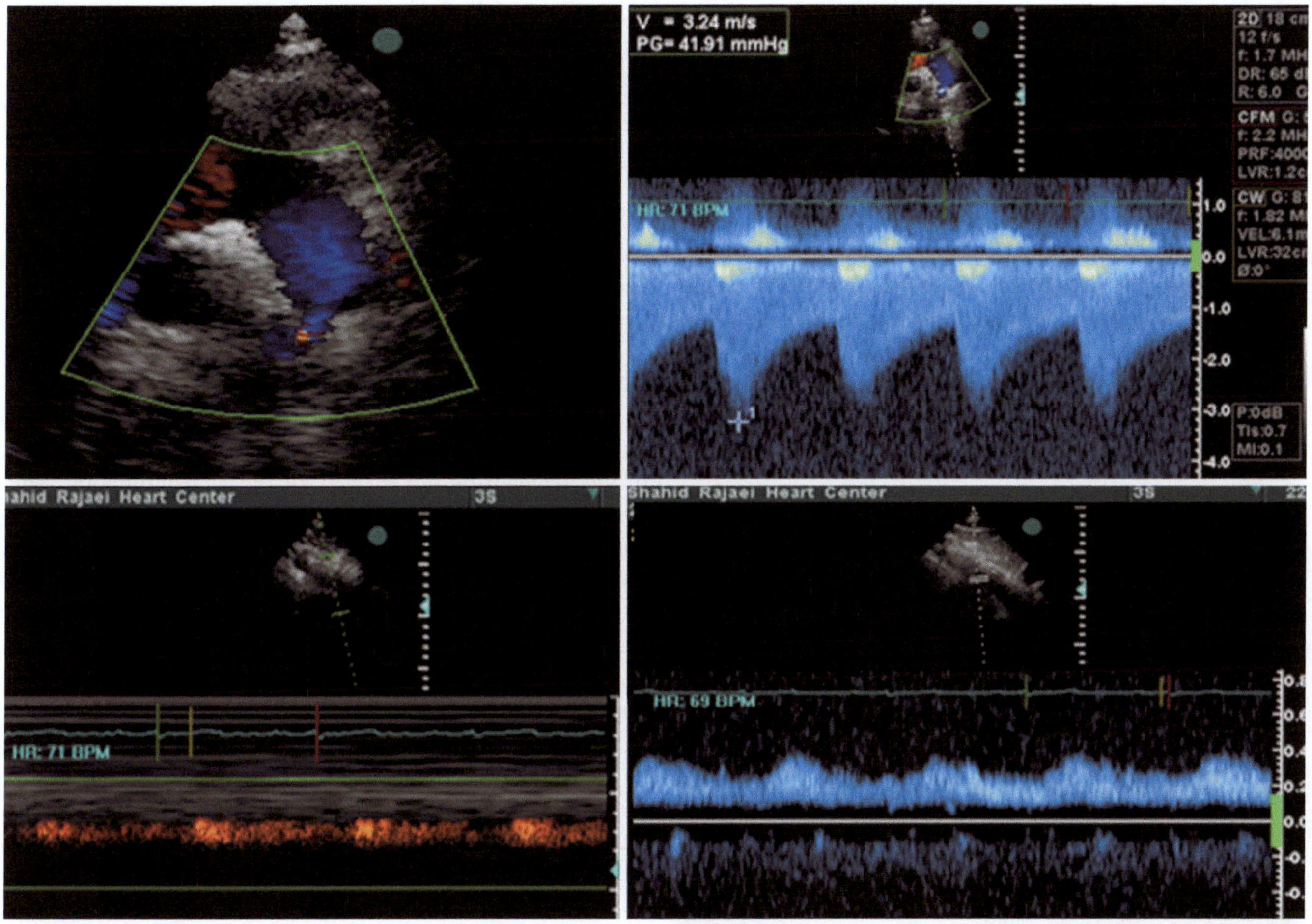

Fig. 28.39 The site of the stenosis may be seen properly in the suprasternal view. In significant coarctation, there is a turbulent flow in the proximal descending aorta and continuous-wave Doppler study will reveal increased velocity through the descending aorta, with a diastolic "tail" (high velocities maintained during diastole). Color Doppler and Doppler flow study of the abdominal aorta demonstrating decreased pulsatility and absence of early diastolic flow reversal in the significant CoA

echocardiography may establish and confirm the diagnosis and delineate the site of obstruction and related lesions. Color-flow Doppler measures the peak pressure gradient across the obstruction. LV dimensions and function are evaluated by 2D echocardiography and M-mode (Fig. 28.39).

Sinus of Valsalva Aneurysms and Fistulae

- 2D and Doppler echocardiographic study may detect the aneurysm and disturbed flow in the CS as well as the site of perforation.
- TEE might provide more precise information. About 90–95% of the congenital aneurysms originate in the right or non-CS of Valsalva and project into the RV or the RA (Figs. 28.40, 28.41, and 28.42). Aneurysms that arise from the non-CS rupture into the RA, and those that arise from the right CS generally communicate to the RV and occasionally to the RA [35, 67, 68].

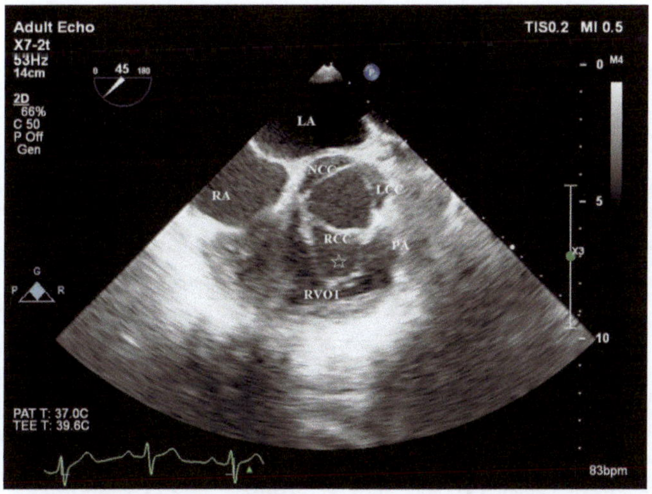

Fig. 28.40 Transthoracic echocardiography in short axis view showing aneurysmal dilation of right sinus of Valsalva with protrusion to the RVOT

Congenital Mitral Stenosis

- 2D and more recently 3D echocardiography, together with color and Doppler study, generally provides a comprehensive study of the anatomy and function in cases with congenital mitral stenosis. The form, shape, and location of the papillary muscles are best seen in the parasternal short-axis view.
- In congenital mitral stenosis, if both papillary muscles are present, frequently they are closer together than is seen in the normal heart. The four-chamber and parasternal long-axis views permit the diagnosis of supravalvular mitral rings.

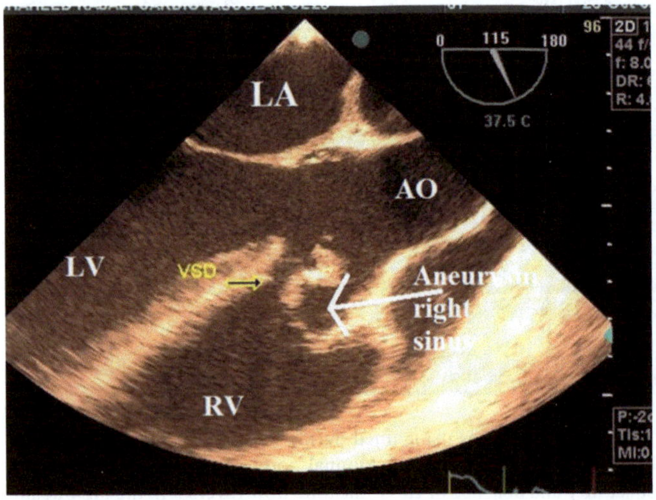

Fig. 28.41 Transesophageal echocardiography in long axis view revealed a "windsock" dilatation of the right sinus of Valsalva which is ruptured to the RVOT (white arrow) and associated VSD (yellow arrow)

- Color-flow Doppler helps determine the level of stenosis and obstruction and also confirms the presence of MV regurgitation. Moreover, Doppler study provides a precise study of the mean gradient and pressure half-time through the MV.

2D TTE in the parasternal short-axis view may determine the number of the papillary muscles and the MV anatomy (Fig. 28.43) [69–73].

Congenital Mitral Regurgitation

Doppler and 2D echocardiography provides a precise study of the mechanism and severity of mitral regurgitation. The cleft of the anterior MV leaflet is best seen in the precordial parasternal short-axis view. Cases with a dysplastic MV have absence mobility of the valve leaflets and shortened chordae. Color Doppler study helps locate the site of mitral regurgitation and evaluate its severity. Nowadays, 3D echocardiography allows a comprehensive and detailed study of the MV apparatus and the mechanisms of regurgitation. Catheterism and MRI are rarely useful in management planning [74, 75].

Pulmonary Valve Stenosis

- Combined 2D echocardiographic and continuous-wave Doppler studies characterize the anatomy of the pulmonary valve and the severity of pulmonary stenosis (Fig. 28.44).
- Essentially, echocardiography has obviated the need for diagnostic cardiac catheterization by measuring the maximum instantaneous gradients.

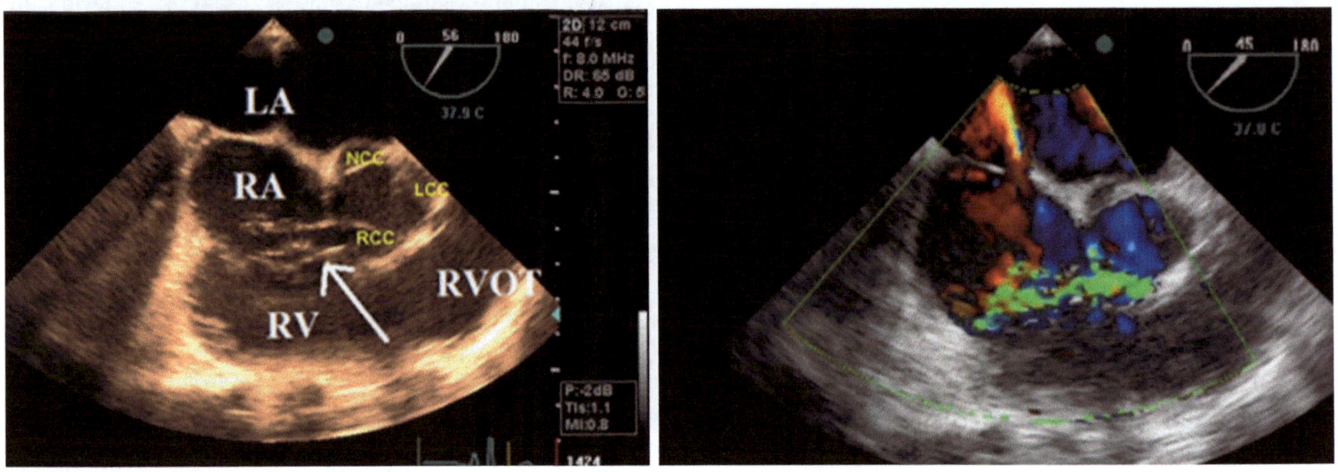

Fig. 28.42 "windsock" dilatation of the right sinus of Valsalva (arrow) which is ruptured to the RA with continuous systolic-diastolic flow in color flow imaging

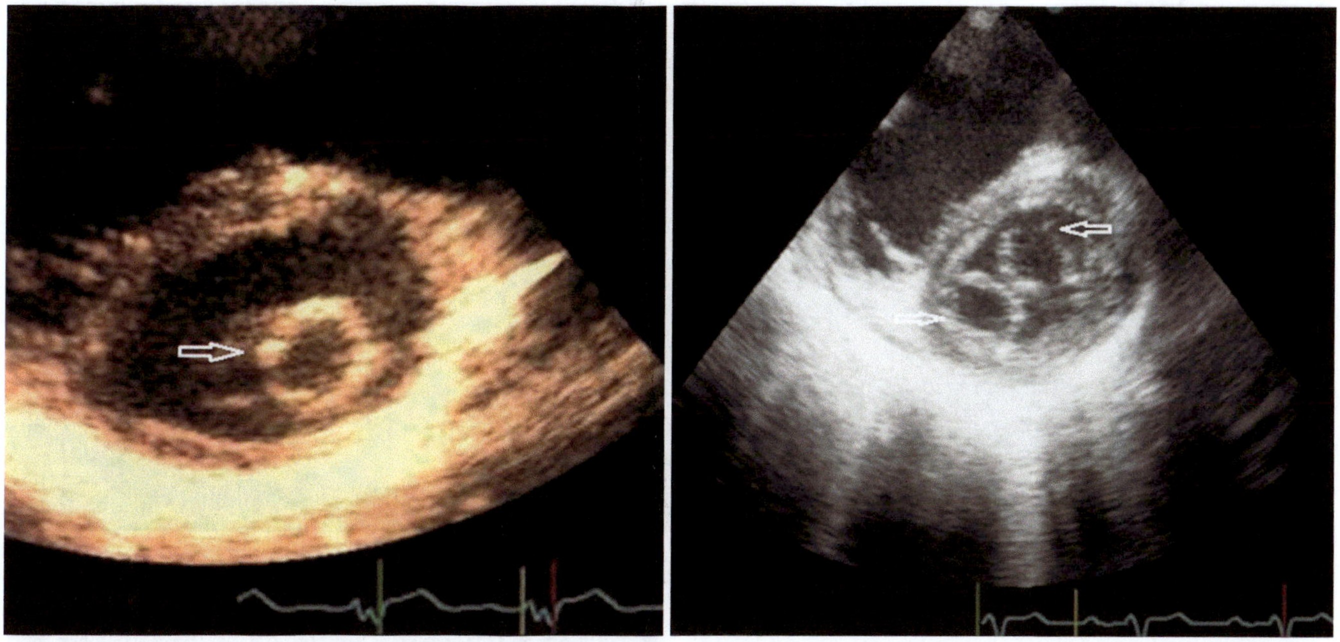

Fig. 28.43 Left: Parachute mitral valve with dominant anterior papillary muscle (arrow). Right Double orifice mitral valve in transthoracic short axis view (double arrow)

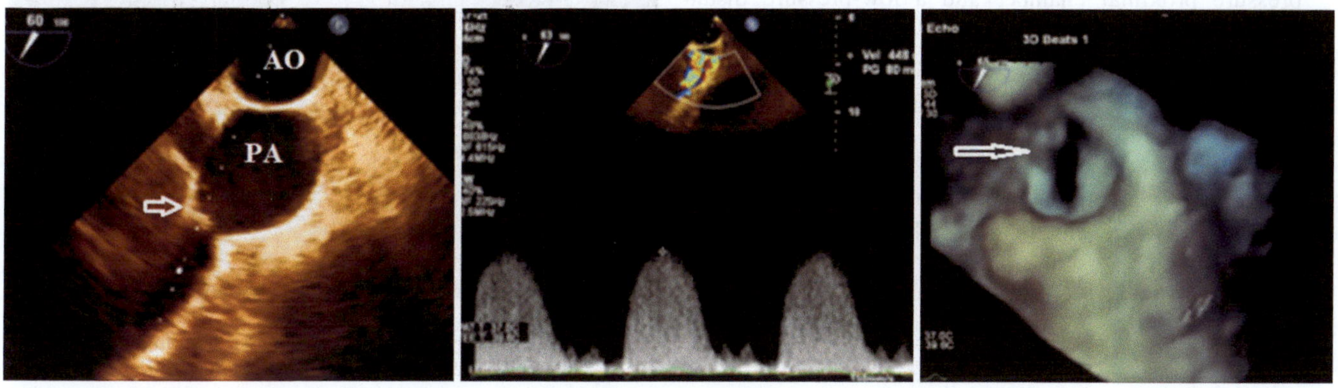

Fig. 28.44 Severe valvular PS in TEE arch view (arrow), by CW Doppler study and bicuspid pulmonary valve in 3D TEE (arrow)

- Recent data suggest that the mean Doppler gradients that correlate better with catheter-derived peak-to-peak gradients and with a value of 50 mmHg are the cut point to start the intervention. Invasive studies are now used for balloon valvuloplasty [20, 76]. RV size, pulmonary artery pressure, TV morphology and function, and status of the interatrial septum may be addressed by echocardiography [21, 76].

Dysplastic Pulmonary Valve Stenosis

Echocardiography proves a thickened plump pulmonary valve, absence of post-stenotic dilation, and varying degrees of supravalvular pulmonary stenosis. Doppler echocardiography may define the severity of the obstruction very well.

The related finding of hypertrophic cardiomyopathy may be confirmed or excluded. If the first echocardiography does not confirm hypertrophic cardiomyopathy, further studies must be undertaken throughout childhood and adolescence, especially in cases with left-axis deviation [76, 77].

Subpulmonary RVOT and Double-Chambered RV

- A DCRV is formed by RV obstruction due to anomalous muscle bundles.
- Echocardiography currently enables diagnosis on a 2D Doppler echocardiogram. The level of subpulmonary obstruction, degree of stenosis, and its relationship with

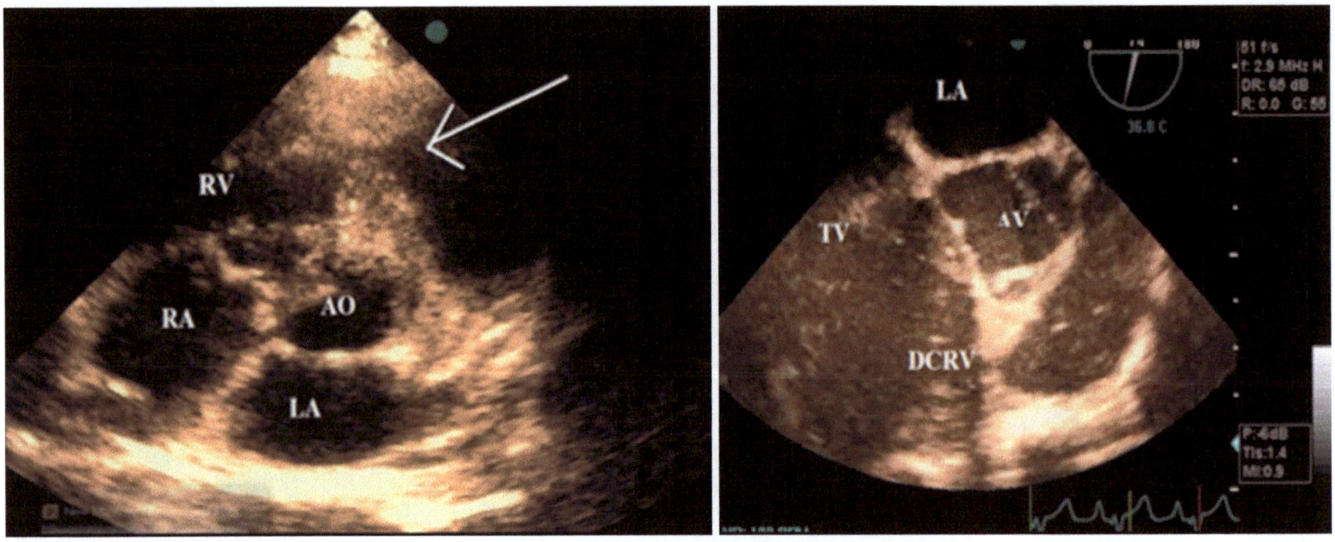

Fig. 28.45 Double-chamber RV (subpulmonary stenosis) with the anomalous muscle bundle (white arrow) in mid portion of RV in TTE and TEE

the VSD are appreciated best in a combination of subcostal right anterior oblique and precordial short-axis views.

- Anomalous muscle bundles divided the RV into a high-pressure proximal chamber and a low-pressure distal chamber (Fig. 28.45).
- Echocardiography may evaluate the presence of possible subaortic stenosis and aortic cusp prolapse. Color-flow, pulsed-wave, or continuous-wave Doppler study frequently allows the differentiation of the VSD flow from that originating from the muscle bundles. Also, this permits an accurate evaluation of the hemodynamic effects of the subpulmonary obstruction. TEE has been used to define structures in older cases with poor windows [78–81].

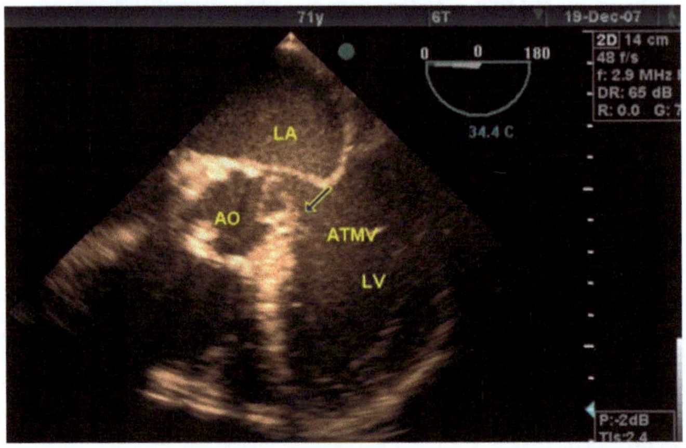

Fig. 28.46 Accessory tissue mitral valve (ATMV) in transesophageal echocardiography 5 chamber view (arrow)

Accessory MV Tissue

- 2D echocardiography, both TTE and TEE, is considered the foremost imaging modality for accessory MV tissue diagnosis, determination of the anatomic characteristics and functional significance, and also the patient's follow-up.
- The accessory MV tissue exhibits an irregular parachute or sail-like feature that is attached to the chordae of the MV, anterior MV leaflet, accessory papillary muscle, or rarely the interventricular septum.
- A large, bulky, and redundant accessory MV tissue folded onto itself may appear as a bulbous, globular, or even cystic mass [82–84]. The recent introduction of 3D echocardiography permits a more realistic characterization of this entity and its related anomalies [85, 86] (Fig. 28.46).

Surgery is indicated only in cases with important LVOT obstruction and in cases undergoing correction of other cardiac malformations and anomalies or exploration of an intracardiac mass [82, 83, 85]. Echocardiography, especially TEE, plays a vital role in the diagnosis, treatment, and follow-up of cases with this rare congenital anomaly [83, 87, 88].

Cor Triatriatum

- Failure of absorption of the common pulmonary vein forms cortriatriatum. This malformation results in a left atrium divided by an abnormal fibromuscular diaphragm into a posterosuperior chamber receiving the pulmonary veins and an anteroinferior chamber containing the left atrial appendage and mitral orifice.

- The diagnosis is established by 2D echocardiography or TEE, with further insight from 3D reconstruction. The obstructive membrane is visualized in the parasternal long-axis, short-axis, and four-chamber views and may be distinguished from a supravalvular mitral ring by its position superior to the LA appendage, which makes part of the distal chamber. Also present is the diastolic fluttering of the mitral leaflets and a high-velocity flow noticed by Doppler examination in the distal atrial chamber and at the mitral orifice [89, 90] (Fig. 28.47).

- Related abnormalities are common and found in 70% of cases. These include ASDs, PFOs, VSDs, persistent left SVCs, partial anomalous pulmonary venous returns, PDAs, and aortic CoA [89].

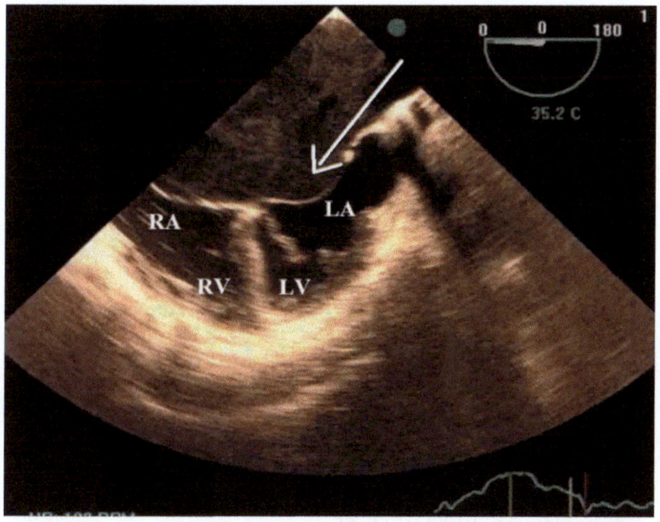

Fig. 28.47 *C*ortriatriatum with a small opening and significant smoky pattern in left atrium in transesophageal echocardiography four chamber view

- TEE may help define the location of the membrane of the fibromuscular diaphragm and the size and number of fenestrations. There are three anatomic types of cor triatriatum: (1) diaphragmatic, (2) hourglass, and (3) tubular. Cor triatriatum may also be classified according to the size of the opening across the membrane as follows:

Group 1, no opening; Group II, one or more openings; and Group III, a wide opening and the size and number of fenestrations in the membrane are variable [91].

Aorto-Pulmonary Window

- Aorto-Pulmonary window is an uncommon congenital anomaly with a defect in the septum between the aorta and pulmonary artery, resulting in a communication between the two arteries.
- Echocardiography may accurately diagnose the main and related anomalies. The LA, LV, and pulmonary artery are dilated. The RV might be hypertrophied. The semilunar valves frequently have normal relation and function.
- The "T" artifact at the edges of the defect is the distinguishing sign from normal dropout. Color-flow Doppler may show the flow through the defect. Spectral Doppler illustrates an abnormal, continuous forward flow in the pulmonary arteries. Important diastolic flow reversal is found in both the proximal aortic arch and the descending aorta. Pulmonary arterial hypertension may also be detected by echocardiography (Fig. 28.48).

Coronary Arteriovenous Fistulae

- Coronary arteriovenous fistula (AVF) is a communication between the coronary arteries and a cardiac chamber or vein. In about 55% of patients, the right coronary artery

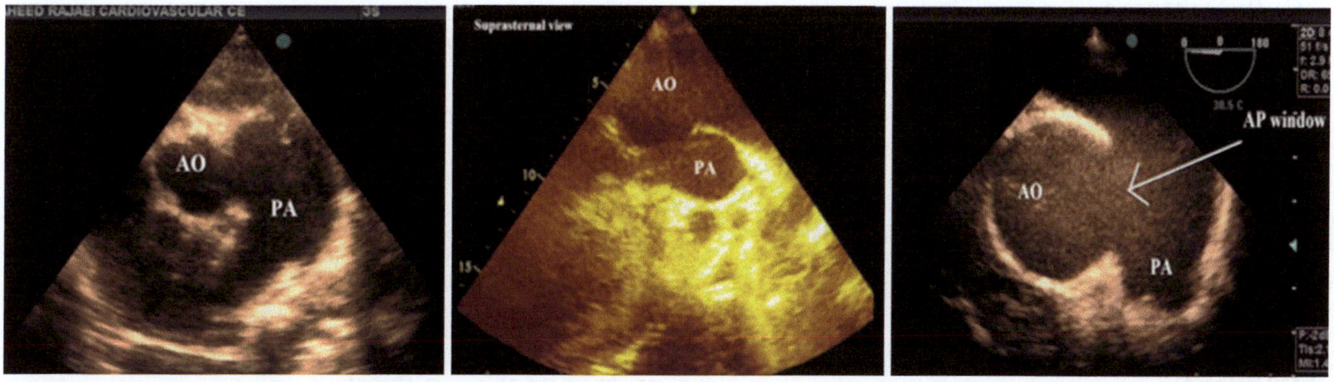

Fig. 28.48 Transthoracic echocardiography in short axis view showing T" artifact at the edges of the defect suggestive for Aortopulmonary septal defect that was confirmed by color flow imaging Aortopulmonary septal defect in transthoracic echocardiography in suprasternal view Aortopulmonary septal defect in transesophageal echocardiography

(RCA) and in nearly 35% of cases left coronary artery (LCA) are the site of the fistula.

- Among the chambers, the right ventricle (RV) is the most involved one, followed by the right atrium (RA) and to a lesser extent the coronary sinus and pulmonary artery (PA).
- In echocardiography, an importantly engorged feeding coronary artery might be noticed. In addition, the entire course, entry site, and exit vessel or chamber might be found by Doppler and color-flow echocardiography.

Multi-plane TEE may also be useful in this context. If echocardiography proves an important coronary arteriovenous fistula, a hemodynamic study via cardiac catheterization is required. Additionally, coronary angiography may be employed to assess the size and the anatomic characteristics of the fistula [92–96].

Questions

1. The ostium primum type accounts for …. of all the types of atrial septal defects.
   A. 10%
   B. 20%
   C. 30%
   D. 40%

2. Dysplastic pulmonary valve stenosis in echocardiography shows all of the following except:
   A. Thickened pulmonary valve
   B. Post-stenotic dilation
   C. Varying degrees of supravalvular pulmonary stenosis
   D. Plump pulmonary valve

3. Echocardiography in aorto-pulmonary window reveals the dilation of the following chambers except for:
   A. Left atrium
   B. Left ventricle
   C. Right ventricle
   D. Pulmonary artery

Answers

1. B
2. B
3. C

References

1. Li W, Henein M, Gatzoulis MA. Echocardiography in adult congenital heart disease. New York City: Springer; 2013.
2. Gatzoulis MA, Webb GD, Broberg CS, Uemura H. Cases in adult congenital heart disease. Philadelphia: Churchill Livingstone; 2010.
3. Bonow RO, Mann DL, Zipes DP, Libby P. Braunwald's heart disease: a textbook of cardiovascular medicine. 9th ed. Philadelphia: Elsevier—Health Sciences Division; 2015. Congenital heart disease chapter.
4. Allen HD, Driscoll DJ, Shaddy RE. Moss and Adams' heart disease in infants, children, and adolescents: including the fetus and young adults. 7th ed. Philadelphia: Lippincott Williams & Wilkins; 2008.
5. Warnes CA. Adult congenital heart disease, AHA clinical series. Hoboken: American Heart Association; 2009. p. 9–24. Chapter 2.
6. Pai RG. Echocardiography in patients with adult congenital heart disease. Echocardiography. 2014;32(s2):s109. https://doi.org/10.1111/echo.12337.
7. Eidem BW, Cetta F, Oleary P. Echocardiography in pediatric and adult congenital heart disease. Philadelphia: Lippincott Williams & Wilkins; 2010.
8. Snider AR, Serwer GA, Ritter SB. Echocardiography in pediatric heart disease. 2nd ed. St. Louis: Mosby; 1997.
9. Perloff J, Marelu A. Perloff's clinical recognition of congenital heart disease. 6th ed. Philadelphia: WB Saunders; 2013.
10. Sadeghpour A, Kiavar M, Alizadehasl A. Comprehensive approach to adult congenital heart disease. London: Springer-Verlag; 2014.
11. Warnes C, Williams RG, Bashore TM, et al. ACC/AHA, guidelines for the management of adults with congenital heart disease. JACC. 2008;52(23):2008.
12. Baumgartner H, Bonhoeffer P, De Groot NM, et al. ESC Committee for Practice Guidelines (CPG). ESC Guidelines for the management of grown-up congenital heart disease (new version 2010). Eur Heart J. 2010;31:2915–57.
13. Lewim MB, Stout K. Echocardiography in congenital heart disease. Philadelphia: Saunders/Elsevier; 2012.
14. Oh JK, Seward JB, Tajik AJ, editors. The echo manual. 3rd ed. Philadelphia: Lippincott Williams & Wilkins; 2007.
15. Den Ven AE, Robbers-Visser D, Krenning BJ, et al. Real-time transthoracic three-dimensional echocardiographic valuation of LV volume and ejection fraction in congenital heart disease. J Am Soc Echocardiogr. 2006;19:1.
16. Lang RM, et al. EAE/ASE recommendations for image acquisition and display using three- dimensional echocardiography. J Am Soc Echocardiogr. 2012;25:3–46.
17. Grewal J, Majdalany D, Syed I. Three-dimensional ultrasound was comparable with MRI in determining RV size and function in most cases with complex congenital heart disease. J Am Soc Echocardiogr. 2010;23:127–33.
18. Li W, Henein M, Gatzoulis MA. Echocardiography in Adult Congenital Heart Disease. Philadelphia: Springer; 2013.
19. Gatzoulis MA, Webb GD, Broberg CS, Uemura H. Cases in adult congenital heart disease. Philadelphia: Churchill Livingstone; 2010.
20. Warnes C, Williams RG, Bashore TM, et al. ACC/ AHA, guidelines for the management of adults with congenital heart disease. JACC. 2008;52(23):2008.
21. Bonow RO, Mann DL, Zipes DP, Libby P. Braunwald's heart disease: a textbook of cardiovascular medicine. 9th ed. Philadelphia: Elsevier—Health Sciences Division; 2015. Congenital heart disease chapter
22. Allen HD, Driscoll DJ, Shaddy RE. Moss and Adams' heart disease in infants, children, and adolescents: including the fetus and young adults. 7th ed. Philadelphia: Lippincott Williams & Wilkins; 2008.
23. Warnes CA. Adult congenital heart disease, AHA clinical series. Hoboken: American Heart Association; 2009. p. 9–24. Chapter 2.
24. Pai RG. Echocardiography in patients with adult congenital heart disease. 2014;32:S109. https://doi.org/10.1111/echo.12337.
25. Oliver JM, Gallego P, Gonzalez A, et al. Sinus venosus syndrome: atrial septal defect or anomalous venous connection? A multiplane transoesophageal approach. Heart. 2002;88(6):634–8.
26. Baumgartner H, Bonhoeffer P, De Groot NM, et al. ESC guidelines for the management of grown-up congenital heart disease (new version 2010). Eur Heart J. 2010;31(23):2915–57.

27. Perloff JK. The clinical recognition of congenital heart disease. 5th ed. Philadelphia: WB Saunders; 1994. p. 300–25.
28. Keane JF, Lock JE, Fyler DC, Nadas AS, editors. Nadas' pediatric cardiology. 2nd ed. Philadelphia: WB Saunders; 2006.
29. Ritter S, Tani LY, Shaddy RE, et al. An unusual variant of total anomalous pulmonary venous connection with varices and multiple drainage sites. Pediatr Cardiol. 2000;21(3):289–91.
30. Sievert H, Taaffe M. Patent foramen ovale: the jury is still out. Eur Heart J. 2004;25(5):361–2.
31. Maffe S, Dellavesa P, Zenone F, et al. Transthoracic second harmonic two- and three-dimensional echocardiography for detection of patent foramen ovale. J Am Coll Cardiol Intv. 2010;3(9):968–73.
32. Shanks M, Manawadu D, Vonder Muhll I, Khan K, Becher H, Choy J. Detection of patent foramen ovale by 3D echocardiography. JACC Cardiovasc Imaging. 2012;5(3):329–31.
33. Becker TE, Ensing GJ, Darragh RK, et al. Doppler derivation of complete pulmonary artery pressure curves in patent ductus arteriosus. Am J Cardiol. 1996;78:1066–9.
34. Bartelings MM, Gittenberger-de Groot AC. Morphogenetic considerations on congenital malformations of the outflow tract. Part 1: Common arterial trunk and tetralogy of Fallot. Int J Cardiol. 1991;32(2):213–30.
35. Snider AR, Serwer GA, Ritter SB. Echocardiography in pediatric heart disease. 2nd ed. St. Louis: Mosby; 1997.
36. Shina A, Seward J, Tajik J, et al. Two-dimensional echocardiographic-surgical correlation in Ebstein's anomaly: preoperative determination of patients requiring tricuspid valve plication vs replacement. Circulation. 1983;68(3):534–44.
37. Otto CM. The practice of clinical echocardiography. 3rd ed. Philadelphia: W.B. Saunders/Elsevier; 2007.
38. Cohen MS, Anderson RH, Cohen MI, et al. Controversies, genetics, diagnostic assessment, and outcomes relating to the heterotaxy syndrome. Cardiol Young. 2007;17(Suppl 2):29–43.
39. Sadeghpour A, Saadatifar H, Kiavar M, et al. Doppler echocardiographic assessment of pulmonary prostheses: a comprehensive assessment including velocity time integral ratio & prosthesis effective orifice area. Congenit Heart Dis. 2008;3:415–21.
40. Tsang FH, Li X, Cheung YF, et al. Pulmonary valve replacement after surgical repair of tetralogy of Fallot. Hong Kong Med J. 2010;16(1):26–30.
41. Kyavar M, Sadeghpour A, Madadi S, et al. Echocardiographic assessment of adults with repaired tetralogy of Fallot: a cardiovascular magnetic resonance comparison study. IHJ. 2012;12:2.
42. Sadeghpour A, Kyavar M, Javani B, et al. Mid-term results of mechanical pulmonary prostheses in adults with congenital heart disease: importance of anticoagulation. Circulation. 2012;125(19):163.
43. Naderi N, Haghighi ZO, Pezeshki S, Alizadehasl A. Quantitative assessment of right atrial function by strain imaging in adult patients with totally corrected tetralogy of Fallot. Arch Cardiovas Imaging. 2013;1(1):8–12.
44. Sadeghpour A, Javani B, Peighambari M, et al. Midterm follow-up of pulmonary valve bioprostheses in adults with congenital heart disease. Anadolu Kardiyol Derg. 2012;12:434–6.
45. Sadeghpour A, Kyavar M, Madadi S, et al. Dopplerderived strain and strain rate imaging assessment of right ventricular systolic function in adults late after tetralogy of Fallot repair: an observational study. Anadolu Kardiyol Derg. 2013;13:536–42.
46. Lev M, Bharati S, Meng CC, et al. A concept of double-outlet right ventricle. J Thorac Cardiovasc Surg. 1972;64:271–81.
47. Warnes CA. Congenital heart disease for the adult cardiologist. Transposition of the great arteries. Circulation. 2006;114:2699–709.
48. Bruneau BG, Logan M, Davis N, et al. Chamberspecific cardiac expression of Tbx5 and heart defects in Holt-Oram syndrome. Dev Biol. 1999;211(1):100–8.
49. Takeuchi JK, Ohgi M, Koshiba-Takeuchi K, et al. Tbx5 specifies the left/right ventricles and ventricular septum position during cardiogenesis. Development. 2003;130(24):5953–64.
50. Van der Bom T, Winter MM, Groenink M, et al. Right ventricular end-diastolic volume combined with peak systolic blood pressure during exercise identifies patients at risk for complications in adults with a systemic right ventricle. J Am Coll Cardiol. 2013;62(10):926–36.
51. Warnes CA. Adult congenital heart disease. Chichester: Wiley-Blackwell; 2009. p. 128–37. Chapter 9.
52. Lai WW, Mertens LL, Cohen M, et al. Echocardiography in pediatric and congenital heart disease. Chichester: Wiley-Blackwell; 2010. p. 398–14. Chapter 24.
53. Agnetti A, Carano N, Cavalli C, et al. Long-term outcome after Senning operation for transposition of the great arteries. Clin Cardiol. 2004;27:611–4.
54. Wells WJ, Blackstone E. Intermediate out-come after Mustard and Senning procedures: a study by the Congenital Heart Surgeons Society. Semin Thorac Cardiovasc Surg Pediatr Card Surg Annu. 2000;3:186–97.
55. Nihoyannopoulos P, Kisslo J. Echocardiography. Dordrecht: Springer; 2009. p. 552. Chapter 28.
56. Armestrong WF, Ryan T. Feigenbaum's echocardiography. 7th. Lippincott Williams & Wilkins; 2010.p. 629–630.; chapter 20.
57. Maganti K, Rigolin VH, Enriquez-Sarano M, Bonow RO. Heart valve disease: diagnosis and management. Mayo Clin Proc. 2010;85:453.
58. Lewin MB, Otto CM. The bicuspid aortic valve: adverse outcomes from infancy to old age. Circulation. 2005;111:832.
59. Braverman AC. The bicuspid aortic valve. In: Otto CM, Bonow RO, editors. Valvular heart disease: a companion to Braunwald's heart disease. Philadelphia: Saunders/Elsevier; 2009. p. 169–86.
60. Freedom RM. The long and the short of it: some thoughts about the fixed forms of left ventricular outflow tract obstruction. J Am Coll Cardiol. 1997;30:1843.
61. Karamlou T, Gurofsky R, Bojcevski A, et al. Prevalence and associated risk factors for intervention in 313 children with subaortic stenosis. Ann Thorac Surg. 2007;84:900.
62. Binet JP, Losay J, Demontoux S, et al. Subvalvular aortic stenosis: long-term surgical results. Thorac Cardiovasc Surg. 1983;31:96.
63. Vogt J, Dische R, Rupprath G, et al. Fixed subaortic stenosis: an acquired secondary obstruction? A twenty-seven year experience with 168 patients. Thorac Cardiovasc Surg. 1989;37:199.
64. Bonow RO, Carabello BA, Chatterjee K, et al. ACC/AHA 2006 guidelines for the management of patients with valvular heart disease: a report of the American College of Cardiology/American Heart Association Task Force on Practice Guidelines (Writing Committee to Revise the 1998 Guidelines for the Management of Patients with alvular Heart Disease) developed in collaboration with the Society.
65. Otto CM, editor. Textbook of clinical echocardiography. 4th ed. Philadelphia: Saunders/Elsevier; 2009.
66. Rosenhek R, Baumgartner H. Aortic stenosis. In: Otto CM, Bonow RO, editors. Valvular heart disease: a companion to Braunwald's heart disease. Philadelphia: Saunders/Elsevier; 2009. p. 127–54.
67. Davidavicius G, Subkovas E, Abraitis V, et al. Coronary anomalies: single center experience. Semin Cardiol. 2004;10:208–13.
68. Child JS. Echocardiographic evaluation of the adult with postoperative congenital heart disease. In: Otto CM, editor. The practice of clinical echocardiography. 3rd ed. Philadelphia: W. B. Saunders/Elsevier; 2007. p. 1083–109.
69. Del Nido PJ, Baird C. Congenital mitral valve stenosis: anatomic variants and surgical reconstruction. Semin Thorac Cardiovasc Surg Pediatr Card Surg Annu. 2012;15(1):69–74.
70. Delmo Walter EM, Komoda T, Siniawski H, et al. Long-term surgical outcome of mitral valve repair in infants and children with Shone's anomaly. Eur J Cardiothorac Surg. 2013;43(3):473–81; discussion 481-2.
71. Brown JW, Fiore AC, Ruzmetov M, et al. Evolution of mitral valve replacement in children: a 40-year experience. Ann Thorac Surg. 2012;93(2):626–33.
72. Chauvaud S. Congenital mitral valve surgery: techniques and results. Curr Opin Cardiol. 2006;21(2):95–9.

73. Karaci AR, Aydemir NA, Harmandar B, et al. Surgical treatment of infective valve endocarditis in children with congenital heart disease. J Card Surg. 2012;27(1):93–8.
74. Rahimtoola SH. The mitral valve is a complex structure. Foreword. Curr Probl Cardiol. 2009;34(3):89.
75. Macnab A, Jenkins NP, Ewington I, et al. A method for the morphological analysis of the regurgitant mitral valve using three dimensional echocardiography. Heart. 2004;90:771.
76. Silvilairat S, Cabalka AK, Cetta F, et al. Echocardiographic assessment of isolated pulmonary valve stenosis: which outpatient Doppler gradient has the most clinical validity? J Am Soc Echocardiogr. 2005;18:1137.
77. Gikonyo BM, Lucas RV, Edwards JE. Anatomic features of congenital pulmonary valvar stenosis. Pediatr Cardiol. 1987;8(2):109–16.
78. Nagashima M, Tomino T, Satoh H, et al. Doublechambered right ventricle in adulthood. Asian Cardiovasc Thorac Ann. 2005;13(2):127–30.
79. Vogel M, Freedom RM, Brand A, et al. Ventricular septal defect and subaortic stenosis: an analysis of 41 patients. Am J Cardiol. 1983;52(10):1258–63.
80. Animasahun BA, Ekure EN, Njokanma OF. Doublechambered right ventricle: an uncommon congenital heart disease. Case report and literature review. Cardiovasc J Afr. 2011;22(5):274–7.
81. Romano MM, Furtado RG, Dias CG, et al. Doublechambered right ventricle in an adult patient diagnosed by transthoracic echocardiography. Cardiovasc Ultrasound. 2007;5:2.
82. Eiriksson H, Midgley FM, Karr SS, et al. Role of echocardiography in the diagnosis and surgical management of accessory mitral valve tissue causing left ventricular outflow tract obstruction. J Am Soc Echocardiogr. 1995;8:105–7.
83. Willens HJ, Levy R, Perez A. Diagnosis of accessory mitral valve tissue by transesophageal echocardiography. Echocardiography. 1994;11:39–45.
84. Prifti E, Frati G, Bonacchi M, Vanini V, Chauvaud S. Accessory mitral valve tissue causing left ventricular outflow tract obstruction (case reports and literature review). J Heart Valve Dis. 2001;10:774–8.
85. Yetkin E, Turhan H. Recurrence of cerebrovascular thromboembolic event in a woman with accessory mitral valve during puerperium period. Int J Cardiol. 2005;105:102–3.
86. Popescu BA, Ghiorghiu I, Apetrei E, et al. Subaortic stenosis produced by accessory mitral valve: the role of echocardiography. Echocardiography. 2005;22:39–41.
87. Garrett HE, Spray TL. Accessory mitral valve tissue (an increasingly recognized cause of left ventricular outflow tract obstruction). J Cardiovasc Surg. 1990;31:225–30.
88. Yoshimura N, Yamaguchi M, Oshima Y, Oka S, Ootaki Y, Tei T, et al. Clinical and pathological features of accessory valve tissue. Ann Thorac Surg. 2000;69:1205–8.
89. Thakrar A, Shapiro MD, Jassal DS, et al. Cor triatriatum: the utility of cardiovascular imaging. Can J Cardiol. 2007;23(2):143–5.
90. Vallakati A, Nerella N, Chandra P, et al. Incidental diagnosis of cor triatriatum in 2 elderly patients. J Am Coll Cardiol. 2012; 59(22):e43.
91. Schluter M, Langenstein BA, Thier W, et al. Transesophageal two-dimensional echocardiography in the diagnosis of cor triatriatum in the adult. J Am Coll Cardiol. 1983;2(5):1011–5.
92. Schamroth C. Coronary artery fistula. J Am Coll Cardiol. 2009;53(6):523.
93. Liberthson RR, Sagar K, Berkoben JP, et al. Congenital coronary arterio-venous fistula. Report of 13 patients, review of the literature and delineation of management. Circulation. 1979;59(5): 849–54.
94. Weymann A, Lembcke A, Konertz WF. Right coronary artery to superior vena cava fistula: imaging with cardiac catheterization, 320-detector row computed tomography, magnetic resonance imaging, and transesophageal echocardiography. Eur Heart J. 2009;30(17):2146.
95. Pouraliakbar H, Sadeghpour A, Alizadehasl A, Firoozi A, Homightoun K, Alborzi N, et al. Large coronary-cameral fistulas in an adult patient: a rare coronary anomaly with concealed clinical findings (case report and literature review). Arch Cardiovasc Imaging. 2016;25:e40954. https://doi.org/10.5812/acvi.40954.
96. Sadeghpour A, Kiavar M, Alizadehasl A. Comprehensive approach to adult congenital heart disease. London: Springer-Verlag; 2014.

Perioperative Transesophageal Echocardiography

29

Anita Sadeghpour and Azin Alizadehasl

Abstract

This chapter explains the role of perioperative transesophageal echocardiography in the care and treatment of an unstable surgical patient. Although it may encompass a broad range of anatomic imaging, noninvasive monitoring should focus on the cardiac causes of hemodynamic or ventilatory instability—including ventricular size and function, valvular anatomy and function, volume status, pericardial abnormalities, and complications from invasive procedures—as well as the clinical impact or the etiology of pulmonary dysfunction. Indeed, a basic perioperative transesophageal echocardiography examination is not designed to prepare practitioners for the use of the full diagnostic potential of transesophageal echocardiography, but sometimes it is needed to provide an advanced examination with detailed data on issues outside the scope of practice as defined within the related guidelines. We will, therefore, review its rules in detail.

Keywords

Perioperative transesophageal echocardiography
Unstable surgical patient · Right ventricular function
Hypovolemia · Air embolism during surgery
Pericardial effusion

Electronic Supplementary Material The online version of this chapter (https://doi.org/10.1007/978-3-319-67691-3_29) contains supplementary material, which is available to authorized users.

A. Sadeghpour, MD, FACC, FASE
Professor of Cardiology, Echocardiography Research Center, Rajaie Cardiovascular Medical and Research Center, Iran University of Medical Science, Tehran, Iran

A. Alizadehasl, MD, FACC, FASE (✉)
Associate Professor of Cardiology, Echocardiologist, Echocardiography and Cardiogenetic Research Centers, Cardio-Oncology Department, Rajaie Cardiovascular Medical and Research Center, Tehran, Iran

Abbreviations

ALPM	Anterolateral papillary muscle
ASA	American society of anesthesiologists
ASC	Ascending
ASD	Atrial septal defect
ASE	American society of echocardiography
AV	Aortic valve
CABG	Coronary artery bypass graft surgery
CHDs	Complex congenital heart diseases
CT	Computed tomography
DESC	Descending
IVC	Inferior vena cava
LAX	Long axis
LE	Lower esophageal
LV	Left ventricular
MRI	Magnetic resonance imaging
PA	Pulmonary artery
PFO	Patent foramen ovale
PPM	Posteromedial papillary muscle
PO-TEE	Perioperative transesophageal echocardiography
PV	Pulmonic valve
RVOT	Right ventricular outflow tract
SAM	Systolic anterior motion
SAX	Short axis
TTE	Transthoracic echocardiography

- Perioperative transesophageal echocardiography (PO-TEE) is an art and science with its own rules. It is performed in the care and treatment of an unstable surgical patient, for complex cardiac surgeries, and for valvular repair procedures. One of the principal goals of a basic PO-TEE study is intraoperative monitoring. While this might encompass a broad range of anatomic imaging, noninvasive monitoring should focus on cardiac causes of hemodynamic or ventilatory instability such as ventricular size and function, valvular anatomy and function, volume status, pericardial abnormali-

A. Sadeghpour, A. Alizadehasl (eds.), *Case-Based Textbook of Echocardiography*, https://doi.org/10.1007/978-3-319-67691-3_29

ties, and complications from invasive procedures, as well as on the clinical impact or the etiology of pulmonary dysfunction. However, sometimes advanced PO-TEE is needed by the full diagnostic potential of TEE [1].

Basics of PO-TEE

Practical Points Before Initiating Image Acquisition

- Good communication with and being respectful to other colleagues in the operating room is very important.
- Knowing the patient's sex, age, weight, height, body surface area, reason for surgery, previous echocardiography data including transthoracic echocardiography (TTE) and TEE, heart catheterization, and other imaging data such as computed tomography (CT) and magnetic resonance imaging (MRI) are crucial for pre- and postoperative decision making.
- PO-TEE starts after the induction of anesthesia, endotracheal intubation, and esophageal intubation (cared by anesthesiologists).
- PO-TEE means performing a complete **pre-pump TEE (just before surgery) in the operating room. In postoperative TEE, immediately after surgery, the patient has been separated from the cardiopulmonary pump but the chest still is opened.** It is important to perform a complete TEE examination prior to surgery, and not just a postsurgical examination.
- Obtaining data should begin as soon as possible to extend the available time of image acquisition and interpretation the images before the surgery starts since when the surgery begins, the noise of the electrocautery will inevitably affect the image quality.
- First the unresolved question regarding cardiac surgery should be addressed. The necessary data from the intraoperative TEE should be obtained from the surgeon and be addressed first.
- PO-TEE is relatively safe and has been related with mortality rates of fewer than 1 per 10,000 cases and morbidity of 2–5 per 1000 cases. Probe manipulation—comprising positioning, turning, rotation, and imaging planes—has been previously extensively described in the comprehensive document of the American Society of Echocardiography (ASE) (See Chap. 3).
- TEE probe is the same as is introduced in Chap. 3, but the probe can be on the left side in the gastric region of the patient for extended periods of time. However, it is more advisable to shut down the echo machine or freeze the probe in the stomach [1–6].

  Precise attention to the vital signs specially the blood pressure just before and during the PO-TEE study is obligatory. Dynamic changes of blood pressure and heart rate may affect the valvular and ventricular function.

Indications for PO-TEE

1. Most cardiac defects ***requiring repair under cardiopulmonary bypass*** are a ***category 1*** indication for ***PO-TEE***, including pre-cardiopulmonary and post-cardiopulmonary imaging. (***Category 1*** means there is **evidence and/or general agreement** that shows PO-TEE will improve the clinical outcomes.)

   Based on the guidelines, for adult patients without contraindications, PO-TEE should be used ***for all open heart surgeries (particularly in all valve repairs) and thoracic aortic surgeries provided that*** appropriate technology and expert certified physicians are available [1, 2].

2. TEE is used as a diagnostic and monitoring imaging modality. It is useful in detecting residual shunts, valvular regurgitation, obstruction, and myocardial dysfunction
3. PO-TEE should be considered in patients candidated for coronary artery bypass graft surgery (CABG) for confirming preoperative diagnoses, detecting new or unsuspected pathologies, adjusting the surgery plans, and assessing the results of surgery.
4. American Society of Anesthesiologists (ASA) practice guidelines recommend basic PO-TEE when the nature of the planned surgery or the patient's known or suspected cardiovascular pathology might result in severe hemodynamic, pulmonary, or neurologic compromise. In addition, when available, basic PO-TEE must be used when unexplained life-threatening circulatory instability persists despite corrective therapy [1, 2, 5, 6].
5. Usefulness of TEE has been documented in:

(a) Neurosurgery when there is a risk of venous air embolism and patent foramen ovale (PFO)
(b) Lung transplantation
(c) Liver transplantation (detecting compression in the cardiac chambers and pericardial effusion)
(d) Major vascular surgery or other major noncardiac surgeries in which unstable hemodynamic is present or threatened [5, 6]

6. These recommendations for performing PO-TEE are subject to modifications based on the institutional facilities, policies, and expertise.

Contraindications and Complications of PO-TEE

- Contraindications and complications of PO-TEE are almost the same as TEE. However, TEE can be considered in a patient with esophageal disease, if the benefit of the data achieved by PO-TEE outweighs the potential risk of TEE considering the possibility of need for other imaging modalities (e.g., epicardial echocardiography), asking for gastroenterology consultation, and doing PO-TEE by the most expert physician [2, 5, 6].

Role of Pre-bypass TEE in the Operating Room

1. Pre-pump TEE examination allows a final check and confirms the pathology, anatomy, and physiology.
2. Pre-pump TEE examination helps find new associated anomalies or unappreciated lesions which may change the surgical plans.
3. Surgeons often like a ***last-minute "update"*** of the anatomy and physiology prior to beginning the surgical operation.
4. PO-TEE facilitates the placement of the central venous catheters, extracorporeal membrane oxygenation, and intra-aortic balloon pumps.
5. It helps the use of preoperative inotrope support by demonstrating the ventricular size and function.
6. Lack of knowledge of pre-bypass findings may lead to the misinterpretation of post-repair findings and their management.

Caveats: A number of things ***may change under anesthesia***:

- Following intubation and ventilation, it is common to find smaller tricuspid regurgitation jet color displays—with a lower peak velocity—due to lower pulmonary resistance in the anesthetized state.
- Cardiac output may be reduced under anesthesia, leading to lower peak velocities through obstructions and decreased severity of mitral regurgitation jets. Thus, PO-TEE should not be used for making a particular surgical decision this crucial decision of whether or not to proceed a surgical repair/replacement for a particular lesion should be made in euvolemia state not in the operating room.

Comprehensive PO-TEE Examination

- Comprehensive PO-TEE examination requires the acquisition of 20 views in the performance of a comprehensive intraoperative multi-plane TEE study.
- Current guideline believes that although a basic PO-TEE echocardiologist should be familiar with the technical skills needed to acquire these 20 views, it is nonetheless a realistic expectation that a basic PO-TEE study focus on encompassing the 11 most relevant views—which may provide the necessary information to use basic PO-TEE echocardiography as a tool for diagnosing the general etiology of hemodynamic instability in surgical cases (Figs. 29.1 and 29.2).

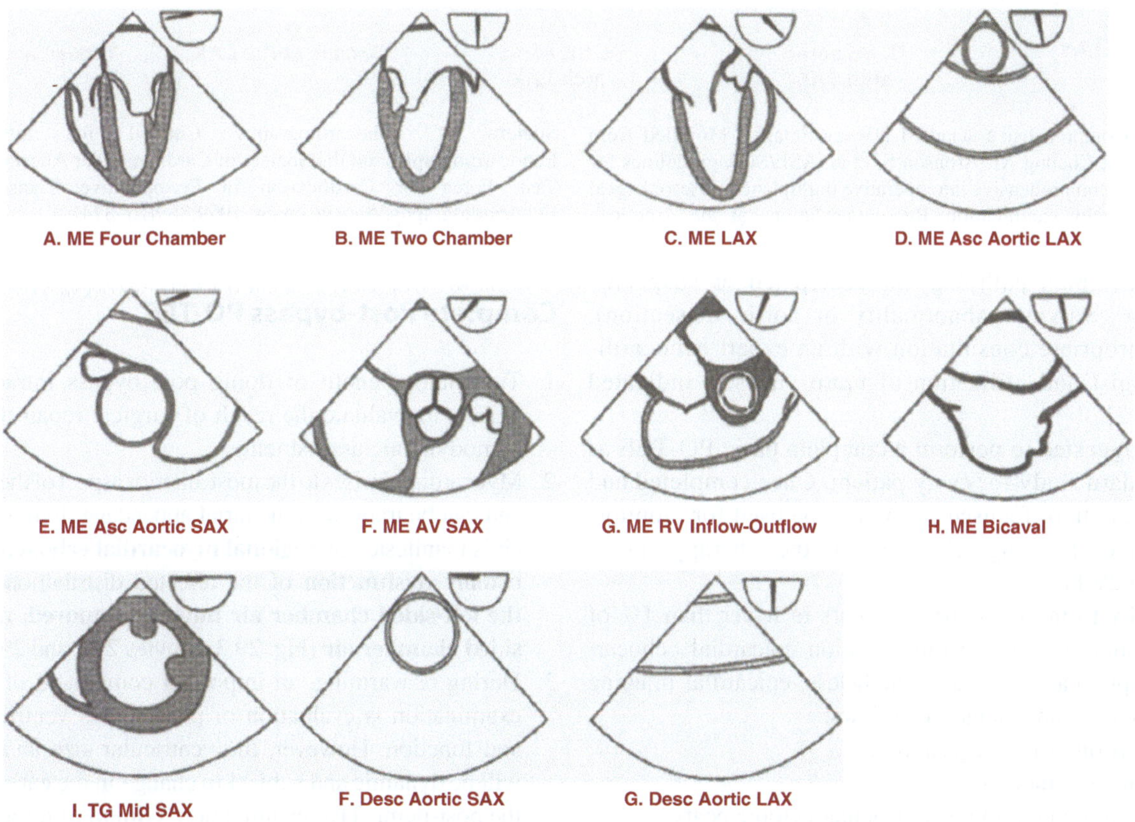

Fig. 29.1 American Society of Echocardiography and Society of Cardiovascular. Anesthesiologists have recommended 11 basic postoperative transesophageal echocardiography (PO-TEE) views. The basic PO-TEE study starts in the mid-esophageal 4-chamber view and continues at transgastric and upper-esophageal levels. *ME* Mid esophageal, *LAX* Long axis view, *SAX* Short axis view, *AV* Aortic valve, *RV* Right ventricle, *TG* Trans gastric

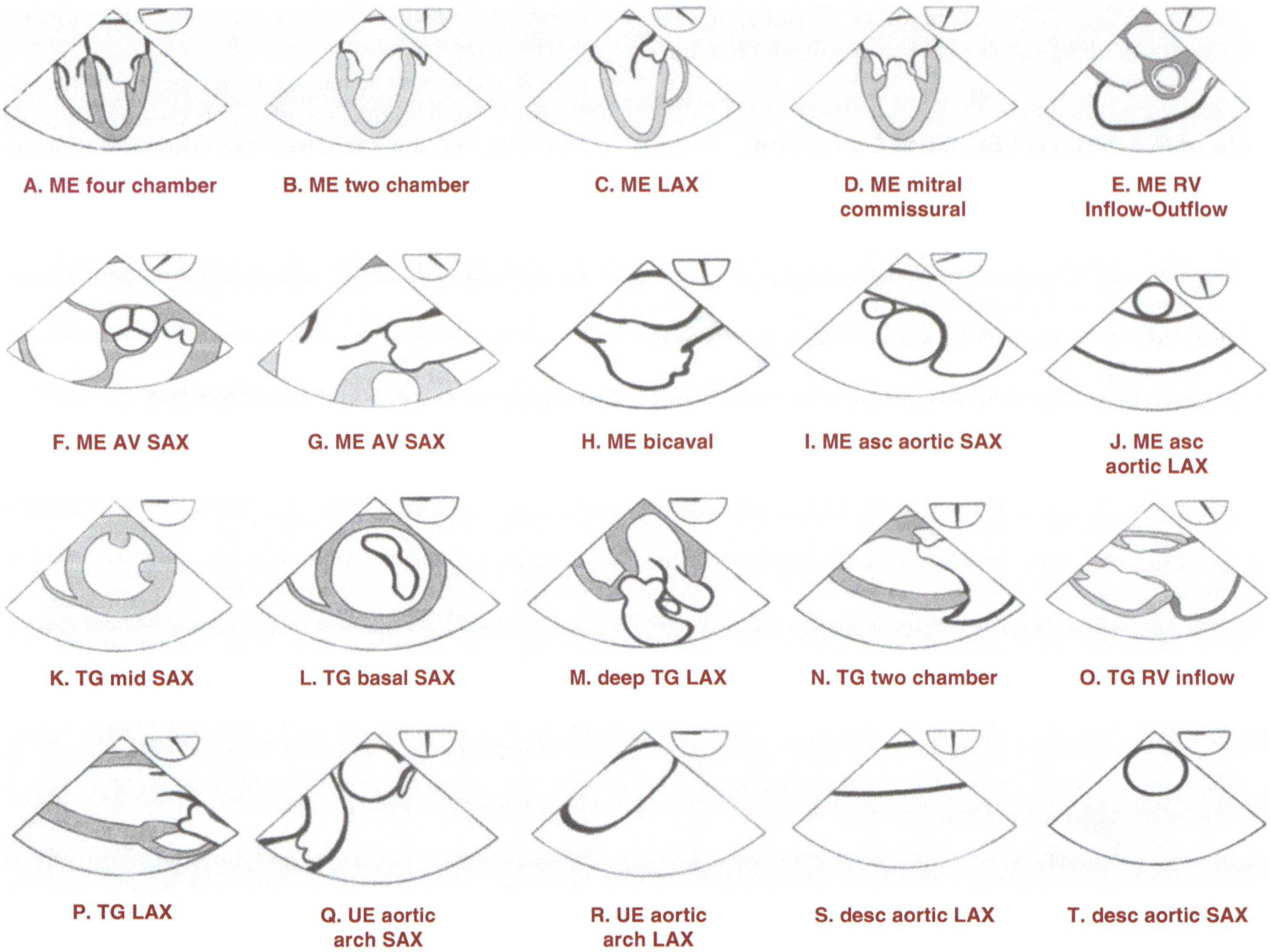

Fig. 29.2 Comprehensive standard 20-view images. Modified from Shanewise JS, Cheung AT, Aronson S, et al. ASE/SCA guidelines for performing a comprehensive intraoperative multiplane transesophageal echocardiography examination: Recommendations of the American Society of Echocardiography Council for Intraoperative Echocardiography and the Society of Cardiovascular Anesthesiologists Task Force for Certification in Perioperative Transesophageal Echocardiography. Anesth Analg. 1999;88:870–874

  - If complex pathology is anticipated or suspected (e.g., valvular abnormality or aortic dissection), appropriate consultation with an expert echocardiologist and utilization of more views is indicated [1, 2].
- It is suggested to perform a complete basic PO-TEE as a standard study for every patient. Once completed and stored, a more focused study may be used for monitoring and tracking changes in the therapy [1–3] (Table 29.1).
- Inability to insert the probe occurs in fewer than 1% of TEE attempts, and in this situation epicardial echocardiography can be used. Nonetheless, epicardial imaging has some disadvantages as follows:
  - Invasion of the surgical field
  - Limited windows
  - Possible induction of ventricular ectopic beats
  - Possible transient hypotension [1, 4, 5].

Complete Post-bypass PO-TEE

1. The major benefit of doing post bypass intraoperative TEE is to evaluate the result of surgical repair and guide hemodynamic assessment.
2. Myocardial air rises to the most anterior aspect of the chamber and can be trapped in the atrial appendage. Intramyocardial air is manifested by **regional myocardial echogenicity and usually dysfunction** of the affected distribution. **Indeed, the left-sided chamber air must be removed, not right-sided chamber air** (Fig. 29.3, Movies 29.1 and 29.2).
3. During re-warming, an important component of the TEE examination is evaluation of post-bypass ventricular size and function. However, the ventricular size and function will be dynamic and subject to change in the early phase of the post-pump TEE examination. **Global and** regional left ventricular function should be evaluated by using transgas-

Table 29.1 Further details on a complete set of postoperative transesophageal echocardiography (PO-TEE) pictures

ME four-chamber view • Angle: ~ 0–10° • Sector depth: ~ 12–14 cm Probe adjustments: Neutral-retroflexed Imaged structures: • LA, LV, MV, RA, RV and TV	Diagnostic uses: • Chamber enlargement/dysfunction • Left ventricular (LV) regional wall motion (inferoseptal and anterolateral walls) • Mitral and tricuspid valve disease • Detection of intracardiac air/mass including thrombosis and atrial septal defect	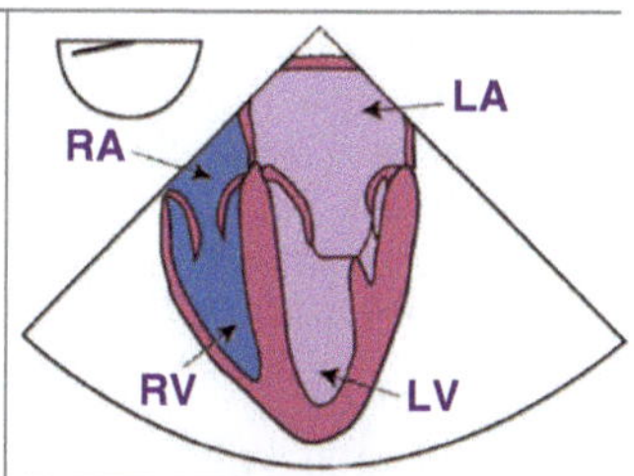
ME mitral commissural view Required structures: • LA, LV, Mitral valve Image settings: Angle: ~ 60–75° • Sector depth: ~12 cm	Diagnostic uses: • LV regional wall motion • Mitral valve disease	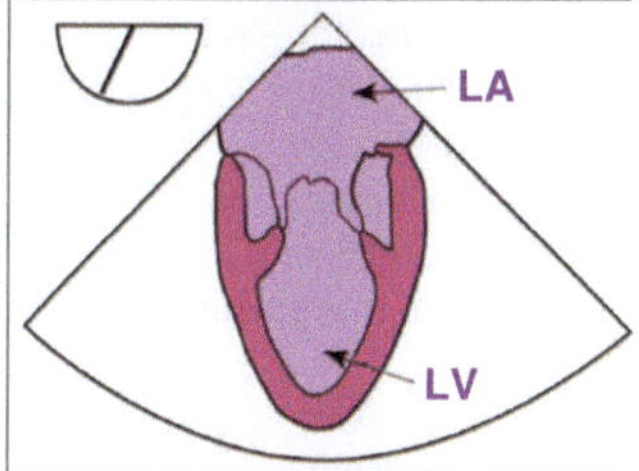
ME two-chamber view Required structures: • Left atrium appendage • Mitral valve • LV apex (maximum LV length) Settings: • Angle: ~ 80–100° • Sector depth: ~12–14 cm	Diagnostic uses: • Left atrial appendage mass or thrombus • LV apex pathology • LV systolic dysfunction • LV regional wall motion (anterior and inferior walls)	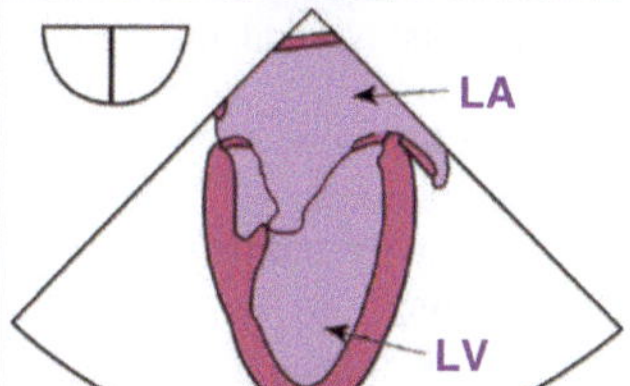
ME LV long axis (LAX) view Imaged structures: • LA, Mitral valve • LV, LV outflow tract • Aortic valve (AV) and proximal ascending (ASC) aorta Settings: • Angle: ~ 110–130° • Sector depth: ~12–14 cm	Diagnostic uses: • Mitral valve and LV outflow tract pathology including SAM • LV ventricular wall motion (anteroseptal and inferolateral walls)	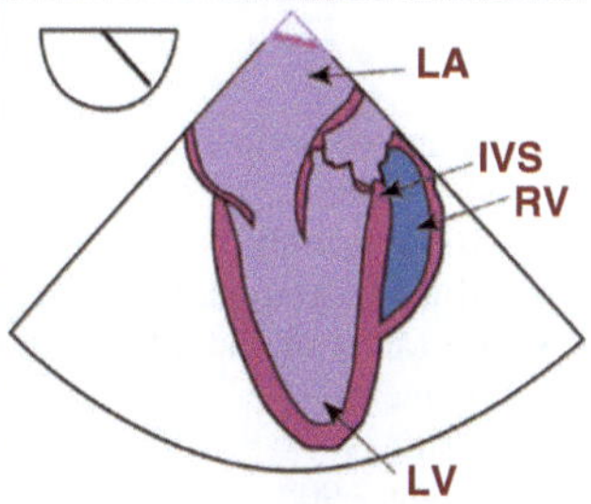
ME AV short axis (SAX) view Imaged structures: • AV leaflets and commissures • Coronary arteries Image settings: • Angle: ~25–40° • Sector depth: ~10–12 cm	Primary diagnostic uses: • AV morphology • Aortic stenosis/regurgitation • Coronary arteries	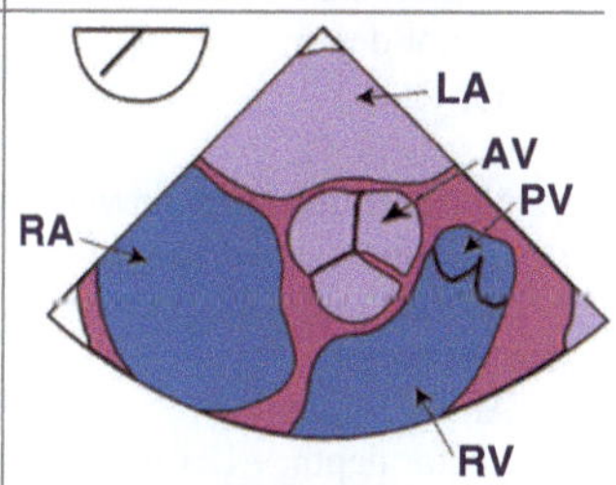
ME RV inflow-outflow Imaged structures: • PV, TV, Main PA (at least 1 cm distal to the PV) • RV inflow-outflow from TV to PV Image settings: • Angle: ~50–70° • Sector depth: ~10–12 cm	Primary diagnostic uses: • Pulmonic valve (PV) and main pulmonary artery (PA) pathology • Right ventricular outflow tract (RVOT) lesion (e.g., subvalvular stenosis)	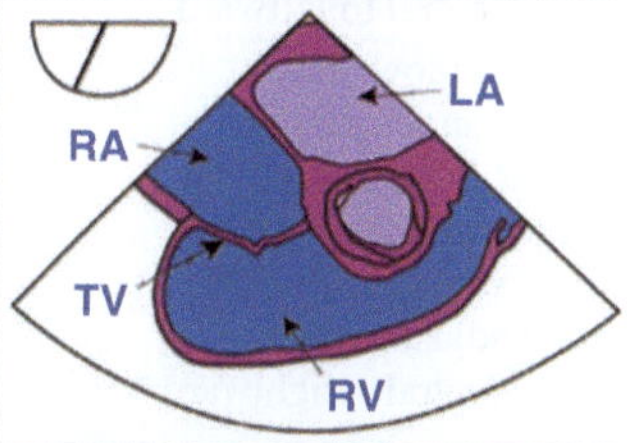
ME AV LAX view Imaged structures: • LVOT, AV, ASC aorta Image settings: • Angle: ~115–130° • Sector depth: ~6–10 cm	Primary diagnostic uses: • Left ventricular outflow tract (LVOT) pathway, AV and ASC aortic pathology	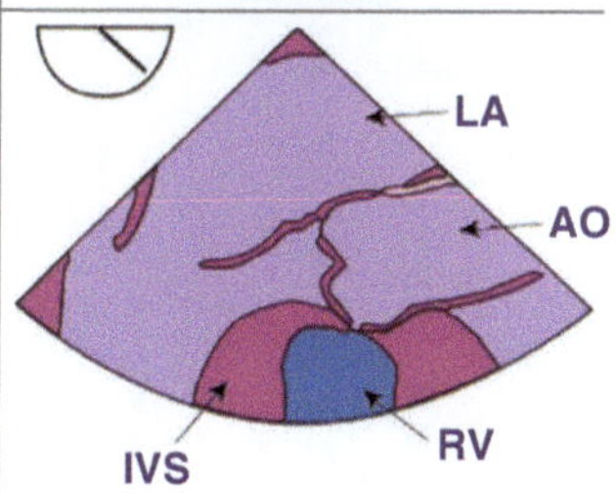

(continued)

Table 29.1 (continued)

ME bicaval view Imaged structures: • Right atrial free wall and appendage, Superior venal cava • Interatrial septum • Inferior vena cava (IVC) • LA Settings: • Angle: ~100–110° • Sector depth: ~8–10 cm • Rotating probe toward right	Diagnostic uses: • Atrial septal defect • Patent foramen ovale Right atrial mass	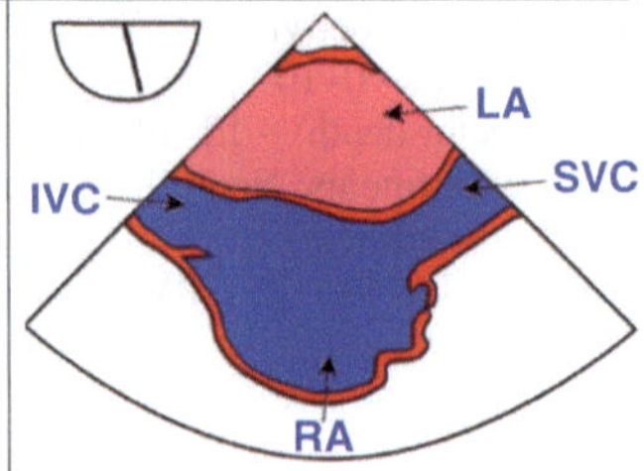
TG basal SAX view Imaged structures: • Mitral leaflets • LV (basal segments) Settings: • Angle: ~0° • Sector depth: ~12 cm Adjustments: Neutral and anteflex	Primary diagnostic uses: • LV systolic dysfunction (basal segments) Mitral valve pathway	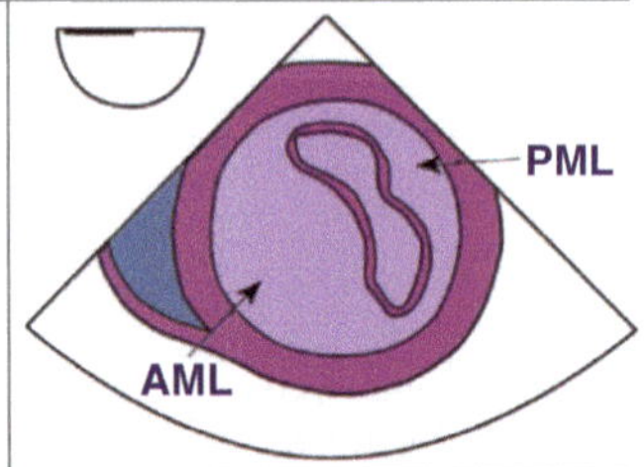
TG mid SAX view Imaged structures: • LV cavity and myocardial segments Image settings: • Angle: ~0° • Sector depth: ~12 cm • Anteflexed	Diagnostic uses: • Hemodynamic instability • Hypovolemia (volume status), LV preload • LV systolic dysfunction and regional wall motion	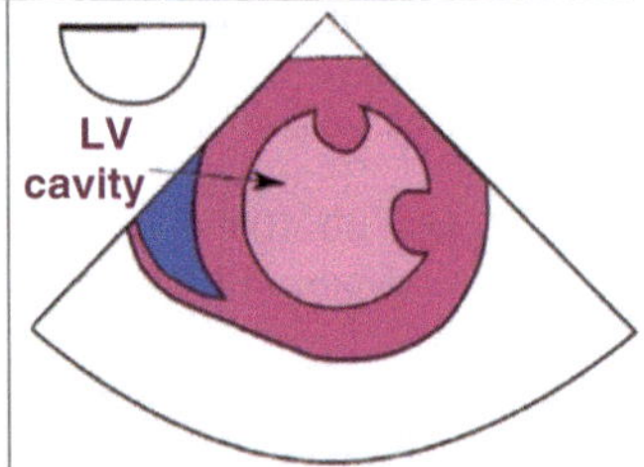
TG two-chamber view Imaged structures: • Mitral leaflets • Mitral subvalvular apparatus • LV (anterior and inferior walls: basal and mid segment) Image settings: • Angle: ~90° • Sector depth: ~12 cm	Primary diagnostic uses: • LV systolic function (anterior and inferior walls) • Mitral subvalvular pathology	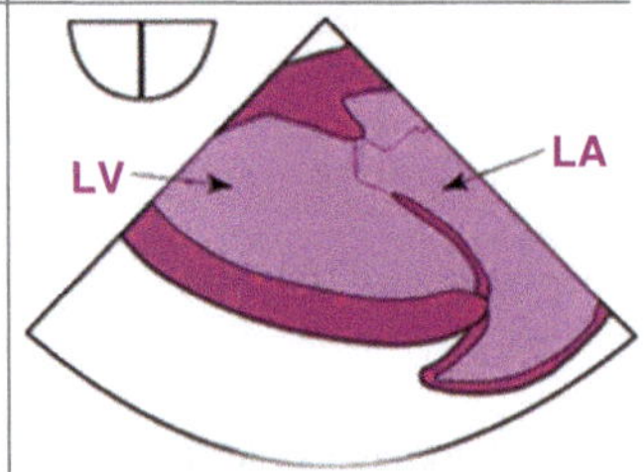
TG LAX view Imaged structures: • Mitral leaflets and subvalvular apparatus • LV (anteroseptal and inferior wall), LV outflow tract, AV and proximal ASC aorta Image settings: • Angle: ~110–130° • Sector depth: ~12 cm • Neutral to leftward	Primary diagnostic uses: • LV systolic dysfunction (anteroseptal and inferolateral walls) Doppler interrogation of AV	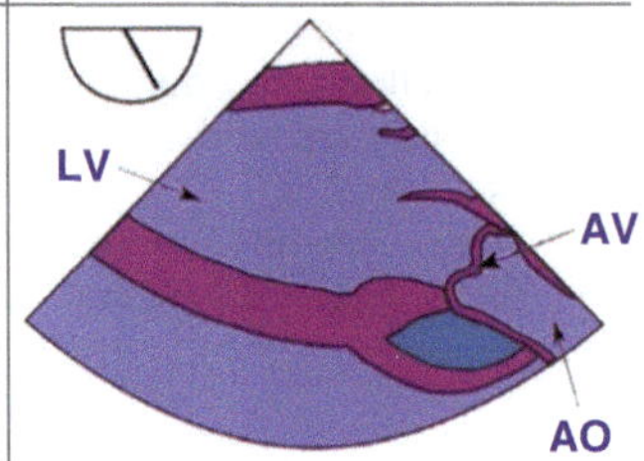
TG RV inflow view Imaged structures: • RA,TV, RV Image settings: • Angle: ~110–130° Probe adjustments: • Neutral—rightward	Diagnostic uses: • RV systolic dysfunction • TV pathology	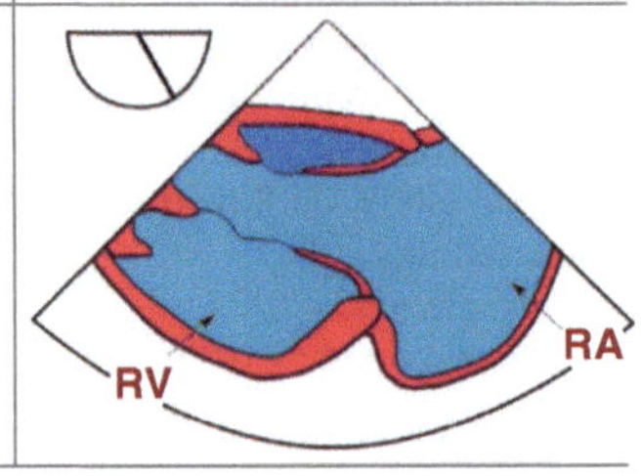

Deep TG LAX view Imaged structures: • LV, AV, ASC aorta Image settings: • Angle: ~0° • Sector depth: ~16 cm • Anteflexed	Primary diagnostic uses: • AV pathology • LVOT pathology Doppler interrogation of AV and LV outflow	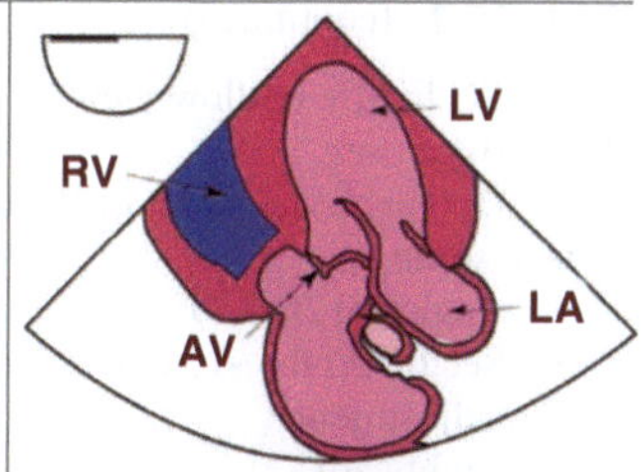
Descending (DESC) aorta SAX view Imaged structures: • DESC aorta in cross-section in the transverse plane (0°) Settings: • Angle: ~0° • Sector depth: ~6 cm • Turning probe toward left until DESC aorta is seen in SAX	Diagnostic uses: • Aortic atherosclerosis plaques • Aortic dissection • Coarctation of Aorta	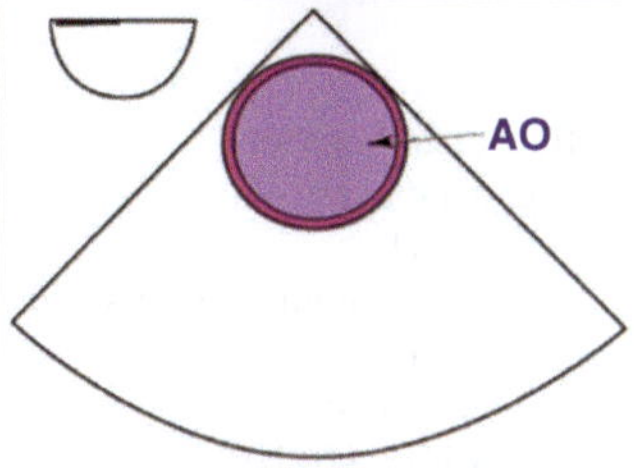
UE aortic SAX view Imaged structures: • Short axis aortic arch and main PA and left subclavian artery Image settings: • Angle: ~ 90° • Sector depth: ~10 cm	Primary diagnostic uses: • Aortic dissection • Diagnosis of patent ductus arteriosus, pulmonary stenosis and measurement of gradient across the pulmonary valve	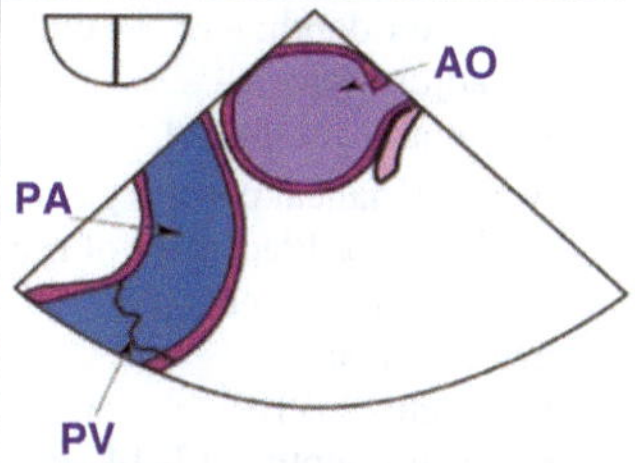
Additional views ME modified bicaval view Primary diagnostic uses: • TV pathology • Doppler interrogation of TV Image settings: • Angle: ~110° • Sector depth: ~8–10 cm Probe adjustments: • Probe rotated toward right as in bicaval view	Primary diagnostic uses: • Right atrium • LA • Interatrial septum • Coronary sinus • TV	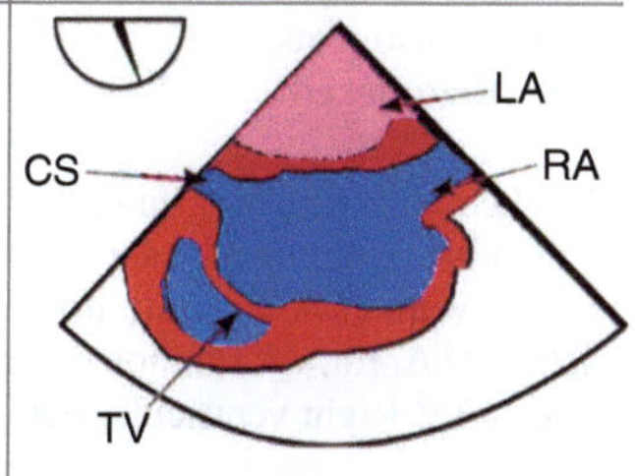
Lower esophageal (LE) hepatic view Primary diagnostic uses: • Inferior vena cava collapsibility and diameter • Hepatic venous flow velocity Image settings: • Angle: ~20° • Sector depth: ~10–12 cm Probe adjustments: • Rightward	Primary diagnostic uses: • Right atrium • Hepatic vein • IVC	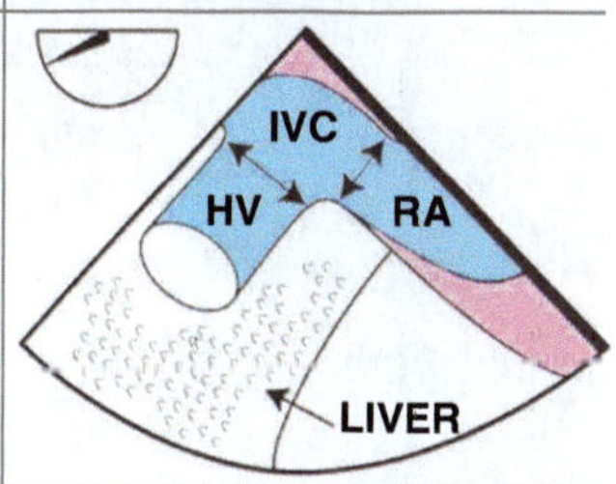
Deep TG RV LAX Primary diagnostic uses: • Doppler assessment across RVOT • RVOT Image settings: • Angle: ~110–130° • Sector depth: ~16 cm Probe adjustments: • Rightward	Primary diagnostic uses: • RV • Pulmonary valve • PA	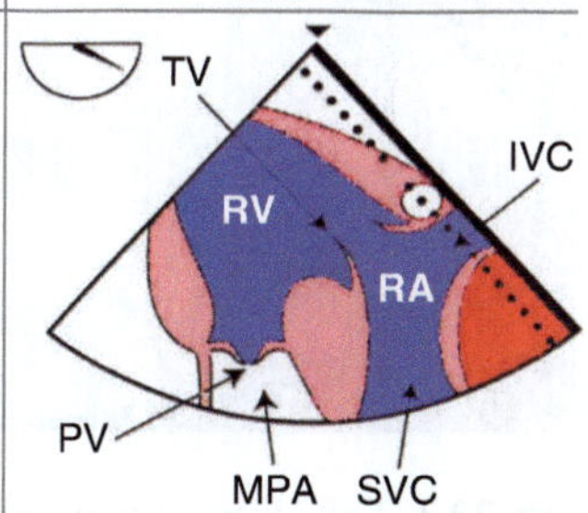

(continued)

Table 29.1 (continued)

Deep TG inflow-outflow view Diagnostic uses: • Doppler assessment of PA flow Image settings: • Angle: ~120–140° • Sector depth: ~16 cm Probe adjustments: • Rightward	Primary diagnostic uses: • RV, PV, PA	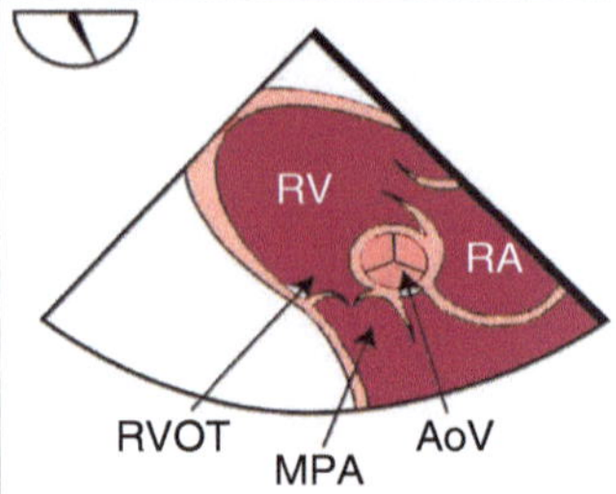
ME 5-chamber view Diagnostic uses: • LVOT • Aortic regurgitation/stenosis by color flow Doppler Image settings: • Angle: ~0–10° • Sector depth: ~12–14 cm Probe adjustments: • Neutral-retoflexed	Primary diagnostic uses: • LA, MV, LV outflow tract, LV • RA, RV, TV	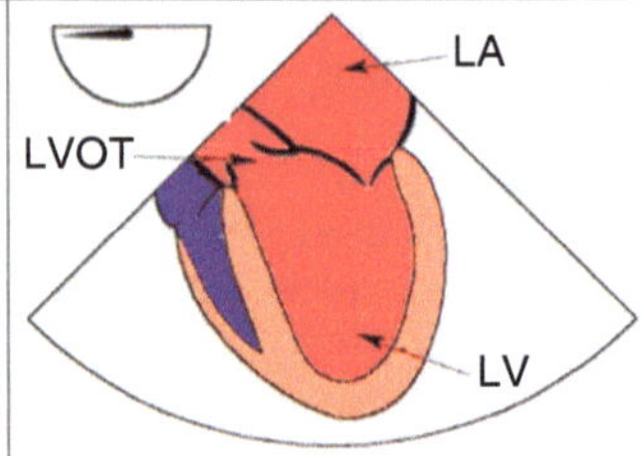
Lower esophageal coronary sinus view • Good for Placement of retrograde cardioplegia cannula Image settings: • Angle: ~0–10° • Sector depth: ~12–14 cm Probe adjustments: • Retroflexed	Primary diagnostic uses: • RA, Hepatic vein, IVC	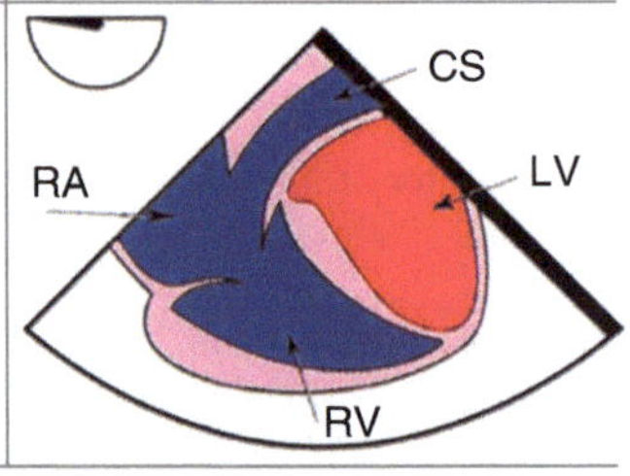

Modified from Kanchi Muralidhar et al.'s practice guidelines for perioperative transesophageal echocardiography: Recommendations of the Indian association of cardiovascular thoracic anesthesiologists. Ann Cardiac Anaesth. 16:4, Oct–Dec-2013. *AV* Aortic valve, *SVC* Superior vena cava, *IVC* Inferior vena cava, *LA* Left atrium, *RA* Right atrium, *PML* Posterior mitral leaflet, *AML* Anterior mitral leaflet, *LV* Left ventricle, *RV* Right ventricle, *AO* Aorta, *PA* Pulmonary artery, *CS* Coronary sinus, *TV* Tricuspid valve, *PV* Pulmonary valve, *MPA* Main pulmonary artery, *HV* Hepatic vein, *RVOT* Right ventricular outflow tract, *LVOT* Left ventricular outflow tract, *TV* Tricuspid valve

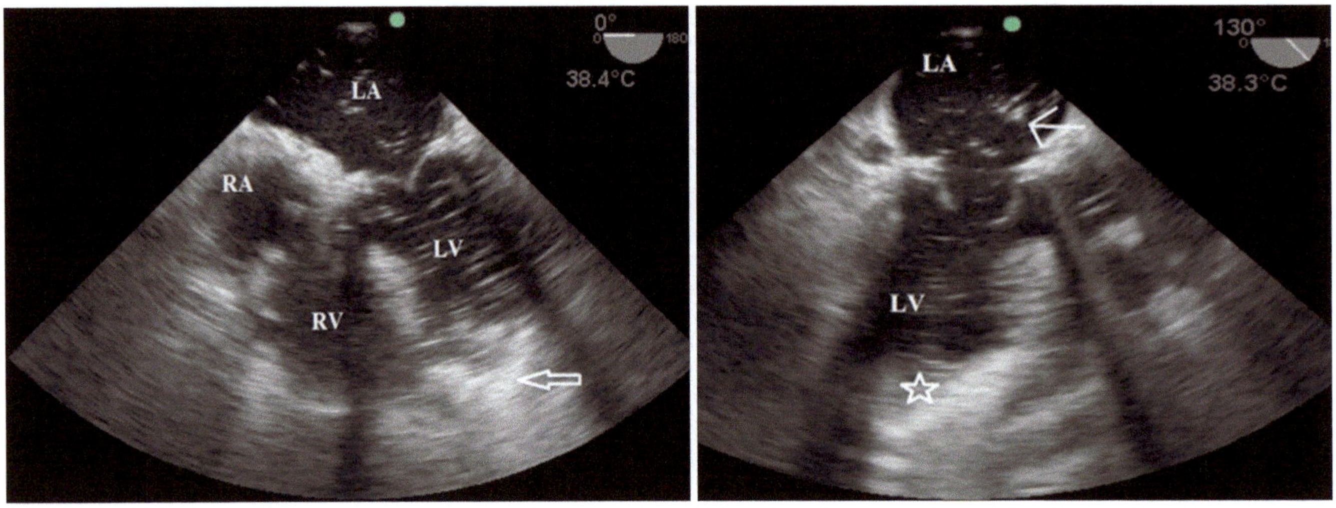

Fig. 29.3 Left-sided intracavitary air with intramyocardial air as is manifested by apical myocardial echogenicity and brightness. Left: Four-chamber view (arrow), Right: Long-axis view (star) and arrow

tric mid-papillary short-axis, mid-esophageal 4-chamber, mid-esophageal 2-chamber, and mid-esophageal long-axis views (Fig. 29.4) to correctly estimate the left ventricular global and regional systolic function and ejection fraction by visual assessment [2]. Postoperative wall motion abnormalities can be seen ***adjacent to the surgical sites of repair.***

4. **As the right coronary artery origin is anterior on the aortic root, myocardial air emboli is more commonly encountered in the distribution of the right coronary artery and is associated with right ventricular dysfunction, left ventricular regional wall motion abnormality, and/or ECG changes.**

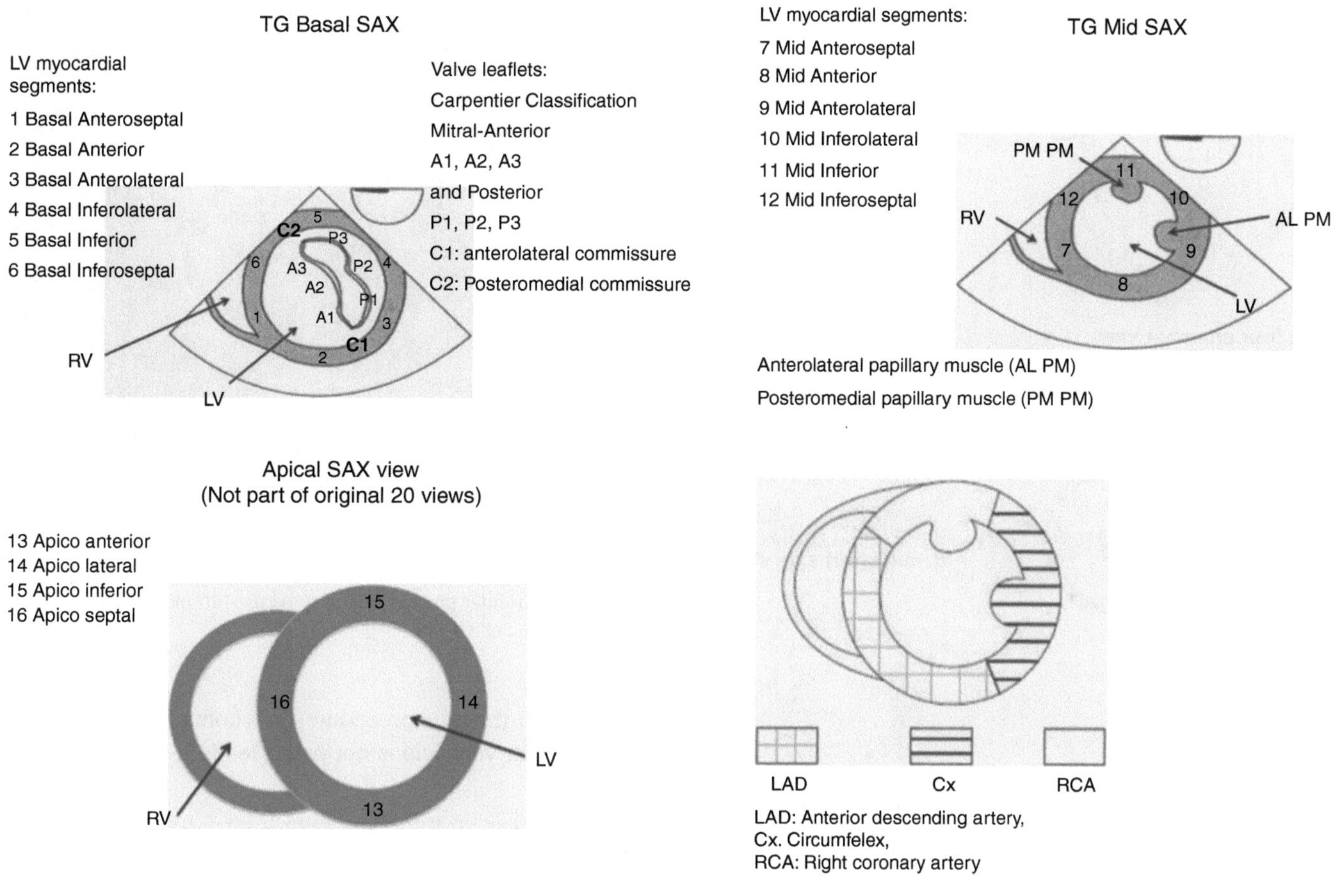

Fig. 29.4 Seventeen-segment model of the left ventricle in the short-axis view with the corresponding coronary territories

5. PO-TEE is useful for evaluating the hypovolemia state, which is a common cause of hemodynamic instability in the perioperative period.
6. Considering right ventricular dysfunction as a cause for refractory hypotension, PO-TEE is useful for evaluating the right ventricular function [2, 4, 6].

Global and Regional Left Ventricular Function

- Determination of the global left ventricular systolic function is one of the most common indications of the PO-TEE study.
- Most basic echocardiologists rely on qualitative, visual estimation of the systolic function. This method is far from precision but allows a basic echocardiologist to identify those cases who might benefit from inotropic therapies. Multiple publications support the use of TEE in cases with severe hemodynamic disturbances and unknown ventricular functions. Regional wall motion analysis using a 17-segment wall motion score described in the ASE guidelines may be performed via the mid-esophageal 4-chamber, mid-esophageal 2-chamber, and mid-esophageal long-axis views (Fig. 29.5). However, visualization of six mid-papillary segments from the transgastric mid-papillary short-axis view may suffice and has been shown to have prognostic importance.
- Transgastric mid-papillary short-axis view provides important diagnostic information pertaining to the regional and global ventricular functions in the hemodynamically unstable patient. Nonetheless, it is the recommendation of the last guidelines that a physician trained in basic PO-TEE echocardiography also use the mid-esophageal 4-chamber, mid-esophageal 2-chamber, and mid-esophageal long-axis views for a more comprehensive evaluation and monitoring of the global and regional left ventricular functions [1, 4, 7, 8].

Right Ventricular Function

- Several techniques for acquiring the quantitative measures of the global right ventricular systolic function have been well described. Nonetheless, most basic echocardiologists rely on a qualitative, visual estimation of the systolic function.

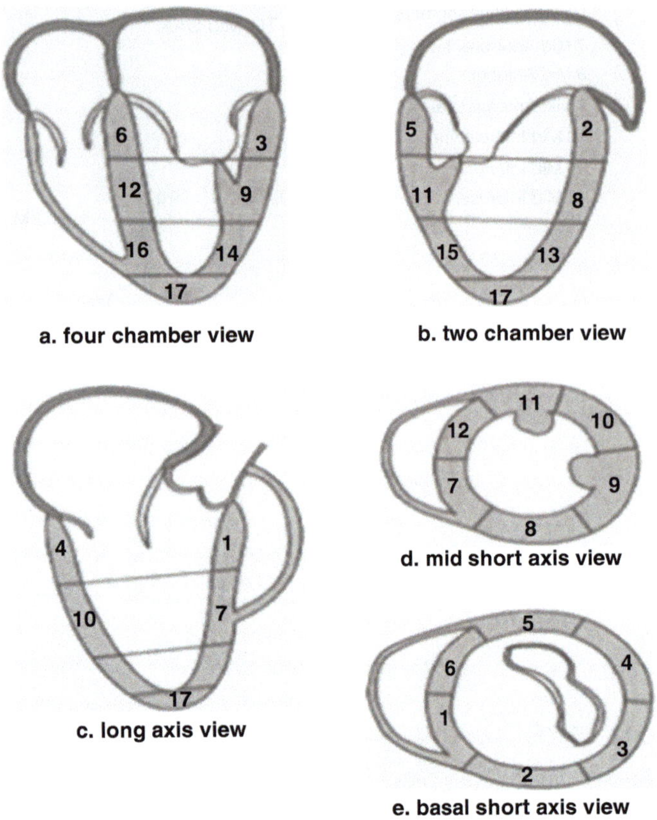

Basal Segments	Mid Segments
1 = Basal Anteroseptal	7 = Mid Anteroseptal
2 = Basal Anterior	8 = Mid Anterior
3 = Basal Anterolateral	9 = Mid Anterolateral
4 = Basal Inferolateral	10 = Mid Inferolateral
5 = Basal Inferior	11 = Mid Inferior
6 = Basal Inferoseptal	12 = Mid Inferoseptal

Fig. 29.5 Practical transesophageal echocardiography views for a more comprehensive evaluation of the global and regional left ventricular functions

Evaluation of the right ventricular function should be routinely performed in hypotensive cases. For example, cases undergoing liver transplantation are at increased risk for hypotension secondary to right ventricular failure. Patients undergoing liver transplantation with pulmonary hypertension have additional risk for right ventricular dysfunction secondary to acute changes in pulmonary pressures related to volume shifts and acid-base disturbances during transplantation. The use of basic PO-TEE echocardiography in this population allows rapid determination of the cardiac status and offers therapeutic advantages over invasive monitoring alone.

- It is recommended that a physician trained in basic PO-TEE echocardiography evaluate the right ventricle in cases of refractory hypotension and that basic PO-TEE monitoring be considered for cases at high risk for right ventricular dysfunction—in particular those cases undergoing non-thoracic procedures in whom direct inspection of the right ventricle is not possible [1, 2, 6–8].

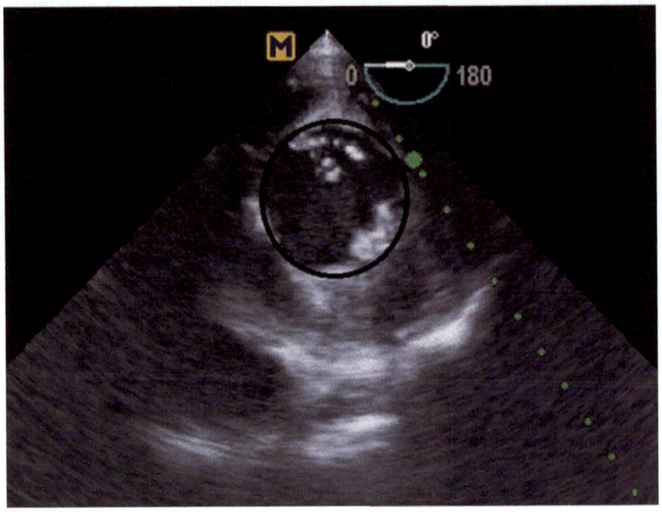

Fig. 29.6 Compared with baseline imaging, measurements of the left ventricular end-diastolic area may be used as an indirect measurement of the left ventricular preload and may be used to monitor response to fluid therapy (black circle)

Hypovolemia

- Hypovolemia is a common cause of hemodynamic instability in the perioperative period. The most common echocardiographic parameters used to diagnose hypovolemia are left ventricular end-diastolic diameter and left ventricular end-diastolic area obtained in the transgastric mid-papillary short-axis view (Fig. 29.6).
  - Compared with the more invasive pulmonary artery catheterization, TEE has been shown to provide a better index of the left ventricular preload in cases with a normal left ventricular function. More advanced Doppler-derived data may also be obtained, but this is time-consuming, requires advanced training, and might have limited accuracy in anesthetized cases.
  - Relative changes between the baseline status and the critical event, however, remain useful in detecting acute changes in the left ventricular preload. The use of basic PO-TEE echocardiography as a monitor includes both intermittent acquisition of images and ongoing live imaging, particularly by obtaining the transgastric mid-papillary short-axis view.
  - A certified echocardiologist (basic or advanced) should be involved in the evaluation of images and its use to effect changes in management, including direct volume resuscitation or pressor administration. It is the recommendation that a physician trained in basic PO-TEE echocardiography use the transgastric mid-papil-

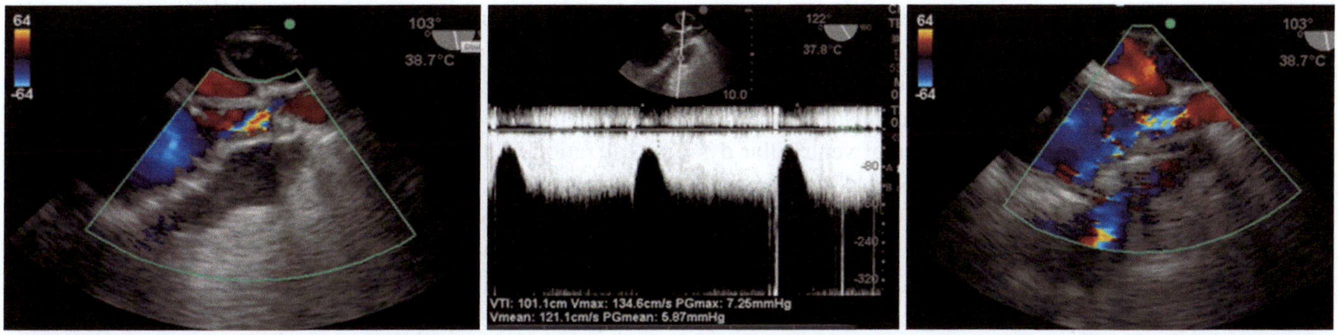

Fig. 29.7 Movies 29.3 and 29.4 Intraoperative transesophageal echocardiography images of an adult patient after sinus venosus type atrial septal defect repair. Left and middle panels show a significant turbulent flow and an increased gradient, suggestive of the superior vena cava to the right atrial junction stenosis. Right panel: Gradient and turbulent flow decreased after fluid therapy

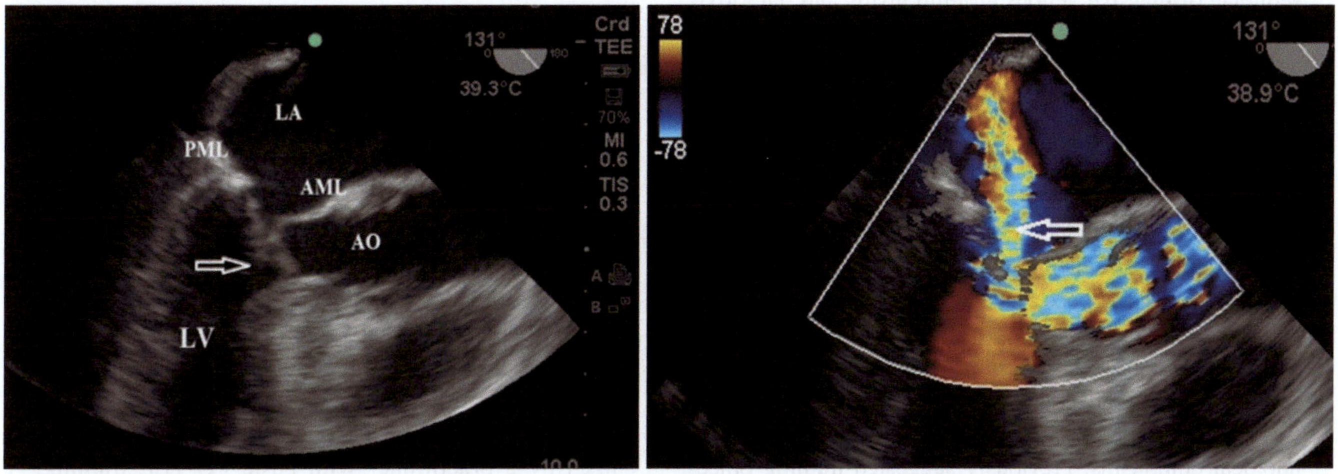

Fig. 29.8 Intraoperative transesophageal echocardiography study in a patient who underwent mitral valve repair shows: Systolic anterior motion (SAM) of the anterior mitral valve leaflet (Left panel) associated with posterior directed mitral regurgitation (Right panel)

lary short-axis view to monitor and guide a hypovolemic patient's response to fluid and blood component therapy (Fig. 29.7) [1, 4, 9].

Basic Valvular Lesions

- Practitioners of basic PO-TEE echocardiography should be familiar with basic valvular lesions. This includes knowledge of color-flow Doppler assessment of valvular regurgitation. Caution should be exercised when assessing the severity of eccentric jets. The mechanism of any regurgitant jet might require consultation with a physician with advanced PO-TEE capabilities (Fig. 29.8).
- Rapid assessment of possible stenotic valvular lesions may be done by visualizing the leaflet motion and using continuous-wave Doppler in any imaging plane in which the blood flow is parallel to the interrogating continuous-wave Doppler beam. Complete assessment of valvular regurgitant and stenotic lesions is outlined in multiple ASE guideline documents. Assessment of prosthetic valve function should be performed by a physician with advanced PO-TEE knowledge.
- It is the recommendation that a physician trained in basic PO-TEE echocardiography use the complete basic PO-TEE study to qualitatively delineate valvular regurgitation and/or stenosis. However, if the valve lesion is considered severe, or if comprehensive quantification is required to ultimately determine the need for intervention, a consultation with an advanced PO-TEE echocardiologist is necessary to confirm the severity and etiology of the valve pathology (Fig. 29.8, Movies 29.5 and 29.6) [1, 2, 10, 11].
- In the previous opinion, the echocardiographic diagnosis of a pulmonary embolism using direct evidence often requires advanced PO-TEE skills. In addition, previously suggested cognitive and technical objectives for basic PO-TEE training have not included pulmonary embolisms. Nonetheless, it is the recommendation that a physician trained in basic PO-TEE echocardiography at least be able to use the mid-

esophageal 4-chamber, mid-esophageal ascending aortic short-axis, and mid-esophageal right ventricular inflow-outflow views to identify indirect echocardiographic findings consistent with a pulmonary embolism such as the presence of thrombi and/or signs of right ventricular dysfunction before the initiation of treatment [1, 4, 12].

Air Embolism During Surgery

- Venous air embolisms commonly occur during craniotomies in the sitting position and have an incidence rate as high as 76%. Although the vast majority of venous air embolisms are small with little clinical significance, the sequelae of massive venous air embolisms and paradoxical embolism across a PFO may be catastrophic. Thus, early detection and treatment are necessary. Basic PO-TEE echocardiography offers the advantage of providing both real-time data and a visual quantification of venous air embolisms. TEE is a more sensitive method for the detection of venous air embolisms than transthoracic. Nevertheless, the detection of these microbubbles can alert the clinician an important issue that may easily be addressed before it becomes problematic.
- Most recent basic PO-TEE echocardiography allows the detection of right-to-left shunts. Diagnosis of a shunt may influence the operative team to avoid the sitting position in this patient population because these cases are prone to paradoxical embolisms. Previously suggested training objectives for basic PO-TEE training included the requirement for knowledge of the echocardiographic presentations of air embolization [4]. It is the recommendation that a physician trained in basic PO-TEE echocardiography use a complete basic PO-TEE study to identify cases at risk for right-to-left shunts and detect intracardiac air promptly [1, 2, 10–12].

Pericardial Effusion

- Echocardiography plays an integral part in the evaluation of trauma involving the thoracic cavity. In trauma, rapid diagnosis and intervention are crucial to optimizing patient outcomes. The value of ultrasonography has long been recognized in the trauma literature, as it is now a part of the Focused Assessment With Sonography in Trauma study. Similarly, TEE is a mobile diagnostic tool that provides a rapid and accurate diagnosis of pericardial effusions, traumatic aortic injuries, and cardiac contusions. Both physical trauma (blunt or penetrating thoracic trauma) and iatrogenic trauma (during invasive procedures) may result in the accumulation of a pericardial effusion. If the effusion accumulates rapidly, hemodynamic instability might ensue, and TEE may facilitate treatment with pericardiocentesis. Many publications support the use of TEE for traumatic aortic injury given the safety, portability, and high diagnostic accuracy of this modality.
- Nonetheless, it is important to keep in mind that the visualization of the distal ascending aorta and the proximal aortic arch is quite limited via TEE. The diagnosis of cardiac contusions might also be difficult and limited in that there is no one diagnostic test for this condition. When used in conjunction with TTE, serial ECG, and serial myocardial enzyme assessment, TEE provides valuable diagnostic information. However, caution must be exercised with the TEE probe placement and manipulation because of a potential coexisting esophageal or cervical spine injury [5, 6].

Simple Adult Congenital Heart Diseases

- TEE assessment of adult cases with complex congenital heart diseases (CHDs) has been used since the late 1980s and usually requires a meticulous sequential evaluation that requires the knowledge and experience of an advanced PO-TEE echocardiologist.
- Although adult CHDs have not previously been included within the scope of basic cognitive echocardiographic skills, several basic congenital lesions might have an impact on intraoperative care (as discussed under "Neurosurgery: Air Embolism") and should be recognized by a practitioner with basic PO-TEE training. A PFO and/or a secundum atrial septal defect (ASD) is generally easily recognized via 2D and color-flow Doppler imaging in the mid-esophageal bicaval view as a defect in the central portion of the interatrial septum and should be considered in cases in whom there is high clinical suspicion of an otherwise unexplainable right-to-left shunt (hypoxia) or left-to-right shunt. However, an advanced PO-TEE echocardiologist should be consulted if further echocardiographic interrogation of the entire interatrial septum is warranted to exclude more complex congenital lesions of the interatrial septum such as smaller secundum ASDs, primum ASDs, or more-difficult-to-visualize sinus venous ASDs.
- Ventricular septal defects are classified on the basis of their location (perimembranous, muscular, double-committed outlet, and inlet) or their pathophysiology (post-infarction) and may be related with important hemodynamic instability.
- Although a basic echocardiologist might perform a basic PO-TEE study with 2D and color-flow Doppler using the mid-esophageal 4-chamber, mid-esophageal 2-chamber, and mid-esophageal aortic valve long-axis views to evaluate a patient for a ventricular septal defect, nowadays it is believed that this type of diagnostic interrogation usually requires advanced PO-TEE skills.

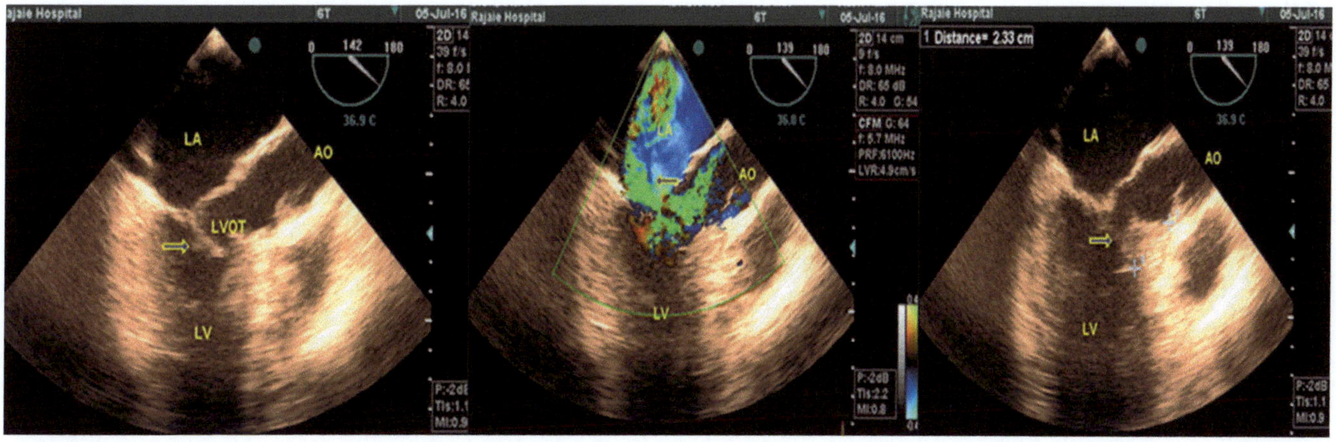

Fig. 29.9 Movie 29.7. Fibromuscular sub-aortic valve stenosis are associated with the systolic anterior motion (SAM) of the anterior mitral valve leaflet and posterior directed mitral regurgitation. Thickness and length of the subvalvular thickening are important as these measurements are useful parameters for estimating the extent of the septomymectomy (Arrows). *LA* Left atrium, *LV* Left ventricle, *AO* Aorta

- Echocardiographic diagnosis and directed intervention for more complex adult CHDs such as ventricular septal defects and less commonly encountered ASDs require consultation with an advanced PO-TEE echocardiologist (Fig. 29.9) [1, 2, 13].

Conclusions

PO-TEE should be considered for most cardiac defects requiring repair under cardiopulmonary bypass. It has been suggested that combined **preoperative and postoperative TEE has a major impact on the diagnostic and treatment plan in about 14% of surgeries.** Needing a return to bypass for further surgery in about 3–8% of bypass cases makes PO-TEE cost-effective [1, 2, 4, 13, 14].

References

1. Reeves ST, Finley AC, Skubas NJ, Swaminathan M, Whitley WS, Glas KE, Hahn RT, Shanewise JS, Adams MS, Shernan SK. Basic perioperative transesophageal echocardiography study: a consensus statement of the American Society of Echocardiography and the Society of Cardiovascular Anesthesiologists. Expert consensus statement. J Am Soc Echocardiogr. 2013;26:443–56.
2. Muralidhar K, Tempe D, Chakravarthy M, Shastry N, Kapoor PM, Tewari P, Gadhinglajkar SV, Mehta Y. Practice guidelines for perioperative transesophageal echocardiography: recommendations of the Indian association of cardiovascular thoracic anesthesiologists. Ann Card Anaesth. 2013;16:4.
3. Labovitz AJ, Noble VE, Bierig M, Goldstein SA, Jones R, Kort S, et al. Focused cardiac ultrasound in the emergent setting: a consensus statement of the American Society of Echocardiography and American College of Emergency Physicians. J Am Soc Echocardiogr. 2010;23:1225–30.
4. Júnior CG, Botelho ESL, dos Santos Diego LA. Intraoperative monitoring with transesophageal echocardiography in cardiac surgery. Rev Bras Anestesiol. 2011;61(4):495–512.
5. Oxorn D. Intraoperative echocardiography. 1st ed. Philadelphia: Saunders, an Imprint of Elsevier Inc; 2012. p. 1–5.
6. American Society of Anesthesiologists and Society of Cardiovascular Anesthesiologists Task Force on Transesophageal Echocardiography. Practice guidelines for perioperative transesophageal echocardiography. An updated report by the American Society of Anesthesiologists and the Society of Cardiovascular Anesthesiologists Task Force on Transesophageal Echocardiography. Anesthesiology. 2010;112:1084–96.
7. Hilberath JN, Oakes DA, Shernan SK, Bulwer BE, D'Ambra MN, Eltzschig HK. Safety of transesophageal echocardiography. J Am Soc Echocardiogr. 2010;23(11):1115–27.
8. Lang RM, Badano LP, Tsang W, Adams DH, Agricola E, Buck T, et al. EAE/ASE recommendations for image acquisition and display using three dimensional echocardiography. J Am Soc Echocardiogr. 2012;25:3–46.
9. Shillcutt SK, Markin NW, Montzingo CR, Brakke TR. Use of rapid "rescue" perioperative echocardiography to improve outcomes after hemodynamic instability in noncardiac surgical cases. J Cardiothorac Vasc Anesth. 2012;26:362–70.
10. Click RL, Abel MD, Schaff HV. Intra-operative transesophageal echocardiography: 5-year prospective review of impact on surgical management. Mayo Clin Proc. 2000;75:241–7.
11. Eltzschig HK, Rosenberger P, Loffler M, Fox JA, Aranki SF, Shernan SK. Impact of intra-operative transesophageal echocardiography on surgical decisions in 12,566 cases undergoing cardiac surgery. Ann Thorac Surg. 2008;85:845–52.
12. Torbicki A, Perrier A, Konstantinides S, Agnelli G, Galie N, Pruszczyk P, et al. Guidelines on the diagnosis and management of acute pulmonary embolism: the Task Force for the Diagnosis and Management of Acute Pulmonary Embolism of the European Society of Cardiology (ESC). Eur Heart J. 2008;29:2276–315.
13. Lopez L, Colan SD, Frommelt PC, Ensing GJ, Kendall K, Younoszai AK, et al. Recommendations for quantification methods during the performance of a pediatric echocardiogram: a report from the Pediatric Measurements Writing Group of the American Society of Echocardiography Pediatric and Congenital Heart Disease Council. J Am Soc Echocardiogr. 2010;23:465–95.
14. Ghavidel AA, Sadeghpour A, Alizadehasl A. A rescue coronary artery bypass grafting in isolated life-threatening right ventricular failure after aortic valve replacement. J Thorac Cardiovasc Surg. 2012;144(6):1538–9. doi:10.1016/j.jtcvs.2012.08.024.

The Role of Echocardiography in Mitral Valve Repair

30

Nishant K. Sekaran, Alina Nicoara, and Zainab Samad

Abstract

Echocardiography is a versatile diagnostic technology integral to the assessment and treatment of mitral regurgitation (MR). MR is broadly classified as primary—resulting from abnormalities of the MV leaflets or apparatus, or secondary—arising from left ventricular dysfunction and subsequent distortion of mitral architecture. While these entities have distinctly different outcomes and treatment strategies, the common therapeutic goal is to reduce MR and improve outcomes through medical management alone or MV repair. MV repair is performed surgically or percutaneously with echocardiography guidance. The echocardiographer can use the full complement of trans-thoracic (TTE) and trans-esophageal (TEE) 2D, 3D, and Doppler techniques to enhance procedural and patient outcomes by (1) performing an integrative assessment of the etiology, mechanism, severity, and hemodynamic impact of the MR, (2) predicting the feasibility and prognosis of MV repair, (3) directly guiding catheter placement, and (4) assessing for complications during or after MV repair.

Keywords

Mitral valve repair · Mitral regurgitation · Trans-thoracic echocardiography · Trans-esophageal echocardiography

Abbreviations

2D	Two-dimensional
3D	Three-dimensional
AP2	Apical 2-chamber
AP3	Apical 3-chamber
AP4	Apical 4-chamber
EF	Ejection fraction
EROA	Effective regurgitant orifice area
FC	Flow convergence
FED	Fibroelastic deficiency
FMR	Functional mitral regurgitation
LA	Left atrium
LAX	Long axis
LV	Left ventricular
LVEDD	Left ventricular end diastolic dimension
LVEF	Left ventricular ejection fraction
LVESD	Left ventricular end systolic dimension
LVH	Left ventricular hypertrophy
LVOT	Left ventricular outflow tract
ME	Mid-esophageal
MR	Mitral regurgitation
MS	Mitral stenosis
MV	Mitral valve
MVP	Mitral valve prolapse
PISA	Proximal isovelocity surface area
PLAX	Parasternal long axis
RF	Regurgitant fraction
RV	Regurgitant volume
SAM	Systolic anterior motion

N. K. Sekaran
Division of General Internal Medicine, University of Michigan Medical School and VA Ann Arbor Healthcare System, Ann Arbor, MI, USA
e-mail: nishants@umich.edu

A. Nicoara
Department of Anesthesiology, Duke University Hospital, Durham, NC, USA

Z. Samad (✉)
Department of Cardiology, Duke University Hospital, Durham, NC, USA
e-mail: zainab.samad@duke.edu

A. Sadeghpour, A. Alizadehasl (eds.), *Case-Based Textbook of Echocardiography*,
https://doi.org/10.1007/978-3-319-67691-3_30

SAX	Short axis
TEE	Trans-esophageal echocardiography
TTE	Trans-thoracic echocardiography
VC	Vena contracta

Introduction

- MV repair is a definitive invasive treatment used to treat or stabilize severe MR arising from primary (e.g. degenerative) or secondary (LV dysfunction) causes, respectively.
- The primary advantages of MV repair compared to MV replacement are lower operative mortality, higher likelihood of preserved LV function, and lower rates of prosthesis-related complications such as thromboembolism, anticoagulation associated bleeding, and endocarditis [1–4].
- MV repair techniques involve surgical or percutaneous approaches. Trans-thoracic (TTE) and trans-esophageal echocardiography (TEE) are integral to the successful performance of both.
- Clinicians must be able to correctly perform and interpret echocardiographic data to facilitate accurate diagnosis, risk stratification, treatment planning, and long-term follow up.

General Classification of MR Lesions Potentially Treated by MV Repair

- MR is defined as **primary** or **secondary** [5].
  - **Primary** MR is caused by abnormalities in the MV leaflets or sub-valvular apparatus (i.e. chordae tendinae or papillary muscles).
  - **Secondary** or "functional" MR results from annular dilation or left ventricular dysfunction with outward displacement of the posterior ventricular wall; this in turn can exert a "tethering effect" on the posterior MV leaflet. The morphology of the leaflets and chordae are normal [3, 6].
- The **Carpentier Functional Classification** classifies MR into etiologic sub-groups based on valve leaflet motion and amount of leaflet tissue [7].
  - Type I has normal leaflet motion; MR is caused by leaflet perforation or annular dilation and the MR jet is centrally directed.
  - Type II has increased leaflet motion resulting from degenerative disease of the leaflets with elongated or ruptured chordae causing valve prolapse or flail and an MR jet directed away from the affected leaflet.
  - Type III has restricted leaflet motion and is sub-categorized into:
    Type IIIa where leaflet motion is restricted during systole and diastole secondary to rheumatic heart disease
    Type IIIb whereby leaflet motion is restricted during systole and is usually caused by ischemic heart disease. There is ventricular dilation, papillary muscle displacement, and leaflet tethering with an eccentric MR jet directed towards the restricted leaflet.
  - Type IVa involves systolic anterior motion of the MV and can be seen, for example, in hypertrophic cardiomyopathy or post-MV repair.
  - Type V involves mixed lesions (e.g. combined rheumatic and endocarditis).

Primary MR, Carpentier Type 1

- **Endocarditis** is an infection of the endocardial layer of the heart that can cause leaflet perforation, valvular abscesses and aneurysms.
  - MV repair may be an option if leaflet destruction is not extensive. These patients demonstrate better early and late prognosis in observational data compared to MV replacement [8] (Fig. 30.1).
- **Cleft MV** is a congenital lesion that can be associated with endocardial cushion defects including atrial septal defect (septum primum) and ventricular septal defect (inlet type) (Fig. 30.2).

Primary MR, Carpentier Type II

- **Degenerative MV** disease is the most common repairable cause of MR in developed countries, and most commonly

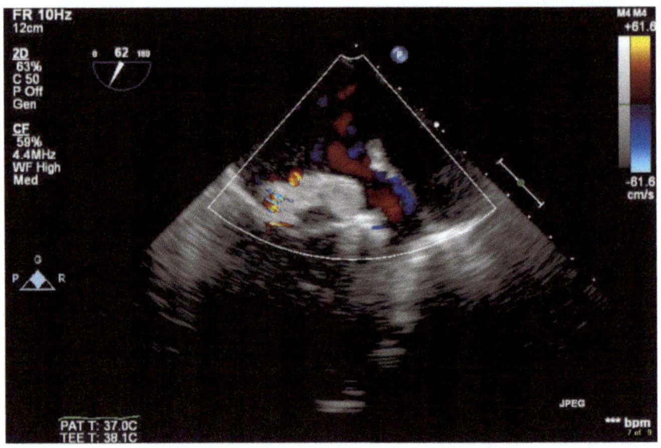

Fig. 30.1 A 2-chamber TEE image from a 41 year old male with fungal endocarditis with a large vegetation on the P3 MV leaflet segment with color Doppler signal through a perforated segment

results from **MV prolapse (MVP)** [9]. **MVP** can be categorized as **myxomatous type** or **fibroelastic deficiency (FED)** (Fig. 30.3); the latter is typically less complex and easier to treat [10].

- **Myxomatous disease** typically occurs in patients <60 years and is characterized by thickening of the leaflets and/or sub-valvular apparatus secondary to accumulation of glycosaminoglycans in the extra-cellular matrix.
- **Fibroelastic deficiency (FED)** typically occurs in patients >60 years and is characterized by chordal elongation or rupture with resultant leaflet prolapse or flail resulting in abrupt MR.

- **MVP** is defined anatomically as superior displacement of the mitral leaflets of more than 2 mm during systole with maximal leaflet thickness of at least 5 mm during diastasis [11].

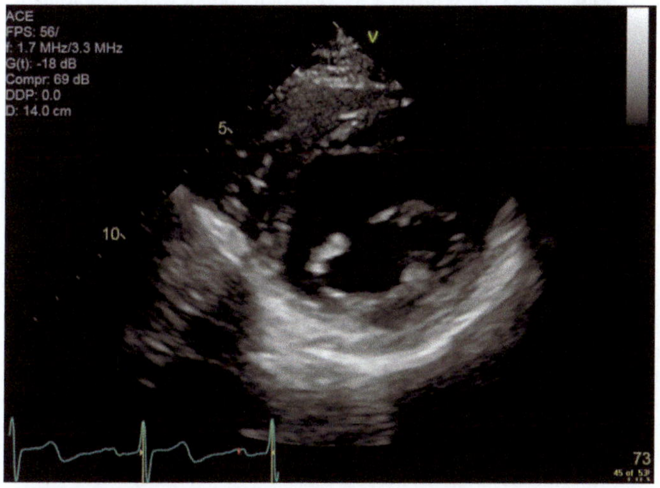

Fig. 30.2 A short-axis 2D TTE image from a 28 year old woman with a history of unrepaired cleft MV. The cleft can be seen in the A2 MV segment

  - One or both thickened MV leaflets typically "bow" or "buckle" in an asymmetric manner past the plane of the mitral annulus during late-systole. As a result, the MR color jet is relatively brief (i.e. not holosystolic).
  - Contemporary prevalence estimates are 2–3% of the population [1].
  - MVP can occur with Marfan's syndrome, which also affects the aortic valve and aortic root.
  - Complications include MR, chordal rupture with flail leaflet, neurologic sequelae, endocarditis, or malignant arrhythmias.
  - This can be captured by M-mode echocardiography or by 2D echocardiography in the parasternal long or AP2 views.

- **Papillary muscle rupture** is a rare entity that can occur with ischemic disease or trauma and result in severe MR.
  - Rupture of the posteromedial papillary muscle occurs more often than rupture of the anterolateral papillary muscle due to a single blood supply from the right coronary or the left circumflex artery [6].
  - MV replacement occurs more commonly than MV repair in this situation.

Primary MR, Carpentier Type IIIa

- **Rheumatic** disease leads to inflammation and results in thickening of the MV leaflets and sub-valvular apparatus. The MV leaflets are restricted and have a characteristic "hockey stick" appearance.
  - Among patients with isolated MV disease referred for surgery, less than 20% of patients with stenotic lesions undergo MV repair [12] (Fig. 30.4).

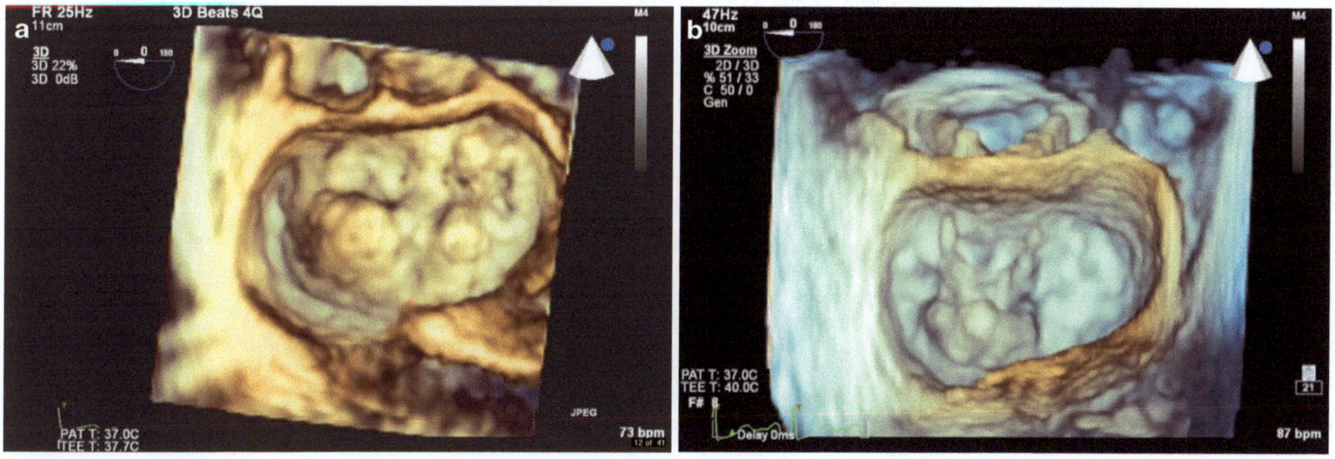

Fig. 30.3 (**a**) A 3D TEE image from a 66 year old woman with a history of degenerative MV (Barlow's) with severe MR. Note annular dilation, myxomatous valve tissue, and multiple prolapsed segments. (**b**) A 3D TEE image from a patient with a history of FED and with flail P2 segment secondary to ruptured chordae

Secondary MR, Carpentier Type IIIb

- **Functional** MR can occur in ischemic or non-ischemic cardiomyopathy and results from apical and lateral displacement of the papillary muscle(s) and "tethering" of the MV apparatus.
  - MV repair is less durable in this context and results in a 20–30% annual failure rate.
  - For patients with ischemic heart disease undergoing coronary bypass surgery, contemporary randomized trial data does not support routine concomitant MV repair for patients with moderate MR [13]. For coronary bypass patients with severe MR, randomized trial data does not support concomitant MV repair over chordal-sparing MV replacement [14] (Table 30.1) (Fig. 30.5).

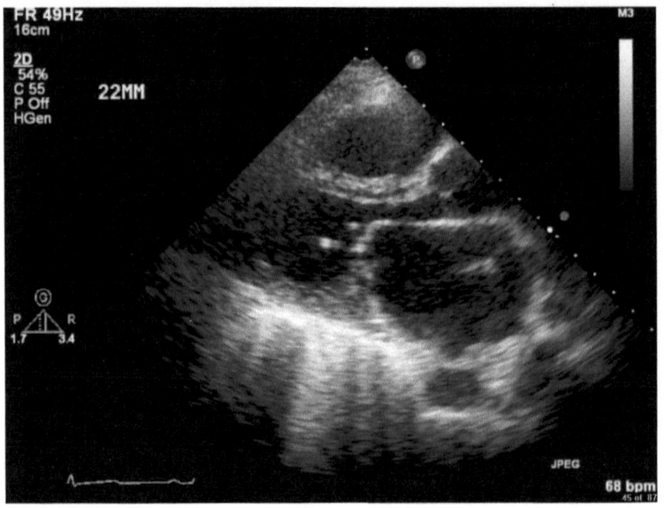

Fig. 30.4 PLAX view from a 39 year old woman with symptomatic rheumatic MV stenosis with associated severe pulmonary hypertension. Note the "hockey stick" appearance of the restricted anterior MV leaflet (arrow)

Table 30.1 MR etiologies that can be potentially treated with MV repair

Condition	Epidemiology	Echocardiographic features	Image acquisition	Repair options
Myxomatous disease (Barlow's)	• Typically <60 years • Longstanding MR • Consider other disease states (e.g. Marfan's disease; assess aortic valve and root)	• Connective tissue accumulation (glycosaminoglycans in the extra-cellular matrix) • Thickening of leaflet segments and sub-valvular apparatus with bileaflet involvement of multiple segments • Buckling of leaflets into LA during (late) systole by ≥2 mm • Increased MV dimensions and abnormal annular dynamics	• Display leaflet thickening and comment on symmetry of prolapse • Correlate prolapse segment with anatomic view; important to demonstrate "bowing" in either PLAX or AP-2 • Correlate diagnosis with timing (late-systole) and color Doppler pattern (eccentric, directed away)	• Complex lesion; posterior repair typically more successful than anterior or bi-leaflet repair • Requires more experienced surgeon
Fibroelastic deficiency (FED)	• Typically >60 years • Abrupt onset MR	• Chordal elongation or rupture causing MV leaflet prolapse or flail • Involvement of multiple segments is rare • Mitral annulus mildly enlarged	• Ensure adequate sweeps and zoom views to capture leaflet morphology (contrast with myxomatous) and attempt to show chordal segments with any associated abnormalities	• Typically less complex than Barlow's type
Functional	• Non-ischemic and ischemic cardiomyopathy • Inferior and posterior infarctions affect posteromedial papillary muscle • Anterior infarctions less likely to cause	• Related to left ventricular remodeling • Papillary muscles are laterally and apically displaced resulting in leaflet systolic "tethering"	• Show abnormal left ventricular wall motion and tethered appearance of the MV	• MV repair less durable for FMR compared to degenerative disease (20–30% recurrent MR at 1 year)
Rheumatic	• Most important form of acquired heart disease in children and young adults in developing world	• Leaflet thickening and retraction, chordal shortening, and commissural fusion • Restricted systolic and diastolic leaflet motion • Exaggerated early trans-mitral gradient relative to mean gradient may indicate concurrent MR. • Assess for secondary attributes (LA enlargement, thrombus in atrial appendage, pulmonary hypertension surrogates)	• Demonstrate the "doming" motion in diastole (restricted leaflet tips with pliable proximal and mid segments) • Sweep through SAX to leaflet tips to enable planimetry measurement • Critically evaluate instrument settings (e.g. gain, power) to avoid "blooming" artifact and distorted appearance • Determine gradient in context of preload, heart rate and rhythm, stroke volume. In atrial fibrillation, obtain multiple cycles	• MV replacement performed more often than MV repair in the United States

Table 30.1 (continued)

Native valve endocarditis	• Associated with structural heart disease, immune compromised, IV drug use, and prosthetic devices	• MR resulting from leaflet perforation or destruction • Aneurysms and abscesses around the MV can occur	• Sweep (with zoom) through valves, prostheses, and adjacent structures looking for an independently mobile vegetation (>2 mm) with low echogenicity and/or abnormal color Doppler signal • Measure vegetation size given the strong association with prognosis (≥10 mm is high risk)	• MV repair an option if leaflet destruction is not extensive
MV cleft	• Typically congenital	• Anterior more common than posterior cleft • Associated with endocardial cushion defects with inlet ventricular septal defect and/or septum primum atrial septal defect	• Sweep through the MV especially in SAX to assess cleft • Look for associated congenital abnormalities including endocardial cushion defects, ventricular septal defect, or septum primum	• Can be repaired
Papillary muscle rupture	• Patients with ischemic disease or trauma presenting with new holosystolic murmur and heart failure	• Posteromedial rupture more common than anterolateral PM due to single vessel supply • Usually portion of PM resulting in partial flail	• TEE easier than TTE to view rupture of PM head • Color flow assessment with eccentric regurgitation directed contralaterally to ruptured PM (+/− normal LA) • Assess for ventricular septal defect/rupture	• Typically MV replacement

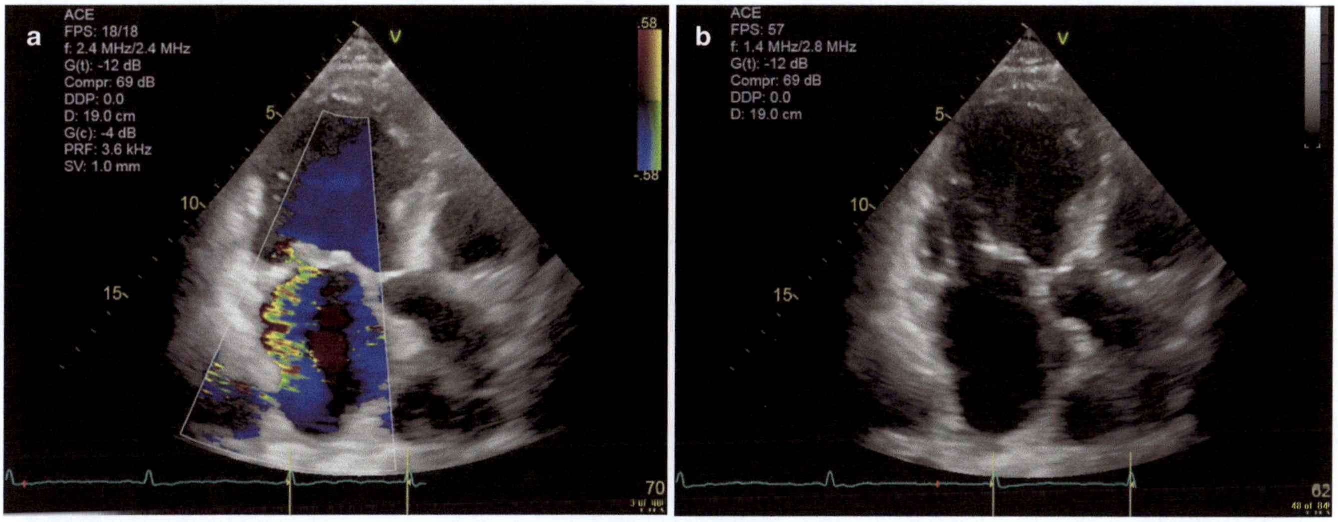

Fig. 30.5 An apical-4 chamber TTE image from a 70 year old male with ischemic cardiomyopathy and severe eccentric functional MR resulting from tethering of the posterior leaflet (P)

General Overview of MV Repair Approaches

- Observational data suggests that MV repair, when performed by an expert surgeon, achieves superior results in terms of operative mortality (<1%), long term survival (equal to age-matched), and durability (95% freedom from reoperation at 15–20 years) compared to MV replacement. Integrative flowcharts for guiding clinical decisions for patients with symptomatic and asymptomatic severe MR (Fig. 30.6). In general, degenerative disease involving the posterior leaflet has better surgical outcomes compared to anterior or bi-leaflet prolapse [5, 10, 15, 16].
- Surgical MV repair technique should be adapted to the pathophysiology of the MV lesion. For degenerative MR, the principles of repair are (1) to ensure normal leaflet motion, (2) to create a large coaptation surface, and (3) to stabilize the annulus.
- Major techniques of surgical MV repair include leaflet resection with rigid or semi-rigid annuloplasty (Carpentier technique) and dynamic non-resectional, fully flexible annuloplasty technique (American Correction) [17].

Indications for MV Repair

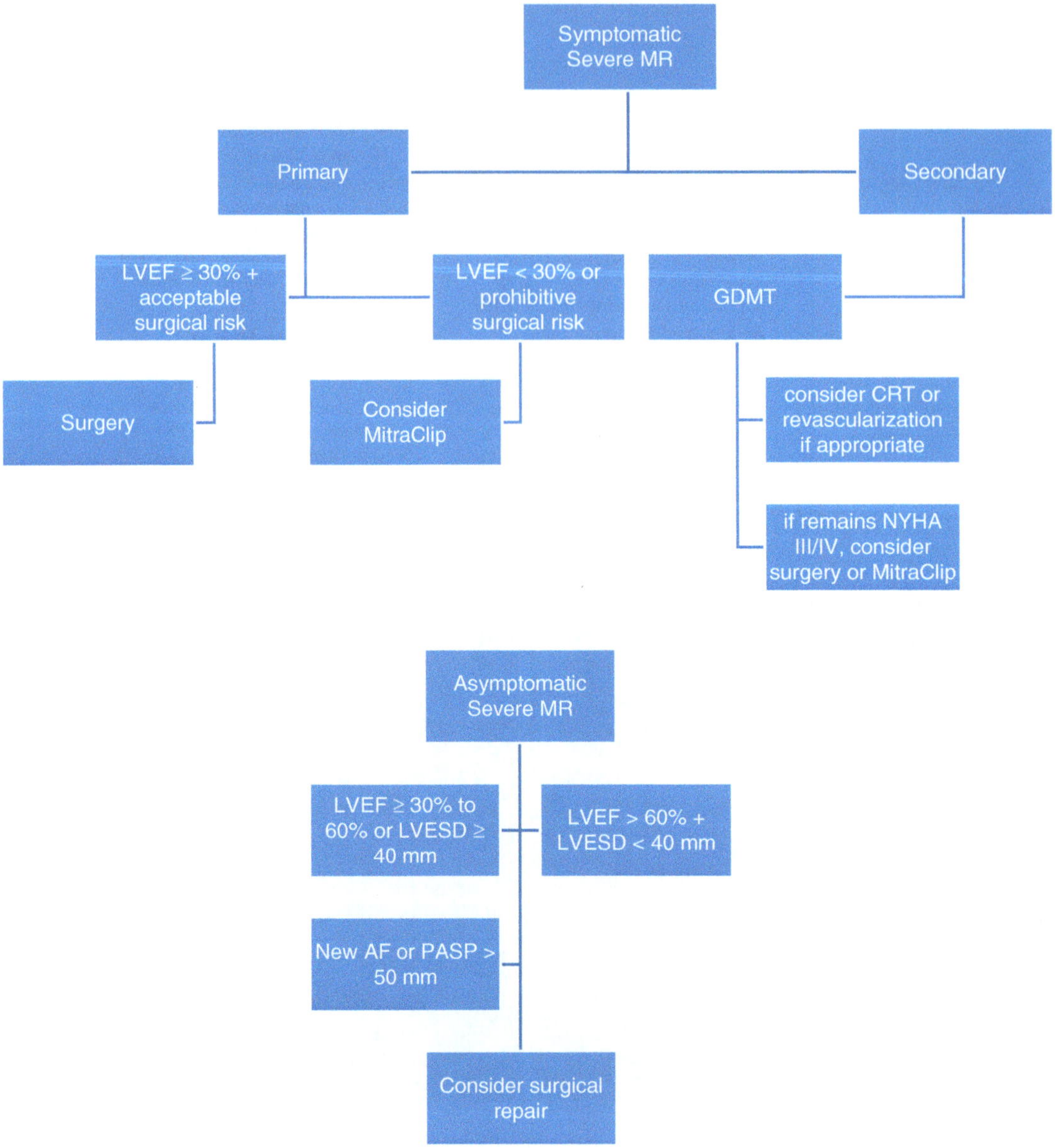

Fig. 30.6 Integrative flowcharts for guiding clinical decisions for patients with symptomatic and asymptomatic severe MR Guideline-directed medical therapy (GDMT) (adapted from 2014 ACC/AHA Valve Guidelines) [5]

- Percutaneous MV repair using an edge-to-edge closure device (i.e. MitraClip) is a reasonable treatment option for patients with symptomatic primary or secondary MR at high surgical risk refractory to goal directed therapies, including cardiac resynchronization or revascularization.

1. **MV annuloplasty** is used to treat annular dilation and is an essential adjunctive component to the long-term durability of MV repair [18].
   - Annuloplasty can be suture or ring, partial or complete, flexible or rigid ring annuloplasty. In general, complete rigid annuloplasty rings are best for functional MR. Flexible or rigid rings can be used for myxomatous valves [19].
2. **Leaflet resection** is used for Carpentier type II lesions, most commonly posterior leaflet prolapse [20].
   - Triangular and quadrangular resection are commonly used effective techniques, especially for P2 prolapse.

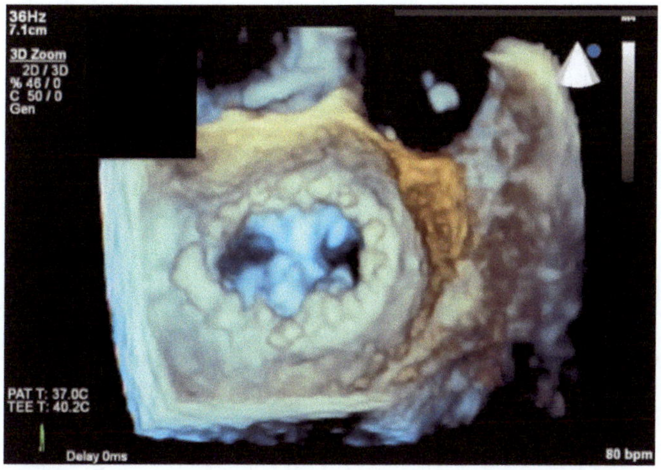

Fig. 30.7 A 3D TEE image of a repaired MV seen from the needs consideration. Left atrium (aortic valve oriented at the top of the image). It shows annuloplasty with a complete ring and edge-to-edge suture (Alfieri stitch) at A2-P2 resulting in a double orifice valve

3. **Chordal replacement** using polytetrafluoroethylene (PTFE) neo-chordae is can be used in all degenerative cases particularly in cases of anterior leaflet prolapse or multiple (or large) segment prolapse.
4. **Papillary muscle shortening** is used to reduce elongated chordae.
5. **Pericardial patch closure** can be used in cases of mitral leaflet perforation or cleft valve.
6. **Edge-to-edge (Alfieri, "Bow Tie", Double Orifice MV Technique)** is used to treat commissural MR secondary to leaflet prolapse or restriction by creating a double orifice MV [21].
7. **Leaflet extension** with autologous pericardium is used to correct Carpentier class IIIa lesions secondary to rheumatic heart disease.
8. **Chordal resection** can be used in Carpentier class IIIa lesions secondary to rheumatic heart disease or ischemic MR where the leaflets may be tethered.
9. **Percutaneous edge to edge MV closure (MitraClip, Abbott Vascular, Chicago, IL)** is used for degenerative or functional MR by using the same principles as the Alfieri edge to edge repair approach to create a double-orifice MV.
10. **Percutaneous annuloplasty and MV replacement** are also in development [25] (Fig. 30.7).

Principles of the Pre-Procedural TTE Examination for MV Repair [21]

- **Two-dimensional echocardiography, Doppler echocardiography, and three-dimensional echocardiography** are complementary techniques for determining severity, hemodynamic consequences, and etiology of MR.
- Assessment of MR includes qualitative and quantitative components that may be problematic to assess in all patients. These data may be internally inconsistent; it is therefore critical to understand the indications and limitations of these parameters, the inter-relationships between parameters, and be able put these data in the appropriate clinical context in order to accurately determine MR severity [26].
- The 2014 ACC/AHA Valvular Heart Disease Guidelines provide lower quantitative thresholds for severe secondary MR (see Table 30.2), compared to primary MR, secondary to worse prognosis in secondary MR and the potential for unreliable (underestimated) quantitative MR measures in this population [5, 27].

Table 30.2 The 2014 ACC/AHA Valvular Heart Disease Guidelines recommendations for MV repair [5]

Indication	Recommendation strength (Level of evidence)[a]
Symptomatic chronic severe primary MR limited to the posterior leaflet	I(B)
Symptomatic chronic severe MR involving the anterior leaflet or both leaflet when a successful and durable repair can be performed	I(B)
Chronic severe MR in the patient undergoing other cardiac surgery	I(B)
Asymptomatic chronic severe MR in an asymptomatic patient (LVEF >60% and LVESD <40 mm) when likelihood of no residual MR and mortality are <95% and <1%, respectively	IIa(B)
Asymptomatic chronic severe MR with LVEF >60% with new onset AF or PASP >50 mmHg	IIa(B)
Chronic moderate MR in a patient undergoing other cardiac surgery	IIa(C)
Symptomatic chronic severe MR with LVEF ≤30%	IIb(C)
Rheumatic valve disease when successful and durable MV repair is possible or anticoagulation reliability is questionable	IIb(B)
Trans-catheter MV repair in patients with NYHA class III/IV heart failure symptoms with reasonable life expectancy but prohibitive surgical risk due to comorbidities	IIb(B)
Chronic moderate secondary MR undergoing other cardiac surgery	IIb(C)

Level of evidence (precision or estimate of uncertainty): A = Multiple populations evaluated (multiple randomized trials or meta-analysis); B = Single population (single randomized trial or non-randomized studies); C = Limited populations (expert opinion)

[a]*Recommendation strength (size of treatment effect):* I = Should be performed; IIa = Reasonable; IIb = May be considered

Two-Dimensional Echocardiography

- Assessment of the architecture of the MV leaflets and sub-valvular apparatus are essential for defining the etiology of MR and whether MV repair is feasible.
- The size and volumes of the LA and LV reflects the extent of remodeling and the burden and chronicity of the MV lesion. Normal LA volume, measured in the apical 4 and 2-chamber views at end-systole, is ≤34 cm^2/m^2. Normal LV end-diastolic volume, indexed to body surface area, is 74 mL/m^2 for men and 61 mL/m^2 for women. Normal LV end systolic volume of 31 mL/m^2 for men and 24 mL/m^2 for women [28].
- Left ventricular function can reflect etiology of MR and the extent of remodeling; the right ventricular function and septal contraction pattern (i.e. bowing in diastole and/or systole) can reflect the impact of pulmonary hypertension.

Three-Dimensional Echocardiography [10, 29]

- Useful for defining the precise location, severity, and mechanism of MR.
- Helpful during surgical and interventional repair procedures for identifying anatomical landmarks and distortions, especially within the commissures, leaflet clefts, and prosthetic devices.
- Volumetric analysis can assist with visualizing complex 3D geometry and measurement. 3D facilitates measurement of the **effective regurgitant orifice area (EROA)** and **vena contracta (VC)**, however, there are presently no published reference standards to compare these measurements to 2D measurements.
- 3D settings must be optimized for both spatial and temporal resolution; interpretation of the associated data must occur within the context of these parameters.

Doppler Echocardiography

- Color flow Doppler (pulse wave) is the primary tool for assessing the presence and severity of MR. Spectral Doppler (continuous wave) plays a confirmatory role and is helpful for determining MR duration and regurgitant flow signal intensity.
- The MR jet, as captured in systole by color Doppler, is described by a region of proximal FC, a narrow region of turbulent flow acceleration (VC), and a regurgitant volume flowing through an orifice into the LA [30].
- Measurement of the MR jet by color Doppler techniques has low inter-observer reliability and have significant drawbacks related to geometric assumptions, measurement errors, imaging technique, and MR timing [27, 28].
- Instrument settings need to be optimized to avoid imaging artifacts that can undermine accurate interpretation: color gain ("blooming"), appropriate Nyquist scale (low pulmonary vein flows, turbulence overestimation), and 2D gain (can obscure color signal) [31] (Table 30.3).

Table 30.3 Echocardiographic parameters of severe MR (adapted from 2003 ASE and 2014 ACC/AHA Guidelines) [5, 21]

Echocardiographic modality	Specific (>90%)	Supportive	Image optimization
2D TTE or TEE	• Flail MV leaflets or ruptured papillary muscle(s)	• Dilated LA and LV size with chronic MR	• Display all segments of mitral leaflets and demonstrate etiology and mechanism; corroborate with 3D assessment • Display cardiac chambers to reflect state of atrial and ventricular remodeling
Continuous wave Doppler		• Dense and triangular shaped MR jet	• Use superior temporal resolution of echocardiography to display timing and duration of MR • Ensure sampling position is parallel to MR jet
Color wave Doppler	• VC width ≥ 0.7 cm *with* jet area > 40% of LA *or* eccentric, wall-impinging jet • Large FC with Nyquist at 40 cm/s		• Ensure "pointing" at the jet, correct sample gating, consider direction of the MR jet relative to transducer position (e.g. eccentric, orthogonal) • Set color gain appropriately to avoid "blooming" • Ensure pulse repetition frequency (2 × Nyquist) is correct
Pulse wave Doppler	• Systolic reversal in pulmonary veins	• Mitral inflow E-wave >1.2 m/s	• See color wave Doppler
Quantitative parameters	• Regurgitant volume ≥ 60 mL/beat in primary MR and ≥30 mL/beat in secondary MR • Regurgitant fraction ≥50%/beat for primary and secondary MR • VC ≥ 0.40 cm^2 in primary MR and ≥0.20 cm^2 in secondary MR		• Need to assess MR severity in the context of dynamic changes in blood pressure, heart rate, LV/LA size and gradient, etiology of MR (e.g. primary vs. secondary, prolapse vs. flail)

Representative Findings of Severe MR Using Doppler Echocardiography [21, 30]

1. **Vena-contracta (VC)** is the narrowest, highest velocity region of the jet flow occurring between the proximal FC region and the region where the jet expands into the LA.
   (a) Ideally measured in PLAX (zoom mode with narrow color flow sector) perpendicular to MV closure at the largest point in systole. Lateral resolution is insufficient for a reliable measurement in the apical view.
   (b) When fixed, VC is independent of flow rate and driving pressure; when dynamic, can change with hemodynamics or cardiac cycle.
   (c) VC < 0.3 cm reflects mild MR and ≥0.7 cm reflects severe MR. The VC diameter can be used to calculate the EROA using the formula πr^2.

2. **Proximal isovelocity surface area (PISA)** is a method that takes advantage of FC to estimate the maximal EROA. Due to issues with inter-rater reliability and the implied geometric assumptions PISA should not be the sole method for determining MR severity (particularly in secondary MR) [26].

   (a) As flow converges, concentric hemispheric shells of uniform velocity form, which are used to solve for EROA. The conservation of mass principle is used to derive the equation EROA = $2(\prod)\, r^2 \times$ aliasing velocity (cm/s)/MR max velocity (cm/s).
   (b) EROA and the MV velocity time index (VTI) can be used to estimate the regurgitant volume (RV) using the eq. RV = EROA x MV VTI.
   (c) The RV is used to estimate the regurgitant fraction (RF) using the eq. RF = RV/forward stroke volume.
   (d) The PISA method assumes that (1) shells are concentric in all dimensions, rather than cylindrical, (2) the base of the hemisphere is a flat 180° (if not, use correction factor of angle/180), (3) the optimal jet timing is in mid-late systole. These assumptions are problematic in secondary MR, (4) maximal EROA given use of peak instantaneous flow rate (Fig. 30.8).

3. **Systolic reversal of pulmonary vein flow** is specific for severe MR (Fig. 30.9).

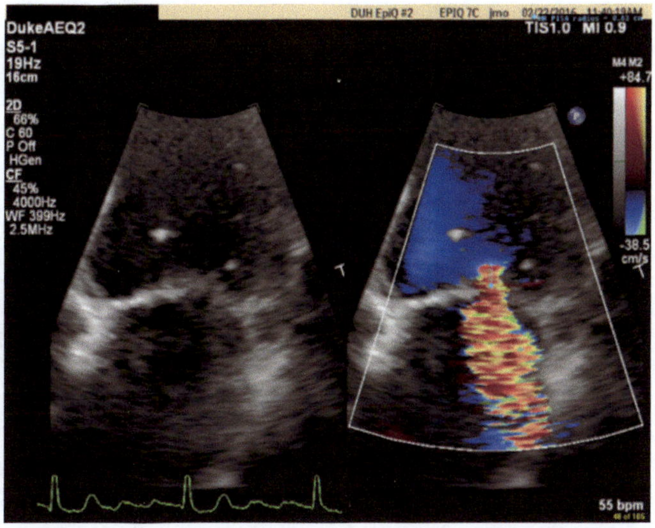

Fig. 30.8 AP-4 view with color Doppler demonstrating a hemispherical PISA shell (P). The sample volume has been placed over the LV, MV, and LA with the aliasing velocity reduced in the direction of the MR. The view was also confirmed in the 2-chamber view

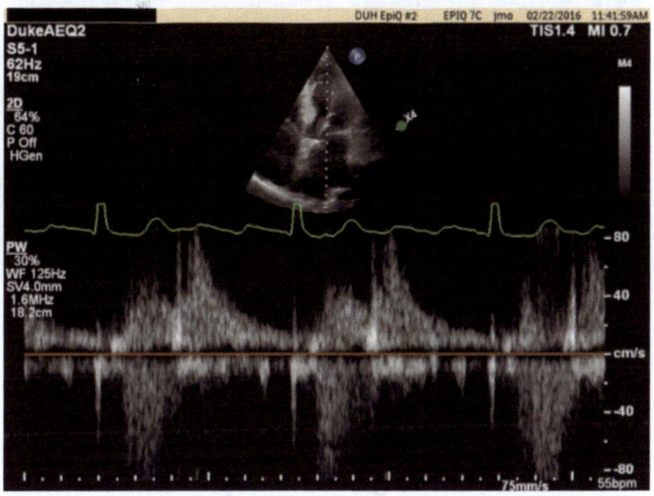

Fig. 30.9 A TTE AP4 view demonstrating systolic reversal of flow in the pulmonary vein by pulse wave Doppler tracing (arrows)

4. **Dense spectral tracing of MR, left atrial enlargement, elevated E wave mitral inflow velocity, and notched pulmonary outflow "W" sign (suggesting pulmonary hypertension)** spectral tracing are supportive signs of severe MR (Fig. 30.10).

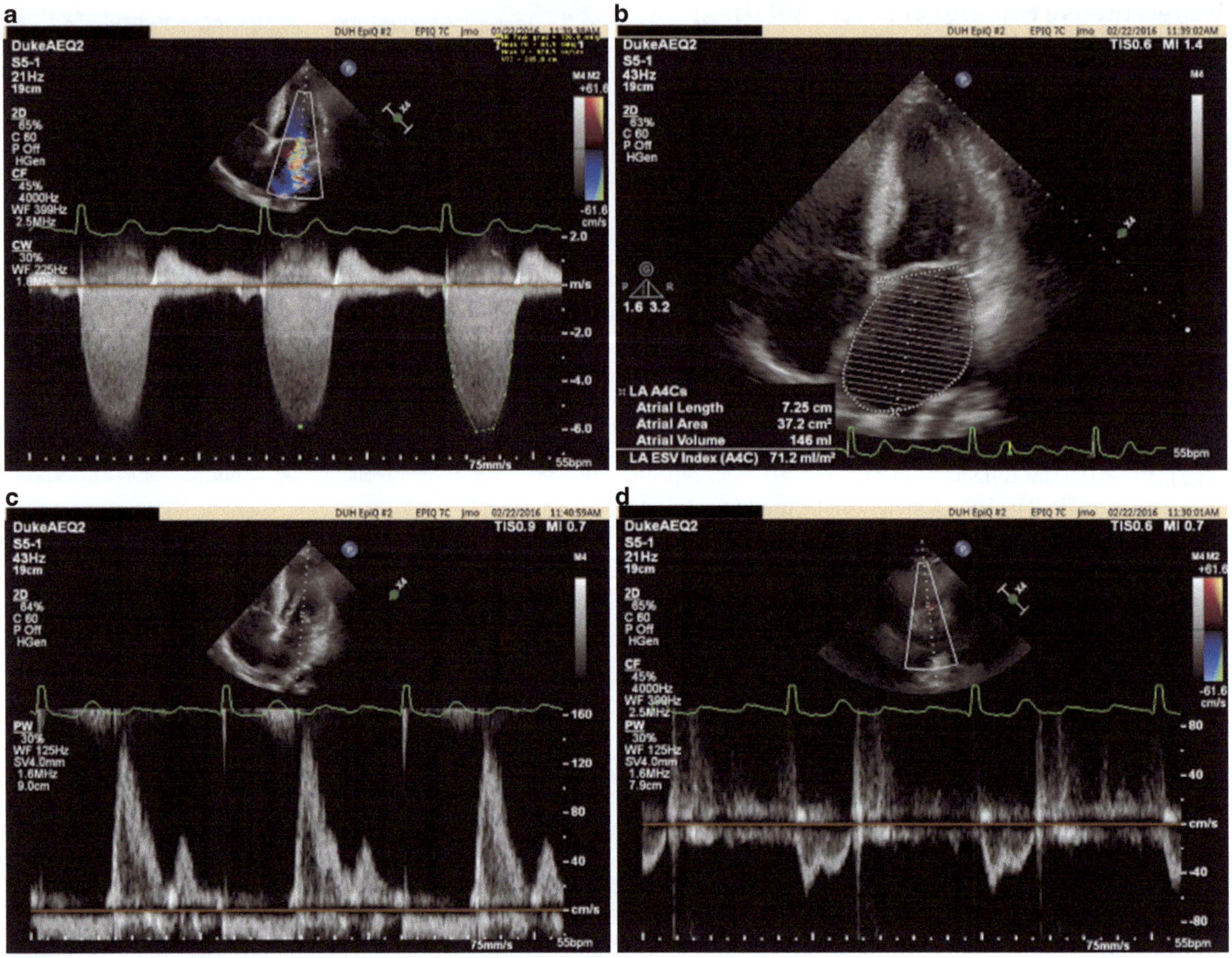

Fig. 30.10 (**a–d**): (**a**) Dense spectral outline of MR, (**b**) LA enlargement, (**c**) an elevated E velocity on the mitral inflow, (**d**) notched RVOT systolic tracing suggesting elevated pulmonary vascular resistance (PVR)

Pre-Procedural TEE Echocardiographic Assessment for Surgical MV Repair [32]

General Principles of Preoperative Trans-esophageal Echocardiography (TEE) for MV Repair

- The 2014 AHA/ACC Valvular Heart Disease Guidelines give class I recommendations for the use of TEE to establish (1) the basis of severe MR if non-invasive imaging provides insufficient data regarding mechanism or severity of MR and/or LV function, and (2) to guide MV repair [3].
- A comprehensive exam of the MV apparatus is essential for understanding the etiology, mechanism, impact, feasibility and prognosis of MV repair. The assessment needs to reflect the movement of the blood pool over the entire cardiac cycle into the left atrium and ultimately across the LVOT.
- Mid-esophageal (ME) views provide the best resolution and information regarding leaflet anatomy. Trans-gastric imaging can provide complementary information about leaflets, papillary muscle and LV anatomy and function in SAX and LAX axes.
  - 3-key ME views are (1) ME 4/5 chamber (0°; advance and retract TEE probe in the esophagus to view entirety of A1/P1 to A3/P3, respectively); (2) mitral commissural view (60–90°; rotate posterior to anterior to view P3-A2-P1 to P3-P2-P1, respectively); and (3) LAX (120–140°; advance and retract along A2-P2 to see all vertical segments).

- Color Doppler patterns are useful for differentiating MR etiology and mechanism. Central jet suggests annular dilation, bi-leaflet tethering, or bi-leaflet myxomatous disease. Eccentric jets will be contralateral to a prolapsed or flail leaflet segment or ipsilateral to a restricted (or tethered) leaflet.
- It is essential to assess MR under optimized hemodynamic conditions. MR severity can be dynamic and influenced by loading conditions (e.g. general anesthesia, volume status, and ventricular function). Patients may require intravenous fluids or vasopressors to correct physiologic distortions.

Specific Principles of Preoperative Transesophageal Echocardiography (TEE) for MV Repair

- Goals of pre-cardiac bypass evaluation are to define the etiology and mechanism of MR; evaluate MR severity under appropriate physiologic conditions; and to identify complementary or ancillary findings including ventricular dysfunction, pulmonary hypertension, pericardial effusion, and tricuspid regurgitation.
- Assess the feasibility and durability of surgical MV repair.

Assessment of Feasibility and Durability of Surgical MV Repair [33]

1. General Principles
   (a) The goal is to have an adequate amount of mobile leaflet tissue covering the coapting area (annular region).
   (b) Feasibility and durability are related to the architecture and integrity of both MV and LV.
2. Degenerative
   (a) The leaflet heights, measured in the ME windows from the annulus to leaflet edges, are useful for guiding repair and predicting outcomes.
      - For A2 and P2, use ME 4/5 chamber or LAX
      - For P1 and P3, use ME mitral commissural
      - Can also use multi-planar reconstruction of a 3D dataset which enables display of different tomographic images from the dataset.

   (b) Anterior leaflet height > 3.0 cm gives the surgeon flexibility to reduce the posterior height to <1.5 cm. If anterior leaflet height < 2.8 cm, less ability to reduce posterior leaflet (Figs. 30.11 and 30.12).
3. Functional
   (a) The goal is to assess leaflet mobility and predict the degree of reversibility of ventricular remodeling. Tethering is a key metric that is inversely related to durability.
      - Assess the impact of left ventricular remodeling on the geometry of the MV by assessing tenting height (distance from the MV annulus to the coaptation point), tenting area (area delineated by the annular plane and leaflet edges), coaptation angles for certain MV scallops (angles between the annular plane and the leaflet insertion) (Figs. 30.13, 30.14, and 30.15).
4. Adverse predictors of difficult repair, recurrent MR, or reoperation [33] (Fig. 30.16) as the following:

Degenerative	Functional
Annular diameter > 5 cm Prolapse/flail of ≥3 segments Bi-leaflet prolapse Atrialization of posterior leaflet insertion Restrictive leaflets Specific measures: Pre-repair posterior leaflet <17 mm; anterior leaflet <25 mm; annular diameter < 35 mm, and short chordae <29 mm Markers of SAM (see below)	Annular diameter > 4 cm Tenting/tethering height (annular plane to coaptation point) > 10 mm Tethering area > 1.6 cm^2 Posterior angle >45° LVEDD >6 cm

5. Risk of systolic anterior motion (SAM) and LVOT obstruction (features that reduce the normal upward and posterior motion of the mitral annulus) [33, 34]
   (a) 14% of degenerative Carpentier type II lesions
   (b) C-sept <2.5 cm; shorter pre-repair distance between coaptation point and interventricular septum
   (c) Larger coapting leaflet heights (AL/PL ratio < 1.4)
   (d) Longer posterior leaflet (>15 mm)
   (e) Thicker ventricular septum (≥15 mm)
   (f) Small LV cavity (<45 mm)
   (g) Larger mitral-aortic angle (intersection of mitral and aortic outflow) > 35° provoked and >65° resting
   (h) Smaller aorto-mitral angle (aortic and mitral annuli at inter-valvular fibrosa) < 120°
   (i) Mitral annular calcification

Perioperative Post-Cardiopulmonary Bypass TEE Exam

- Key aspects are to reassess mechanism and severity of residual MR (with physiologic correction, as needed), assess for mitral stenosis as a consequence of MV repair, assess for **systolic anterior motion** (**SAM**, Fig. 30.17), and assess ventricular function.

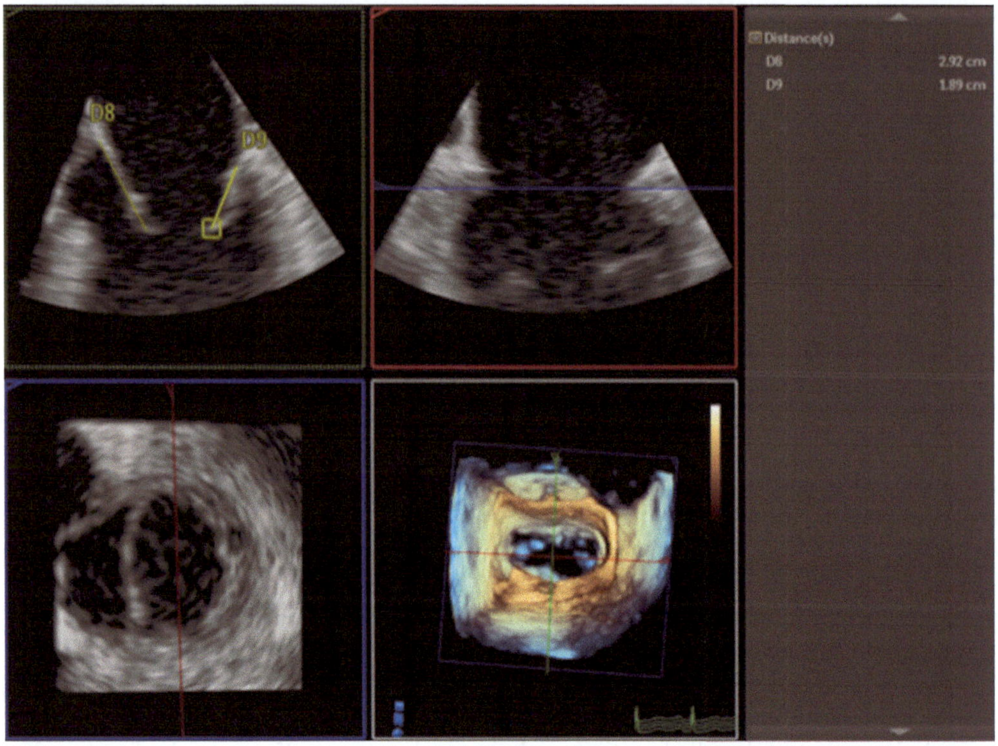

Fig. 30.11 65 year-old patient presents with severe MR due to FED and flail P2 segment. Multi-planar reconstruction of the 3D dataset displays three tomographic views from the dataset: two LAX (green panel, upper left shows the ME LAX view and red plane, upper right shows the ME mitral commissural image) and one short axis at the level of the mitral annulus (blue panel). Measurements of the A2 and P2 segments (shown in diastole) can be made

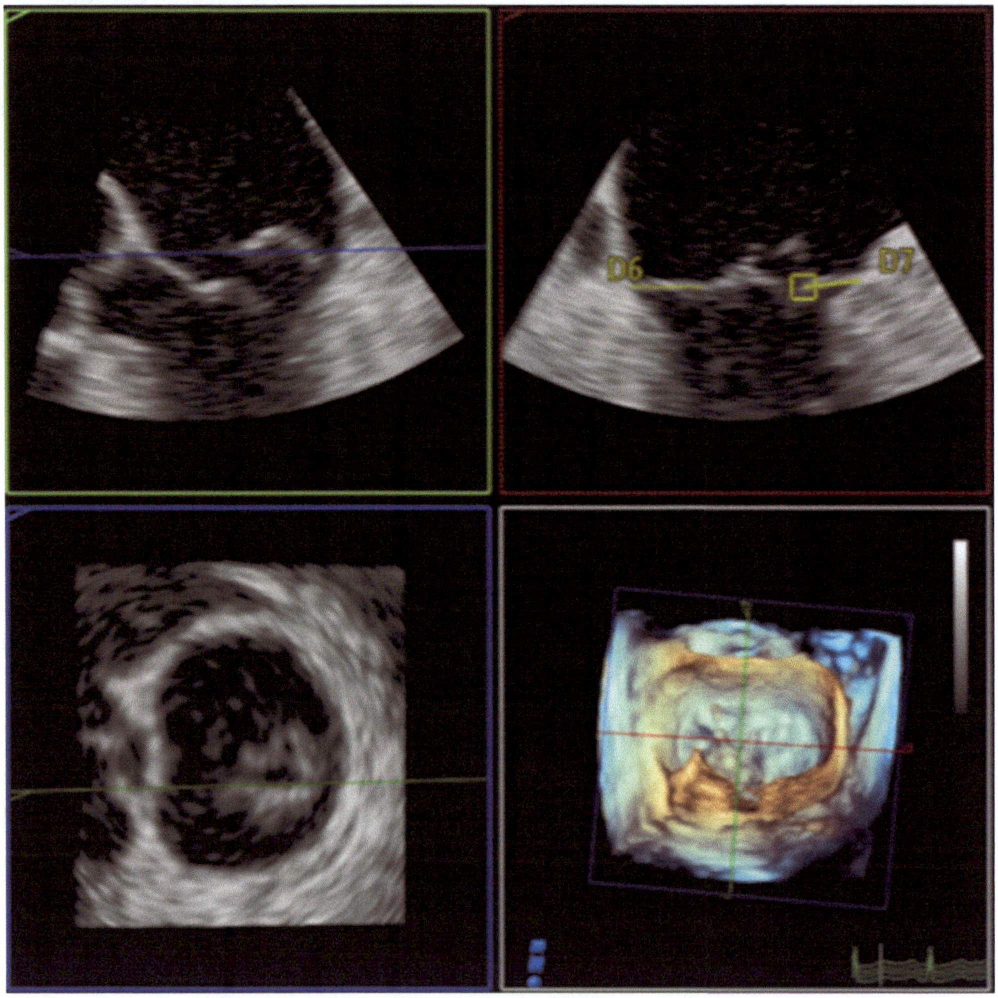

Fig. 30.12 65 year-old patient presents with severe MR due to FED and flail P2 segment. Multi-planar reconstruction of the three-dimensional dataset displays three tomographic views from the dataset: (1) ME LAX view (green panel, upper left); (2) Mid-esophageal mitral commissural view (red plane, upper right); (3) Short-axis at the level of the mitral annulus (blue panel). Measurements of P1 and P3 segments (shown in systole) can be made in the ME mitral commissural view

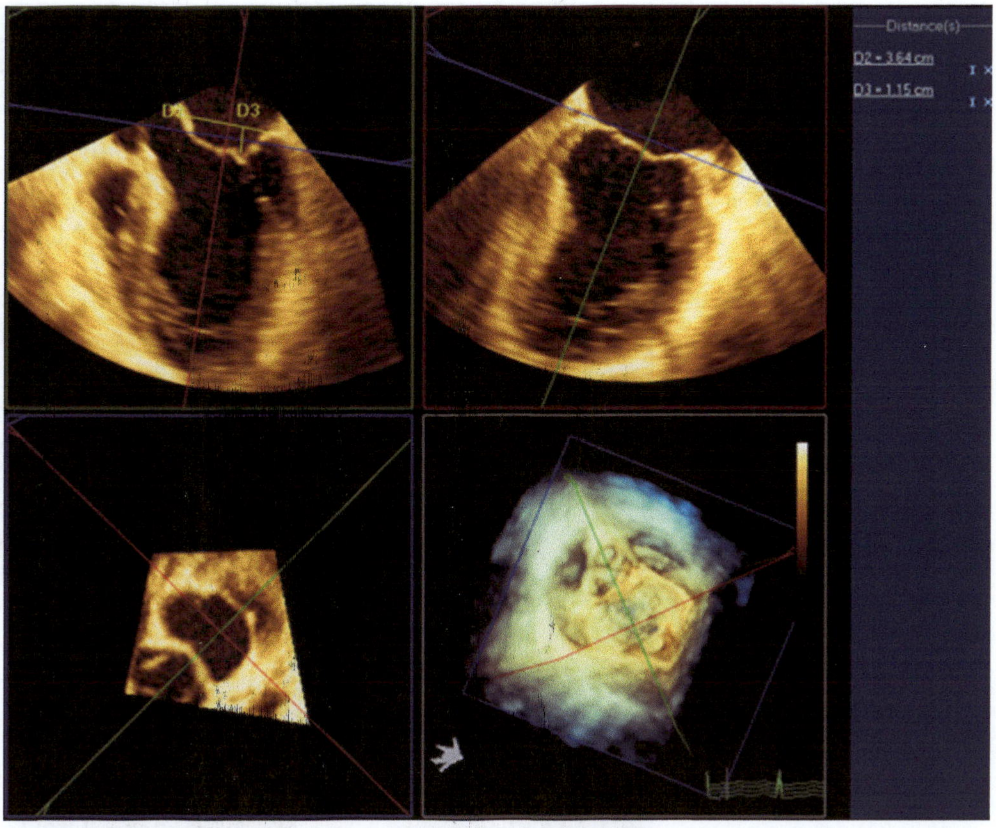

Fig. 30.13 Multi-planar reconstruction of a 3D dataset. The green panel, upper left, shows a tomographic view of the MV from inside the dataset, corresponding to the ME LAX view. The tenting height can be measured from the annulus plane to the coaptation point

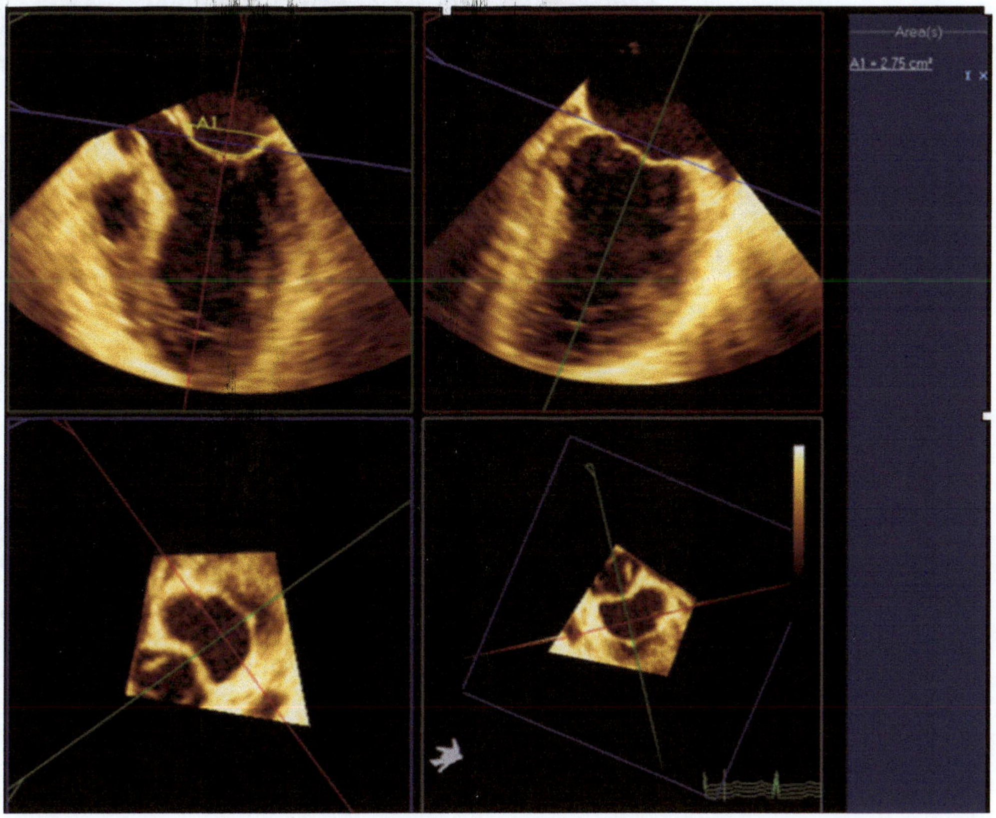

Fig. 30.14 Multi-planar reconstruction of a 3D dataset. The green panel, upper left, shows a tomographic view of the MV from inside the dataset, corresponding to the ME LAX view. The tenting area (TA) can be measured from the annulus plane to the coaptation point

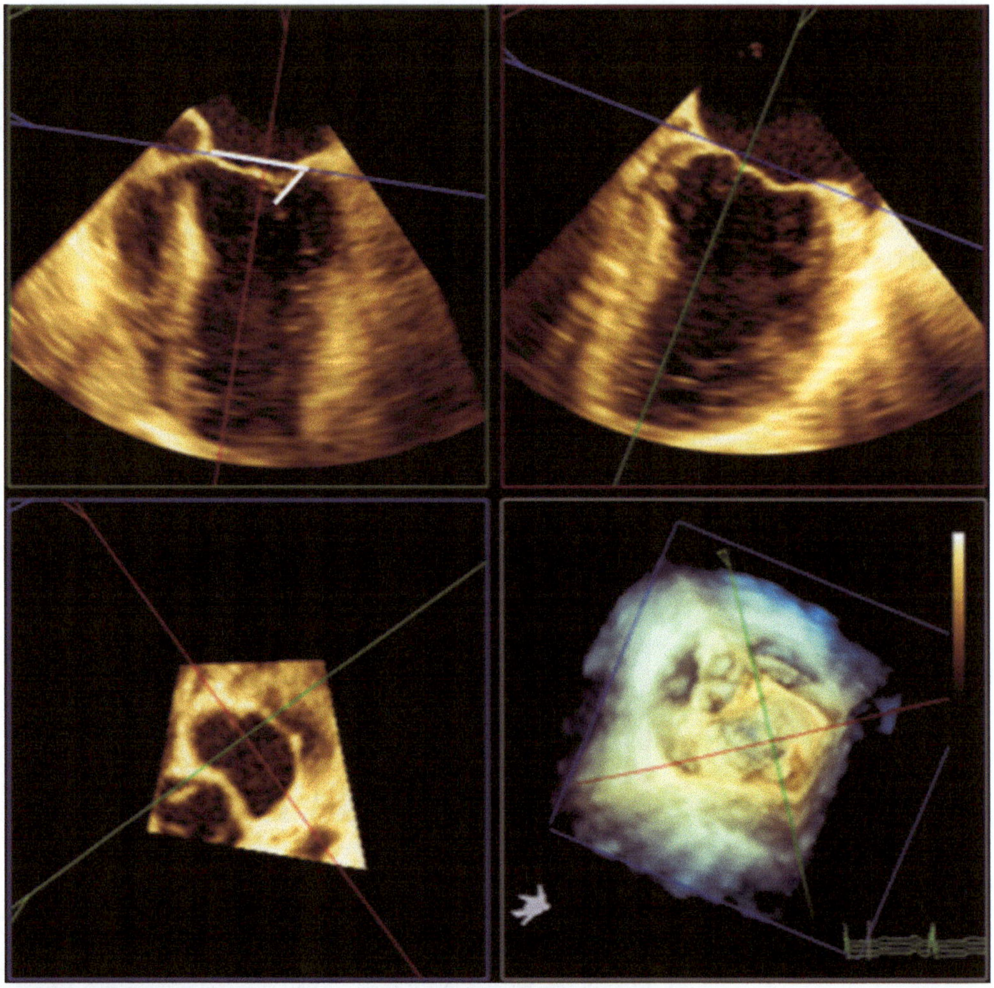

Fig. 30.15 Multi-planar reconstruction of a 3D dataset. As can be seen in the blue panel (lower left), the green plane has been placed at the level of A3-P3 segments. The green panel (upper left) shows the MV in LAX view at the level of A3-P3 segments in systole. The closing angle of the P3 segment can be measured

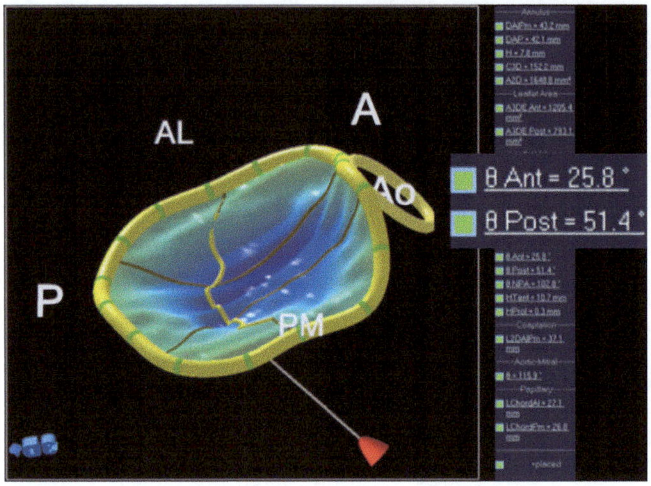

Fig. 30.16 Parametric representation of the MV using specialized software (Philips QLAB, Andover, MA). Specific measurements are generated, including the closing angles for A2 and P 2 segments

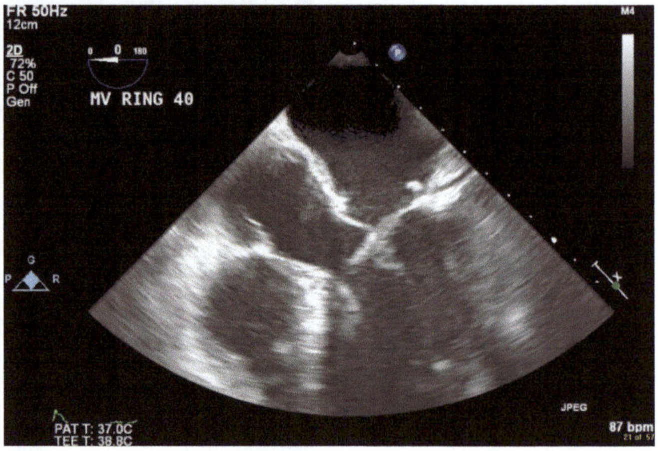

Fig. 30.17 Post-MV repair systolic anterior motion in a patient with bileaflet MVP. Note the movement of the mitral valve towards the LVOT in systole

- The goal is to have no MR or trivial MR. MV repair yielding more than mild MR is not durable and will need to be revised or MV replacement will need to occur after consideration of risks, benefits, and likelihood of procedural success. It is critical to ensure adequate sampling of entire jet through anteflexion/retroflexion and sweeping maneuvers. Additionally, there may need to be recovery time post-bypass to allow for ventricular adaptation.
- Assess for mitral stenosis by assessing LA FC and continuous wave Doppler in the context of the hemodynamic state. Tachycardia can increase mean pressure gradients. Mean gradients <5 mmHg are expected post-MV repair. Mean diastolic gradient ≥7 mmHg may be clinically significant.
- Assess for systolic anterior motion of the MV leaflets. This can occur because of excess leaflet tissue relative to mitral annular size. Blood flow across the left ventricular outflow tract can cause drag on the MV leaflets and create a significant pressure gradient. Clinically significant SAM requiring repair revision occurs when LVOT velocity ≥ 3.5 m/s and at least mild MR.
  - Since SAM is affected by loading conditions it is important to optimize preload, maintain adequate blood pressure, and minimize inotropic agents.
- Assess left and right ventricular function. Ensure adequate flow through the circumflex artery to ensure no iatrogenic injury during MV repair. Right ventricular impairment may occur as a consequence of gas embolus down the right coronary artery secondary to inadequate de-airing maneuvers.

Percutaneous MV Repair

- The EVEREST II (Endovascular Valve Edge-to-Edge Repair Study) clinical trial randomized 279 patients to MitraClip (n = 184) or MV repair or replacement surgery (n = 95) [22].
  - The primary endpoint was a composite of freedom from death, surgery for MV dysfunction, or 3+ or 4+ MR at 12 months
  - The primary endpoint favored the surgery arm (55% vs. 73%, p = 0.007), which was primarily driven by repeat surgery in the percutaneous arm within the first 12 months (20% vs. 2%, p < 0.001). There were no cases of clip dislodgement or mitral stenosis in the percutaneous arm.
  - The primary composite safety endpoint at 30 days favored the percutaneous arm (15% vs. 48%, p < 0.001), which was primarily driven by ≥2 units packed red cell transfusion (13% vs. 45%, p < 0.001).
- The patient selection criteria included patients with moderate (3+) or severe (4+) MR (arising from A2/P2 scallops) who were symptomatic (LVEF ≥ 25% and LVESD ≤ 55 mm) or asymptomatic with LVEF 25–60%, LVESD 40–55 mm, new atrial fibrillation, or pulmonary hypertension.
- There were specific anatomical echocardiographic exclusion parameters (presented below). In commercial use, the MV orifice area < 4 cm^2 is not strictly adhered to [23] (Table 30.4) (Fig. 30.18).

Table 30.4 Specific echocardiographic exclusion parameters specified in EVEREST II [24]

Severe LV dysfunction (EF < 25%) or dilation (LVESD > 55 mm)
Severe leaflet calcification
Flail gap ≥ 10 mm
Flail width ≥ 15 mm
LV end systolic dimension > 55 mm
MV orifice area < 4 cm^2
Leaflet vertical coaptation length < 2 mm and leaflet coaptation depth > 11 mm
Prohibitive anatomy for implantation, positioning or MR reduction: A2 or P2 calcification or cleft, severe prolapse, insufficient chordal support
Active endocarditis or rheumatic disease
Atrial septal defect or symptomatic patent foramen ovale
Other MV prosthesis
Intracardiac mass, thrombus or vegetation

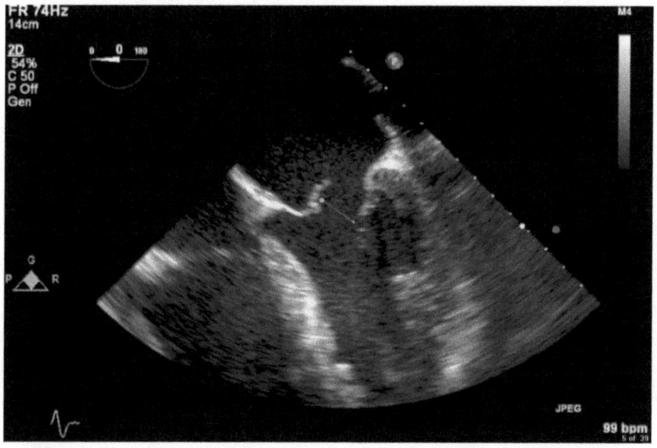

Fig. 30.18 A 0-degree TEE 4-chamber view demonstrating a flail A2 segment. The space between the anterior and posterior leaflets is known as the flail gap (F). The gap measures 16 mm in this patient

Peri-Procedural Echocardiographic Assessment During Percutaneous Approach to MV Repair [35, 36]

The procedure can be conceptually organized into eight distinct steps (see Table 30.5):

Table 30.5 Peri-procedural echocardiographic approach to percutaneous MV repair [35, 36]

Step #	Goal	Echocardiographic views	Notes
1	Intra-atrial (IAS) trans-septal puncture	Bicaval (BCV) Basal short axis (BSAX) Zero degree (measure height)	Assess for IAS defect
2	Introduce steerable catheter into the LA	BSAX	Visualize echo-dense rings at the catheter tip
3	Insert delivery sheath into LA	BSAX	Continuous visualization to ensure the delivery sheath remains in the LA
4	Positioning the open mitral clip above the leaflet target	TEE LAX view (LAX) TEE inter-commissural (IC) view (60) TEE 3D *en face*	LAX shows A-P dimension IC view shows M-L dimension
5	Advancement of the delivery system into the LV	Live 3D TEE Trans-gastric 2D TEE	Shows system moving across coaptation plane
6	Grasping the leaflets	2D TEE LVOT 3D TEE *en face*	Sweep to ensure entire leaflet is within grasping arms Assess diastolic mean MV gradient when grasping arms closed Assess impact of clip on MR reduction by color jets and pulmonary vein profiles
7	Clip release	2D TEE (0, 60, 120) Color Doppler 3D TEE Color Doppler 2D TEE (120) RUPV 2D TEE (30) LUPV TEE trans-gastric LAX 2D TEE (120, bi-caval)	Assess for regurgitant color flow; PV tracings; pericardial effusion; IAS shunt; TR

- Step #1: **Trans-septal puncture** across the **intra-atrial septum** (Fig. 30.19)
- Steps #2 and #3: Introduction of steerable catheter into the LA (LA) and subsequent advancement of the clip delivery system into the LA (Fig. 30.20)
- Step #4: Steering and positioning the MitraClip above the MV (Fig. 30.21)
- Step #5: Advancement of the delivery system into the LV

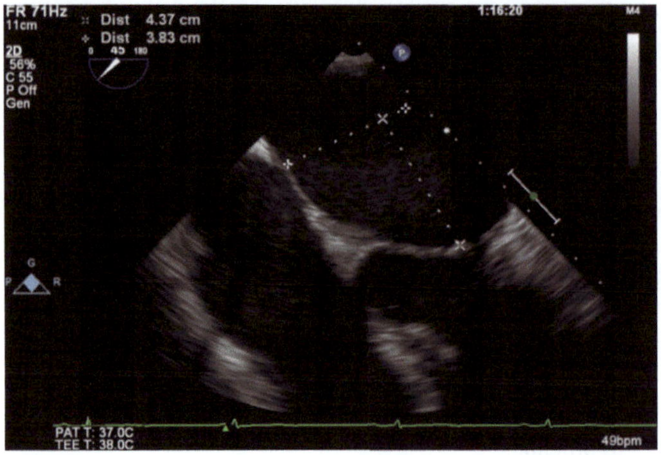

Fig. 30.19 A ME four-chamber (zero degree) view is used to measure the height of the puncture site above the line of mitral leaflet coaptation. This is typically performed approximately 4 cm above the annular plane. Orthogonal TEE views showing the bi-caval and basal short-axis views are then used to identify the posterior and inferior region of the intra-atrial septum

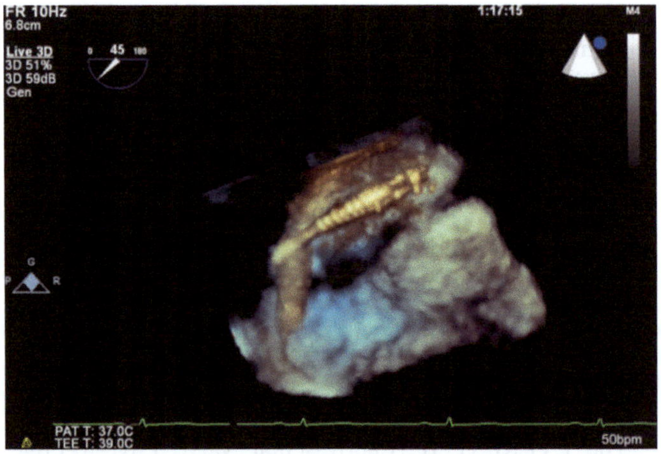

Fig. 30.20 A 3D TEE SAX showing the guide catheter sheath introduced into the LA across the inter-atrial septum. An echo-dense ring can be visualized at the tip of the guide catheter. This needs to be visualized continuously during dilator retraction to ensure that the clip delivery system will be appropriately introduced into the LA

- Step #6: Grasping the leaflets (Figs. 30.22, 30.23, and 30.24)
- Step #7: Clip release (Fig. 30.25)
- Step #8: Assess for post procedural changes and or complications (Fig. 30.26)

Follow Up of MV Repair

- The 2011 Appropriate Use Criteria for Echocardiography (multiple societies) support the use of echocardiography for MV disease when there are new clinical symptoms or

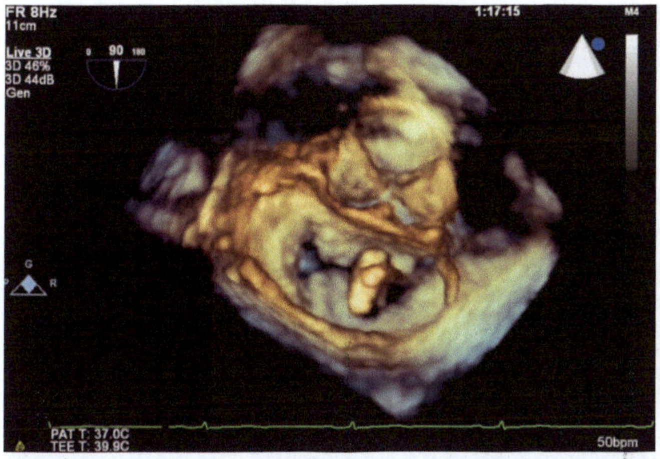

Fig. 30.21 A 3D TEE *en face* view of the MV demonstrates the perpendicular orientation of the open mitral clip to the leaflet targets

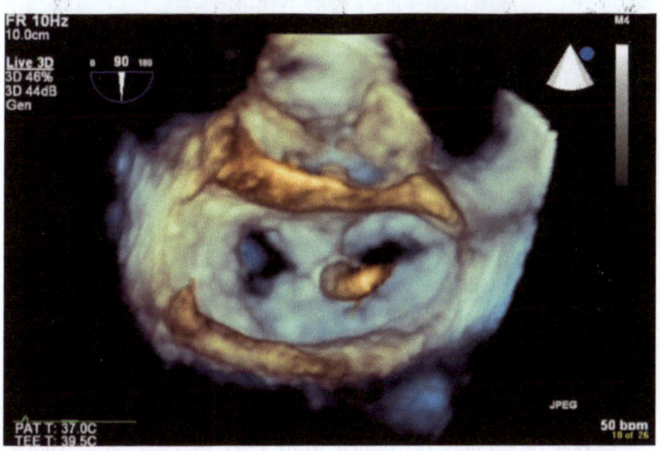

Fig. 30.22 A zoomed 2D left ventricular outflow tract view showing the clip arms perpendicular to the valve leaflets in the anterior and posterior dimensions. Leaflet insertion into the mitral clips should be assessed in multiple views with sweeps to confirm insertion

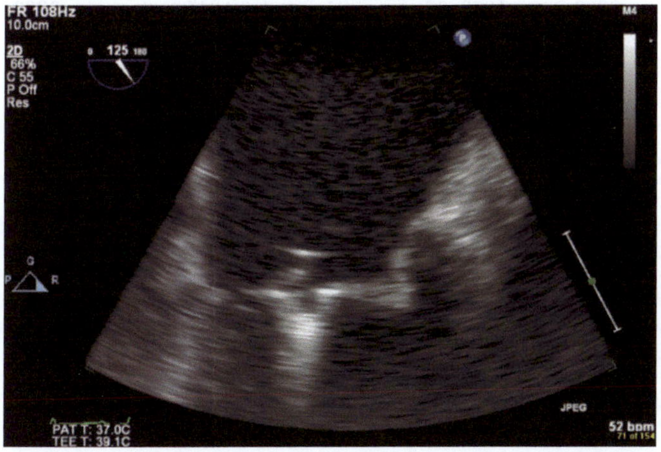

Fig. 30.23 A live 3D-TEE *en face* view demonstrates a double orifice mitral valve with catheter attached to the clip

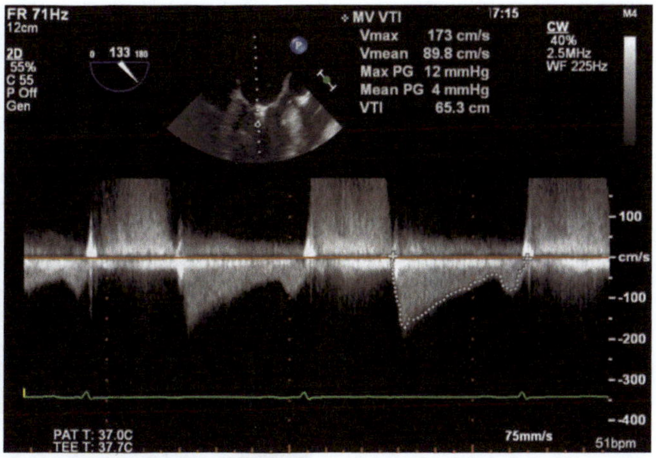

Fig. 30.24 A diastolic MV gradient is assessed to ensure a mean diastolic gradient of 4 mmHg or less

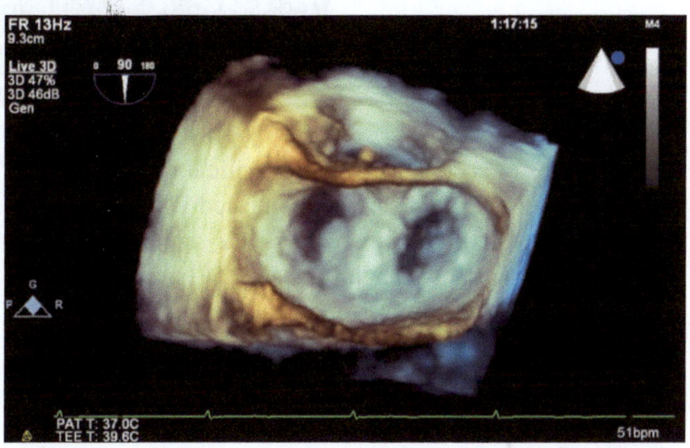

Fig. 30.25 3D TEE *en face* image demonstrating a double orifice MV

clinical changes suggestive of disease progression or complications. There are no specific recommendations pertaining to routine imaging post-MV repair [37]. Many physicians will perform a post-MV repair TTE to assess integrity of repair and features of LV remodeling (or reverse remodeling). For symptomatic patients with prior surgical or percutaneous MV repair, the clinician should follow the principles for pre-procedure and peri-procedural imaging of MV repair.

- Comprehensive echocardiographic assessment of the repaired MV leaflets, integrity of the annuloplasty ring, and sub-valvular apparatus is essential—with particular attention directed to the origin and mechanism of regurgitant jets, presence of mitral stenosis, extent of ventricular remodeling, and surrogates of pulmonary hypertension.
- The prognosis for patients with posterior prolapse repair performed in Centers of Excellence is better than patients with anterior leaflet prolapse, bileaflet prolapse, or ischemic MR [38, 39].

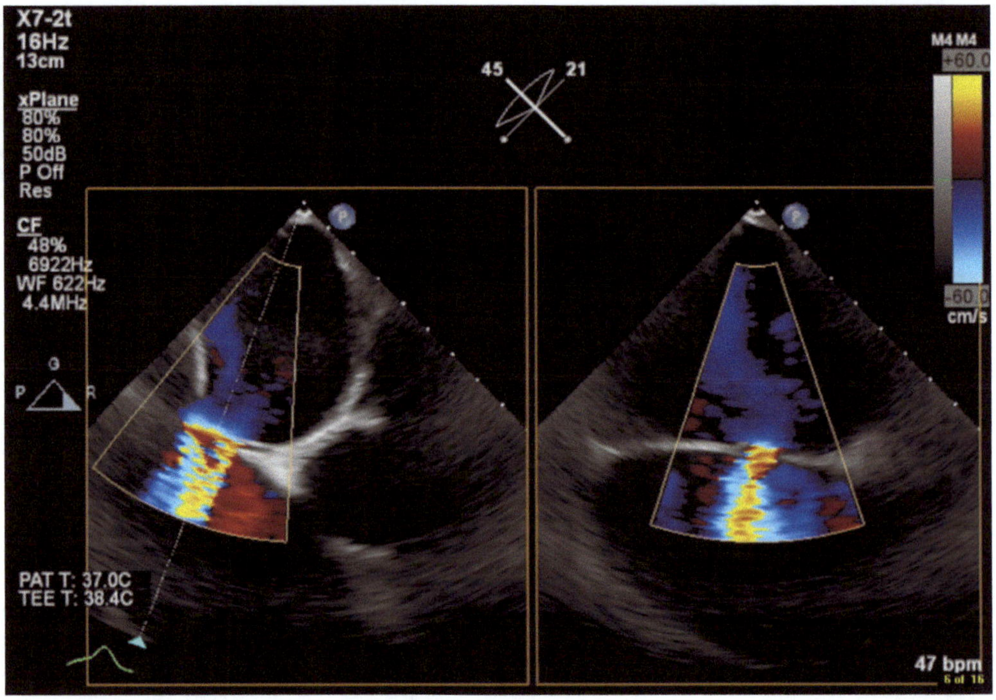

Fig. 30.26 Assessment of the trans-septal puncture site to evaluate for atrial level shunting. High LA pressures can result in an expected left to right shunt (*above*). With severe tricuspid regurgitation, right to left shunting with consequent hypoxemia may occur (not shown). Additional evaluation includes assessment for pericardial tamponade, LV and RV function, and atrial appendage thrombus (not shown)

– In cases of secondary MR, it is critical that the clinical assessment of MR severity be placed in the context of (1) systemic blood pressure; (2) LV size, LV function, and gradient between the LA and LV (peak velocity of MR); (3) goal-directed medical therapy, (4) need for revascularization therapy, and (5) need for resynchronization therapy. These parameters underlie the dynamic nature of MR [26].

Key Summary Points

- MR is classified as being **primary** (caused by abnormalities of the leaflets or sub-valvular apparatus) or **secondary** (caused by abnormalities of the ventricle) each with distinctly different treatment strategies and outcomes.
- MV repair is a surgical or percutaneous correction strategy designed to restore normal coaptation of the MV and thereby reduce mitral regurgitation. In general, the success and durability of MV repair is best for patients with degenerative MV disease and normal left ventricular function.
- TTE and TEE echocardiography are essential for the evaluation and treatment of MV disease through MV repair. The echocardiographer should have three major goals: (1) To understand the etiology, mechanism, severity, and impact of the MR; (2) to determine the feasibility and prognosis of MV repair and to help guide the procedure; (3) to demonstrate a critical understanding of the role of echocardiography in assessing the structural and hemodynamic features of MV disease.

References

1. Gammie JS, Sheng S, Griffith BP, et al. Trends in mitral valve surgery in the United States: results from the Society of Thoracic Surgeons Adult Cardiac Surgery Database. Ann Thorac Surg. 2009;87(5):1431–7. discussion 1437-1439. https://doi.org/10.1016/j.athoracsur.2009.01.064.
2. Badhwar V, Peterson ED, Jacobs JP, et al. Longitudinal outcome of isolated mitral repair in older patients: results from 14,604 procedures performed from 1991 to 2007. Ann Thorac Surg. 2012;94(6):1870–7. discussion 1877-1879. https://doi.org/10.1016/j.athoracsur.2012.05.105.
3. Mick SL, Keshavamurthy S, Gillinov AM. Mitral valve repair versus replacement. Ann Cardiothorac Surg. 2015;4(3):230–7. https://doi.org/10.3978/j.issn.2225-319X.2015.03.01.
4. Daneshmand MA, Milano CA, Rankin JS, et al. Mitral valve repair for degenerative disease: a 20-year experience. Ann Thorac Surg. 2009;88(6):1828–37. https://doi.org/10.1016/j.athoracsur.2009.08.008.
5. Nishimura RA, Otto CM, Bonow RO, et al. 2014 AHA/ACC guideline for the management of patients with valvular heart disease: a report of the American College of Cardiology/American Heart Association Task Force on Practice Guidelines. J Am Coll Cardiol. 2014;63(22):e57–e185. https://doi.org/10.1016/j.jacc.2014.02.536.
6. Rankin JS, Daneshmand MA, Milano CA, Gaca JG, Glower DD, Smith PK. Mitral valve repair for ischemic mitral regurgitation: review of current techniques. Heart Lung Vessels. 2013; 5(4):246–51.
7. Carpentier A, Chauvaud S, Fabiani JN, et al. Reconstructive surgery of mitral valve incompetence: ten-year appraisal. J Thorac Cardiovasc Surg. 1980;79(3):338–48.
8. Feringa HHH, Shaw LJ, Poldermans D, et al. Mitral valve repair and replacement in endocarditis: a systematic review of literature. Ann Thorac Surg. 2007;83(2):564–70. https://doi.org/10.1016/j.athoracsur.2006.09.023.

9. Enriquez-Sarano M, Akins CW, Vahanian A. Mitral regurgitation. Lancet Lond Engl. 2009;373(9672):1382–94. https://doi.org/10.1016/S0140-6736(09)60692-9.
10. Tsang W, Freed BH, Lang RM. The role of 3-dimensional echocardiography in the diagnosis and management of mitral valve disease: myxomatous valve disease. Cardiol Clin. 2013;31(2):203–15. https://doi.org/10.1016/j.ccl.2013.03.002.
11. Freed LA, Levy D, Levine RA, et al. Prevalence and clinical outcome of mitral-valve prolapse. N Engl J Med. 1999;341(1):1–7. https://doi.org/10.1056/NEJM199907013410101.
12. Kim GS, Lee CH, Kim JB, et al. Echocardiographic evaluation of mitral durability following valve repair in rheumatic mitral valve disease: impact of Maze procedure. J Thorac Cardiovasc Surg. 2014;147(1):247–53. https://doi.org/10.1016/j.jtcvs.2012.10.007.
13. Michler RE, Smith PK, Parides MK, et al. Two-year outcomes of surgical treatment of moderate ischemic mitral regurgitation. N Engl J Med. 2016;374(20):1932–41. https://doi.org/10.1056/NEJMoa1602003.
14. Goldstein D, Moskowitz AJ, Gelijns AC, et al. Two-year outcomes of surgical treatment of severe ischemic mitral regurgitation. N Engl J Med. 2016;374(4):344–53. https://doi.org/10.1056/NEJMoa1512913.
15. Kron IL, Acker MA, Adams DH, et al. 2015 The American Association for Thoracic Surgery Consensus Guidelines: ischemic mitral valve regurgitation. J Thorac Cardiovasc Surg. 2016;151(4):940–56. https://doi.org/10.1016/j.jtcvs.2015.08.127.
16. Mathew J, Swaminathan M, Ayoub C. Clinical manual and review of transesophageal echocardiography. 2nd ed. New York: McGraw Hill Professional; 2010.
17. Lawrie GM, Zoghbi W, Little S, et al. One hundred percent reparability of degenerative mitral regurgitation: intermediate-term results of a dynamic engineered approach. Ann Thorac Surg. 2016;101(2):576–84. https://doi.org/10.1016/j.athoracsur.2015.07.029.
18. Bolling SF. Mitral reconstruction in cardiomyopathy. J Heart Valve Dis. 2002;11(Suppl 1):S26–31.
19. Glower DD. Surgical approaches to mitral regurgitation. J Am Coll Cardiol. 2012;60(15):1315–22. https://doi.org/10.1016/j.jacc.2011.11.081.
20. Koprivanac M, Kelava M, Alansari S, et al. Degenerative mitral valve disease-contemporary surgical approaches and repair techniques. Ann Cardiothorac Surg. 2017;6(1):38–46. https://doi.org/10.3978/13327.
21. Zoghbi WA, Enriquez-Sarano M, Foster E, et al. Recommendations for evaluation of the severity of native valvular regurgitation with two-dimensional and Doppler echocardiography. J Am Soc Echocardiogr Off Publ Am Soc Echocardiogr. 2003;16(7):777–802. https://doi.org/10.1016/S0894-7317(03)00335-3.
22. Feldman T, Foster E, Glower DD, et al. Percutaneous repair or surgery for mitral regurgitation. N Engl J Med. 2011;364(15):1395–406. https://doi.org/10.1056/NEJMoa1009355.
23. Sorajja P, Mack M, Vemulapalli S, et al. Initial experience with commercial transcatheter mitral valve repair in the United States. J Am Coll Cardiol. 2016;67(10):1129–40. https://doi.org/10.1016/j.jacc.2015.12.054.
24. Mauri L, Garg P, Massaro JM, et al. The EVEREST II Trial: design and rationale for a randomized study of the evalve mitraclip system compared with mitral valve surgery for mitral regurgitation. Am Heart J. 2010;160(1):23–9. https://doi.org/10.1016/j.ahj.2010.04.009.
25. Blanke P, Naoum C, Webb J, et al. Multimodality imaging in the context of transcatheter mitral valve replacement: establishing consensus among modalities and disciplines. JACC Cardiovasc Imaging. 2015;8(10):1191–208. https://doi.org/10.1016/j.jcmg.2015.08.004.
26. Grayburn PA, Carabello B, Hung J, et al. Defining "severe" secondary mitral regurgitation: emphasizing an integrated approach. J Am Coll Cardiol. 2014;64(25):2792–801. https://doi.org/10.1016/j.jacc.2014.10.016.
27. Grayburn PA, Weissman NJ, Zamorano JL. Quantitation of mitral regurgitation. Circulation. 2012;126(16):2005–17. https://doi.org/10.1161/CIRCULATIONAHA.112.121590.
28. Lang RM, Badano LP, Mor-Avi V, et al. Recommendations for cardiac chamber quantification by echocardiography in adults: an update from the American Society of Echocardiography and the European Association of Cardiovascular Imaging. J Am Soc Echocardiogr Off Publ Am Soc Echocardiogr. 2015;28(1):1–39.e14. https://doi.org/10.1016/j.echo.2014.10.003.
29. Lang RM, Badano LP, Tsang W, et al. EAE/ASE recommendations for image acquisition and display using three-dimensional echocardiography. J Am Soc Echocardiogr. 2012;25(1):3–46. https://doi.org/10.1016/j.echo.2011.11.010.
30. Kisslo J, Rivera JD, Adams DB, Mackenson BG, Jollis JJ, Glower DD. Mitral valve disease. In: Nihoyannopoulos P, Kisslo J, editors. Echocardiography. London: Springer; 2009. p. 135–213. http://link.springer.com/chapter/10.1007/978-1-84882-293-1_8. Accessed 5 Feb 2017.
31. Armstrong WF, Feigenbaum H, Ryan T. Feigenbaum's echocardiography. 7th ed. Philadelphia: Wolters Kluwer Health/Lippincott Williams & Wilkins; 2010.
32. Sidebotham DA, Allen SJ, Gerber IL, Fayers T. Intraoperative transesophageal echocardiography for surgical repair of mitral regurgitation. J Am Soc Echocardiogr. 2014;27(4):345–66. https://doi.org/10.1016/j.echo.2014.01.005.
33. Maslow A. Mitral valve repair: an echocardiographic review: part 1. J Cardiothorac Vasc Anesth. 2015;29(1):156–77. https://doi.org/10.1053/j.jvca.2014.03.007.
34. Maslow A. Mitral valve repair: an echocardiographic review: part 2. J Cardiothorac Vasc Anesth. 2015;29(2):439–71. https://doi.org/10.1053/j.jvca.2014.03.013.
35. Slipczuk L, Siegel RJ, Jilaihawi H, Hussaini A, Kar S. Optimizing procedural outcomes in percutaneous mitral valve therapy using transesophageal imaging: a stepwise analysis. Expert Rev Cardiovasc Ther. 2012;10(7):901–16. https://doi.org/10.1586/erc.12.72.
36. Wunderlich NC, Siegel RJ. Peri-interventional echo assessment for the MitraClip procedure. Eur Heart J Cardiovasc Imaging. 2013;14(10):935–49. https://doi.org/10.1093/ehjci/jet060.
37. American College of Cardiology Foundation Appropriate Use Criteria Task Force, American Society of Echocardiography, American Heart Association, et al. ACCF/ASE/AHA/ASNC/HFSA/HRS/SCAI/SCCM/SCCT/SCMR 2011 appropriate use criteria for echocardiography. a report of the American College of Cardiology Foundation Appropriate Use Criteria Task Force, American Society of Echocardiography, American Heart Association, American Society of Nuclear Cardiology, Heart Failure Society of America, Heart Rhythm Society, Society for Cardiovascular Angiography and Interventions, Society of Critical Care Medicine, Society of Cardiovascular Computed Tomography, Society for Cardiovascular Magnetic Resonance American College of Chest Physicians. J Am Soc Echocardiogr Off Publ Am Soc Echocardiogr. 2011;24(3):229–67. https://doi.org/10.1016/j.echo.2010.12.008.
38. Suri RM, Clavel M-A, Schaff HV, et al. Effect of recurrent mitral regurgitation following degenerative mitral valve repair: long-term analysis of competing outcomes. J Am Coll Cardiol. 2016;67(5):488–98. https://doi.org/10.1016/j.jacc.2015.10.098.
39. Kron IL, Hung J, Overbey JR, et al. Predicting recurrent mitral regurgitation after mitral valve repair for severe ischemic mitral regurgitation. J Thorac Cardiovasc Surg. 2015;149(3):752–761.e1. https://doi.org/10.1016/j.jtcvs.2014.10.120.

Intraprocedural Transesophageal Echocardiography

31

Devin W. Kehl, Florian Rader, and Robert J. Siegel

Abstract

The use of transcatheter approaches in the management of severe valvular heart disease is increasing worldwide. Left atrial appendage closure device implantation for patients with atrial fibrillation is also on the rise. Transesophageal echocardiography (TEE) plays an essential role in proper patient selection and in real-time guidance of these procedures. In the following chapter, we review the role of echocardiography, specifically 2D and 3D TEE, in transcatheter aortic valve replacement (TAVR), mitral valve repair with MitraClip, and left atrial appendage closure with the Watchman device. For each procedure, we review the most important echocardiographic views, measurements, and considerations for pre-procedural patient and device selection, intra-procedural guidance of device placement and positioning, and post-procedural monitoring for complications.

Keywords

Transesophageal echocardiogram · 3D echocardiography · Transcatheter aortic valve replacement · MitraClip · Left atrial appendage occluder device

Abbreviations

CT	Computed tomography
IAS	Inter-atrial septum
LA	Left atrium
LAA	Left atrial appendage
LUPV	Left upper pulmonary vein
LVOT	Left ventricular outflow tract
MDCT	Multidetector computed tomography
ME	Mid-esophageal
MR	Mitral regurgitation
MV	Mitral valve
PVR	Paravalvular regurgitation
TAVR	Transcatheter aortic valve replacement
TEE	Transesophageal echocardiography

Role of Echocardiography in Transcatheter Aortic Valve Replacement (TAVR)

- Assessment of anatomy
  - Aortic annulus sizing (Fig. 31.1)

    Aortic stent-valves are circular in shape. However, the left ventricular outflow tract (LVOT) is oval, not circular, shaped in 90% of patients [1]. The LVOT is often asymmetric in the presence of left ventricular hypertrophy and aortic stenosis

    Oversizing can lead to aortic annulus rupture, and undersizing can lead to paravalvular regurgitation or valve embolization

    Goal is to define the diameter, area, and perimeter of the aortic annulus using transesophageal echocardiography (TEE) to corroborate pre-procedural measurements from computed tomography (CT), or as a sole measurement when CT measurement is not available (Table 31.1)

    3D TEE results in less underestimation of annular size than 2D when compared to CT as gold standard

    2D diameter should be measured as the distance between basal attachments of the right and non-coronary cusps during mid-systole from the mid-esophageal (ME) long axis (110–140°) view

    3D allows for measurement of orthogonal views and is preferred to 2D TEE measurement for aortic prosthesis sizing to reduce the risk of paravalvular regurgitation [2]

D. W. Kehl, MD · F. Rader, MD, MS
R. J. Siegel, MD, FACC (✉)
Cedars-Sinai Heart Institute, Los Angeles, CA, USA
e-mail: siegel@cshs.org

A. Sadeghpour, A. Alizadehasl (eds.), *Case-Based Textbook of Echocardiography*,
https://doi.org/10.1007/978-3-319-67691-3_31

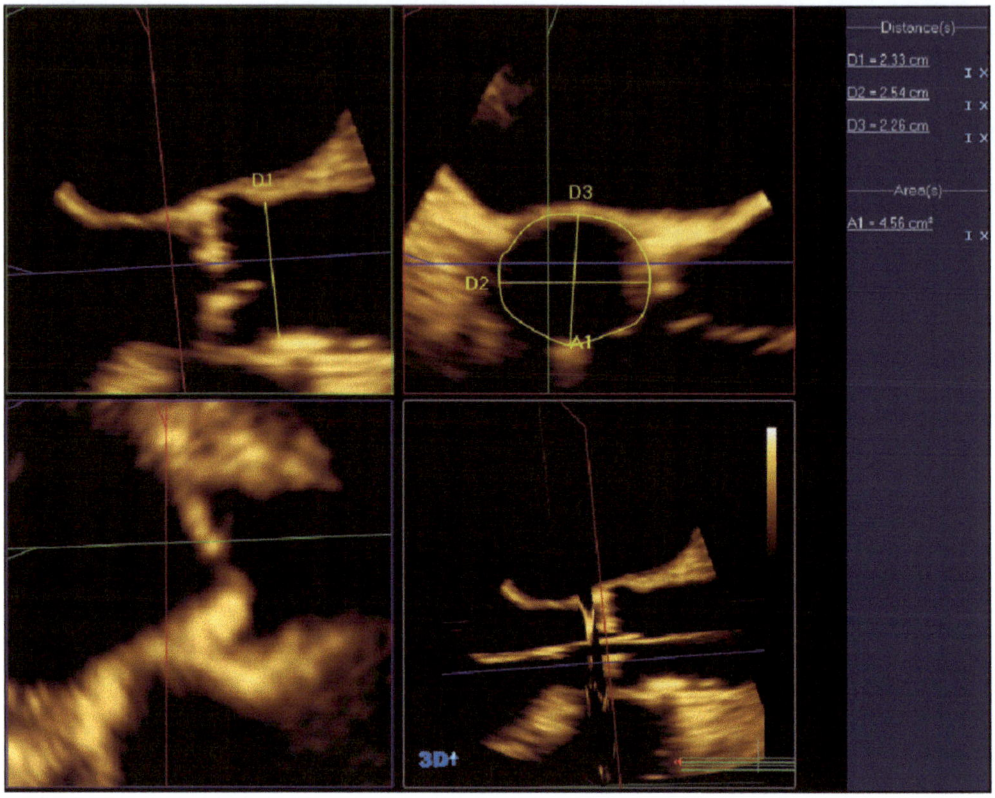

Fig. 31.1 Example of use of 3D TEE for aortic annular sizing. Measurement of the aortic valve annular diameter (D2, D3) and area (A1) and sinotubular junction diameter (D1) using 3D TEE (Qlab, Philips Ultrasound, Bothell, Washington) imaging of the annulus in long axis (top left), short axis (top right), and 3D reconstruction (bottom panels) ensures that measurements are coaxial to the annular plane. Imaging confirmed this patient to be appropriate for implantation of a 26 mm Edwards Sapien S3 balloon-expandable valve

Table 31.1 Evidence-based aortic prosthesis sizing for prediction of paravalvular aortic regurgitation (adapted, with permission, from Jilaihawi et al. 2013) [2]

Evidence basis	Balloon-expandable aortic prosthesis sizing			
Prosthesis				
Diameter, mm	20	23	26	29
Area, cm^2	3.14	4.15	5.31	6.61
Perimeter, mm	62.8	72.3	81.7	91.1
3D–TEE (QLab)				
Mean diameter, mm	15.1–18.1	18.1–21.1	21.1–24.1	24.1–27.1
Area, cm^2	1.96–2.71	2.71–3.59	3.59–4.58	4.58–5.70
Perimeter, mm	50.4–59.3	59.3–68.2	68.2–77.1	77.1–86.0
Cross-sectional CT				
Mean diameter, mm	17.3–20.3	20.3–23.3	23.3–26.3	26.3–29.3
Area, cm^2	2.31–3.20	3.20–4.23	4.23–5.40	5.40–6.72
Perimeter, mm	55.6–65.4	65.4–75.2	75.2–85.0	85.0–94.8
2D–TEE				
Manufacturer-directed sizing, mm	16–19	18–22	21–25	24–27

3D TEE and multidetector CT (MDCT) cross-sectional perimeter and area measurements of the aortic annulus have been strongly correlated [3]. Diameter measurements by 3D-TEE have been shown to underestimate CT-derived diameter by 1–2 mm or ~10% [2]

Aortic prosthesis sizing by 3D-TEE and MDCT have been shown to be equally accurate for prediction of mild or greater paravalvular regurgitation (PVR) [3]; MDCT may be superior to 3D TEE in the detection of moderate or greater PVR [2]

- Coronary height

  Important to measure the distance from the open left aortic cusp to the proximal edge of the left coronary ostium. This can be measured in ME short axis view (30–60°) at the level of the aortic valve. 3D echo reconstruction provides the most reliable estimates. A minimum of 10 mm is generally recommended to proceed safely.

  Important to measure the distance from the aortic annulus to the proximal edge of the right coronary ostium. This is best measured in ME long axis (110–140°). 3D echo reconstruction provides the most reliable estimates.

- Guidance of positioning
  - Although prosthesis positioning is mainly guided by fluoroscopy, adjunctive TEE imaging can be helpful.
  - Depending on the valve type, ideal placement of the ventricular edge of the valve is usually 4 mm below the aortic cusps. The valve will move further antegrade into the LVOT when deployed.

Table 31.2 Grading of aortic valve regurgitation post-TAVR

	Trace	Mild	Mild to moderate	Moderate	Moderate to severe	Severe
Circumferential extent of PVR (%) (color Doppler)	<10	<10	10–20	20–30	>30	>30
Jet width/LVOT diameter (%)	<5	5–15	15–30	30–45	45–60	>60

- After implantation, the valve should be 1–2 mm below the insertion parts of the native aortic valve cusps
- Placement too deep in the left ventricle restricts anterior mitral leaflet opening and is associated with "supraskirtal" PVR
- Placement too high (i.e., shallow) in the aortic sinuses of Valsalva increases risk of coronary ostial obstruction, distal embolization of the valve prosthesis, and PVR below the prosthesis
- Confirm coaxial positioning of the undeployed valve prior to inflation. Poor alignment between the valve and the aortic annulus can also lead to PVR regurgitation post-deployment

• Post-TAVR deployment
- Assessment of aortic regurgitation (Table 31.2)
  Any degree of aortic valve regurgitation has been reported in 88% of post-TAVR cases [1].
  Moderate or greater PVR is reported in ~10% of patients with early generation balloon-expandable valves [2]. Recent generation valves (i.e., S3, Edwards Lifesciences) with enhanced skirt structure have reduced this rate markedly, to 2.9% at 30 days and 2.7% at 1 year [4].
  The presence of moderate or severe regurgitation post-TAVR has been reported to have a 3.79 fold higher risk of 1 year mortality [5]
  No increase in mortality has been demonstrated for mild or less residual aortic regurgitation
  Paravalvular jets are often multiple, irregular, and eccentric. Therefore, a multiparameter assessment is needed to reliably quantify regurgitation.
  The primary semi-quantitative measure of PVR post-TAVR is the circumferential extent of the regurgitant jet by color Doppler interrogation of the aortic annulus short axis. <10% circumferential extent is consistent with mild severity, 10–30% is consistent with moderate severity, and >30% generally indicates severe [6]
  The circumferential extent varies significantly depending on the plane of color Doppler interrogation. Too low a plane (i.e., too deep in the LVOT) may result in overestimation, and too high a plane (i.e., above the stent-valve) may result in an underestimate [6]
  Consistent holodiastolic flow reversal and jet extent into the LVOT beyond the tip of the anterior mitral valve leaflet have been shown to be independent predictors of significant (moderate or greater) PVR post-TAVR [7]
  Significant transvalvular regurgitation is rare (~1%) [8, 9]
  3D TEE features associated with transvalvular aortic regurgitation include large prosthetic expansion, elliptical prosthetic shape, and anti-anatomical position [8]
  Transvalvular regurgitation may also result from underdeployment of a valve cusp and may respond to catheter manipulation [9]
- Identification of complications (Fig. 31.2)
  Other complications include distal embolization, aortic annular rupture, aortic hematoma with or without dissection, pericardial effusion with or without cardiac tamponade, transient LV dysfunction, coronary obstruction due to the prosthesis or displaced aortic valve leaflet or calcium, mitral regurgitation, and systolic anterior motion of the mitral valve

Key Points
- The LVOT is oval but aortic stent-valves are circular in shape. This represents one important anatomical basis for PVR post-TAVR.
- The presence of moderate or greater aortic regurgitation post-TAVR carries an increased risk of post-procedural mortality
- 3D TEE provides more reliable measurements of coronary height than 2D TEE
- TEE imaging is critical to the timely identification of procedural complications

Role of Echocardiography in Percutaneous Mitral Valve Repair with Mitraclip

- Assessment of anatomy and patient selection (Fig. 31.3)
  - FDA approved for treatment of degenerative mitral regurgitation (MR) in high risk patients based on the EVEREST and EVEREST II trials [11, 12]
  - Registry data [13] and observational data [14, 15] support the safety and efficacy of MitraClip for reduction of functional mitral regurgitation in patients at high risk for surgery, with improvement in ejection fraction, left ventricular size, and clinical heart failure [16]. However, a mortality benefit has yet to be demonstrated

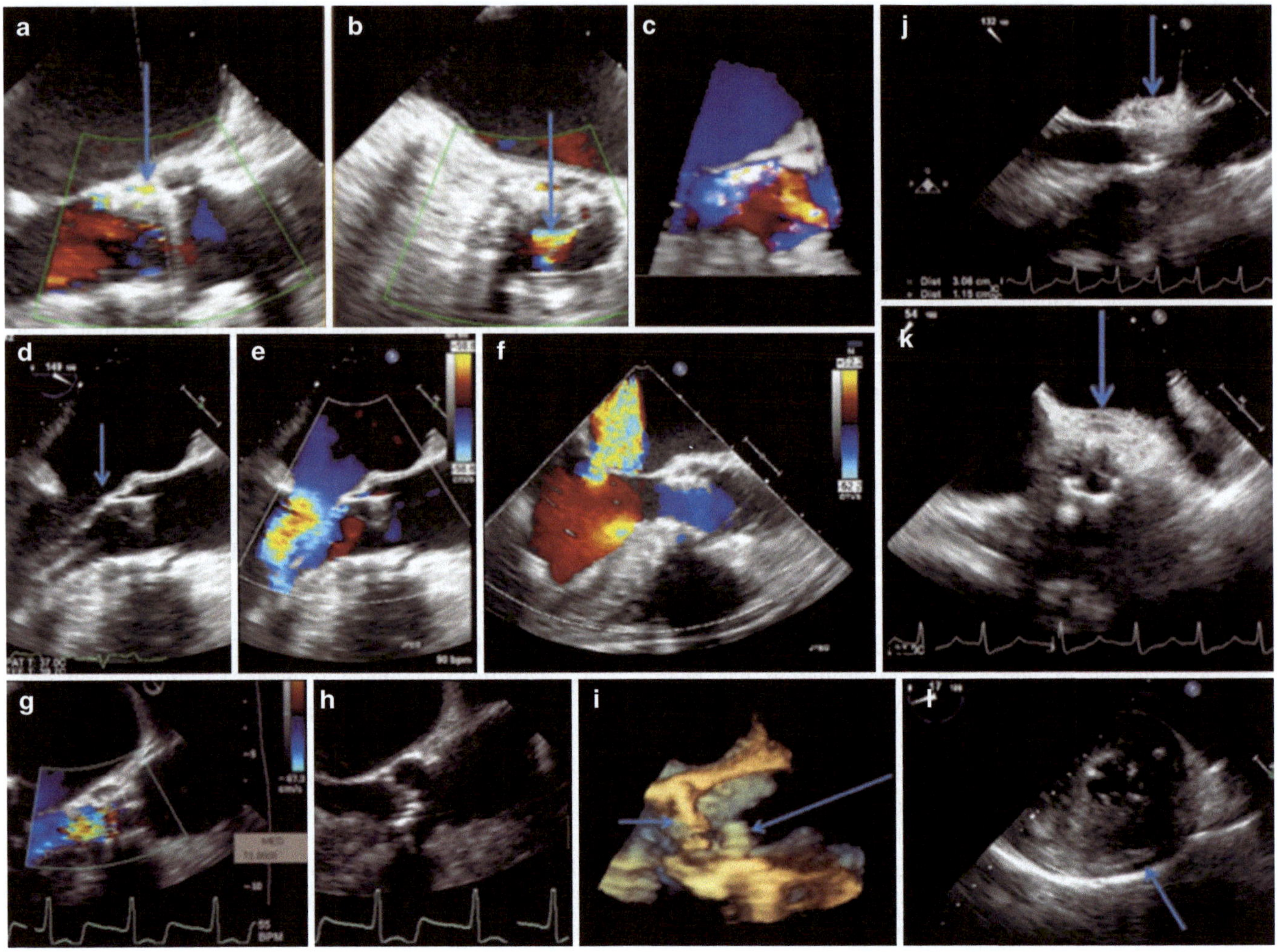

Fig. 31.2 Potential intra-procedure complications of TAVR. Paravalvular (Panel A, long axis view of the aortic valve, blue arrow) or transvalvular (Panel B, short axis of the aortic valve, blue arrow) may be seen following aortic valve deployment. 3D imaging (panel C) can be helpful to characterize the regurgitation. Deployment of the valve too deep in the LVOT can interfere with the mitral valve apparatus (panels D and E, long axis view, blue arrow) and lead to mitral regurgitation (panel F). Deployment of the valve above the level of the aortic annulus (Panels G, long axis view of the aortic valve) can lead to aortic regurgitation and valve embolization (Panel H, same patient post-embolization). The spatial relationship between the bioprosthetic valve and the coronary ostia is important because native leaflet calcium (Panel I, 3D long axis view of the aortic valve, short arrow) or aortic root calcium (Panel I, long arrow) can be dislodged or displaced during valve deployment and lead to coronary artery obstruction. Aortic root hematoma or rupture is a very rare but potentially devastating complication, more common in patients with a heavily calcified aortic annulus or narrow sino-tubular junction. Echocardiographic hallmarks of hematoma include aortic wall thickening on long axis (panel J, blue arrow) or short axis (panel K, blue arrow) of the aortic root. Pericardial effusion (Panel L, transgastric short axis view of the left ventricle, blue arrow) may also occur in this setting and may require emergent drainage

in this cohort. The ongoing COAPT trial randomizes patients with severe functional MR to optimal medical therapy with vs without MitraClip.

- Ideal or unsuitable morphology is summarized in Table 31.3
- Success also achievable with pathology in the P1 or P3 segment, a mitral valve (MV) area between 3 and 4 cm^2 with good leaflet mobility, a mobile posterior leaflet length between 7 and 10 mm, leaflet restriction in systole, and a flail width > 15 mm in patients with large rings allowing for multiple clips to be implanted

• Intra-procedural (Fig. 31.4)

- Trans-septal puncture (Fig. 31.5)

  Proper location of puncture of the interatrial septum (IAS) has a critical effect on the technical ease and success of the procedure

  Optimal site of IAS puncture is posterior and superior

  Use the bicaval view (ME 90–110°) to determine inferior-superior position

  Use the basal short axis view (ME 30–45°) to determine anterior-posterior position. More posterior access is needed for proper alignment along the line of coaptation.

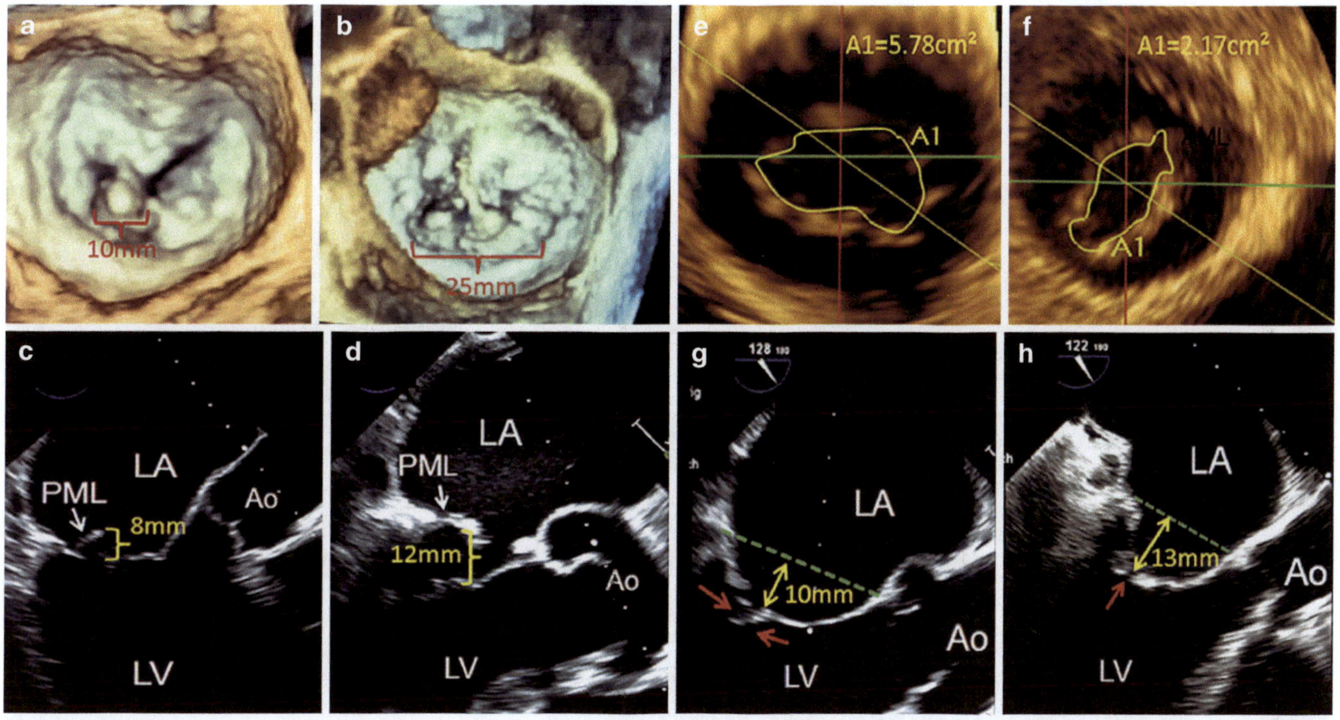

Fig. 31.3 Echocardiographic measurements for determining patient suitability for MitraClip (Borrowed, with permission, from Fig. 5 of Beigel et al. 2014 [10]). Panel A: 3D TEE en face view of the mitral valve in a patient with a flail middle portion of the posterior leaflet. The flail width (red brackets) is relatively narrow and suitable for MitraClip. Panel B: Patients with a large flail width > 15 mm are less suitable for MitraClip. Panels C and D: TEE mid-esophageal long axis views of the mitral valve with measurements of flail gap (yellow brackets). Panel C shows a patient suitable for MitraClip with flail gap <10 mm, and Panel D shows a patient less suitable for MitraClip, with a flail gap >10 mm and calcified posterior leaflet. Panels E and F: Mitral valve area can be measured with 3D TEE (Qlab, Philips Ultrasound). Mitral valve area should exceed 4 cm^2 (panel E) to reduce the risk of mitral stenosis post-deployment. Panels G and H: TEE mid-esophageal long axis view of the mitral valve showing patients with functional mitral regurgitation. The tenting height or coaptation depth (yellow arrows), measured as the distance from the base of the mitral valve (green line) to the leaflet tips in diastole, should optimally be ≤10 mm (panel G) to be suitable for MitraClip

Table 31.3 Morphological characterization for MitraClip eligibility (adapted, with permission, from Wunderlich et al. 2013) [17]

Ideal valve morphology	Unsuitable valve morphology
MR originating from the mid portion of the valve (degenerative or functional etiology)	Perforated mitral leaflets or clefts
Lack of calcification in the grasping area	Lack of primary and secondary chordal support
Mitral valve area > 4 cm^2	Severe calcification in the grasping area
Length of posterior leaflet ≥10 mm	Length of posterior leaflet <7 mm
Non-rheumatic or endocarditic valve disease	Hemodynamically relevant mitral stenosis (mean transmitral pressure gradient ≥4 mmHg or mitral valve orifice area < 30 mm^2)
Flail-width < 15 mm, flail gap <10 mm	Gap between the leaflets >2 mm
Sufficient leaflet tissue for mechanical coaptation: coaptation depth > 11 mm, coaptation length > 2 mm	Rheumatic valve disease—with restriction in systole und diastole or endocarditic valve disease

- Consider the use of x-plane at ME 45° and 90° for simultaneous viewing of both axes

Once tenting of the IAS is seen at the desired position, the four-chamber (ME 0°) view is used to determine height above mitral annulus prior to puncture
- Degenerative MR: Ideal puncture site is 4–5 cm above the mitral annulus, in order to guarantee enough space for adequate catheter and MitraClip maneuvering
- Functional MR: Ideal puncture site is slightly more inferior and closer to the annular plane (~3.5 cm above the annular plane), because the line of coaptation is usually below the plane of the mitral annulus due to tethering

A patent foramen ovale should not be used for transseptal access: this passage through the IAS is too anterior

An atrial septal defect should not be used for transseptal access (even in a superior–posterior position), as the sheath usually cannot be stabilized within the defect

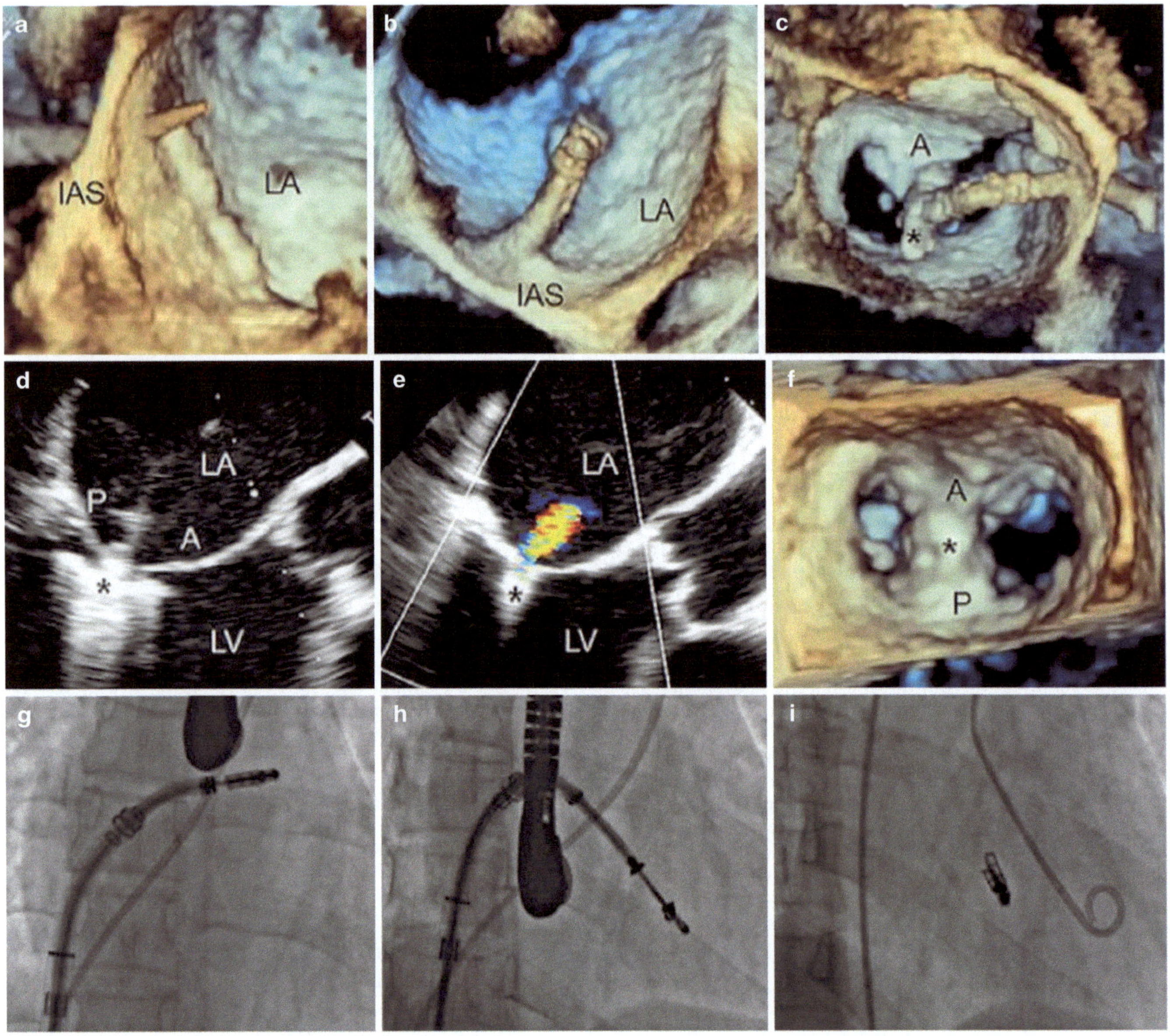

Fig. 31.4 Steps of MitraClip deployment (Borrowed, with permission, from Fig. 4 of Beigel et al. 2014 [10]). 2D and 3D TEE images demonstrating the steps of MitraClip deployment. Panel A: Trans-septal puncture. Panel B: Introduction of the catheter system to the LA through the IAS. Panel C: Advancement of the delivery system and positioning of the MitraClip in between the mitral valve leaflets. Panel D: Positioning of the MitraClip between the anterior and posterior mitral valve leaflets. Panel E: 2D TEE showing mild MR after deployment of the MitraClip. Panel F: 3D TEE en-face view of the mitral valve post-deployment demonstrates a typical double-orifice appearance. Panels G–I: Fluoroscopic images showing the device within the LA (Panel G), advanced towards the left ventricle (Panel H), and post-deployment (Panel I). Asterisk points to the location of the MitraClip

Once the trans-septal sheath has been inserted, a guidewire is placed in the left upper pulmonary vein (LUPV) and should be visualized by TEE to ensure the wire is not placed in the left atrial appendage (LAA)

- Steerable guide catheter insertion and clip delivery system insertion and positioning

  The guide-dilator assembly is advanced into the left atrium until the tip of the guide extends approximately 3 cm in the LA

  3D imaging can identify the radio-opaque tip ring of the guide catheter

  3D imaging can also be helpful to avoid puncture of the LA free wall

- Steering and positioning of the MitraClip device above the valve

  Clip should be positioned over the greatest regurgitant jet and confirmed in orthogonal views

  Medial-lateral displacements should be monitored from ME 60° view (i.e., bi-commissural view). 3D

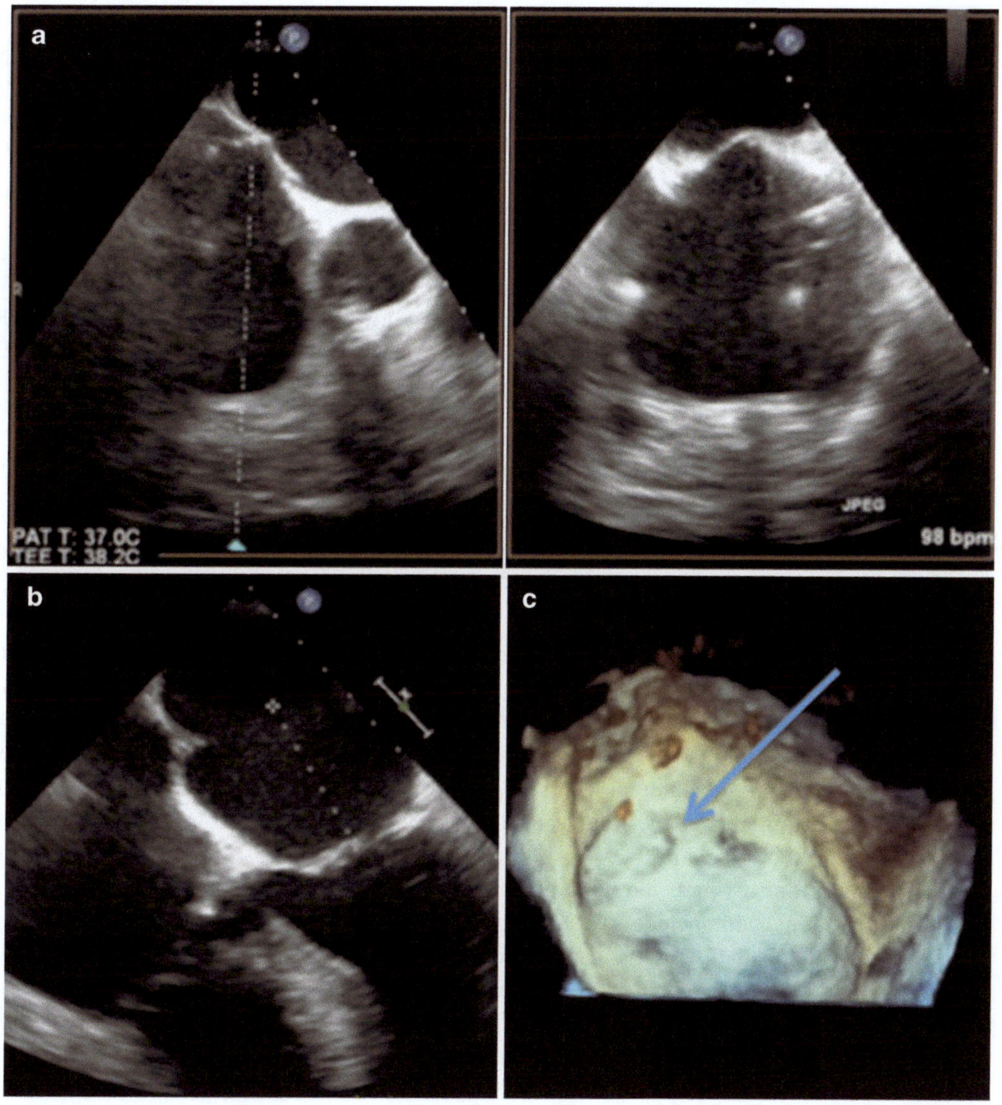

Fig. 31.5 TEE guidance of trans-septal puncture. TEE images of a trans-septal puncture positioned superior and posterior in the IAS. Panel A: 2D X-plane imaging shows simultaneous short axis (left panel) and bicaval (right panel) views of the IAS for optimal positioning superior and posterior on the IAS. Panel B: ME 4-chamber view of the IAS allows for measurement of the height (dotted white line) above the mitral valve annular plane. Panel C: Tenting of the IAS (blue arrow) from the LA side and guidance of optimal positioning of trans-septal puncture can also be confirmed on 3D imaging of the IAS

imaging is helpful to determine true bilateral commissural imaging.

Anterior-posterior displacements should be monitored from the ME long-axis view

Clip arm orientation should be perpendicular to the line of coaptation and should be confirmed using 3D en-face view of the mitral valve, or in a short axis transgastric view

- Positioning of the Clip delivery system in the left ventricle

  X-plane imaging with ME 60° view and ME long-axis view should be used

  Clip arms should be seen in the ME long-axis view but not in the ME 60° view

  2D transgastric short axis or 3D en-face view of the mitral valve from the LA side should be used to reassess orientation of delivery system in relation to the line of coaptation

- Grasping of the leaflets

  Consider use of X-plane at ME 60° view and ME long-axis. Grasping of posterior leaflet best seen in ME long axis

  Ensure that subvalvular chordae tendinae have not been entrapped on the ME 60° view

  Verify insertion of both leaflets and satisfactory grasp by observation of:

  Leaflet tip insertion between the gripper and arms of the clip

  Limited leaflet mobility (systolic and diastolic) relative to the tips of both clip arms

  Adequate MR reduction (see section below)

  Partial closure of the clip is recommended to assess the effect on MR prior to complete closure

  Assessment of residual MR and mitral stenosis (see section below) should be performed prior to clip deployment and following clip deployment

- Post-MitraClip deployment
  - Assessment of residual MR
    There are no validated studies of MR assessment following creation of a double orifice. Therefore, a multimodality approach is needed.
    Multiple small jets are frequently seen and are compatible with mild MR
    Pulmonary vein flow pattern should be assessed. Systolic flow reversal should no longer be present and there should be increased systolic forward flow compared to baseline.
    The proximal isovelocity surface area (PISA) method cannot be used to quantify the MR post-procedure, as is not validated for multiple MR jets which appear frequently after MitraClip implantation, nor for the newly created geometry of the mitral valve with two (or even more) orifices,
    Summation of vena contractae by 2D is not reliable in the presence of multiple jets. However, 3D vena contracta may be used
  - Evaluation for mitral stenosis
    Acceptable post-procedure mean transmitral gradient is ≤5 mmHg by continuous wave Doppler
    MVA by planimetry of the double orifice derived by 3D should be <1.5 mm^2
  - Evaluation for post-procedure complications
    Complications can include partial clip detachment, thrombus formation on the catheter, chordae tendinae entrapment by the MitraClip, pericardial effusion or tamponade, persistent atrial septal defect, cardiac arrhythmias, air embolism, and embolic cerebrovascular complications [10]

Key Points

- Morphologic characterization of the mitral valve with 2D and 3D TEE is critical for proper selection of candidates for mitral valve repair with MitraClip
- Proper location of puncture of the IAS has a critical effect on the technical ease and success of the procedure
- Assessment of pulmonary venous Doppler flow pattern is critical to the assessment of residual mitral regurgitation after MitraClip implantation

Role of Echocardiography in Left Atrial Appendage Closure Device Placement

- Multiple percutaneous LAA closure devices have been developed, including LAA plug devices and occluder devices
- The following discussion will focus on imaging considerations for the Watchman LAA occluder device (Boston Scientific, Natick, Massachusetts).
  - Device sizes include 21, 24, 27, 30, 33 mm

Table 31.4 LAA morphologic subtypes [18]

Windsock	Single long tube-like structure Ideal for Watchman
Chicken wing	Most common morphology Prominent bend in the proximal or middle portion of the dominant lobe Less optimal for Watchman due to an often short proximal portion
Cauliflower	Short length relative to the size of the orifice Less optimal for Watchman
Cactus	Dominant central lobe with secondary lobes extending from the central lobe superiorly and inferiorly

- Pre-procedural
  - Assessment of anatomy
    Confirm absence of thrombus
    Assess the morphologic subtype, number of lobes, and pectinate features
      The impact of the morphologic subtype on procedural outcome is not well described, but some morphologies, such as the windsock, are anatomically more suitable for Watchman placement (Table 31.4)
  - Sizing of landing zone in the LAA ostium (Fig. 31.6)
    Device sizing is of critical importance to procedural success
      Undersizing the device increases the risk of device migration or peridevice leak
      Oversizing the device increases the risk of perforation and pericardial effusion
    The landing zone is measured from the level of the superior edge of the mitral valve annulus (also noted by the circumflex artery) to a point 1–2 cm deep into the LAA from the limbus of the left upper pulmonary vein (LUPV)
    Measure at ME 0°, 45°, 90°, 135°
      Largest dimension is typically noted at 120–135°
    Should be >17 mm, <31 mm
    Device chosen should have 10–20% (2–4 mm) greater diameter than the maximum ostium dimension
  - Measurement of LAA depth
    The Watchman device is as long as it is wide. Therefore, the dominant lobe should be at least as deep as the size of the device chosen
    LAA depth is measured from ostium line to the deepest portion of the dominant lobe, perpendicular to the landing zone measurement
    The device should not protrude >4–7 mm beyond the LAA ostium
- Intra-procedural
  - Guidance of positioning
    Trans-septal puncture
      The optimal position for puncture is in the inferior and posterior portion of the IAS

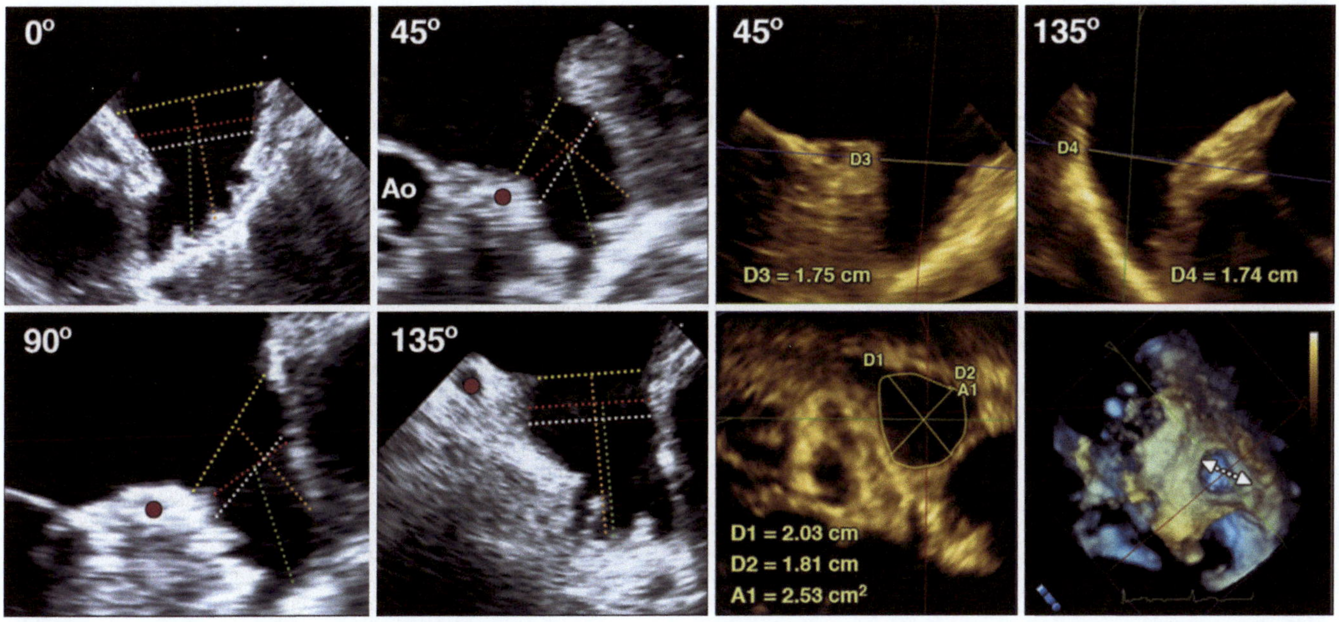

Fig. 31.6 2D and 3D TEE Measurements of LAA Dimensions (Borrowed, with permission, from Fig. 4 of Wunderlich et al. 2015 [19]). Left panel: Landing zone dimensions of the LAA are pictured in 4 imaging planes. The ostial plane (yellow line) and landing zone measurement (red line) for the LAA occluder device (i.e., Watchman) are shown. The landing zone should be measured from the inferior portion of the LAA ostium indicated by the left circumflex artery (red dot) to a point 1–2 cm distal to the rim of the LUPV. The white line indicates the measurement of the landing zone for LAA plug devices (not discussed in this chapter). The depth of the main lobe should be measured perpendicular to the landing zone line for the occluder device (green line) or along the expected axis of the LAA plug devices (orange line). Right panel: 3D measurements of the LAA landing zone, including diameter (D1–D4) and area (A1)

ME 90° view (bicaval view) may be used to verify positioning along superior-inferior axis, in the mid to inferior portion

ME 45° view (short axis view) at the aortic valve level may be used to verify positioning along the anterior-posterior axis, away from the aortic valve

Device positioning

Following trans-septal puncture the access sheath is advanced into the left atrium and into the LUPV. The sheath is then pulled back from the LUPV and advanced to the LAA.

- Post-Watchman deployment

Verify position, anchor, size, and seal

Plane of the maximum diameter of the device should be at or just distal to the ostium and should span the entire LAA ostium

Anchoring is verified by the procedural cardiologist by the tug test

Maximum diameter of the device should be measured at all angles. Expect a 10–20% smaller diameter in situ than original device size

Color Doppler should be used to verify appropriate seal

Despite a dearth of definitive data, recommendations call for continuation of anticoagulation only for peri-device leaks >5 mm in diameter [20]. Therefore, peri-device leaks ≤5 mm are generally acceptable and do not require device repositioning

- Complications

LA or LAA perforation—5.2% [20, 21]

During the entire procedure the pericardium should be continually assessed for the presence of any pericardial effusion, which could indicate traumatic hemopericardium

Device embolization—0–2.7% [20, 21]

Thrombus formation on the device—4.2% [20, 21]

Residual flow into the LAA (>5 mm)—8% at 6 months [20]

Persistent atrial septal defect—11% at 6 months [22]

- Post-procedural follow-up
  - Repeat TEE 45 days post procedure

    Visualize Watchman at 0°, 45°, 90°, 135° with 2D and color Doppler

    Verify absence of peri-device leaks >5 mm

    Verify absence of thrombus

Key Points

- The ostium of the left atrial appendage should be measured a multiple orthogonal angles for proper sizing of the occluder device.
- The landing zone of the Watchman occluder device should be measured from the level of the superior edge of the mitral valve annulus to a point 1–2 cm from the limbus of the left upper pulmonary vein
- Proper device sizing (diameter 10–20% larger than landing zone diameter) by TEE is critical to procedural success

Questions

1. Which of the following echocardiographic features of the mitral valve is least compatible with successful percutaneous repair with MitraClip?
   A. Flail gap of 9 mm
   B. Flail width of 9 mm
   C. Mitral valve area 4.2 cm^2
   D. Severe mitral leaflet calcification
   E. Severe mitral annular calcification

2. Which of the following locations on the inter-atrial septum is the optimal puncture site for placement of the Watchman left atrial appendage occluder device?
   A. Posterior and inferior
   B. Posterior and superior
   C. Anterior and inferior
   D. Anterior and superior

3. Which of the following is not a useful method of assessment of paravalvular regurgitation after TAVR?
   A. Assessment of holodiastolic flow reversal in the descending thoracic aorta
   B. Circumferential extent of the regurgitant jet by color Doppler assessment of the short axis view of the aortic valve
   C. Degree of extension of the color Doppler jet into the LVOT
   D. All of the above are useful methods

Answers

1. D
2. A
3. D

References

1. Saitoh T, Shiota M, Izumo M, et al. Comparison of left ventricular outflow geometry and aortic valve area in patients with aortic stenosis by 2-dimensional versus 3-dimensional echocardiography. Am J Cardiol. 2012;109(11):1626–31.
2. Jilaihawi H, Doctor N, Kashif M, et al. Aortic annular sizing for transcatheter aortic valve replacement using cross-sectional 3-dimensional transesophageal echocardiography. J Am Coll Cardiol. 2013;61(9):908–16.
3. Khalique OK, Kodali SK, Paradis JM, et al. Aortic annular sizing using a novel 3-dimensional echocardiographic method: use and comparison with cardiac computed tomography. Circ Cardiovasc Imaging. 2014;7(1):155–63.
4. Herrmann HC, Thourani VH, Kodali SK, et al. One-year clinical outcomes with SAPIEN 3 transcatheter aortic valve replacement in high-risk and inoperable patients with severe aortic stenosis. Circulation. 2016;134(2):130–40.
5. Tamburino C, Capodanno D, Ramondo A, et al. Incidence and predictors of early and late mortality after transcatheter aortic valve implantation in 663 patients with severe aortic stenosis. Circulation. 2011;123(3):299–308.
6. Pibarot P, Hahn RT, Weissman NJ, Monaghan MJ. Assessment of paravalvular regurgitation following TAVR: a proposal of unifying grading scheme. JACC Cardiovasc Imaging. 2015;8(3):340–60.
7. Mihara H, Shibayama K, Jilaihawi H, et al. Assessment of post-procedural aortic regurgitation after TAVR: an intraprocedural TEE study. JACC Cardiovasc Imaging. 2015;8(9):993–1003.
8. Shibayama K, Mihara H, Jilaihawi H, et al. 3D assessment of features associated with transvalvular aortic regurgitation after TAVR: a real-time 3D TEE study. JACC Cardiovasc Imaging. 2016;9(2):114–23.
9. Ng AC, Delgado V, van der Kley F, et al. Comparison of aortic root dimensions and geometries before and after transcatheter aortic valve implantation by 2- and 3-dimensional transesophageal echocardiography and multislice computed tomography. Circ Cardiovasc Imaging. 2010;3(1):94–102.
10. Beigel R, Wunderlich NC, Kar S, Siegel RJ. The evolution of percutaneous mitral valve repair therapy: lessons learned and implications for patient selection. J Am Coll Cardiol. 2014;64(24):2688–700.
11. Feldman T, Wasserman HS, Herrmann HC, et al. Percutaneous mitral valve repair using the edge-to-edge technique: six-month results of the EVEREST phase I clinical trial. J Am Coll Cardiol. 2005;46(11):2134–40.
12. Feldman T, Foster E, Glower DD, et al. Percutaneous repair or surgery for mitral regurgitation. N Engl J Med. 2011;364(15):1395–406.
13. Whitlow PL, Feldman T, Pedersen WR, et al. Acute and 12-month results with catheter-based mitral valve leaflet repair: the EVEREST II (endovascular valve edge-to-edge repair) high risk study. J Am Coll Cardiol. 2012;59(2):130–9.
14. Grayburn PA, Foster E, Sangli C, et al. Relationship between the magnitude of reduction in mitral regurgitation severity and left ventricular and left atrial reverse remodeling after MitraClip therapy. Circulation. 2013;128(15):1667–74.
15. Maisano F, Franzen O, Baldus S, et al. Percutaneous mitral valve interventions in the real world: early and 1-year results from the ACCESS-EU, a prospective, multicenter, nonrandomized post-approval study of the MitraClip therapy in Europe. J Am Coll Cardiol. 2013;62(12):1052–61.
16. Taramasso M, Maisano F, Latib A, et al. Clinical outcomes of MitraClip for the treatment of functional mitral regurgitation. EuroIntervention. 2014;10(6):746–52.
17. Wunderlich NC, Siegel RJ. Peri-interventional echo assessment for the MitraClip procedure. Eur Heart J Cardiovasc Imaging. 2013;14(10):935–49.
18. Di Biase L, Santangeli P, Anselmino M, et al. Does the left atrial appendage morphology correlate with the risk of stroke in patients with atrial fibrillation? Results from a multicenter study. J Am Coll Cardiol. 2012;60(6):531–8.
19. Wunderlich NC, Beigel R, Swaans MJ, Ho SY, Siegel RJ. Percutaneous interventions for left atrial appendage exclusion: options, assessment, and imaging using 2D and 3D echocardiography. JACC Cardiovasc Imaging. 2015;8(4):472–88.
20. Holmes DR, Reddy VY, Turi ZG, et al. Percutaneous closure of the left atrial appendage versus warfarin therapy for prevention of stroke in patients with atrial fibrillation: a randomised non-inferiority trial. Lancet. 2009;374(9689):534–42.
21. Reddy VY, Holmes D, Doshi SK, Neuzil P, Kar S. Safety of percutaneous left atrial appendage closure: results from the Watchman left atrial appendage system for embolic protection in patients with AF (PROTECT AF) clinical trial and the Continued Access Registry. Circulation. 2011;123(4):417–24.
22. Singh SM, Douglas PS, Reddy VY. The incidence and long-term clinical outcome of iatrogenic atrial septal defects secondary to transseptal catheterization with a 12F transseptal sheath. Circ Arrhythm Electrophysiol. 2011;4(2):166–71.

Echocardiography in the Critical Care Unit

32

Anita Sadeghpour and Azin Alizadehasl

Abstract

Transthoracic echocardiography (TTE) has been incorporated effectively into patient care in 90% of critically ill patients. However, despite its advantages in terms of its noninvasive nature, the quality of the images may be insufficient-particularly in chest traumas and intrathoracic surgery. That is why transesophageal echocardiography (TEE) has replaced TTE in the intensive care unit (ICU), especially in patients with an endotracheal tube. Even now, there is a broad range of echo applications available to ICU physicians to enhance and improve their care of critically ill patients, with many new applications on their way.

Keywords

Transthoracic echocardiography (TTE) · Transesophageal echocardiography (TEE) · Critical Care Unit · Intensive care unit (ICU) · Cardiac arrest · Aortic dissection · Tamponade · Pulmonary emboli

Abbreviations

CO	Cardiac output
CPR	Cardiopulmonary resuscitation
EF	Ejection fraction
ICU	Intensive care unit
LV	Left ventricular
LVED	Left ventricular end-diastolic
LVES	Left ventricular end-systolic
LVOT	Left ventricular outflow tract
PTE	Pulmonary thromboembolism
RV	Right ventricular
RVOT	Right ventricular outflow tract
SAM	Systolic anterior motion
SV	Stroke volume
TEE	Transesophageal echocardiography
TTE	Transthoracic echocardiography
VTI	Velocity time integral

Impact of Echocardiography

- Echocardiography has a central role in critically ill patients as a diagnostic and hemodynamic monitoring tool.
- It has been suggested that echocardiography can change therapeutic management in about 25% of critically ill patients who are mechanically ventilated.
- TEE, albeit semi-invasive, is a completely safe procedure—with the incidence of esophageal perforation and mortality reported in 1 out of 5000 and in 1 out of 10,000 cases, correspondingly.
- Limited or highly focused bedside echocardiography in the ICU for differential diagnosis is very important and useful.
- As a general rule, whenever diagnostic information may change the management of the patient and TTE cannot obtain sufficient data, TEE should be considered [1–8].
- The deployment of TTE and TEE is category 1 indication in unstable patients with unexplained hemodynamic disturbances, suspected valve disease, or thromboembolic problems.
- There is a strong agreement regarding the use of TEE in persistent unexplained hypotension and hypoxemia [9, 10].

Electronic Supplementary Material The online version of this chapter (https://doi.org/10.1007/978-3-319-67691-3_32) contains supplementary material, which is available to authorized users.

A. Sadeghpour, MD, FACC, FASE
Professor of Cardiology, Echocardiography Research Center, Rajaie Cardiovascular Medical and Research Center, Iran University of Medical Science, Tehran, Iran

A. Alizadehasl, MD, FACC, FASE (✉)
Associate Professor of Cardiology, Echocardiologist, Echocardiography and Cardiogenetic Research Centers, Cardio-Oncology Department, Rajaie Cardiovascular Medical and Research Center, Tehran, Iran

A. Sadeghpour, A. Alizadehasl (eds.), *Case-Based Textbook of Echocardiography*,
https://doi.org/10.1007/978-3-319-67691-3_32

Hypotensive State

- Circulatory failure is a common complication in the emergency department and the ICU setting. Consequently, physical examination, cardiac ultrasonography, and hemodynamic monitoring traditionally provide invaluable information on the proper management [11, 12].

Left Ventricular Function

- The evaluation of left ventricular (LV) function plays a crucial role in hypotensive patients who are in shock inasmuch as a quick evaluation of global LV function can determine whether the state of shock is correlated with the poor ventricular function.
- Moreover, other causes such as hypovolemia or sepsis should be ruled out.
- It is widely accepted that for critical care physicians, a focused echocardiographic interpretation of LV function and the cardiac index is necessary.
- Regional wall motion can be identified by echocardiography and assist physicians in selecting their next approach (e.g., inserting an intra-aortic balloon pump, performing coronary angiography, or proceeding to revascularization).

Right Ventricular Function

- The assessment of right ventricular (RV) function is of particular interest in critical care. It is estimated that approximately 25% of patients with acute respiratory distress syndrome have RV dysfunction and pulmonary hypertension. Importantly, RV failure is independently associated with mortality in critically ill patients.
- A subjective assessment of RV area compared to LV area in the apical 4-chamber view may be used instead. The RV should be smaller than the LV, and an RV:LV end-diastolic area ratio > 0.6 indicates a dilated RV. Additionally, RV dilatation is often allied to LV underfilling and a poor cardiac output [11–16].

Preload Assessment

- Hypovolemia is a common finding in patients with an unstable hemodynamic state.
- Intracardiac volume status can be assessed by left ventricular end-diastolic (LVED) and left ventricular end-systolic (LVES) areas in LV short-axis imaging. Hypovolemia is commonly associated with a hyperdynamic LV—with a reduced end-diastolic volume and kissing papillary muscles in systole—indicating an amplified ejection fraction (EF) with empty ventricles during diastole. This is reflected in M-mode imaging (Table 32.1).
- Patients with sepsis have a tendency to gain a low afterload, which is reflected in a normal LVED area and a low LVES area.
- Patients with dilated left cardiac chambers suffering from chronic cardiac failure may be hypovolemic and have a greater LVED area [11, 13–15, 17].
- RA pressure can be evaluated by echocardiography (Table 32.2, Fig. 32.1).

Table 32.1 Common findings in hypovolemia state

1. Reduced left ventricular end-diastolic volume
2. Systolic kissing papillary muscles
3. Empty ventricles with an exaggerated ejection fraction

Table 32.2 Evaluation of right atrial pressure by echocardiography (Fig. 32.1) [17]

Inferior vena cava size (cm)	Collapsibility	Right atrial pressure (mm Hg)
Size ≤2.1	collapses >50% during sniff	0–5
Size >2.1	collapses >50% during sniff	5–10
Size >2.1	collapses <50% during sniff	10–20

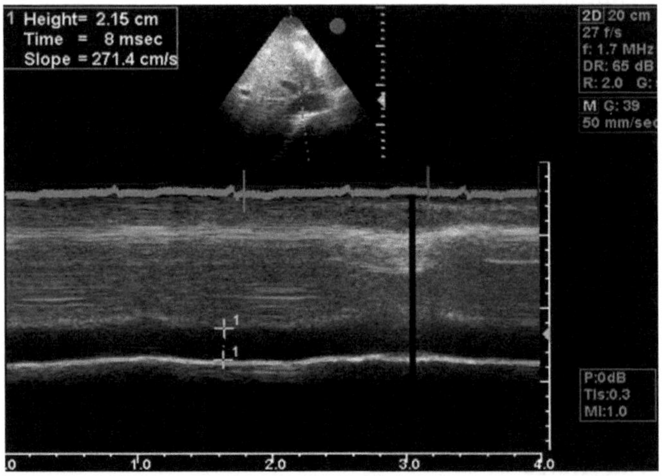

Fig. 32.1 Subcostal view shows a dilated inferior vena cava with a < 50% respiratory collapse, suggestive of a high right atrial pressure

Cardiac Tamponade

- Cardiac tamponade is a clinical diagnosis, and the patient should be promptly transferred to the operating room.
- Echocardiography can be of great help with the typical findings of compressed cardiac chambers with significant pericardial liquid collection (Fig. 32.2, Movie 32.1) and classic RV free wall diastolic collapse (Fig. 32.3).
- Pericardial effusion ≥1 cm can be considered significant; however, this may not accurately reflect the pressure

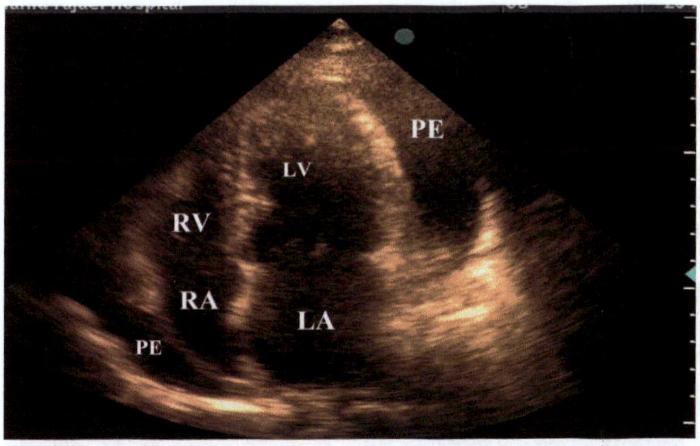

Fig. 32.2 (Movie 1) Large circumferential pericardial effusion

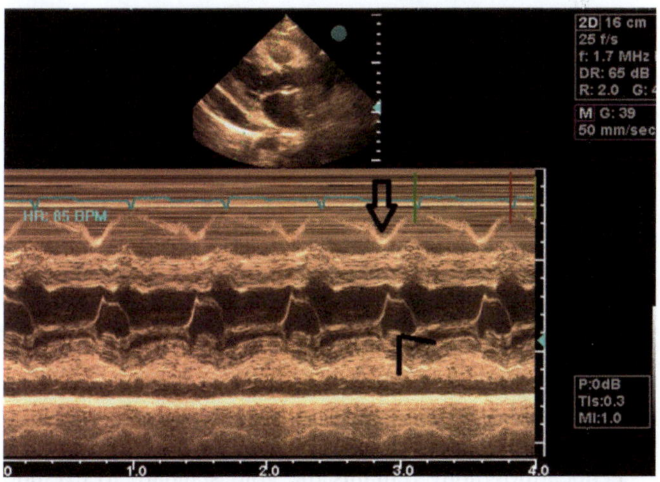

Fig. 32.3 Right ventricular outflow tract diastolic collapse in M-mode study (black arrow) in the parasternal long-axis view (arrow head) shows the opening of the mitral valve in diastole

within the pericardial space, which is of increasing clinical significance [18–20].

Thromboembolic Disease

- Echocardiography is not a sensitive method for the detection of pulmonary thromboembolism (PTE); nonetheless, in an emergent situation in an unconscious patient who cannot be transferred to the radiology unit, echocardiography can be used for diagnosis.
- Uncommonly, a thrombus in the right atrium can be found by TTE.
- Eighty percent of patients who are in shock and suffer from PTE present signs of RV strain such as dysfunction and dilatation.
- Left atrial appendage or LV apical thrombus can clarify the source of systemic emboli and may precipitate anticoagulation [21, 22].

Valvular Disease

- TEE has a unique ability in the evaluation of valvular heart disease, post-cardiac surgery valve function, and paravalvular leakage-as well as in the detection of vegetation, abscess, and other complications of infective endocarditis [12, 14, 15].

Left Ventricular Outflow Tract Obstruction

- Systolic anterior motion (SAM) of the mitral valve commonly happens when there is a complex of some disorders such as hypovolemia, LV hypertrophy with increased myocardial contractility, and vasodilatation.
- Under these circumstances, a rise in the velocity of the blood flow in the left ventricular outflow tract (LVOT) combines with a quick systolic time and attracts the anterior mitral valve leaflet through the LVOT.
- This dynamic obstacle leads to cardiovascular collapse, requiring a prompt diagnosis by echocardiography for proper management. The treatment includes the use of intravenous fluids, vasopressors, and beta-blockers [7–9, 23].

Aortic Dissection

- Contrast computed tomography angiography is the gold-standard method for the diagnosis of acute aortic dissection. Nonetheless, TEE has a significant role in diagnosis of aortic valve incompetence, pericardial effusion, and coronary artery involvement as indicated by regional wall motion abnormalities.
- In some centers, patients with acute aortic dissection are transferred directly to the operating room, where TEE is performed as the first investigation of choice (Fig. 32.4, Movie 32.2) [24–27].

Septic Patients

- During the last decade, the management of severe sepsis and septic shock in the emergency department and the ICU has improved significantly.
- This requires an assessment of LV function and volume status.
- Sepsis has a variety of cardiac involvements, ranging from diffuse myocardial suppression to LV hyperdynamism. Hyperdynamic LV function can be detected by echocardiography in patients in the emergency department, which supports the diagnosis of sepsis.
- Based on the literature, more than one-third of patients with septic shock had myocardial suppression, while the rest suffered from hyperdynamic function. Such documented data underscore the invaluable role of echocar-

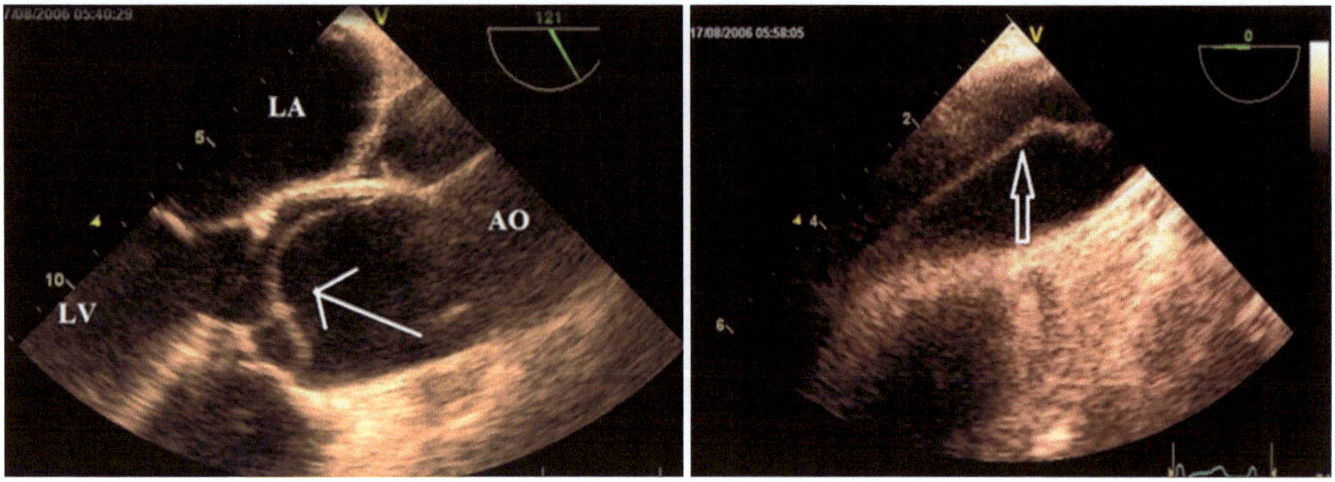

Fig. 32.4 (Movie 2) Left panel: Dissecting flap (arrow) in the ascending aorta, interfering with the aortic valve. Right panel: Extending dissecting flap to the distal of the ascending aorta and aortic arch (arrow)

diography in patients with sepsis who have hypotension or need fluid resuscitation.

- Of course, there are various therapeutic modalities to treat such patients; they include inotropes in patients with myocardial suppression and vasoconstrictors in patients with hyperdynamic LV function [28, 29].

Trauma

- Injuries to the thorax comprise one-quarter of the deaths ascribed to traumas. A swift concentrated echocardiographic assessment can detect pericardial effusion, myocardial contusion, hematoma of the mediastinum, aortic intramural hematomas, dissection and transection of the aorta, and also pleural effusion (please refer to Trauma chapter) [30–32].

Cardiac Arrest

- Focused and limited echocardiography in cardiac arrest can promptly provide the clinician with both diagnostic and also prognostic information, which should be done in a quick way in 10-second pulse checks to minimize cardiopulmonary resuscitation (CPR) disruption.
- Many previously published articles have demonstrated that the absence of cardiac motion at any stage of the resuscitation denotes no chance for the return of spontaneous circulation. However, echocardiography should not be used as a base for ceasing the CPR.
- Recent documents appropriately increase the concern that the routine use of TTE for cases in cardiac arrest can contribute to inappropriate interruptions in CPR [33–37].

Echocardiography in the Mechanically Ventilated Patient

- While the majority of mechanically ventilated patients can be satisfactorily imaged via TTE, significant failure rates occur in post-cardiac surgery patients. So, in addition to providing reliable high resolution images for all critically ill patients, TEE has offered a new way to evaluate cardiac function in positive pressure ventilation [7, 38, 39].
- In addressing unexplained hypoxemic respiratory failure, echocardiography remains the gold standard to exclude the right-to-left shunts. Nonetheless, an imaging assessment of respiratory failure in most ICUs should also include echocardiography [40, 41].
- Also, echocardiography confers a reliable tool to measure changes in global and regional LV functions in response to therapeutic maneuvers like inotropic or volume therapy [42, 43].
- As a final point, echocardiography can be of use in mechanically ventilated patients who cannot be weaned and separated from the ventilator machine. Myocardial ischemia can happen in response to increased respiratory workload [43, 44].

Advanced Applications of Echocardiography in the ICU

- The decreasing use of pulmonary artery catheters in most institutions has encouraged a search for less invasive methods to estimate cardiac filling pressures and hemodynamics (Tables 32.3 and 32.5) [17].

Table 32.3 Methods by which critical monitoring parameters are assessed with a PA catheter versus serial echocardiographic measurements

Monitoring technique	PA catheter	Echocardiography	Advantage[a]
Filling pressure	RAP, PCWP, directly measured	RAP, PCWP indirectly measured	PA catheter
Cardiac output	Thermodilution	Doppler-derived	Equal
Valve assessment	Not possible	Anatomic/Doppler	Echocardiography
Systolic/diastolic function	Estimated form PCWP/CO	Table 32.5 parameters	Echocardiography
Risks	Invasive technique	Noninvasive	Echocardiography
Speed of assessment	Immediate changes detected	Operator dependent	PA catheter

PA pulmonary artery, *RAP* right atrial pressure, *PCWP* pulmonary capillary wedge pressure, *CO* cardiac output
[a]*Advantage* refers to which monitoring parameter the writing group considered more suitable for the particular application

Table 32.4 Indications for echocardiography in critically care setting

Evaluation of hemodynamic failure
Hypotension in post-cardiac surgery
Unexplained hypoxemia
Identification of aortic dissection, tamponade, central pulmonary emboli, and valvular heart disease
Cardiac arrest
Preload assessment
Evaluation of ventricular function
Guiding the therapeutic intervention (transvenous pacemaker and Intra-aortic balloon pump)

Table 32.5 Echocardiographic parameters for LAP assessment

Monitoring parameter	Specific values to use while guiding interventions
Transmitral E/e′	E/e′ < 8; normal LVEF = normal LAP
	E/e′ ≥ 13; normal LVEF = increased LAP E/A > 2; DT <150 ms; depressed LVEF = increased LAP E/A < 1 and E < 50 cm/s; depressed LVEF = normal LAP

LAP left atrial pressure, *LVEF*, left ventricular ejection fraction, *E* mitral inflow peak early filling velocity, *e′* early diastolic annular velocity, *A* late diastolic filling velocities

- Tissue Doppler imaging, which is a method for measuring the velocity of myocardial tissue, is a key component in the valuation of diastolic function in echocardiography labs.

Although filling pressures are traditionally measured via TTE, the accuracy of a TEE-derived estimation of filling pressures in critically ill patients has been shown to be acceptable when compared to the gold-standard invasive measures. Also, a standard 2D valuation of the inferior vena cava is an effective way to gauge fluid status in the ICU and the emergency department [45–47].

- An accurate and noninvasive study of cardiac output (CO) and stroke volume (SV) is often considered the best goal in hemodynamic monitoring and may be estimated both by TTE and TEE. Although the quantification of CO has not ever been shown to improve the patient outcome, it is nevertheless used in many wards to aid in the titration of fluids, inotropes, and vasopressors. The estimation of CO by echocardiography is done by the hydraulic orifice formula, multiplying the cross-sectional area of any valve by the flow velocity (velocity time integral [VTI]) across it [17, 48].
- Since an accurate measurement of LVOT and right ventricular outflow tract (RVOT) may be difficult in critically ill patients, RVOT VTI can be used to show RV SV and LVOT VTI can be used to show LV SV.
- LVOT VTI >18 cm has been suggested for a normal LV SV.
- It has been suggested that if LVOT VTI increases >12.5% during passive leg elevation in critically ill patients, SV will increase by intravenous fluid administration-with 77% sensitivity and 100% specificity [17, 49].
- TTE is pleasing due to its noninvasiveness and the ease with which parallel alignment with LVOT and RVOT may be achieved, while TEE offers augmented accuracy in the measurement of the cross-sectional area—a key source of mistake in the calculation of CO.
- Although ultrasound has gained widespread recognition for its ability and facility to improve safety in central venous catheter insertion, the use of ultrasound to guide pericardiocentesis has also been broadly studied-with utmost complications being reasonably minor.
- Accordingly, the use of ultrasound can offer improved safety and comfort for emergent pericardiocentesis in the presence of pericardial fluid in hemodynamically unstable patients [46, 47, 50–53].
- In summary: echocardiography has a central role in critically ill patients as a diagnostic and hemodynamic monitoring tool that can guide therapeutic interventions (Table 32.6) [17].

Table 32.6 Specific clinical settings where echocardiography can guide therapeutic interventions

	Specific clinical settings	Needed monitoring parameters
Critical Clinical problems	Hypotension	IVC collapsibility index, regional wall motion LVOT VTI response to passive leg raising
	CHF	IVC collapsibility Transmitral E/e' RV s' TAPSE Regional wall motion
	Sepsis	IVC collapsibility index LVIDD, LVIDS Regional wall motion
	Respiratory failure Possible pulmonary embolus	IVC collapsibility index RVs′ TAPSE Doppler PASP RVOT VTI Regional wall motion RVIDd/LVIDd ratio
	Pericardial effusion/ tamponade	Pericardial effusion size Right ventricular diastolic collapse IVC collapsibility index
	Prosthetic valve dysfunction	Transvalvular gradient
Trauma	Blunt trauma Aortic trauma Myocardial contusion	IVC collapsibility LVIDd, LVIDs Pericardial effusion size Regional wall motion
	Burns	IVC collapsibility index LVIDd, LVIDs Transmitral E/A ratio, E/e′

IVC inferior vena cava, *LVOT* left ventricular outflow tract, *VTI* velocity time integral, *E* mitral inflow peak early filling velocity, *e′* early diastolic annular velocity, *RV s′* tricuspid annular velocity, *A* late diastolic filling velocities, *TAPSE* tricuspid annular plane systolic excursion, *PASP* pulmonary artery systolic pressure, *RVIDd* right ventricular internal dimension in diastole, *LVIDd* left ventricular internal diameter in diastole, *LVIDs* left ventricular internal dimension in systole

Questions

1. In a patient with hemodynamic failure, which of the following statements is suggestive of hypovolemia state?
   A. Reduced LV end-diastolic volume
   B. Normal LV end-diastolic volume
   C. Normal LV end-systolic volume
   D. Reduced LV end-systolic volume
2. In which of the following settings in the ICU, echocardiography is not an appropriate imaging modality?
   A. Patients with unexplained hypoxemia
   B. Post-cardiac surgery patients with hypotension
   C. Patients with deep vein thrombosis and suspected small pulmonary emboli
   D. Patients in cardiac arrest
3. In a hypotensive patient with the SAM of the mitral valve and significant LVOT obstruction, which medication should be discontinued?
   A. Vasopressors
   B. B-blockers
   C. Inotropes
   D. IV fluid administration

Answers

1. A
   Hypovolemia is commonly associated with a hyperdynamic LV—with a reduced end-diastolic volume and kissing papillary muscles in systole.
2. C
   Echocardiography is not a sensitive method for the detection of PTE, unless in a patient with large massive saddle emboli.
3. C
   The treatment for SAM includes the use of intravenous fluids, vasopressors, and beta-blockers. Inotropes exacerbate SAM.

References

1. Royse CF, Seah JL, Donelan L, Royse AG. Point of care ultrasound for basic haemodynamic assessment: novice compared with an expert operator. Anaesthesia. 2006;61:849–55.
2. Lemola K, Yamada E, Jagasia D, Kerber RE. A hand-carried personal ultrasound device for rapid evaluation of left ventricular function: use after limited echo training. Echocardiography. 2003;20:309.
3. Stewart WJ, Douglas PS, Sagar K, Seward JB, Armstrong WF, Zoghbi W, Kronzon I, Mays JM, Pearlman AS, Schnittger I, St Vrain JA, Kerber RE. Echocardiography in emergency medicine: a policy statement by the American Society of Echocardiography and the American College of Cardiology. The Task Force on Echocardiography in Emergency Medicine of the American Society of Echocardiography and the Echocardiography TPEC Committees of the American College of Cardiology. J Am Soc Echocardiogr. 1999;12:82–4.
4. Kallmeyer IJ, Collard CD, Fox JA, Body SC, Shernan SK. The safety of transesophageal echocardiography: a case series of 7200 cardiac surgical patients. Anesth Analg. 2001;92:1126–30.
5. Benjamin E, Griffin K, Leibowitz AB, et al. Goal-directed transesophageal echocardiography performed by intensivist to assess left ventricular function: comparison with pulmonary artery catheterization. J Cardiothorac Vasc Anesth. 1998;12:10–5.
6. Karski JM. Transesophageal echocardiography in the intensive care unit. Semin Cardiothorac Vasc Anesth. 2006;10:162–6.
7. Vignon P, Mentec H, Terré S, Gastinne H, Gueret P, Lemaire F. Diagnostic accuracy and therapeutic impact of transthoracic and transesophageal echocardiography in mechanically ventilated patients in the ICU. Chest. 1994;106(6):1829–34.
8. Chew MS. Haemodynamic monitoring using echocardiography in the critically Ill: a review. Cardiol Res Pract. 2012;2012:139537. https://doi.org/10.1155/2012/139537.

9. Mayo PH, Narasimhan M, Koenig S. Critical care transesophageal echocardiography. Chest. 2015;148(5):1323–32. https://doi.org/10.1378/chest.15-0260.
10. Thys DM, Abel M, Brooker RF, Cahalan MK, Connis R, Duke P, et al. Practice guidelines for perioperative transesophageal echocardiography. Anesthesiology. 2010;112:1084–96.
11. Rivers E, Nguyen B, Havstad S, et al. Early goal-directed therapy in the treatment of severe sepsis and septic shock. N Engl J Med. 2001;345(19):1368–77.
12. Randazzo M, Snoey E, Levitt M, Binder K. Accuracy of emergency physician assessment of left ventricular ejection fraction and central venous pressure using echocardiography. Acad Emerg Med. 2003;10(9):973–7.
13. Mann H, Nolan P. Update on the management of cardiogenic shock. Curr Opin Crit Care. 2006;2(5):431–6.
14. Melamed R, Sprenkle M, Ulstad V, Herzog C, Leatherman J. Assessment of left ventricular function by intensivists using hand-held echocardiography. Chest. 2009;135(6):1416–20.
15. Moore C, Rose G, Tayal V, Sullivan D, Arrowood J, Kline J. Determination of left ventricular function by emergency physician echocardiography of hypotensive patients. Acad Emerg Med. 2002;9(3):186–93.
16. Gunst M, Ghaemmaghami V, Sperry J, et al. Accuracy of cardiac function and volume status estimates using the bedside echocardiographic assessment in trauma/critical care. J Trauma. 2008;65(3):509.
17. Porter T, Shillcutt S, Adams M, Desjardins G, Glas K, Olson J, et al. Guidelines for the use of echocardiography as a monitor for therapeutic intervention in adults: a report from the American Society of Echocardiography. J Am Soc Echocardiogr. 2015;28:40–56.
18. Guberman B, Fowler N, Engel P, Gueron M, Allen J. Cardiac tamponade in medical patients. Circulation. 1981;64(3):633–40.
19. Mandavia D, Hoffner R, Mahaney K, Henderson S. Bedside echocardiography by emergency physicians. Ann Emerg Med. 2001;38(4):377–82.
20. Blaivas M. Incidence of pericardial effusion in patients presenting to the emergency department with unexplained dyspnea. Acad Emerg Med. 2001;8(12):1143–6.
21. Wells P, Anderson D, Rodger M, et al. Excluding pulmonary embolism at the bedside without diagnostic imaging: management of patients with suspected pulmonary embolism presenting to the emergency department by using a simple clinical model and d-dimer. Ann Intern Med. 2001;135(2):98–107.
22. Ceylan N, Tasbakan S, Bayraktaroglu S, et al. Predictors of clinical outcome in acute pulmonary embolism. Correlation of CT pulmonary angiography with clinical, echocardiography and laboratory findings. Acad Radiol. 2011;18(1):47–53.
23. Kapoor MC. Systolic anterior motion of the mitral valve in hypovolemia and hyper-adrenergic states. Indian J Anaesth. 2014;58(1):7–8.
24. Nienaber C, von K, Nicolas V, Siglow V, Piepho A, Brockhoff C, et al. The diagnosis of thoracic aortic dissection by noninvasive imaging procedures. N Engl J Med. 1993;328(1):1–9.
25. Budhram G, Reardon R. Diagnosis of ascending aortic dissection using emergency department bedside echocardiogram. Acad Emerg Med. 2008;15(6):584.
26. Perkins A, Liteplo A, Noble V. Ultrasound diagnosis of type A aortic dissection. J Emerg Med. 2010;38(4):490–3.
27. Vignon P, Spencer K, Rambaud G, et al. Differential transesophageal echocardiographic diagnosis between linear artifacts and intraluminal flap of aortic dissection or disruption. Chest. 2001;119(6):1778–90.
28. Jones A, Craddock P, Tayal V, Kline J. Diagnostic accuracy of left ventricular function for identifying sepsis among emergency department patients with nontraumatic symptomatic undifferentiated hypotension. Shock. 2005;24(6):513–7.
29. Vieillard-Baron A, Prin S, Chergui K, Dubourg O, Jardin F. Hemodynamic instability in sepsis: bedside assessment by Doppler echocardiography. Am J Respir Crit Care Med. 2003;168(11):1270–6.
30. Meyer D, Jessen M, Grayburn P. Use of echocardiography to detect occult cardiac injury after penetrating thoracic trauma: a prospective study. J Trauma. 1995;39(5):902–7.
31. Speight J, Sanders M. Pericardial tamponade with a positive abdominal FAST scan in blunt chest trauma. J Trauma. 2006;61(3):743.
32. Baxa M. Cardiac rupture secondary to blunt trauma: a rapidly diagnosable entity with two-dimensional echocardiography. Ann Emerg Med. 1991;20(8):902–4.
33. Blaivas F. Outcome in cardiac arrest patients found to have cardiac standstill on the bedside emergency department echocardiogram. Ann Emerg Med. 2001;8(6):616–21.
34. Testa A, Cibinel G, Portale G, et al. The proposal of an integrated ultrasonographic approach into the ALS algorithm for cardiac arrest: the PEA protocol. Eur Rev Med Pharmacol Sci. 2010;14(2):77–88.
35. Hernandez C, Shuler K, Hannan H, Sonyika C, Likourezos A, Marshall J. CAUSE: Cardiac arrest ultra-sound exam—a better approach to managing patients in primary non-arrhythmogenic cardiac arrest. Resuscitation. 2008;76(2):198–206.
36. Morrison L, Deakin C, Morley P, et al. Part 8: advanced life support: 2010 International Consensus on Cardiopulmonary Resuscitation and Emergency Cardiovascular Care Science with Treatment Recommendations. Circulation. 2010;122(Suppl 2):S345–421.
37. Blyth L. Bedside focused echocardiography as predictor of survival in cardiac arrest patients: a systematic review. Acad Emerg Med. 2012;19(10):1119–26.
38. Parker M, Cunnion R, Parrillo J. Echocardiography and nuclear cardiac imaging in the critical care unit. JAMA. 1985;254(20):2935–9.
39. Vieillard-Baron A, Qanadli SD, Antakly Y, et al. Transesophageal echocardiography for the diagnosis of pulmonary embolism with acute cor pulmonale: a comparison with radiological procedures. Intensive Care Med. 1998;24(5):429–33.
40. Jardin F, Vieillard-Baron A. Right ventricular function and positive pressure ventilation in clinical practice: from hemodynamic subsets to respirator settings. Intensive Care Med. 2003;29(9):1426–34.
41. Yeh YL, Liu CK, Chang WK, Chan KH, Li JY, Tsai SK. Detection of right to left shunt by transesophageal echocardiography in a patient with postoperative hypoxemia. J Formos Med Assoc. 2006;105(5):418–21.
42. Michard F, Teboul JL. Using heart-lung interactions to assess fluid responsiveness during mechanical ventilation. Crit Care. 2000;4(5):282–9.
43. Gernoth C, Wagner G, Pelosi P, Luecke T. Respiratory and haemodynamic changes during decremental open lung positive end-expiratory pressure titration in patients with acute respiratory distress syndrome. Crit Care. 2009;13(2):R59.
44. Lamia B, Maizel J, Ochagavia A, et al. Echocardiographic diagnosis of pulmonary artery occlusion pressure elevation during weaning from mechanical ventilation. Crit Care Med. 2009;37(5):1696–701.
45. Nagueh SF, Middleton KJ, Kopelen HA, Zoghbi WA, Quiñones MA. Doppler tissue imaging: a noninvasive technique for evaluation of left ventricular relaxation and estimation of filling pressures. J Am Coll Cardiol. 1997;30(6):1527–33.
46. Ommen SR, Nishimura RA, Appleton CP, et al. Clinical utility of Doppler echocardiography and tissue Doppler imaging in the estimation of left ventricular filling pressures: clinical investigation and reports. Circulation. 2000;102:1788–94.
47. Bouhemad B, Nicolas-Robin A, Benois A, Lemaire S, Goarin JP, Rouby JJ. Echocardiographic Doppler assessment of pulmonary capillary wedge pressure in surgical patients with postoperative circulatory shock and acute lung injury. Anesthesiology. 2003;98(5):1091–100.

48. Nagueh SF, Appleton CP, Gillebert TC, Marino PN, Oh JK, Smiseth OA, et al. Recommendations for the evaluation of left ventricular diastolic function by echocardiography. J Am Soc Echocardiogr. 2009;22:107–33.
49. Lamia B, Ochagavia A, Monnet X, Chemia D, Richard C, Teboul JL. Echocardiographic prediction of volume responsiveness to critically ill patients with spontaneous breathing activity. Intensive Care Med. 2007;33:1125–32.
50. Vignon P, AitHssain A, François B, et al. Echocardiographic assessment of pulmonary artery occlusion pressure in ventilated patients: a transoesophageal study. Crit Care. 2008;12(1):R18.
51. Poelaert J, Schmidt C, Van Aken H, Hinder F, Mollhoff T, Loick HM. A comparison of transoesophageal echocardiographic Doppler across the aortic valve and the thermodilution technique for estimating cardiac output. Anaesthesia. 1999;54(2):128–36.
52. Pinsky MR. Assessment of indices of preload and volume responsiveness. Curr Opin Crit Care. 2005;11(3):235–9.
53. Vieillard-Baron A, Chergui K, Rabiller A, et al. Superior vena caval collapsibility as a gauge of volume status in ventilated septic patients. Intensive Care Med. 2004;30(9):1734–9.

Echocardiography and Pulmonary Hypertension

33

Maude Limoges and Lawrence Rudski

Abstract

Transthoracic echocardiography (TTE) should be done as an initial test for individuals suspected of having pulmonary hypertension. If the peak TR velocity is above 2.8 m/s or if secondary signs of pulmonary hypertension are present, further investigations should be considered.

Normal systolic pulmonary artery value varies with age and body mass index. Systolic, diastolic and mean pulmonary artery pressures can be evaluated through tricuspid regurgitation, pulmonary regurgitation, ventricular septal defect and right ventricular outflow tract acceleration time. The values obtained reliably estimate the pulmonary pressure if there is no right ventricular outflow tract obstruction.

A pre- versus post-capillary etiology for pulmonary hypertension can be determined by looking at pulmonary vascular resistance, left sided systolic and diastolic functions, left atrial size, left sided valvular heart disease and by using a scoring system such as the Opotowsky or D'Alto criteria. The right ventricle is a structure with an unique geometry which makes it more challenging to image. Therefore, the right ventricular function should be evaluated by using multiple views showing its different segments using a combination of quantitative parameters and qualitative assessment. Progressive tricuspid regurgitation (TR), the presence of a new, at least moderate, pericardial effusion, decreased right ventricular (RV) function as illustrated by abnormal myocardial performance index (MPI), tricuspid annular plane systolic excursion (TAPSE) and RV strain, increased right atrial size and pressure are all features associated with poor prognosis in the context of pulmonary arterial hypertension (PAH). The frequency at which TTE should be repeated is determined by the underlying cause for the PH. Patients with class 1, 3 or 4 PH should generally be referred to a center with expertise in investigation and management of PH.

Keywords

Pulmonary hypertension · Pulmonary arterial hypertension
Pre-capillary pulmonary hypertension
Post-capillary pulmonary hypertension

Abbreviations

2D	Two dimensional
ASD	Atrial septal defect
ASE	American Society of Echocardiography
AT	Acceleration time
BMI	Body mass index
BMPR2	Bone morphogenetic protein receptor type 2
CT	Computed tomography
CTEPH	Chronic thromboembolic pulmonary hypertension
CW	Continuous wave Doppler
dPG	Diastolic pressure gradient
E	Peak E-wave velocity of the mitral valve
E′	Tissue Doppler index of the mitral valve annulus
EACVI	European Association of Cardivascular Imaging
EI	Eccentricity index
HIV	Human immunodeficiency virus
IVC	Inferior vena cava
LA	Left atrium
LHC	Left sided heart catheterization
LV	Left ventricle
mPAP	Mean pulmonary artery pressure
MPI	Myocardial performance index
MS	Mitral stenosis
PA	Pulmonary artery
PADP	Pulmonary artery diastolic pressure
PAEDP	Pulmonary artery end diastolic pressure

M. Limoges, MD · L. Rudski, MD, FRCPC, FACC, FASE (✉)
Azrieli Heart Center, Division of Cardiology, Department of Medicine, Center for Pulmonary Vascular Diseases, Jewish General Hospital and McGill University, Montreal, QC, Canada
e-mail: maude.limoges@mail.mcgill.ca; lrudski@jgh.mcgill.ca

A. Sadeghpour, A. Alizadehasl (eds.), *Case-Based Textbook of Echocardiography*,
https://doi.org/10.1007/978-3-319-67691-3_33

PAH	Pulmonary arterial hypertension
PCWP	Pulmonary capillary wedge pressure
PFT	Pulmonary function test
PH	Pulmonary hypertension
PISA	Proximal isovelocity surface area
PLAX	Parasternal long axis
PR	Pulmonary regurgitation
PREDV	Pulmonary regurgitation end diastolic velocity
PSAX	Parasternal short axis
PVR	Pulmonary vascular resistance
PW	Pulsed wave Doppler
RA	Right atrium
RAP	Right atrial pressure
RHC	Right heart catheterization
RV S′	Tissue Doppler index of the tricuspid valve annulus
RV	Right ventricle
RVOT	Right ventricular outflow tract obstruction
RVSP	Right ventricular systolic pressure
sPAP	Systolic pulmonary artery pressure
TAPSE	Tricuspid annular plane systolic excursion
TR	Tricuspid regurgitation
TTE	Transthoracic echocardiography
TVI	Time velocity integral
V/Q	Ventilation - perfusion
VSD	Ventricular septal defect

Introduction

Pulmonary hypertension (PH) is a complex condition that can result from various pathophysiological processes. While it is divided typically into five classes, it is often classified into pre-capillary versus post-capillary PH. It can happen as a consequence of lung diseases such as emphysema or sleep apnea, heart diseases including dilated and restrictive cardiomyopathies as well as valvulopathies, congenital heart anomalies, connective tissue diseases and liver disease. A small but important sub-group of PH is idiopathic PH. Yet, independently of the etiology, it can lead to significant morbidity and premature death. It is important to be able to identify/recognize this disease entity and be able to assess mechanisms and markers of prognosis in order to guide optimal management. Echocardiography plays an important role in reaching these goals.

Diagnosis and Initial Evaluation

- **Mean pulmonary artery pressure (mPAP) ≥ 25 mmHg measured by right heart catheterization (RHC) is diagnostic of pulmonary hypertension, independent of the etiology.**
  - Further measurements of the pulmonary capillary wedge pressure (PCWP), pulmonary vascular resistance (PVR) and diastolic pressure gradient (DPG), define whether there is isolated or combined pre or post capillary PH [1].
- **A TTE should always be performed in the initial evaluation of a patient suspected of having PH** [1].
  - *Peak tricuspid regurgitation velocity* (measured by continuous wave Doppler)
    Use the highest value obtained from the multiple imaging windows
    Convert to sPAP using the simplified Bernoulli equation (see below)
    Can be underestimated in cases of severe TR leading to laminar flow through the tricuspid valve and associated marked elevation in right atrial pressure.
    Used in European guidelines to suggest PH, as opposed to systolic pulmonary artery pressure since it does not rely on the more subjective assessment of right atrial pressure
  - *Secondary signs of pulmonary hypertension* (routinely obtained during TTE study) (Fig. 33.1) [2, 3]:
    Flattening (D-shape) of the interventricular septum in systole +/− diastole in the PSAX,
    Right ventricle to left ventricle basal diameter ratio > 1,
    Mid-systolic notching of the Doppler envelope when pulsing the RVOT (a sign of pre-capillary PH, which is thought to be due to decreased compliance/increased stiffness of the pulmonary vascular bed leading to premature systolic pulmonary artery reflection wave),
    Early diastolic pulmonary regurgitation velocity > 2.2 m/s,
    IVC diameter > 21 mm with decreased respiratory collapse
    Right atrial area > 18 cm^2
    Right ventricular hypertrophy.

- *The probability of having PH is suggested by:*

Peak tricuspid requrgitation velocity (m/s)	Presence of other echo 'PH signs'[a]	Echocardiographic probability of pulmonary hypertension
≤2.8 or not measurable	No	Low
≤2.8 or not measurable	Yes	Intermediate
2.9–3.4	No	
2.9–3.4	Yes	High
>3.4	Not required	

[1]

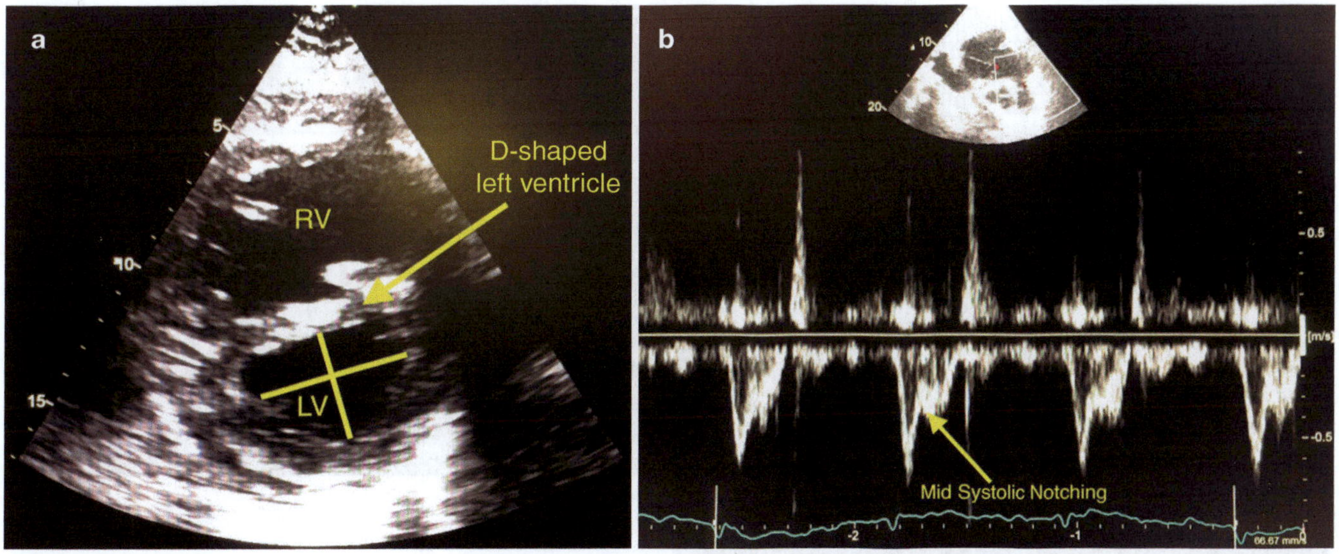

Fig. 33.1 (**a**) Prominent D-shaped left ventricle. When it is present during diastole only, it is a sign of right ventricular volume overload; when it is present during systole, it is a sign of pressure overload. The eccentricity index (EI), which is a way of reflecting an abnormal motion of the interventricular septum, can be determined by measuring the length of the LV in 2 perpendicular axis in the short axis view. The EI is then determined by doing the ratio of these values obtained at both end-systole and end-diastole. (**b**) Prominent mid-systolic notching obtained by PW Doppler through the right ventricular outflow tract

- The resting and physiologic **sPAP vary according to age and body mass index.**
  - >50 year old or body mass index (BMI) > 30 kg/m^2 — > sPAP ≦ 40 mmHg normal [4].
- Classifying **degree of severity of PH** by echo
  - No standard consensus but rough estimates are as follows:
  - Mild PH— > sPAP between 40 and 50 mmHg,
  - Moderate PH— > sPAP between 50 and 69 mmHg and,
  - Severe— > sPAP > = 70 mmHg.

One should always remember that sPAP is a function of stroke volume, according to the equation P = Q × R where P is pressure, Q is flow, and R is resistance. As PH becomes very severe and the RV decompensates, the PAP may actually fall due to the fall in stroke volume. Similarly, in cirrhosis (high cardiac output), the sPAP may be elevated despite normal resistance. Documenting the overall stroke volume (obtained by the continuity equation, measuring the cross-sectional area of the outflow tract and the velocity time integral through that outflow tract) might be helpful in the initial assessment when evaluating the etiology. Stroke volume or cardiac output may also be helpful during follow up when mentioning the sPAP in the context of RV systolic function.

Measurements of Pulmonary Artery Pressure [5]

- **Systolic pulmonary artery pressure estimated based on the tricuspid regurgitation velocity**.
  - Most commonly used method
  - The maximum TR velocity is obtained by continuous wave Doppler and through the simplified Bernoulli equation (Pressure = 4v^2), the velocity is converted to a pressure. This represents the pressure difference between the right ventricle and the right atrium. To obtain the right ventricular systolic pressure (RVSP), this pressure gradient is added to the right atrial pressure. If there is no significant gradient across the pulmonic valve, the RVSP = sPAP.
- **Important points to note regarding the TR flow signal**:
  - Assessment of the TR jet must be done in multiple views in order to obtain the maximal velocity. As the Doppler shift principal is used, the maximal TR velocity will be measured when the ultrasound beam will be most parallel with the TR jet (Figs. 33.2a and 33.2c).
  - Ensure that the TR envelope is complete and with appropriate gain for adequate measurement. If the envelope is not complete, an estimate of sPAP should not be reported. Don't "overgain" the Doppler envelope, as this will lead to an overestimate, particularly at higher pressures, since the velocity is squared (Fig. 33.2b).
  - When there is severe TR, the TR velocity cannot be reliably assessed by the simplified Bernoulli equation, due to the presence of laminar flow across the tricuspid valve. The RA and RV approach acting as a single chamber and therefore there is little pressure gradient (Fig. 33.2).

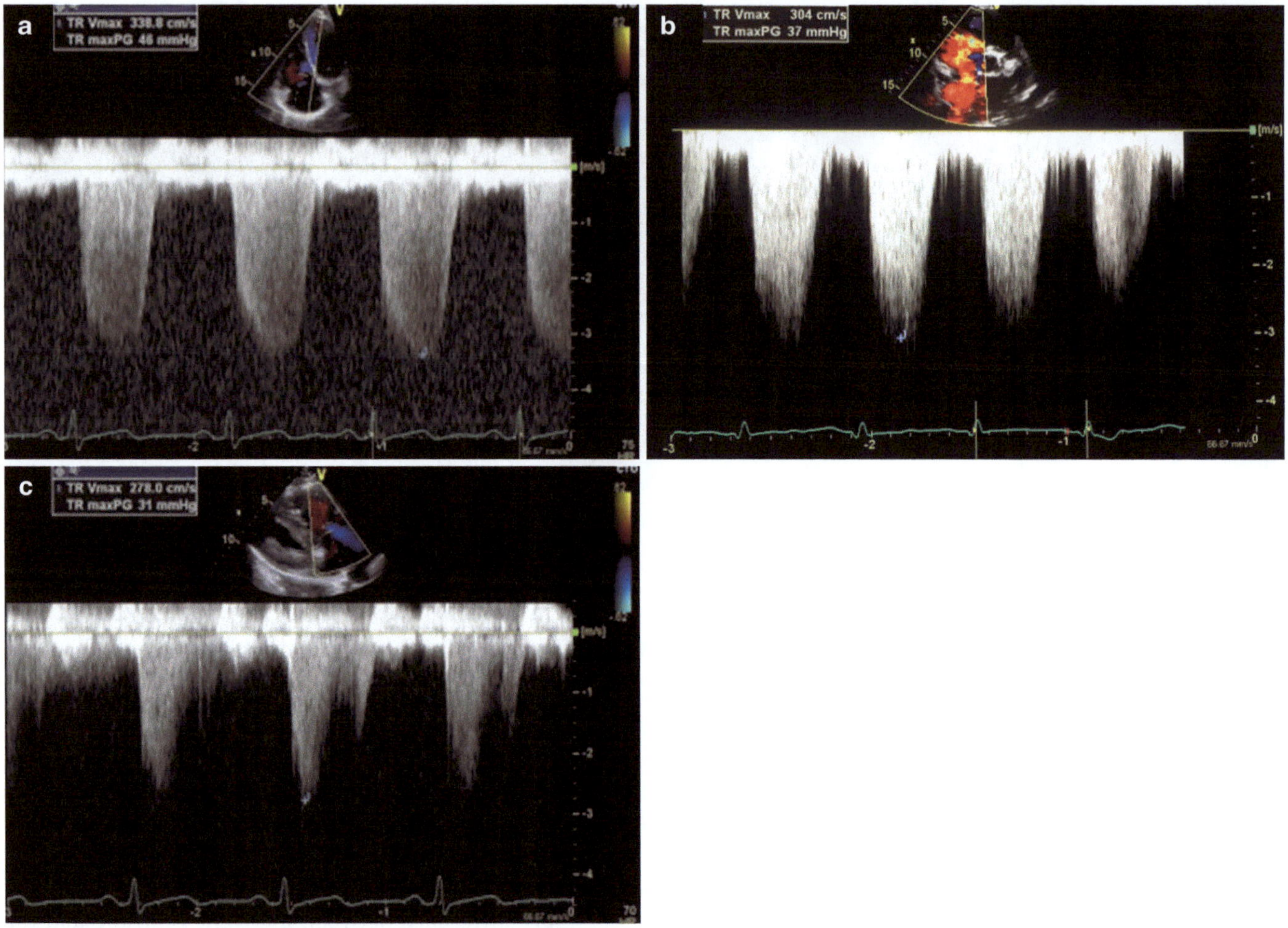

Fig. 33.2 These 3 images showing TR signal illustrate the importance of adequate technique for reliable data acquisition. (**a**) When measuring the TR velocity, it is important to be properly aligned with the direction of the regurgitant jet and to use the appropriate gain in order to obtain a well defined and complete TR envelope. (**b**) It is also important not to maximize the gain as it can lead to overestimation of the velocity. Any error in the velocity measurement will be magnified by the second order due to the relationship between the velocity and the derived pressure in the Bernoulli equation. (**c**) Figure 33.2c shows an incomplete TR envelope (due to inadequate alignment with the TR jet) from which a reliable value cannot be obtained

- **The RAP is estimated by looking at the dimension of the IVC and its relative change in size during respiration.**

IVC dimension (mm)	Inspiratory collapse (%)	Estimated RAP (mmHg)
<21	>50	3
<21	<50	8
>21	>50	8
>21	<50	15

– *Limitation*

This method of assessing the RAP, although simple, might underestimate the true RAP especially in cases of severe RV dysfunction or severe TR where the RAP can be much higher than 15 mmHg (the maximal value obtained by this method). Recently, there has been some data supporting indexing IVC dimension to body surface area in a select patient population [6].

- **The RV systolic pressure is a reliable estimate of the systolic pulmonary artery pressure only if there is no obstruction in the right ventricular outflow tract.**
  – To obtain a real estimate of the sPAP from the RVSP, there need to be unimpeded flow between the RV and the PA.
  – If there is subvalvular obstruction, pulmonary artery stenosis or pulmonary valve stenosis, the obtained RVSP will overestimate the true sPAP. Many people simply subtract the trans-pulmonic valve peak gradient from the RVSP obtained by the TR gradient in order to estimate the sPAP. This correction, however, has not been well validated, and often leads to an underestimation of the sPAP
  – In order to appropriately assess the RVOT for any significant abnormalities, it is best to obtain a short axis view at the level of the aorta. A superiorly

angulated PLAX view may be helpful as well. The RVOT and pulmonic valve are occasionally well visualized in a subcostal short axis imaging plane, or subcostal long-axis anteriorly angulated view, particularly in thin subjects and pediatric patients.

- **Estimate the sPAP when a ventricular septal defect (VSD) is present.**
  - The maximal velocity obtained across the VSD can be converted into a pressure gradient through the simplified Bernoulli equation. That pressure now represents the pressure difference between the left ventricle and the right ventricle. The systolic left ventricular pressure is usually very similar to the systolic arterial pressure, if no left ventricular outflow tract obstruction exists. Subtract the pressure (obtained through measurement of flow velocity across the VSD) from the systolic blood pressure measurement (obtained by measurement with a blood pressure cuff on the arm). This provides the RVSP.
  - Once again, if no RVOT obstruction exists, the RVSP reflects the sPAP.
- **Estimation of mean pulmonary artery pressure (mPAP)**

  The definition of PH is made based on a mean PAP, as determined by RHC. There are several methods of estimating mPAP by echo, several of them with excellent correlation with RHC.

  - *MPAP through measurement of tricuspid regurgitation velocity*

    In a technique similar to that used to obtain mean gradient across the aortic valve, the complete TR jet envelope can be traced, giving TR TVI and yielding a mean RV-RA pressure gradient. Adding an estimated RAP as described above yields an estimated mPAP. This method has the attraction of being most physiologically sound [7].
  - *MPAP through measurement of peaked pulmonary regurgitation velocity*

    MPAP derived from peak early diastolic pulmonary regurgitation velocity

    mPAP = 4 × Peak PR velocity^2+ RAP.
  - *MPAP through measurement of the right ventricular outflow tract flow acceleration.*

    A pulsed wave Doppler is obtained at the level of the pulmonary valve in the parasternal short axis view. Then, the time interval between the beginning of flow through the pulmonary valve and its peak velocity is measured. This is called the acceleration time. The Mahan's equation is then used to obtain the mPAP.

    Mahan's equation: mPAP = 79–0.45(AT).

    Principle = Acceleration time of the forward flow through the pulmonary valve will become shorter with increasing pulmonary artery pressure. This is dependent on the heart rate and the cardiac output.
  - *MPAP through measurement of the systolic pulmonary artery pressure*

    Regression equation whereby mPAP is closely approximated by the simple relationship mPAP = 0.62 × sPAP + 1.95, simplified to mPAP = 0.6 × sPAP [8]. The sPAP used is derived from the peaked TR velocity as described earlier in this chapter.

    This relationship was tested against RHC in a large series of subjects and showed a very low rate of misclassification.
  - *MPAP calculated from the systolic and diastolic pulmonary artery pressures*

    mPAP = 2/3 dPAP + 1/3 sPAP

    These values can be filled in based on sPAP measured from TR jet and dPAP measured from PR jet as indicated below.
- **Method to obtain diastolic pulmonary artery pressure**
  - *dPAP derived from end diastolic pulmonary regurgitation velocity*

    A continuous wave Doppler is obtained through the pulmonary valve in the parasternal short axis view.

    End diastolic velocity is measured and converted to a pressure gradient through the Bernoulli equation ($P = 4v^2$). The pressure gradient obtained represents the change in pressure between the pulmonary artery and the right ventricle. And at the end of diastole, the RVEDP should be equal to the right atrial pressure. Thus, dPAP = 4 × PREDV^2 + RAP (Fig. 33.3).

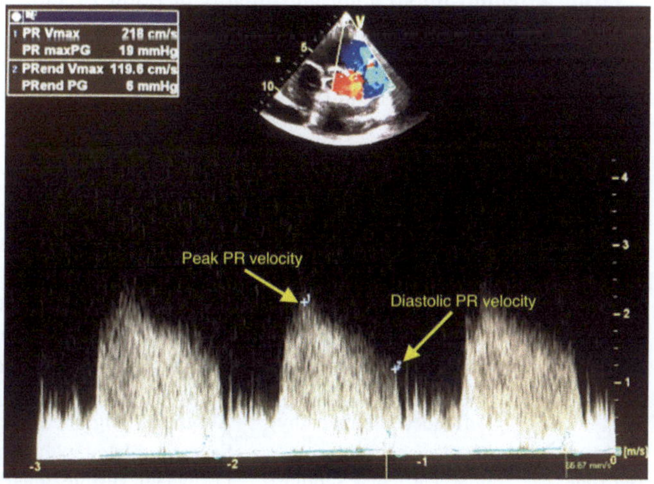

Fig. 33.3 Illustration of where the peaked and diastolic pulmonary regurgitation velocity are obtained in order to derive the mean pulmonary artery pressure and the diastolic pulmonary artery pressure respectively

Pulmonary Vascular Resistance (PVR)

- PVR = (mPAP - PCWP)/CO.
- By echo — > *Abbas formula: 10 x (Peak TR velocity/ RVOT TVI) + 0.16* [9]. One often drops the factor of 0.16. The RVOT TVI is measured by pulsed Doppler in the distal RVOT.
  - Calculating the PVR is relevant when an elevated PAP is obtained in order to eliminate a high flow state influencing the calculations. Increased flow through the pulmonary valve (PV) will lead to an increased PAP without intrinsic pulmonary vascular disease.
    High flow state conditions
    Cirrhosis
    Paget's disease
    Anomalies leading to left to right sided shunting.

Evaluation of Pulmonary Hypertension Etiologies

- Nice classification system of PH [10]
  - Class 1: Pulmonary arterial hypertension (PAH)
  - Class 2: PH due to left sided heart disease
  - Class 3: PH due to chronic lung disease and/or hypoxemia
  - Class 4: PH due to chronic thromboembolic pulmonary hypertension
  - Class 5: PH with unclear and/or multifactorial mechanisms
- Determining the etiology of pulmonary hypertension requires a thorough evaluation which includes history, physical examination, bloodwork, serology and multimodality imaging and testing.
- From a diagnostic strategy and treatment point of view, the various causes of pulmonary hypertension can be divided into 2 large categories: pre-capillary (which includes classes 1, 3, 4 and 5) and post capillary (which includes class 2).
- *Distinguishing pre vs post capillary pulmonary hypertension* (Table 33.1).
  - **Opotowsky et al. Criteria published in 2012** [11]
    Left atrial anterior-posterior dimension < 3.2 cm (+1 point)
    Presence of mid-systolic notch or acceleration time < 80 ms (+1 point)
    Lateral mitral E:e' > 10 (−1 point)
    Left atrial anterior-posterior dimension > 4.2 cm (−1 point)
    = > The score obtained by those 4 criteria varies between −2 and +2. The higher the score, the higher the probability of having PH resulting from pulmonary vascular disease, meaning a pre-capillary etiology. A score ≥ 0 had a sensitivity of 100% and a specificity of 62%.
  - **D'Alto et al. Criteria published in 2015** [12]
    More refined prediction rule to determine if pre-capillary PH is present.
    If the score is < 5 points, a pre-capillary etiology is unlikely to be present (PPV 68%; NPV 78%)
    5 Criteria
    Right heart chamber larger than the left
    Left ventricular eccentricity index > 1.2
    Dilated IVC without inspiratory collapse
    E/e' ratio < = 10
    Right ventricle forming the heart apex
  - **Important facts**
    These 2 prediction rules are not diagnostic but can help in the diagnosis.
    Echocardiography remains an important starting point for establishing the presence and severity of pulmonary hypertension and to determine etiology, but many other investigations (RHC, PFTs, high resolution CT chest, V/Q scan, sleep study, LHC, serology for autoimmune diseases, HIV, … etc.) have to be completed prior to initiation of any type of therapy.

Table 33.1 Distinguishing pre-capillary vs post capillary pulmonary hypertension

	Parameters	Favors pre-capillary PH (pulmonary arterial hypertension)	Favors post-capillary PH (pulmonary venous hypertension)
Left ventricle	LV size/systolic function	Normal or small/normal-low normal	Dilated/reduced
	LA volume	Normal or small	Moderate—severely dilated
	Left ventricular diastolic function	Normal or Mild impairment; E:E′ < 8	Pseudonormal/restrictive with increased filling pressures (E:E′ > 15)
	Left-sided valvulopathy	Absent/non-significant	Moderate/severe aortic or mitral disease
Right ventricle	RV size/shape	Severely dilated with rounded RV apex	Normal or mildly dilated
	Interventricular Septum	D-shape in systole or early diastolic septal shift	Normal shape
Pulmonary artery	RVOT flow/pulmonary valve motion	Mid-systolic notching of PW Doppler envelope/ notching of M-mode valve tracing	Absence of notching
	Pulmonary vascular resistance	Increased	Normal
	PA acceleration time	<80 ms	>80 ms

Be careful with disease entities that have a mixed pathophysiology (ex: scleroderma), because there might be a combination of both pre and post capillary processes contributing.

- *Evaluation for left sided heart disease is a critical component of the echocardiographic exam (more suggestive of post capillary etiology)*
  - Assessment of left sided diastolic function
  - Assessment of left sided systolic function
  - Assessment of left atrial volume
  - Assessment of mitral and/or aortic valvulopathies
- *Evaluation of left to right sided shunt*
  - Important to R/O atrial septal defect in all patients with elevated sPAP by echo since a shunt can lead to pulmonary arterial hypertension in a small subset of patients, particularly with certain genetic predisposition (abnormal BMPR2 haplotype).

    2D imaging with the use of colour Doppler flow crossing the interatrial septum

    Agitated contrast saline to detect such a defect (if 2D Colour Doppler flow imaging is negative).

    Transesophageal echocardiography (especially for sinus venosus ASD) to detect ASD if TTE uncertain, or to establish size and margins of defect to determine if candidate for closure by device.

Assessment of Right Ventricle

- Complex anatomy
- No single dedicated view
- Indices from all the views where RV can be observed have to be used to best determine RV size and function.

Parasternal Long Axis View (Fig. 33.4)

- Visualization of the right ventricular outflow tract.
- Tilting of the probe inferomedially allows for visualization of the right ventricular inlet

  The anterior and inferior RV walls can be visualized as well as the tricuspid valve leaflets (the anterior and either the posterior or the septal leaflets) (Fig. 33.4).

Parasternal Short Axis View

- The anterior and inferior RV walls can be visualized as well as the tricuspid valve leaflets (the anterior and either the posterior or the septal leaflets).
  - Visualization of the right ventricular body at the distal, mid and basal levels.
  - Interventricular septum

    Normally circular shape toward the right ventricle.

    If flattens (confers a D-shaped form to the left ventricle) in diastole only — > right ventricular volume overload.

    If flattens in both systole and diastole — > right ventricular pressure overload. The RV systolic pressure and end diastolic pressure always approximate or exceed the left ventricular systolic and diastolic pressures, respectively. An early diastolic septal shift

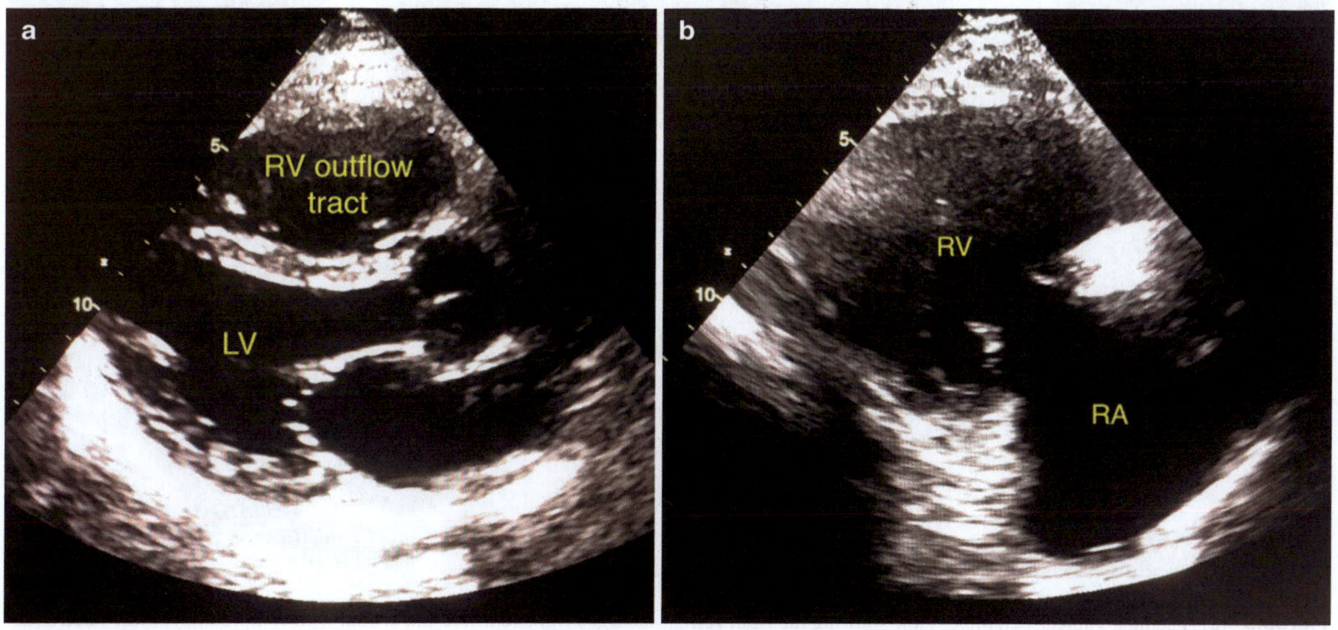

Fig. 33.4 (**a**) A standard parasternal long axis view allowing visualisation of the proximal right ventricular outflow tract. (**b**) Visualisation of the right ventricular inlet obtained by tilting the probe inferomedially while in the standard PLAX view

suggests a pre-capillary etiology, as the RV diastolic pressure is higher than the LV diastolic pressure. The exception to this "rule of thumb" is in PH related to severe mitral stenosis (MS), where the LV diastolic pressure is relatively "protected" by the MS.

Apical 4 Chamber View

- Visualization of the right ventricular cavity and its free wall, the right atrium and the tricuspid valve leaflets.
- RV focused apical 4-chamber is usually preferred to measure RV size as compared to the standard apical 4 chamber.
  Obtained with the probe kept over the cardiac apex, and the position of the transducer slightly rotated towards the RV and tilted to obtain adequate visualization of the RV free wall.
- Standard apical 4-chamber is often used to judge the relative size of the RV to the LV. In PAH, the RV often appears markedly larger than the LV with the LV having the appearance of being compressed. The LA has a similar appearance relative to the RA, with the interatrial septum bulging into the LA, suggesting a RA pressure that exceeds LA pressure (Fig. 33.5). These findings are often absent in post-capillary PH whereby the RV size and shape may be preserved despite severe PH. This is the result of high filling pressures in the left sided chambers.

Subcostal Window

- Right ventricle, RV free wall, the right atrium, the interatrial septum and the inferior vena cava (Fig. 33.6).

Right Ventricular Size and Function [2]

Prognosis in pulmonary hypertension is strongly related to the right heart's ability to compensate for the increased afterload. Initially, changes are adaptive, but ultimately the RV dilates and fails. The right ventricle must therefore be carefully assessed by echocardiography. A guideline-based approach to assess RV size and systolic function is important. The ASE/EACVI's recommendations for size and function normal cut-offs are designed to differentiate normal versus abnormal values and were not specifically designed to determine normalcy in pulmonary hypertension. As such, cut-off values for prognostication may be different in the PH population.

A few clinical pearls and comments specifically related to PH are outlined below. A complete discussion of ASE/

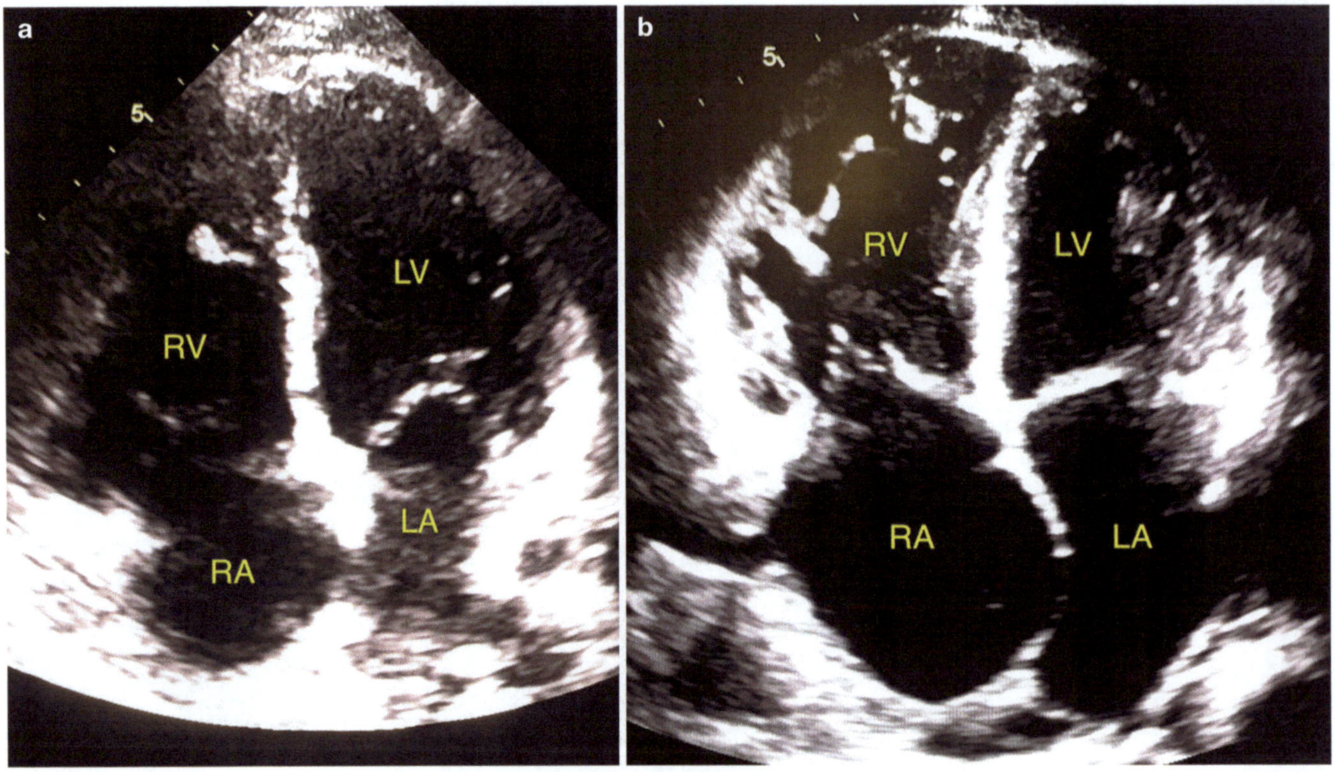

Fig. 33.5 (**a**) A standard apical 4 chamber view showing the right ventricle and the right atrium in direct comparison with the left ventricle and left atrium. (**b**) An apical 4 chamber view showing significantly enlarged right ventricle and atrium with compression of left sided structures. This will lead to a decrease in left sided cardiac output

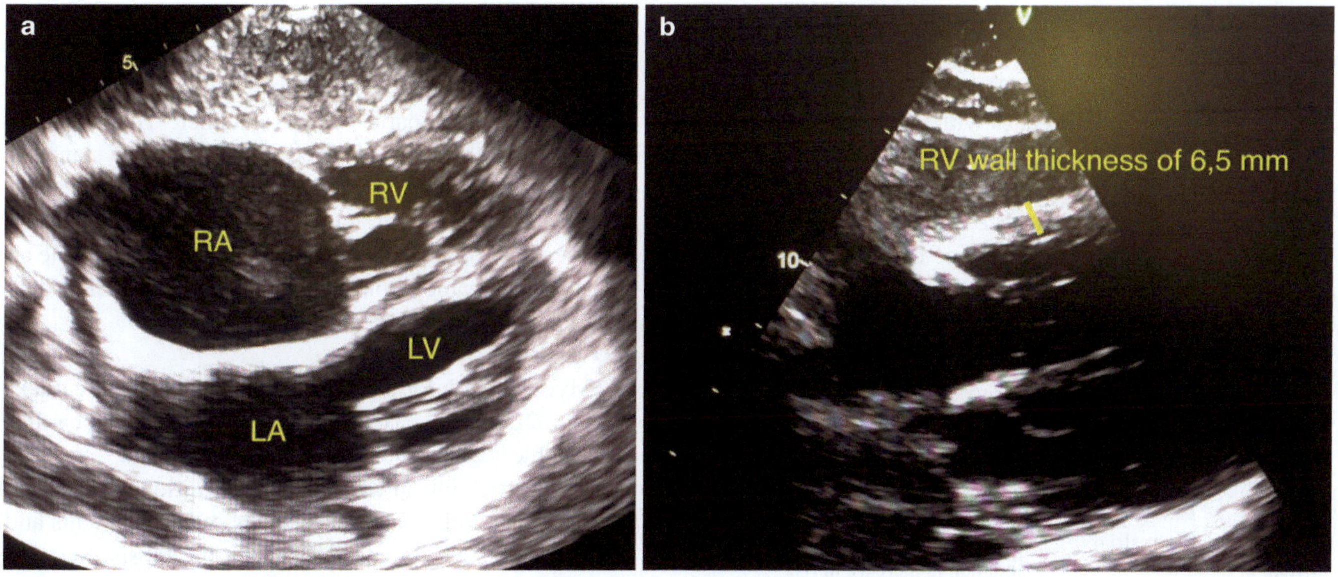

Fig. 33.6 (**a**) A standard subcostal view showing the right sided cardiac chambers in relation to the left sided structures. (**b**) This is also the view to measure the thickness of the right ventricular wall at end diastole at the level of the tip of the anterior tricuspid valve leaflet. If the wall thickness is > 5 mm, it suggests right ventricular hypertrophy, which may indicate chronicity in the setting of PH

EACVI recommendations for the assessment of the right heart is covered in Chap. 12.

Prognosis

- Overall, prognosis associated with the diagnosis of pulmonary hypertension varies depending on the etiology of the pulmonary hypertension, the functional class and the comorbidities of the patient.

By echo, there are some findings that are associated with a more unfavourable outcome. These have been mainly studied in and hence, used for pulmonary arterial hypertension (Table 33.2).

Of note, the pulmonary artery pressure (measured by TTE), despite being important to follow up and to grade the severity of PH, has not been demonstrated to have prognostic value [13, 14].

- ***Presence of a pericardial effusion***
  - Normally, drainage of fluid occurs through a venous and lymphatic network located within the subepicardium and draining into the right atrium. When right sided pressure are elevated, there is compression of those channels and hence, impaired fluid resorption which in turn, leads to accumulation of fluid in the pericardial sac.
  - Several studies have correlated the presence of a pericardial effusion with adverse prognosis [13, 15, 16].
  - A recent large study demonstrated that only moderate and large incident (new) pericardial effusion tend to be strongly associated with increased mortality [17].
- ***Increased indexed right atrial area***
  - Right atrial enlargement results from increased RAP which can be due to right sided diastolic dysfunction resulting from RV failure or functional TR.
  - Multiple studies have shown its prognostic value in individual patients with PH [15, 16, 18–20]
  - A value of > 18 cm^2/m^2 (measured in the apical-4 chamber view at the end of systole) has been used as the cutoff value after which the risks of morbidity and mortality increase. Further dilatation of the right atrium seems to correlate even more with adverse prognosis [18, 20].
- ***Inferior vena cava***
  - Another echocardiographic marker of elevated RA pressure, as assessed by the standard echocardiographic study, is the presence of a dilated and non-collapsing IVC. In a large study of PAH patients, an estimated RAP > 15 mmHg by echo was a strong predictor of mortality—even stronger than echocardiographic measures of right ventricular function [21].
- ***Degree of septal shift toward the left ventricle in diastole***
  - Any shift of the inter ventricular septum, whether during diastole and/or systole reflects an abnormal pressure gradient between the LV and RV. This is also reflected by the eccentricity index [13, 15, 16, 20]. It seems to be predictive of mortality and/or need for transplantation.
- ***RV myocardial performance index***
  - Studies, over the years, have shown benefits of determining the RV MPI to better assess the chance of hav-

ing an adverse outcome, including death and/or need for transplantation. There is also some data suggesting benefits in following RV MPI over time and that changes in MPI correlates with change in clinical status [14, 16, 22, 23].

- ***Tricuspid annular plane systolic excursion and RV S′***
  - The prognostic significance of these 2 findings is controversial. They are markers of the longitudinal function of the RV. Different diseases involving the RV can lead to various types of systolic dysfunction. However, it seems that when they are severely reduced, there is an increased risk of adverse outcomes [24].
  - RV dysfunction does not appear to be uniformly distributed in all parts of the chamber. The RV base appears to be affected much more in the late stages of the disease, such that S'and TAPSE only become "abnormal" at late stages. As such, a normal value does not correlate well with normal function, while an abnormal value strongly suggests significant RV dysfunction, and imparts a poorer prognosis.
- ***2D Strain***
  - Myocardial deformation imaging by 2D speckle tracking "2D strain" has gained prominence in echocardiographic assessment of RV function and in prognostication in a variety of conditions. 2D Strain has been studied in a large series of PAH patients and has been strongly correlated with prognosis. Survival is significantly reduced with RV strain values of < 20% (less negative than −20%) [25] (Fig. 33.7).
- ***Progressive TR***
  - Chronic PH leads to tricuspid valve tenting, reduced leaflet coaptation surface and resultant TR. This leads to RV remodeling [26] which in turn leads to further RV dilatation.
  - By itself, the severity of the tricuspid regurgitation correlates with mortality [27–29]. Recently, the progression of TR has been directly correlated with increased RV remodeling and with all cause mortality.
  - TR severity is best assessed using a composite method of visual assessment, proximal isovelocity surface area (PISA) or vena contracta and presence of reversal in the hepatic veins.

Table 33.2 Summary of prognostic factors

	Factors	Findings associated with poor prognosis (mortality +/− transplantation)
Right atrium	Right atrial area	RAA ≥ 18 cm²/m² Incremental increase in risk especially if > 27–32 cm²/m². Bustamante-Labarta et al. [30]; Salach et al. [18]
	Inferior vena cava (reflecting right atrial pressure)	Right atrial pressure ≥ 15 mmHg (IVC diameter more than 21 mm and collapsibility index < 50%) Austin et al. [21]; Brierre et al. [13]
Right ventricle	Abnormal septal curvature/ eccentricity index	An abnormal end-diastolic septal curve [13] Abnormal EI [17]. Brierre et al. [13]; Raymond et al. [17]
	Myocardial performance index	An elevated Tei index seems to be associated with an increased risk of mortality. The cut off value to predict poor outcome is unclear. In one study it was ≥ 0.83 [14] and in another one, it was ≥0.98 [13]. Yeo et al. [14]; Brierre et al. [13]
	TAPSE	Clinical trials have been inconsistent in showing that this marker is a good prognostic indicator; a normal TAPSE value is not associated with a better outcome. However, a low TAPSE, (a cutoff value of ≤ 15 cm might be used [24]) appears to confer an increased risk of mortality [13]. Forfia et al. [24]; Brierre et al. [13]
	2D strain	GLS ≤ −15% [25] Increased risk with further decline in strain, especially if ≤ −12.5% [31] Sachdev et al. [31]; Fine Nowell et al. [25]
Other parameters	Pericardial effusion	Incidental development of moderate to large pericardial effusion Shimony et al. [17]; Raymond et al. [16]
	Progressive TR	Progressive TR Medvedofsky et al. [29]; Nath et al. [27]; Bustamante-Labarta et al. [30]

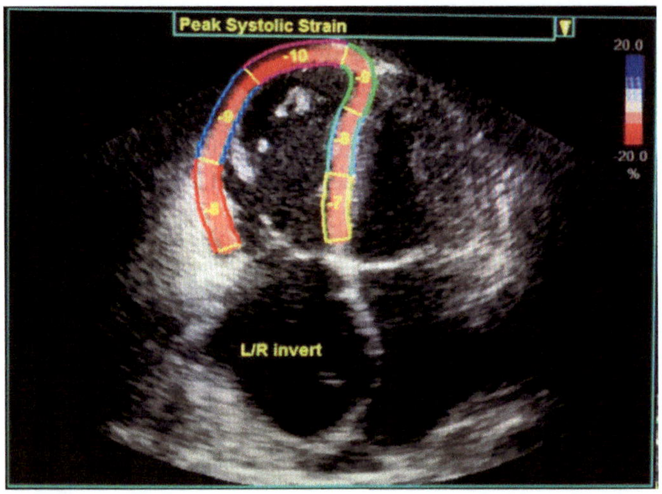

Fig. 33.7 This figure illustrates "2D" strain of the right ventricle. The RV free wall is mainly affected with an averaged global longitudinal strain of—9%

- **Screening and follow up**

PH, being a complex condition with different etiologies leading to various hemodynamic progression overtime, needs individualized follow up.

A follow up has to include history, re-evaluating symptoms, how they have been progressing in response to a new treatment or a change in treatment and physical examination. Depending on the evolution of these elements, clinical follow up will be adjusted. When a comprehensive assessment needs to be done, this will also include the need for repeat transthoracic echocardiography.

- *Pulmonary arterial hypertension (General)*
- For individuals with pulmonary arterial hypertension:
  Full TTE at baseline and subsequently every 6–12 months.
  Repeat a TTE in case of clinical worsening or 3 to 6 months after a change in therapy.

The study should include evaluation of the right atrial size, right ventricular dimension and function (using various parameters explained in Chap. 12), pulmonary artery pressure, IVC dimension and magnitude of tricuspid regurgitation [1].

For family members of individuals with documented PAH, a formal TTE should be done at least once to evaluate for PH. TTE should also be repeated if symptoms appear.

If a genetic mutation associated with PH is present (e.g., BMPR2 mutation), yearly TTE is recommended [32]. These individuals should be referred to centers with expertise in pulmonary vascular disease.

Connective tissue disease

For individuals with systemic sclerosis, mixed connective tissue disease and other connective tissue disease with scleroderma features, a TTE should be done at the time of diagnosis and annually thereafter, though the data upon which this recommendation is made is relatively scant. Additionally, if any new signs or symptoms become present, a repeat TTE should be done, as new significant dyspnea is often a marker of incident PAH. Approximately 15% of individuals with scleroderma will develop PH. PH in scleroderma patients can be due to a primary vascular disease, as a consequence of left sided heart disease or restrictive lung disease, all of which are related to their underlying connective tissue disease [33].

Portopulmonary hypertension

Individuals with portopulmonary hypertension (1–5%), independent of the underlying cause, are at risk of developing PH. TTE is only recommended if symptoms suggestive of PH are present. It is not routinely recommended. However, a TTE should always be done to assess for PH in individuals being evaluated for liver transplantion, irrespective of symptoms [1].

Human Immunodeficiency Virus (HIV)

The prevalence of HIV related PAH is < 1%. Routine TTE is not recommended in HIV infected individuals that are asymptomatic. However, TTE should be done if there is unexplained dyspnea or other signs suggestive of PH [1].

Congenital heart disease

The incidence of PAH in individuals with congenital heart disease varies depending on the baseline congenital defects present, the palliative and corrective procedures done. Those with known non corrected systemic to pulmonary shunts are at risk of developing PH during their lifetime and should have TTE done at the time of diagnosis. If no correction of the underlying defect is done, TTE should be repeated at regular interval to assess for development of PH.

For those who develop Eisenmenger syndrome, referral to centers with expertise in both congenital heart disease and pulmonary vascular disease should be done.

- *PH secondary to left sided heart disease*
- For individuals with PH secondary to left sided heart disease, the frequency at which a TTE should be repeated is mainly determined by the underlying left sided pathology involved.
- *PH secondary to lung disease or chronic thromboembolic disease*
- Individuals with underlying lung disease should have a TTE if the dyspnea is out of proportion to the severity of the lung disease as determined by clinical evaluation and pulmonary function test [1].
- There is no recommendation for screening for chronic thromboembolic disease in individuals with history of acute pulmonary embolism. Indeed, a significant number of individuals with CTEPH have no history of thromboembolic disease [1].
- Once a diagnosis of PH secondary to lung disease or chronic thromboembolic disease is established, TTE should be repeated in accordance with the recommendations for individuals with class 1 PH.

Patients with class 1, 3 or 4 pulmonary hypertension should usually be referred to a center with expertise in pulmonary hypertension, where there is also experience in the interpretation of various echocardiographic parameters.

Questions

1. Which of the following echocardiographic parameters is not a secondary sign of pulmonary hypertension:
   A. Right ventricle to left ventricle basal diameter ratio > 1
   B. Mid-systolic notching of the Doppler envelope when pulsing the RVOT
   C. Early diastolic pulmonary regurgitation velocity > 2.2 m/s,
   D. Right atrial area > 15 cm^2

2. Which phrase is wrong about classifying the degree of severity of PH by echo:
   A. Mild PH —> is suggested by sPAP between 40 and 50 mmHg,
   B. Moderate PH —> is suggested by sPAP between 50 and 69 mmHg
   C. Severe —> is suggested by sPAP >=70 mmHg
   D. None of them.

3. What is the mean PA pressure in patient with TR velocity of 3 m/s, PR end diastolic pressure of 2m/s and RAP of 10 mmHg?
   A. Mean PAP=28mmHg
   B. Mean PAP=33mmHg
   C. Mean PAP=43mmHg
   D. Mean PAP=25mmHg

4. What is the mean PA pressure with TR velocity of 4 m/s, peak velocity of PR is 3m/s and RAP of 10 mmHg?
   A. Diastolic PAP= 46 mmHg
   B. Diastolic PAP= 55 mmHg
   C. Diastolic PAP= 64 mmHg
   D. Diastolic PAP= 74 mmHg

Answers

1. D
2. D
3. B
4. A

References

1. Galliè N, et al. Guidelines for the diagnosis and treatment of pulmonary hypertension. Eur Heart J. 2015;10:1–58.
2. Rudski LG, et al. Guidelines for the echocardiographic assessment of the right heart in adults: a report from the American Society of Echocardiography. J Am Soc Echocardiogr. 2010;23:685–713.
3. Lang RM, et al. Recommendations for cardiac chamber quantification by echocardiography in adults: an update from the American Society of Echocardiography and the European Association of Cardiovascular Imaging. Eur Heart J Cardiovasc Imaging. 2015;16:233–71.
4. McQullian BM, et al. Clinical correlates and reference intervals for pulmonary artery systolic pressure among echocardiographically normal subjects. Circulation. 2001;104:2797–802.
5. Oh JK, et al. The echo manual. 3rd ed. Philadelphia, PA: Lippincton Williams and Wilkins; 2006.
6. Taniguchi T, et al. Impact of body size on inferior vena cava parameters for estimating right atrial pressure: a need for standardization? J Am Soc Echocardiogr. 2015;28:1420–7.
7. Aduen JF, et al. An alternative echocardiographic method to estimate mean pulmonary artery pressure: diagnostic and clinical implications. J Am Soc Echocardiogr. 2009;22(7):814–9.
8. Steckelberg RC, et al. Derivation of mean pulmonary artery pressure from noninvasive parameters. J Am Soc Echocardiogr. 2013;26(5):464–8.
9. Abbas A, et al. A simple method for noninvasive estimation of pulmonary vascular resistance. J Am Coll Cardiol. 2003;41:1021–7.
10. Simonneau G, et al. Clinical classification of pulmonary hypertension. J Am Coll Cardiol. 2004;43(Suppl 1):S5–S12.
11. Opotowsky AR, Ojeda J, Rogers F, Prasanna V, Clair M. A simple echocardiographic prediction rule for hemodynamics in pulmonary hypertension. Circ Cardiovasc Imaging. 2012;5:765–75.
12. D'Alto M, et al. Echocardiographic prediction of pre-versus post capillary pulmonary hypertension. J Am Soc Echocardiogr. 2015;28:108–15.
13. Brierre G, et al. New echocardiographic prognostic factors for mortality in pulmonary arterial hypertension. Eur J Echocardiogr. 2010;11:516–22.
14. Yeo TC, et al. Value of a Doppler-derived index combining systolic and diastolic time intervals in predicting outcome in primary pulmonary hypertension. Am J Cardiol. 1998;81:1157–61.
15. Bossone E, et al. Echocardiography in pulmonary arterial hypertension: from diagnosis to prognosis. J Am Soc Echocardiogr. 2013;26:1–14.
16. Raymond RJ, et al. Echocardiographic predictors of adverse outcomes in primary pulmonary hypertension. J Am Coll Cardiol. 2002;39:1214–9.
17. Shimony A, et al. Incidence and significance of pericardial effusion in patients with pulmonary arterial hypertension. Can J Cardiol. 2013;29:678–82.
18. Sallach JA, Tang WHW, Borowski AG, Tong W, Porter T, Martin MG, et al. Right atrial volume index in chronic systolic heart failure and prognosis. JACC Cardiovasc Imaging. 2009;2:527–34.
19. Fukuda Y, et al. Utility of combining assessment of right ventricular function and right atrial remodelling as a prognostic factor for patients with pulmonary hypertension. Int J Cardiovasc Imaging. 2014;30:1269–77.
20. Ryan T, et al. An echocardiographic index for separation of right ventricular volume and pressure overload. J Am Coll Cardiol. 1985;5:918–24.
21. Austin C, et al. Echocardiographic assessment of estimated right atrial pressure and size predicts mortality in pulmonary arterial hypertension. Chest. 2015;147(1):198–208.
22. Tei C, Dujardin KS, Hodge DO, Bailey KR, McGoon MD, Tajik AJ, et al. Doppler echocardiographic index for assessment of global right ventricular function. J Am Soc Echocardiogr. 1996;9:838–47.
23. Sebbag I, Rudski LG, Therrien J, Hirsch A, Langleben D. Effect of chronic infusion of epoprostenol on echocardiographic right ventricular myocardial performance index and its relation to clinical outcome in patients with primary pulmonary hypertension. Am J Cardiol. 2001;88:1060–3.
24. Forfia PR, et al. Tricuspid annular displacement predicts survival in pulmonary hypertension. Am J Respir Crit Care Med. 2006;174:1034–41.

25. Fine Nowell M, et al. Outcome prediction by quantitative right ventricular function assessment in 575 subjects evaluated for pulmonary hypertension. Circ Cardiovasc Imaging. 2013;6:711–21.
26. Topilsky Y, et al. Clinical context and mechanism of functional tricuspid regurgitation in patients with and without pulmonary hypertension. Circ Cardiovasc Imaging. 2012;5:314–23.
27. Nath J, et al. Impact of tricuspid regurgitation on long term survival. J Am Coll Cardiol. 2004;43:405–9.
28. Lee J-W, et al. Long-term prognosis of isolated significant tricuspid regurgitation. Circ J. 2010;74:375–80.
29. Medvedofsky D, et al. Tricuspid regurgitation progression and regression in pulmonary arterial hypertension: implications for right ventricular and tricuspid valve apparatus geometry and patients outcome. Heart J Cardiovasc Imaging. 2017;18(1):86–94.
30. Bustamante-Labarta M, et al. Right atrial size and tricuspid regurgitation severity predict mortality or transplantation in primary pulmonary hypertension. J Am Soc Echocardiogr. 2002;15:1160–4.
31. Sachdev A, et al. Right ventricular strain for prediction of survival in patients with pulmonary arterial hypertension. Chest. 2011;139:1299–309.
32. McLaughlin V, et al. ACCF/AHA 2009 expert consensus document on pulmonary hypertension a report of the American College of Cardiology Foundation Task Force on Expert Consensus Documents and the American Heart Association developed in collaboration with the American College of Chest Physicians; American Thoracic Society, Inc.; and the Pulmonary Hypertension Association. J Am Coll Cardiol. 2009;53:1573–619.
33. Khanna D, et al. Recommendations for screening and detection of connective-tissue disease associated pulmonary arterial hypertension. Arthritis Rheum. 2013;65(12):3194–201.

Echocardiography in Heart Transplantation

34

Nehzat Akiash, Anita Sadeghpour, and Azin Alizadehasl

Abstract

Orthotopic Heart Transplantation (OHT) is an appropriate treatment for patients with end-stage heart failure, as the beating heart is taken from a donor and will implanted in the normal place of the recipient who has a high chance for post-transplantation recovery, improvement in quality of life, and survival. In recent decades, significant progress has been made in measures needed to control and assess transplant rejection and post-transplantation infections (Stengel et al., Heart 86(4):432–437, 2001).

The first heart transplant surgery technique, described by Shumway, Lower, and Stofer, is known as biatrial anastomosis technique (BAAT) (Bolman, Oper Tech Thorac Cardiovasc Surg 4(2):98–113, 1999; Kitamura et al., Circ J 73(7):1235–1239, 2009), which was later replaced by bicaval anastomosis technique (BCAT) (Locali et al., Arq Bras Cardiol 94(6):829–840, 2010). Other methods such as modified bicaval anastomosis technique (mBCAT) were developed by a group of Japanese heart surgeons as an appropriate heart transplant method (Bolman, Oper Tech Thorac Cardiovasc Surg 4(2):98–113, 1999). In first year after OHT, graft rejection and infections are more common cause of death, and often allograft vasculopathy and malignancy occur 5 year after cardiac transplant, whereas survival rate of patients following OHT has shown dramatic progress due to advances in surgical methods and improvements in management of patients after OHT.

Keywords

Echocardiography · Heart transplantation · Biatrial anastomosis technique · Bicaval anastomosis technique · Coronary artery disease · Cardiac allograft vasculopathy · Doppler tissue imaging

Abbreviations

2D	Two-dimensional
2DE	Two-dimensional echocardiography
3D	Three-dimensional
3DE	Three-dimensional echocardiography
BAAT	Biatrial anastomosis technique
BCAT	Bicaval anastomosis technique
CAD	Coronary artery disease
CAV	Cardiac allograft vasculopathy
DTI	Doppler tissue imaging
EF	Ejection fraction
HF	Heart failure
HT	Heart transplantation
HTN	Hypertension
IVRT	Isovolumic relaxation time
IVUS	Intravascular ultrasound
LA	Left atrial
LV	Left ventricular
OHT	Orthotopic heart transplantation
PH	Pulmonary hypertension
PVR	Pulmonary vascular resistant
RA	Right atrial

Electronic Supplementary Material The online version of this chapter (https://doi.org/10.1007/978-3-319-67691-3_34) contains supplementary material, which is available to authorized users.

N. Akiash, MD
Assistant Professor of Cardiology, Atherosclerosis Research Center, Ahvaz Jundishapur University of Medical Sciences, Ahvaz, Iran

A. Sadeghpour, MD, FACC, FASE (✉)
Professor of Cardiology, Echocardiography Research Center, Rajaie Cardiovascular Medical and Research Center, Iran University of Medical Science, Tehran, Iran

A. Alizadehasl, MD, FACC, FASE
Associate Professor of Cardiology, Echocardiologist, Echocardiography and Cardiogenetic Research Centers, Cardio-Oncology Department, Rajaie Cardiovascular Medical and Research Center, Tehran, Iran

A. Sadeghpour, A. Alizadehasl (eds.), *Case-Based Textbook of Echocardiography*,
https://doi.org/10.1007/978-3-319-67691-3_34

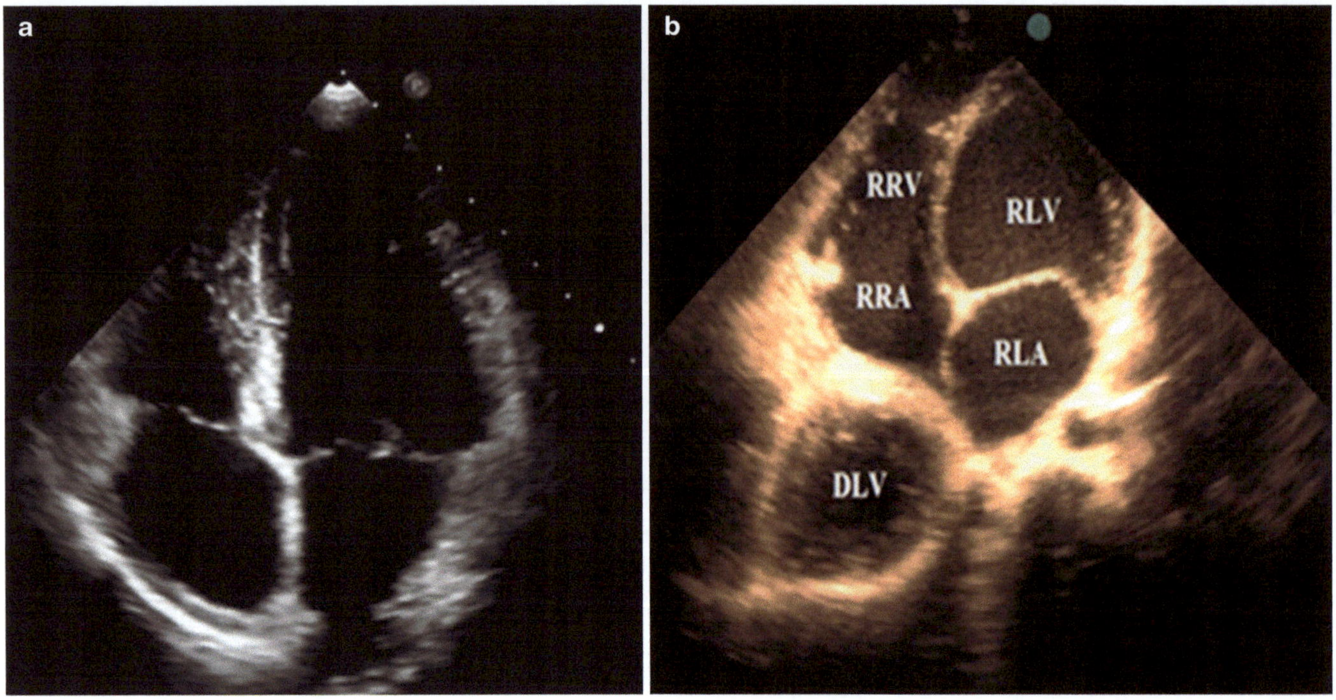

Fig. 34.1 (**a**) Orthotopic Heart Transplantation (OHT) as the donor heart is implanted in the normal place of the recipient and recipient heart is removed. (**b**) Heterotopic heart transplantation means the donor heart is placed in an ectopic place and patient native heart is preserved [1]. *RRV* recipient right ventricle, *RLV* recipient left ventricle, *RRA* recipient right atrium, *RLA* recipient left atrium, *DLV* donor left ventricle

RV	Right ventricular
TDI	Tissue Doppler imaging
TNF-α	Tumor necrosis factor-α
TR	Tricuspid regurgitation
TTE	Transthoracic echocardiography

Introduction

Although the orthotopic heart transplantation (OHT) is the standard method of heart transplantation, "heterotopic heart transplantation" is rare techniques which place the donor heart in an ectopic place without removing the patient native heart. This technique has restricted indication which includes patients who are not candidate for OHT, patients with significant recipient-donor mismatch and patients with severe irreversible pulmonary hypertension (Figs. 34.1 and 34.2) (Movies 34.1, 34.2, and 34.3)

- Nowadays, the most common surgical procedures for implanting the donor heart are biatrial and the bicaval techniques.
- In the United States (US), bicaval anastomosis is the preferred method with this idea that bicaval anastomosis will:
  - Preserve atrial form
  - Preserve physiologic conduction pathway
  - Result in less systemic arterial embolism
  - Result less tricuspid regurgitation (TR).

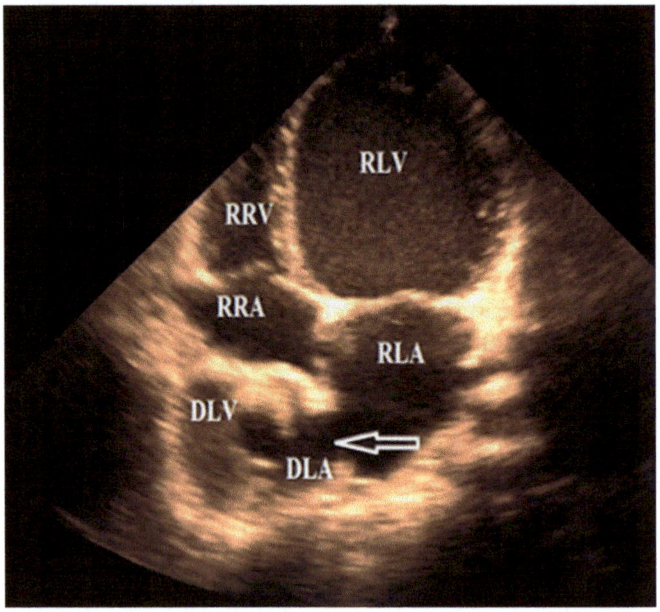

Fig. 34.2 Heterotopic heart transplantation. *RRV* recipient right ventricle, *RRA* recipient right atrium, *RLV* recipient left ventricle, *RLA* recipient left atrium, *DLV* donor left ventricle, *DLA* donor left atrium. Atrial-atrial anastomosis (white arrow)

- It has been shown that in patients with bicaval anastomosis the need for permanent pacemakers is less when compared to the biatrial anastomosis [2, 3].
- Bicaval anastomosis in orthotopic Heart Transplantation (OHT) needs five anastomosis sites including: Pulmonary artery, Aorta, left atrium, superior vena cava and inferior vena cava (Fig. 34.3).

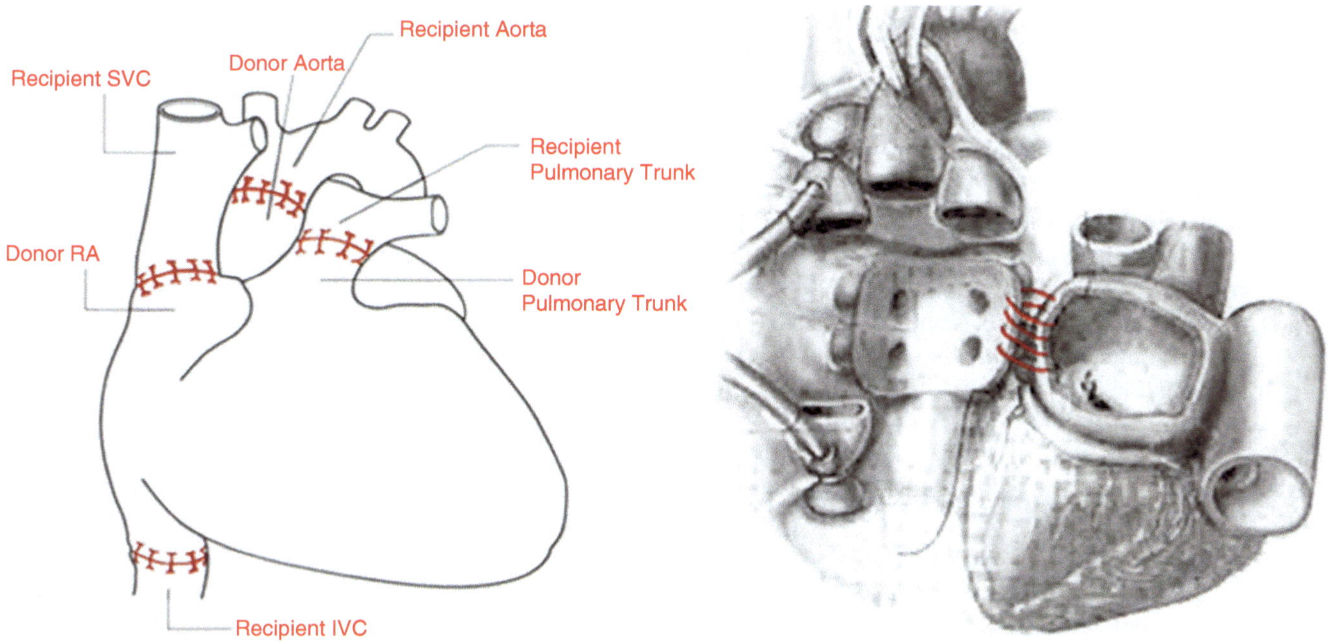

Fig. 34.3 Bicaval anastomosis method in orthotopic Heart Transplantation (OHT) needs five anastomosis sites: Pulmonary artery, Aorta, left atrium, superior vena cava and inferior vena cava (red sutures). *RA* right atrium, *SVC* superior vena cava, *IVC* inferior vena cava

Prognosis of patients following OHT has shown dramatic progress over the past two decades [4]. Data from the International Society for Heart and Lung Transplantation has shown 1 year survival rate 87% in first-time recipients in adult heart transplantation and 10-year survival rate of 50% [5].

Since coronary arteries are involved in some patients with heart failure (HF), they have greater mortality rates compared to patients with non-ischemic congestive HF. Thus, when clinical and hemodynamic variables are the same in both recipients, priority for heart transplantation is given to patients with coronary artery disease (CAD) [6].

Donor Selection in Cardiac Transplantation

- The ideal cardiac donor for transplantation was initially the heart from a person younger than 40 years old with normal cardiac function and no past medical history that had suffered brain-death. However, due to the shortage of transplant hearts, the heart from older people was used, but the concern about the outcome of using older donor persisted, especially risks of CAD and graft vasculopathy in donor heart. Currently, donors up to 60–65 years olds can be accepted [3, 7].
- Transthoracic echocardiography (TTE) was first used as a method for screening cardiac donor in 1988. TTE can be used as a non-invasive and highly accurate method to achieve successful transplantation outcome.
- TTE can exclude donor hearts from transplantation list because of severe left ventricular dysfunction and severe valvular heart disease with high accuracy [8].
- However, some studies have shown that some echocardiographic abnormalities in the donor heart can be resolved after transplantation with no adverse effects on short-term and long-terms survival. For example, the autonomic storm that occurs in some donors following brain-death and manifests as arterial hypertension, tachycardia, and increased workload on the heart, changes myocardial function in the donor heart, which is actually an echocardiographic abnormality before transplantation, and disappears afterwards [9]. In donors with no cardiac structural abnormalities, but with LVEF <40%, a number of evaluations including hormonal resuscitation and hemodynamic treatments are performed, and the transplant criteria should be reassessed [10].

Pre-transplantation Echocardiographic Assessment of the Recipient

- Assessment of regional wall motion abnormalities, Global systolic function
- Valvular abnormalities
- Congenital abnormalities
- Presence of LVH (if associated with long ischemic time or older age of donor can increase mortality) [11]
  - One of the pre-transplantation assessments is a series of indices related to pulmonary artery pressure using echocardiography (see Chap. 33).
  - Pulmonary hypertension (PH) occurs in up to 70% of patients with moderate to severe HF. Pulmonary hypertension and increased pulmonary vascular resistance (PVR) in patients who candidate for cardiac transplan-

tation are considered as a risk factor for right ventricular (RV) failure following heart transplantation [12].
  - Pulmonary vascular resistance (PVR) can be calculated using pulsed Doppler pulmonary systolic flow [13].
  - Echocardiographic calculation of PVR may be useful in reducing the number of serial right heart catheterizations in patients who are candidates for OHT; however it may have less accuracy in patients with borderline PVR (2–4 Wood units) [14, 15].
  - Therefore, patients with resistant PH after pharmacological testing are not suitable candidates for heart transplantation [12].

Post-Transplantation Assessments

Ventricular Systolic and Diastolic Function

- Increased LV wall thickness and LV end diastolic volume can take place at early post-transplantation.
- The mechanisms of hypertrophy are still unknown, but it can lead to diastolic dysfunction. One of the factors that can explain such changes is immune system disorders or cytokines produced in response to allograft. In fact, increases in cytokines and Tumor necrosis factor-α (TNF-α) can provide the ground for development of cardiac cells growth [16]. Furthermore, use of immunosuppressive medications such as cyclosporine can induce arterial hypertension (HTN), resulting in ventricular hypertrophy.
- Failure to control blood pressure in the first few months after transplantation leads to left ventricular hypertrophy, with no evidence of transplant rejection and medical treatment can regress LV hypertrophy with no changes in the size of cardiac chambers or ventricular function [17].
- In the uncomplicated HT, ventricular systolic function remains normal even in 10–15 years after transplantation [14].

Diastolic Function

- Increased LV filling pressures early after OHT can be seen mostly due to impaired bi-ventricular function and usually improves after a few weeks to months or over years.
- Post-transplantation diastolic dysfunction can be a manifestation of transplant rejection. Following acute heart transplant rejection, lymphocyte infiltration, inflammation of myocardial tissue and impaired left ventricle filling occur before increased myocardial wall-thickness [18].

Finding Restrictive physiology in early after OHT can be suggestive of:

- Ischemic myocardial injury
- Recipient pulmonary hypertension
- Volume overload

Persistent restrictive physiology can be suggestive of:

- Systemic hypertension
- Rejection
- Ischemic fibrosis
  - Diastolic dysfunction (impaired myocardial relaxation or increased stiffness) may result from the edema, myocyte damage and inflammation which are seen in graft rejection or Cardiac allograft vasculopathy (CAV) [14, 19].

Doppler Tissue Imaging (TDI), Strain and Strain Rate Imaging

- Doppler tissue imaging (TDI) is a method for assessment of diastolic function. Many studies have shown that early diastolic mitral annular velocity significantly reduces with increasing transplant rejection grade [20].
- TDI has high specificity but poor sensitivity, due to the effect of recipient's atrial contraction time on ventricular early filling and also sinus tachycardia, which can cause overlapping of A and E. In fact, maintaining morphology of the left atrium (LA) in bicaval technique leads to normal dynamics of the left ventricle filling [4].
- Endo-myocardial biopsy in assessing transplant rejection is an invasive method; therefore, cardiac ultrasound as a non-invasive method is first used for its detection, in which ventricular filling dysfunction should be examined, among other indices. In the rejection process, cellular infiltration causes abnormality in myocardial contractions.
- Measurement of regional strain and strain rate is a widely used modality for assessment of regional ventricular function and systolic deformation and can show early and subclinical changes (before changes in conventional echocardiography) in regional systolic function.
- Strain and strain rate are used as a modality for monitoring and detecting rejection and also for reducing the number of biopsies.
- Generally, structural and functional changes that occur in a cardiac allograft include post-transplantation hypertrophy and remodeling that happen in the context of HTN and systolic and diastolic dysfunction may occur during acute and chronic rejection (Table 34.1) [21].

Evidence of transplant rejection in patients includes:

- Reduced Tissue-Doppler velocities (Fig. 34.4)
- Reduced stroke volume (SV) and left ventricular ejection fraction (LVEF)
- Increased LV posterior wall thickness
- Pericardial effusion

- Reduced isovolomic relaxation time (IVRT)
- Mitral inflow E/A > 1.7
- Reduced systolic and diastolic circumferential and radial strains
  - Reduced global longitudinal strain (GLS) with absolute value of less than 14.8% has significant association with increased risk of treatment-requiring rejection (grade 1B or higher rejection).
  - Santos et al. suggested high sensitivity and specificity (85.7%, 81.4%) and 98.8% negative predictive value in Average LV longitudinal strain <15.5% and 85.7% sensitivity, 91% specificity for RV free wall longitudinal strain <17% in patients with Acute cellular rejection ≥2R [22, 23].
  - Till now, there is no single echocardiography parameter to be used alone for reliable diagnosis of acute cardiac allograft rejection. Multiple echocardiographic parameters with serial follow up besides clinical presentations should be used for diagnosis of cardiac allograft rejection [24].

Table 34.1 Echocardiographic assessment of the recipient after heart transplantation

Increase LV wall thickness and LV end diastolic volume	May be seen early after OHT
Ventricular systolic function	Usually remain normal in uncomplicated HT
Increased LV filling pressures immediately after cardiac transplantation	Usually improves after a few weeks to months or over years
Paradoxical septal motion (post operation septum)	Common finding after HT
RV enlargement and tricuspid regurgitation	Severity are parallel to secondary pulmonary hypertension
Increase LV wall thickness and LV end diastolic volume	Seen in biatrial anastomosis

Rejection is categorized to three types:

- Hyperacute rejection (occurs within minutes to hours after heart transplantation)
- Acute rejection (occur from the first week to several years after transplantation)
- Chronic rejection or late graft failure, which occurs months to years after transplantation, is mediated by antibodies. Sometimes chronic ischemia occurs due to progressive graft loss from ischemia.

Major concern in Heart transplant patients:

- Rejection
- Complications of Biopsy
- Cardiac allograft vasculopathy (CAV) [19]

Left and Right Atrium

- In heart transplant surgery using BAAT, anastomosis is performed between donor and recipient atrial tissues. Hence, echocardiography reveals biatrial enlargement.
- Left and right atria enlargement can be estimated in apical views, and sometimes a high-density edge is seen in 4-chamber view in the mid part of atrium, which indicates the site of anastomosis of donor and recipient tissues. In this technique, atrial enlargement increases the

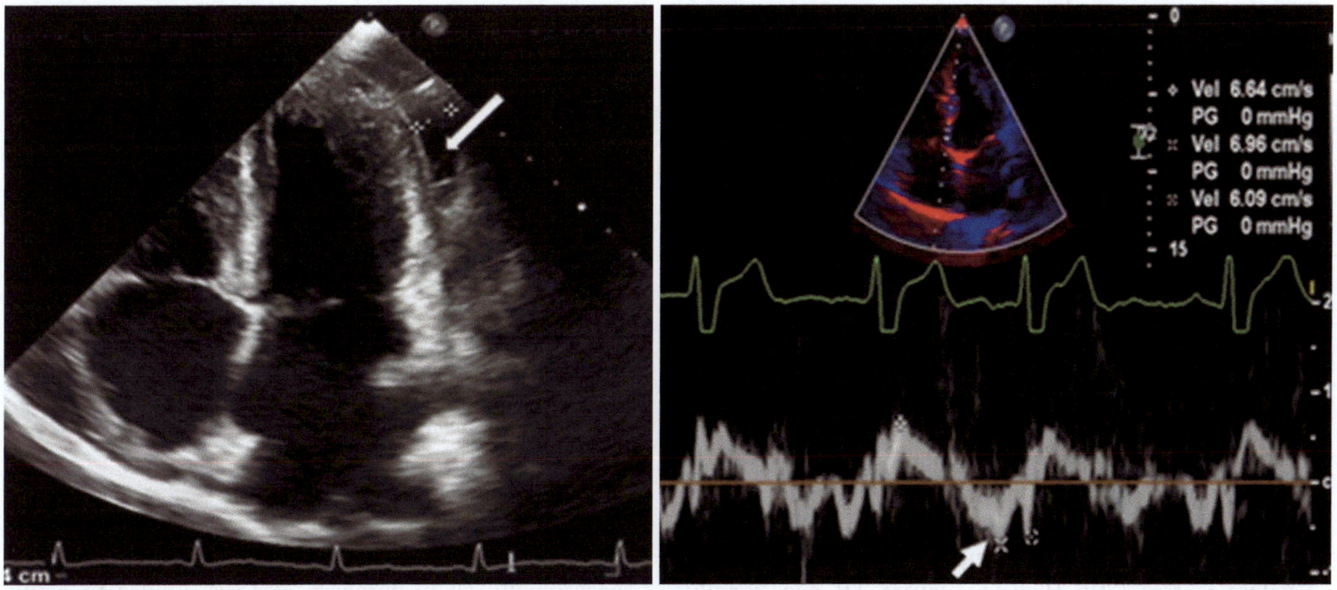

Fig. 34.4 New pericardial effusion and reduced Tissue-Doppler velocities after heart transplantation can be suggestive for transplant rejection

risk of atrial thrombosis [4]. Atrial anatomy is better preserved with BCAT approach, with negligible increase in longitudinal diameter and no clear change in atrium shape [25].

- In most patients, the RV is subjected to an increased pulmonary pressure immediately after transplantation, with the risk of acute right ventricular failure due to the afterload mismatch.
- Surgery techniques that maintain function of the right atrium (RA) can have beneficial effects on the function and stroke volume of the RV. In bicaval approach, where anatomy and size of RA are better preserved, RA will have a better contraction pattern, but in the standard OHT method, an asynchronous contraction is common between donor and recipient atrium [26].

Heart Valves

- The most common valve disorder following transplantation is tricuspid regurgitation (TR) seen in 19–84% of cases.
- Post-transplantation TR is dynamic in nature with two types of anatomical TR and functional TR.

Functional TR:

- Occurs due to impaired atrioventricular annulus geometry and annulus dilatation which ultimately leads to malcoaptation of the tricuspid valve (TV) leaflets and central jet TR.
- Etiologies of functional TR:
  - Biatrial anastomosis of donor and recipient,
  - RV dysfunction due to allograft rejection
  - Mismatch of recipient pericardial cavity and donor heart.
  - Transplant rejection rate corresponds with higher risk of TR.

Anatomical TR:

- Occurs due to disruption in TV apparatus, which includes rupture of chordae or leaflets. One of the most important causes of TR is endomyocardial biopsy, which predisposes the tricuspid valve to rupture or flail [27].
- Severity and prevalence of TR increase over the time after cardiac transplantation.
- Patients with moderate to severe TR have more RV dysfunction and symptoms compared to those with mild TR [28].
- Despite RV dysfunction and presence of TR in patients following transplantation, symptomatic right sided heart failure is rare [29]. However, severe TR occasionally causes developing RV dysfunction, and ultimately reduces cardiac index [30]. Sometimes patients will require Tricuspid valve surgery [29].
  - Atrioventricular valve regurgitation after heart transplantation is a common finding, which usually occurs early after transplantation due to such causes as poor lymphatic drainage and edema of transplanted heart that often disappears in the first 3 months following transplantation.
  - In some cases, myxomatous changes in donor valve or endocarditis cause atrioventricular regurgitation. In biatrial anastomosis method, there will be some degrees of Mitral regurgitation (MR) and TR due to mismatch in atrioventricular size, and ultimately dilatation of annulus of tricuspid and mitral valve [31–33].

Importance of Echocardiography in Endomyocardial Biopsy

- Acute allograft rejection is one of the main causes of post-transplantation mortality, which is estimated 13% in the first year following transplantation [34].
- An important measure that should be considered in heart transplant patients is transplant rejection assessments, where the gold standard for detecting rejection is myocardial biopsy of the right ventricle and histopathologic examination of samples [35].
- Endomyocardial biopsy is performed under fluoroscopic or echocardiographic guide or both with some limitation for both methods. Fluoroscopy does not show soft tissues and sometimes by echocardiography, it is difficult to find the tip of bioptome, and biopsy should be performed cautiously.
- More advanced techniques such as three-dimensional echocardiography (3DE) may allow visualization of the biopsy equipment and cardiac structures better then two-dimensional echocardiography (2DE) [36].
- Biopsy from various sites such as septum, apex, and right ventricular free wall is possible if guided by echocardiography. Echocardiography reduces biopsy complications such as TV damage and ventricular perforation. Furthermore, echocardiography facilitates assessment of biopsy complications such as pericardial effusion [37].

Coronary Artery Vasculopathy Following Heart Transplantation

- Coronary artery vasculopathy is clearly different from native coronary artery atherosclerosis. Although allografts occasionally show coronary stenosis similar to native coronary artery, in most cases, vasculopathy is diffuse in transplanted heart and causes concentric stenosis of large epicardial and small endocardial arteries [38].

- Cardiac allograft vasculopathy (CAV) is a rapidly progressive disease of coronary arteries that often manifests as intimal proliferation in early stages and luminal stenosis of coronary arteries in later stages, and ultimately leads to ischemia and myocardial infarction. CAV is one of the causes of death in early years following heart transplantation.
- The pathogenesis of vasculopathy of transplanted heart is complex and heterogeneous. Immunological and non-immunological factors cause endothelial damage and ultimately coronary artery disease. However, there is a risk of a potential interaction between donor heart and recipient's risk factors in patients with history of ischemic cardiomyopathy. Immunologic factors appear to be vitally important in CAV pathogenesis, especially in the first year following transplantation [39].
- Detection of donor CAV is performed using:
  - Angiography which is invasive methods
  - Intravascular ultrasound (IVUS), still considered as a sensitive method which allows direct observation of vessel wall morphology, and also a method for assessing early stages of CAV. IVUS cannot assess all epicardial coronary arteries [40].
  - Non-invasive technique: dobutamine stress echocardiography (DSE).
- Stress echocardiography with exercise in heart transplant recipients has limited accuracy, due to reduced chronotropic response to physiological exercise in these patients [41]. Sometimes, wall motion abnormalities are observed in stress echocardiography, while visible lesion cannot be seen in epicardial arteries, which may be due to involvement of small arteries or endothelial dysfunction. Moreover, the absence of collateral arteries may cause functional abnormalities [40].
- DSE is a valuable method for detecting CAV compare to IVUS as a gold standard method with high sensitive and specificity in detecting CAV [14].
- Ultimately, the results of IVUS and dobutamine stress echocardiography have prognostic value in recipients [40].
- Current consensuses suggest that both stress echocardiography and myocardial perfusion imaging may be useful in detection of CAV in patients who are not candidate for invasive evaluation.

Questions

1. Each of the following conditions can result in persistent restrictive physiology after cardiac transplant EXCEPT
   A. Systemic hypertension
   B. Severe mitral regurgitation
   C. Ischemic fibrosis
   D. Transplant rejection
2. Each of the following statements regarding cardiac transplant rejection is true EXEPT
   A. Reduced stroke volume
   B. Reduced LV posterior wall thickness
   C. Reduced systolic circumferential strains
   D. Reduced global longitudinal strain
3. Which of the following is the most common valve disorder after cardiac transplantation?
   A. Tricuspid valve regurgitation
   B. Aortic valve regurgitation
   C. Pulmonary valve regurgitation
   D. Mitral valve regurgitation
4. All of the following conditions are associated with functional TR after orthotopic heart transplantation EXCEPT
   A. RV dysfunction due to allograft rejection
   B. Mismatch of recipient pericardial cavity and donor heart
   C. Biatrial anastomosis of donor and recipient
   D. Flail of tricuspid valve due to endomyocardial biopsy

Answers

1. B
2. B
3. A
4. D

References

1. Kadner A, Chen RH, Adams DH. Heterotopic heart transplantation: experimental development and clinical experience. Eur J Cardiothorac Surg. 2000;17(4):474–81.
2. Davies RR, Russo MJ, Morgan JA, Sorabella RA, Naka Y, Chen JM. Standard versus bicaval techniques for orthotopic heart transplantation: an analysis of the United Network for Organ Sharing database. J Thorac Cardiovasc Surg. 2010;140(3):700–8, 8.e1-2.
3. Mann D, Zipes D, Libby P, Bonow R. Braunwald's heart disease: a textbook of cardiovascular medicine, Single Volume. 10th ed. Philadelphia: Elsevier/Saunders; 2014. p. 2040.
4. Mondillo S, Maccherini M, Galderisi M. Usefulness and limitations of transthoracic echocardiography in heart transplantation recipients. Cardiovasc Ultrasound. 2008;6:2.
5. Stehlik J, Edwards LB, Kucheryavaya AY, Benden C, Christie JD, Dipchand AI, et al. The Registry of the International Society for Heart and Lung Transplantation: 29th official adult heart transplant report—2012. J Heart Lung Transplant. 2012;31(10):1052–64.
6. Costanzo MR, Augustine S, Bourge R, Bristow M, O'Connell JB, Driscoll D, et al. Selection and treatment of candidates for heart transplantation. A statement for health professionals from the Committee on Heart Failure and Cardiac Transplantation of the Council on Clinical Cardiology, American Heart Association. Circulation. 1995;92(12):3593–612.
7. Brock MV, Salazar JD, Cameron DE, Baumgartner WA, Conte JV. The changing profile of the cardiac donor. J Heart Lung Transplant. 2001;20(9):1005–9.

8. Venkateswaran RV, Bonser RS, Steeds RP. The echocardiographic assessment of donor heart function prior to cardiac transplantation. Eur J Echocardiogr. 2005;6(4):260–3.
9. Sopko N, Shea KJ, Ludrosky K, Smedira N, Hoercher K, Taylor DO, et al. Survival is not compromised in donor hearts with echocardiographic abnormalities. J Surg Res. 2007;143(1):141–4.
10. Kilic A, Emani S, Sai-Sudhakar CB, Higgins RSD, Whitson BA. Donor selection in heart transplantation. J Thorac Dis. 2014;6(8):1097–104.
11. Wever Pinzon O, Stoddard G, Drakos SG, Gilbert EM, Nativi JN, Budge D, et al. Impact of donor left ventricular hypertrophy on survival after heart transplant. Am J Transplant. 2011;11(12):2755–61.
12. Kettner J, Dorazilova Z, Netuka I, Maly J, Al-Hiti H, Melenovsky V, et al. Is severe pulmonary hypertension a contraindication for orthotopic heart transplantation? Not any more. Physiol Res. 2011;60(5):769–75.
13. Temporelli PL, Scapellato F, Eleuteri E, Imparato A, Giannuzzi P. Doppler echocardiography in advanced systolic heart failure: a noninvasive alternative to Swan-Ganz catheter. Circ Heart Fail. 2010;3(3):387–94.
14. Otto CM. The practice of clinical echocardiography. 5th ed. Philadelphia: Saunders; 2017. p. 577–95.
15. Kuppahally SS, Michaels AD, Tandar A, Gilbert EM, Litwin SE, Bader FM. Can echocardiographic evaluation of cardiopulmonary hemodynamics decrease right heart catheterizations in end-stage heart failure patients awaiting transplantation? Am J Cardiol. 2010;106(11):1657–62.
16. Stetson SJ, Perez-Verdia A, Mazur W, Farmer JA, Koerner MM, Weilbaecher DG, et al. Cardiac hypertrophy after transplantation is associated with persistent expression of tumor necrosis factor-alpha. Circulation. 2001;104(6):676–81.
17. Angermann CE, Spes CH, Willems S, Dominiak P, Kemkes BM, Theisen K. Regression of left ventricular hypertrophy in hypertensive heart transplant recipients treated with enalapril, furosemide, and verapamil. Circulation. 1991;84(2):583–93.
18. Corcos T, Tamburino C, Léger P, Vaissier E, Rossant P, Mattei M-F, et al. Early and late hemodynamic evaluation after cardiac transplantation: a study of 28 cases. J Am Coll Cardiol. 1988;11(2):264–9.
19. Mann DL, Zipes DP, Libby P, Bonow RO. Braunwald's heart disease: a textbook of cardiovascular medicine. 10th ed. Philadelphia: Saunders; 2014. p. 575–88.
20. Stengel SM, Allemann Y, Zimmerli M, Lipp E, Kucher N, Mohacsi P, et al. Doppler tissue imaging for assessing left ventricular diastolic dysfunction in heart transplant rejection. Heart. 2001;86(4):432–7.
21. Bellenger NG, Marcus NJ, Davies C, Yacoub M, Banner NR, Pennell DJ. Left ventricular function and mass after orthotopic heart transplantation: a comparison of cardiovascular magnetic resonance with echocardiography. J Heart Lung Transplant. 2000;19(5):444–52.
22. Mingo-Santos S, Monivas-Palomero V, Garcia-Lunar I, Mitroi CD, Goirigolzarri-Artaza J, Rivero B, et al. Usefulness of two-dimensional strain parameters to diagnose acute rejection after heart transplantation. J Am Soc Echocardiogr. 2015;28(10):1149–56.
23. Sera F, Kato TS, Farr M, Russo C, Jin Z, Marboe CC, et al. Left ventricular longitudinal strain by speckle-tracking echocardiography is associated with treatment-requiring cardiac allograft rejection. J Card Fail. 2014;20(5):359–64.
24. Lu W, Zheng J, Pan X, Sun L. Diagnostic performance of echocardiography for the detection of acute cardiac allograft rejection: a systematic review and meta-analysis. PLoS One. 2015;10(3):e0121228.
25. Thorn EM, de Filippi CR. Echocardiography in the cardiac transplant recipient. Heart Fail Clin. 2007;3(1):51–67.
26. Aziz T, Burgess M, Khafagy R, Hann AW, Campbell C, Rahman A, et al. Bicaval and standard techniques in orthotopic heart transplantation: medium-term experience in cardiac performance and survival. J Thorac Cardiovasc Surg. 1999;118(1):115–22.
27. Wong RC, Abrahams Z, Hanna M, Pangrace J, Gonzalez-Stawinski G, Starling R, et al. Tricuspid regurgitation after cardiac transplantation: an old problem revisited. J Heart Lung Transplant. 2008;27(3):247–52.
28. Kalra N, Copeland JG, Sorrell VL. Tricuspid regurgitation after orthotopic heart transplantation. Echocardiography. 2010;27(1):1–4.
29. Wilhelmi M, Pethig K, Wilhelmi M, Nguyen H, Struber M, Haverich A. Heart transplantation: echocardiographic assessment of morphology and function after more than 10 years of follow-up. Ann Thorac Surg. 2002;74(4):1075–9. discussion 9.
30. Chan MC, Giannetti N, Kato T, Kornbluth M, Oyer P, Valantine HA, et al. Severe tricuspid regurgitation after heart transplantation. J Heart Lung Transplant. 2001;20(7):709–17.
31. Bouma W, Brugemann J, Hamer IJ, Klinkenberg TJ, Koene BM, Kuijpers M, et al. Mitral valve repair and redo repair for mitral regurgitation in a heart transplant recipient. J Cardiothorac Surg. 2012;7:100.
32. Fernandez J, Babadjanov D, Farivar RS. Mitral and tricuspid valve repair 21 years after cardiac transplantation. J Thorac Cardiovasc Surg. 2010;140(1):e3–4.
33. Wijburg ER, Balk AH, van Herwerden LA. Double valve repair in a transplanted heart. J Thorac Cardiovasc Surg. 1998;115(1):250–1.
34. Doering LV, Hickey K, Pickham D, Chen B, Drew BJ. Remote noninvasive allograft rejection monitoring for heart transplant recipients: study protocol for the novel evaluation with home electrocardiogram and remote transmission (NEW HEART) study. BMC Cardiovasc Disord. 2012;12:14.
35. Roshanali F, Mandegar MH, Bagheri J, Sarzaeem MR, Chitsaz S, Alaeddini F, et al. Echo rejection score: new echocardiographic approach to diagnosis of heart transplant rejection. Eur J Cardiothorac Surg. 2010;38(2):176–80.
36. From AM, Maleszewski JJ, Rihal CS. Current status of endomyocardial biopsy. Mayo Clin Proc. 2011;86(11):1095–102.
37. Nguyen CT, Lee E, Luo H, Siegel RJ. Echocardiographic guidance for diagnostic and therapeutic percutaneous procedures. Cardiovasc Diagn Ther. 2011;1(1):11–36.
38. Smart FW, Ballantyne CM, Cocanougher B, Farmer JA, Sekela ME, Noon GP, et al. Insensitivity of noninvasive tests to detect coronary artery vasculopathy after heart transplant. Am J Cardiol. 1991;67(4):243–7.
39. Guddeti RR, Matsuo Y, Matsuzawa Y, Aoki T, Lennon RJ, Lerman LO, et al. Ischemic cardiomyopathy is associated with coronary plaque progression and higher event rate in patients after cardiac transplantation. J Am Heart Assoc. 2014;3(4):e001091.
40. Spes CH, Klauss V, Rieber J, Schnaack SD, Tammen AR, Uberfuhr P, et al. Functional and morphological findings in heart transplant recipients with a normal coronary angiogram: an analysis by dobutamine stress echocardiography, intracoronary Doppler and intravascular ultrasound. J Heart Lung Transplant. 1999;18(5):391–8.
41. Spes CH, Mudra H, Schnaack SD, Klauss V, Reichle FM, Uberfuhr P, et al. Dobutamine stress echocardiography for noninvasive diagnosis of cardiac allograft vasculopathy: a comparison with angiography and intravascular ultrasound. Am J Cardiol. 1996;78(2):168–74.
42. Bolman RM III. Heart Transplantation Technique. Oper Tech Thorac Cardiovasc Surg. 1999;4(2):98–113.
43. Kitamura S, Nakatani T, Kato T, Yanase M, Kobayashi J, Nakajima H, et al. Hemodynamic and echocardiographic evaluation of orthotopic heart transplantation with the modified bicaval anastomosis technique. Circ J. 2009;73(7):1235–9.
44. Locali RF, Matsuoka PK, Cherbo T, Gabriel EA, Buffolo E. Should biatrial heart transplantation still be performed?: a meta-analysis. Arq Bras Cardiol. 2010;94(6):829–40.
45. Stehlik J, Edwards LB, Kucheryavaya AY, Aurora P, Christie JD, Kirk R, et al. The Registry of the International Society for Heart and Lung Transplantation: twenty-seventh official adult heart transplant report—2010. J Heart Lung Transplant. 2010;29(10):1089–103.

Echocardiography in Patients with Ventricular Assist Devices

35

Anita Sadeghpour and Azin Alizadehasl

Abstract

Cardiac assist devices and mechanical circulatory supports (MCSs) play an important role in the management of end-stage heart disease.

MCSs are mechanical pumps to support or replace the ventricular heart function.

In patients who are candidate for MCSs implantation: echocardiography is the first-line imaging modality for patient selection, pre implantation, during implantation and after implantation to optimize the device settings. In this chapter, we will review role of echocardiography in patients who are candidate for ventricular assist devices (VADs) implantation.

Keywords

Echocardiography · Ventricular assist devices · Biventricular assist devices · Right ventricular assist devices · Left ventricular assist devices (LVADs) · Inflow-cannula abnormality · Pump malfunction · Pump arrest

Abbreviations

ASE	American society of echocardiography
AV	Aortic valve
CFI	Color flow imaging
FDA	Food and drug administration
LVAD	Left ventricular assist device
LVADs	Left ventricular assist devices
LVEF	Left ventricular ejection fraction
LVIDd	Left ventricular internal diameter
MCSs	Mechanical circulatory supports
MR	Mitral regurgitation
MV	Mitral valve
PFO	Patent foramen ovales
RV	Right ventricular
TEE	Transesophageal echocardiography
TTE	Transthoracic echocardiography
VADs	Ventricular assist devices

Cardiac assist devices and mechanical circulatory supports (MCSs) play an important role in the management of end-stage heart disease.

MCSs are mechanical pumps to support or replace the ventricular heart function. The following indications for MCS implantation have been approved: bridge to recovery, bridge to transplantation and destination therapy. In patients who are candidate for MCSs implantation: echocardiography is the first-line imaging modality for patient selection, pre implantation, during implantation and after implantation to optimize the device settings. Comprehensive echocardiography should be perform in patients who are candidate for ventricular assist devices (VADs) implantation, to evaluate any structural and/or functional abnormalities which may exclude LVAD implantation or need more intervention before surgical planning.

- Cardiac assist devices and mechanical circulatory supports (MCSs) play an important role in the management of end-stage heart disease.
- MCSs are mechanical pumps to support or replace the ventricular heart function. Usually, short-term devices are located outside the body (extracorporeal) and durable long-term devices are intracorporeal and implanted in the body.
- U.S. Food and Drug Administration (FDA) has approved the following indications for MCSs [1, 2]:
  1. **Bridge to recovery** (one of the most common indications of MCSs): Recommended in patients with reversible myocardial injury, including:

A. Sadeghpour, MD, FACC, FASE
Professor of Cardiology, Echocardiography Research Center, Rajaie Cardiovascular Medical and Research Center, Iran University of Medical Science, Tehran, Iran

A. Alizadehasl, MD, FACC, FASE (✉)
Associate Professor of Cardiology, Echocardiologist, Echocardiography and Cardiogenetic Research Centers, Cardio-Oncology Department, Rajaie Cardiovascular Medical and Research Center, Tehran, Iran

A. Sadeghpour, A. Alizadehasl (eds.), *Case-Based Textbook of Echocardiography*,
https://doi.org/10.1007/978-3-319-67691-3_35

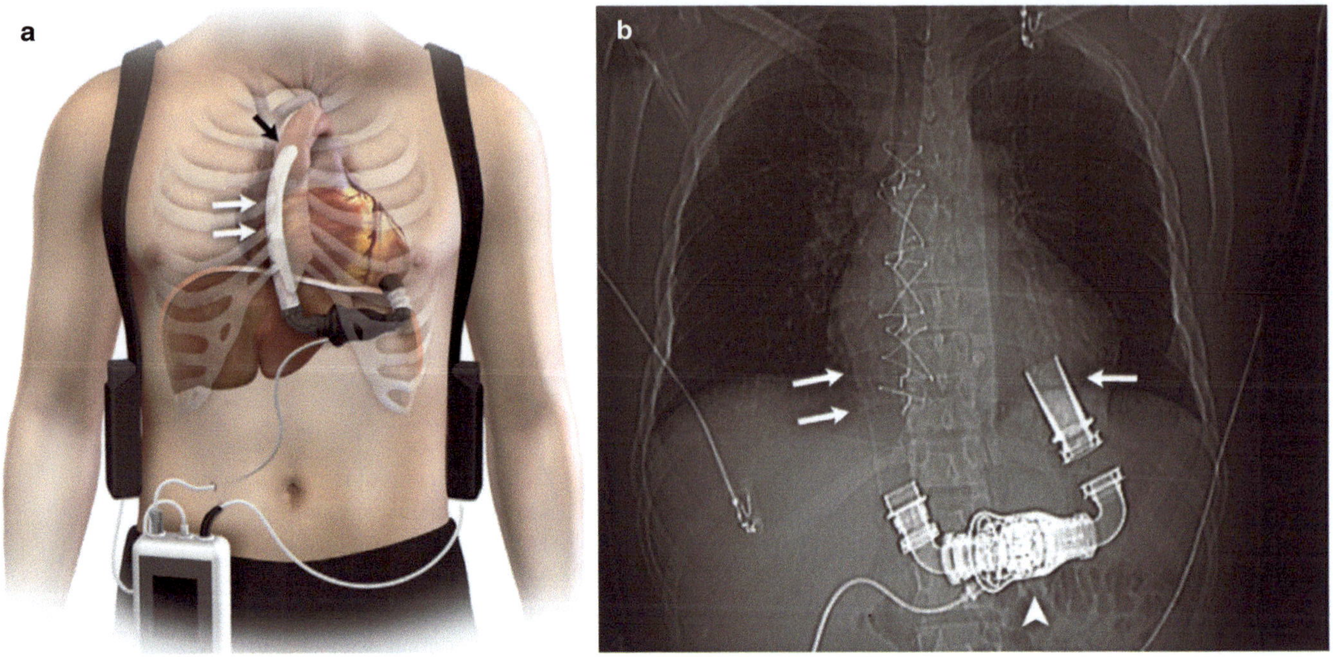

Fig. 35.1 (**a**) Drawing of the HM-II LVAD, showing the subdiaphragmatic pump location, right parasternal outflow-graft position (double white arrows), and outflow graft-to-ascending aorta anastomosis (black arrow). (**b**) X-ray CT scout image showing the anatomic relationship between the left ventricle and the device inflow cannula (single arrow), impeller housing (arrowhead), and outflow graft (double arrows), controller (white box), battery packs (black boxes). Permission from Stainback R, Estep JD, Agler DA, Birks EJ, Bremer M, Hung J et al. Echocardiography in the management of patients with left ventricular assist devices: recommendations from the American Society of Echocardiography. J Am Soc Echocardiogr. 2015;28:853–909

   (a) Acute myocarditis
   (b) Acute myocardial infarction
   (c) Post cardiac cardiogenic shock
2. **Bridge to transplantation**: Indicated in patients with advanced heart failure, low probable reversible myocardial injury, and candidates for heart transplantation such as those with chronic valvular, ischemic, or idiopathic conditions.
3. **Destination therapy**: Indicated in patients with chronic irreversible heart failure and refractory symptoms who meet the following criteria:
   (a) Stable hemodynamic
   (b) No manifestations of significant organ injury, debilitation, or cachexia
   (c) Not candidated for heart transplantation
   (d) Significant functional limitations (NYHA FC IIIB or IV) in the past 45 days despite optimal tolerated medical treatment
   (e) Left ventricular ejection fraction (LVEF) < 25%
   (f) Peak exercise oxygen consumption (peak VO_2) $\leq$ 14 mL/kg/min

- MCSs or ventricular assist devices (VADs) have been classified as:
  1. Biventricular assist devices
  2. Right ventricular (RV) assist devices
  3. Left ventricular assist devices (LVADs)
- Most implanted VADs consist of inflow cannula, outflow cannula, pump, power supply, and controller.
  1. There are 2 FDA-approved continuous flow LVADs in adults: the Heart Mate II (HM-II) (Fig. 35.1) and the HVAD (Heart Ware), which have 3 components:
     (a) LV inflow cannula (most often connected to the LV apex)
     (b) Outflow graft cannula (most often attached to the ascending aorta)
     (c) Mechanical impeller
- Following hemodynamic criteria associated with acute myocardial injury have been suggested for implanting MCSs [1, 2]:
  1. Cardiac index <1.8 to 2.2 L/min/m^2
  2. Systolic blood pressure < 90 mmHg
  3. Pulmonary capillary wedge pressure > 20 mmHg
  4. Right atrial pressure > 18–20 mmHg
  5. Evidence of poor tissue perfusion (renal, hepatic, and brain dysfunction), despite optimal medical management
     - Different types of assist devices can provide *bridge to recovery*; they include:
       – Intra-aortic balloon pumps
       – VADs
       – Extracorporeal membrane oxygenation
- Recently, the American Society of Echocardiography (ASE) has published a new guideline focusing on the role of echocardiography in LVADs [3].

Echocardiography is the Key Imaging Modality in the Following of Different Stages

A. Patient selection and pre implantation of MCSs
B. During implantation: To guide proper surgical insertion and to optimize the initial device settings
C. After implantation: To evaluate the native heart, subclinical device dysfunction, and device settings
D. At follow-up: To evaluate the causes of device alarms and ventricular function.
   - Generally, transthoracic echocardiography (TTE) is the 1st-line imaging modality for screening VAD candidates.
   - In acute and emergency situations or inadequate TTE findings, transesophageal echocardiography (TEE) can be performed.
   - Echocardiography should be performed by an expert echocardiographer, who is familiar with MCSs, advanced heart failure, and hemodynamic assessment.

- **Patient selection and pre implantation assessment:**
  - Patients who are candidate for LVADs need comprehensive echocardiography for any structural and/or functional abnormalities which may exclude LVAD implantation or which may need more intervention before surgical planning. The following high-risk parameters require particular attention and consideration [2, 3] (Table 35.1):

    I. **Ventricular function**
      - Majority of patients who are candidated for LVADs have severe LV systolic dysfunction, and an LVEF below 25% is the cut point for destination therapy in many centers.
      - LV size, LVEF, and cardiac output should be measured by the most accurate available method in the echo lab such as 3D echocardiography if it is available or the modified Simpson method by 2D echocardiography. Enhancing endocardial definition by contrast agents should be strongly considered for precise LVEF measurement [4, 5].
      - Measurement of the end-diastolic left ventricular internal diameter (LVIDd) by 2D echocardiography in the parasternal long-axis view is an important parameter for LVAD candidates.
      - Small LV cavity defined as an LVIDd smaller than 63 mm has been suggested as a predictor for a worse outcome after LVAD implantation [6].
      - Comparison of the LVIDd between pre and post LVAD implantation helps to assess the degree of LVAD-mediated of LV unloading.

Table 35.1 Preimplantation TTE/TEE "red-flag" findings

Left ventricle and interventricular septum
Small LV size, particularly with increased LV trabeculation
LV thrombus
LV apical aneurysm
Ventricular septal defect
Right ventricle
RV dilatation
RV systolic dysfunction
Atria, interatrial septum, and inferior vena cava
Left atrial appendage thrombus
PFO (Patent foramen ovales) or atrial septal defect
Valvular abnormalities
Any prosthetic valve (especially mechanical AV or MV)
> mild AR
≥moderate MS
≥ moderate TR or > mild TS
> mild PS; ≥ moderate PR
Other
Any congenital heart disease
Aortic pathology: aneurysm, dissection, atheroma, coarctation
Mobile mass lesion
Other shunts: patent ductus arteriosus, intrapulmonary

AR aortic regurgitation, *AV* aortic valve, *LV* left ventricular, *MS* mitral stenosis, *MV* mitral valve, *PFO* patent foramen ovale, *PR* pulmonary regurgitation, *PS* pulmonary stenosis, *RV* right ventricle, *TR* tricuspid regurgitation, *TS* tricuspid regurgitation

Permission from Stainback R, Estep JD, Agler DA, Birks EJ, Bremer M, Hung J et al. Echocardiography in the management of patients with left ventricular assist devices: recommendations from the American Society of Echocardiography. J Am Soc Echocardiogr. 2015;28:853–909

    II. **Intracardiac thrombi**
      - Presence of intracardiac thrombi increases the risk of embolic stroke during the LV apex cannulation, which can be removed by the implanting surgeon.

    III. **Right ventricular dysfunction**
      - Assessment of RV systolic function is critically important as the RV failure can cause significant morbidity and mortality (about 10–30%) in LVAD-implanted patients.
      - Quantitative evaluation of the RV size and systolic function and at a minimum, qualitative assessment besides the evaluation of tricuspid regurgitation severity should be done (Chap. 14).
      - Preoperative diagnosis of the RV systolic dysfunction may change the plan of LVAD implantation to the biventricular VAD for better outcomes [7].
      - RV enlargement and systolic dysfunction, high right atrial pressure based on a dilated inferior vena cava size and reduced collapsibility, and moderate or more tricuspid regurgitation are the echocardiographic keys of the RV dysfunction.

IV. **Valve stenosis**
  - Moderate or severe mitral stenosis should be corrected before LVAD insertion as it can prevent a sufficient flow through the cannula inflow.
  - Conversely, any degree of aortic stenosis can be tolerated as the LVAD bypasses the LV outflow tract.

V. **Valve regurgitation**
  - Assessment of aortic regurgitation severity before LVAD implantation is critically important.
  - Significant aortic regurgitation creates a "blind" loop as the flow enters the LVAD from the LV apex and is pumped into the ascending aorta. However, in patients with significant aortic regurgitation, the flow reverses into the LV and again into the LVAD.
  - It is important to know that, in the setting of advanced heart failure, reduced LV stroke volume, and high LV end-diastolic pressure, the accurate estimation of aortic regurgitation severity is not easy and color Doppler study may be unimpressive. So whenever possible, the regurgitant fraction should be calculated.
  - **Mitral regurgitation** Any degree of mitral regurgitation, even when it is significant, is acceptable and markedly improves after LVAD implantation. LVADs reduce the LV filling pressures and the LV size and improve mitral coaptation [3].
  - **Tricuspid regurgitation** In contrast to mitral regurgitation, the presence of at last moderate tricuspid regurgitation can be a marker of the RV dysfunction and surgical repair should be considered at the time of LVAD implantation [8].
  - **Pulmonary regurgitation**

- Significant pulmonary regurgitation can be tolerated in the setting of a good RV function and successful LVAD implantation, but it will require repair before the implantation of right ventricular assist devices.

VI. **Prosthetic valves**
  - Even normally functioning mechanical prosthetic aortic valves should be replaced with a bioprosthesis because the LVAD support will reduce the forward flow through the aortic valve prosthesis and will increase the risk of thrombosis and thromboembolic events.

VII. **Congenital heart disease**
  - Any type of congenital heart disease, even the complex one, is not a contraindication for VAD implantation. However, patent foramen ovales, ventricular septal defects, and other intracardiac shunts can cause arterial oxygen desaturation after VAD implantation and should be repaired at the time of VAD implantation.
  - For the evaluation of ventricular septal defects using color flow study and patent foramen ovales, intravenous agitated saline with provocative maneuvers such as the Valsalva is necessary.

VIII. **Acute and active endocarditis**

- Any mobile mass suggestive of vegetation and acute infective endocarditis is a high-risk finding and can be an absolute contraindication for VADs [8].

Intraprocedural TEE

- Comprehensive perioperative TEE is necessary to evaluate and confirm the undiagnosed or underappreciated abnormal findings with more focus on
  - Aortic regurgitation severity, tricuspid regurgitation severity, and RV function
  - Intracardiac shunts and patent foramen ovales
  - Presence of intracardiac thrombi

Intraoperative TEE During LVAD Implantation

TEE detects intracardiac air that occurs during LVAD implantation and is useful for establishing successful de-airing maneuvers (Table 35.2).

Inflow cannula: The inflow cannula is implanted in the LV apex toward the mitral valve Fig. 35.2; however, some angulation toward the interventricular septum may be seen.

Using simultaneous X-plane imaging and real-time 3D echocardiography can be helpful in positioning the LV inflow cannula. Proper alignment of the inflow cannula should be confirmed by color flow imaging and pulsed-wave study, which shows a low-velocity laminar systolic dominant flow usually equal to or smaller than 1.5 m/s [9].

Outflow graft: The distal part of the outflow graft to the aorta anastomosis can be seen by color flow imaging in the majority of the patients. The flow from the outflow graft into the aorta can be visualized by color flow imaging at the right pulmonary artery level. A peak systolic velocity of more than 2 m/s by continuous-wave Doppler study needs more investigation as an abnormal finding.

Pump speed: The optimization of the pump speed is not easy and the selection of the optimal speed setting differs between the centers, with some centers optimizing the pump speed that minimizes the LV end-diastolic volume and/or the LVIDd with intermittent aortic valve opening and others optimizing the speed to maximize the LV unloading and

Table 35.2 Post LVAD implantation complications detected by echocardiography

Pericardial effusion with or without cardiac tamponade including RV compression
LV failure secondary to partial LV unloading
RV failure
Inadequate LV filling or excessive LV unloading (small LV dimensions typically <3 cm and/or marked deviation of interventricular septum towards LV) may be due to RV failure and/or pump speed too high for loading conditions
LVAD suction with induced ventricular ectopy
LVAD-related continuous aortic insufficiency clinically significant—at least moderate and possibly severe—characterized by an AR proximal jet-to-LVOT height ratio > 46%, or AR vena contracta ≥3 mm; increased LV size
LVAD-related mitral regurgitation
a. Primary: inflow cannula interference with mitral apparatus
b. Secondary: MR-functional, related to partial LV unloading/persistent heart failure
Intracardiac thrombus
Inflow-cannula abnormality: high-velocity color or spectral Doppler at inflow orifice
Results from malposition, suction event/other inflow obstruction: aliased color-flow Doppler, CW Doppler velocity > 1.5 m/s
Low-velocity inflow (markedly reduced peak systolic and nadir diastolic velocities) may indicate internal inflow-cannula thrombosis or more distal obstruction within the system
Pump malfunction/pump arrest:
a. Reduced inflow-cannula or outflow-graft flow velocities on color and spectral Doppler or, with pump arrest, shows diastolic flow reversal
b. Signs of worsening HF: including dilated LV, worsening MR, worsened TR, and/or increased TR velocity

2D two-dimensional, *3D* three-dimensional, *A* mitral valve late peak diastolic velocity, *AR* aortic regurgitation, *AV* aortic valve, *BP* blood pressure, *CW* continuous-wave, *E* mitral valve early peak diastolic velocity, mitral annular velocity, *HVAD* HeartWare ventricular assist device, *IVC* inferior vena cava, *LV* left ventricular, *LVAD* left ventricular assist device, *LVOT* left ventricular outflow tract, *MR* mitral regurgitation, *MV* mitral valve, *RAP* right atrial pressure, *RV* right ventricular, *RVOT* right ventricular outflow tract, *SV* stroke volume, *TR* tricuspid regurgitation

Adopted and modified from Estep et al. permission from Stainback R, Estep JD, Agler DA, Birks EJ, Bremer M, Hung J et al. Echocardiography in the management of patients with left ventricular assist devices: recommendations from the American Society of Echocardiography. J Am Soc Echocardiogr. 2015;28:853–909

leaving the aortic valve closed, which is best assessed by M-mode echocardiography [3].

Surveillance Echocardiography

Patients with successful LVAD implantation need follow-up echocardiography at certain scheduled intervals: before hospital discharge or approximately 2 weeks after implantation, followed by surveillance TTE at 1, 3, 6, and 12 months after device implantation and then every 6–12 months [3, 10].

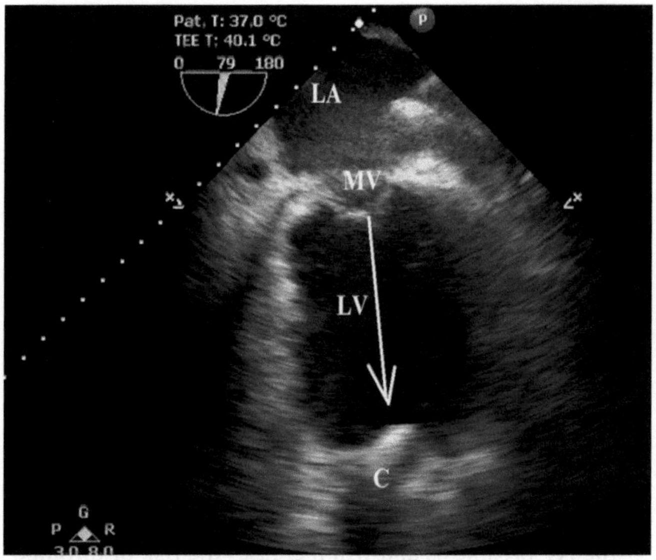

Fig. 35.2 Abnormal implanted inflow cannula in the LV apex (the orientation is not toward the MV inflow) and should be re positioned toward MV inflow. *LA* left atrium, *LV* left ventricle, *MV* mitral valve, *C* cannula

Questions

1. In evaluation of a patient with past medical history of heart valve replacement and now is candidate for left ventricular assist device (LVAD) implantation, which of the following strategy is the best management:
   A. In normally functioning Mitral valve (MV) mechanical prostheses, replacement with a bioprosthesis should be considered.
   B. In normally functioning Aortic valve mechanical prostheses, replacement with a bioprosthesis should be considered.
   C. In abnormal functioning Mitral valve (MV) prostheses with significant MR replacement with a bioprosthesis should be considered.
   D. Abnormal functioning aortic valve bioprostheses with significant AR do not require AV replacement.

2. In pre implantation left ventricular assist device (LVAD) evaluation, which of the following abnormality do not require any therapeutic intervention:
   A. Ventricular septal defect
   B. Patent foramen ovale (PFO)
   C. Moderate mitral stenosis
   D. Moderate mitral regurgitation(MR)

3. Which of the following findings in post LVAD implantation is abnormal:

A. Position of inflow cannula in the LV apex towards the MV with mild angulation to the inter ventricular septum
B. High velocity flow through the inflow cannula detected by Doppler study
C. LV unloading with continuous closed aortic valve
D. LV unloading with intermittent AV opening

Answers

1. B
   Even normally functioning mechanical prosthetic aortic valve (AV) should be replaced with a bioprosthesis, since the LVAD support will reduce the forward flow through the AV prosthesis and will increases the risk of thrombosis and thromboembolic events.
2. D
   Any degree of MR even significant MR is acceptable and markedly improves after LVAD implantation. LVAD reduces LV filling pressures, LV size and improves mitral coaptation.
3. B
   Proper alignment of the inflow cannula should be confirmed by Color flow imaging (CFI) and pulse wave study which shows a low-velocity laminar systolic dominant flow usually ≤1.5 m/s.

References

1. Bonow RO, Mann DL, Zipes DP, Libby P. Braunwald's heart disease: a textbook of cardiovascular medicine. Philadelphia: Elsevier Health Sciences; 2011.
2. Otto CM. The practice of clinical echocardiography. 5th ed. Philadelphia, PA: Elsevier Health Sciences; 2017.
3. Stainback RF, Estep JD, Agler DA, Birks EJ, Bremer M, Hung J, et al. Echocardiography in the management of patients with left ventricular assist devices: recommendations from the American Society of Echocardiography. J Am Soc Echocardiogr. 2015;28(8):853–909.
4. Lang RM, Badano LP, Mor-Avi V, Afilalo J, Armstrong A, Ernande L, et al. Recommendations for cardiac chamber quantification by echocardiography in adults: an update from the American Society of Echocardiography and the European Association of Cardiovascular Imaging. J Am Soc Echocardiogr. 2015;28(1):1–39. e14
5. Porter TR, Abdelmoneim S, Belcik JT, McCulloch ML, Mulvagh SL, Olson JJ, et al. Guidelines for the cardiac sonographer in the performance of contrast echocardiography: a focused update from the American Society of Echocardiography. J Am Soc Echocardiogr. 2014;27(8):797–810.
6. Topilsky Y, JK O, Shah DK, Boilson BA, Schirger JA, Kushwaha SS, et al. Echocardiographic predictors of adverse outcomes after continuous left ventricular assist device implantation. J Am Coll Cardiol Img. 2011;4(3):211–22.
7. Fitzpatrick JR, Frederick JR, Hiesinger W, Hsu VM, McCormick RC, Kozin ED, et al. Early planned institution of biventricular mechanical circulatory support results in improved outcomes compared with delayed conversion of a left ventricular assist device to a biventricular assist device. J Thorac Cardiovasc Surg. 2009;137(4):971–7.
8. Feldman D, Pamboukian SV, Teuteberg JJ, Birks E, Lietz K, Moore SA, et al. The 2013 International Society for Heart and Lung Transplantation Guidelines for mechanical circulatory support: executive summary. J Heart Lung Transplant. 2013;32(2):157–87.
9. Ammar KA, Umland MM, Kramer C, Sulemanjee N, Jan MF, Khandheria BK, et al. The ABCs of left ventricular assist device echocardiography: a systematic approach. Eur Heart J Cardiovasc Imaging. 2012;13(11):885–99.
10. Raina A, Vaidya A, Gertz ZM, Chambers S, Forfia PR. Marked changes in right ventricular contractile pattern after cardiothoracic surgery: implications for post-surgical assessment of right ventricular function. J Heart Lung Transplant. 2013;32(8):777–83.

36 Cardiac Masses and Tumors

Azin Alizadehasl and Anita Sadeghpour

Abstract

Primary tumors of the heart are infrequent across all age groups, with a described prevalence of 0.001–0.03% in autopsy series. Secondary involvement of the heart by extracardiac tumors is 20–40 times more common than that by primary cardiac tumors.

When cardiac tumors are considered in the differential diagnosis, the most ideal initial method of evaluation is echocardiography, either transthoracic (TTE) or transesophageal (TEE)—depending on the clinical circumstances. The sensitivity of TTE and TEE for the detection of a cardiac mass is 93% and 97%, respectively. Therefore, TEE is more comprehensive and accurate than TTE in the evaluation of such masses. Moreover, TEE is particularly advantageous in evaluating right atrial tumors. Three-dimensional echocardiography can assess the size of cardiac masses and define the complex anatomy of the heart. If a cardiac lesion is identified, chest computed tomography with contrast enhancement and cardiac magnetic resonance imaging with contrast are superior modalities for the characterization of the lesions and the description of the extent of tumor involvement. They may also help exclude the possibility of the direct cardiac extension of a tumor, created by the adjacent mediastinal structures.

In this chapter, we will explain other masses such as thrombi, vegetations, cysts, normal structures, and artifacts.

Electronic Supplementary Material The online version of this chapter (https://doi.org/10.1007/978-3-319-67691-3_36) contains supplementary material, which is available to authorized users.

A. Sadeghpour, MD, FACC, FASE
Professor of Cardiology, Echocardiography Research Center, Rajaie Cardiovascular Medical and Research Center, Iran University of Medical Science, Tehran, Iran

A. Alizadehasl, MD, FACC, FASE (✉)
Associate Professor of Cardiology, Echocardiologist, Echocardiography and Cardiogenetic Research Centers, Cardio-Oncology Department, Rajaie Cardiovascular Medical and Research Center, Tehran, Iran

Keywords

Cardiac masses · Cardiac tumors · Transesophageal echocardiography · Transthoracic echocardiography · Myxoma Rhabdomyoma

Abbreviations

ASA	Atrial septal aneurysm
ASE	American society of echocardiography
Avs	Aortic valves
CE	Cardiac echinococcosis
CV	Cardiovascular
DVT	Deep venous thrombosis
IAS	Inter-atrial septum
IVC	Inferior vena cava
LA	Left atrium
LAA	Left Atrial appendage
MR	Magnetic resonance
MV	Mitral valve
MVs	Myxomatous valves
PFO	Patent foramen ovale
RA	Right atrium
RV	Right ventricle
TB	Tuberous sclerosis
TEE	Transesophageal
TTE	Transthoracic

Introduction

- Cardiac masses are infrequent echocardiographic findings. The differential diagnosis is wide, however can be narrowed down by basic features and characterisation based on location, appearance and size. The main groups

A. Sadeghpour, A. Alizadehasl (eds.), *Case-Based Textbook of Echocardiography*, https://doi.org/10.1007/978-3-319-67691-3_36

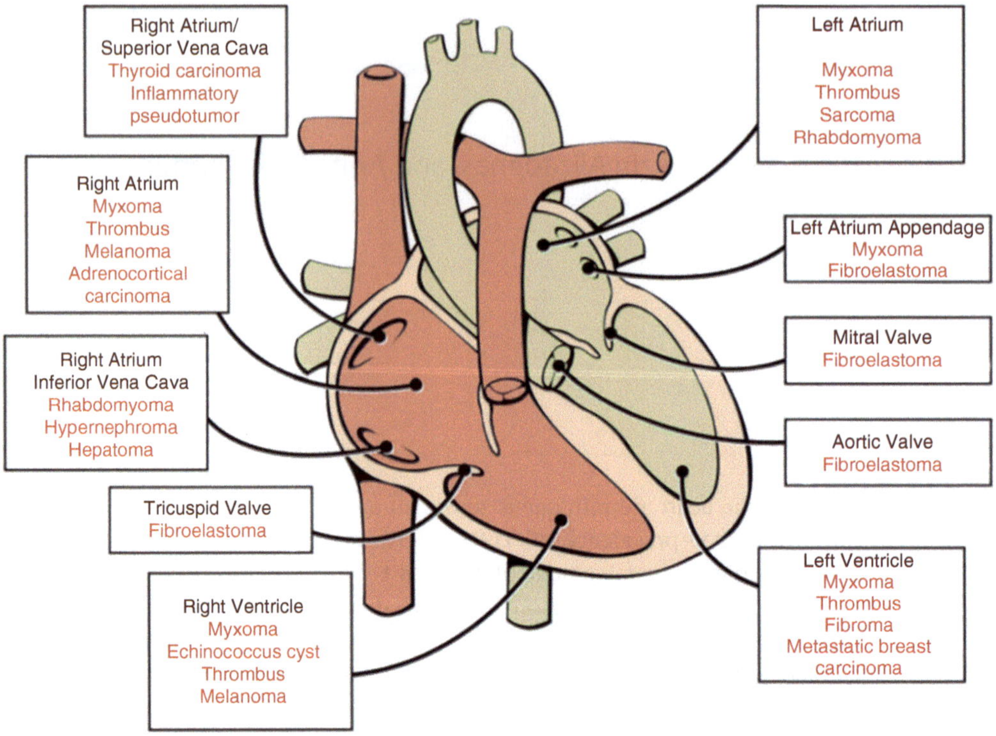

Fig. 36.1 Cardiac masses classification according to intra-cardiac attachment site. Modified figure from [1]. Charles J Bruce. Cardiac tumours: diagnosis and management. Heart 2011;97:151e160

Table 36.1 Cardiac masses

Neoplastic				
Primary		**Secondary**	**Non-neoplastic**	**Other**
Benign	Malignant	Direct extension	Hamartomas	Thrombus
Myxoma	Sarcoma	Breast	Rhabdomyoma	Vegetation
PFE*	Lymphoma	Lung	Fibroma	CAT*
Lipoma		Oesophagus	PFE	Normal structure
		Mediastinal tumour	**Age-related growths**	Image artefact
		Haematogenous	Lipomatous hypertrophy	
		Melanoma	**Reactive proliferation**	
		Lung	Llambl's excrescence	
		Breast	PFE	
		Genitourinary		
		Gastrointestinal		
		Venous		
		Renal		
		Adrenal		
		Thyroid		
		Lung		
		Hepatoma		
		Lymphatic		
		Lymphoma		
		Leukaemia		

**CAT* calcified amorphous tumour, *PFE* papillary fibroelastoma
Modified table from 1. Charles J Bruce. Cardiac tumours: diagnosis and management. Heart. 2011;97:151e160

of diagnosis are neoplasms, thrombus, vegetations, normal structures and artefacts.

- A absolute diagnosis cannot usually be made from echocardiography appearance alone, and a combination of clinical findings, other imaging modalities and also biopsy is needed to reach a conclusion [1–3] (Fig. 36.1 and Table 36.1).

Primary Neoplasms

Benign Tumors

Pericardial Cysts

- Pericardial cysts are benign fluid filled masses of the parietal pericardium and are supposed to be a congenital anomaly. They might be solitary or multi-locular, and some have been recognized to grow hugely (even >20 cm) size. They account for about 20% of benign primary cardiac tumors and usually happen near the cardio-phrenic borders (right more than left). This creates the appearance of cardiomegaly on chest radiographies and an encapsulated echo-lucent area in echocardiography. 75% of cases are asymptomatic. Though, if large they might cause atypical chest pain, atrial fibrillation, breathlessness, cough, or mechanical problems like RVOT obstruction. Sporadic cases of cardiac tamponade secondary to intra-pericardial rupture and also hemorrhage have reported [4, 5].

Atrial Myxoma

- The "atrial myxoma" is the commonest primary cardiac tumor, however even so is an infrequent diagnosis. Although, myxoma most commonly arises in the left atrium (LA) from the inter-atrial septum on the region of the fossa ovalis, it can arise from any cardiac chamber or even from the mitral or tricuspid valves. They are frequently solitary, however multiple myxomas happen in familial cases. Rarely recurrence happens after surgical removal of tumor.
- Atrial myxoma can result valvular stenosis or obstruction due to tumor prolapsing through the mitral valve (MV). Also, emboli can happen, due to either tumor breaking off or thrombus development on the tumor. The look of a myxoma needs to be distinguished from a large atrial clot or thrombus. Characteristically, myxoma is attached to the inter-atrial septum and has a heterogeneous and gelatinous texture, frequently with evidence of cavitation. But, thrombus more frequently arises in the LA appendage or LA roof and usually is homogeneous [1–3, 6] (Figs. 36.2, 36.3 and 36.4).

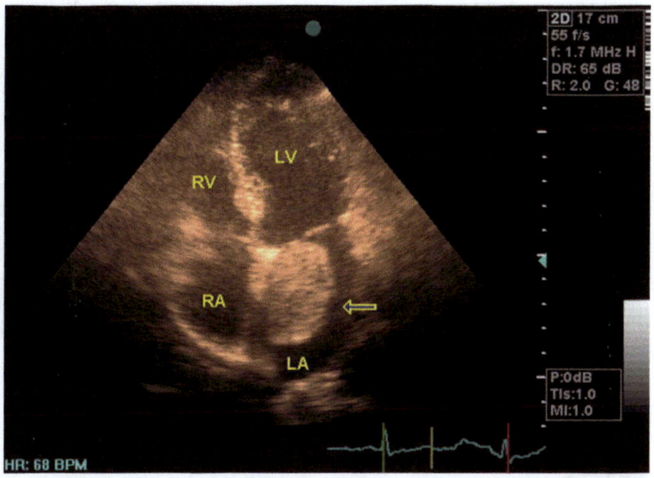

Fig. 36.2 Movie 36.1: Transthoracic echocardiography, apical for chamber view, large LA myxoma (arrow). *LV* left ventricle, *LA* left atrium, *RV* right ventricle, *RA* right atrium

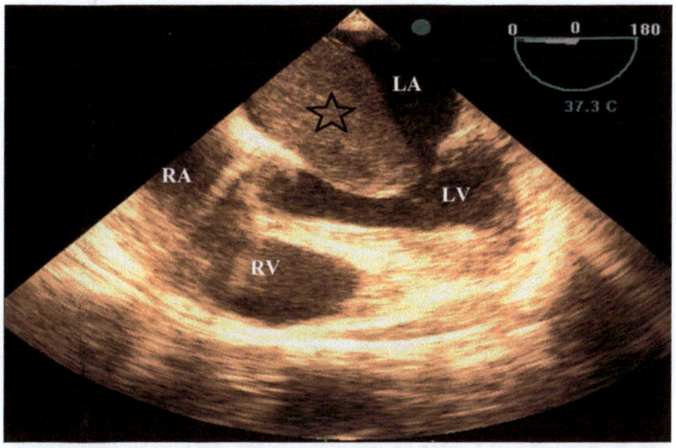

Fig. 36.3 Movie 36.2: Tranesophageal echocardiography, mid esophageal 0° view, large LA myxoma (star). *LV* left ventricle, *LA* left atrium, *RV* right ventricle, *RA* right atrium

Papillary Fibroelastomas

- Papillary fibroelastomas are the next most-common cardiac benign tumors and also the most common valvular tumor. About 80% are found on left sided (aortic or mitral) valves, though any valve might be affected, and 9% are showed as multiple lesions. They have a trend to appear on either side of the aortic valve or on the atrial side of the mitral valve. Less commonly, they have also been seen on mitral chordae or papillary muscles. On echocardiography they appear round, oval, or irregular in shape and also homogeneous in texture. Nearly half have a short stalk, that confers more mobility [1, 7, 8] (Figs. 36.5 and 36.6).

Lipoma

- Lipomas are composed of benign adipose tissue and most of them rise in the sub-endocardium with a wide range of size. On echocardiography study, lipomas tend to be immobile, broad based, without a pedicle and well circumscribed. They are homogenous without calcification, hyper-echoic in the cardiac cavity Fig 36.8 but hypo-echoic at the pericardium. Commonly lipomas are asymptomatic, but might cause arrhythmias or valvular dysfunction. Sub-epicardial lipomas can cause compression of the coronary arteries, leading to chest pain [1–3].

Rhabdomyoma

- This is truly a non-neoplastic disease (hamartoma) of striated muscles growth. Most cases happen in children and are related with tuberous sclerosis (TB). They arise anyplace in the heart (intra-mural or intra-cavitary) and are frequently multiple. The effects of the tumor on cardiac function depend on size and place (valve obstruction, arrhythmia, …). The echocardiographic features are frequently small, lobulated, hyper-echoic and homogeneous tumors [1–3, 9] (Figs. 36.7 and 36.8).

Fibroma

- Fibromas are primary benign cardiac tumor, that most commonly involve LV and intrerventricular septum. It has an abnormal texture and calcification is a frequent finding in the tumor. It can cause ventricular arrhythmias and heart failure [1, 2].

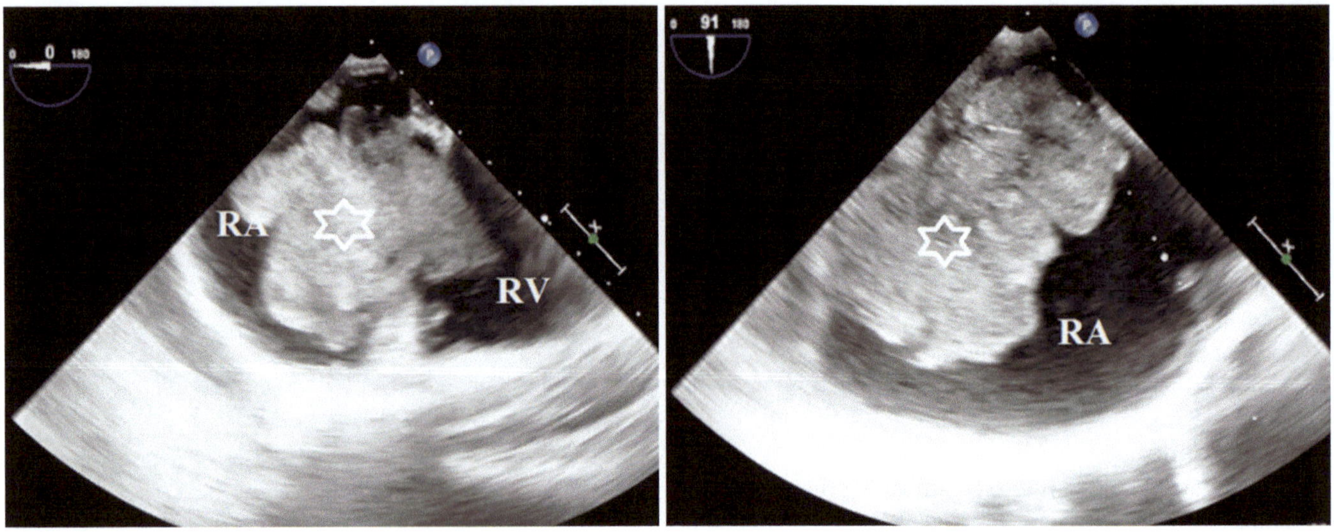

Fig. 36.4 Tranesophageal echocardiography, mid esophageal 4 chamber view (left) and bicaval view (right), large multi-lobulated RA myxoma (star). *RV* right ventricle, *RA* right atrium

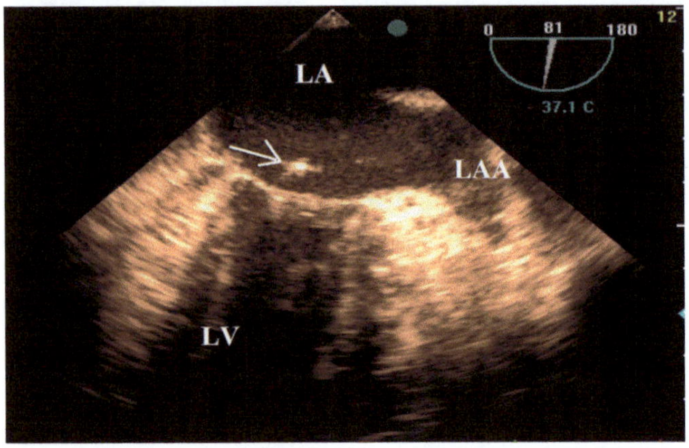

Fig. 36.5 Movie 36.3 Tranesophageal echocardiography, mid esophageal 80° view, mitral valve papillary fibroelastoma (arrow). *LV* left ventricle, *LA* left atrium, *LAA* left atrium appendage

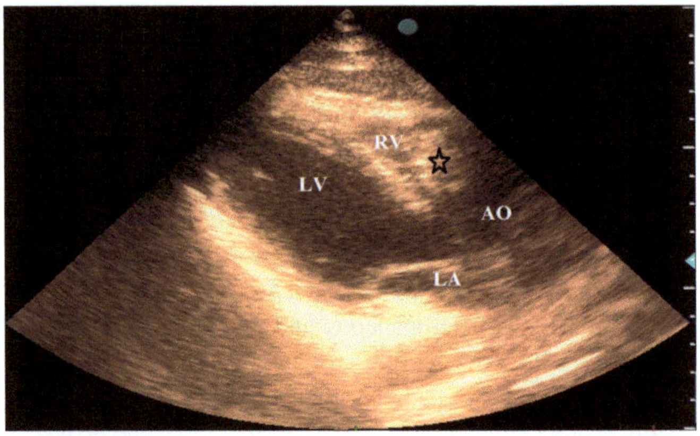

Fig. 36.7 Movie 36.5: Transthoracic echocardiography para-esternal long axis view. RV round and solid mass that diagnosed by pathology as rhabdomyoma (star). *LV* left ventricle, *LA* left atrium, *RV* right ventricle, *AO* aorta

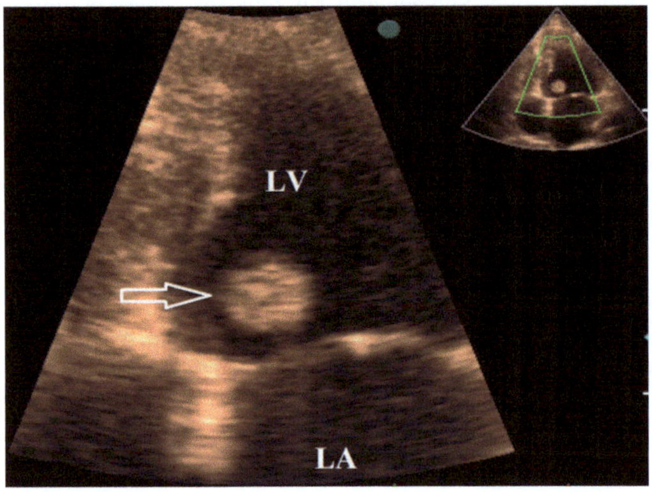

Fig. 36.6 Movie 36.4: Transthoracic echocardiography, apical 4 chamber view, mitral valve papillary fibroelastoma (arrow). *LV* left ventricle, *LA* left atrium

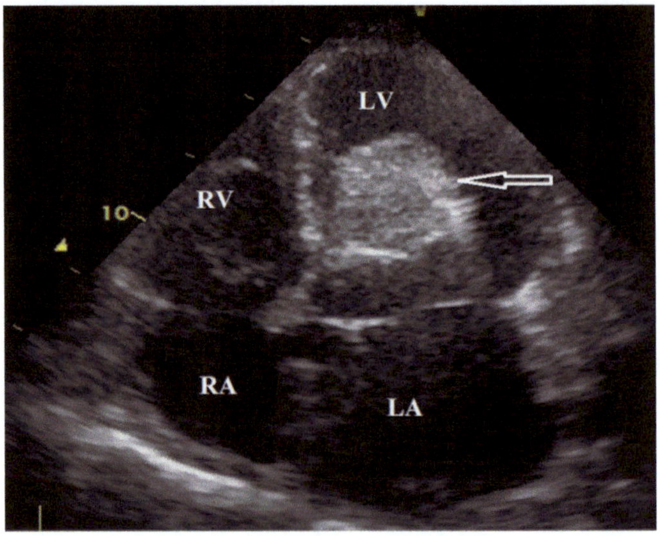

Fig. 36.8 Movie 36.6: Transthoracic echocardiography, apical 4 chamber view, benign tumor of LV that diagnosed by pathology as lipoma (arrow). *LV* left ventricle, *LA* left atrium, *RV* right ventricle, *RA* right atrium

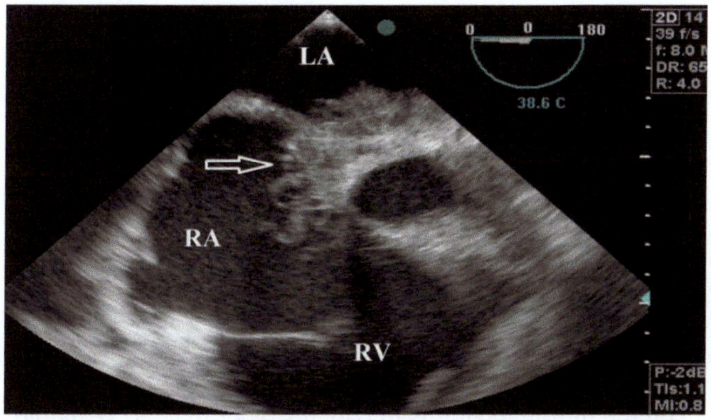

Fig. 36.9 Tranesophageal echocardiography, mid esophageal 0° of f-axis view, malignant hemangio sarcoma around the aortic valve (arrow). *RV* right ventricle, *LA* left atrium, *RA* right atrium

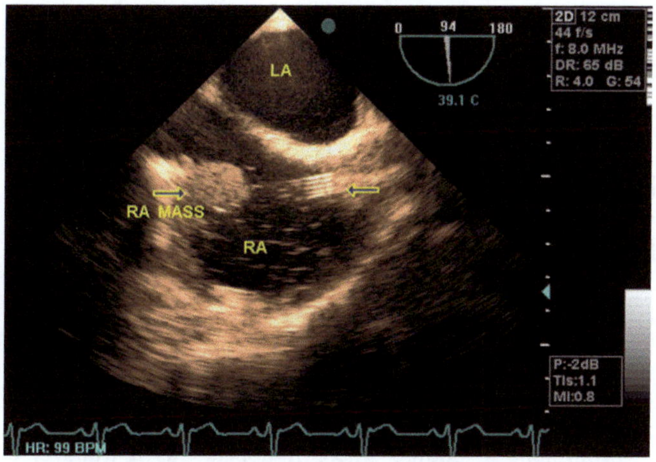

Fig. 36.10 Movie 36.7: Tranesophageal echocardiography, mid esophageal 90° view, RA mass (Thrombus) adjacent the port of chemotherapy. *RV* right ventricle, *LA* left atrium, *RA* right atrium

Malignant Tumors

- The most common primary malignant tumors of the heart are sarcomas, and these typically arise in the right ventricle (RV). They might be diffusely infiltrative, or sometimes a discrete polypoid or sessile mass that extend into the pericardium or ventricular cavity. Primary malignant cardiac lymphomas on the other hand have been seen with increasing frequency in the immuno-compromised host, like HIV and post-transplant patients. These masses are mostly diffuse large B-cell lymphomas. On echocardiography, they may appear as homogeneous, infiltrating masses leading to 'wall thickening' and restrictive hemodynamics or as nodular masses intruding into the cardiac chambers, preferably the right heart chambers and specially the RA. Distant metastases are frequently present, and the prognosis is so poor (1.10) (Fig. 36.9).

Secondary Neoplasms

- Spread of tumor to the heart from other sites (metastases) is more common than primary cardiac neoplasms. The most common sites of origin contain lung, breast, melanoma and also lymphoma. Spread is via the blood, or directly through the pericardium, and tumor deposits might involve any structure in the heart. The echocardiographic texture of the tumor is frequently discrete from surrounding cardiac muscle.
- Renal cell carcinoma is a special example case of metastatic spread to the heart. It typically invades the renal vein and inferior vena cava (IVC). In advanced cases the tumor ascends the IVC and reaches the right atrium (RA) or even further, causing stenotic and embolic complications. It might resemble a RA myxoma [1, 2, 9, 10].

Thrombus

- Intra-cardiac thrombus is more likely to happen if there is stasis of blood, damaged endothelium or abnormal coagulation. In the absence of any predisposing factors for clot formation, another diagnoses must be considered.
- The appearance of thrombus may be globular or pedunculated and mobile, or sometimes laminated, immobile and echo-dense. It should be considered that dilated cardiomyopathy and recent trans-mural myocardial infarction can be related with mural thrombus at sites of akinesis. In this condition laminated thrombus may be mistaken from akinetic myocardium.
- Atrial fibrillation and also mitral stenosis typically lead to thrombus formation in the LA appendage, although other sites in the LA can be affected. Transoesophageal echocardiography study is required if definitive exclusion of LA thrombus is necessary [1–3] (Fig. 36.10).

Vegetations

- Mobile discrete masses that are attached to valves are more probably to be vegetation, particularly if clinical and laboratory signs of infective endocarditis are existent, and symptoms of valvular regurgitation are of recent onset see chap. 19. Of course, myxomatous MV must also be distinguished from vegetation and tumors [1–3].

Intravascular Devices

- Permanent pacemaker or implantable cardioverter defibrillator leads can frequently be seen in the right side of the heart as very echogenic, thin and linear structures, however frequently only a small portion is visualised at once so the appearance may firstly be confusing. Occasionally reverberation artefact is seen. Pacing leads may also be seen in the coronary sinus of cases with biventricular pacemakers for congestive heart failure.
- Devices are also used for closure of atrial and ventricular septal defects. These are structurally like an umbrella,

with metallic supports radiating from the center of the device, which is deployed flat against the septum. The final look is rather like a rivet [1–3, 9].

Normal Structures Simulating Tumors

Intracardiac

- In the right atrium, the Eustachian valve (also known as the valve of the IVC) is a ridge of tissue that extends from the entry of the IVC to the inter-atrial septum. In fetal life, this valve directs blood to the fossa ovalis. It can remain prominent in adults, where it appears as a transverse linear echo running approximately parallel to the tricuspid annulus across the posterior RA in RV inflow views, or in subcostal views.
- The Chiari network is similarly an embryonic remnant of the sinus venosus, which extends from and is continuous with the Eustachian valve. It persists in 2–3% of normal adults (confirmed by autopsy), and appears on ultrasound as a lacy weblike or fenestrated membranous echogenic mass with a characteristic chaotic, undulating motion independent from that of the tricuspid valve and right heart. On parasternal long- or short-axis views, bulging of the interatrial septum into the RA, owing to an interatrial septal aneurysm or LA volume overload, can be mistaken for a "tumor" when the scanning plane cuts tangentially across the septum. Careful inspection of both atria from all windows must clarify this misdiagnosis [1–3].
- Annular calcification, particularly of the mitral apparatus, and fat deposition, often seen around the tricuspid annulus and interatrial septum (interatrial septal lipomatous hypertrophy) can also simulate intracardiac masses. Calcific deposits tend to be very echobright and irregular, whereas fat usually appears as a less echodense, homogenous mass with smoother edges.
- Myxomatous MV, when severely thickened, have been mistaken for tumors. Within the LA appendage, pectinate muscles appear as small multiple pyramidal structures with their bases continuous with the myocardial wall. Unlike masses and thrombi, the pectinate muscles are not independently mobile from appendage contractions. Small short linear echodensities known as "Lambl's excrescences" are often noted at the tips of the aortic valve leaflets, on both the left ventricular outflow tract and aortic side, as well as on the mitral apparatus in patients older than 50 years old. Pathological studies have revealed these to be long fibrin strands, although the larger and more developed strands may contain cellular elements of papillary fibroelastoma.
- Within the left ventricle, prominent left ventricle trabeculations, false tendons, aberrant muscle bands or bridges, and subaortic membranes must be distinguished from tumors. Delineation of the origins and insertions of these structures, a cylindrical or linear morphology, and the presence of thickening during systole can aid in the differential diagnosis. Within the right ventricle, the moderator band can appear quite thick, however its location extending from the apical free wall to the midseptum is characteristic [1–3, 6, 9, 10].

Extracardiac

- An epicardial fat pad usually appears as a discrete "soft" or deformable mildly granular echogenic mass lying adjacent to pericardium, typically anterior to the right heart and/or adjacent to the atrioventricular groove. A useful clue for distinguishing pericardial fat is the identification of the echolucent cylindrical lumen of the cor-

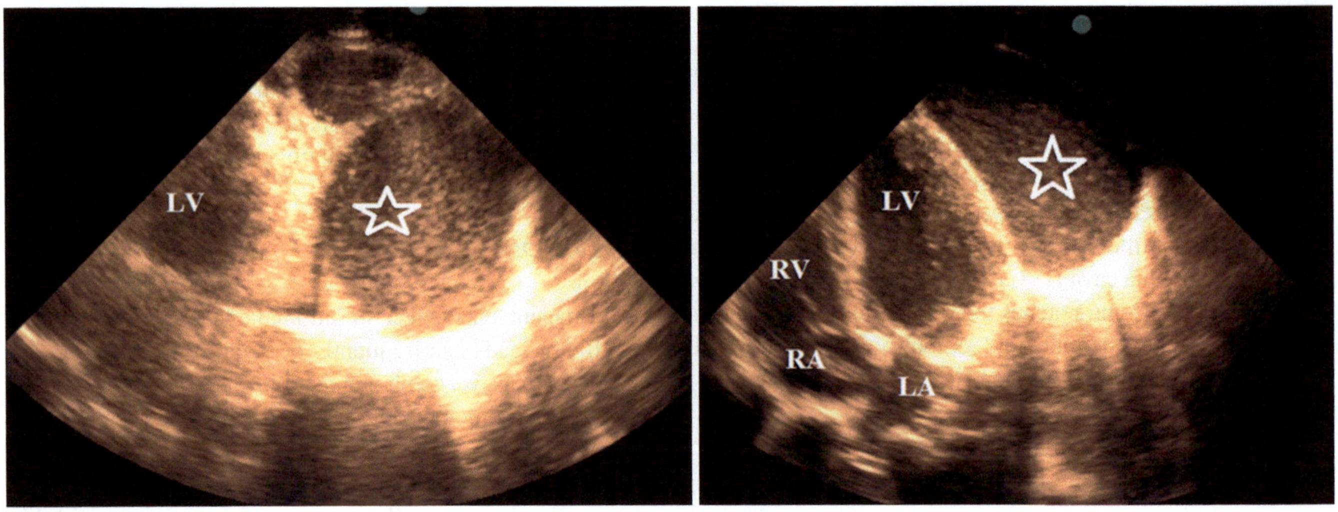

Fig. 36.11 Movie 36.8: Transthoracic echocardiography off –axis (left) and apical 4 chamber (right) views, large extra cardiac mass that was diagnosed by pathology as Hodjkin lymphoma (star). *LV* left ventricle, *LA* left atrium, *RV* right ventricle, *RA* right atrium

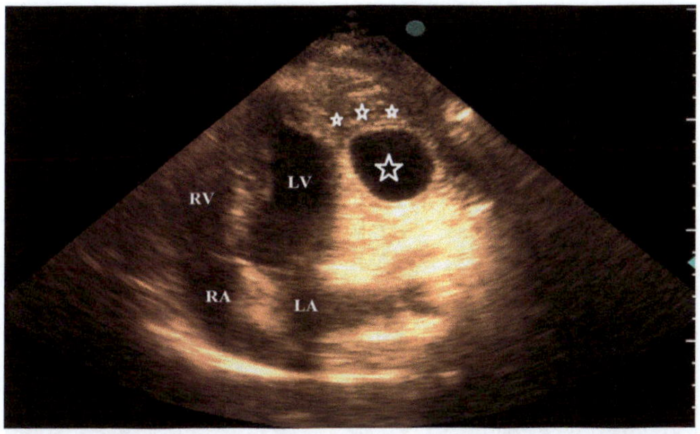

Fig. 36.12 Movie 36.9: Transthoracic echocardiography, apical 4 chamber view, large intra-myocardial septated cyst in lateral of LV diagnosed as hydatid cyst (star). *LV* left ventricle, *LA* left atrium, *RV* right ventricle, *RA* right atrium

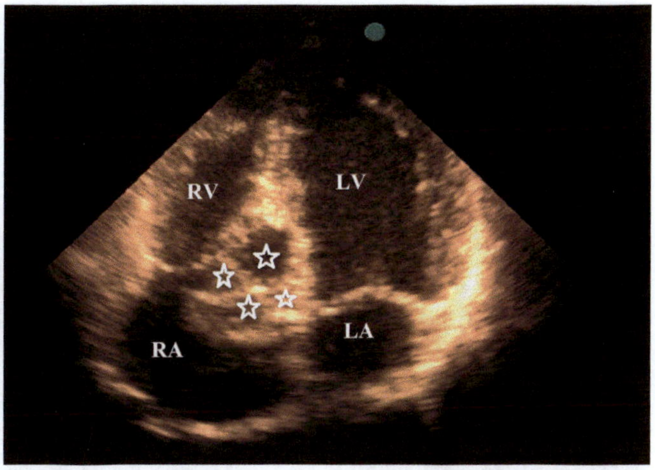

Fig. 36.13 Movie 36.10: Transthoracic echocardiography, apical 4 chamber view, large intra-myocardial IVS of LV cyst diagnosed as hydatid cyst (stars). *LV* left ventricle, *LA* left atrium, *RV* right ventricle, *RA* right atrium, *IVS* inter-ventricular septum

onary artery running within it. However, epicardial fat pads may be distrihowevered anywhere around the heart. They tend to increase in size with age or in patients with longstanding steroid use. Pleural effusions and ascites are occasionally confused with pericardial effusions. Proper identification must avoid the occasional misdiagnosis of echogenic collapsed lung segments, fibrin, or thrombus within the pleural or abdominal cavities, which can appear similar to tumor masses [1–3, 9] (Fig. 36.11).

Cardiac Hydatid Cyst

Echocardiography is an extremely valuable tool for diagnosing Cardiac Echinococcosis (CE). Classic cystic CE lesions appear as well-defined echolucent structures on echocardiographic images, whereas those that have become solidified, calcified, or degenerated can be hyperechogenic and, thus, mimic semisolid or solid mass lesions [11].

Echinococcus Granulosus

The worm completes its life cycle in two hosts.

Primary or the most common definite host is dog while the secondary or intermediate host are sheep, horse, goat, and man.

- The eggs are swallowed by the intermediate host and through intestinal wall to reach the portal circulation from where they are carried to the liver.
- The liver act as the first filter.
- Some of the embryos pass through the hepatic capillaries, enter the pulmonary circulation to reach the lungs.

World Health Organization 2001 classification of hepatic hydatid cysts. This classification was proposed by WHO in 2001 and at the time of writing (July 2016) remains the most widely used classification for hydatid cyst.

- Simple cysts with well-defined borders and uniform anechoic contents are not pathognomonic for echinococcal cysts (nonparasitic cysts have the same appearance).
- Cysts with a visible split wall inside (floating membrane or water lily sign) are pathognomonic.
- Septated cysts, or cysts with a honeycomb pattern, are likely to be echinococcal.
  - A solid heterogeneous mass is difficult to differentiate from granulomas or tumors, although calcification suggests echinococcal cyst [11].

Differential diagnosis (Figs. 36.12, 36.13 and 36.14):

- Complex pyogenic abscess.
- Hemorragic or simple cyst
- Infected cyst
- Cystic metastases

Questions

1. What is the most common tumor in left atrial auricle?
   A. hemangioma
   B. rhabdomyoma
   C. fibroelastoma
   D. lipoma

2. Which of the following statement about Papillary fibroelastomas is not correct?
   A. Papillary fibroelastomas are the second most common cardiac benign tumors.
   B. About 80% of Papillary fibroelastomas are found on right-sided valves.
   C. Nine percent of patients with Papillary fibroelastomas exhibit multiple lesions.

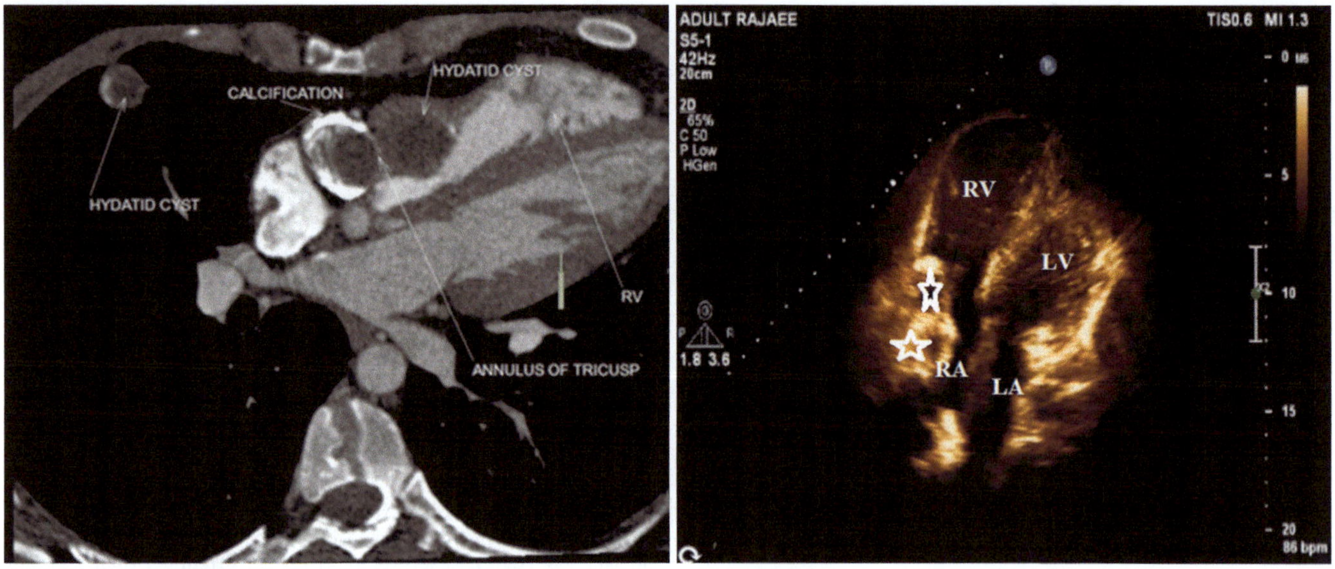

Fig. 36.14 Cardiac CT (left) and transthoracic apical 4 chamber view (right) showing hydatid cyst of RV free wall adjacent to the TV annulus (Star). *LV* left ventricle, *LA* left atrium, *RV* right ventricle, *RA* right atrium, *TV* tricuspid valve

   D. On echocardiography, papillary fibroelastomas appear round, oval or irregular in shape and also homogeneous in texture.

3. What is wrong about cardiac sarcomas?
   A. They are the most common primary malignant tumors of the heart.
   B. They typically arise in the right atrium.
   C. Distant metastases are frequently present.
   D. The prognosis is very poor.
4. A 7-year-old boy with a history of a seizure disorder and developmental delay is found to have cortical tubers on brain magnetic resonance imaging. If tuberous sclerosis is suspected, which of the following cardiac tumors is the likely to develop?
   A. Left atrial myxoma
   B. Cardiac sarcoma
   C. Rhabdomyoma
   D. Cardiac lymphoma

Answers

1. C
2. B
3. B
4. C

References

1. Bruce CJ. Cardiac tumours: diagnosis and management. Heart. 2011;97:151e160. https://doi.org/10.1136/hrt.2009.186320.
2. Peters PJ, Reinhardt S. The echocardiographic evaluation of intracardiac masses: a review. J Am Soc Echocardiogr. 2006;19:230.
3. Kirkpatrick JN, Wong T, Bednarz JE, et al. Differential diagnosis of cardiac masses using contrast echocardiographic perfusion imaging. J Am Coll Cardiol. 2004;43:1412.
4. Maisch B, Seferovic PM, Ristic AD, et al. The task force on the diagnosis and management of pericardial diseases of the European Society of Cardiology. Guidelines on the diagnosis and management of pericardial diseases: executive summary. Eur Heart J. 2004;25:587.
5. Patel J, Park C, Michaels J, et al. Pericardial cyst: case reports and a literature review. Echocardiography. 2004;21:269.
6. Burke A, Jeudy J Jr, Virmani R. Cardiac tumours: an update. Heart. 2008;94:117.
7. Sun JP, Asher C, Yang XS, et al. Clinical and echocardiographic characteristics of papillary fibroelastomas: a retrospective and prospective study in 162 patients. Circulation. 2001;103:2687.
8. Silbiger JJ, Bazaz R, Trost B. Lipomatous hypertrophy of the interatrial septum revisited. J Am Soc Echocardiogr. 2010;23:789.
9. Butany J, Leong SW, Carmichael K, et al. A 30-year analysis of cardiac neoplasms at autopsy. Can J Cardiol. 2005;21:675.
10. Abraham KP, Reddy V, Gattuso P. Neoplasms metastatic to the heart: review of 3314 consecutive autopsies. Am J Cardiovasc Pathol. 2009;3:195.
11. Tufekcioglu O, Birincioglu CL, Arda K, Fansa I, Saritas A, Karahan M. Echocardiography findings in 16 cases of cardiac echinococcosis: proposal for a new classification system. J Am Soc Echocardiogr. 2007;20:895–904.

Evaluation of Cardiac Sources of Emboli by Echocardiography

37

Azin Alizadehasl and Anita Sadeghpour

Abstract

An embolus is an intra-vascular mass that generally includes a thrombus and atheromatous or cellular matter that has entered the circulation and creates symptoms by lodging at the end of the arteries and disturbing the blood flow to the organs. Emboli from the venous system might enter the right side of the heart and cause pulmonary emboli, while those created on the left side of the heart and great arteries may create infarcts in the brain, kidneys, intestine, and skin. Though, small strokes and transient ischemic attacks are frequently caused by atheromatous debris from the aorta or major cerebral arteries. A paradoxical embolus is a systemic infarct in which the source of the embolus is supposed to be from the venous system; it bypasses the pulmonary circulation by means of an intra-cardiac shunt and goes across into the arterial circulation.

Keywords

Sources of emboli · Deep venous thrombosis (DVT) · Embolic strokes · Lambl's excrescences · Patent foramen ovale (PFO) · Intra-cardiac thrombus · Atrial fibrillation · Thromboembolism

Abbreviations

ASA	Atrial septal aneurysm
ASE	American society of echocardiography
Avs	Aortic valves
CV	Cardiovascular
DVT	Deep venous thrombosis
IAS	Inter-atrial septum
LA	Left atrial
LAA	Left atrial appendage
MR	Magnetic resonance
MV	Mitral valve
PFO	Patent foramen ovale
RA	Right atrium
RV	Right ventricle
TEE	Transesophageal echocardiography
TTE	Transthoracic echocardiography

An embolus is an intra-vascular mass that generally includes a thrombus and atheromatous or cellular matter that has entered the circulation and creates symptoms by lodging at the end of the arteries and disturbing the blood flow to the organs. Emboli from the venous system might enter the right side of the heart and cause pulmonary emboli, while those created on the left side of the heart and great arteries may create infarcts in the brain, kidneys, intestine, and skin. Though, small strokes and transient ischemic attacks are frequently caused by atheromatous debris from the aorta or major cerebral arteries. A paradoxical embolus is a systemic infarct in which the source of the embolus is supposed to be from the venous system; it bypasses the pulmonary circulation by means of an intra-cardiac shunt and goes across into the arterial circulation [1].

Electronic Supplementary Material The online version of this chapter (https://doi.org/10.1007/978-3-319-67691-3_37) contains supplementary material, which is available to authorized users.

A. Alizadehasl, MD, FACC, FASE
Associate Professor of Cardiology, Echocardiologist, Echocardiography and Cardiogenetic Research Centers, Cardio-Oncology Department, Rajaie Cardiovascular Medical and Research Center, Tehran, Iran

A. Sadeghpour, MD, FACC, FASE (✉)
Professor of Cardiology, Echocardiography Research Center, Rajaie Cardiovascular Medical and Research Center, Iran University of Medical Science, Tehran, Iran

A. Sadeghpour, A. Alizadehasl (eds.), *Case-Based Textbook of Echocardiography*, https://doi.org/10.1007/978-3-319-67691-3_37

Epidemiology

- Embolic strokes are typically occurred by the sudden onset of symptoms in the middle or anterior cerebral artery territories, or multiple events in the peripheral territories. These must be distinguished from lacunar or hemorrhagic strokes, which are secondary to intrinsic cerebro-vascular disease or hypertension.
- In elderly cases (>55 years old), atherosclerosis of the great arteries and the internal carotid arteries is supposed to account for 20–60% of embolic strokes. These cases frequently have coexisting cardio-aortic disease and internal carotid artery disease; it is, thus, difficult to recognize which vessel is the culprit source of the embolus in many cases.
- AF with related thrombus forming in the left atrial appendage (LAA) is also one of the most frequent causes of embolic strokes.
- Younger cases (<55 years old) with embolic strokes are less likely to have substantial atheromatous disease and more likely to have cardiogenic sources of emboli or hyper-coagulable states. Approximately 40% of strokes are of an undecided origin (cryptogenic), of which up to half have been correlated with various cardiac abnormalities, which are noticeable by echocardiography. Other systemic emboli-those targeting the eye, kidney, spleen, or skin-are frequently the result of vegetations or thrombi shed from an abnormal or prosthetic cardiac valve or the result of atheromatous debris dislocated by intraarterial catheter procedures. A pulmonary embolus is the result of a deep venous thrombosis (DVT), which has broken free and moved to the lung bed [1–3].

Etiology

- Transthoracic echocardiography (TTE) may detect the potential cardio-embolic reasons of systemic emboli. The predominance of cardiac abnormalities disposing to emboli varies in different ages of the patient.
- In older cases, important findings might contain the following: atheroma might be seen as irregular thickening of the aortic wall in the aortic root, ascending, arch, and also descending abdominal aorta. Calcified plaques tend to seem very jagged and echo dense, and the related thrombus might appear as tethered however mobile elements.
- Plaques that are more than 4 mm in thickness or contain mobile or protruding elements are related with a higher risk of stroke. Atheroma is better imaged on transesophageal echocardiography (TEE) Fig. 37.1, Movie 37.1 and when coronary artery bypass graft surgery is planned in cases with important aortic root disease, TEE or "epi-aortic scanning" regularly assists in guiding bypass pump cannula placement and reduces the risk of stroke by the dislocated plaque in the punctured area.
- The presence of AF, predominantly in the presence of rheumatic heart disease, raises the risk of atrial thrombus formation. Left atrial (LA) thrombi frequently happen in relationship with spontaneous echo contrast (Fig. 37.2, Movie 37.2 and Fig. 37.3) which is thought to represent high fibrin and red blood cells in the early stages of coagulation. Though TTE frequently does not fully visualize the LAA, thrombi might rarely be seen in the body of the LA or right atrium (RA).

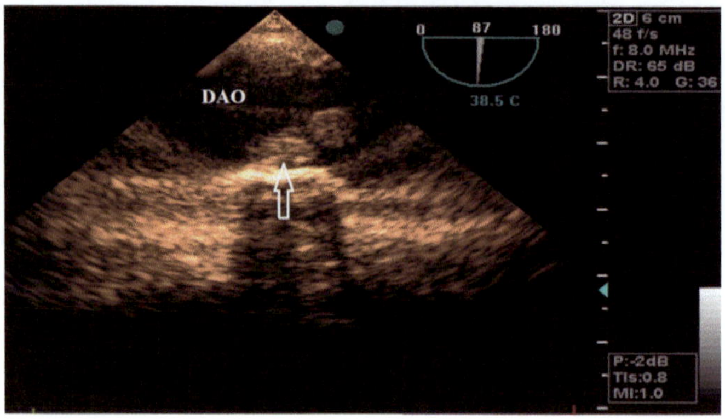

Fig. 37.1 Movie 37.1. Transesophageal echocardiography, long axis view showing complex atherosclerotic plaque in descending thoracic aorta (arrow)

- The presence of dys-kinetic or aneurysmal areas of the left ventricle (LV) in a case with a history of myocardial infarction must always prompt assessment for a related intra-mural thrombus, which may differ greatly in shape and mobility (Fig. 37.4 and Movies 37.3 and 37.4). Mitral valve (MV) stenosis, stranding, and MV annular calcification have all been recommended to be allied to the risk of emboli, though there are frequently confusing risk factors. MV prolapse was historically implicated as a risk factor, however this appears to be an artifact of the over-diagnosis of MV prolapse in this population, rather than including a true etiological substrate [1, 3–5].
- Vegetations are more likely to happen on abnormal native valves like bicuspid aortic valves (AVs) or myxomatous MVs. On mechanical prosthetic valves, the masses (thrombi or vegetations) might not be clearly imaged since of acoustic shadowing with the prosthesis, and TEE must be performed for this pathology (Fig. 37.5 and Movie 37.5).
- Marantic endocarditis is a disease related with cancer, hyper-coagulable states, and inflammatory situations and creates continuous fibrin and thrombus formation on the valves, which may be a source of emboli. Other sources commonly found in old cases that might increase the risk of stroke include aortic sclerosis (irregular tissue thickening of the AV leaflet edges), Lambl's excrescences (fibrin comprising strands found on the leaflet edges and rarely in the LV outflow tract), and papillary fibroelastomas (Fig. 37.6 and Movie 37.6). More hardly, echocardiography may distinguish aortic dissections with the intimal flap extending to obstruct a carotid artery. Sub-costal views of the IVC rarely detect previously un-suspected deep vein thromboses [2–5].

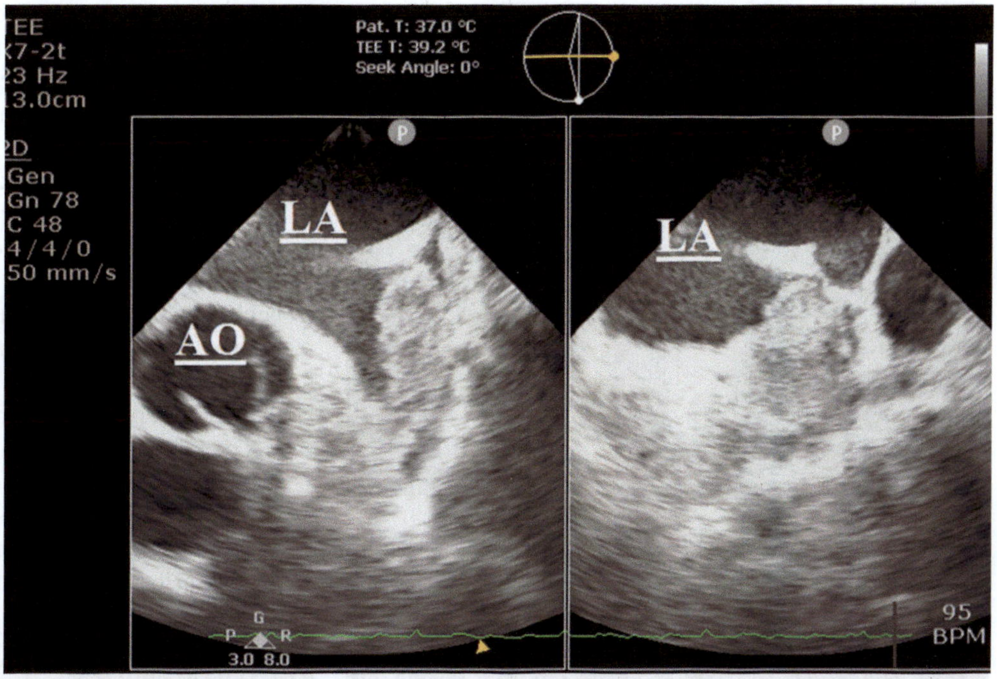

Fig. 37.2 Movie 37.2. Transesophageal and echocardiography, x-plain view showing large fresh left atrial appendage clot associated with spontaneous contrast in LA

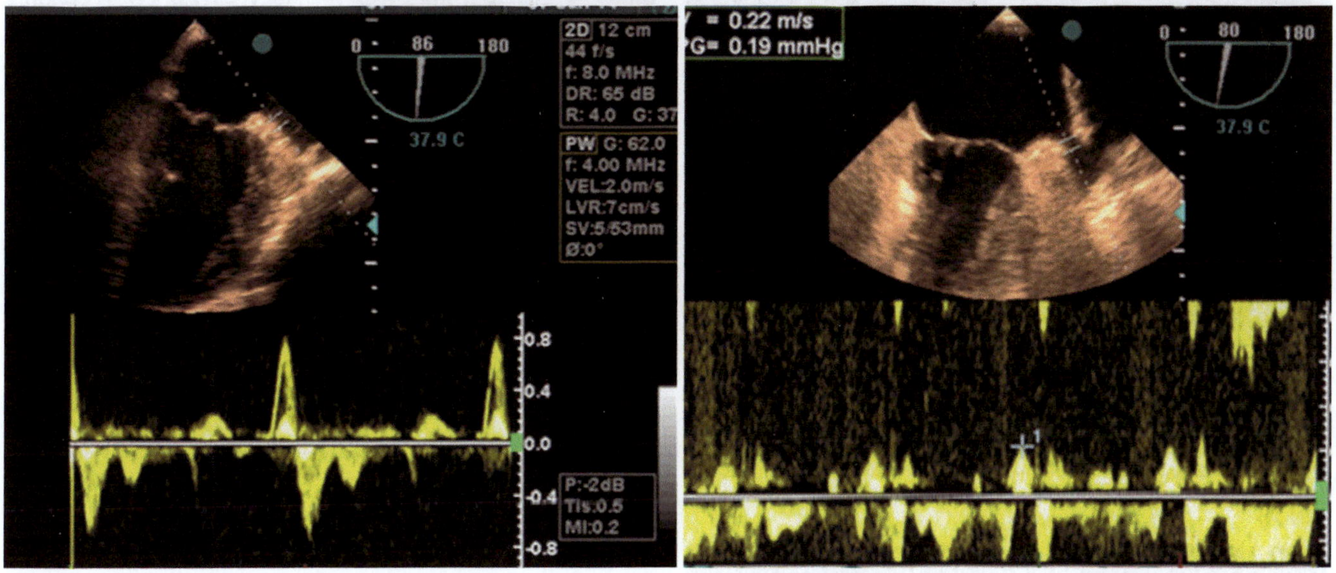

Fig. 37.3 Left panel: Normal LAA velocity in Transesophageal echocardiography, Right panel: Reduced LAA velocity in patient with paroxysmal AF

Young and Elderly Cases, Different approaches

- The epidemiology of cardiogenic emboli in younger cases is dissimilar from that of older cases. Those with abnormal native valves like myxomatous or prolapsed MVs or bicuspid AVs are vulnerable to infective endocarditis and resultant vegetations, which might embolize.
- Vegetations longer than 10 mm are at the highest risk for causing embolic problems. Among intra-cardiac tumors, myxomas are also more frequently found in younger cases owing to embolization.
- Paradoxical emboli constitute a well-known risk of CHD with intra-cardiac shunts, as in the case of inter-atrial or inter-ventricular septal defects. The existence of a dilated RA and- or right ventricle (RV) in the absence of other reasons must prompt a diligent search for intra-cardiac shunts by both 2D imaging and color Doppler.
- Patent foramen ovale (PFO) is a disorder in which the ostium primum rises from the LA side and spans the fossa ovalis; nevertheless, it does not fuse totally with the opposing ostium secundum. PFO is basically a normal variant, happening in 25–30% of the population. Under situations in which the RA pressure exceeds the LA pressure, PFO may permit a right-to-left intra-cardiac flow to happen (similar to a trapdoor or a flap) (Fig. 37.7, Movie

37.7). A cautious color Doppler scan of a sector zoomed in on the inter-atrial septum (IAS), mostly in the subcostal window, may rarely detect the flow across the PFO as a narrow red jet of a transient left-to-right flow. The flow is classically greatest in late systole and in early diastole.

- A "bubble study" or injection of intravenous saline that has been agitated with air to produce echo contrast is an echocardiographic method used to identify PFO (Fig. 37.8, Movie 37.8). The appearance of echogenic bubbles in the left side of the heart closely (within 6 beats of opacifying the RA) is indicative of a right to left shunt (see Chap. 9). Since the LA pressure is usually higher than the RA pressure, maneuvers that briefly increase the RA pressure like the Valsalva, sniffing, coughing, abdominal compression, and leg elevation may increase the sensitivity of a bubble contrast study for identifying PFO.
- PFO may permit paradoxical emboli from the venous system to lodge in the systemic arteries. The incidence of PFO seems

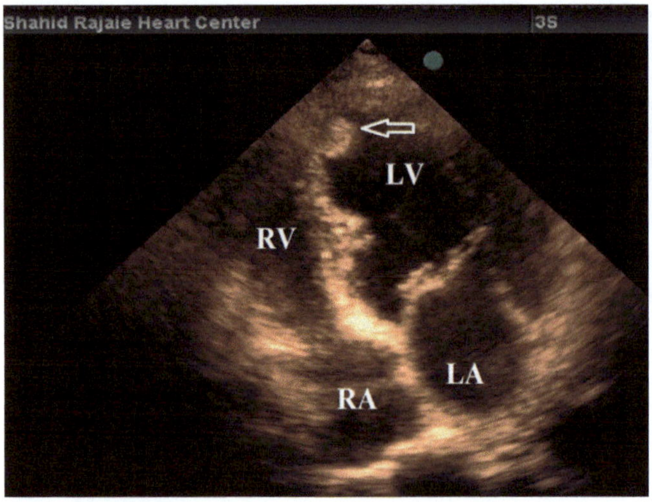

Fig. 37.4 Movies 37.3 and 37.4. Off axis 4 chamber view showing dys-kinetic apicoseptal segment with apical thrombus

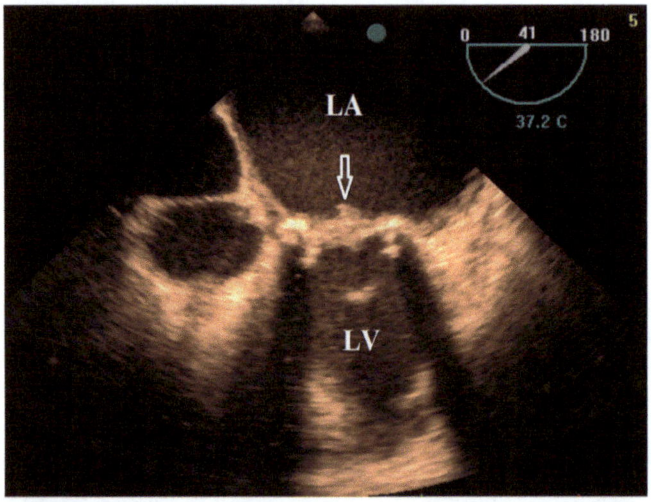

Fig. 37.5 Movie 37.5. Vegetation on mitral bioprostheses visualized in TEE (arrow)

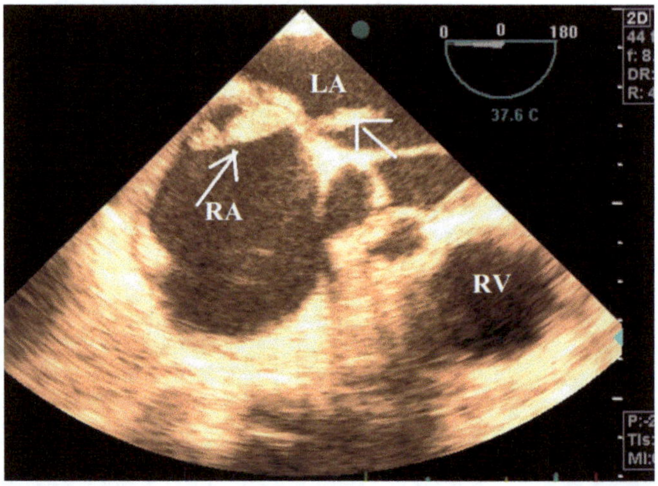

Fig. 37.7 Movie 37.7. Transesophageal echocardiography, mid esophageal 0′ view showing thrombus in transit via patent foramen ovale. *RA* right atrium, *LA* left atrium, *RV* right ventricle

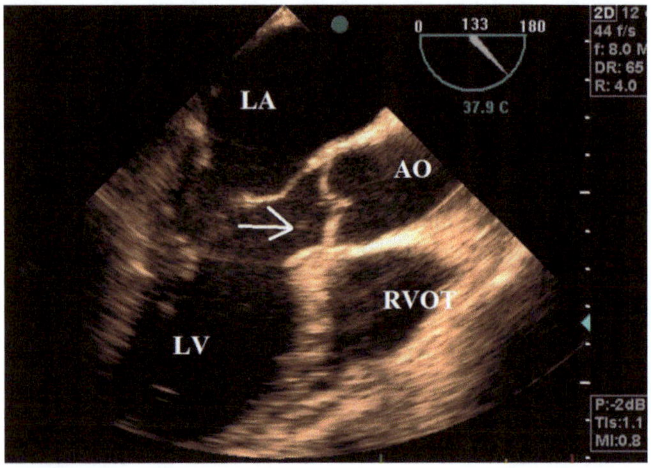

Fig. 37.6 Movie 37.6. Transesophageal echocardiography, mid esophageal 130′ view showing lambl's excrescence of aortic valve that can be a source of emboli (arrow). *LV* left ventricle, *LA* left atrium, *AO* aorta, *RVOT* right ventricular outflow tract

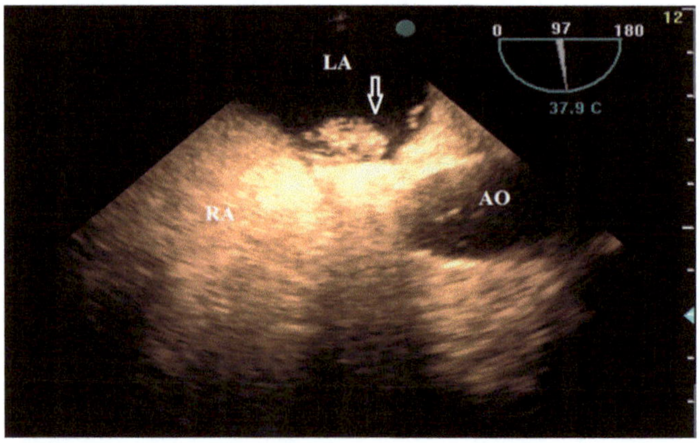

Fig. 37.8 Movie 37.8. Transesophageal echocardiography, mid esophageal 97′ view showing large patent foramen ovale with some bubble passage in contrast study. *RA* right atrium, *LA* left atrium, *AO* aorta

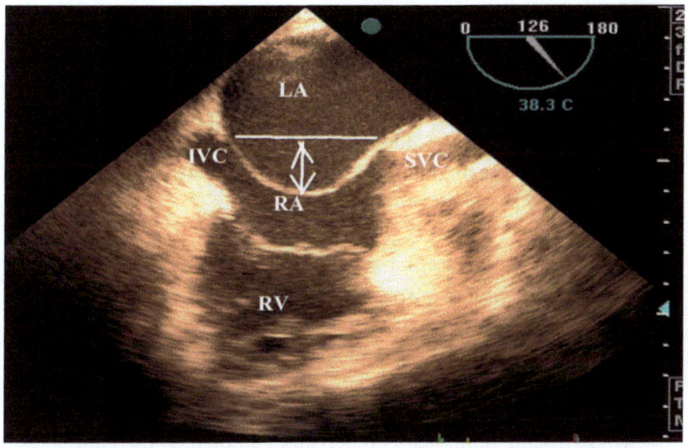

Fig. 37.9 Movie 37.9. Transesophageal echocardiography, mid esophageal 120′ modified bicaval view showing inter-atrial septum aneurysm (arrow). *RA* right atrium, *RV* right ventricle, *LA* left atrium, *IVC* inferior vena-cava, *SVC* superior vena cava

to be higher in cases with the ischemic type of stroke, more than threefold higher in cases younger than 55 years old.

- An atrial septal aneurysm (ASA) is a disproportionately redundant hypermobile area of the IAS, which may be seen on echocardiography. It is very commonly related to PFO and typically involves the area of the fossa ovalis; nevertheless, it may extend to contain the surrounding limbic areas or even the entire IAS. The criteria for the diagnosis of ASA are dissimilar, however it is mostly accepted that maximal excursion of the IAS more than 10 mm from the center line describes an ASA (Fig. 37.9, Movie 37.9). Localized thrombi have been found on an anecdotal basis nestled within ASAs, and ASAs are 3–6 times more frequent in cases with ischemic stroke-again with the highest incidence in the younger population. The incidence of both a PFO and an ASA is noticeably increased in cases with embolic strokes, more than 15-fold in a meta-analysis. Cases younger than 55 years of age with a PFO alone seem not to be at higher risk of stroke than the overall population. Nonetheless, the presence of both PFO and ASA appears to confer a higher risk of a recurrent ischemic event, despite treatment with aspirin (Fig. 37.10, Movie 37.10). A large amount of right to left shunting may also confer an increased risk of paradoxical emboli. Decisions for therapy and secondary risk prevention at this point include aspirin, plus additional anticoagulation and the closure of the PFO by surgery or trans-catheter devices [1–3, 5–7].

Workup for the Source of the Embolus

- Precise and specific guidelines are provided for each category of embolic sources, including the LA and LAA, LV, heart valves, cardiac tumors, and also thoracic aorta. Additionally, there are recommendations regarding pulmonary embolism and embolism related to cardiovascular (CV) surgery and percutaneous procedures.

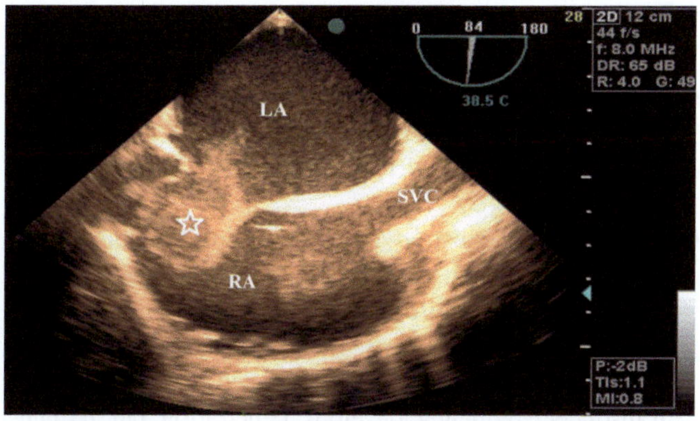

Fig. 37.10 Movie 37.10. Transesophageal echocardiography, mid esophageal 80′ bicaval view showing inter-atrial septum aneurysm with significant smoke pattern (*star*). *RA* right atrium, *LA* left atrium, *IVC* inferior vena-cava, *SVC* superior vena cava

Table 37.1 Echocardiographic predictors of embolic risk in cases with AF

Left ventricular systolic dysfunction (ejection fraction < or = 35%)
Complex aortic plaques
Left atrial appendage (LAA) thrombi or spontaneous echo contrast
LAA dysfunction (emptying blood flow velocities ≤20 cm/s or reduced contraction at M-mode)

- The utility of echocardiography in searching for a supposed cardiac source of emboli will vary with the patient's age and co-morbidities.
- Echocardiography is more likely to be useful in younger cases or in those with known disposing cardiac circumstances. In contrast, the workup of most elderly cases with a stroke must start with an imaging modality of the internal carotid arteries (either carotid duplex ultrasound, angiographic computed tomography CT study, or magnetic resonance (MR) imaging or MR angiography).

When is TEE indicated in the examination of stroke?

- If there is a high doubt as to the cardiac source of the embolus and TTE earnings inadequate information to rule out a cardiac source, TEE is indicated provided that the results would impact the therapy.
- The sensitivity of TEE has been revealed to be superior for the LAA thrombi (closely 100% vs 39–63% for TTE), ascending aortic atheroma, and also vegetations (88–100% sensitivity vs 44–60% for TTE). TEE is better able to assess prosthetic valves, predominantly MVs, which frequently cause much acoustic shadowing artifact on TTE studies. TEE is also more sensitive (89% vs <50% for TTE by using contrast) and 100% specific for identifying the abnormalities of the IAS. Though, it is only moderately better (11% vs 4% for TTE) for identifying intra-cardiac masses, and there is no incremental finding about extra-cardiac masses (containing thrombi) in cases without CV disease and a negative TTE (Table 37.1; Fig. 37.1) [1–3, 6–8].

TTE in Competition with TEE

- The quality of TTE varies among patients and depends on body habitus, size of the intercostal spaces, presence of chest deformities, and lung diseases such as pulmonary emphysema.
- Even with the most advanced echocardiographic equipment, TTE imaging might still be suboptimal or even unobtainable. Because the ultrasound beam loses energy as it travels through the tissue, structures that are far from the chest wall may not be well imaged by TTE. A lower transducer frequency develops penetration but reduces image resolution.
- As a result, structures that might be important sources of embolism such as *the posteriorly situated LA and its appendage, the IAS, and the thoracic aorta may be sub optimally imaged by TTE.* With the transducer in the esophagus in TEE, there is close proximity between the transducer and the posterior aspect of the heart. This shorter distance enables the use of higher frequency transducers [1, 2, 8–10].
- TEE can provide images of higher resolution and disclose findings that might be responsible for cardiac and aortic sources of embolism. In many echocardiography labs, assessment for a source of embolism is the most common indication for TEE. Though TEE is typically safe, it is still considered a semi-invasive procedure. Complications are rare, but the most severe one is esophageal perforation (reported incidence ranging from 0.01% to 0.09% of all studies done). Other complications include damage to the oral cavity, teeth, pharynx, and trachea, as well as complications related to topical anesthesia and sedation. Performance of TEE must follow suitable American Society of Echocardiography (ASE) guidelines.
- Unless there are clinical findings that suggest conditions that explain the embolic event such as atrial fibrillation, mitral stenosis, and infective endocarditis, the results of TTE are often negative. It has been consequently suggested that TTE may be needless in patients with cryptogenic stroke and negative clinical assessment. TTE might also be needless when TEE is already planned (e.g., for the evaluation of intra-cardiac masses, prosthetic valves, and the thoracic aorta or when TEE is used to guide a percutaneous procedure related to the cardiac source of embolism). Others believe that TTE might occasionally provide information not well seen on TEE (such as LV apical thrombi) or might even eliminate the need for the more invasive and expensive TEE (Tables 37.2 and 37.3) [1, 4, 7, 9, 10].

Table 37.2 Appropriate use criteria for echocardiography in the evaluation of cardiac sources of emboli

Appropriate use: transthoracic echocardiography (TTE)
Symptoms or conditions potentially related to suspected cardiac etiology, including but not limited to chest pain, shortness of breath, palpitations, transient ischemic attack, stroke, and peripheral embolic event
Suspected cardiac mass
Suspected cardiovascular source of the embolus
Initial evaluation of suspected infective endocarditis with positive blood culture results or new murmur
Reevaluation of infective endocarditis at high risk for progression or complication or with a change in clinical status or cardiac examination results
Known acute pulmonary embolism to guide therapy (e.g., thrombectomy and thrombolytic therapy)
Reevaluation of known pulmonary embolism after thrombolysis or thrombectomy for the assessment of change in RV function and/or pulmonary artery pressure
Appropriate use: TEE
As the initial or supplemental test for the evaluation for the cardiovascular source of the embolus with no identified noncardiac source
As the initial or supplemental test to diagnose infective endocarditis with a moderate or high pretest probability (e.g., staph bacteremia, fungemia, prosthetic heart valve, or intracardiac device)
As the initial test for evaluation to facilitate clinical decision-making with regard to anticoagulation, cardioversion, and/or radiofrequency ablation
Uncertain indication for use: TEE
Evaluation for the cardiovascular source of the embolus with a previously identified non-cardiac source
Inappropriate use: TTE
Transient fever without evidence of bacteremia or new murmur
Transient bacteremia with a pathogen not typically associated with infective endocarditis and/or a documented nonendovascular source of infection
Routine surveillance of uncomplicated infective endocarditis when no change in management is contemplated
Suspected pulmonary embolism to establish diagnosis
Routine surveillance of prior pulmonary embolism with normal RV function and pulmonary artery systolic pressure
Inappropriate use: TEE
Evaluation for the cardiovascular source of the embolus with a known cardiac source in which TEE would not change management
Routine use of TEE when diagnostic TTE is reasonably anticipated to resolve all diagnostic and management concerns
Surveillance of prior TEE findings for interval change (e.g., resolution of the thrombus after anticoagulation and resolution of the vegetation after antibiotic therapy) when no change in therapy is anticipated
To diagnose infective endocarditis with low pretest probability (e.g., transient fever, known alternative source of infection, negative blood culture results, and atypical pathogen for endocarditis)
Evaluation when a decision has been made to anticoagulate and not to perform cardioversion

Table 37.3 TEE and TTE: recommended techniques for visualization of sources of embolism

Cardio-embolic source	TTE	TEE
Atrial arrhythmias	• Sweeps of atria and atrial appendages from multiple perspectives (PLAX, PSAX, apical views; two-chamber view for LAA) • High-frequency imaging • Trans-pulmonary contrast	• Sweeps of atria and atrial appendages from multiple perspectives • Multi-plane (biplane) imaging • 3D imaging high light atrial anaotomy and structures • Trans-pulmonary contrast • High-frequency imaging
Valvular disease: • mechanical valve prosthesis • rheumatic heart disease	• Fundamental imaging • Sweeps, anteriorly posteriorly/superiorly and inferiorly of valve (s) • 3D imaging may require nonstandard imaging windows for better resolution • Color Doppler (with sweeps)	• Fundamental imaging • Sweeps, anteriorly posteriorly/superiorly and inferiorly of valve (s) • 3D imaging to assess/better define valvular structure and related anatomy • Color Doppler (with sweeps)
Endocarditis	• High frequency and fundamental imaging • Sweeps, anteriorly and posteriorly/superior and inferiorly of valve(s) • 3D imaging, preferably from parasternal perspective for better resolution • Color Doppler	• High-frequency and fundamental imaging • Sweeps, anteriorly and posteriorly/superiorly and inferiorly of valve(s) • 3D imaging (for point of attachment and sizing) • Color Doppler
Non-ischemic and ischemic cardiomyopathies	• High-frequency and fundamental imaging (with sweeps) • Sweeps, anteriorly and posteriorly/superiorly and inferiorly from multiple perspectives with and without harmonics • 3D and multi-plane imaging • Trans-pulmonary contrast • Color Doppler (in aneurysmal wall cases and for VSD checks)	• Sweeps, anteriorly and posteriorly/superiorly and inferiorly from multiple perspectives, especially gastric views for LV/RV focus • Trans-pulmonary contrast • 3D and multi-plane imaging • Color Doppler (in aneurysmal wall cases and for VSD checks)
Cardiac masses		
Intra-cardiac thrombus, vegetations (marantic or infective)	• High-frequency and fundamental imaging (with sweeps) • Sweeps, anteriorly and posteriorly/superiorly and inferiorly from multiple perspectives with and without harmonics • Off-axis/nonstandard views(to better show and define location) • 3D and Multiplan imaging • Trans-pulmonary contrast	• High-frequency and fundamental imaging (with sweeps) • Sweeps, anteriorly and posteriorly/superiorly and inferiorly from multiple perspectives • 3D and multi-plane imaging • Trans-pulmonary contrast
Intra-cardiac tumors, fibroelastoma	• Sweeps, anteriorly and posteriorly/superiorly and inferiorly from multiple perspectives with and without harmonics • 3D and multi-plane imaging (for point of attachment, and for size and shape) • Trans-pulmonary contrast (to assist in border definition and check for vascularization)	• Sweeps, anteriorly and posteriorly/superiorly and inferiorly from multiple perspectives • 3D and multi-plane imaging (for point of attachment) • Trans-pulmonary contrast (to assist in border definition and check for vascularization)
Thromboembolism from the thoracic aorta	• Additional 2D views such as right parasternal and high left parasternal, short-axis perspective of suprasternal notch • Sweeps, anteriorly and posteriorly/superiorly and inferiorly /lateral and medial with and without harmonics • Trans-pulmonary contrast • 3D and multi-plane imaging • High-frequency and fundamental imaging	• Sweeps, anteriorly and posteriorly/superiorly and inferiorly of aorta from multiple views with without harmonics • 3D and multi-plane imaging (for point of attachment) • Trans-pulmonary contrast
Aortic arch atheromatous plaque	• 3D and multi-plane imaging • High-frequency and fundamental imaging	• 3D and multi-plane imaging • High-frequency and fundamental imaging

(continued)

Table 37.3 (continued)

Cardio-embolic source	TTE	TEE
Intra-cardiac shunt	• Color Doppler with appropriate Nyquist shift to show shunt (low for inter-atrial septal shunts and large VSDs, high for small VSD) • Off-axis/nonstandard views • Agitated saline contrast study (as appropriate)	• Color Doppler with appropriate Nyquist shift to show shunt (low for inter-atrial septal shunts and large VSDs, high for small VSD) • Agitated saline contrast study (as appropriate)
Intra-pulmonary shunt	• Agitated saline contrast study (as appropriate)	• Agitated saline contrast study (as appropriate)
Trans-catheter device	• High-frequency and fundamental imaging (with sweeps) • Sweeps, anteriorly and posteriorly/superiorly and inferiorly from multiple perspectives with and without harmonics • 3D and multi-plan imaging	• High-frequency and fundamental imaging (with sweeps) • Sweeps, anteriorly and posteriorly/superiorly and inferiorly from multiple perspectives with and without harmonics • 3D and multi-plan imaging

Modified table from Muhamed Saric, Alicia C. Armour, M. Samir Arnaout, Farooq A. Chaudhry, Richard A. Grimm, DO, Itzhak Kronzon, Bruce F. Landeck, II, Kameswari Maganti, Hector I. Michelena and Kirsten Tolstrup. Guidelines for the Use of Echocardiography in the Evaluation of a Cardiac Source of Embolism. ASE GUIDELINES AND STANDARDS. J Am Soc Echocardiogr. 2016;29:1–42

Multi-Plane and 3D Imaging

3D and multi-plane imaging has opened up echocardiography to new techniques of interrogating and evaluating cardiac structure and function. Though standard 2D imaging is still used for the majority of studies, 3D and multi-plane imaging can highlight areas frequently missed or overlooked as well as identify areas of interest when it comes to the sources of cardiac, aortic, and also pulmonary emboli. For example in the standard 2D image, the LA myxoma is revealed moving through the MV orifice, while the 3D image displays not only the LA myxoma as it moves in the LA and MV but also the point of connection on the IAS (Table 37.3) [1, 4].

Trans-Pulmonary Contrast and Saline

The suitability and use of transpulmonary contrast for endocardial border delineation as well as Doppler enhancement is well defined in the "2014 ASE contrast guidelines." Further uses of trans-pulmonary contrast can contain border and structure definition of thrombi and masses as well as viewing if a structure is vascularized (e.g., cardiac magnetic resonance). Although color Doppler can sometimes identify intra-cardiac shunts, the use of agitated saline contrast yields higher incidence of findings (Table 37.3) [1, 7–10].

Conclusion

During the past 2 decades, vast progress has been made in the noninvasive diagnosis of cardio-embolic events. A potential cardiac source of embolism must be considered in all cases presenting with stroke or transient ischemic attack. In this regard, echocardiography is a potent tool not only for the assessment of the cardio-embolic sources of stroke, but also for the establishment of recommendations for the primary and secondary prevention of cardio-embolic strokes.

MCQ

1. Echocardiographic predictors of embolic risk in cases with AF are as follow except for:
   A. Left ventricular systolic dysfunction (ejection fraction < or = 45%)
   B. Complex aortic plaques
   C. left atrial appendage (LAA) thrombi or spontaneous echo contrast
   D. LAA dysfunction (emptying blood flow velocities ≤20 cm/s or reduced contraction at M-mode)

2. What is the pathology in the following figure?

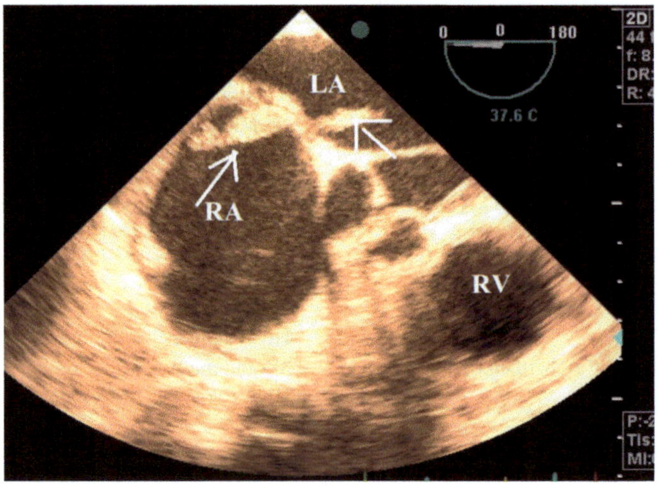

A. Thrombus in transit via patent foramen ovale
B. No pathology
C. Lead in RA and LA
D. Artifact

3. The incidence of PFO seems to be higher in cases with the ischemic type of stroke, more than ... fold higher in cases younger than 55 years old.
A. 2
B. 3
C. 4
D. 5

Answers

1. A
2. A
3. B

References

1. Saric M, Armour AC, Samir Arnaout M, Chaudhry FA, Grimm RA, Kronzon I, Landeck BF II, Maganti K, Michelena HI, Tolstrup K. Guidelines for the use of echocardiography in the evaluation of a cardiac source of embolism. ASE guidelines and Standards. J Am Soc Echocardiogr. 2016;29:1–42.
2. Pepi M, Evangelista A, Nihoyannopoulos P, Flachskampf FA, Athanassopoulos G, Colonna P, Habib G, Bernd Ringelstein E, Sicari R, Zamorano JL. Recommendations for echocardiography use in the diagnosis and management of cardiac sources of embolism. Eur J Echocardiogr. 2010;11:461–76.
3. Senior R, Becher H, Monaghan M, Agati L, Zamorano J, Vanoverschelde JL, et al. Contrast echocardiography: evidence-based recommendations by European Association of Echocardiography. Eur J Echocardiogr. 2009;10:194–212.
4. Kurt M, Shaikh KA, Peterson L, Kurrelmeyer KM, Shah G, Nagueh SF, et al. Impact of contrast echocardiography on evaluation of ventricular function and clinical management in a large prospective cohort. J Am Coll Cardiol. 2009;53:802–10.
5. American Heart Association & American Stroke Association. Cryptogenic stroke initiative. http://www.strokeassociation.org/STROKEORG/boutStroke/TypesofStroke/CryptogenicStrokesofUnknownCause/Cryptogenic-Stroke-initiative_UCM_471631_article.Jsp#.VjD9L7erR9M. Accessed 28 Oct 2015.
6. Douglas PS, GarciaMJ HDE, Lai WW, Manning WJ, Patel AR, et al. ACCF/ ASE/ AHA/ ASNC/HFSA/HRS/SCAI/SCCM/SCCT/ SCMR 2011 appropriate use criteria for echocardiography. A report of the American College of Cardiology Foundation Appropriate Use CriteriaTask Force, American Society of Echocardiography, American Heart Association, American Society of Nuclear Cardiology, Heart Failure Society of America, Heart Rhythm Society, Society for Cardiovascular Angiography and Interventions, Society of Critical Care Medicine, Society of Cardiovascular Computed Tomography, Society for Cardiovascular Magnetic Resonance American College of Chest Physicians. J Am Soc Echocardiogr. 2011;24:229–67.
7. Pepi M, Evangelista A, Nihoyannopoulos P, Flachskampf FA, Athanassopoulos G, Colonna P, et al. Recommendations for echocardiography in the diagnosis and management of cardiac sources of embolism. Eur J Echocardiogr. 2010;11:461–76.
8. Ustrell X, Pellise A. Cardiac workup of ischemic stroke. Curr Cardiol Rev. 2010;6:175–83.
9. Lang RM, Badano LP, Tsang W, Adams DH, Agricola E, Buck T, et al. EAE/ASE recommendations for image acquisition and display using three-dimensional echocardiography. J Am Soc Echocardiogr. 2012;25:3–46.
10. Porter TR, Abdelmoneim S, Belcik JT, McCulloch ML, Mulvagh SL, Olson JJ, et al. Guidelines for the cardiac sonographer in the performance of contrast echocardiography: a focused update from the American Society of Echocardiography. J Am Soc Echocardiogr. 2014;27:797–810.

Disease of the Aorta

38

Azin Alizadehasl and Anita Sadeghpour

Abstract

Echocardiography plays an essential role in the diagnosis, management plans, and follow-up of aortic diseases. Study of the aorta is a routine part of the standard echocardiographic examination. Transthoracic echocardiography (TTE) permits adequate assessment of several aortic segments, mainly the aortic root and the proximal ascending aorta. Transesophageal echocardiography (TEE) overcomes the limitations of TTE in the evaluation of the thoracic aorta. TEE must be used in a complementary manner. Echocardiography is useful and valuable for assessing the size, biophysical properties, and atherosclerotic involvement of the thoracic aorta. Although TEE is a useful method in the diagnosis of aortic dissection, TTE may be used as the initial modality in the emergency setting. Intimal flap in the proximal ascending aorta, pericardial effusion/tamponade, and left ventricular function can be easily visualized by TTE. Nonetheless, a negative TTE does not rule out aortic dissection and other imaging modalities should be considered. TEE must define entry tear location, mechanisms and severity of aortic regurgitation, and also true lumen compression. Additionally, echocardiography is crucial in selecting and monitoring surgical and endovascular treatment and in noticing possible complications. Even though other imaging techniques such as computed tomography and magnetic resonance imaging have a greater field of view and can yield complementary information, echocardiography is accurate, portable, rapid, and cost-effective in the diagnosis, management plans, and follow-up of most aortic diseases.

Keywords

Aortic diseases · Transesophageal echocardiography
Transthoracic echocardiography · Aneurysm of aorta
Aortic dissection · Intramural hematoma (IMH)
Coarctation (COA) · Pseudoaneurysms

Abbreviations

AV	Aortic valve
BSA	Body surface area
COA	Coarctation
CT	Computed tomography
IMH	Intramural hematoma
MRI	Magnetic resonance imaging
STJ	Sinotubular junction
TEE	Transesophageal echocardiography
TTE	Transthoracic echocardiography

Anatomy

- The aorta is the main artery of the body and is divided into thoracic and abdominal parts by the diaphragm. The thoracic aorta is subdivided into ascending, arch, and descending portions with the innominate and left subclavian arteries, correspondingly. The aortic arch consequently gives off all the main vessels to the head and upper limbs.
- The aortic root contains the aortic annulus, sinuses of Valsalva, and sinotubular junction (STJ). The course of the thoracic aorta starts on the anterior mediastinum, in

Electronic Supplementary Material The online version of this chapter (https://doi.org/10.1007/978-3-319-67691-3_38) contains supplementary material, which is available to authorized users.

A. Alizadehasl, MD, FACC, FASE (✉)
Associate Professor of Cardiology, Echocardiologist, Echocardiography and Cardiogenetic Research Centers, Cardio-Oncology Department, Rajaie Cardiovascular Medical and Research Center, Tehran, Iran

A. Sadeghpour, MD, FACC, FASE
Professor of Cardiology, Echocardiography Research Center, Rajaie Cardiovascular Medical and Research Center, Iran University of Medical Science, Tehran, Iran

A. Sadeghpour, A. Alizadehasl (eds.), *Case-Based Textbook of Echocardiography*,
https://doi.org/10.1007/978-3-319-67691-3_38

the pericardium to the right side of the midline. It bends in front of the trachea, arches across to the left, and then lands on the posterior mediastinum-in front of the thoracic vertebrae and behind the esophagus [1].

- Like all the arteries, the aorta is made up of three histologically different layers: the intima, media, and adventitia. The intima is a thin inner layer of endothelium and subendothelial connective tissue. The media is a thick muscular layer that provides the majority of elasticity and strength. Lastly, the adventitia is a fibrous protecting outer layer [1].
- Echocardiographic assessment of the aorta and also the main pulmonary artery is a routine part of the standard echocardiographic study. For imaginative purposes, the aorta is divided into the following segments, beginning at the aortic valve (AV):
  - Aortic annulus
  - Sinuses of Valsalva
  - STJ
  - Ascending aorta
  - Aortic arch
  - Descending thoracic aorta
  - Proximal abdominal aorta [1–3]
- The term "aortic root" has a different explanation, which can lead to mistakes in communication. In the study of genetic connective tissue disorders, the aortic root frequently refers to the aortic sinuses-from the AV level to the STJ. Nonetheless, a surgical aortic root replacement classically extends from the aortic annulus to the mid ascending aorta. Accordingly, when the aorta is abnormal, more precise specific terms for labeling the anatomic position are preferred [2, 3].
- The aortic root and the proximal ascending aorta are typically seen on the parasternal long-axis view. Part of the descending thoracic aorta is also seen behind the left atrium in this view.
- The right parasternal view is used to precisely image the ascending aorta, whereas the suprasternal windows determine the aortic arch and its branches (Fig. 38.1). The subcostal window can be employed to evaluate the suprarenal abdominal aorta [2–4].
- Imaging the thoracic aorta with transthoracic echocardiography (TTE) differs between patients. More often than not, images are suboptimal and it is not possible to diagnose or eliminate the aortic pathology with confidence. Consequently, if aortic pathology is supposed, other forms of imaging such as transesophageal echocardiography (TEE), computed tomography (CT), and magnetic resonance imaging (MRI) are typically essential to reach a firm diagnosis [2–4].

The aortic root dimensions must be measured in every examination. Dimensions must be made at the AV annulus (among the hinge points of the AV cusps), sinus of Valsalva, and STJ. Additionally, direct measurements from 2D images are now suggested.

- The thoracic aorta can be characterized as having three major segments. The ascending aorta extends from the annulus to the innominate artery and includes the three sinuses of Valsalva, the three cusps of the aortic valve, the sinotubular junction, the ostia of the coronary arteries, and the proximal ascending aorta. The arch extends from a left innominate to the ligamentum arteriosum and includes the great vessels arising off of the arch. The descending thoracic aorta extends from the ligamentum arteriosum to the level of the diaphragm (Fig. 38.2).
- TEE provides a considerably wider window to the aortic anatomy. The aorta can be imaged from the AV annulus through the ascending aorta, arch, and descending thoracic aorta to the level of the gastroesophageal connection [4–6].

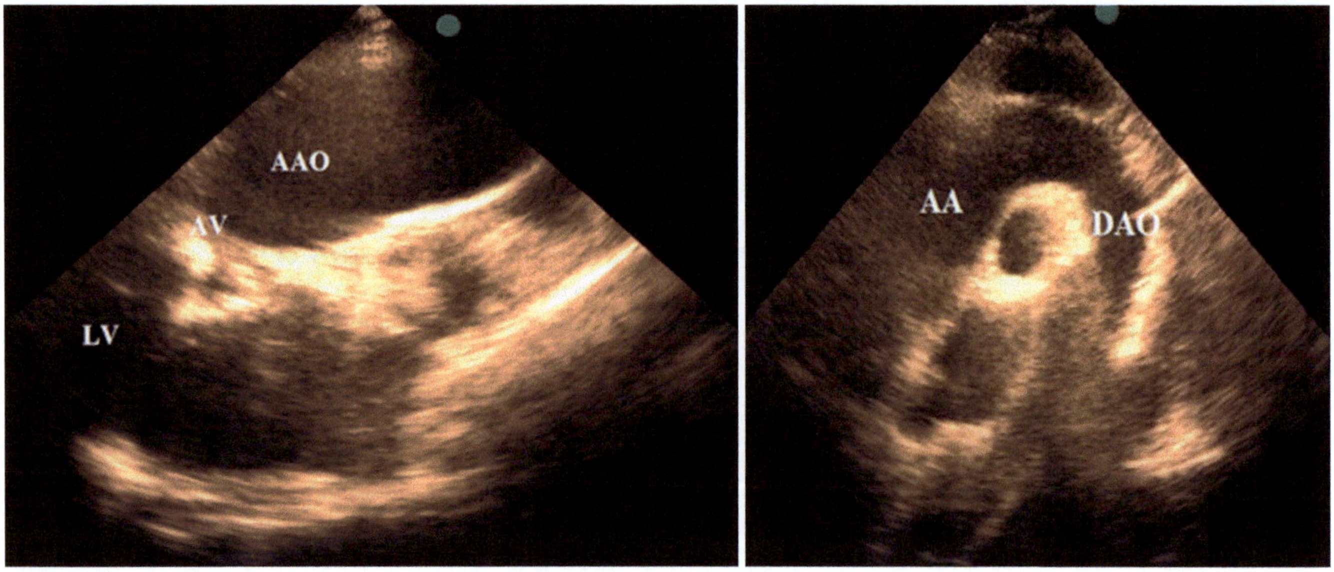

Fig. 38.1 Left: transthoracic echocardiography, right parasternal view for better imaging the ascending aorta Right: transthoracic echocardiography suprasternal view for imaging the aortic arch

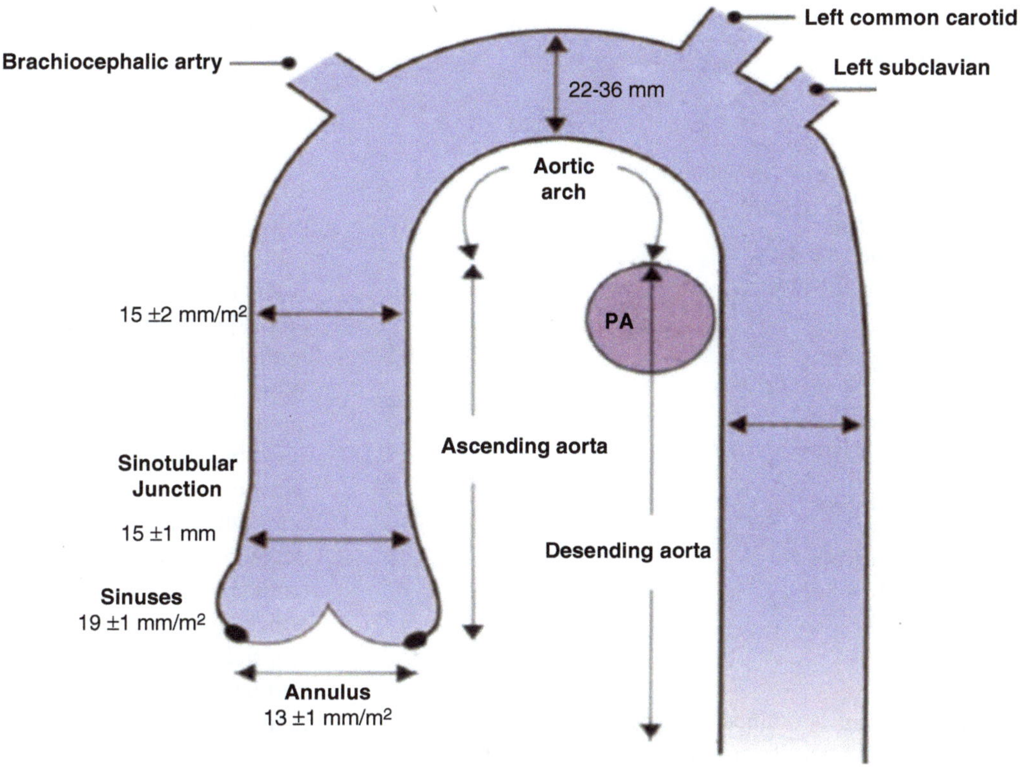

Fig. 38.2 The normal dimensions of the aorta are noted in the schematic and vary with location. Dimensions are given both indexed to body surface area (BSA) and as the range anticipated in routine adult echocardiography. PA, right pulmonary artery. Modified figure of: Echocardiography in aortic diseases: EAE recommendations for clinical practice. Eur J Echocardiogr. 2010 Sep; 11(8):645–58

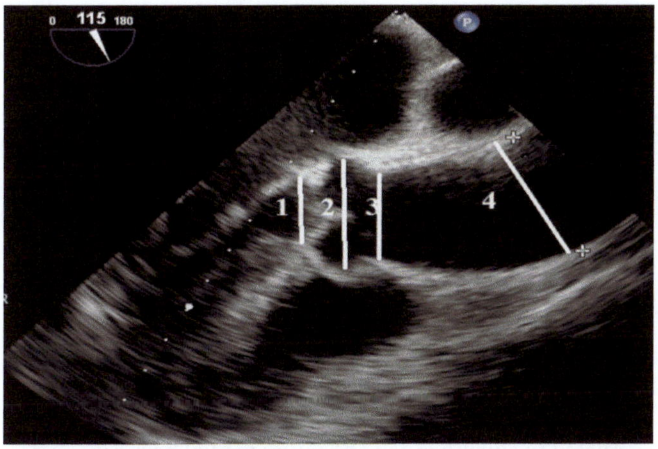

Fig. 38.3 Transthoracic echocardiography long axis view for precise measurement of the (1) Aortic Valve annulus, (2) sinus of Valsalva, (3) sinotubular junction, (4) Asc aorta

- Mostly, the proximal 5–10 cm of the ascending aorta can be imaged by scanning at a 120° imaging plane of TEE (Fig. 38.3).

It has been suggested to measure the aortic root diameter perpendicularly to the axis of the proximal aorta, several times, at end-diastole using the leading edge-to-leading edge technique and consider the largest diameter [2]. Measurement should be done when the closure line is in the centre of the aortic root.

By rotating the imaging plane to 40–60°, a series of short-axis views of the proximal part of the ascending aorta can be achieved-containing a short-axis view of the AV closure.

The descending thoracic aorta is imaged by inserting the probe deeper toward the gastroesophageal connection site, and scanning at a 0° plane. The probe can then be gradually withdrawn along the length of the aorta and a series of short-axis views of the thoracic aorta achieved. At any point along the aorta, the image can be rotated to a 90° plane to obtain a longitudinal view of the aorta [2, 4–6].

Aortic Dilation and Aneurysm

- Dilation of the aorta can happen at any point alongside its course. It is important to know that documentation of disease in one part of the aorta must prompt assessment of the full extent of the aorta because many of them have manifestations in other areas as a part of a global pathology. Main aortic abnormality are categorized in Table 38.1. When aortic diameter exceeds the Z score ≥ -2 is considered dilated [2].

Table 38.1 Main aortic abnormalities

• Dilation
• Aneurysms
• Aortic dissection
• Intramural hematoma (IMH)
• Thrombi
• Atheromas
• Coarctation (COA)
• Pseudoaneurysms
• Traumas
• Takayasu's arteritis
• Infections of the aorta

Table 38.2 Causes of aortic aneurysms

Weakened wall
Atherosclerosis
Aortitis
Takayasu's arteritis
Ankylosing spondylitis and other spondyloarthritis
Giant cell arteritis
Collagen disorders
Marfan's syndrome
Ehlers-Danlos syndrome
Infection
Syphilis
Tuberculosis
Salmonella
Post-traumatic
Deceleration injuries
Catheter injury
Increased wall stress
Hypertension
Post aortic stenosis
Bicuspid AV
Aortic coarctation

- An aneurysm is defined as expansion to more than 1.5 times the normal dimension for that feature of the aorta. Dilation of the aorta can either be isolated or related to other cardiovascular diseases such as hypertension or AV disease.
- Primary aortic dilation happens with cystic medial necrosis, as characterized by Marfan's syndrome. Nonetheless, it is also seen in other connective tissue diseases. Secondary dilation of the aorta can happen in volume or pressure overload states such as aortic insufficiency or hypertension. Post-stenotic dilation happens in cases with valvular aortic stenosis and possibly represents simultaneous primary disease of the aorta, rather than being secondary to any hemodynamic abnormality [1, 4, 6].
- Ascending aortic aneurysms have a tendency to be caused by diseases that lead to cystic necrosis of the media. This is mainly related to Marfan's syndrome and other hereditary aortic syndromes. However, it can also happen with ageing and hypertension. The aneurysms of the descending aorta are more often due to atherosclerosis (Table 38.2).
- TTE (in the parasternal long-axis view) is valuable for noticing ascending aortic aneurysms, mainly those involving the aortic root and the STJ. This modality is, however, less reliable at identifying aneurysms at other places.
- The echocardiographic appearance of an aneurysm is a region of dilatation that enlarges in systole. The maximal internal diameter must be measured and referenced to the patient's age and body surface area. Dilatation of the aortic root can disrupt the AV leaflets and cause aortic insufficiency [1, 2, 4].

Sinus of Valsalva Aneurysms

- The sinuses of Valsalva are the outpouchings of the aorta at the level of the AV cusps, from which the coronary arteries rise. They are not typically seen very well in TTE. Aneurysmal dilatation of the sinuses happens most usually as a congenital heart disease, correlated with a ventricular septal defect.
- Aneurysms rising from the right Valsalva sinus classically protrude into the right atrium, where they are frequently initially imaged as a filamentous or "windsock" structure. When imaged in the short axis view, they may resemble a circular mobile structure mimicking a cystic mass. A sinus of Valsalva aneurysm rising from the non-coronary sinus can dissect inferiorly into the interventricular septum, where it is noticed as a cystic structure. It can also develop in patients with aortic root pathology, and after cardiac surgery. A rare complication is aneurysm rupture, which usually causes aortic insufficiency into the right ventricle or the other cardiac chambers, depending on the particular sinus involved. Rarely, a sinus of Valsalva aneurysm might thrombose and mimic an intracardiac mass [1–4].

Aortic Dissection

- Aortic dissection is a situation in which the intima shears apart from the rest of the aortic wall, creating a flap of tissue and a false lumen.
- The aortic dissection can propagate along the aortic wall and re-enter the true lumen at a distal location or cause occlusion of the aorta and its branches. When the aortic root is involved, acute severe aortic insufficiency, coronary artery obstruction, and pericardial effusion can happen. Rupture into a pleural space rarely happens. The underlying reason mirrors that of aortic aneurysms, and it is mainly related to situations causing cystic medial necrosis.
- Unequivocal echocardiographic evidence of aortic dissection needs demonstration of a mobile dissection flap, a false lumen, and an entry or exit points among the true and false lumens. Most of the time, however, the findings on TTE are more confusing such as aortic root dilatation, acute aortic insufficiency, AV cusp prolapse, pericardial effusion, and pleural effusion (Figs. 38.4 and 38.5). Because TTE images only a limited area of the ascending aorta, normally it is not considered a sufficient diagnostic tool for the exclusion of aortic dissection.
- Nevertheless, when an intimal flap is detected on TTE imaging, a dissection of the proximal aorta is most likely present. However, to confirm the diagnosis and distinguish an intimal flap from artefacts, the flap should be seen in more than one view and off axis view would be useful.

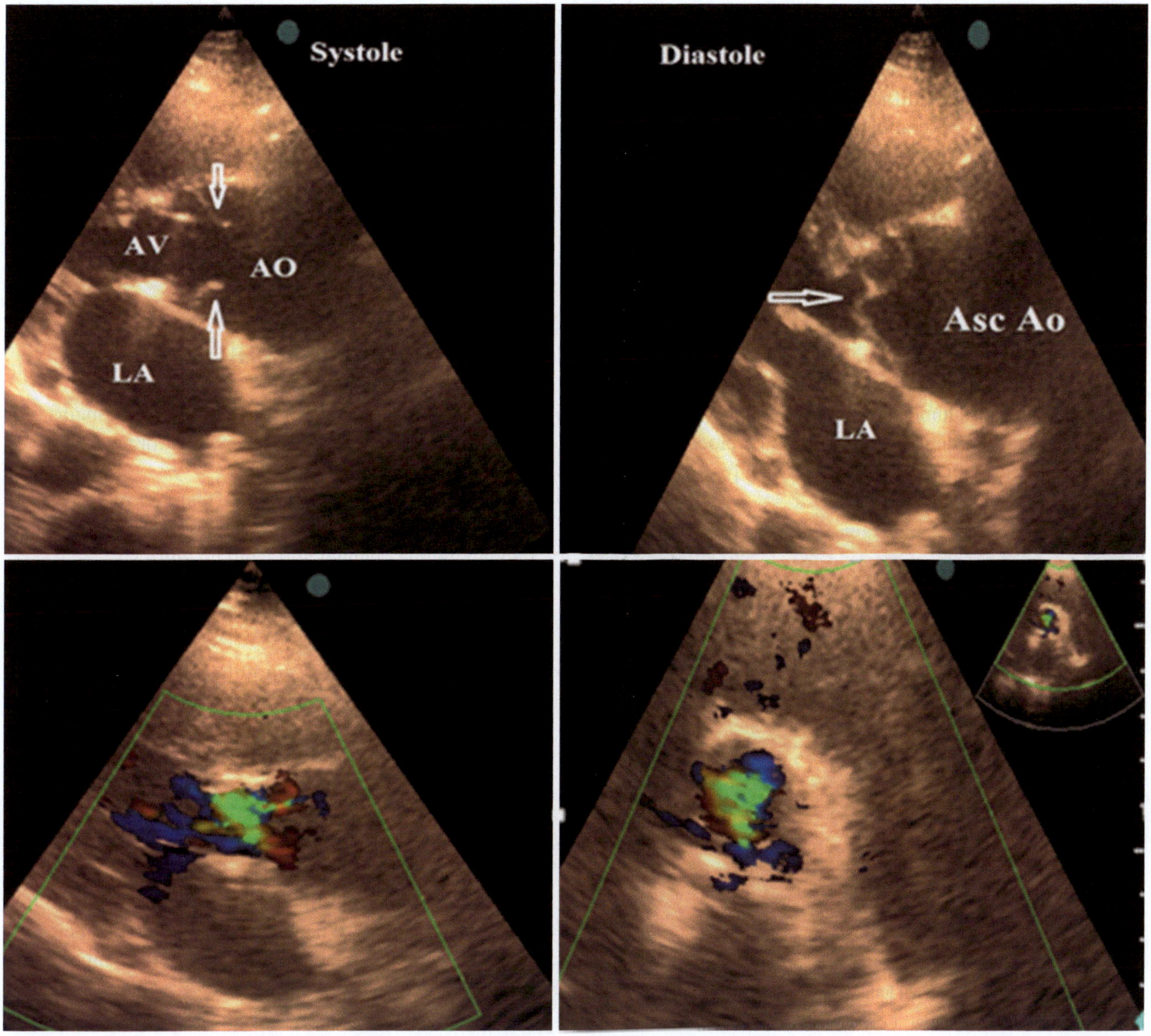

Fig. 38.4 Mobile dissecting flap obviously is visible in transthoracic echocardiography in systole and diastole that interfere with Aortic valve closure resulting sever aortic regurgitation in long axis and short axis view of transthoracic echocardiography

The dissecting flap should have an independent motion regarding the aortic walls and usually is associated with AR and pericardial effusion (Movies 38.1 and 38.2).

Other imaging methods such as TEE, CT, and MRI will be needed to fully characterize its extent [6–8].

- TEE has emerged as a primary diagnostic tool in the revealing of aortic dissection, and large series have suggested that it is used in nearly two-thirds of patients with supposed acute aortic dissection It can be done in critically ill cases in intensive care units, emergency departments, and operating rooms and provides a decisive diagnostic methodology (Figs. 38.6, 38.7, 38.8, Movie 38.5) In addition, complications such as pericardial effusion, aortic insufficiency, pseudoaneurysm, adventitial hematoma, and rupture can all be recognized (Movies 38.3 and 38.4).
- A skilled echocardiographer should not have trouble in separating artifacts from aortic dissection. Clues to artifact versus true aortic dissection include random mobility of a true dissection flap as opposed to a more rigid and fixed position with respect to the aortic wall realized in the artifact. Not rarely, artifacts will arise as a side lobe from the STJ and their intensity will gradually reduce in the lumen, while a true dissection flap will not lose its echo intensity along its course. Color-flow imaging can

be valuable for demonstrating the margination of the flow by a true dissection flap, while an artifact will not affect the distribution of the color flow signal [7–9].

- Sometimes, it can be difficult to distinguish the true from the false lumen. Several clues, however, enable a precise distinction of the two. In the ascending aorta, there is typically little confusion because one can appreciate the outlet of blood through the AV, which-by classification-will be into the true lumen. Clues that enable an accurate identification, especially in the descending aorta of the true lumen, include the fact that it will expand with systole as blood is ejected into it. It frequently has a more regular shape, which might be either circular or oval. Particularly in the descending thoracic aorta, the true lumen is the smaller of the two lumens. The false lumen is often filled with swirling homogeneous echoes, demonstrating stasis of blood, or rarely with frank thrombi (Figs. 38.9 and 38.10) [6–9].

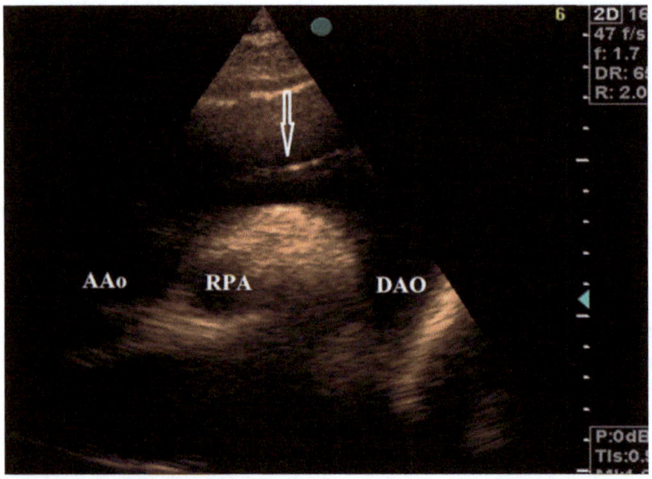

Fig. 38.5 Dissecting flap in aortic arch confirms the aortic dissection that was seen in the parasternal long axis view

- Lastly, the shearing of the intima from the media often results in small fibrinous tags of tissue in the false lumen, characterizing small muscle remnants where the intima has been sheared from the media.
- In skilled hands, the accuracy of TEE for the detection of aortic dissection is remarkably high and equivalent to that of competing procedures such as CT and MRI. Aortic dissection may also involve the coronary arteries, causing acute myocardial infarction, with evidence of regional wall motion abnormalities [8–10].

Intramural Hematoma (IMH)

- Aortic IMH is an accumulation of blood that remains limited within the aortic media; it accounts for nearly 5–20% of acute aortic syndromes.
- In the IMH, the typical imaging features of the classic aortic dissection are absence which means: No dissection flap, no double channel aorta and no entry site.
- Typical features of IMH is a crescentic or concentric pattern thickening of the aortic wall with more than 0.5 cm thickness (Table 38.3) [2].
- On TEE, it appears as a smooth, homogenously echogenic bulge within the medial layer of the aortic wall. It is hypothesized to rise from (A) rupture of a penetrating atherosclerotic ulcer, (B) spontaneous rupture of the vasa vasorum, or more frequently (C) blunt traumas.
- IMH is distinguished from the classically focal, echo-bright, and irregular plaque in the aortic wall in that it extends smoothly and longitudinally along the aorta. On cross-sectional views, it appears as a crescentic or circular area of homogeneous thickening around the central aortic lumen (Figs. 38.11 and 38.12).

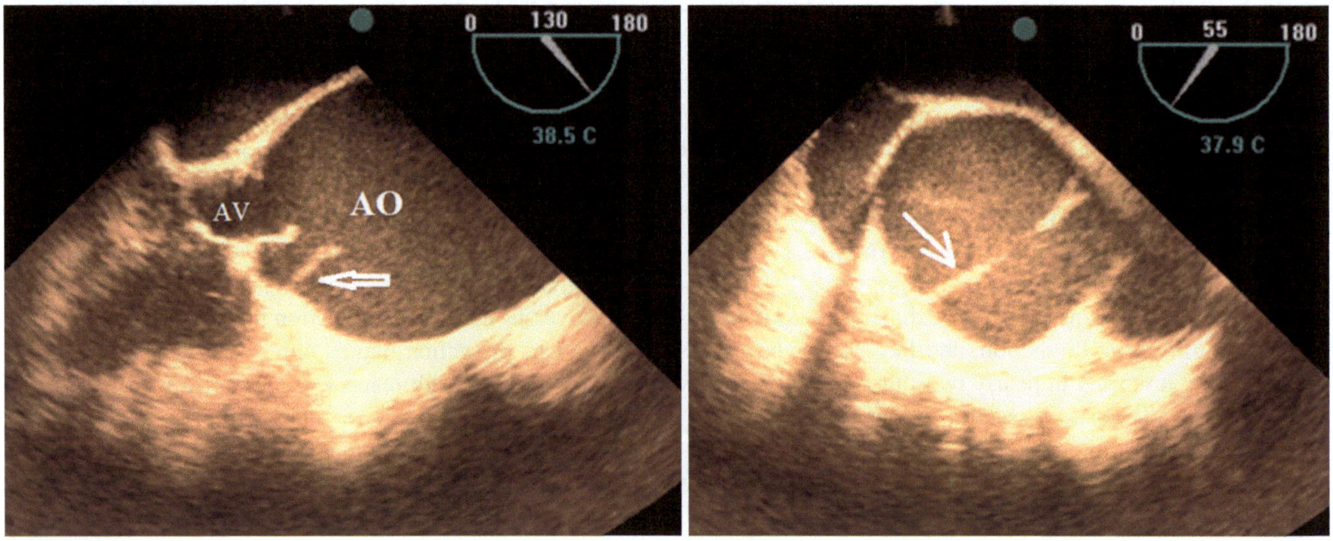

Fig. 38.6 Confirming the dissecting flap in two orthogonal views (arrow)

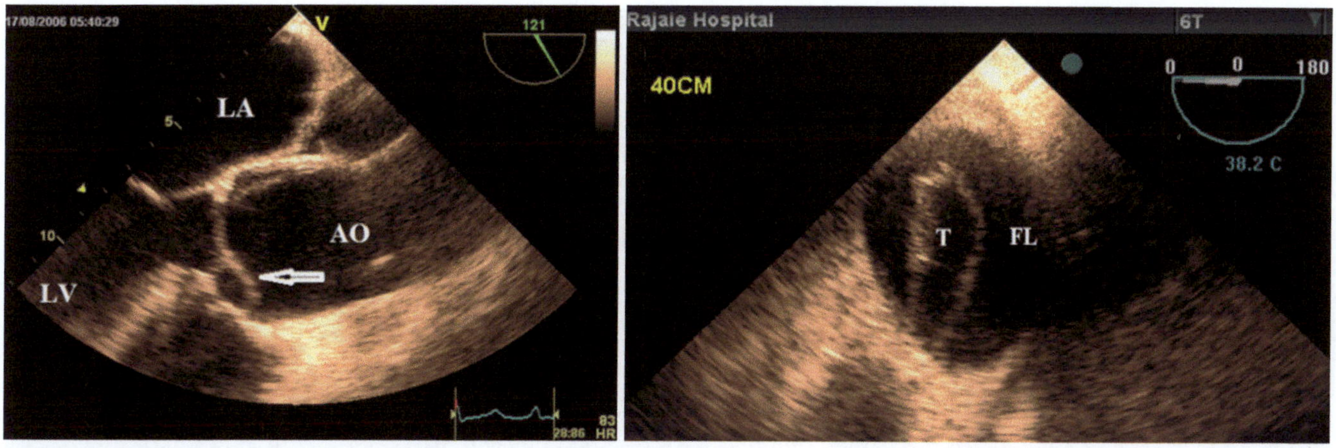

Fig. 38.7 Left panel: thin, mobile linear echogenicity in the artic root (arrow) with interference with Aortic valve closure suggesting for acute type A acute aortic dissection. Right panel: Large false lumen (fl) with smoke pattern and small true lumen (T) in descending thoracic aorta (Movie 38.5)

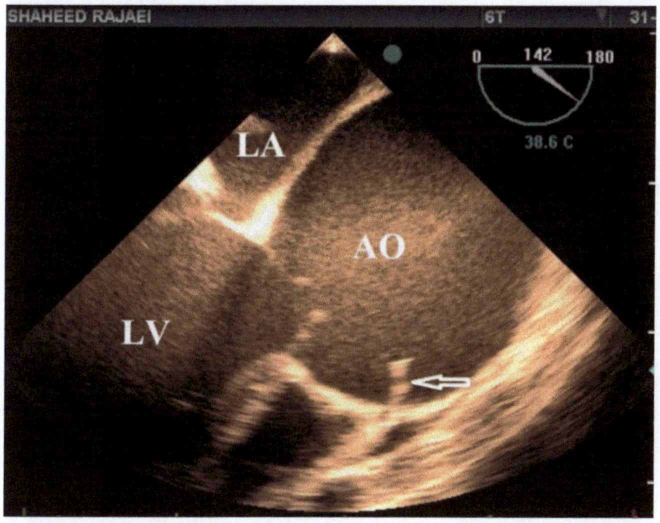

Fig. 38.8 Thick and fixed linear echogenicity associated with aneurysmal dilatation of aortic root in a Marfan syndrome suggestive of chronic dissecting flap (Movie 38.6)

- Unlike aortic dissection, the intimal layer is still intact and is not mobilized; thus, there is no detectable intimal tear and no blood flow communication with the aortic lumen. If the IMH is fairly small, additional imaging with CT or MRI may be necessary to definitively recognize the hematoma and distinguish it from the differential diagnoses of plaques or periaortic fat. IMH can rise in either ascending or descending sites and may enlarge or progress to frank aortic dissection [2, 10–12].

Aortic Thrombi

- In rare cases, a mobile thrombus can form within the aortic lumen. This is more common in the proximal descending thoracic aorta and frequently has been related to peripheral embolization. Such thrombi are noted as highly mobile echo-dense masses within the lumen, which often appear to be attached to the aortic wall by an equally thin stalk. Suitable therapy for intra-aortic thrombi is controversial, and the relative roles of aggressive anticoagulation versus surgical removal have not been fully clarified [2–4].

Aortic Atheromas

- Atherosclerosis can affect the aorta, like other major arteries, and frequently coexists with coronary atherosclerotic disease. Atheromas appear as a thickening of the arterial wall, which can be focal or generalized, and might be related to calcification. Severe atheromas (>4 mm thickness) or complex lesions such as protruding or mobile atherosclerosis may be a cause of stroke and systemic embolism (Table 38.4). Aortic atheromas are most common in older cases or in individuals with a history of tobacco use, hypertension, and high cholesterol. Moreover, they can be an integral component of atherosclerotic aneurysms. Not rarely, they are also encountered in patients in whom a cardiovascular source of emboli is suspected. Atheromas of the aorta are considered by their locations and topographic appearances. They are most prevalent in the descending thoracic aorta and arch, and they are far less frequently encountered in the ascending aorta. Recognition is far more reliable with TEE than TTE (Fig. 38.13, Movie 38.7) [2–4, 13, 14].

Coarctation of the Aorta (COA)

This is a narrowing of the aorta due to abnormal embryonic development. COA is localized to the descending thoracic aorta distal to the origin of the left subclavian artery, near

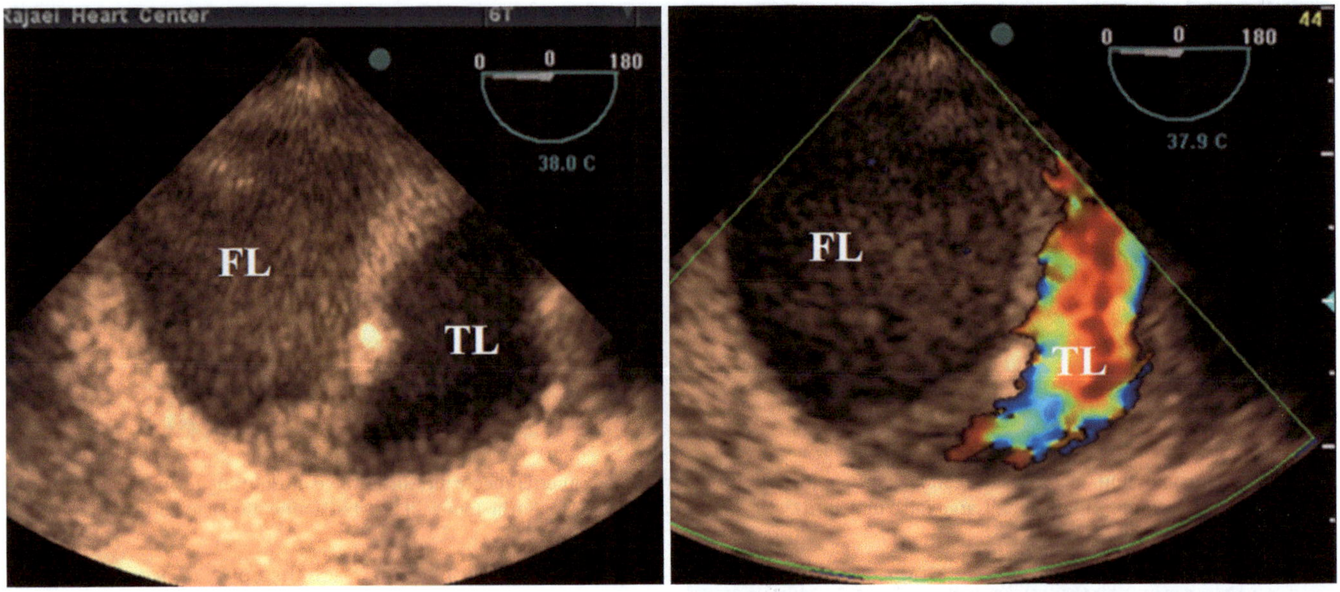

Fig. 38.9 Dissecting flap in descending thoracic aorta. Left: Smoke and stagnant flow in the larger lumen is suggestive for false lumen. Right: Turbulent color Doppler study of the small lumen is suggestive for true lumen

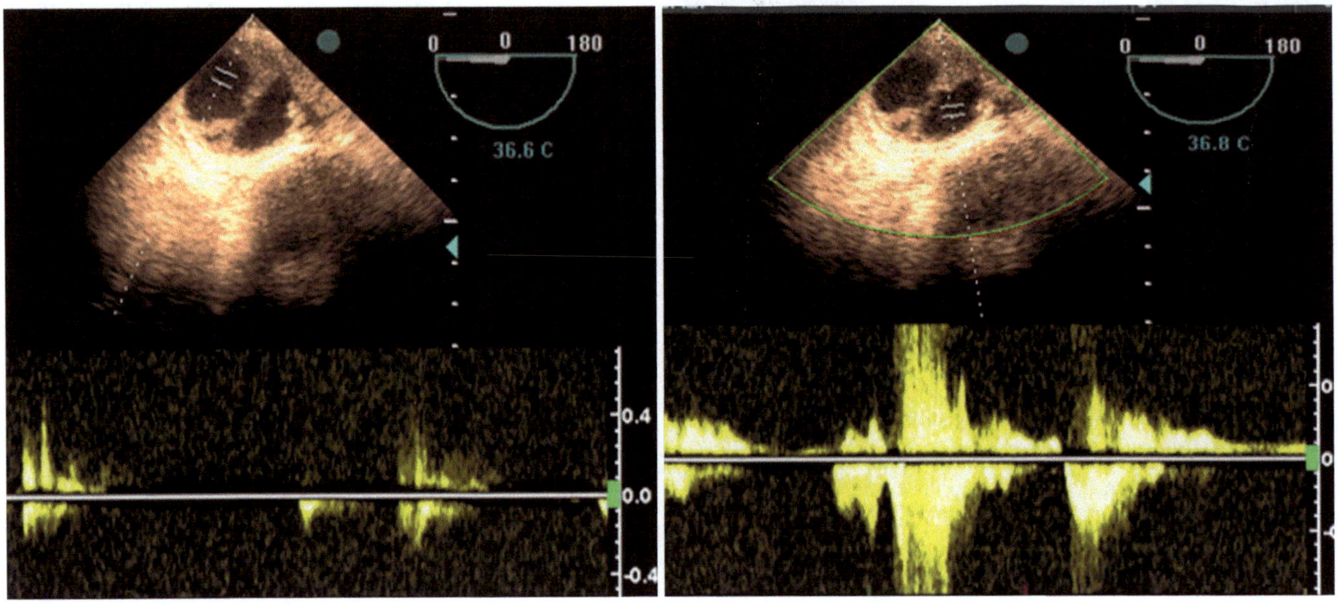

Fig. 38.10 Dissecting flap in descending thoracic aorta. Left: PW Doppler study of the larger lumen showing weak and delayed flow suggestive for false lumen. Right: PW Doppler study of the small lumen showing dense flow signal suggestive for true lumen

the ligamentum arteriosus. It can occur in isolation or in relation to other congenital heart diseases, most especially a bicuspid AV. It has a specific association with Turner's syndrome. The majority of cases are detected in infants, although rare cases may present in adulthood with complications such as hypertension, aortic dissection, aortic aneurysm, infective endocarditis, heart failure, and cerebral hemorrhage.

Table 38.3 Imaging features of Intramural Hematoma (IMH)

1	Focal aortic wall thickening (crescentic > concentric)
2	Preserved luminal shape with smooth luminal border
3	Absence of dissection flap and false lumen
4	Echolucent regions may be present in the aortic wall
5	Central displacement of intimal calcium

From Goldstein S, Evangelista A, Abbara S, Arai A, Asch F, Badano L et al. Multimodality Imaging of Diseases of the Thoracic Aorta in Adults. Am Soc Echocardiogr 2015

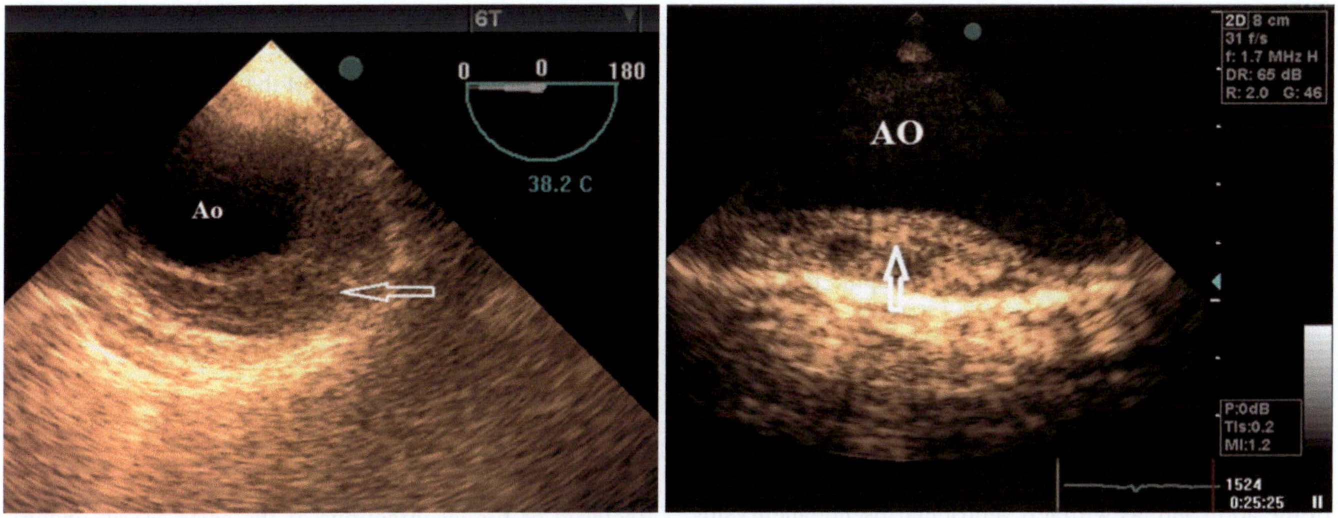

Fig. 38.11 Intramural hematoma in short axis and long axis of the descending thoracic aorta (arrows)

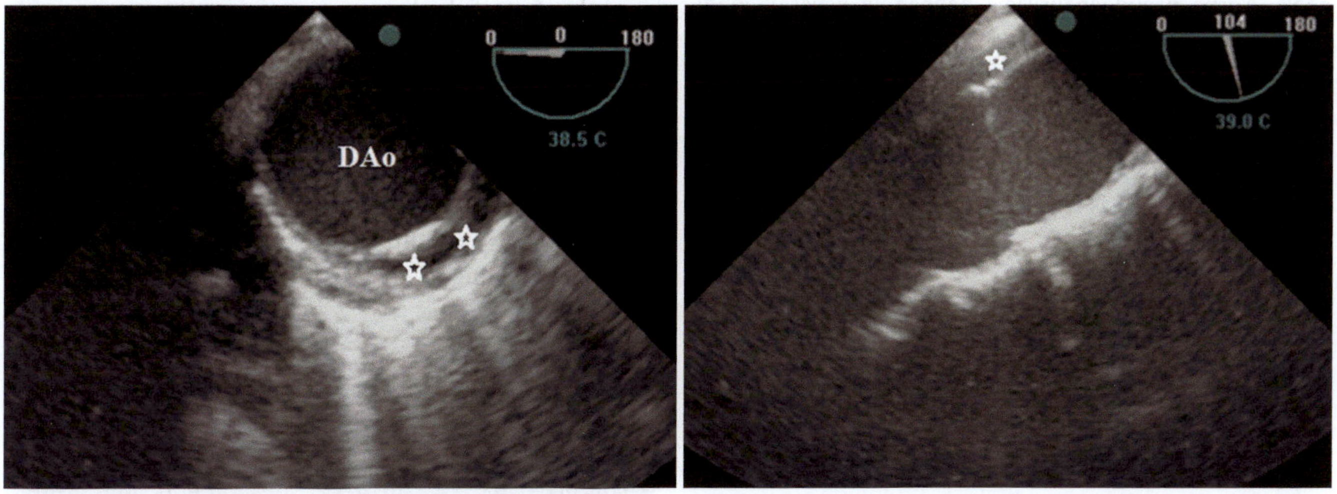

Fig. 38.12 Intramural hematoma in short axis and long axis view of transthoracic echocardiography (star)

Table 38.4 Grading system for severity of aortic atherosclerosis

Grade	Severity (atheroma thickness)	Description
1	Normal	Intimal thickness <2 mm
2	Mild	Mild (focal or diffuse) intimal thickening of 2–3 mm
3	Moderate	Atheroma >3–5 mm (no mobile/ ulcerated components)
4	Severe	Atheroma >5 mm (no mobile/ ulcerated components)
5	Complex	Grade 2, 3, or 4 atheroma plus mobile or ulcerated components

From Goldstein S, Evangelista A, Abbara S, Arai A, Asch F, Badano L et al. Multimodality imaging of diseases of the thoracic aorta in adults. Am Soc Echocardiogr. 2015

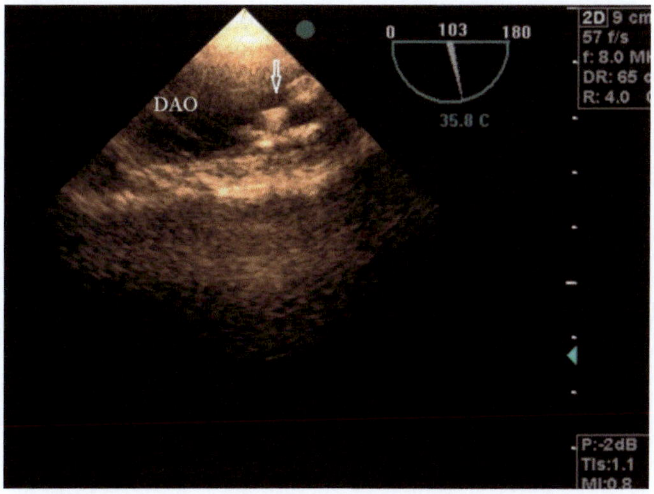

Fig. 38.13 Complex atherosclerotic plaque of descending thoracic aorta

In the suprasternal view, COA appears as a ridge-like constricting of the descending thoracic aorta, allied to a turbulent high-velocity flow. Less frequently, a long tubular constriction happens. Continuous-wave Doppler is utilized to evaluate the severity of the gradient across the COA using Bernoulli's equation. In catheterism, a gradient more than 25 mm Hg is considered severe enough to warrant intervention, either by surgery or by percutaneous balloon dilatation. Such cases need echocardiographic follow-up to identify re-stenosis [2–6].

Aortic Pseudoaneurysms

Aortic pseudoaneurysms characterize a contained rupture of the aorta and, as with left ventricular pseudoaneurysms, are distinguished by an extraluminal aneurysmal sack communicating with the true lumen with a relatively narrow neck. Aortic pseudoaneurysms happen in several conditions such as spontaneous rupture of an aortic aneurysm with consequent sealing off of the hemorrhage or as a sequela of aortic dissection. Pseudoaneurysms can also result from traumas or iatrogenic injury. Because they are outside the contour of the normal aorta, imaging may be problematic and CT is frequently necessary to make a decisive diagnosis [2–4].

Aortic Traumas

Aortic transection is a catastrophic sequela of blunt chest injuries, classically after a high-speed impact injury such as that experienced by an unrestrained passenger involved in a motor vehicle accident. The characteristic injury is partial or complete transection of the descending thoracic aorta, characteristically at the area of the ligamentum arteriosum. Complete aortic transection is a nearly instantaneously fatal event, for which there is rarely time for diagnostic imaging. Partial transection may allow survival and arrival to an emergency department for evaluation. In most trauma centers, chest CT is the primary diagnostic modality.

TEE has substantial promise for the detection of aortic traumas. It should be emphasized that there are several manifestations of aortic traumas, many of which may be subtle. Because most patients with complete or closely complete aortic transection do not survive, it is uncommon to document this fatal complication. For aortic traumas in which there has been at least partial disruption through the media into the adventitia, periadventitial hematoma is often present [2–6].

Takayasu's Arteritis

This is an inflammatory disease of the aorta and its proximal branches. By definition, Takayasu's arteritis happens in cases younger than 40 years. It results in marked, irregular intimal thickening and accumulation of inflammatory tissue in the proximal aorta and the ostia of the major branches, including the coronary arteries. Echocardiographically, its appearance is similar to that of atherosclerotic disease. On very rare occasions, other forms of arteritis such as giant cell arteritis can involve the aorta [2, 15].

Infections of the Aorta

Bacterial or fungal infections of the aorta are an uncommon subset of infective endocarditis (Fig. 38.14). They typically will rise at an area of atherosclerotic involvement or at the area of the ligamentum arteriosum on the aortic side of a patent ductus arteriosus. They will manifest as a pedunculated mobile mass, for which the differential obviously contains complex mobile atherosclerotic disease. The infectious nature of the mass may be recommended by the overall clinical condition but obviously only proven by direct inspection. Infrequently encountered in contemporary practice is syphilitic aortitis, which results in inflammatory thickening of the proximal aorta [2, 4, 15–20].

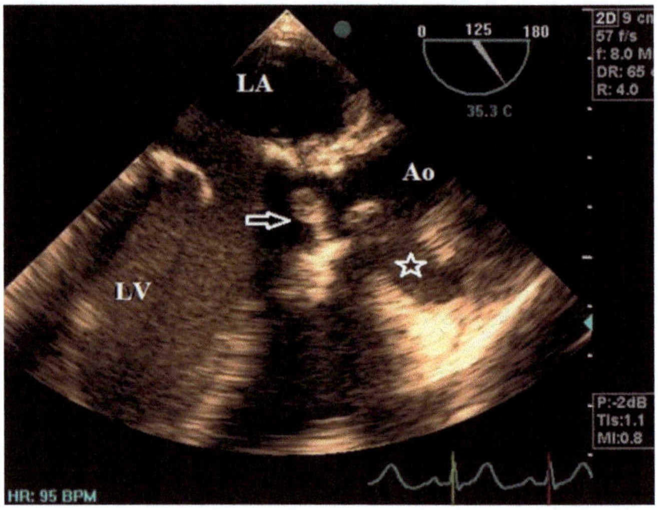

Fig. 38.14 Long axis view in TEE in a patient after bio-prostheses Aortic Valve Replacement and Mitral Valve Replacement showing large pedunculated mass associated with mycotic aneurysm of the aortic root diagnosed as Fungal (Aspergilosis) infective endocarditis

Questions

1. Aortitis includes all of the following diseases except for:
   A. Takayasu's arteritis
   B. Ankylosing spondylitis and other spondyloarthritis
   C. Giant cell arteritis
   D. Marfan Syndrome

2. Imaging features of Intramural Hematoma (IMH) are as follow except for:
   A. Focal aortic wall thickening (concentric > crescentic)
   B. Preserved luminal shape with smooth luminal border
   C. Absence of dissection flap and false lumen
   D. Central displacement of intimal calcium

3. What is wrong regarding the grading of the severity of aortic atherosclerosis:
   A. Mild: Mild (focal or diffuse) intimal thickening of 2–3 mm
   B. Moderate: Atheroma >3–5 m (no mobile/ulcerated components)
   C. Severe: Grade 2, 3, or 4 atheroma plus mobile or ulcerated components
   D. Normal: Intimal thickness <2 mm

4. What is the Star?

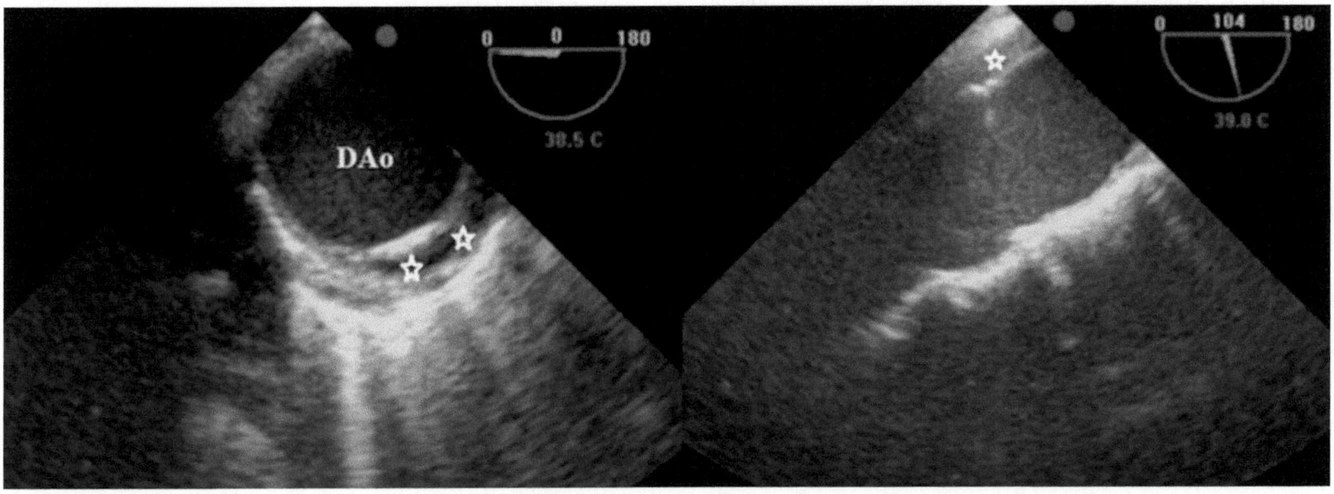

   A. Intramural hematoma in short axis and long axis view of Transthoracic Echocardiography.
   B. Intraluminal hematoma in short axis and long axis view of Transthoracic Echocardiography.
   C. Intramural hematoma in short axis and long axis view of Transesophageal echocardiography.
   D. Intraluminal hematoma in short axis and long axis view of Transesophageal echocardiography.

Answers

1. D
2. A
3. C
4. D

References

1. Kuzmik GA, Sang AX, Elefteriades JA. Natural history of thoracic aortic aneurysms. J Vasc Surg. 2012;56:565.
2. Goldstein S, Evangelista A, Abbara S, Arai A, Asch F, Badano L, et al. Multimodality imaging of diseases of the thoracic aorta in adults. Am Soc Echocardiogr. 2015;28:119–82.
3. Evangelista A, Flachskampt FA, Erbel R, Antonini-Canterin F, Vlachopoulos C, Rocchi G, Sicari R, Nihoannopoulos P, Zamorano J; European Association of Echocardiography; Document Reviewers: Pepi M, Breithardt OA, Plonska-Gosciniak E. Echocardiography in aortic diseases: EAE recommendations for clinical practice. Eur J Echocardiogr. 2010;11(8):645–58.
4. Hiratzka LF, Bakris GL, Beckman JA, et al. ACCF/AHA/AATS/ACR/ASA/SCA/SCAI/SIR/STS/SVM guidelines for the diagnosis and management of patients with thoracic aortic disease: A report of the American College of Cardiology Foundation/American Heart Association Task Force on Practice Guidelines, American Association for Thoracic Surgery, American College of Radiology, American Stroke Association, Society of Cardiovascular

Anesthesiologists, Society for Cardiovascular Angiography and Interventions, Society of Interventional Radiology, Society of Thoracic Surgeons, and Society for Vascular Medicine. Circulation. 2010;e266(2010):121.

5. Evangelista A, Flachskampf F, Lancellotti P, Badano L, Aguilar R, Monaghan M, et al. European Association of Echocardiography for standardization of performance, digital storage and reporting of echocardiographic studies. Eur J Echocardiogr. 2008;9:438–48.
6. Orihashi K, Matsuura Y, Sueda T, Watari M, Okada K, Sugawara Y, et al. Aortic arch branches are no longer a blind zone for trans-esophageal echocardiography: a new eye for aortic surgeons. J Thorac Cardiovasc Surg. 2000;120:466–72.
7. Roberts WC, Vowels TJ, Ko JM, et al. Comparison of the structure of the aortic valve and ascending aorta in adults having aortic valve replacement for aortic stenosis versus for pure aortic regurgitation and resection of the ascending aorta for aneurysm. Circulation. 2011;123:896.
8. Braverman AC. Acute aortic dissection: clinician update. Circulation. 2010;122:184.
9. Tsai TT, Trimarchi S, Nienaber CA. Acute aortic dissection: perspectives from the International Registry of Acute Aortic Dissection (IRAD). Eur J Vasc Endovasc Surg. 2009;37:149.
10. LeMaire SA, McDonald ML, Guo DC, et al. Genome-wide association study identifies a susceptibility locus for thoracic aortic aneurysms and aortic dissections spanning FBN1 at 15q21.1. Nat Genet. 2011;43:996.
11. Hagan PG, Nienaber CA, Isselbacher EM, et al. The International Registry of Acute Aortic Dissection (IRAD): New insights into an old disease. JAMA. 2000;283:897.
12. Estrera A, Miller C III, Lee TY, et al. Acute type A intramural hematoma: analysis of current management strategy. Circulation. 2009;120:S287.
13. Eggebrecht H, Plicht B, Kahlert P, et al. Intramural hematoma and penetrating ulcers: indications to endovascular treatment. Eur J Vasc Endovasc Surg. 2009;38:659.
14. Bischoff MS, Geisbusch P, Peters AS, et al. Penetrating aortic ulcer: defining risks and therapeutic strategies. Herz. 2011;36:498.
15. Nathan DP, Boonn W, Lai E, et al. Presentation, complications, and natural history of penetrating atherosclerotic ulcer disease. J Vasc Surg. 2012;55:10.
16. Soto ME, Espinola-Zavaleta N, Ramirez-Quito O, Reyes PA. Echocardiographic follow-up of patients with Takayasu's arteritis: five-year survival. Echocardiography. 2006 May;23(5):353–60.
17. Hsu RB, Lin FY. Infected aneurysm of the thoracic aorta. J Vasc Surg. 2008;47:270.
18. Sedivy P, Spacek M, El Samman K, et al. Endovascular treatment of infected aortic aneurysms. Eur J Vasc Endovasc Surg. 2012;44:385.
19. Laser A, Baker N, Rectenwald J, et al. Graft infection after endovascular abdominal aortic aneurysm repair. J Vasc Surg. 2011;54:58.
20. Restrepo CS, Betancourt SL, Martinez-Jimenez S, et al. Aortic tumors. Semin Ultrasound CT MR. 2012;33:265.

Role of Echocardiography in Arrhythmia

39

Azin Alizadehasl and Anita Sadeghpour

Abstract

Simultaneous evaluation of electrical activity and functional and anatomical cardiac changes by echocardiographic examination provides criteria for the diagnosis of arrhythmias and their hemodynamic consequences.

Structural echocardiography views the kinetics of atrial and ventricular walls and the behavior of the valve apparatus during the cardiac cycle, establishing morphological and functional parameters which might identify atrial and ventricular arrhythmias.

Changes in transvalvular systolic and diastolic flow velocities or tissue velocities in conjunction with simultaneous analysis of the temporal relationship between ventricular and atrial activity provide criteria for a positive and differential diagnosis of arrhythmias. In the same situation provided by arrhythmias, echocardiography can measure and quantify the hemodynamic parameters of ventricular function.

Keywords

Transesophageal echocardiography (TEE) · Arrhythmia Ventricular arrhythmias · Supraventricular arrhythmias Atrial fibrillation (AF) · Direct cardioversion (DC) Implantable cardioverter-defibrillator (ICD)

A. Alizadehasl, MD, FACC, FASE
Associate Professor of Cardiology, Echocardiologist, Echocardiography and Cardiogenetic Research Centers, Cardio-Oncology Department, Rajaie Cardiovascular Medical and Research Center, Tehran, Iran

A. Sadeghpour, MD, FACC, FASE (✉)
Professor of Cardiology, Echocardiography Research Center, Rajaie Cardiovascular Medical and Research Center, Iran University of Medical Science, Tehran, Iran

Abbreviations

ACCF	Appropriateness criteria of the american college of cardiology foundation
AF	Atrial fibrillation
ASE	American society of echocardiography
ATRAMI	Autonomic tone and reflexes after myocardial infarction
DC	Direct cardioversion
ICD	Implantable cardioverter-defibrillator
INR	International normalized ratio
LGE/CMR	Late gadolinium enhancement/ Cardiovascular magnetic resonance
LVEF	Left ventricular ejection fraction
MADIT-II	Multicenter automatic defibrillator implantation trial II
SCD-HeFT	Sudden cardiac death in heart failure trial
TEE	Transesophageal echocardiography

Echocardiography plays an important role in the management of arrhythmia. In this chapter, we discuss this issue in three aspects: echocardiography and supraventricular tachycardia, echocardiography and ventricular arrhythmia, and new modalities of echocardiography in this matter.

Echocardiography and Supraventricular Tachycardia

- Atrial fibrillation (AF) is not only the most common cardiac arrhythmia in the US, but also has an increasing prevalence over the upcoming decades [1].
- Direct cardioversion (DC) constitutes an essential treatment modality for atrial fibrillation (AF); there, however, remains a substantial risk of stroke and other systemic thromboembolic events in the use of DC. Conventionally, this risk is ameliorated by keeping patients anticoagulated

A. Sadeghpour, A. Alizadehasl (eds.), *Case-Based Textbook of Echocardiography*, https://doi.org/10.1007/978-3-319-67691-3_39

and attaining an international normalized ratio (INR) of 2–3 for 3 weeks leading up to DC.

- The occurrence of thromboembolic complications in the absence of demonstrable left atrial thrombi and spontaneous echocardiographic contrast in relation with transient atrial dysfunction (stunning) caused by cardioversion indicate that cardioversion is likely to give rise to new thrombus creation. In such cases, it is mandatory that all patients receive full anticoagulant therapy at the time of cardioversion.
- More recently, conducting transesophageal echocardiography (TEE) prior to DC has proven as effective as conventional anticoagulation in preventing stroke. In addition, it is known to speed up DC itself. TEE-guided cardioversion may be deemed a more desirable option than conventional therapy in certain patients such as those who are highly symptomatic, hemodynamically compromised, recently diagnosed with AF, or have a high risk of stroke [2, 3].
- In tandem with DC, TEE is also regularly employed before the ablation of atrial flutter and other supraventricular arrhythmias to detect atrial or atrial auricle thrombi with a view to identifying the risk of systemic embolism both in patients with initial episodes of atrial flutter and in those with prior episodes of atrial flutter with inadequate anticoagulation. This treatment strategy has been extrapolated from the current guidelines on AF [3, 4].
- There is a paucity of information as regards the prevalence and the clinical relationship between atrial thrombi and spontaneous echocardiographic contrast in patients with AF or atrial flutter. It is widely believed that both atrial thrombi and spontaneous echocardiographic contrast embody important risk factors for systemic embolization.
- Echocardiography is utilized to determine left ventricular ejection fraction (LVEF), left atrial size Doppler flow and M-mode of MV inflow (of course, transthoracic echocardiography [TTE] may be done for these reasons (Fig. 39.1).
- Presence of left atrial thrombi or sludge, or spontaneous echocardiographic contrast. Echoes that are smoke-like (i.e., swirling and dynamic) and have an optimal gain throughout the cardiac cycle are termed “spontaneous echocardiographic contrast”. Sludge is an echo-density that is not only dynamic but also gelatinous and precipitous; it lacks a discrete mass and is present through the cardiac cycle (Fig. 39.2). A thrombus is an intracavity mass that is consistently echo-dense; in addition, it is constrained, present in more than one imaging plane, and is dissimilar to the underlying left atrium or the left atrial appendage endocardium and pectinate muscle (Fig. 39.3) [2–5].

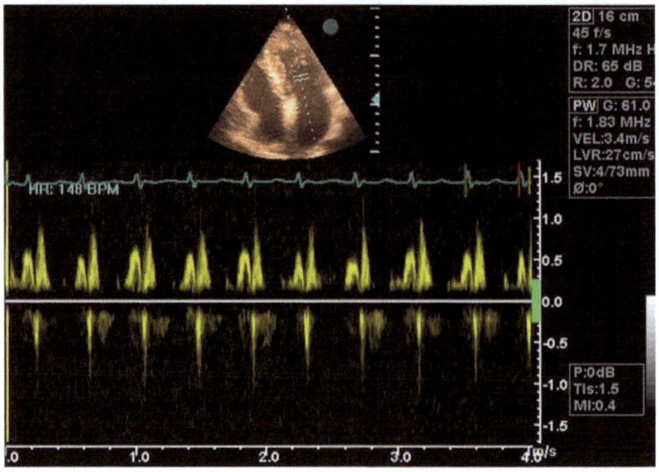

Fig. 39.1 Transthoracic echocardiography, Apical 4-Chamber view, Doppler flow pattern of MV inflow in 2:1 atrial Flutter

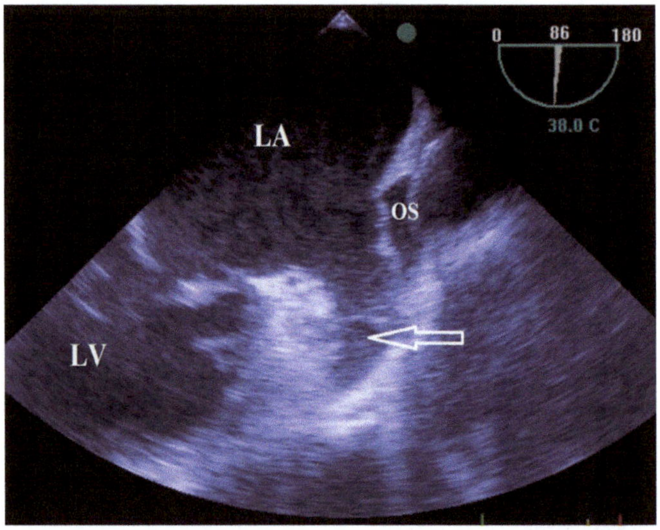

Fig. 39.2 Transesophageal echocardiography (TEE), mid esophageal view, severe smoke and sludge in Left atrial appendage (arrow)

- TEE is an ideal imaging modality in evaluation of Left atrial appendage velocity in normal and tachyarrhythmia (Figs. 39.4 and 39.5). LAA contraction velocity is about 60 ± 14 cm/s and the filling velocity was 52 ± 13 cm/s [6]. Reduced LAA velocity will lead stasis and contribute to thrombus formation (Velocities <40 cm/sec has significant association with risk of stroke) and very low emptying Left atrial appendage flow velocities (shown above the baseline) less than 20 cm/s have been associated with increased risk for clot formation in the Left atrial appendage and consequently increased risk of embolic events [7].
- The LA diameter, however, can underestimate atrial dilation, especially when dilation occurs in an asymmetric fashion. The American Society of Echocardiography (ASE) advocates the use of a 2D–derived LA volume

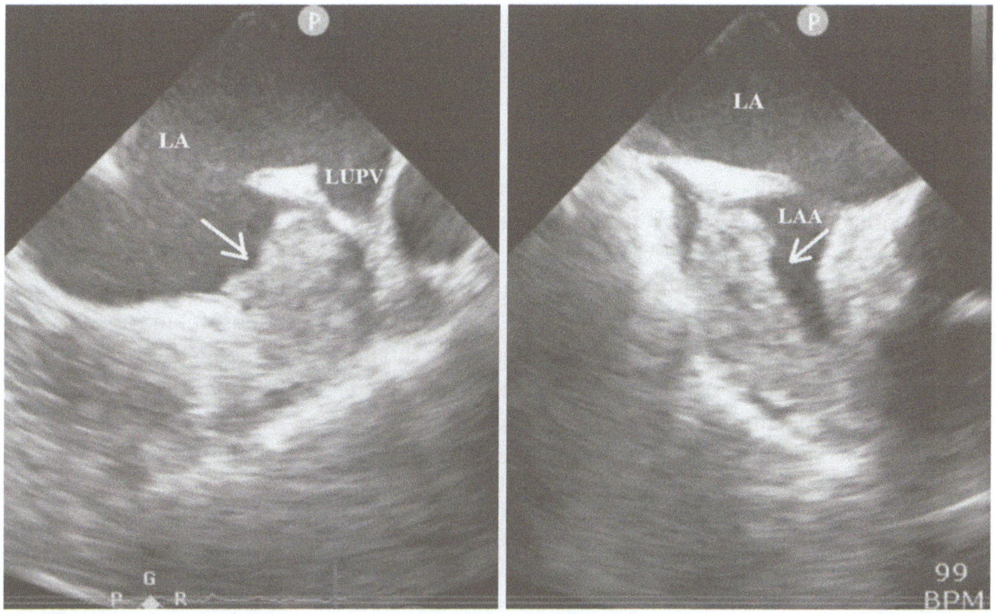

Fig. 39.3 Transesophageal echocardiography (TEE), mid esophageal, biplane views of Left atrial appendage with large clot

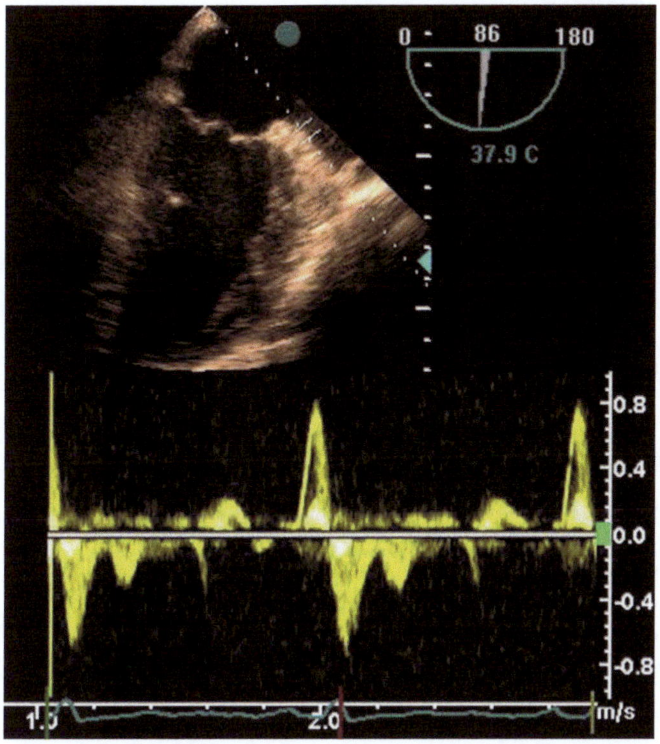

Fig. 39.4 Transesophageal echocardiography (TEE), Mid esophageal, normal Doppler flow velocity of Left atrial appendage

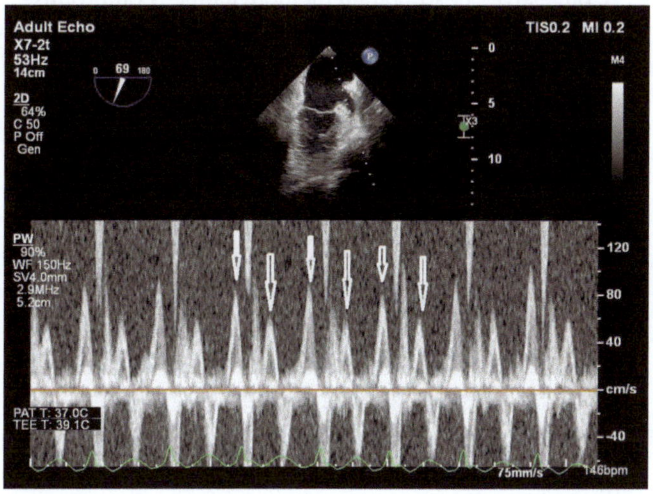

Fig. 39.5 Transesophageal echocardiography (TEE), mid esophageal, Doppler flow pattern of left atrial appendage in 2:1 atrial flutter

using either the Simpson or biplane method from the apical four-chamber and two-chamber views Common measures used to assess [7].

- 4 consecutive weeks of adequate oral anticoagulation can be used instead of TEE-guided cardioversion in symptomatic patient with tolerable arrhythmia [8].

Left atrial function contain the height of the A wave, which may be used to calculate atrial contraction force, and the atrial emptying fraction, which is derived from the calculated minimum (end of ventricular diastole) and maximum (end of ventricular systole) atrial volumes. The magnitude of the A wave depends on the loading situations and is regularly absent when the echocardiogram is done during Atrial fibrillation, causing important limitations to this method of evaluating atrial function. 2D strain of the LA uses two-dimensional speckle tracking strain imaging for the quantification of regional and global left atrial deformation [7, 9].

Indications for and Descriptions of Transesophageal Echocardiography in Atrial Fibrillation/Atrial Flutter

- Checking for TEE indications requires a meticulous review of patient charts. According to the 2011 Appropriateness Criteria of the American College of Cardiology Foundation/American Society of Echocardiography (ACCF/ASE), these indications are classified as "appropriate", "inappropriate", and "unclassifiable". Accordingly, "unclassifiable" data that should be excluded from further analysis are those considered inadequately documented. Indications are additionally classified according to the principal indication for the use of TEE into 7 "appropriate" categories and 4 "inappropriate" categories [5, 10, 11].

Appropriate

1. "Congestive heart failure/hemodynamic compromise" consists of patients with current congestive heart failure exacerbation or hemodynamic instability. This indication does not contain patients with a history of congestive heart failure currently well compensated for.
2. "Symptomatic" is comprised of patients having significant symptoms of AF—including palpitations, chest pain, dyspnea, fatigue, lightheadedness, and syncope. This indication does not contain patients already hospitalized or those diagnosed for the first time with AF.
3. "Hospitalized and symptomatic" incorporates patients hospitalized for a reason other than AF who have developed symptomatic AF during admission.
4. "New-onset AF" encompasses patients who are diagnosed for the first time with AF and are in AF for more than 48 h.
5. "High stroke risk" comprises patients with a history of stroke, previous left atrial thrombi, transient ischemic attack, hypertrophic obstructive cardiomyopathy, or rheumatic fever.
6. "Subtherapeutic anticoagulation" is composed of patients who are undergoing conventional anticoagulation but have a documented INR less than 2 at any point in the preceding 3 weeks and who do not already have one of the indications defined here.
7. "Miscellaneous" involves patients undergoing TEE for a cause unrelated to AF that is found elsewhere in the appropriateness criteria such as evaluation of valve function or endocarditis. The timing of TEE coincidentally helps expedite DC [10–12].

Inappropriate

1. "Stable with therapeutic anticoagulation >3 weeks" comprises patients who are hemodynamically stable and are therapeutically anticoagulated for at least 3 weeks. These patients have completed the conventional method of risk reduction for thromboembolism and do not need TEE.
2. "AF < 48 h" involves patients who have no history of AF and are in AF for less than 48 h. It is assumed that TEE is not useful inasmuch as the time for thrombus formation is inadequate.
3. "Permanent AF" is comprised of patients in whom sinus rhythm cannot be sustained after cardioversion or in whom the physician and patient opt to accept AF. These patients are not indicated for TEE or DC.
4. "Hospitalized but asymptomatic" consists of patients who are hospitalized and are in AF but do not have symptoms, congestive heart failure exacerbation, or hemodynamic compromise. These patients can be managed with 3 weeks of anticoagulation.

Often, patients have more than one indication for TEE.

Accordingly, to determine the main indication, we rank the categories as follows:

(a) Congestive heart failure/hemodynamic compromise
(b) Hospitalized and symptomatic
(c) New onset
(d) Symptomatic
(e) Subtherapeutic anticoagulation
(f) Miscellaneous
(g) High stroke risk

All these criteria can be used for the management of other forms of supraventricular arrhythmias requiring cardioversion or ablation.

Allowing for multiple comparisons, the significant markers of the risk for systemic embolization can be obtained only from TEE. For all the interesting clinical and echocardiographic associations studied in many investigations, none is strong enough to obviate the need for TEE [10–15].

Echocardiography and Ventricular Arrhythmia

- Since the emergence of the implantable cardioverter-defibrillator (ICD) approximately a quarter of a century ago, the number of indications for implantation has increasingly risen, so much so that currently diverse cardiac conditions are taken into consideration. The LVEF constitutes the most applicable quantifiable parameter when selecting candidates for ICD implantation. For some time now, there has been a consensus over the use of ICDs in patients having survived a life-threatening ventricular arrhythmia as a secondary prevention of sudden cardiac death. Be that as it may, studies such as the Sudden Cardiac Death in Heart Failure Trial (SCD-HeFT) and the Multicenter Automatic Defibrillator Implantation Trial II (MADIT-II) have demonstrated the clinical utility of prophylactic ICD implantation in patients with a reduced LVEF as the primary prevention of sudden cardiac death as well. ICD therapy is also employed in patients with ischemic cardiomyopathy (e.g., patients with prior myocardial infarction with residual scar tissue) for the prevention of sudden cardiac death.

- In the European Autonomic Tone and Reflexes After Myocardial Infarction (ATRAMI) study, which recruited 1284 patients after myocardial infarction, less than half of the study population whose deaths were attributed to sudden cardiac death in the 21-month follow-up period had an LVEF less than 35% [15–17].
- Although TTE helps analyze myocardial function in patients with suspected cardiomyopathy, much of the information obtained from echocardiography is more often than not ignored in the risk assessment of future adverse cardiac events. Research has shown that certain structural parameters, most notably LV internal dimensions and left atrial size, may serve as surrogate markers alongside LVEF to predict which patients may benefit from ICD therapy or to help alter ICD parameters or adjunctive antiarrhythmic pharmacotherapy in patients who already have an ICD. Patients with LV internal dimensions greater than 4 cm are over twice more likely to experience ventricular tachycardia than patients with normal LV systolic dimensions (HR = 2.5) [16–18].

New Modalities of Echocardiography and Arrhythmia

Defined as the standard deviation of time to peak negative strain from the 16 LV segments, mechanical dispersion as assessed by strain echocardiography is thought to be able to predict arrhythmic events independently of the LVEF in patients after myocardial infarction. Following myocardial infarction—not least in patients with LVEFs greater than 35% who do not fulfill the current ICD indications—patient selection for ICD therapy may be augmented by a combination of mechanical dispersion, which reflects myocardial contraction heterogeneity, and global strain.

- In patients not fulfilling the current ICD criteria with global longitudinal strain worse than 16%, mechanical dispersion should be analyzed. What should be borne in mind is that a value greater than 75 ms may act as a threshold. Literature review shows that a combination of these two new parameters improves the positive predictive value of arrhythmic events to 21% from 11% by the LVEF alone. This strategy is likely to better post-myocardial infarction patient selection for primary ICD therapy [11–13].
- In hypertrophic cardiomyopathy, mechanical dispersion, global longitudinal strain, wall thickness, and fibrosis by late gadolinium enhancement/cardiovascular magnetic resonance (LGE/CMR) are mentioned as the markers of ventricular arrhythmias and sudden cardiac death. Mechanical dispersion is a strong and independent predictor of arrhythmic events and is related to the amount of fibrosis. Global longitudinal strain is allied to ventricular arrhythmias and the presence of fibrosis despite a normal EF. Patients with global longitudinal strain worse than −15.0% (log-rank $P = 0.04$), mechanical dispersion greater than 67 ms (log-rank $P = 0.02$), and greater than 2% LGE on CMR (log-rank $P < 0.001$) more frequently have ventricular arrhythmias and sudden cardiac death [18, 19].
- In arrhythmogenic right ventricular dysplasia, right ventricular mechanical dispersion is present in asymptomatic mutation carriers and may assist in risk stratification. Contraction duration in 6 right ventricular and 16 LV segments is measured as the time from onset R on ECG to maximum myocardial shortening in each segment. The standard deviation of contraction duration is defined as mechanical dispersion. Mechanical dispersion is more pronounced in arrhythmogenic right ventricular dysplasia patients with arrhythmias than in asymptomatic mutation carriers and healthy individuals in the right ventricle (52 [41,63] vs. 35 [23,47] vs. 13 [9,19] ms; $P < 0.001$) [20].
- Also, when ventricular fibrillation occurs, TEE shows that the heart abruptly reduces end-diastolic LV volume and assumes a systolic configuration, whereas myocardial contractions are still observed—although they are ineffective. Furthermore, their rapid succession does not allow diastolic ventricular expansion. A dense spontaneous echocardiographic contrast with a smoke-like appearance quickly occupies the left atrium. After the interruption of the ventricular fibrillation and the onset of the basic rhythm, the dense spontaneous echocardiographic contrast is flushed away completely with just a few cardiac contractions [16–18].

- Mechanical dispersion in arrhythmia can be assessed by strain and twist echocardiography. The LV synchronous contraction is significantly related to LV strain twist mechanics (Fig. 39.6).
- Valuation of LA strain using two-dimensional speckle tracking strain imaging has been recently presented for the quantification of regional and global left atrial deformation. Longitudinal deformation of the atrial wall is evaluated in the mid-septal and mid-lateral walls in the apical 4-chamber view. Wall strain and strain rate versus time curves are created from these areas of interest. Global peak atrial longitudinal strain of 42.2% ± 6.1% and global time to peak longitudinal strain of 368 ± 30 ms have been reported as reference indices of normal atrial myocardial deformation [21].
- Additionally, in a study, we investigated whether phase analysis applied to two-dimensional echocardiographic cine loops in apical and basal rotation and LV twist objectively identifies these focal areas and can be used to localize ventricular insertion sites of accessory pathways. We were able to obtain angle-independent information on torsion (or contraction), which we applied to assess the site of first contraction and the extent of premature ventricular contraction associated with the accessory pathway. In this patient, we used angle-independent 2-D speckle tracking echocardiography which recently has been validated. Based on literature review, this is one of the monitory reports on localization of the accessory pathway and determination the extent of ventricular preexcitation using LV torsion and twist (Figs. 39.7, 39.8 and 39.9).

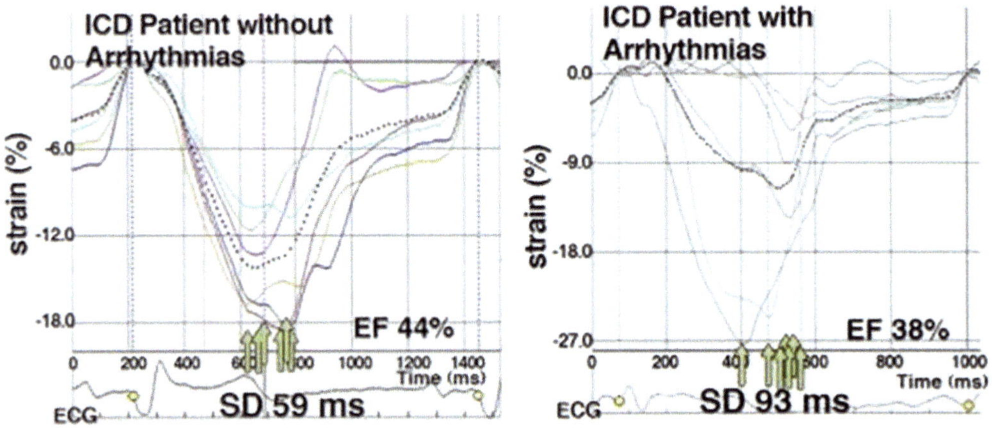

Fig. 39.6 Mechanical dispersion by strain echocardiography in ICD patient with and without arrhythmias during follow-up. Longitudinal Strain echocardiography curves in the 4-chamber view from a post-MI ICD patient without arrhythmic events (left panel), and a post-MI ICD case with recurrent arrhythmias (right panel). Green arrows indicate the timing of maximum myocardial shortening in each segment. Myocardial shortening is reduced in right panel, and the timing of shortening is dispersed compared with left panel. ICD, Implantable cardioverter-defibrillator, SD, Standard deviation of time to maximum myocardial shortening, MI, Myocardial infarction. Haugaa KH et al. Mechanical dispersion assessed by myocardial strain in patients after myocardial infarction for risk prediction of ventricular arrhythmia. JACC Cardiovasc Imaging 2010;3:247–56

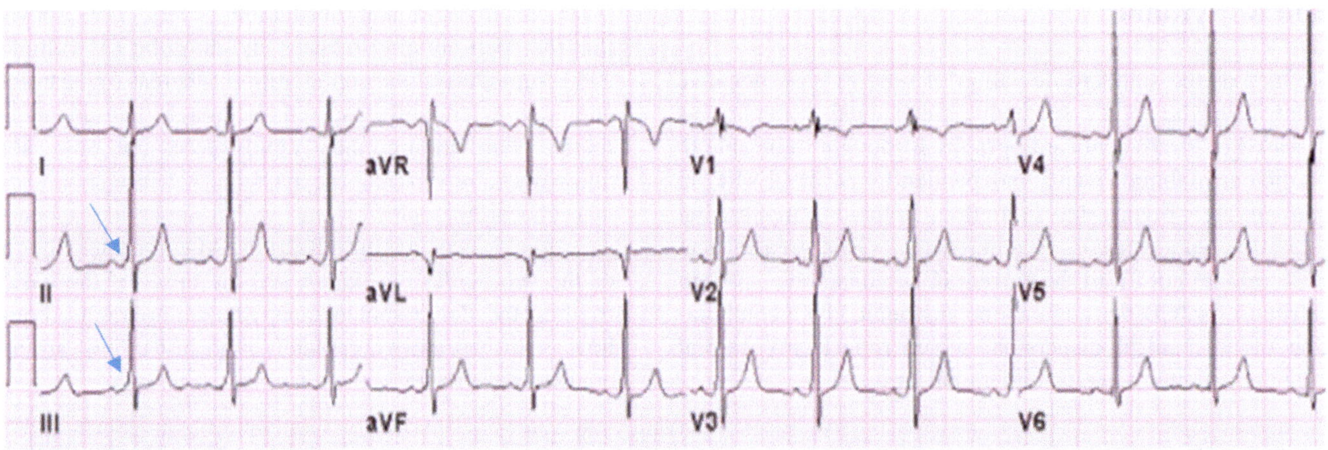

Fig. 39.7 Twelve leads ECG shows a typical pattern of preexcitation, suggestive of a left lateral accessory pathway (blue arrows)

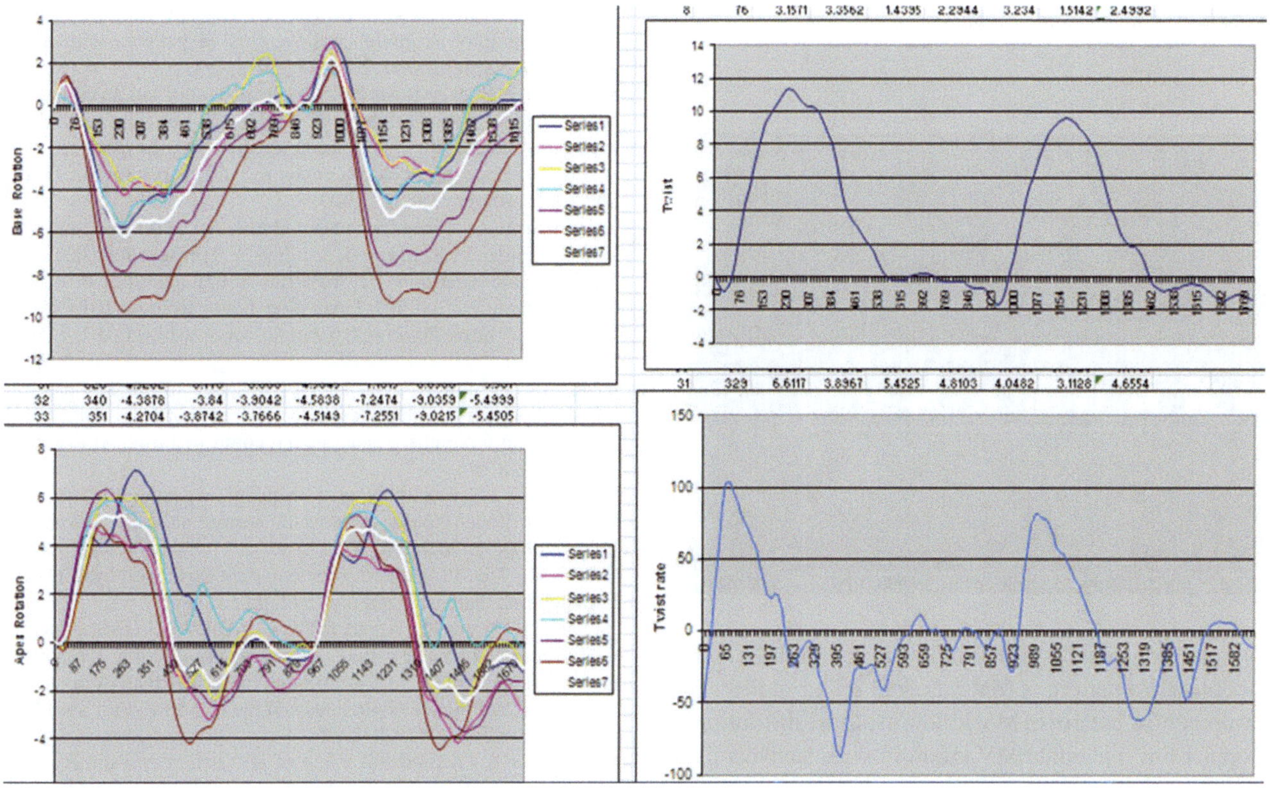

Fig. 39.8 LV rotation curves (left) shows discordant base and apex rotation as a clue to determine the site of first contraction peak (apico lateral, basolateral and posterolateral graphs) and the extent of pre excited ventricular contraction. Twist and twist rate curves reveal some deformation (right)

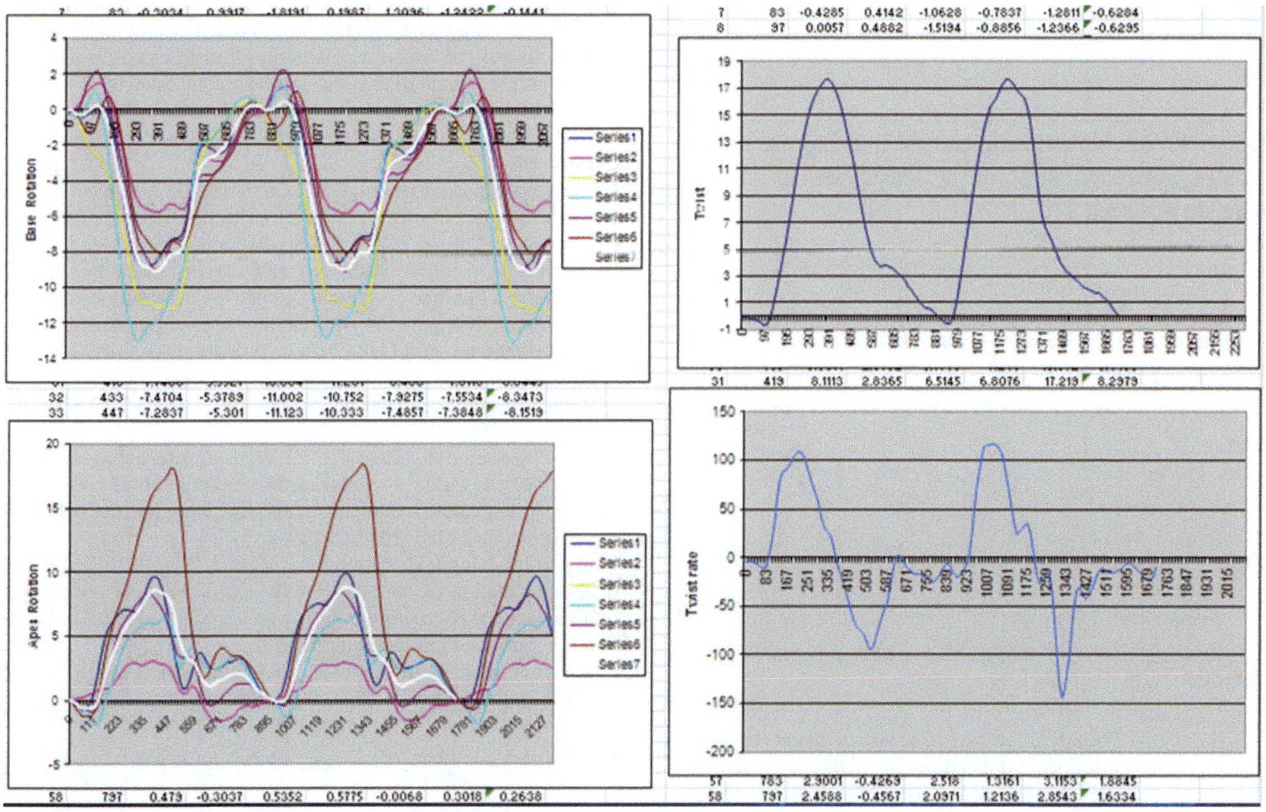

Fig. 39.9 LV apical and basal rotation (left) and twist, twist rate (right) curves after successful ablation reveals concordant and normalized base and apex rotation, twist and twist rate

Questions

1.

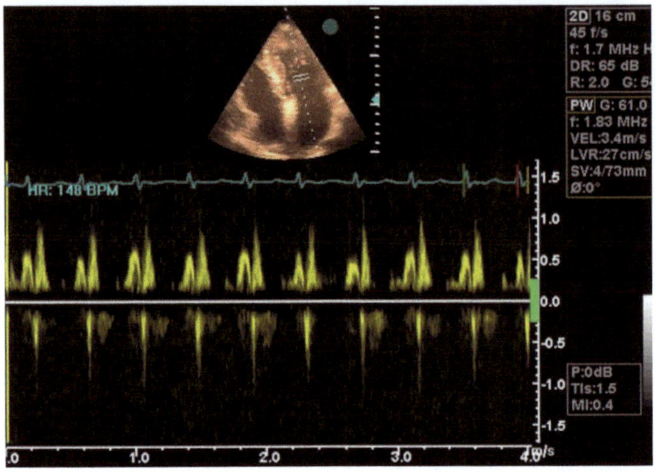

A. Doppler flow pattern of MV inflow in 1:1 atrial Flutter.
B. Doppler flow pattern of MV inflow in 2:1 atrial Flutter.
C. Doppler flow pattern of MV inflow in atrial Fibrillation.
D. Doppler flow pattern of MV inflow in sinus tachycardia.

2. Reduced LAA velocity will lead stasis and contribute to thrombus formation (Velocities <**?** cm/s has significant association with risk of stroke):
   A. 60
   B. 50
   C. 40
   D. 70

3. Patients who are hemodynamically stable and are therapeutically anticoagulated for at least**?** weeks. These patients do not need TEE.
   A. 2
   B. 3
   C. 4
   D. 1

Answers

1. B
2. C
3. B

References

1. Go AS, Hylek EM, Phillips KA, et al. Prevalence of diagnosed atrial fibrillation in adults: national implications for rhythm management and stroke prevention: the AnTicoagulation and Risk Factors in Atrial Fibrillation (ATRIA) Study. JAMA. 2001;285:2370–5.
2. Klein AL, Grimm RA, Murray RD. Use of transesophageal echocardiography to guide cardioversion in patients with atrial fibrillation. N Engl J Med. 2001;344:1411–20.
3. Kleemann T, Becker T, Strauss M. Prevalence of left atrial thrombus and dense spontaneous echo contrast in patients with short-term atrial fibrillation <48 hours undergoing cardioversion: value of transesophageal echocardiography to guide cardioversion. J Am Soc Echocardiogr. 2009;22:1403–8.
4. Alyeshmerni D, Pirmohamed A, Barac A, Smirniotopoulos J, Xue E, Goldstein S, Mazel J, Lindsay J. Transesophageal echocardiographic screening before atrial flutter ablation: is it necessary for patient safety? J Am Soc Echocardiogr. 2013;26(9):1099–105. https://doi.org/10.1016/j.echo.2013.05.017. Epub 2013 Jul 11.
5. Klein AL, Grimm RA, Jasper SE. Efficacy of transesophageal echocardiography-guided cardioversion of patients with atrial fibrillation at 6 months: a randomized controlled trial. Am Heart J. 2006;151:380–9.
6. Tabata T, Oki T, Fukuda N, et al. Influence of aging on left atrial appendage flow velocity patterns in normal subjects. J Am Soc Echocardiogr. 1996;9:274–80.
7. Otto CM. The practice of clinical echocardiography. 5th ed. Philadelphia: Saunders; 2017. p. 577–95.
8. January CT, Wann LS, Alpert JS, et al. AHA/ACC/HRS guideline for the management of patients with atrial fibrillation: a report of the American College of Cardiology/American Heart Association Task Force on Practice Guidelines and the Heart Rhythm Society. J Am Coll Cardiol. 2014;64:e1–76.
9. Sadeghpour A. Incremental value of left atrium two-dimensional strain in patients with heart failure. Arch Cardiovasc Imaging. 2013;1(2):49–50. https://doi.org/10.5812/acvi.15896.
10. Douglas PS, Garcia MJ, Haines DE. ACCF/ASE/AHA/ASNC/HFSA/HRS/SCAI/SCCM/SCCT/SCMR 2011 appropriate use criteria for echocardiography. A report of the American College of Cardiology Foundation Appropriate Use Criteria Task Force, American Society of Echocardiography, American Heart Association, American Society of Nuclear Cardiology, Heart Failure Society of America, Heart Rhythm Society, Society for Cardiovascular Angiography and Interventions, Society of Critical Care Medicine, Society of Cardiovascular Computed Tomography, and Society for Cardiovascular Magnetic Resonance. J Am Coll Cardiol. 2011;57:1126–66.
11. Fuster V, Ryden LE, Cannom DS. ACC/AHA/ESC 2006 guidelines for the management of patients with atrial fibrillation: a report of the American College of Cardiology/American Heart Association task force on practice guidelines and the European Society of Cardiology committee for practice guidelines (writing committee to revise the 2001 guidelines for the management of patients with atrial fibrillation). J Am Coll Cardiol. 2006;48:e149–246.
12. Wazni OM, Tsao HM, Chen SA. Cardiovascular imaging in the management of atrial fibrillation. J Am Coll Cardiol. 2006;48(10):2077–84.
13. Asher CR, Klein AL, The ACUTE Trial. Transesophageal echocardiography to guide electrical cardioversion in atrial fibrillation. Assessment of cardioversion using transesophageal echocardiography. Cleve Clin J Med. 2002;69:713–8.
14. Mansour IN, Lang RM, Furlong KT, Ryan A, Ward RP. Evaluation of the application of the ACCF/ASE appropriateness criteria for transesophageal echocardiography in an academic medical center. J Am Soc Echocardiogr. 2009;22:517–22.
15. Nagarakanti R, Ezekowitz MD, Oldgren J. Dabigatran versus warfarin in patients with atrial fibrillation: an analysis of patients undergoing cardioversion. Circulation. 2011;123:131–6.
16. Catanzaro JN, Makaryus JN, Makaryus AN, Sison C, Vavasis C, Fan D, Jadonath R. Echocardiographic predictors of ventricular tachycardia. Clin Med Insights Cardiol. 2014;8(Suppl 4):37–42.

17. Haugaa KH, Grenne BL, Eek CH, Ersbøll M, Valeur N, Svendsen JH, et al. Strain echocardiography improves risk prediction of ventricular arrhythmias after myocardial infarction. JACC Cardiovasc Imaging. 2013;6(8):841–50.
18. Haugaa KH, Smedsrud MK, Steen T, Kongsgaard E, Loennechen JP, Skjaerpe T, et al. Mechanical dispersion assessed by myocardial strain in patients after myocardial infarction for risk prediction of ventricular arrhythmia. JACC Cardiovasc Imaging. 2010;3:247–56.
19. Haland TF, Almaas VM, Hasselberg NE, Saberniak J, Leren IS, Hopp E, Edvardsen T, Haugaa KH. Strain echocardiography is related to fibrosis and ventricular arrhythmias in hypertrophic cardiomyopathy. Eur Heart J Cardiovasc Imaging. 2016;17(6):613–21. https://doi.org/10.1093/ehjci/jew005. Epub 2016 Feb 11.
20. Sarvari SI, Haugaa KH, Anfinsen OG, Leren TP, Smiseth OA, Kongsgaard E, et al. Right ventricular mechanical dispersion is related to malignant arrhythmias: A study of patients with arrhythmogenic right ventricular cardiomyopathy and subclinical right ventricular dysfunction. Eur Heart J. 2011;32:1089–96.
21. Esmaeilzadeh M, Vakilian F, Maleki M, Amin A, Taghavi S, Bakhshandeh H. Evaluation of left atrial two-dimensional strain in patients with systolic heart failure using velocity vector imaging. Arch Cardiovasc Imaging. 2013;1(2):51–7.

Echocardiography in Systemic Diseases

40

Azin Alizadehasl and Anita Sadeghpour

Abstract

Cardiovascular disorders are a vital manifestation of systemic diseases and lead to substantial mortality and morbidity. Echocardiography has emerged as a useful noninvasive modality for the screening and evaluation of cardiac involvement in these cases. The technological developments in echocardiographic techniques and their concomitant advances in the recognition of subclinical diseases have ushered in a greater appreciation of the nature and prevalence of cardiac involvement in this group of patients. The present review explains cardiac involvement in patients with systemic lupus erythematosus, antiphospholipid antibody syndrome, Takayasu arteritis, and ankylosing spondylitis and introduces the role of different echocardiographic modalities in their evaluation.

Keywords

Systemic diseases · Echocardiography · Systemic lupus erythematosus · Antiphospholipid antibody syndrome · Takayasu arteritis · Ankylosing spondylitis

Abbreviations

APS	Antiphospholipid syndrome
AV	Aortic valve
CAD	Coronary artery disease
MR	Mitral regurgitation
MV	Mitral valve
PH	Pulmonary hypertension
RA	Rheumatoid arteritis
SLE	Systemic lupus erythematosus
TA	Takayasu arteritis
TEE	Transesophageal echocardiography
TTE	Transthoracic echocardiography

Rheumatologic diseases are chronic systemic inflammatory diseases with common involvement of cardiovascular system. Echocardiography provide a comprehensive cardiac assessment in these patients.

Systemic Lupus Erythematosus

- Cardiovascular system is involved in systemic lupus erythematosus (SLE) in different ways. There may be substantial crossover among many of the connective tissue diseases such as mixed connective tissue disease, SLE, Raynaud phenomenon, and scleroderma. Valvular heart disease from SLE may range from mild valvular thickening with normal function to overt valvulo-pathy with vegetations and severe regurgitation or stenosis [1, 2].

SLE affects all parts of the cardiovascular system including (Table 40.1):

- Libman-Sacks vegetations
- Leaflet fibrosis
- Valve regurgitation
- Pericarditis
- Asymptomatic effusion
- Myocarditis/cardiomyopathy
- Coronary artery disease (CAD)
- Atherosclerotic
- Arteritis,
- Pulmonary hypertension

Electronic Supplementary Material The online version of this chapter (https://doi.org/10.1007/978-3-319-67691-3_40) contains supplementary material, which is available to authorized users.

A. Alizadehasl, MD, FACC, FASE (✉)
Associate Professor of Cardiology, Echocardiologist, Echocardiography and Cardiogenetic Research Centers, Cardio-Oncology Department, Rajaie Cardiovascular Medical and Research Center, Tehran, Iran

A. Sadeghpour, MD, FACC, FASE
Professor of Cardiology, Echocardiography Research Center, Rajaie Cardiovascular Medical and Research Center, Iran University of Medical Science, Tehran, Iran

A. Sadeghpour, A. Alizadehasl (eds.), *Case-Based Textbook of Echocardiography*, https://doi.org/10.1007/978-3-319-67691-3_40

Table 40.1 Cardiac abnormalities in SLE

Site of involvement	Prevalence (%)
Pericarditis/effusion	11–54
Myocarditis	7–10
Valvular heart disease	15–75
Coronary artery disease	6–10

Modified from Doria A, et al. Cardiac Involvement in systemic lupus erythematosus

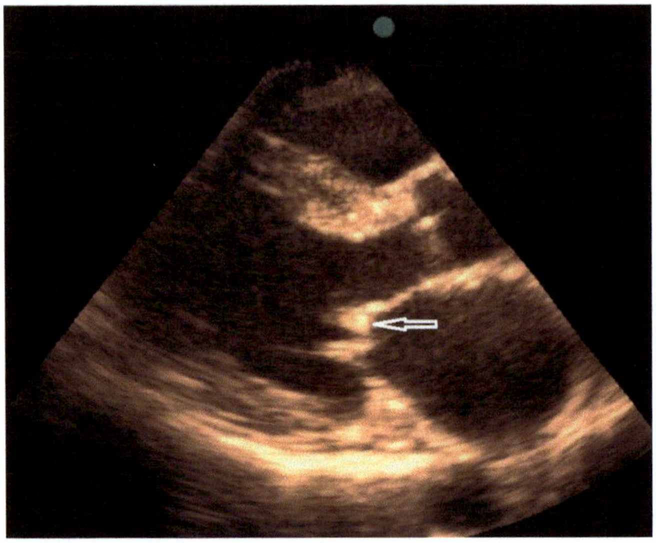

Fig. 40.1 LV long axis view showing thickened MV leaflets especially at their tips

- Echocardiography plays an essential role in the diagnosis, monitoring, and also management of SLE related cardiac disease [2–5].
- A classic lesion encountered in cases with SLE is non-infectious endocarditis with the so-called Libman-Sacks vegetation. Transthoracic echocardiography (TTE) is able to distinguish SLE related vegetations (Libman-Sacks endocarditis) with a sensitivity of 63% and a specificity of 58%. Transesophageal echocardiography (TEE) is superior to TTE in assessing SLE related valve disease. These are most frequently encountered on the mitral valve (MV) and more often are on the atrial side of the leaflet. They tend to be less mobile than infectious vegetations. They might have an inflammatory component that may result in leaflet deformity and variable degrees of valvular regurgitation (Fig. 40.1, Movies 40.1 and 40.2). When encountered on the aortic valve (AV), they are frequently on the arterial side. They might resolve with successful therapy of the underlying disease (Table 40.2).
- Another manifestations of SLE contain coronary vasculitis which may result in regional or global dysfunction and thereby mimic either an acute coronary syndrome or cardiomyopathy [2–4].
- The occurrence of SLE-related pulmonary hypertension (PH) is low; thus, screening echocardiography is not currently suggested for asymptomatic cases.

Table 40.2 Mechanisms of valvular heart disease in SLE

Mechanism	Clinical consequence
Healing of verrucous valvular lesions, leading to leaflet retraction	Valvular regurgitation, and rarely, stenosis
Large valvular verrucous lesion	Obstruction of valvular orifice leading to stenosis or malcoaptation of leaflets leading to regurgitation
Infective endocarditis	Due to underlying abnormal valve or immunosuppression
Chordal rupture in presence of verrucae	Valvular regurgitation
Papillary muscle dysfunction due to acute myocardial infraction	Valvular regurgitation
Mitral valve prolapse	Valvular regurgitation

Modified from Roberts WC, High ST. The heart in systematic lupus erythematosus. Curr Probl Cardio 1999; 24 (1):1–56

- The potential incremental diagnostic value of real time three dimensional TEE in this disease remains to be defined, cause there are only case reports of its use in this object.
- A final sign of SLE might be acute pericarditis. There are no typical features of the pericarditis or pericardial infusion seen in SLE. On rare circumstance, SLE has been related with PH, though this association is far more common with scleroderma.
- In summary, SLE affects all parts of the cardiovascular system. Echocardiography plays an essential role in the diagnosis, monitoring, and also management of SLE related cardiac disease [2–5] (Figs. 40.1 and 40.2; Movies 40.1–40.3).

Antiphospholipid Antibody Syndrome

- Antiphospholipid antibody syndrome is closely related to many connective tissue diseases and has been reported as an integral part of systemic lupus. This syndrome results in a variably hyper-coagulable state with a tendency toward both venous and arterial thrombosis. In addition, cases with the antiphospholipid antibody syndrome develop sterile valvular vegetations similar to those seen in systemic lupus. Though not basically destructive, they might result in valvular regurgitation. They might resolve with successful treatment of the underlying systemic illness and systemic anticoagulation. In all likelihood, some individuals formerly diagnosed with Libman-Sacks vegetative lesions might have had sterile vegetations related to the antiphospholipid antibody syndrome. Large, mobile valvular masses or vegetations may be seen in 10–40% of cases and might be difficult to distinguish from infective vegetations. In addition to valvular vegetations, focal or diffuse thickening of valve leaflets has been detected (Table 40.3).

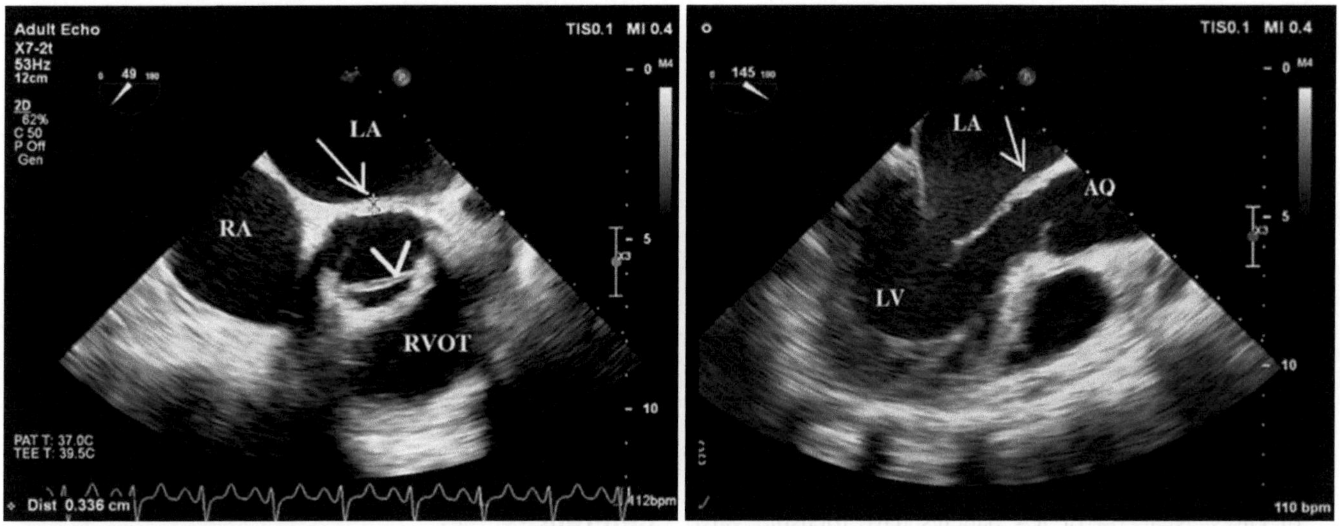

Fig. 40.2 Left: Thickened tricuspid aortic valve. Right: Thickened aortic wall suggestive of aortitis

Table 40.3 Valvular involvement in anti-phospholipid antibody syndrome

Valvular thickness > 3 mm
Localized thickening of proximal and middle portion of the valve leaflets
Nodules on the atrial surface of the mitral valve and/or the aortic surface of the aortic valve
Rheumatic valvular disease and infective endocarditis should be excluded

Modified from Miyakis S, Lockshin MD, Atsumi T, et al. international consensus statement on an update of the classification criteria for definite antiphospholipid syndrome (APS). J Thromb Haemost 2006; 4(2):295–306

- On rare circumstances, a catastrophic antiphospholipid antibody syndrome develops with acute severe multi-organ system failure related to micro-thrombosis of arterial and venous circuits. Myocardial necrosis might be a part of this syndrome. From an echocardiographic perspective, it will present as acute vegetative lesions and-or myocardial necrosis with instances of isolated papillary muscle rupture having been described [2, 6, 7].

Scleroderma and Raynaud Phenomenon

- Many other connective tissue diseases may have cardiovascular manifestations. Diseases closely related to SLE such as mixed connective tissue disease characterize a crossover category for' which all the different manifestations of SLE might be seen. Cases with Raynaud phenomenon or with the full complex of scleroderma have a greater than natural prevalence of pulmonary arterial hypertension. In cases with scleroderma, PH anatomically and physiologically is similar to primary PH with an increase in pulmonary vascular resistance at the arteriolar level. Concurrent pericardial effusion might be more common in scleroderma than in PH of other etiologies and is not necessarily an indicator of end stage disease [2, 8].

Takayasu Arteritis (TA)

- TA, a granulomatous panarteritis, affects the aorta and its major branches, characteristically before the age of 40 years. The disease predominates in women, with a female-to-male ratio of up to 10:1. Cause the diagnosis is often delayed, considerable arterial injury accrues. The current diagnostic criteria depend on detection of established stenotic disease and do not yet reflect the increasing sensitivity of noninvasive imaging.
- By Echo-Doppler study aortic arch branch vessels are often affected and the carotid artery can have diffuse, homogeneous wall thickening, known as the 'macaroni sign'. The descending aorta can be stenotic with 'pseudo-coarctation'.
- So, echocardiography, a noninvasive technique, shows a great utility in detection and follow-up of cardiovascular manifestations in cases with TA. New techniques, more sensitive toward detecting the early stages of left ventricular dysfunction, are promising to limit left ventricular hypertrophy development. Also, aortic valve involvement may cause aortic regurgitation in some patients with Takayasu arteritis and that aortic regurgitation is more common than previously believed.
- Additionally, high-resolution ultrasound, CMR, MRA, CTA, and PET have all been studied. Though the potential of these techniques is not in doubt, their specificity and sensitivity in the management of TA remain to be determined. 18F-FDG-PET-CT may reveal evidence of active arteritis and lead to early detection of pre-stenotic disease. A current consensus review has suggested that this technique is particularly useful for the detection of active arteritis in cases

not receiving immunosuppressive therapy. Demonstration of arterial wall enhancement, edema, or thickening on MRA and CTA may facilitate the diagnosis of pre-stenotic disease, and stenoses and aneurysms can be readily identified and monitored. Color duplex ultrasound is of specific use in assessing the common carotid and proximal subclavian arteries in TA. Homogeneous, bright concentric arterial wall thickening is a typical finding in affected common carotid arteries [9–11].

Rheumatoid Arteritis (RA)

- By echocardiography, Mitral regurgitation (MR) is evidenced in 80% of RA. Aortic regurgitation is found in 1/3 of cases. Near 1/4 of RA patients have tricuspid valve abnormalities. Pericarditis is found in about 10% of cases. 1/3 of RA patients has evidence of cardiomyopathy and about 40% has atheroma of the aorta. Rarely, echo-generating nodules are seen on a mitral or aortic valve [12].

Ankylosing Spondylitis

- Cases with ankylosing spondylitis and cardiac abnormalities were older, had a longer disease duration, and more peripheral joint disease than those without cardiac abnormalities. Doppler echocardiography is a useful method in the assessment of cardiac disease in ankylosing spondylitis and might detect aortic valve disease at an early preclinical stage [13].

Questions

1. Which Sentence is wrong in SLE:
   A. SLE mimics either an acute coronary syndrome or cardiomyopathy.
   B. The occurrence of SLE-related pulmonary hypertension is high.
   C. A final sign of SLE might be acute pericarditis.
   D. There are no typical features of the pericarditis or pericardial infusion seen in SLE.

2. Valvular involvement in Anti-phospholipid Antibody Syndrome are except for:
   A. Valvular thickness >3 mm
   B. Localized thickening of proximal and middle portion of the valve leaflets.
   C. Nodules on the ventricular surface of the mitral valve and the aortic valve.
   D. Rheumatic valvular disease and infective endocarditis should be excluded.

3. Which Sentence is wrong in RA:
   A. Mitral regurgitation (MR) is evidenced in 80% of RA.
   B. Aortic regurgitation is found in 1/3 of cases.
   C. Near 1/4 of RA patients have tricuspid valve abnormalities.
   D. Pericarditis is found in about 50% of cases.

Answers

1. B
2. C
3. D

References

1. Cauduro KGM, Tsang TSM, et al. Clinical and echocardiographic characteristics of hemodynamically significant pericardial effusions in cases with systemic lupus erythematosus. Am J Cardiol. 2003;92(11):1370–2.
2. Lang RM, Goldstein SA, Kronzon I, et al. ASE's comprehensive echocardiography. Philadelphia: Elsevier; 2015. Chapters 175 and 176.
3. Yu H, Li Y-N. Echocardiographic abnormalities in a cohort of Chinese cases with systemic lupus erythematosus. J Clin Ultrasound. 2011;39(9):519–26.
4. Pieretti J, Roman MJ, Devereux RB, et al. Systemic lupus erythematosus predicts increased left ventricular mass. Circulation. 2007;116(4):419–26.
5. Zawadowski M, Klarich KW, Moder KG, et al. A contemporary case series of lupus myocarditis. Lupus. 2012;21(13):1378–84.
6. Gleason CB, Stoddard MF, Wagner SG, et al. A comparison of cardiac valvular involvement in the primary antiphospholipid syndrome versus anticardiolipin-negative systemic lupus erythematosus. Am Heart J. 1993;125(4):1123–9.
7. Zuily V, Regnault C, Selton-Suty C, et al. Increased risk for heart valve disease related with antiphospholipid antibodies in cases with systemic lupus erythematosus: meta-analysis of echocardiographic studies. Circulation. 2011;124(2):215–24.
8. Lambova S. Cardiac manifestations in systemic sclerosis. World J Cardiol. 2014;6(9):993–1005.
9. Soto ME, Espinola-Zavaleta N, Ramirez-Quito O, Reyes PA. Echocardiographic follow-up of patients with Takayasu's arteritis: five-year survival. Echocardiography. 2006;23(5):353–60.
10. Mann DL, Zipes DP, Libby P, Bonow RO. Braunwald's heart disease a textbook of cardiovascular medicine (Chapter 14). 10th ed. Philadelphia: Elsevier; 2015.
11. Hashimoto Y, Oniki T, Aerbajinai W, Numano F. Aortic regurgitation in patients with Takayasu arteritis: assessment by color Doppler echocardiography. Heart Vessels Suppl. 1992;7:111–5.
12. C G, Bianchi-Fior P, Cormier B, Barthelemy B, Rat AC, Boissier MC. Cardiac manifestations of rheumatoid arthritis: a case-control transesophageal echocardiography study in 30 patients. Arthritis Rheum. 2001;45(2):129–35.
13. O'Neill TW, King G, Graham IM, Molony J, Bresnihan B. Echocardiographic abnormalities in ankylosing spondylitis. Ann Rheum Dis. 1992;51(5):652–4.

Echocardiography in End-Stage Renal Disease

41

Azin Alizadehasl and Anita Sadeghpour

Abstract

The population of End-stage renal disease (ESRD) is increasing with higher mortality due to cardiovascular disease which is the leading cause of death in these cases. Valvular heart disease, pericardial effusion, systolic and diastolic dysfunction and pulmonary hypertension are common cardiac abnormality in these patients.

Keywords

Echocardiography · End-stage renal disease · Pericardial effusion · Pulmonary hypertension · Mitral annulus calcification · Dialysis-related pericarditis

Abbreviations

AV	Aortic valve
CATs	Calcified amorphous tumors
ESRD	End-stage renal disease
HTN	Hypertension
LVH	Left ventricular hypertrophy
MAC	Mitral annulus calcification
PH	Pulmonary hypertension

- End-stage renal disease (ESRD) population is increasing. More importantly cardiovascular disease is the leading cause of death in ESRD cases. Cardiovascular mortality is 5–30 times greater in dialysis cases than in individuals from the general people who are the same sex, age, and also race.
- Cases with ESRD often have renal disease owing to hypertension (HTN) or diabetes. In addition to premature coronary artery disease, strokes, and peripheral emboli, the metabolic derangement in ESRD such as hyperparathyroidism results in ectopic calcification, mainly of the fibrous skeleton of the heart. This is most often manifested as the calcification of the mitral valve annulus called mitral annulus calcification (MAC).
- The degree of annular calcification is related to the magnitude of hyperparathyroidism and may range from small focal deposits to extensive circumferential deposits of calcium at the annulus Fig. 41.1). In advanced cases and extensive calcification, Calcinosis and even mobile calcified masses can be seen in ESRD. The calcification my invades the proximal mitral valve leaflets and might create functional mitral stenosis. Subgroups of Calcified amorphous tumors (CATs) are echogenic spindle shaped mobile masses which arise from the mitral valve and are frequently attached to bulky MACs in patients with ESRD called termed "MAC-related CAT" [1–4].

Valvular Heart Disease

Indeed, valvular heart disease is common in cases with chronic renal disease.

Based on epidemiological data, it is estimated that in cases undergoing dialysis:

- Mitral annular calcification (MAC) is present in 10–50% of cases.
- Aortic valve calcification occur in 25–60% of cases. AV calcification in dialysis cases happens 10–20 years earlier compare to the general population [1, 5, 7].
- Aortic stenosis is the most common valvular stenosis in these cases. It progresses more quickly, with a predictable incidence of 3.3% per year.
- Yearly echocardiography has been recommended for renal cases with aortic stenosis [2].

A. Alizadehasl, MD, FACC, FASE (✉)
Associate Professor of Cardiology, Echocardiologist, Echocardiography and Cardiogenetic Research Centers, Cardio-Oncology Department, Rajaie Cardiovascular Medical and Research Center, Tehran, Iran

A. Sadeghpour, MD, FACC, FASE
Professor of Cardiology, Echocardiography Research Center, Rajaie Cardiovascular Medical and Research Center, Iran University of Medical Science, Tehran, Iran

A. Sadeghpour, A. Alizadehasl (eds.), *Case-Based Textbook of Echocardiography*,
https://doi.org/10.1007/978-3-319-67691-3_41

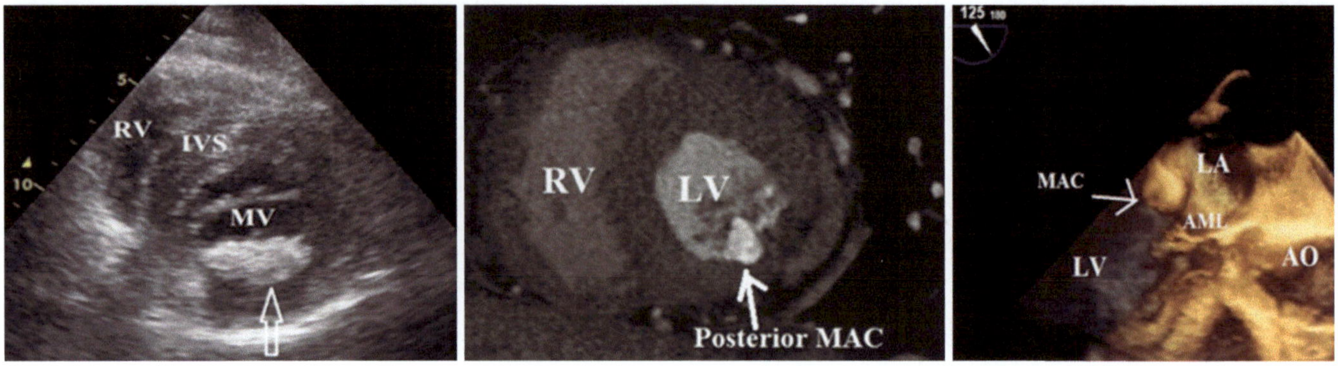

Fig. 41.1 Large bulky posterior mitral annulus calcification (MAC) with some extension to the body of posterior Mitral leaflet (white arrow) in a patient with ESRD, Short-axis view in Transthoracic echocardiography (Left panel), in cardiac computed tomography (middle panel) Right panel: Mitral annulus calcification (MAC) of the posterior mitral valve in 3D transesophageal echocardiography long axis view

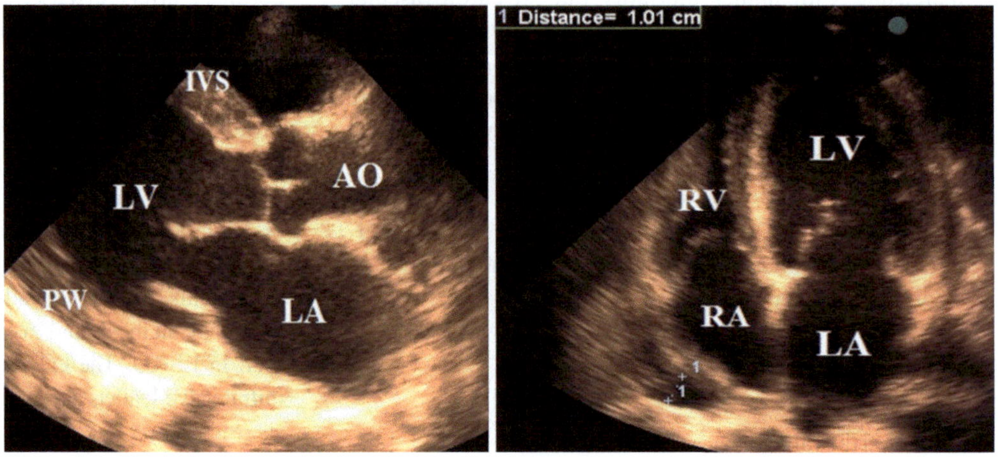

Fig. 41.2 Left ventricular hypertrophy (left) and pericardial effusion (Right) in a patient with ESRD

- Regurgitant lesions are also common and the severity is influenced by hypertension and the volume status of the patient.
- Nearly 40% of dialysis cases have moderate or severe mitral regurgitation and 18% moderate-to-severe tricuspid regurgitation.
- Aortic regurgitation happens less often; merely 4% of the cases having been studied had moderate aortic regurgitation [2, 6, 7].

Myocardial Involvement

- Secondary features of ESRD include left ventricular hypertrophy (LVH) due to HTN, chronic volume overload and anemia and abnormal texture of the hypertrophied myocardium that mimics cardiac amyloid.
- LVH has a prevalence of nearly 32% in cases with ESRD and rises to nearly 75% at the time of the initiation of dialysis therapy. Kidney transplantation has been suggested to cause LVH regression.

Pericardial Involvement

Renal failure is allied to:

- Pericardial effusion,
- Pericarditis,
- Chronic constrictive pericarditis.

Up to 20% of cases with renal failure may develop pericardial disease and echocardiography is the diagnostic test of choice for pericardial effusion detection (Fig. 41.2).

- There are two major types of chronic renal failure-related pericardial disease.
  1. **Uremic pericarditis** happens in 6–10% of cases with renal failure before dialysis begins or afterward mainly due to inflammation of pericardium correlated to the severity of azotemia.
  2. **Dialysis-related pericarditis** has been detected in up to 13% of cases who are on maintenance dialysis.

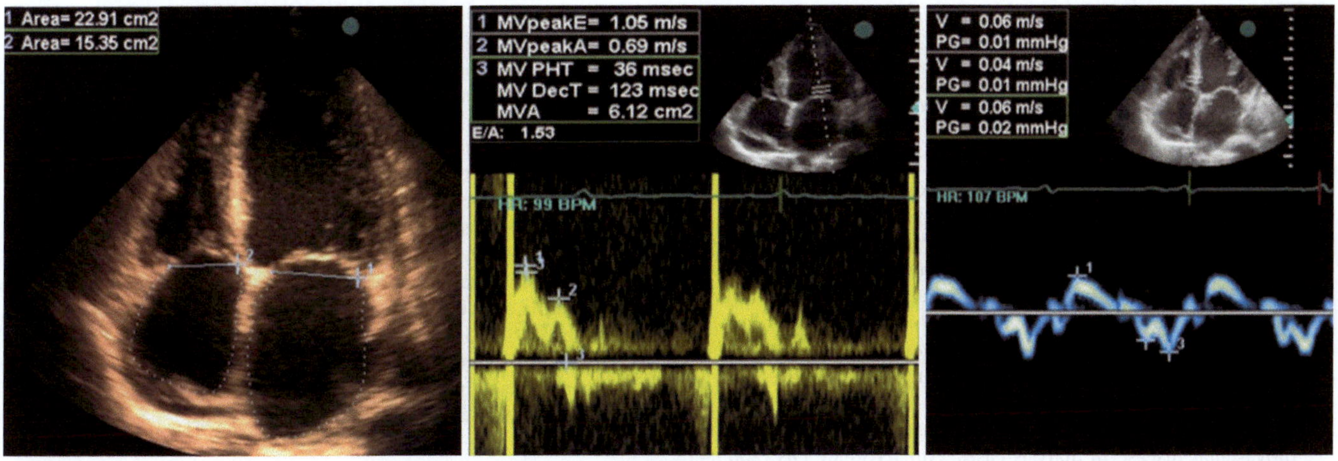

Fig. 41.3 Diastolic dysfunction in a patient with ESRD regarding to left atrial enlargement, LA maximum volume index 38 cc/m^2(left) and psuedonormal pattern (middle) of Mitral inflow and reduced tissue velocity of mitral annulus

The etiologies include inadequate dialysis or fluid overload, that should be managed by intensive hemodialysis.

- Serial follow up echocardiography is recommended [2].

Pulmonary Hypertension (PH)

- In cases with ESRD, the frequency of finding PH is increasing, mostly due to: chronic fluid overload, HTN, myocardial stiffness, and placement and use of arteriovenous fistulae [2, 3, 6, 7].

Systolic and Diastolic Function

- Ischemic heart disease and HTN can lead to systolic dysfunction and reduced contractility. On occasion, cases with ESRD develop systolic and diastolic dysfunction, which may not be related to uncontrolled HTN, coronary artery disease, or other identifiable factors. The presumed etiology of the dysfunction is accumulation of metabolic products such as metalloproteinases in the myocardium.
- Indeed, LV diastolic dysfunction is a common finding in cases with ESRD (Fig. 41.3).
- Diastolic dysfunction is correlated with the development of congestive heart failure and increased mortality. Myocardial fibrosis is one of the etiologies for the development of diastolic dysfunction. Many cases have been reported in which systolic function improves after the institution of more aggressive dialysis or renal transplantation.
- ESRD cases develop congestive heart failure and other cardiovascular disorders because of cardio-renal syndromes. Cardio-renal syndromes are disorders of the heart and kidneys, in which acute or chronic dysfunction in one organ might induce acute or chronic dysfunction in the other [2, 5, 8–10].

Questions

1. Which of the following sentences is correct regarding the valvular heart disease in ESRD patients:
   A. Mitral stenosis due to mitral annulus calcification (MAC) is the most common valve stenosis in these patients.
   B. Mitral regurgitation and tricuspid regurgitation are not a common finding in these patients.
   C. Aortic valve (AV) stenosis due to AV calcification is the most common valve stenosis in these patients.
   D. Aortic regurgitation is a common finding in these patients.

2. Which of the following abnormality is not a common finding in patients with hypertension and ESRD:
   A. LVH
   B. Diastolic dysfunction
   C. Pulmonary hypertension
   D. Significant AR

Answers

1. C
2. D

References

1. Park M, Hsu CY, Li Y, et al. Associations between kidney function and subclinical cardiac abnormalities in CKD. J Am Soc Nephrol. 2012;23:1725–34.
2. Goldberger M. End-stage renal disease (Chapter 172). In: Lang RM, Goldstein SA, Kronzon I, et al., editors. ASE's comprehensive echocardiography. Philadelphia: Elsevier; 2015.
3. Masuda S, Motoyoshi N, Ito K, Hayatsu Y, Akiyama M, Kawamoto S, et al. Surgical removal of calcified amorphous tumor localized to mitral valve leaflet without mitral annular calcification. Surgical Case Rep. 2015;1:39.
4. Sadeghpour A, Alizadehasl A, Nojoomizadeh L, Pouraliakbar H, Bayati P. CASE: Cardiovascular Imaging Case Report Elsevier publishing company, June 2017;1(3): 96–98 2017.
5. K/DOQI Workgroup. K/DOQI clinical practice guidelines for cardiovascular disease in dialysis cases. Am J Kidney Dis. 2005;45 (4 Suppl 3):S1–S153.
6. London GM, Pannier B, Marchais SJ, et al. Calcification of the aortic valve in the dialyzed patient. J Am Soc Nephrol. 2000;11:778–83.
7. Sarnak MJ, Levey AS, Schoolwerth AC, Coresh J, Culleton B, Hamm LL, PA MC, et al. Kidney disease as a risk factor for development of cardiovascular disease. Circulation. 2003;108:2154–69.
8. Cheung AK, Sarnak MJ, Yan G, et al. Atherosclerotic cardiovascular disease risks in chronic hemodialysis cases. Kidney Int. 2000;58:353–62.
9. Foley RN, Parfrey PS, Harnett JD, et al. Clinical and echocardiographic disease in cases starting end-stage renal disease therapy. Kidney Int. 1995;47:186–92.
10. Tonelli M, Bohm C, Pandeya S, et al. Cardiac risk factors and use of cardioprotective medications in cases with chronic renal insufficiency. Am J Kidney Dis. 2001;37:484–9.

42 Echocardiography in Pregnancy

Atousa Mostafavi

Abstract

Approximately, 2% of pregnancies occur in females with cardiovascular diseases, and this is associated with increased maternal and fetal risk. Profound changes that take place in the maternal circulation during this period (e.g., blood volume and heart rate increase and thus stress the heart) tend to complicate the condition of the mother-to-be.

Labor and delivery is another issue that adds to the heart's workload, and a mother who has tolerated the pregnancy may become complicated. The risk depends on the nature and severity of the underlying heart disease.

Minor abnormalities of the heart's shape and function as well as hemodynamic changes happen in pregnancy. Although they are not normally deemed a cause for concern, they may pose life-threatening risks to mother and fetus in women with a history of cardiovascular disease.

Keywords

Echocardiography · Pregnancy · Congenital heart diseases · Aortic diseases · Mitral stenosis · Pulmonary hypertension · Peripartum cardiomyopathy

Abbreviations

LA	Left atrial
LV	Left ventricular
LVOT	Left ventricular outflow tract
NYHA	New York heart association
PTMC	Percutaneous transvenous mitral commissurotomy
RA	Right atrium
RV	Right ventricle
TEE	Transesophageal echocardiography
VTI	Velocity time integral

A. Mostafavi
Echocardiography Research Center, Rajaie Cardiovascular Medical and Research Center, Iran University of Medical Sciences, Tehran, Iran

Changes in the Normal Heart During Pregnancy

Hemodynamic Changes

Hemodynamic changes occur at two time periods in a pregnant woman:

1. during pregnancy
2. during labor and delivery

During Pregnancy

- Blood volume increases by about 50% above the baseline.
- Heart rate increases by about 20% above the baseline.
- Cardiac output increases by 20–30% above the baseline.
- Peripheral arterial resistance rises and there is a slight drop in blood pressure.
- Venous pressure rises in the lower extremities.

During Labor and Delivery

The hemodynamic changes during this period are abrupt and profound.

- With each uterine contraction, about 500 mL of blood is transfused into the circulation.
- Cardiac output is increased by about 50% during labor and even higher during delivery.
- There is blood loss of about 400 mL during vaginal delivery and 800 mL during cesarean section.
- There is an abrupt rise in venous return during delivery.
- There are also changes in physical examination and imaging modality in normal pregnancy [1].

A. Sadeghpour, A. Alizadehasl (eds.), *Case-Based Textbook of Echocardiography*,
https://doi.org/10.1007/978-3-319-67691-3_42

Echocardiography in Pregnancy

Echocardiography, which is an ultrasound of the heart, is safe during pregnancy. A routine modality for the evaluation of the heart and the diagnosis of its problems, echocardiography can distinguish between cardiac problems and problems associated with a normal pregnancy.

There are some changes in echocardiographic findings in a normal pregnancy.

Changes in the Chamber Size

- Left atrial (LA) size increases by about 10%–15%. (LA volume during pregnancy is about 48.7 ± 13.9 mL.)
- Left ventricular (LV) size increases by about 5%–10%. (LV volume in the 3rd trimester is about 104.6 ± 21 mL.)
- LV mass increases. (The mass during pregnancy is about 134.5 ± 31 g.)
- Mass/ volume ratio remains normal.
- Left ventricular outflow tract (LVOT) diameter increases. (The diameter during pregnancy is about 2.0 ± 0.1 cm.)
- Dilation of the right atrium (RA) and the right ventricle (RV) is more obvious than that in the left-sided chambers.
- RA area increases. (The area during pregnancy is about 14.3 ± 2.3 cm^2.)
- -RV diastolic area increases. (The area during pregnancy is about 18.3 ± 3 cm^2.) [2]

Changes in Systolic and Diastolic Functions

- Stroke volume is increased. (Stroke volume during pregnancy is about 63.7 ± 14 m.)
- There is a rise in the heart rate with a resulting increase in the cardiac index (3.0 ± 0.7 mL/min/m^2) [2].
- Parameters of LV systolic function, including ejection fraction, shortening fraction, and tissue Doppler velocity, have been variously described as decreased, increased, or remained unchanged. The cause most probably is due to the load dependency of these parameters and the variations of the loading condition during pregnancy [3].
- There have been reports of decreased global longitudinal and circumferential strain, global area strain, and radial strain in late pregnancy [3].
- In the evaluation of diastolic function, there is an increased peak early transmittal inflow velocity (E wave) in the 1st trimester, which is subsequently decreased throughout pregnancy [4]. The peak of the A wave increases during the 2nd trimester. The E/A ratio increases significantly in the 1st trimester and subsequently decreases due to augmented A-wave velocity [4–6].
- In the evaluation of diastolic function by tissue Doppler imaging, there have been reports of an increased peak early diastolic (Em) velocity in the 2nd trimester and a decline in the 3rd trimester. Late diastolic (Am) velocity decreases as pregnancy progresses and subsequently there will be a decline in the Em/Am ratio and the E/Em ratio throughout pregnancy [5]. Pulmonary vein flow: Pulmonary venous peak systolic velocity increases, peaking in the 2nd trimester. The velocity time integral (VTI) of diastolic velocity decreases from the 1st to the 2nd trimester. The peak of the reverse flow velocity of atrial contraction increases, but the duration remains unchanged. In late pregnancy, due to the compression of the enlarged uterus, there is a pseudo wall motion abnormality in the posterior wall [7].

Changes in the Valvular Shape and Function

The increase in stroke volume and cardiac output can result in some changes.

- Any valvular regurgitation can be accentuated.
- Velocity across the LVOT and the RVOT increases, mimicking an increase in the valve gradient [8].
- Sometimes, mild valvular dysfunction before pregnancy causes acute regurgitation such as acute mitral regurgitation due to chordal rupture in a myxomatous mitral valve and acute aortic insufficiency due to aortic dissection [9]. Some instances of valvular dysfunction become less apparent during pregnancy such as mitral valve prolapse and regurgitation due to the ideal coaptation of the leaflets, secondary to an increase in LV volume.

Changes in the Pericardium

- Hydropericardium is the most frequent form of pericardial involvement.
- Typically, the amount of fluid is small.
- Pericardial effusion is clinically silent.
- It is present in the 3rd trimester.
- If the pericardial effusion is associated with compressive effects on the heart chambers as well as with significant symptoms or ECG changes, the pathologic condition should be considered [10].

Cardiovascular Disease in Pregnancy

Changes in the Echocardiographic Findings of Different Valve Diseases

Mitral Stenosis

Although the frequency of rheumatic heart diseases has decreased worldwide, these diseases are still encountered, with mitral stenosis being the most common.

Patients with mild mitral stenosis can tolerate pregnancy well, but those with severe mitral stenosis (mitral valve area<1.5 cm^2) have high morbidity and even mortality.

The gradient across the mitral valve depends on the mitral valve area, flow volume, and heart rate. The pregnancy-induced rise in the cardiac output leads to an increase in the pressure gradient and, as a result, pulmonary atrial and venous hypertension will develop [11] (Figs. 42.1 and 42.2, Table 42.1).

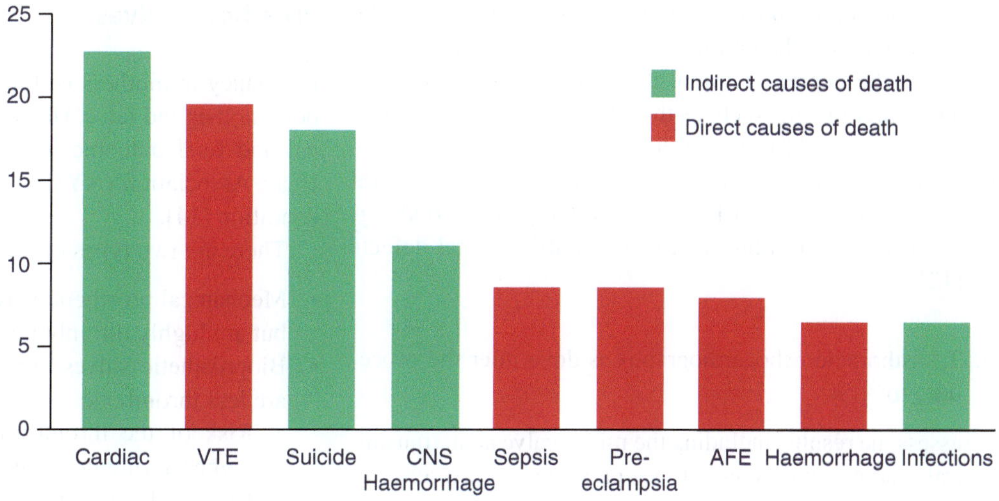

Fig. 42.1 Overall death rates per million maternities

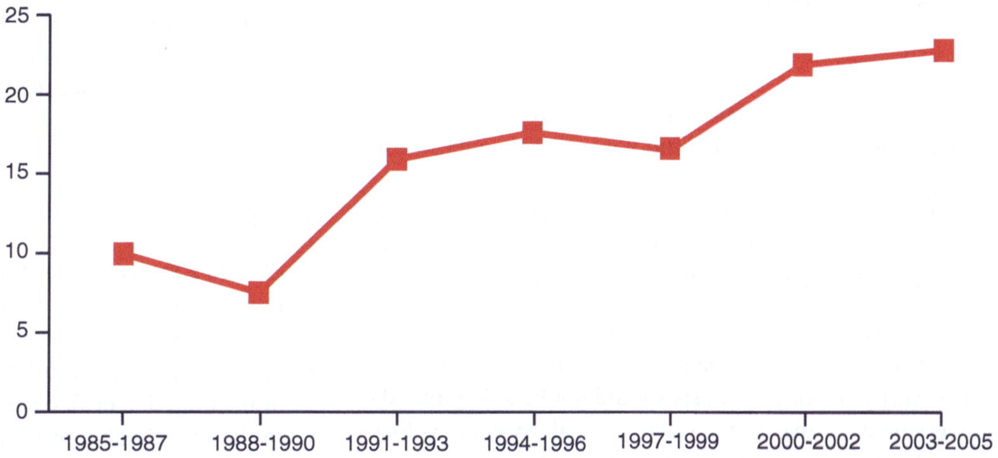

Fig. 42.2 Evolution of maternal mortality from heart disease in the UK

Table 42.1 Cardiovascular disease in pregnancy includes

Heart disease during pregnancy
• Congenital heart disease – Most frequent cause of cardiac complications in industrialise countries (70–80%), rare in developing countries (10–20%)
• Valvular disease: – Most frequent cause of cardiac complications in developing countries (50–90%), 15% in industrialised countries.
• Cardiomyopathies: – Rare but severe
• Coronary heart disease: – Rare but increasing frequency

Key point: Transmitral valve gradient dose not correlate accurately with the severity of mitral stenosis. The gradient may be overestimated in pregnancy. Nonetheless, the mitral valve area is not influenced by pregnancy and should be measured.

In patients with severe mitral stenosis and feasible valve anatomy, pre pregnancy percutaneous transvenous mitral commissurotomy (PTMC) should be performed. If the disease is discovered in pregnancy and the patient has persistent symptoms despite optimal medical therapy, this procedure should be performed in the 2nd trimester with good safety and result.

Echocardiography before and during Percutaneous Transvenous Mitral Commissurotomy in Pregnancy

1. Echocardiography is done before the procedure to....

- reduce the fluoroscopic time.
- calculate the mitral valve area and the Wilkins score with a view to checking the feasibility of PTMC.
- assess the severity of mitral regurgitation. (More-than-mild mitral regurgitation is an exclusion criterion.)
- measure the transmittal gradient and pulmonary arterial pressure.

2. Transesophageal echocardiography (TEE) is done to exclude LA appendage clot.

- TEE or transthoracic echocardiography (the former being the superior modality) is done during the procedure to:

- facilitate septal puncture and determine the position of the guide wire and the balloon before and during inflation.
- assess the degree of mitral regurgitation after each balloon inflation and to check the adequacy of the procedure versus the need for further dilation.
- look for the complications of PTMC like severe mitral regurgitation, pericardial effusion, tamponade, dislodgment of the thrombus, and residual atrial septal defects [12].

3. Transthoracic echocardiography is done after the procedure to:

- assess the results, including the mitral valve area, transmitral gradient, pulmonary artery pressure, and presence or worsening of mitral regurgitation.
- look for complications.

Aortic stenosis

- Two common etiologies of aortic valve stenosis in this age group are bicuspid aortic valve and rheumatic aortic stenosis.
- Patients with mild or moderate aortic stenosis (aortic valve area >1.5 cm^2) can tolerate pregnancy well, whereas those with severe aortic stenosis have high morbidity and mortality.

Key points: The high cardiac output state in pregnancy leads to the overestimation of the gradient across the aortic valve. The severity of aortic stenosis should not be solely based on the gradient of the aortic valve or peak systolic velocity. Instead, the aortic valve area should be calculated.

- Patients with bicuspid aortic valves have some degree of aortopathy. On echocardiography before pregnancy, the ascending aorta should be measured accurately. If the ascending aorta is >50 mm, pre pregnancy aortic surgery should be considered [13].

Mitral and Aortic Regurgitation

Patients with severe regurgitation and normal LV function tolerate pregnancy well.

Pre pregnancy evaluation by echocardiography should consist of the following data:

- LV size and ejection fraction
- Severity of regurgitation
- Pulmonary artery pressure

In patients with aortic insufficiency, the size of the ascending aorta should be measured.

Key point: The severity of regurgitation may be overestimated in pregnancy.

Prosthetic Valves

Pregnancy in mothers with prosthetic valves carries risk for both mother and fetus. However, there may be a good maternal and fetal outcome in patients with a good New York Heart Association (NYHA) function class and stable heart condition [14].

There are two types of prostheses:

- Mechanical prosthetic valves, which have long durability but are highly thrombotic.
- Bioprosthetic valves, which have less longevity and but are less thrombotic.
  - Risk of the thrombosis of the mechanical valve is higher during pregnancy.
  - Risk of the degeneration of the bioprosthetic valve is higher during pregnancy.
  - Transprosthetic valve gradient is higher during pregnancy due to high output state.
- Pre pregnancy echocardiography is crucial; it will serve as a reference for subsequent examinations.

Data which should be obtained by echocardiography are as follows:

- LV and RV size and systolic function
- Function of the native valves and estimation of pulmonary artery pressure
- Pressure gradient across the prosthesis and determination of the effective orifice area
- In the mitral valve prosthesis, the determination of pressure half time and the Doppler velocity index
- In the aortic valve prosthesis, the determination of the acceleration time and the Doppler velocity index [15]
  - Effective orifice area is calculated via the continuity equation, and it can differentiate patient prosthetic mismatch from that of true stenosis.

High Gradient in the Aortic Valve Prosthesis Is Due to 1 or More of the Following Etiologies:

1. Valve obstruction owing to either valve dysfunction, pannus formation, or patient prosthetic mismatch
2. Subvalvular obstruction
3. High output state (The Doppler velocity index is helpful in this setting.)
4. Pressure recovery [16]

High Gradient in the Mitral Valve Prosthesis Is Due to 1 or More of the Following Etiologies:

1. Valve obstruction due to valve dysfunction, pannus formation, and patient prosthetic mismatch
2. High output state

Table 42.2 Congenital heart disease (specific defects)

Specific defect	Maternal and fetal risk, management and delivery
ASD, VSD, AVSD, CoA, PST, AVST	Low to moderate risk, WHO I or II
Fallot, Ebstein's anomaly	Should be repaired before pregnancy: WHO II
Transposition of great arteries	WHO III Irreversible decline in maternal cardiac function in 10% of pregnancies
Congenitally corrected TGA	WHO III, Fetal loss increased, pregnancy contraindicated if EF <40%

Congenital Heart Diseases with Pregnancy

Congenital heart diseases are classified as follows:

1. Acyanotic heart diseases with left-to-right shunting (atrial septal defects, ventricular septal defects, and patent ductus arteriosus)
2. Cyanotic heart diseases with right-to-left shunting (tetralogy of Fallot, tricuspid atresia, transposition of the great arteries, and total anomalous pulmonary venous connection)
3. Cyanotic heart diseases without shunting
4. Diseases of the aorta [8] (Table 42.2)

Evaluation Before Pregnancy

- Identifying the risk to the mother
- Identifying the potential risk to the fetus, including the risk of inheritance
- Evaluating the mother's ability to tolerate the pregnancy
- Evaluating high-risk patients with contraindications to pregnancy (including cyanotic heart disease and the Eisenmenger syndrome)
- In repaired lesions, evaluating for residual hemodynamic lesions or sequelae of palliative procedures
- Exercise test for the evaluation of function capacity in selected cases [8]

When Is the Exercise Test Considered Abnormal?

1. When the patient cannot achieve 70% of the predicted workload.
2. When there is a fall in O_2 saturation.
3. When there is a drop in blood pressure.
4. When there is an abnormal chronotropic response and exercise-induced arrhythmia [17].

What should be reported in the echocardiographic evaluation of a shunt lesion? [18]

- Size and function of the chambers
- Size of the defect and its location
- Magnitude of the gradient
- Magnitude and direction of the shunt flow
- Pulmonary artery pressure

Table 42.3 Patients who have undergone previous successful surgical repair for congenital heart disease tolerate pregnancy often well if:

No mechanical valve is implanted
The exercise tolerance is good
The ventricular function is normal

- Secondary manifestation of the shunt lesion (e.g., the mitral annular dilation secondary to post tricuspid shunt may lead to mitral regurgitation.)
- Distance to the adjacent structure (when considering for device closure)
- Definition of the operability

Key point: The shunt flow may be modified by the presence of distal obstruction or by associated shunts.

- Associated aortic stenosis or coarctation of the aorta exaggerates the shunt through ventricular septal defects.
- Mitral stenosis may be masked in the presence of an atrial septal defect.
- Significant mitral regurgitation may become unmasked after the closure of an atrial septal defect.
- Atrial septal defects may exaggerate the severity of pulmonary stenosis.

General rules

- Patients with small shunts and a normal pulmonary artery pressure can tolerate pregnancy well (Table 42.3).
- Pregnancy in patients with the Eisenmenger syndrome is contraindicated.
- Any shunt with pulmonary hypertension should be repaired before pregnancy.
- Cyanosis leads to high mortality and morbidity for mother and fetus.

No risk CHD patients:

- Mild PS
- Small VSD
- Small PDA
- Repaired ASD, VSD, PDA, PAPVC
- Isolated PAC, PVC

So much High risk CHD patients:

- Mechanical valves.
- Systemic RV.
- Fontan physiology.
- Cyanotic or complex CHD.
- Severe PAH.

Aortic Diseases

- Aortic dilation is rare and can be catastrophic during pregnancy.

Table 42.4 Increased risk of dissection during pregnancy May lead to consider prophylactic surgery

	Risk of dissection
Marfan syndrome	Ascending aorta >45 mm
Bicuspid aortic valve	Lower risk than Marfan
Ehlers Danlos type IV	Even in non-dilated aorta
Turner syndrome	Consider body size indexed aortic root >27 mm/m^2 BSA

Table 42.5 Ascending aorta diameter and delivery type

• <40 mm	Vaginal delivery is favoured
• 40–45 mm	Decision on individual basis
• >45 mm	Caesarean delivery should be considere

- Most common reasons for aortic diseases are the bicuspid aortic valve and the Marfan, Loeys–Dietz, Ehlers–Danlos, and Turner syndromes [19].
- In the Marfan syndrome, prophylactic aortic replacement should be performed if the diameter is >40 mm, based on the 2010 thoracic aortic disease guideline, and >45, based on the European guideline. In other diseases, prophylactic surgery should be performed if the aortic diameter is >50 mm [20].
- In patients with the Marfan syndrome and a normal aortic diameter, echocardiography should be done in each trimester.
- In all pregnant women with aortic dilation, monthly or bimonthly echocardiography should be done for the detection of expansion.
- Aortic diameters <40 mm are rarely associated with complications [21]. The risk of dissection in the Marfan syndrome varies from 1% in aortic diameters <40 mm to 10% in aortic diameters >40 mm [22] (Tables 42.4 and 42.5).

Peripartum Cardiomyopathy

Peripartum cardiomyopathy is a rare and life-threatening cardiovascular complication with the following features:

- It is a non-familial idiopathic form of cardiomyopathy.
- It is a heart failure with a reduced ejection fraction.
- It begins in the last month of pregnancy or at 5 months post partum.
- It is categorized as dilated cardiomyopathy, but the LV may be non-dilated.
- Nearly always, the LV ejection fraction is <45% [23].

Echocardiography is the most important tool for the diagnosis of peripartum cardiomyopathy.

Differentiation from Other Causes of Cardiomyopathy

1. ***Hypertensive disorder in pregnancy***
   - Cardiac involvement in preeclampsia is predominantly diastolic dysfunction, and systolic function is normal.
   - Systolic dysfunction has been reported in preterm preeclampsia, with proteinuria, edema, and abnormal hepatic, cerebral, and hematologic functions [23].
2. ***Genetic form of cardiomyopathy***
   - It is not easy to distinguish peripartum cardiomyopathy from the genetic form. Careful family history taking can be helpful.
3. ***Cardiomyopathy triggered by pathogens (viral infection)***
   - It is distinguishable from peripartum cardiomyopathy. Cardiac biopsy can be useful, but it is rarely used during pregnancy [23].

Pregnancy and Pulmonary Hypertension

1. Interaction between the hemodynamic consequences of PH and the normal hemodynamic profile of pregnancy produce an excessive mortality to both the mother and fetus.
2. **Definition**: Mean PAP >25 mm Hg at rest Sys PAP > 35–40 mm Hg
3. **Classification:**
   - IPAH
   - Post-capillary PH (PCWP > 15 mmHg- PH due to LV disease
   - PAH associated with lung disease
   - CTEPH
   - Miscellaneous

Hemodynamic Effects of PH on Pregnancy and Delivery

- Excessive volume burden on a compromised pressure overloaded RV
- RV failure and RV ischemia
- Exacerbation of LV diastolic impairment
- Restriction of the ability of blood flow to increase in response to gestation
- Systemic hypotension
- Inadequate perfusion pressure to vital organs and fetus
- In situ thrombosis
- During labour and delivery: Hypotension, Tachycardia, Metabolic acidosis, and sometimes difficult or impossible to reverse

Complications:

1. Maternal mortality: **36%** for Eisenmenger syndrome,30% for idiopathic PAH,56% for PH related to a variety of underlying causes
2. Most maternal deaths occurred within 30 days
3. The most common reason of death resistant RV failure and cardiogenic shock
4. SCD due to malignant arrhythmia, PTE and dissection and rarely rupture of PA
5. Half of all deliveries occur prematurely
6. 1/3 of all infants have IUGR
7. Better neonatal survival ≠ 90%

Pregnancy and PH Management Issues

Pregnancy and PH management issues

- Pregnancy prevention
- Elective termination
- Prenatal management
  admission
  anticoagulation
  liberal oxygen supplementation
- Management of delivery
  cesarean section. General anesthesia, volume repletion
- Postpartum management
  ICU admission
  Bed rest
  Anticoagulation [23, 24]

Conclusion

So the following situations are very important and with so much risk during pregnancy (Table 42.6):

Severe PAH for any reason.
LVEF <30%.
NYHA class III or IV.
Severe LV obstruction.
Marfan with aortic root >4.5 cm.
PPCMP with any degree of LV impairment.
Cyanotic or complex CHD.

Table 42.6 Specific maternal high risk conditions WHO (III–IV)

Condition	Expected outcome
Pulmonary hypertension	Neonatal survival 87–89%
Eisenmenger syndrome	Maternal mortality of 20–50% Life birth 12% if O_2 saturation <85%
Cyanotic HD without PH	Depends on maternal oxygen saturation Life birth 12% if O_2 saturation <85%
Severe LVOTO	Should be treated before pregnancy. If not, discourage pregnancy.

Questions

1. So much High risk CHD patients for pregnancy are all of the following items except for:
   A. Mechanical valves.
   B. Systemic RV.
   C. Severe RV obstruction.
   D. Cyanotic or complex CHD.

2. Which sentences is wrong about pregnancy and PAH:
   A. Most maternal deaths occurred within 30 days
   B. The most common reason of death is resistant RV failure and cardiogenic shock
   C. 1/3 of all deliveries occur prematurely
   D. 1/3 of all infants have IUGR

3. Which sentences is wrong :
   A. Associated aortic stenosis or coarctation of the aorta exaggerates the shunt through the ventricular septal defects.
   B. Mitral stenosis may be masked in the presence of an atrial septal defect.
   C. Significant mitral regurgitation may become unmasked after the closure of an atrial septal defect.
   D. Atrial septal defects may diminish the severity of pulmonary stenosis.

4. Which sentences is wrong in pregnancy:
   A. Left atrial (LA) size increases by about 10%–15%. (LA volume during pregnancy is about 48.7 ± 13.9 mL)
   B. Left ventricular (LV) size increases by about 5%–10%. (LV volume in the 3rd trimester is about 104.6 ± 21 mL)
   C. LV mass increases (The mass during pregnancy is about 134.5 ± 31 g)
   D. Mass/ volume ratio increases.

Answers

1. C
2. C
3. D
4. D

References

1. Mann DL, Zipes DP, Libby P, Bonnw RO. Braunwald's heart disease: a textbook of cardiovascular medicine. 10th ed. London: Elsevier Health Sciences; 2011. p. 1755–70.
2. Tso G, Lee J, Lui G, Trivedi H, Cohen M, Bernstein P, Taub C. Range of echocardiographic parameter during normal pregnancy. J Am Coll Cardiol. 2012;59(13s):1.

3. Cong J, Fan T, Yang X, Squires JW, Cheng G, Zhang L, Zhang Z. Structural and functional changes in maternal left ventricle during pregnancy: a three-dimensional speckle—tracking echocardiography study. Cardiovasc Ultrasound. 2015;13:6.
4. Kametas NA, MCAuliffe F, Hancock J, Chambers J, Nikolaides KH. Maternal left ventricular mass and diastolic function during pregnancy. Ultrasound Obstet Gynecol. 2001;18(5):460–6.
5. Fok WY, Chan LY, Wong JT, Yu CM, Lau TK. Left ventricular diastolic function during normal pregnancy: assessment by spectral tissue Doppler imaging. Ultrasound Obstet Gynecol. 2006;28: 789–93.
6. Mesa A, Jessurun C, Hernandez A, Adam K, Brown D, Vaughn WK, Wilansky S. Left ventricular diastolic function in normal human pregnancy. Circulation. 1999;99:511–7.
7. Armstrong W, Ryan T. Feigenbaum's echocardiography. 7th ed. Philadelphia: Wolters Kluwer Health; 2011.
8. Harris IS. Management of pregnancy in patients with congenital heart disease. Prog Cardiovasc Dis. 2011;53(4):305–11.
9. Stout KK, Otto CM. Pregnancy in woman with valvular heart disease. Heart. 2007;93:552–8.
10. Ristic AD, Seferovic PM, Ljubic A, Jovanovic I, Ristic G, Pankuweit S, Ostojic M, Masch B. Pericardial effusion in pregnancy. Herz. 2003;28(3):209–15.
11. Karamermer Y, Roos-Hesselink JW. Mitral stenosis before, during and after pregnancy. Iran Cardiovasc Res J. 2007;1(1).
12. Silvestry FE, Kerber RE, Brook MM, Carroll JD, Eberman KM, Goldstein SA, Herrmann HC, Homma S, Mehran R, Packer DL, Parisi AF, Pulerwitz T, Seward JB, Tsang TS, Wood MA. Echocardiography-guided interventions. J Am Soc Echocardiogr. 2009;22(3):213–31.
13. Nanna M, Stergiopoulos K. Pregnancy complicated by valvular heart disease: an update. J Am Heart Assoc. 2014;3(3):e000712.
14. Khalil AA, Mohyuddin S, Akhtar K. Pregnancy outcome in women with prosthetic heart valves. Pak J Med Health Sci. 2012;6(3):519–24.
15. Christian S. Management and follow up of prosthetic heart valves. Heart. 2014;90:818–24.
16. Bach DS. Echo-Doppler evaluation of hemodynamics after aortic valve replacement: principles of interrogation and evaluation of high gradients. JACC Cardiovasc Imaging. 2010;3(3):296–304.
17. Lui GK, Silversides CK, Khairy P, Fernandes SM, Valente AM, Nickolause MJ, Earing MG, Aboulhosn JA, Rosenbaum MS, Cook S, Kay JD, Jin Z, Gersony DR. Heart rate response during exercise and pregnancy outcome in women with congenital heart disease. Circulation. 2011;125(30):242–8.
18. Awasthy N, Radhakrishnan S. Stepwise evaluation of left to right shunt by echocardiography. Iran Heart J. 2013;65(2):201–18.
19. Bons LR, Roos-Hesselink JW. Aortic disease and pregnancy. Curr Opin Cardiol. 2016;31(6):611–7.
20. Mulder BJ, Meijboom LJ. Pregnancy and Marfan syndrome: an ongoing discussion. J Am Coll Cardiol. 2012;60(3):230–1.
21. Hiratzka LF, Bakris GL, Beckman JA, Bersin RM, Carr VF, Casey DE Jr, Eagle KA, Hermann LK, Isselbacher EM, Kazerooni EA, Kouchoukos NT, Lytle BW, Milewicz DM, Reich DL, Sen S, Shinn JA, Svensson LG, Williams DM. Guidelines for diagnosis and management of patients with thoracic aortic disease. JACC J. 2010;55(14):1509–44.
22. Carboni S, Capucci R, Pivato E, Poggi A, Patella A. Marfan's syndrome and pregnancy:good maternal and fetal outcome. J Prenatal Med. 2013;7(2):21–4.
23. Hilfiker-Kleiner D, Haghikia A, Nonhoff J, Bauersachs J. Peripartum cardiomyopathy: current management and future perspectives. Eur Heart J. 2015;36(18):1090–7.
24. Pieper PG, Hoendermis ES. Pregnancy in women with pulmonary hypertension. Neth Heart J. 2011;19(12):504–8.

Echocardiography in Trauma

43

Azin Alizadehasl and Anita Sadeghpour

Abstract

Transthoracic and transesophageal echocardiography, both, have been proposed as methods to monitor volume status and also regional and global systolic function in a wide variety of traumatic settings; and they have proved useful in the immediate assessment of left and right ventricles, both, systolic function, volume status, and detection of significant pericardial, valvular or aortic pathology too.

Based on the mechanism of injury, cardiac trauma can be categorized to the Penetrating and Non penetrating (blunt) trauma. The non penetrating or blunt trauma has replaced the previous term of "cardiac contusion" and which the severity ranges from minor bruises of the myocardial rupture. Blunt chest trauma which portends cardiac injury should be managed appropriately with TEE guide in order to hasten the diagnosis and make it more precise and safe.

Keywords

Transthoracic echocardiography · Transesophageal echocardiography · Blunt trauma · Stab wound · Chordal rupture · Aortic trauma

Electronic Supplementary Material The online version of this chapter (https://doi.org/10.1007/978-3-319-67691-3_43) contains supplementary material, which is available to authorized users.

A. Alizadehasl, MD, FACC, FASE (✉)
Associate Professor of Cardiology, Echocardiologist, Echocardiography and Cardiogenetic Research Centers, Cardio-Oncology Department, Rajaie Cardiovascular Medical and Research Center, Tehran, Iran

A. Sadeghpour, MD, FACC, FASE
Professor of Cardiology, Echocardiography Research Center, Rajaie Cardiovascular Medical and Research Center, Iran University of Medical Science, Tehran, Iran

Abbreviations

TAR	Traumatic aortic rupture
TEE	Transesophageal echocardiography
TTE	Trans thoracic echocardiography

In the United States trauma is the third cause of death in under 40 years population, Blunt trauma is a conventional mechanism. For instance, generally 25% of all mortalities emanate from chest trauma in the United States. Actually serious accidents e.g. motor vehicle accidents or falls commonly lead to blunt trauma. Blunt trauma resulting direct transfer of energy to the heart or cause compression of the heart between the vertebral column and the sternum. One of the rare consequences of blunt trauma is cardiac rupture; however it is substantially uncommon, it provokes tremendously high mortality [1–4].

- Two retrospective review studies declare data which claim varied outcomes in comparison with each other. 5% and 40.6% Right atrial rupture, left atrial rupture 10% and 25%, right ventricular rupture 15% and 31.3% and left ventricular rupture 10% and 12.5%, respectively [3].
- Echocardiography specially transesophageal echocardiography (TEE), has a key role in precise assessment of patients with precordial or transthoracic injuries (Fig. 43.1, Movies 43.1 and 43.2).
- Trans thoracic echocardiograpohy (TTE) may be suboptimal in blunt chest trauma (as most patients have chest wall injury, and makes "subcostal view" the more useful view in these patients. TEE in expert hand has a high diagnostic accuracy with sensitivity (91–100%)and specificity 98–100% respectively. TEE detects more subtle abnormalities, such as valvular insufficiency, Cardiac septal defects and wall motion abnormality [1, 5–11].
- By deployment of ultrasound in the setting of acute trauma valuably identifying intra-thoracic injuries during the triage would be implemented earlier. Furthermore

A. Sadeghpour, A. Alizadehasl (eds.), *Case-Based Textbook of Echocardiography*,
https://doi.org/10.1007/978-3-319-67691-3_43

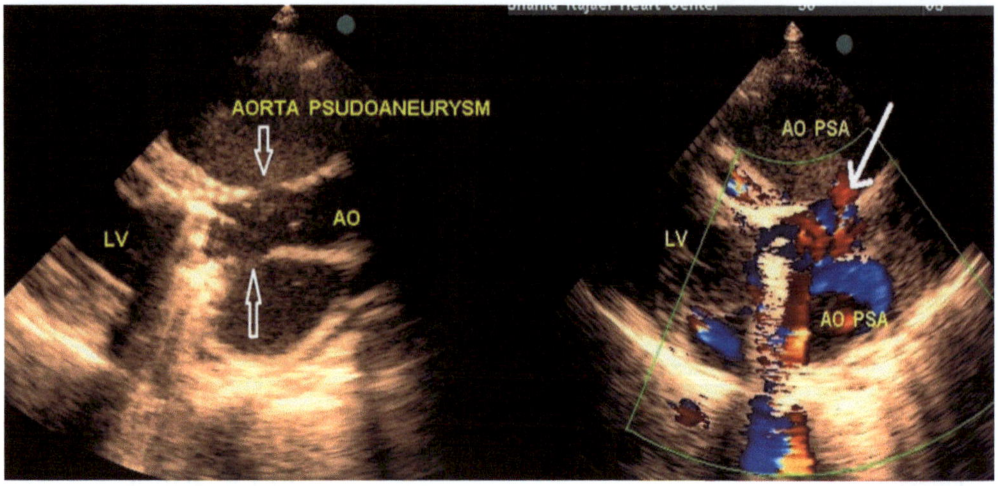

Fig. 43.1 Aortic transection in a patient with history of Aortic valve replacement a few years ago and falling down and chest pain from the steps 2 weeks before admission, Parasternal long axis view in TTE shows large echo free space around ascending aorta that flow goes through it via a narrow neck (arrows). *Ao* Aorta, *PSA* Psudoaneurysm

combination of electrocardiogram and echocardiography decreases admissions in intensive care unit to monitor the heart following to blunt chest trauma.

- One of the most conventional form of blunt trauma is cardiac contusion meaning the injury of myocyte of the heart, incidentally now it is an issue which encompasses considerable debate. There are obstacles to make an exact diagnosis of cardiac contusion due to the lack of any gold standards or obvious definition. Valve, septum or ventriculu-septal and atrial wall rupture and also cardiac wall motion abnormalities need crucial conservative observation by echocardiography. Massive trauma other than chest might elevate the troponin level as a diagnostic criteria [4, 5].
- It should be mentioned that cardiac rupture due to blunt cardiac injury is one of the most obliterating condition virtually patients with ruptured chamber(s) of heart never reach the emergency department alive. In fact, ruptured chamber of heart is primarily termed in autopsy sequences [5–12].
- TEE is suitable for various indications such as penetrating wounds to the precordium, traumatic aortic dissection, retrieval of a foreign body, valvular trauma, and postoperative evaluation of cardiac repair to assess patients with trauma to the heart or great vessels. TEE as a diagnostic test is invaluable, safe beneficial, and precise [13–15].
- Traumatic aortic rupture (TAR) is a life- threatening injury ensuing usually in the isthmus of aorta (area between subclavian and the first intercostal arteries), unrestrained frontal collisions or by side-impact crashes produce a shear stress which causes TAR. The rupture of adventitia is a crucially a risk of TAR that typically poses lethal hemorrhage [15].
- Currently CT and TEE are gold standards to diagnose TAR however, previously aortography furnishes TAR diagnosis. Unequivocally a profit of TEE attributable to its capacity to do the procedure retrievably and portably. Even it is highly useful for patients at bedside position with several traumatic injuries.
- An irregular and thick intraluminal flap crosses the lumen of the isthmus of aorta in the transverse view due to the fact that this lesion disrupts intimal and medical layers of the aorta, it should be seen as a medial flap in longitudinal view. Medial flap is almost perpendicular to the wall of aorta so that traumas most of the time are restricted and limited to a few centimeters [15–21].
- In fact, TEE is preferable other than various imaging techniques for diagnosing aortic trauma. It is capable of diagnosing managing conditions such as aortic rupture pseudo-aneurysm, traumatic aortic dissection, and intramural hematoma and makes the diagnosis more precise, quick and safe [21–23].
- Overall, according to our knowledge by the use of TEE, the diagnosing and managing of all heart structures in trauma -such as mitral and specially tricuspid leaflets chorda rupture with severe regurgitation—become easier, accurate and will be world spread in near future (Fig. 43.2).
- The most common sites of tearing in VSD is the membranous and muscular parts of the septum.
- Cardiac rupture has a worse prognosis with a survival rate of approximately 20%. In the blunt trauma of the chest, septal rupture most frequently occur near the apex while the injury occurs in late diastole or early systole.
- The autopsy data has shown that ventricular rupture due to blunt cardiac trauma mostly involves the LV followed by the RV, but right atrial disruption is more common in patients who arrive alive to the hospital [11, 24].

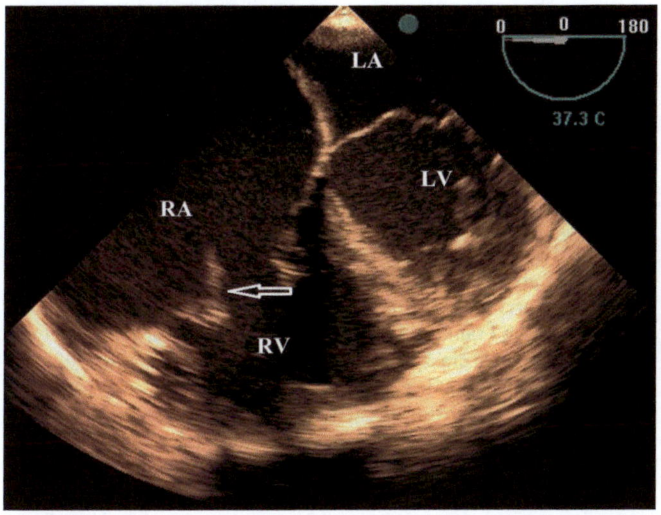

Fig. 43.2 Tricuspid valve flail in a young girl detected after 10 years of blunt chest trauma, resulting severe RV and RA enlargement

Penetrating Cardiac Trauma

The overall mortality related to the penetrating cardiac trauma has not changed significantly which shows that penetrating trauma are highly lethal. Any penetrating wounds to the epigastrium and precordium needs more investigation for possible cardiac injury.

Indeed, up to 80% of stab wounds that cause heart injury ultimately will lead to tamponade which is contrary to the gunshot wounds of the heart that more frequently is associated with haemorrhage rather than tamponade. The treatment of choice is surgical exposure via median sternotomy or anterior thoracotomy to control the hemorrhage and relief the tamponade [11].

- The wounds injuries of the RV (which has thicker wall) seals more readily than the wounds involves the RA.

Penetrating injuries of the coronary arteries resulting a rapid onset tamponade and cardiac ischemia.

Iatrogenic Heart Injury

- Iatrogenic cardiac injury can be seen in cardiac catheterization (coronary arteries or cardiac perforation and aortic dissection), insertion of central venous line, cardiac massage, etc. Even appropriate technique can be associated with complications which may lead to emergency intervention such as cardiac surgery. As little as 60–100 mL of blood in the pericardium may lead to clinical tamponade (Fig. 43.3, Movie 43.3).

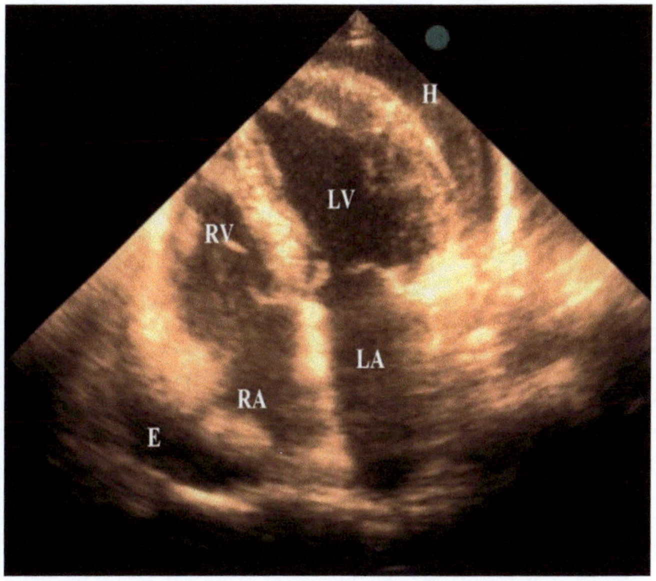

Fig. 43.3 Hemo-pericardium and clinically tamponade after cardiac catheterization. Fresh hematoma(H), Pericardial effusion (E)

Questions

1. In a patient with severe chest wall injury, which of the following views are more appropriate for evaluation the cardiac injury in Transthoracic echocardiography?
   A. Apical views
   B. Parasternal views
   C. Subcostal views
   D. There is no difference between windows

2. In the acute setting of the hemopericardium due to cardiac perforation, what is the minimum blood volume which can results clinical tamponade?
   A. 50–100 cc
   B. 100–200 cc
   C. 200–300 cc
   D. At least 500 cc

3. All of the following sentences regarding the cardiac injury are correct except:
   A. In blunt cardiac trauma the anterior structure such as RV and RA are involved more commonly than posterior structures such as LA.
   B. About 80% of stab wounds that cause heart injury ultimately will lead to haemorrhagic shock.

C. Most injuries in gunshot wounds of the heart causing tamponade rather than haemorrhage.
D. The most common site of tearing in VSD is the inlet part of the septum

Answers

1. C
2. A
3. D

   The most common sites of tearing in VSD is the membranous and muscular parts of the septum. Indeed, up to 80% of stab wounds that cause heart injury ultimately will lead to tamponade which is contrary to the gunshot wounds of the heart that more frequently is associated with haemorrhage rather than tamponade

References

1. Porter TR, Shillcutt SK, Adams MS, Desjardins G, Glas KE, Olson JJ, Troughton RW. Guidelines for the use of echocardiography as a monitor for therapeutic intervention in adults: a report from the American Society of Echocardiography. J Am Soc Echocardiogr. 2015;28:40–56.
2. Jennings SB, Rice J. Supporting the early use of echocardiography in blunt chest trauma. Crit Ultrasound J. 2012a;4(1):7.
3. Jennings SB, Rice J. Supporting the early use of echocardiography in blunt chest trauma. Crit Ultrasound J. 2012b;4(1):7.
4. Elie MC. Blunt cardiac injury. Mt Sinai J Med. 2006a;73:542.
5. Martin M, Mullenix P, Rhee P, et al. Troponin increases in the critically injured patient: mechanical trauma or physiologic stress? J Trauma. 2005;59:1086.
6. Sangalli F, Galbiati L, Fumagalli R. Chest trauma—echocardiography in cardiovascular thoracic injuries. In: Sarti A, Lorini FL, editors. Echocardiography for intensivists and other ultrasound techniques in the ICU. Milan: Springer; 2012. https://doi.org/10.1007/978-88-470-2583-7_37.
7. Türk EE, Tsokos M. Blunt cardiac trauma caused by fatal falls from height: an autopsy-based assessment of the injury pattern. J. Trauma. 2004;57:301.
8. Rozycki G, Ballard R, Feliciano D, Schmidt J, Pennington S. Surgeonperformed ultrasound for the assessment of truncal injuries: lessons learned from 1540 patients. Ann Surg. 1998;228(4):557–67.https://doi.org/10.1097/00000658-199810000-00012.
9. Holanda MS, Domínguez MJ, López-Espadas F, López M, et al. Cardiac contusion following blunt chest trauma. Eur J Emerg Med. 2006;13:373.
10. Elie MC. Blunt cardiac injury. Mt Sinai J Med. 2006b;73:542.
11. Zipes D, Libby P, Bonow R. Braunwald's heart disease: a textbook of cardiovascular medicine, 10th edn. Philadelphia: Elsevier, 2011, p. 1658–63.
12. Parmley LF, Mattingly TW, Manion WC, Jahnke EJ Jr. Nonpenetrating traumatic injury of the aorta. Circulation. 1958;17:1086.
13. Fisher RG, Hadlock F. Laceration of the thoracic aorta and brachiocephalic arteries by blunt trauma. Report of 54 cases and review of the literature. Radiol Clin North Am. 1981;19:91.
14. Fitzharris M, Franklyn M, Frampton R, et al. Thoracic aortic injury in motor vehicle crashes: the effect of impact direction, side of body struck, and seat belt use. J Trauma. 2004;57:582.
15. Fabian TC, Richardson JD, Croce MA, et al. Prospective study of blunt aortic injury: Multicenter Trial of the American Association for the Surgery of Trauma. J Trauma. 1997;42:374.
16. Duwayri Y, Abbas J, Cerilli G, et al. Outcome after thoracic aortic injury: experience in a level-1 trauma center. Ann Vasc Surg. 2008;22:309.
17. Collier B, Hughes KM, Mishok K, et al. Is helical computed tomography effective for diagnosis of blunt aortic injury? Am J Emerg Med. 2002;20:558.
18. Cinnella G, Dambrosio M, Brienza N, et al. Transesophageal echocardiography for diagnosis of traumatic aortic injury: an appraisal of the evidence. J Trauma. 2004;57:1246.
19. Vignon P, Lang RM. Use of Transesophageal echocardiography for the assessment of traumatic aortic injuries. Echocardiography. 1999;16:207.
20. Patel NH, Stephens KE Jr, Mirvis SE, et al. Imaging of acute thoracic aortic injury due to blunt trauma: a review. Radiology. 1998;209:335.
21. Hiratzka LF, Bakris GL, Beckman JA, et al. 2010 ACCF/AHA/AATS/ACR/ASA/SCA/SCAI/SIR/STS/SVM guidelines for the diagnosis and management of patients with thoracic aortic disease: a report of the American College of Cardiology Foundation/American Heart Association Task Force on Practice Guidelines, American Association for Thoracic Surgery, American College of Radiology, American Stroke Association, Society of Cardiovascular Anesthesiologists, Society for Cardiovascular Angiography and Interventions, Society of Interventional Radiology, Society of Thoracic Surgeons, and Society for Vascular Medicine. Circulation 2010;121:e266.
22. Hainer C, Böckler D, Bernhard M, et al. Blunt traumatic aortic injury: importance of transesophageal echocardiography. Anaesthesist. 2008;57:262.
23. Marty B, Tozzi P, Ruchat P, et al. An IVUS-based approach to traumatic aortic rupture, with a look at the lesion from inside. J Endovasc Ther. 2007;14:689.
24. Vougiouklakis T, Peschos D, Doulis A, et al. Sudden death from contusion of the right atrium after blunt chest trauma: case report and review of the literature. Injury. 2005;36:213.

Aging Changes in Echocardiography

44

Paulina Wejner-Mik, Piotr Lipiec,
and Jarosław D. Kasprzak

Abstract

The progressive growing of the elderly population has become one of the most challenging global public health issues. Aging is a natural process where irreversible damage to the intracellular exceed the possibility of self-repair. The aging process is associated with degenerative processes on the heart valves, especially aortic and mitral. Age related changes include calcifications and amyloid deposition of both mitral and aortic valve; in advanced form it can lead to damage to the valves. The aorta dilates and tilts rightward on the interventricular septum. It is important to differentiate the cardiac manifestations of normal aging which do not require medical treatment of heart disease in an older patient and situations where the changes are considered pathologic and no longer "normal aging".

Keywords

Echocardiography · Elderly · Valve sclerosis Degeneration

Abbreviations

2D	Two dimensional
3D	Three dimensional
Ao Asc	Ascending Aorta
AV	Aortic valve
CAD	Coronary artery disease
E	Peak E-wave velocity of the mitral valve (cm/s)
E′	TDI of the mitral annulus
EF	Ejection fraction
LA	Left atrium
LV	Left ventricle
LVEF	Left ventricular ejection fraction
MAC	Mitral annulus calcification
RA	Right ventricle
RV	Right ventricle
STE	Speckle-tracking echocardiography
TDI	Tissue Doppler imaging

Introduction

- Cutoff for the achievement of old age is arbitrary. Most developed countries have accepted the chronological age of 65 years or older.
- Currently, the population aging is a generalized process across Western Europe and North America. The older population numbered 46.2 million in 2014 (the latest year for which data is available); they represented 14.5% of the U.S. population. People 65 or older are expected to grow to be 21.7% of the population by 2040. By 2060, there will be about 98 million elderly persons, more than twice their number in 2014 [1].
- The prevalence of CVD, including hypertension, CHD, HF, and stroke, increases from about 40% in men and women 40–59 years of age, to 70–75% in persons 60–79 years of age, and to 79–86% among those aged 80 years or older [2].
- The prevalence of cardiovascular disease in this (demographically increasingly important) population convinces of the need to know the morphological and physiological changes associated with aging, the ability to recognize and distinguish between pathology [3].

P. Wejner-Mik, MD, PhD (✉) · P. Lipiec · J. D. Kasprzak
Department of Cardiology, Medical University of Lodz, Lodz, Poland
e-mail: mik@ptkardio.pl

A. Sadeghpour, A. Alizadehasl (eds.), *Case-Based Textbook of Echocardiography*,
https://doi.org/10.1007/978-3-319-67691-3_44

Common Echocardiographic Changes in Elderly

- Aging is a natural process where irreversible damage to the intracellular exceed the possibility of self-repair. The repair processes are largely impaired due to telomere shortening, altered and inflammation gene expression, oxidative stress, UV. The cellular senescence is associated with the formation of the characteristic morphological changes in the myocardium, such as: cellular accumulation of lipofuscin, an increase in fibroblast number and collagen deposition.
- The increase in interstitial myocardial fibrosis and infiltration of amyloid deposits cause adverse ventricular geometry remodeling—the most severe within the septum. Isolated calcification its upper part, near the AV node—characteristic of old age—can lead to atrioventricular block.
- A decrease in myocyte number with an increase in myocyte size and a significant increase in the share of connective tissue leads to increased ventricular mass and to ventricular stiffening with the decrease in diastolic filling. The consequence of these changes is impaired left ventricular diastolic function.
- Left and right ventricular systolic function is not altered by aging in subjects without coronary artery disease.
- Reduced number of myocyte with their hypertrophy is also associated with the decreased responsiveness to catecholamines. This results in a progressive reduction of maximum heart rate during exercise.
- Age related changes include calcifications and amyloid deposition of both mitral and aortic valve; in advanced form it can lead to damage to the valves.
- The aorta dilates and tilts rightward on the interventricular septum.

Valve Sclerosis

- The aging process is associated with degenerative processes on the heart valves, especially aortic and mitral. To a certain extent these changes may be considered as physiological aspects of the aging process of the heart and may belong to a "broad standard" image of the heart in an elderly patient.
- Over the years the diameter of the valve annulus increases progressively throughout an adult life, although this trend was greater for semilunar than for atrioventricular valves [4].
- Aging is also associated with thickening, fibrosis and gradual calcification of aortic valve leaflets and mitral annulus (Fig. 44.1).
- Early sign of age-related degeneration of aortic valve is nodular thickening of one or more of the aortic cusps; it is usually located at the nodule of Arantius or the base of the commissures (Fig. 44.1c).
- In contrast to the mitral valve - aortic valve calcification often contributes to development hemodynamically significant stenosis. Mild aortic stenosis occurs in 40%, significant in 13% of the elderly [5].
- Aortic valve cusp calcification are sometimes accompanied by calcification of the sinotubular junction above the aortic valve. This calcification is usually benign and clinically silent (Fig. 44.2).
- Many elderly patients have deposits of calcium within the aortic valve cusps, mitral annulus and the epicardial coronary arteries—this triad is called "senile calcification syndrome". The presence of intracardiac calcifications particularly stenotic, calcified aortic valve is considered a marker of the severity of atherosclerosis and an independent predictor of stroke [6].
- Mitral Annular Calcification (MAC) is a common finding in the hearts of elderly patients, particularly females (Fig. 44.1a, b). It concerns nearly 20% of people in seven

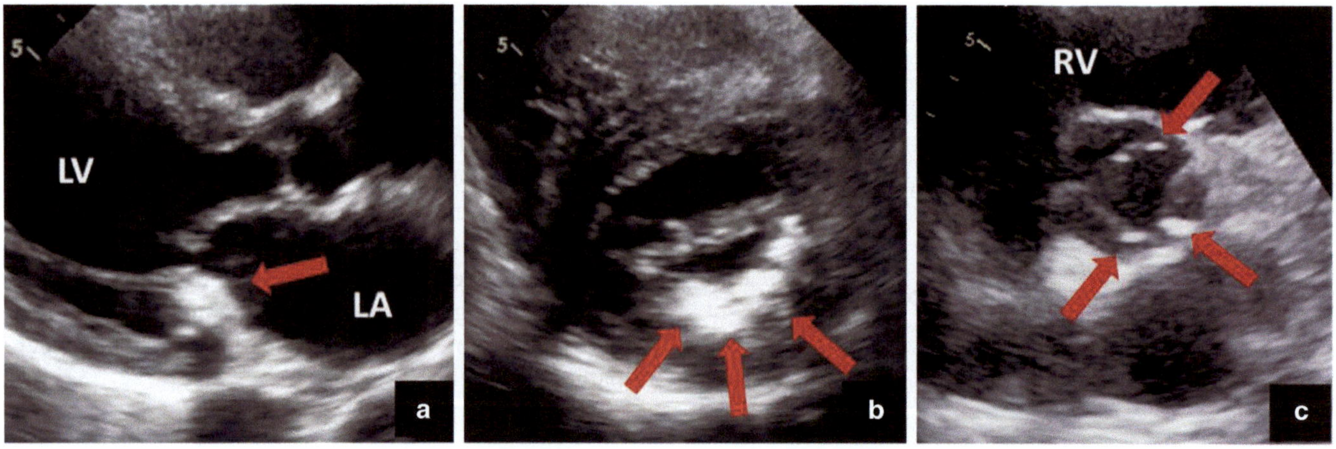

Fig. 44.1 Thickening, fibrosis and calcification of mitral annulus with large MAC at the base of the posterior mitral leaflet (**a, b**). Nodular calcification of aortic valve leaflets with a nodule of the base of the commissures (**c**). Parasternal long axis view (**a**), short axis view (**b, c**)

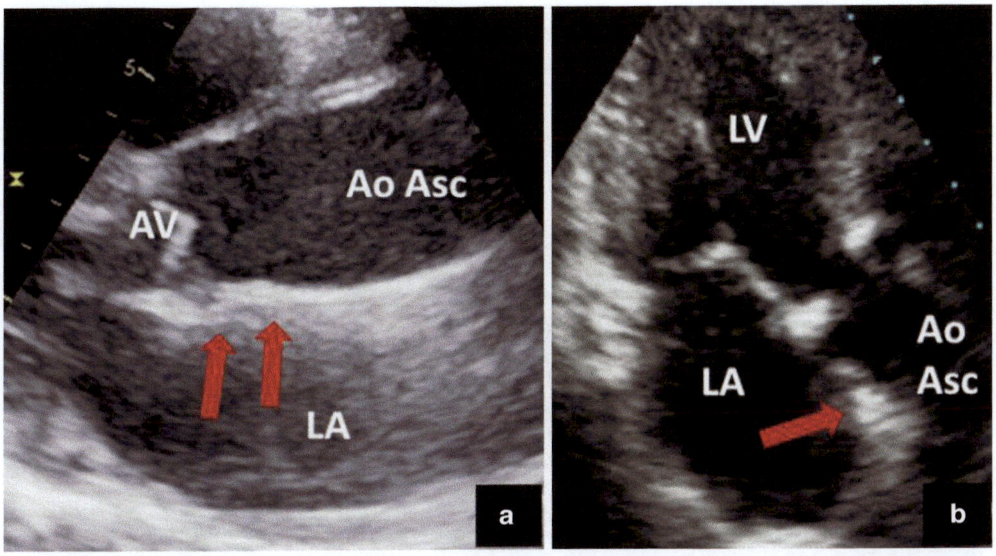

Fig. 44.2 Calcification of the sinotubular junction above the aortic valve. Parasternal long axis view (**a**) and apical long axis view (**b**)

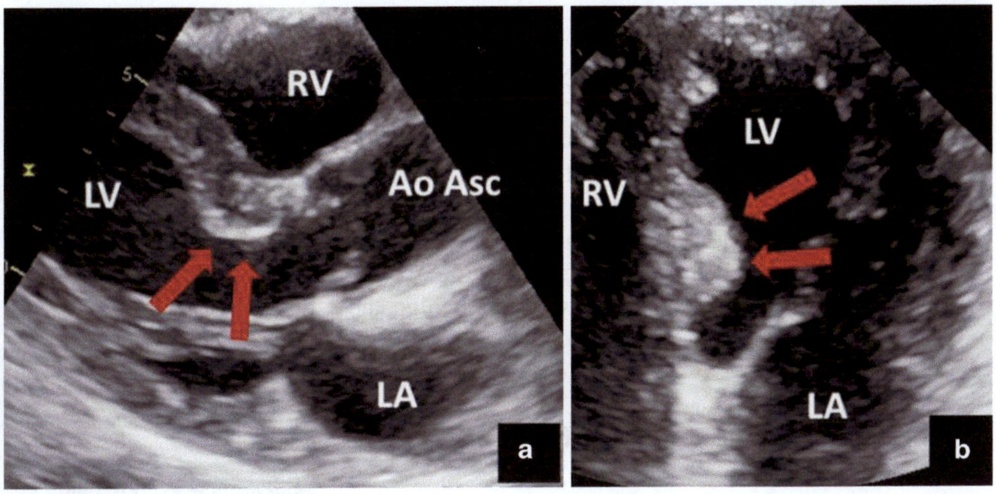

Fig. 44.3 Hypertrophy of proximal intraventricular septum contributing to a sigmoidal shape of the left ventricle outflow tract. Parasternal long axis view (**a**), and apical four-chamber view (**b**)

decade of life, and after 90 years of age occurs in near 90%. MAC is usually a lump calcification at the base of the posterior mitral leaflet, less often calcification surround the valve. Sometimes it can mimic a valvular mass/tumor.

- MAC may also restrict the posterior leaflet motion and leading to valve regurgitation, generally mild, usually eccentrically toward the back wall of the atrium.
- Calcification of the mitral valve can sometimes restrict the leaflet motion, but usually does not cause clinically significant stenosis.

Chamber Changes in the Eldery

- Aging increases slightly wall thickness and left ventricular mass. The increase in left ventricular mass in a healthy elderly is related to the increase in wall thickness. The volume of the left ventricle decreases [7].
- The angle between the ascending aorta and the left ventricular outflow tract increases, often combined with a hypertrophy of proximal intraventricular septum resulting in a sigmoidal shape of the left ventricle outflow tract (Fig. 44.3). It can cause a small area of turbulence during echocardiographic color Doppler assessment, usually without a significant increase in gradient in the left ventricular outflow.
- With age, the left atrium increases in volume. In the eighth decade of life in patients with preserved systolic function, without valvular defect, the left atrial diameter may increase up to 45 mm [8].
- However, the upper limit of normal value of maximum left atrial volumes index (maxLAVi) is independent of age and sex and is 34 mL/m^2 [9].
- In older subjects without any evidence for structural cardiac disease, an age-dependent increase of right atrial and right ventricular size should be assumed [10].
- In people after 80 years of age, amyloid may be found in any chamber, the coronary arteries, the valves and the

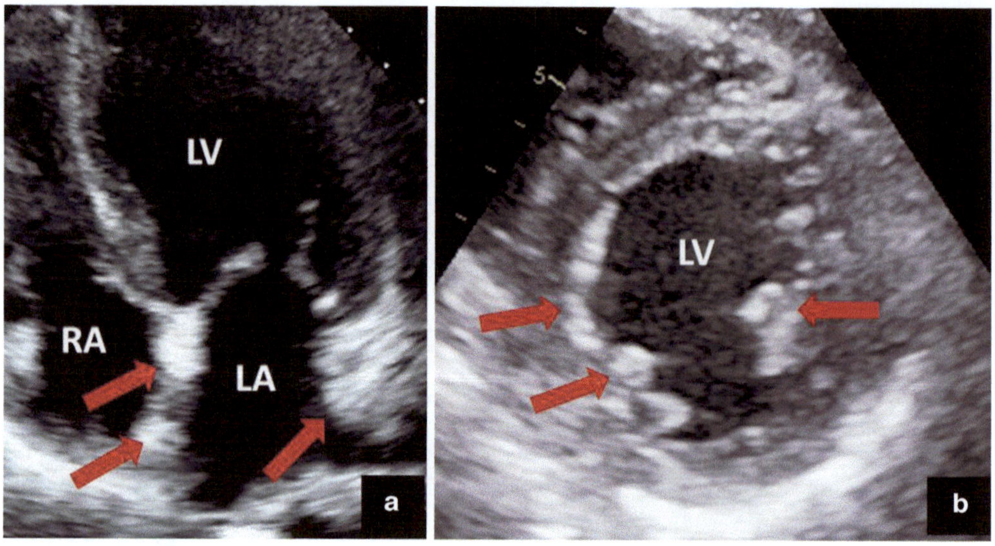

Fig. 44.4 Amyloid deposition—thickening of the heart wall and interatrial septum. Apical four-chamber view (**a**) and parasternal short axis view (**b**)

pericardium. Echocardiography may reveal bolding of leaflets valves, thickening of the heart wall and interatrial septum (Fig. 44.4). Amyloid deposition may cause stiffening and contribute to diastolic dysfunction [11, 12].

- Lambl's excrescences represent a common valvular degenerative lesion, probably due to wear and tear [13]. They can cause turbulence during echocardiographic color Doppler assessment but usually they are benign and clinically silent.

Systolic and Diastolic Function of the Left Ventricle

- The prevalence of clinical CHF increases from 6.6% in patients 65–69 years of age, to 14% in patients 85 years or older. Of patients with clinical CHF, 80% has normal or mildly reduced systolic function.
- Aging process may be accompanied by the impairment of the right ventricular diastolic function and small alterations of right ventricle systolic function [14], however, usually right ventricular systolic function remains normal (Fig. 44.5).
- Age is strongly associated with diastolic parameters - the mitral inflow velocity profile changes with a progressive decrease of the peak of early passive filling velocity (E wave) and deceleration time (DT), and the increase of the the late active diastolic filling velocity (A wave). Thereby, the ratio of early to late filling (E/A) decreases. An abnormal relaxation pattern should be anticipated in responses to normal aging of the heart, but more advanced diastolic filling (E/A > 1) should be considered abnormal [15].
- TDI measurement is also age-dependent. It has been observed a decrease of early diastolic velocity (e′) of approximately 1 cm/s per decade and an increase of the

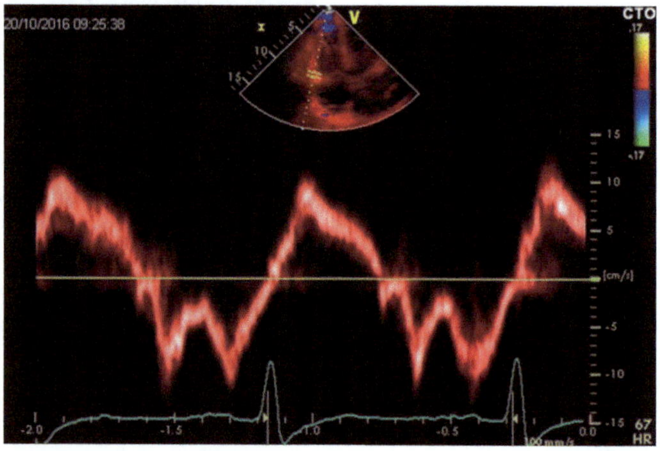

Fig. 44.5 TDI of the basal right ventricle wall shows normal systolic velocity (S′ = 0.12 cm/s) in 88 year old woman

ratio of early filling to diastolic velocity (E/e′) in elderly patients [16] (Fig. 44.6).

- 2D speckle tracking echocardiography provides quantitative assessment of global and segmental ventricular function. Studies on cohort of asymptomatic patients showed a difference in strain between younger and older subjects, resulting in a slightly lower longitudinal strain in elderly patients [17–19] (Fig. 44.7).
- Similarly, the evaluation of 3D speckle-tracking echocardiography shows age-related differences of left ventricular twist. The apical and basal twist increases during the aging process, leading to an increase LV twist value. The mean peak twist in young participants was about 12°, whereas the value for older participants was nearly 19°. Older age increases global systolic LV twist and decreases the untwist velocity. The cause of this fact can be subendocardial fibrosis and weakening of the subendocardial fibres [20].

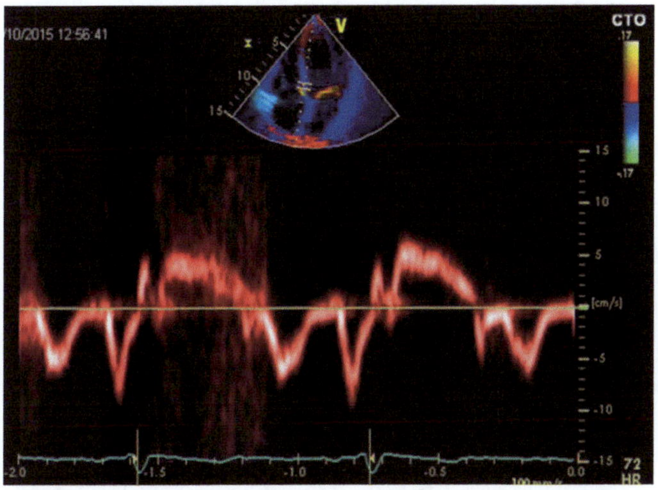

Fig. 44.6 Tissue Doppler Imaging (TDI) measurement. Normal value of early diastolic velocity (e′ = 7 cm/s) in 74 year old man

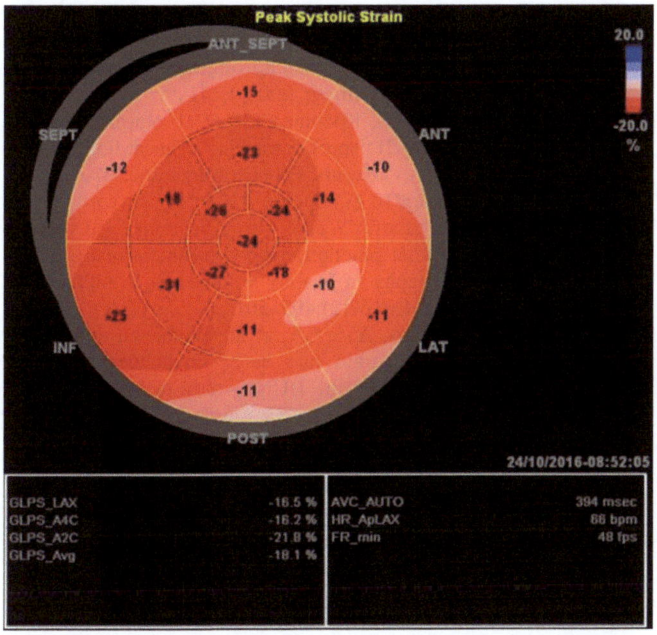

Fig. 44.7 2D speckle tracking echocardiography. Slightly reduced value of longitudinal strain in 88 year old women. Global longitudinal strain (GLS) with value −18%

Questions

1. So called: "senile calcification syndrome" means:
   A. deposits of calcification of the aortic valve cusps, mitral annulus and the epicardial coronary arteries
   B. deposits of calcification of the aortic valve cusps, annulus and mitral annulus
   C. deposits of calcification of the aortic valve cusps, mitral annulus and the sinotubular junction of the aorta above the aortic valve
   D. deposits of intracardiac calcifications particularly stenotic, calcified aortic valve.

2. MAC:
   A. means calcifications and amyloid deposition of both mitral and aortic valve.
   B. is usually located at the base of the anterior mitral leaflet.
   C. usually restricts the leaflet motion.
   D. usually does not cause clinically significant stenosis.

3. Which of the following findings the age-related change?:
   A. Hypertrophy of proximal intraventricular septum usually without increase in gradient in the left ventricular outflow.
   B. Hypertrophy of proximal intraventricular septum usually with increase in gradient in the left ventricular outflow.
   C. Hypertrophy of middle segments of the left ventricle.
   D. Hypertrophy of apical segments of the left ventricle.

4. Select the true statement: The aging process is associated with degenerative processes on the heart valves:
   A. thickening and gradual calcification typically concerns aortic annulus and mitral valve leaflets
   B. in contrast to the aortic valve - mitral valve calcification often contribute to development hemodynamically significant stenosis
   C. the diameter of the valve annulus increased progressively throughout adult life, although this trend was greater for atrioventricular than for semilunar valves.
   D. the diameter of the valve annulus increases progressively throughout adult life, although this trend is greater for semilunar than for atrioventricular valves.

5. Which of the change of following parameters is typical in the elderly?
   A. Systolic velocity of the mitral annulus slightly increases.
   B. Strain rate of the basal segments slightly increases.
   C. Global longitudinal strain (GLS) slightly decreases.
   D. Systolic twist or torsion slightly decreases.

Answers

1. A
   "Senile calcification syndrome" means deposits of calcification of the aortic valve cusps, mitral annulus and the epicardial coronary arteries.
2. D
   MAC is usually located at the base of the anterior mitral leaflet, does not cause clinically significant stenosis.
3. A
   Hypertrophy of proximal intraventricular septum is the age-related change, does not increase in gradient in the left ventricular outflow.

4. D

The aging process is associated with degenerative processes on the heart valves: the diameter of the valve annulus increases progressively throughout adult life, although this trend is greater for semilunar than for atrioventricular valves.

5. C

Typically in the elderly, global longitudinal strain (GLS) slightly decreases, systolic twist or torsion slightly increases.

References

1. www.aoa.acl.gov/Aging_Statistics/index.aspx.
2. Lloyd-Jones D, Adams R, Carnethon M, et al. Heart disease and stroke statistics-2009 update: a report from the American Heart Association Statistics Committee and Stroke Statistics Subcommittee. Circulation. 2009;119(3):e21–181.
3. Yazdanyar A, Newman AB. The burden of cardiovascular disease in the elderly: morbidity, mortality, and costs. Clin Geriatr Med. 2009;25(4):563–vii.
4. Kitzman DW, Sihloz DH, Hagen PT. Age-related changes in normal human hearts during the first 10 decades of life. A quantitative anatomic study of 765 specimens from subjects 20 to 99 years old. Mayo Clin Proc. 1988;63:137–46.
5. Lindroos M, Kupari M, Heikkila J, Telvis R. Prevalence of aortic valve abnormalities in the elderly. J Am Coll Cardiol. 1993;21:1220–4.
6. Nemcsik J, Farkas K, Kolossváry E, et al. Intracardiac calcification is a marker of generalized atherosclerosis. Angiology. 2007;58:413–9.
7. Chopra HK (ed), CSI Cardiology Update 2014: Echocardiographic evaluation in elderly: what is new? 2015 Jaypee Brothers Medical Piblishers. ISBN 978-93-5152-618-6.
8. Takemoto Y, Barnes ME, Seward JB, et al. Usefulness of left atrial volume in predicting first congestive heart failure in patients > or = 65 years of age with well-preserved left ventricular systolic function. Am J Cardiol. 2005;96:832–6.
9. Lang RM, Badano LP, Mor-Avi V, et al. Recommendations for cardiac chamber quantification by echocardiography in adults: an update from the American Society of Echocardiography and the European Association of Cardiovascular Imaging. J Am Soc Echocardiogr. 2015;16:233–71.
10. Laszlo R, Baumann T, Konz H. Echocardiographic B-mode evaluation of the right heart in older people: the ActiFE Study. Arch Gerontol Geriatr. 2016;67:145–52.
11. Desai HV, Aronow WS, Peterson SJ, Frishman WH. Cardiac amyloidosis: approaches to diagnosis and management. Cardiol Rev. 2010;18:1–11.
12. Nucci EM, Lisi M, Cameli M, et al. The role of 3D and speckle tracking echocardiography in cardiac amyloidosis: a case report. Eur Rev Med Pharmacol Sci. 2014;18(1):74–7.
13. Dumaswala B, Dumaswala K, Hsiung MC, et al. Incremental value of three-dimensional transesophageal echocardiography over two-dimensional transesophageal echocardiography in the assessment of Lambl's excrescences and nodules of Arantius on the aortic valve. Echocardiography. 2013;30(8):967–75.
14. Laszlo R, Baumann T, Konz H, et al. Right ventricular function assessed by tissue Doppler echocardiography in older subjects without evidence for structural cardiac disease. Aging Clin Exp Res. 2017;29(3):557–62.
15. Dugo C, Rigolli M, Rossi A, Whalley GA. Assessment and impact of diastolic function by echocardiography in elderly patients. J Geriatr Cardiol. 2016;13(3):252–60.
16. Innelli P, Sanchez R, Marra F, et al. The impact of aging on left ventricular longitudinal function in healthy subjects: A Pulsed Tissue Doppler study. Eur J Echocardiogr. 2008;9:241–9.
17. Menting ME, McGhie JS, Koopman LP, et al. Normal myocardial strain values using 2D speckle tracking echocardiography in healthy adults aged 20 to 72 years. Echocardiography. 2016;33(11): 1665–75. https://doi.org/10.1111/echo.13323.
18. Sun JP, Lee AP, Wu C, Lam YY, et al. Quantification of left ventricular regional myocardial function using two-dimensional speckle tracking echocardiography in healthy volunteers—a multi-center study. Int J Cardiol. 2013;167(2):495–501.
19. Dalen H, Thorstensen A, Aase SA, et al. Segmental and global longitudinal strain and strain rate based on echocardiography of 1266 healthy individuals: the HUNT study in Norway. Eur J Echocardiogr. 2010 Mar;11(2):176–83.
20. Tavakoli V, Sahba N. Assessment of age-related changes in left ventricular twist by 3-dimensional speckle-tracking echocardiography. J Ultrasound Med. 2013;32(8):1435–41.

Echocardiography in Obesity

45

Karina Wierzbowska-Drabik and Jarosław D. Kasprzak

Abstract

Beyond the influence on acquisition and quality of echocardiographic images obesity is connected with remodeling and functional impairment of cardiac function. To the most common belong concentric hypertrophy of left ventricular muscle, diastolic dysfunction, left atrial dilatation and hypertrophy of right ventricular wall. Moreover, recent studies reported subclinical deterioration of left ventricular and right ventricular systolic function detected mainly with tissue Doppler and strain analysis. To the typical findings in obese patients belong thickened layer of epicardial adipose tissue (EAT) which was recognized as predictor of atherosclerosis advancement and cardiovascular events.

Keywords

Obesity · Left ventricular hypertrophy · Diastolic dysfunction · Strain · Left ventricular function · Right ventricular function · Epicardial adipose tissue Pericardial adipose tissue

Abbreviations

2D	Two dimensional
3D	Three dimensional
A	Peak velocity of the mitral (or tricuspid) valve atrial wave inflow (cm/s)
a′	Peak velocity of the mitral (or tricuspid) annulus atrial phase motion (cm/s)
BMI	Body mass index
CFR	Coronary flow reserve
CT	Computed tomography
E	Peak velocity of the mitral (or tricuspid) valve early wave inflow (cm/s)
E/A	Ratio of early to atrial inflow velocity (respectively mitral or tricuspid)
E/e′	Ratio of early inflow velocity to early annulus velocity (respectively mitral or tricuspid)
e′	Peak velocity of the mitral (or tricuspid) annulus early phase motion (cm/s)
e′/a′	Ratio of early to atrial phase of annulus velocity (respectively mitral or tricuspid)
EAT	Epicardial adipose tissue
ECG	Electrocardiogram
GLS	Global longitudinal strain
HbA1C	Glycosylated hemoglobin
IL1; 6;16	Interleukin 1, 6;16
IMT	Intima-media thickness
LA	Left atrium
LDL	Low density lipoprotein
LV	Left ventricular
MRI	Magnetic resonance imaging
NAFLD	Non-alkoholic fatty liver disease
PAT	Pericardial adipose tissue
PET	Positrone emission tomography
QT	QT interval in ECG
RA	Right atrium
RV	Right ventricle
TAPSE	Tricuspid annular plane systolic excursion
TNF α	Tumor necrosis factor α

Introduction

- Obesity is related to higher cardiovascular risk and associated with development of diastolic heart failure [1, 2]. It was estimated that **11% of heart failure in men and 14% in women may be caused by obesity alone with predominance of heart failure with preserved ejection fraction** [3]. Obesity promotes development of

K. Wierzbowska-Drabik, MD, PhD (✉)
J. D. Kasprzak MD, PhD
Chair and Department of Cardiology, Medical University of Lodz, 1/5 Kniaziewicza Street, Lodz, Poland
e-mail: wierzbowska@ptkardio.pl

A. Sadeghpour, A. Alizadehasl (eds.), *Case-Based Textbook of Echocardiography*,
https://doi.org/10.1007/978-3-319-67691-3_45

hypertension, coronary artery disease with prominent microvascular dysfunction [4, 5] and is related to increased risk of arrhythmia due to augmented myocardial heterogeneity, hypertrophy and fibrosis of the heart muscle, QT interval prolongation and eccentric remodeling of cardiac chambers [6–8].

- However, the bulk of evidence suggests that early detection of myocardial dysfunction in isolated obesity requires detailed echocardiographic assessment with the incorporation of novel techniques. On the other hand, obesity may deteriorate the quality of transthoracic images and often imposes additional challenges for echocardiographer.

Specific Technical Issues During the Examination of Obese Patient

- The intuitive observation that obesity, especially severe, **deteriorates image quality** of transthoracic examination was recently documented in several studies. On the other hand contemporary echocardiographic tools and techniques (high sensitivity transducers with improved field depth, harmonic imaging and contrast agents) offer sufficient potential to overcome these limitations in the majority of obese patients.
- Big body habitus may impede high quality recording of typical views. Siadecki et al. showed that correct determination of both pericardial- myocardial interface and left ventricular endocardial border was significantly impaired in subgroup of patients with BMI (body mass index) between 30–39 kg/m^2 and ≥40 kg/m^2 in comparison to non-obese subjects during bedside focused examination [9].
- The accurate assessment of left ventricular endocardial border is especially important during **echocardiographic stress test**. Whereas some authors proposed transesophageal approach in severe obesity for avoiding of poor transthoracic acustic window the others tested widely used contrast enhancement [10]. Shah and al. described excellent feasibility of echocardiographic stress test assessment (treadmill exercise or dobutamine) with contrast used in 96% of cases in obese patients with BMI >35 kg/m^2 (SUMO study- Stress Ultrasonography in Morbid Obesity) [11]. Similarily, in the study of Lerakis et al. contrast enhancement enabled acquisition of diagnostic images in 97% [12]. Thus, the demand for contrast agent utilization may be higher in this group of patients.
- Echocardiographic **assessment of coronary flow reserve (CFR)** poses especial technical difficulties related to registration of flow in small and relocating distal part of coronary artery. Despite this limitation Olsen et al. achieved high feasibility of 97% and good correlation with PET assessment for CFR measured in left anterior descending artery in obese patients. Interestingly, the application of contrast agent in this study reached only 14% [13].
- **Typical echocardiographic findings** in obese patients include **epicardial fat** mimicking pericardial effusion and **lipomatous hypertrophy** caused by fat deposition in the interatrial septum which should be differentiated with tumors and other masses. Fat (mature and fetal/brown) deposition in the interatrial septum (dumbbell shape due to sparing of fossa ovalis region) may hamper transseptal puncture increasing the risk of tamponade [14].

The Impact of Obesity on Conventional and Deformation Parameters of Left Ventricle (LV), Left Atrium (LA), LV Mass and Function

Pathomechanisms

- From hemodynamic point of view obesity may be considered as **a chronic volume overload and proinflammatory state** with hyperinsulinemia which adds significantly to **myocardial hypertrophy** and **diastolic dysfunction** development. Since the obesity is typically related with coexistence of other cardiovascular risk factors (hypertension, prediabetic state or diabetes, dyslipidemia) separation of specific impact of uncomplicated obesity on cardiac function is often difficult.
- **Blood pressure control** is also often poorer in obese and pressure values, even retained in normal limits, are typically higher than in lean subjects.
- Beyond the hemodynamic effects **the accumulation of adipose tissue** in direct vicinity of heart vessels and muscle exerts metabolic effects by secretion of active adipokines and triglycerides storage in nonfat cells causes cell dysfunction because of lipotoxicity [15].

Structural Remodeling

- The increase of adipose tissue and body mass raises the metabolic demand which is achieved mainly by increase **in stroke volume**. This causes **left atrial and ventricular dilatation** to accommodate the increased venous return and developing of eccentric hypertrophy pattern [16, 17].
- The increase in **left ventricular mass** is more prevalent and was observed both in adults and children using echocardiography or MRI [18]. The synergistic action of obesity, hypertension and insulin resistance may lead to severe hypertrophy in patients with metabolic syndrome, see Fig. 45.1.

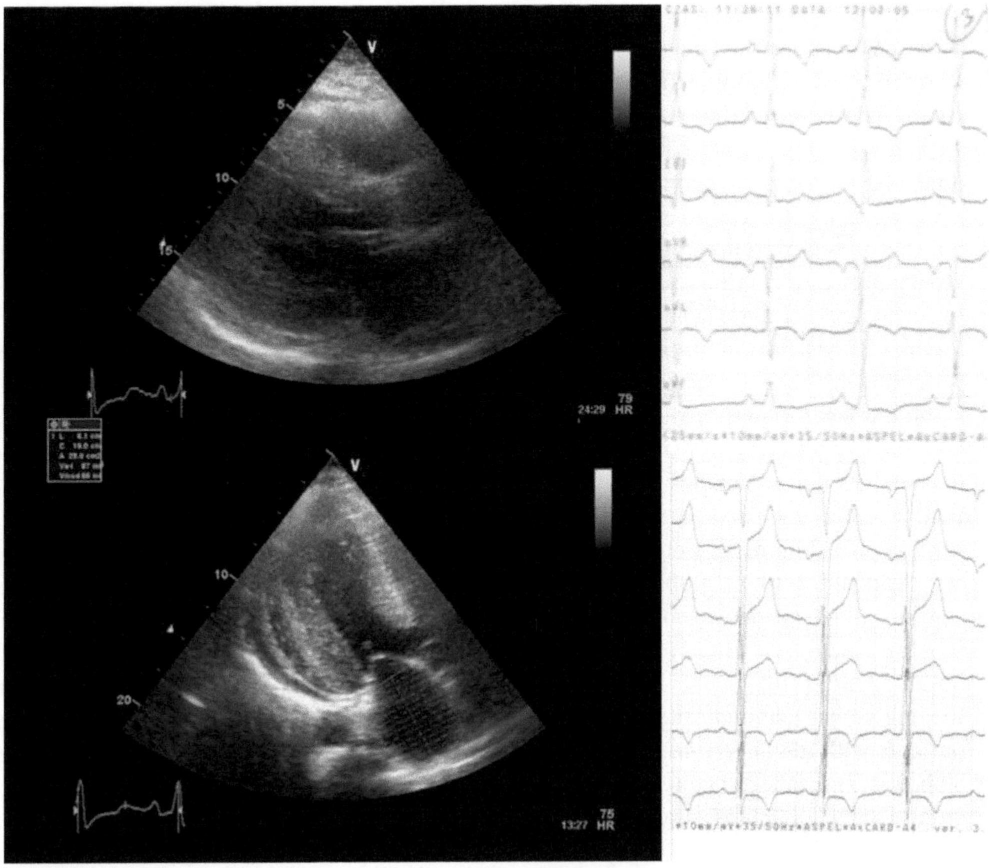

Fig. 45.1 Severe hypertrophy of the left ventricle and significant enlargement of the left atrium in young 43-year-old male patient with morbid obesity (BMI 45 kg/m^2) and metabolic syndrome in echocardiography and 12-lead ECG. LV mass index 332 g/m^2, LA volume index 35 mL/m^2. *BMI* body mass index, *ECG* electrocardiogram, *LV* left ventricle, *LA* left atrium

- In the study of Owan et al. [19] **reduction of BMI by an average 15 kg/m^2 after bariatric surgery resulted in LV mass diminution of 30 g on average.**
- Many obese patients without known cardiovascular disease present with normal echocardiograms. Some older studies underlined the absence of association between BMI and global indices of left ventricular (LV) systolic function as fractional shortening or ejection fraction or postulated even some compensatory changes [20–22].

Diastolic Dysfunction

- Most studies demonstrated **prolonged relaxation even in mild obesity** and there are data revealing diastolic dysfunction also in overweighted patients [23, 24]. The **increase of left ventricular filling pressure** may be observed **firstly during exercise** even if it is normal at rest and diastolic dysfunction is accompanied with hyperkinetic systole. In further stages of the disease the resting **diastolic dysfunction increases** and systolic deterioration develops.
- There is also the possibility that **the impact of BMI on diastolic function may be different among ethnicities.** Lee SL et al. [25] in the large group of 788 Japanese subjects documented that the risk of diastolic dysfunction in overweight and obese subgroup was higher than observed previously in Western populations.
- Successful **weight reduction is related to the improvement of diastolic function** and exercise tolerance in severe obesity which was documented by Fenk et al. in 188 obese subjects with mean BMI 40.2 ± 8.6 kg/m^2. After 1-year weight reduction program with success defined as 8% of weight loss, improvement of ≥2 conventional parameters of diastolic function (e′, e′/a′, E/A, E/e′, atrial reversal duration of pulmonary flow) was observed in 30% of patients and median 6- min walk distance prolongation reached 65 m [26].

Systolic Function

- Crendal et al. reported **left ventricular hypertrophy, diastolic dysfunction** and **attenuated longitudinal strain and strain rate** in group of 92 patients with metabolic syndrome in age from 50 to 70 years. **The severity of reduction in longitudinal deformation correlated with the increased number of risk factors composing metabolic syndrome and abdominal obesity**, TNF-α, HbA1C levels and systolic dyssynchrony explained 48% of strain impairment. Other parameters of left ventricular systolic function: ejection fraction, maximal systolic velocity of mitral annulus, circumferential strain and twist remained in that study preserved [27].

- **Reduction of global left ventricular longitudinal strain, preserved radial strain and decreased of some segmental values of circumferential strain** were observed in group of normotensive obese children and adolescents by Binnetoglu et al. [28].
- Wang et al. **reported preclinical diastolic and systolic left ventricular dysfunction** (expressed as lower longitudinal strain and greater dyssynchrony) in obese subjects regardless the coexistence of metabolic syndrome, although in patients with other features of metabolic syndrome **diastolic dysfunction, left atrial enlargement and left ventricular hypertrophy** were more pronounced [29].
- In small group of patients with morbid obesity (mean BMI 44 ± 9 kg/m^2) and type 2 diabetes mellitus bariatric surgery providing mean weight loss of 28 ± 16 kg caused also **improvement of global longitudinal strain** from significantly depressed to normal values (−13.2 ± 3.7% at baseline and −19.7 ± 2.2% after achieving mean BMI 35 ± 6 kg/m^2) [30].
- Resting global longitudinal strain may be near normal **in patients with less severe obesity or only overweight** with diabetes. The detection of preclinical dysfunction may require detailed analysis with stress echocardiography especially during recovery phase [31]. Karimian and al. **did not report on significant impairment of left ventricular longitudinal systolic strain nor radial strain in severely obese patients nor register any impact of weight loss achieved with 12 weeks on low-caloric diet** causing decrease of mean BMI in studied group from 38.6 ± 6.2 to 31.5 ± 5.3 kg/m^2 on left ventricular systolic function. Left atrial and ventricular dimensions were unchanged in that study, despite reduction in blood pressure and heart rate. **Nevertheless these negative results may be related to small number of examined subjects** [32].
- Vitarelli and al. applied the widened spectrum of deformation analysis in their study including 80 children and adolescents with hypercholesterolemia (40 obese) in age from 6 to 18 years [33]. **Left ventricular global longitudinal strain and global area strain** (the combination of longitudinal and circumferential strain vectors) were lower in dyslipidemic children and further reduced in obese patients. Described left ventricular deformation parameters correlated with LDL cholesterol levels and body mass index.
- Interestingly, **the influence of obesity on LV systolic myocardial function which may be detected with 2D speckle tracking method was reported even in the field of prenatal echocardiography**. In fetuses of mothers with obesity examined in 25 week of gestation age a significant reduction of left ventricular global longitudinal strain (−21.1 ± 7.5% vs. −27 ± 5.2%) and averaged circumferential strain rate (−1.3 [−1.8 ÷ 1.1] s^{-1} vs. −1.6 [−2.1 ÷ −1.3] s^{-1}) was reported in comparison to control group [34]. Remarkable, the average values of above mentioned parameters were close to those measured in fetuses of mothers with diabetes mellitus.

Key Points for LV/LA Structure and Function in Obesity

1. **Left ventricular hypertrophy and enlargement**, with positive correlation of LV mass-to-volume ratio with body mass index and waist circumference which indicates on concentric type of remodeling in more severe obesity
2. **Left atrial dilatation** related to volume overload was observed both in adults and children [35]
3. **Left ventricular diastolic dysfunction** which correlates with duration of obesity and diminishes after successful weight reduction, presenting as reduced early diastolic mitral annular velocities and mitral inflow E/A ratio
4. Left ventricular ejection fraction is usually preserved and may decrease as a late sign in morbid obesity but along with the wide implementation of the deformation analysis **the evidence of subtle, subclinical impairment of systolic myocardial function related to obesity is growing**.
5. The most prevalent changes in myocardial deformation parameters include **impairment of longitudinal systolic strain and systolic and diastolic strain rate** with stepwise deterioration related to the number of coexisting metabolic risk factors, equivocal and limited data concerning circumferential strain and usually preserved radial left ventricular function and rotation parameters

The Impact of Obesity on Conventional and Deformation Parameters of Right Ventricle (RV)

Pathomechanisms and Structural Remodeling of RV

- In comparison to LV mass and function data concerning the influence of obesity on RV are less numerous. On the right side of the heart there is also an **increase of pulmonary vascular resistance and filling pressure** which may be related to sleep apnea/hypoventilation syndrome, recurrent thromboembolism or left ventricular dysfunction.
- Tadic M et al. [36] observed **higher RV volume indexes based on three-dimensional echocardiography in obese patients with uncontrolled hypertension** in comparison with normal-weight subjects. **RV remodeling**

detected with advanced echocardiographic techniques correlated with blood pressure variability in 127 hypertensive patients and was significantly affected by obesity.

- The greater **RV free wall thickness and chamber volumes** were documented in the study of Wong et al. although RV ejection fraction did not differ between obese and normal-weight subjects [37]. Increased **RV end-diastolic volume and mass** was confirmed also with cardiac MRI in MESA-right ventricle study [38]. Moreover, RV mass increase correlated with BMI growth and exceeded the increase in RV end-diastolic volume.
- In the study of Rider et al. [39] in group of 739 normotensive, normoglycaemic and normocholesterolaemic subjects examined with MRI **moderately strong positive correlation was observed between BMI and RV mass** with 0.8 g increase in RV mass in men and 1.0 g in women for each additional BMI point. Moreover, some sex-specific differences were detected **with concentric remodeling of RV in men** and **mixed pattern of eccentric and concentric remodeling in women** (with correlation between BMI and RV end-diastolic volume observed only in women). Furthermore, typical for obesity LV diastolic dysfunction was associated with the concentric RV remodeling.
- In the study of Sokmen et al. [40] obese patients presented **enlarged diameters of right atrium (RA), RV and RV wall thickness** as well as **decreased tricuspid E/A ratio** in transtoracic echocardiography.

RV Function in Obesity: Classical and Deformation Parameters

- In patient with mild obesity in above cited study **tissue Doppler parameters of RV function** (e′/a′, isovolumetric relaxation time and myocardial performance index) were impaired in comparison to controls and observed changes deepened in the subgroup with a BMI ≥35 kg/m^2. **In severely obese group also systolic velocity of tricuspid annulus motion was decreased.**
- In our study young, severely obese patients (mean age 37 ± 9, BMI 46 ± 6 kg/m^2) had similar LV ejection fraction and TAPSE as the controls **but the systolic and early diastolic velocities measured with pulsed tissue Doppler as well as left ventricular circumferential and radial strain were significantly lower in obese subjects indicating on early functional impairment of both ventricles** [41]. Figure 45.2 presents the typical constellation of echocardiographic findings in obese patient.
- On the other hand, Zeller J and al. compared the parameters of both left and right ventricular (LV/RV) function between 153 obese subjects with average BMI 41.2 ± 8.7 kg/m^2 and 38 controls matched according to sex and age with average BMI 25.5 ± 3.3 kg/m^2 at baseline and after 1 year of weight reduction program [42]. Obese patients presented with significantly diminished LV systolic and diastolic function (lower ejection fraction 66 ± 6% vs. 69 ± 6%, p = 0.004 and higher E/E′ 7.4 ± 2.5 vs. 6.3 ± 2.6, p = 0.01) but **the parameters of RV function and geometry (TAPSE, systolic velocity of tricuspid annulus- RV S′ and Tei index for RV) did not differ between compared groups.** Similarly, weight reduction did not influence in this study the RV function.
- In the cited study of Vitarelli et al. [33] **obese subjects in comparison with control group displayed reduced global and free-wall right ventricular strain.**
- According to data from Utah obesity study (Owan et al., [19]) bariatric surgery and **successful weight reduction resulted in decrease of RV chamber area and increase of RV fractional area changing.**

Key Points for RV/RA Structure and Function in Obesity

1. **The right ventricular hypertrophy (in both sexes) and enlargement (better documented in women**, with positive correlation of RV mass with body mass index
2. **The right atrial dilatation** related to volume overload
3. **Right ventricular diastolic dysfunction** presenting as reduced early diastolic tricuspid annular velocities and E/A ratio of tricuspid inflow
4. **Subclinical right ventricular systolic dysfunction** which may be revealed mainly with tissue Doppler or strain imaging

Epicardial Adipose Tissue: Clinical Significance

- Additional diagnostic challenge in obese patients is related to the differentiation between **epicardial fat** (also known as subepicardial [43], located between the outer wall of the myocardium and the visceral layer of pericardium and sharing the same microcirculation with myocardium) and **pericardial fat** (located anteriorly to epicardial fat and parietal pericardium; named also as subxiphoid in radiology). Both layers are histologically different and only epicardial layer is predictive of metabolic syndrome, visceral adiposity and insuline resistance [44]. On the other hand both described adipose layers are sometimes named "pericardial fat" in opposition to intramyocardial fat and in such conceptualization they are correlated with diminution of left ventricular systolic function e.g. decrease in stroke volume and cardiac index in healthy subjects (mean age 29 ± 10 years., mean BMI 23 ± 3 kg/m^2) [45].

- **Epicardial adipose tissue (EAT) is a part of visceral fat** which occupies particularly atrioventricular and interventricular grooves, environs coronary arteries and antecedes right ventricle free wall [46]. **EAT similarly to intraabdominal mass originates from brown fat tissue during embryogenesis, has endocrine and inflammatory activities** (produces cytokines: IL-1, IL-6, IL-16, soluble IL-6 receptor, TNF α, angiotensinogen, leptin, resistin and visfatin) and its thickness correlates with waist circumference [30].
- Since thickness of EAT is the highest in the anterior aspect of the right ventricular wall and ultrasound beam is directed perpendicularly allowing better axial resolution during measurements **the proposed reference areas of EAT measurement encompass parasternal long and short axis windows** [47].
- **EAT presents as echo-lucent area** (see space signed by d letter in Fig. 45.3) **above the right ventricular outer wall surface** (signed as b) **and below visceral layer of pericardium** (a in Fig. 45.3 indicating adherent visceral and parietal layers of pericardium) and **should be measured at the thickest level**. Averaging of measurements from minimum three cycles encompassing both long and short axis views is recommended and evaluation during diastole reassures consistency with standard CT and MRI assessment. As far as timing of measurement is concerned it should be remember that the EAT thickness is greater during systole than diastole [48].

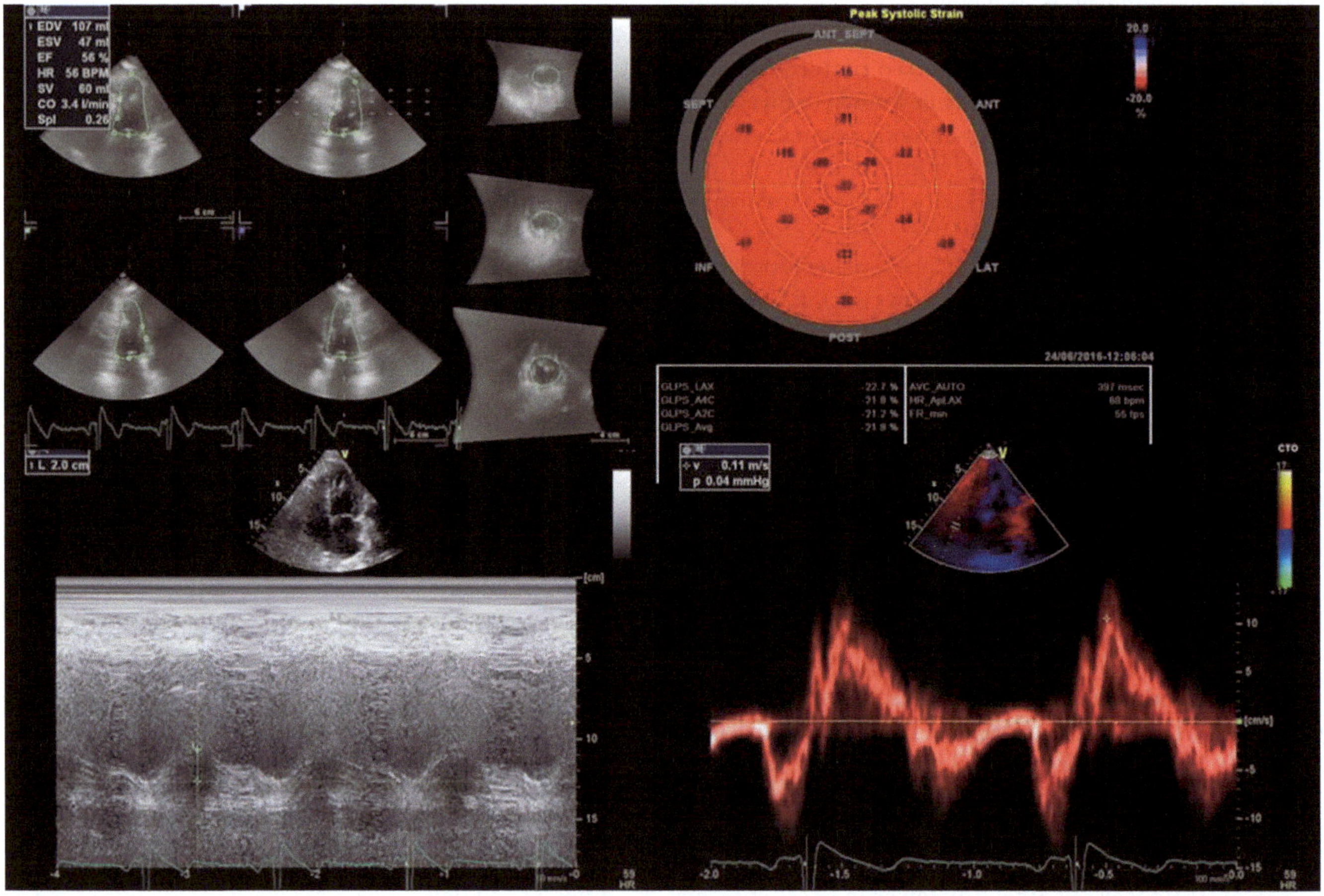

Fig. 45.2 *Upper panel*: preserved systolic function of left and right ventricle in female patients with BMI 34 kg/m^2. Left ventricular ejection fraction 56%, global longitudinal strain 21.9%, TAPSE 20 mm, S′ of tricuspid annulus 11 cm/s. *BMI* body mass index, *TAPSE* tricuspid annular plane systolic excursion, *S′* maximal systolic velocity of tricuspid annulus motion. *Middle panel*: enlarged left atrium (LA) expressed as increased LA a-p diameter in long axis view 54 mm and LA volume in apical four-chamber view 71 mL. *a-p* antero-posterior. *Lower panel*: Tissue Doppler and mitral inflow analysis of an obese patient showing decreased maximal early diastolic velocity e′ measured in septal and lateral part of mitral annulus: 6 cm/s and 7 cm/s, respectively. Delayed relaxation mitral profile with E/A ratio < 1 (I stadium of diastolic dysfunction), prolonged mitral inflow early wave deceleration time of 254 ms and lowered early inflow propagation velocity of 32 cm/s (slope measurement indicated with arrows) are also displayed

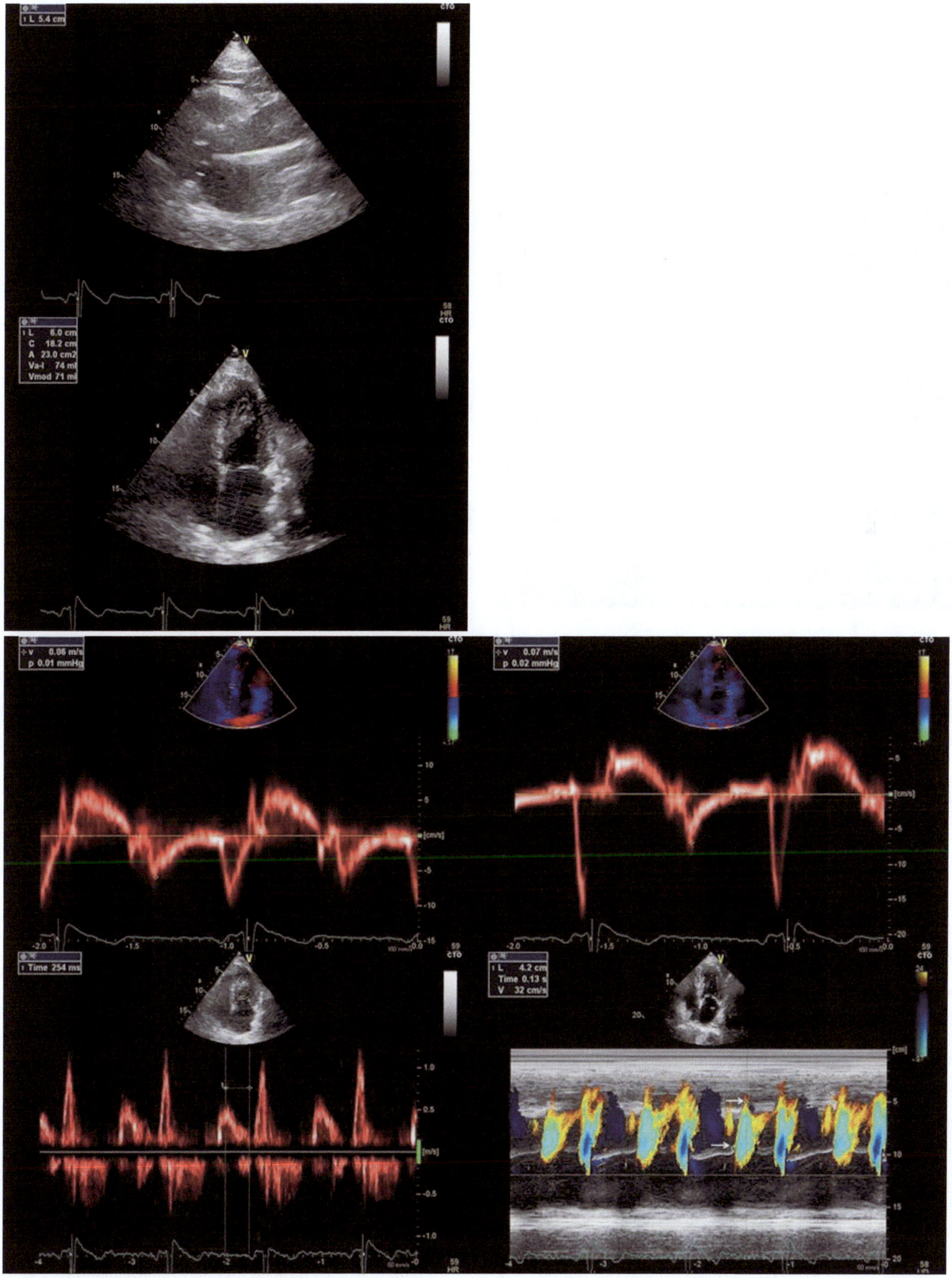

Fig. 45.2 (continued)

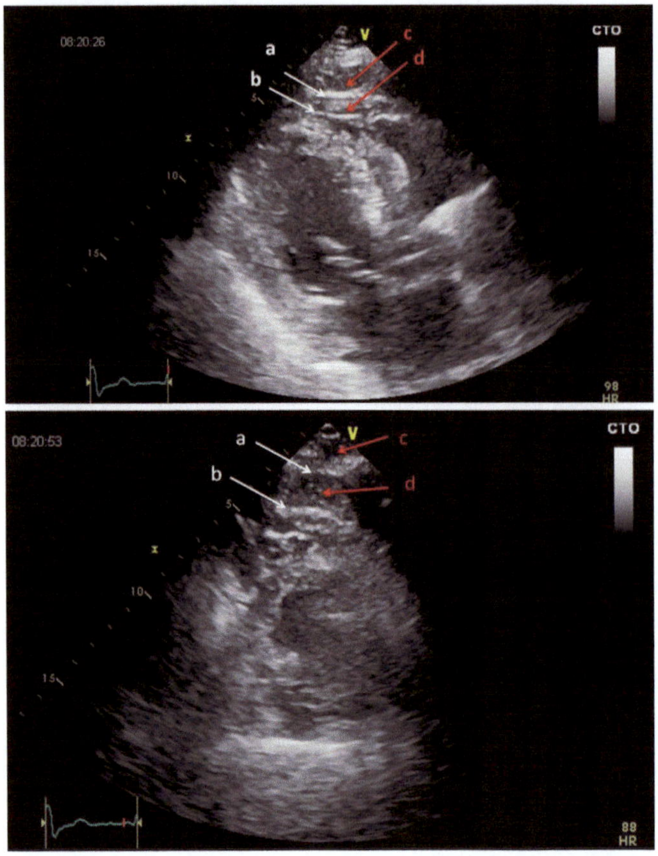

Fig. 45.3 Anatomic relations between pericardial layers and epicardial and pericardial adipose tissue in transthoracic echocardiography. *Upper panel*: Parasternal long axis view; *Lower panel*: Parasternal short axis view; (**a**) adherent parietal and visceral layers of pericardium before the right ventricle in the settings of the physiological amount of fluid in pericardial sac, (**b**) outer surface of right ventricular wall, (**c**) pericardial adipose tissue (PAT), d-epicardial adipose tissue (EAT)

- Contrarily, **pericardial adipose tissue (PAT) does not change its thickness during heart cycle**, has different embryonic origin and biomolecular features and should be differentiated from EAT (see hypoechoic area signed by c letter in Fig. 45.3). To the evident limitations of echocardiographic EAT measurement belong partial character and lower reproducibility in comparison with CT or MRI measurements.
- The thickness of epicardial fat layer seems to correlate rather with the amount of visceral fat than with anthropometric measurements and was postulated as the marker of metabolic risk. Moreover, the positive correlation with the insuline resistance, hypertension and presence and severity of coronary artery disease has been recently documented [49–52]. Erkan et al. documented strong **correlation of EAT thickness with Gensini and Syntax score** ($r = 0.82$, $p < 0.001$ and $r = 0{,}825$, $p < 0.001$ respectively). The authors divided studied group of 183 patients according to coronary artery lesions advancement into normal, noncritical disease (≥1 coronary lesion with <70% stenosis) and critical disease (≥1 coronary lesion with ≥70% stenosis). The cutoff thickness value for EAT to predict critical disease was established as >5.75 mm [53].
- In turn in the recently published study of Kocaman et al. **EAT thickness correlated significantly with intima-media thickness (IMT) of carotid arteries** ($r = 0.623$, $p < 0.001$) being independent predictor for both IMT and presence of carotid plaque [54]. In patients >65 years correlation between amount of epicardial adipose tissue located mainly in arterial grooves of coronaries and mitral **annular calcifications and aortic valve calcifications** were recently documented and in MRI based study of Homsi R et al. epicardial fat volume correlated significantly with **aortic stiffness** expressed as aortic pulse wave velocity [55, 56]. In addition to morphologic lesions increased epicardial fat volume >149 cm^3 assessed with computed tomography was found as a predictor for ergonovine-induced **coronary artery spasm** [57].

Key Points: Epicardial Adipose Tissue as Novel Risk Marker

1. EAT located between visceral pericardium and myocardium shares microcirculation with the heart muscle, produces numerous proinflammatory mediators, correlates positively with age, diabetes and hypertension and may promote progression of atherosclerosis especially in coronary arteries.
2. According to literature review **threshold for EAT thickness having prognostic significance for cardiac abnormalities and indicating on clinically significant atherosclerosis advancement oscillates around 5 mm.** Higher values were proposed as criteria for increased amount of epicardial fat which may be considered as novel cardiometabolic risk factor that predict the presence of complex and critical coronary artery disease [58].

Conclusions

- Transthoracic echocardiographic examination of obese subjects imposes specific challenges on echocardiographer but with contemporary echo tools, contrast and novel techniques in the majority of cases provides sufficient information.
- Typical remodeling related with obesity involves concentric myocardial hypertrophy of both ventricles walls, left atrial dilatation and diastolic dysfunction of left ventricle whereas the detection of right ventricular dysfunction and impairment of systolic function of both ventricles requires usually novel techniques with volumetric assessment and deformation analysis.

- Epicardial adipose tissue, often prominent in obese patients, may be measured in transthoracic echocardiography and represents a novel prognostic cardiovascular marker.

Questions

1. To the proposed factors involved in heart remodeling in obesity belong:
   A. volume overload related mainly to central fat accumulation
   B. proinflammatory state
   C. left ventricular diastolic dysfunction and increase of pulmonary pressure
   D. all above mentioned

2. Indicate the answer which do not present changes typical for isolated obesity:
   A. left ventricular hypertrophy
   B. visually assessed regional contractility i mpairment
   C. left atrial dilatation
   D. diastolic dysfunction

3. 45 year-old male patient with BMI 39 kg/m^2 with a such constellation of parameters: LVMI 150 g/m^2; EF 60%, E/A 0.4; E = 48 cm/s, e′ in septal part of mitral annulus = 6 cm/s and global longitudinal strain of LV, GLS = −16% presents:
   A. myocardial hypertrophy; I stadium of diastolic dysfunction, completely normal LV systolic function
   B. normal mass index of LV, II stadium of diastolic dysfunction, normal longitudinal deformation
   C. myocardial hypertrophy, I stadium of diastolic dysfunction, preserved LV ejection fraction
   D. myocardial hypertrophy, normal diastolic function, subclinical systolic dysfunction of LV

4. To the sex-specific differences of the obesity impact on right ventricle belongs:
   A. the lack of right ventricular hypertrophy in women
   B. the faster progression of RV dilatation in men
   C. higher increment of RV mass on each point of BMI progression in women
   D. exclusively eccentric RV hypertrophy in men

5. Which answer displays correct description of EAT:
   A. accumulation of fat in the region of fossa ovalis
   B. located subepicardially metabolically active adipose tissue
   C. located subepicardially metabolically inactive fat tissue
   D. located on the outer surface of pericardium brown fat tissue

Answers

1. D
   All mentioned factors may play the role in the pathomechanism of heart remodeling in obesity. Volume overload are related more with central adipose tissue than peripheral fat accumulation because of greater blood flow through metabolically active central fat. Proinflammatory state are connected with cytokines excretion from adipose tissue including but not limited to EAT activity. Correlation between LV diastolic dysfunction and RV hypertrophy in obese subjects was documented in the literature and illustrates some aspect of ventricular interdependence mediated with pulmonary artery hypertension reliant on LV diastolic dysfunction.
2. B
   Visually assessed regional contractility impairments as well as lowering of LV EF are not typical for isolated obesity but, when present, are usually related to ischemic heart disease.
3. C
   Presented obese patient had myocardial hypertrophy (defined for males as LVMI >115 g/m^2 and for females as LVMI > 95 g/m^2 in case of linear measurements and >102 g/m^2 for males and >88 g/m^2 for females in case of 2D measurement [59]), I stadium of diastolic dysfunction (since the delayed relaxation profile with E/A $\leq$ 0.8 with E $\leq$ 50 cm/s, and e′ in septal part of mitral annulus <7 cm/s according to recent ASE/EACVI guidelines for diastolic dysfunction- Nagueh SF et al. [60]) and normal LV EF (52–72% indicating normal range for males and 54–74% for females).
4. C
   According to recent study of Rider et al. [39] based on large group of subjects with wide range of BMI (15.3–59.2 kg/m^2) women revealed higher increase of RV mass per each point of BMI increase (+1.0 g vs. +0.8 g in men) and only women exhibited RV cavity dilatation (+ 1.0 mL of RV end-diastolic volume per BMI point increase) in MRI-based assessment.
5. B
   EAT is located subepicardially and metabolically active adipose tissue.

References

1. Flegal KM, Carrol MD, Ogden CL, Johnson CL. Prevalence and trends in obesity among US adults, 1999-2000. JAMA. 2002;288:1723–7.
2. Ku CS, Lin SL, Wang DJ, Chang SK, Lee WJ. Left ventricular filling in young normotensive obese adults. Am J Cardiol. 1994;73:613–5.
3. Kenchaiah S, Evans JC, Levy D, et al. Obesity and the risk of heart failure. N Engl J Med. 2002;347:305–13.

4. Selthofer-Relatic K, Bosnjak I, Kibel A. Obesity related coronary microvascular dysfunction: from basic to clinical practice. Cardiol Res Pract. 2016;2016:7. https://doi.org/10.1155/2016/8173816.
5. Bagi Z, Broskova Z, Feher A. Obesity and coronary microvascular disease- implications for adipose tissue-mediated remote inflammatory response. Curr Vasc Pharmacol. 2014;12:453–61.
6. Brown CD, Higgins M, Donato KA, et al. Body mass index and the prevalence of hypertension and dyslipidemia. Obes Res. 2000;8:605–19.
7. Kannel WB, Plehn JF, Cupples LA. Cardiac failure and sudden cardiac death in the Framingham study. Am Heart J. 1988;115:869–75.
8. Esposito K, Nicolletti G, Marzano S, et al. Autonomic dysfunction associates with prolongation of QT interval and blunted night BP in obese women with visceral obesity. J Endocrinol Investig. 2002;25:RC32–5.
9. Siadecki SD, Frasure SE, Lewiss RE, Saul T. High body mass index is strongly correlated with decreased image quality in focused bedside echocardiography. J Emerg Med. 2016;50:295–301.
10. Bhat G, Daley K, Dugan M, Larson G. Preoperative evaluation for bariatric surgery using transesophageal dobutamine stress echocardiography. Obes Surg. 2004;14:948–51.
11. Shah BN, Zacharias K, Pabla JS, Karogiannis N, Calicchio F, et al. The clinical impact of contemporary stress echocardiography in morbid obesity for the assessment of coronary artery disease. Heart. 2016;102(5):370.
12. Lerakis S, Kalogeropoulos AP, El-Chami MF, Georgiopoulou VV, Abraham A, et al. Transthoracic dobutamine stress echocardiography in patients undergoing bariatric surgery. Obes Surg. 2007;17:1475–81.
13. Olsen RH, Pedersen LR, Snoer M, Christensen TE, Ghotbi AA, et al. Coronary flow velocity reserve by echocardiography: feasibility, reproducikility and agreement with PET in overweight and obese patients with stable and revascularized coronary artery disease. Cardiovasc Ultrasound. 2016;14:22.
14. Laura DM, Donnino R, Kim EE, Benenstein R, Freedberg RS, Saric M. Lipomatous atrial septal hypertrophy: a review of its anatomy, pathophysiology, multimodality imaging, and relevance to percutaneous interventions. J Am Soc Echocardiogr. 2016;29:717–23.
15. Zhou YT, Grayburn P, Karim A, et al. Lipotoxic heart disease in obese rats: implications for human obesity. Proc Natl Acad Sci U S A. 2000;97:1784–9.
16. Kaltman AJ, Goldring RM. Role of circulatory congestion in the cardiorespiratory failure of obesity. Am J Med. 1976;60:645–53.
17. Mathew B, Francis L, Kayalar A, Cone J. Obesity: effects on cardiovascular disease and its diagnosis. J Am Board Fam Med. 2008;21:562–8.
18. Friberg P, Allandsdotter JA, Ambring A, et al. Increased left ventricular mass in obese adolescens. Eur Heart J. 2004;25:987–92.
19. Owan T, Avelar E, Morley K, Jiji R, Hall N, Krezowski J, et al. Favorable changes in cardiac geometry and function following gastric bypass surgery: 2-year follow-up in the Utah obesity study. J Am Coll Cardiol. 2011;57:732–9.
20. Movahed MR, Saito Y. Lack of association between obesity and left ventricular systolic function. Echocardiography. 2009;26:128–32.
21. Turkbey E, McClelland RL, Kronmall RA, et al. The impact of obesity on the left ventricle. The Multi-Ethnic Study of Atherosclerosis (MESA). JACC Cardiovasc Imaging. 2010;3:266–74.
22. Di Bello V, Santini F, DiCori A, et al. Obesity cardiomyopathy: Is it a reality ? An ultrasonic tissue characterization study. J Am Soc Echocardiogr. 2008;21:151–6.
23. Aurigemma GP, de Simone G, Fitzgibbons TP. Cardiac remodeling in obesity. Circ Cardiovasc Imaging. 2013;6:142–52.
24. Russo C, Jin Z, Homma S, Rundek T, Elkind MS, Sacco RL, di Tullio MR. Effect of obesity and overweight on left ventricular diastolic function: a community-based study in an elderly cohort. J Am Coll Cardiol. 2011;57:1368–74.
25. Lee SL, Daimon M, DiTullio MR, Homma S, Nakao T, et al. Relationship of left ventricular diastolic function to obesity and overweight in a Japanese population with preserved left ventricular ejection fraction. Circ J. 2016;80:1951–6.
26. Fenk S, Fischer M, Strack C, Schmitz G, Loew T, Lahmann C, Baessler A. Successful weight reduction improves left ventricular diastolic function and physical performance in severe obesity. Int Heart J. 2015;56:196–202.
27. Crendal E, Walther G, Vinet A, Dutheil F, Naughton G, Lesourd B, Chapier R, Rupp T, Courteix D, Obert P. Myocardial deformation and twist mechanics in adults with metabolic syndrome: impact of cumulative metabolic burden. Obesity. 2013;21:E679–86.
28. Binnetoglu FK, Yildrim S, Topaloglu N, Tekin M, Kaymaz N, Aylanc H, Karakurt H. Early detection of myocardial deformation by 2D speckle tracking echocardiography in normotensive obese children and adolescents. Anatol J Cardiol. 2015;15:151–7.
29. Wang YC, Liang CS, Gopal DM, et al. Preclinical systolic and diastolic dysfunction in metabolically healthy and unhealthy obese individuals. Circ Heart Fail. 2015;8:897–904.
30. Leung M, Xie M, Durmush E, Leung DY, Wong VW. Weight loss with sleeve gastrectomy in obese type 2 diabetes mellitus: impact on cardiac function. Obes Surg. 2016;26:321–6.
31. Wierzbowska-Drabik K, Hamala P, Kasprzak JD. Delayed longitudinal myocardial function recovery after dobutamine challenge as a novel presentation of myocardial dysfunction in type 2 diabetic patients without angiographic coronary artery disease. Eur Heart J Cardiovasc Imaging. 2015;16:676–83.
32. Karimian S, Stein J, Bauer B, Teupe C. Impact of severe obesity and weight loss on systolic left ventricular function and morphology: assessment by 2-dimensional speckle tracking echocardiography. J Obes. 2016;2016:6. https://doi.org/10.1155/2016/2732613.
33. Vitarelli A, Martino F, Capotosto L, Martino E, Colantoni C, et al. Early myocardial deformation changes in hypercholesterolemic and obese children and adolescents. Medicine. 2014;93:e71.
34. Kulkarni A, Li L, Craft M, Nanda M, Lorenzo JM, et al. Fetal myocardial deformation in maternal diabetes mellitus and obesity. Ultrasound Obstet Gynecol. 2016;49(5):630–6. https://doi.org/10.1002/uog.15971.
35. Azza MA, Ragab SH, Ismail NA, Awad MAM, Kandil ME. Echocardiographic assessment of epicardial adipose tissue in obese children and its relation to clinical parameters of the metabolic syndrome. J Clin Basic Cardiol. 2011;14:7–11.
36. Tadic M, Cuspidi C, Vukomanovic V, Kocijanic V, Celic V, Stanisavlievic D. The association between obesity, blood pressure variability and right ventricular function and mechanics in hypertensive patients. J Am Soc Echocardiogr. 2016;29(8):802–11. https://doi.org/10.1016/j.echo.2016.04.001.
37. Wong CY, O'Moore-Sullivan T, Leano R, Hukins C, Jenkins C, Marwick TH. Association of subclinical right ventricular dysfunction with obesity. J Am Coll Cardiol. 2006;47:611–6.
38. Chahal H, McClelland RL, Tandri H, Jain A, Turkbey EB, Hundley WG, et al. Obesity and right ventricular structure and functions: the MESA-right ventricle study. Chest. 2012;141:388–95.
39. Rider OJ, Lewis AJM, Lewandowski AJ, Ntusi N, Nethononda R, et al. Obese subjects show sex-specific differences in right ventricular hypertrophy. Circ Cardiovasc Imaging. 2014;8(1):pii: e002454. https://doi.org/10.1161/CIRCIMAGING.114.002454.
40. Sokmen A, Sokmen G, Acar G, Akcay A, Koroglu S, Koleoglu M, Yalcintas S, Aydin MN. The impact of isolated obesity on right ventricular function in young adults. Arq Bras Cardiol. 2013;101:160–8.
41. Wierzbowska-Drabik K, Chrzanowski Ł, Kapusta A, Uznańska-Loch B, Płońska E, Krzemińska-Pakuła M, Kurpesa M, Rechciński T, Trzos E, Kasprzak JD. Severe obesity impairs

systolic and diastolic heart function - the significance of pulsed Doppler, strain and strain rate parameters. Echocardiography. 2013;30:904–11.
42. Zeller J, Strack C, Fenk S, Mohr M, Loew T, Schmitz G, Maier L, Fischer M, Baessler A. Relation between obesity, metabolic syndrome, successful long-term weight reduction and right ventricular function. Int Heart J. 2016;57:441–8.
43. Iacobellis G, Pellicelli AM, Sharma AM, et al. Relation of subepicardial adipose tissue to carotid intima-media thickness in patients with human immunodeficiency virus. Am J Cardiol. 2007;99:1470–2.
44. Iacobellis G. Epicardial and pericardial fat: close but very different. Obesity. 2009;17:625.
45. Wolf P, Winhofer Y, Smajis S, Jankovic D, Anderwald CH, et al. Pericardial rather than intramyocardial fat is independently associated with left ventricular systolic heart function in metabolically healthy humans. PLoS One. 2016;11:e0151301. https://doi.org/10.1371/journal.pone.0151301.
46. Bertaso AG, Bertol D, Duncan BB, Foppa M. Epicardial fat: definition, measurement and systematic review of main outcomes. Arq Bras Cardiol. 2013;101:e418–28.
47. Iacobellis G, Assael F, Ribaudo MC, Zappaterreno A, Alessi G, Di Mario U, et al. Epicardial fat from echocardiography: a new method for visceral adipose tissue prediction. Obes Res. 2003;11:304e310.
48. Iacobellis G, Willens HJ, Barbaro G, Sharma AM. Threshold values of high-risk echocardiographic epicardial fat thickness. Obesity. 2008;16:887–92.
49. Iacobellis G, Leonetti F. Epicardial adipose tissue and insuline resistance in obese subjects. J Clin Endocrinol Metab. 2005;90:6300–2.
50. Dicker D, Atar E, Kornowski R, Bachar GN. Increased epicardial adipose tissue thickness as a predictor for hypertension: a cross-sectional observational study. J Clin Hypertens (Greenwich). 2013;15:893–8.
51. Sinha SK, Thakur R, Jha MJ, Goel A, Kumar V, Kumar A, Mishra V, Varma C, Krishna V, Singh AK, Sachan M. Epicardial adipose tissue thickness and its association with the presence and severity of coronary artery disease in clinical setting: a cross-sectional observational study. J Clin Med Res. 2016;8:410–9.
52. Eroglu S. How do we measure epicardial adipose tissue thickness by transthoracic echocardiography? Anatol J Cardiol. 2015;15:416–9.
53. Erkan AF, Tanindi A, Kocaman SA, Ugurlu M, Tore HF. Epicardial adipose tissue thickness is an independent predictor of critical and complex coronary artery disease by Gensini and Syntax scores. Tex Heart Inst J. 2016;43:29–37.
54. Kocaman SA, Baysan O, Cetin M, Kayhan Altuner T, Polat Ocakli E et al. An increase in epicardial adipose tissue is strongly associated with carotid intima-media thickness and atherosclerotic plaque but LDL only with plague. Anatol J Cardiol. 2016; doi: https://doi.org/10.14744/AnatolJCardiol.2016.6885.
55. Alnabelsi TS, Alhamshari Y, Mulki RH, Codolosa JN, Koshkelashvili N, Goykhman I, Pressman GS, Romero-Corral A. Relation between epicardial adipose and aortic valve and mitral annular calcium determined by computed tomography in subjects aged ≥65 years. Am J Cardiol. 2016;118:1088–93. https://doi.org/10.1016/j.amjcard.2016.07.012.
56. Homsi R, Thomas D, Gieseke J, Meier-Schroers M, Dabir D, et al. Epicardial fat volume and aortic stiffness in healthy individuals: a quantitative cardiac magnetic resonance study. Rofo. 2016;188:853–8.
57. Ito T, Fujita H, Ichihashi T, Ohte N. Impact of epicardial adipose tissue volume quantified by non-contrast electrocardiogram-gated computed tomography on ergonovine-induced epicardial coronary artery spasm. Int J Cardiol. 2016;221:877–80.
58. Mookadam F, Goel R, Alharthi MS, Jiamsripong P, Cha S. Epicardial fat and its association with cardiovascular risk: a cross-sectional observational study. Heart Views. 2010;11:103–8.
59. Lang R, Badano LP, Mor-Avi V, Aifilalo J, Armstrong A, et al. Recommendations for cardiac chamber quantification by echocardiography in adults: an update from the American Society of Echocardiography and the European Association of Cardiovascular Imaging. J Am Soc Echocardiogr. 2015;28:1–39.
60. Nagueh SF, Smiseth OA, Appleton CP, Byrd BF, Dokainish H, et al. Recommendations for the evaluation of left ventricular diastolic function by echocardiography: an update from the American Society of Echocardiography and the European association of Cardiovascular Imaging. J Am Soc Echocardiogr. 2016;29:277–314.

Full Schematic Echocardiographic Formulas and Points

46

Azin Alizadehasl and Anita Sadeghpour

Abstract

In this chapter the echocardiography formulas are listed to provide an understanding of useful and practical, basic and advanced echocardiographic calculations and measurements. The required parameters of these formulas are included in the echocardiographic machine software, so the operator need an understanding of the principles involved these quantifications and it is necessary to be aware of the indications and limitations of their use.

Keywords

Echocardiographic Formulas · Calculation in echocardiography · Points of Echocardiography · Stroke volume · Cardiac Output · Ejection Fraction · Myocardial performance index

Abbreviations

AO	Aortic opening
AVA	Aortic valve area
AVR	Aortic valve replacement
CSA	Cross-sectional area
CW	Continuous wave
DD	Diastolic dysfunction
DF	Diastolic function
DTI	Doppler tissue imaging
ET	Ejection time
HOCM	Hypertrophic obstructive cardio myopathy
HV	Hepatic vein
IVCT	Isovolumic contraction time
IVRT	Isovolumic relaxation time

A. Alizadehasl, MD, FACC, FASE (✉)
Associate Professor of Cardiology, Echocardiologist, Echocardiography and Cardiogenetic Research Centers, Cardio-Oncology Department, Rajaie Cardiovascular Medical and Research Center, Tehran, Iran

A. Sadeghpour, MD, FACC, FASE
Professor of Cardiology, Echocardiography Research Center, Rajaie Cardiovascular Medical and Research Center, Iran University of Medical Science, Tehran, Iran

This Chapter is a collection of educative figures with gathering of echocardiographic formulas with courtesy to all of references' authors.

A. Sadeghpour, A. Alizadehasl (eds.), *Case-Based Textbook of Echocardiography*,
https://doi.org/10.1007/978-3-319-67691-3_46

LA	Left atrium	RAP	RA pressure
LPA	Left atrial pressure	RUPV	Right upper pulmonary vein
LVOT	Left ventricular outflow tract	RVFAC	Right ventricular fractional area change
LVOT VTI	LVOT Sub-valvular velocity time integral	RVOT	Right ventricular outflow tract diameter
MR	Mitral regurgitation	RVOT VTI	RVOT Sub-valvular velocity time integral
MV	Mitral valve	RVSP	Right ventricular systolic pressure
MVA	Mitral valve area	RWT	Relative wall thickness
PHT	Pressure half-time	SPAP	Systolic pulmonary artery pressure
PISA	Proximal isovelocity surface area	TCO	Tricuspid valve opening time
PW	Pulsed wave	Vp	Propagation velocity

Variable	Definition
LVEDD	**Left ventricular end-diastolic dimension (mm)**
LVESD	**Left ventricular end-systolic dimension (mm)**
FS	**Fractional Shortening (%)**
Normal	**>25% (M-Mode)**
	>18% (Direct 2-D measurement)

Fig. 46.1 **Left ventricular fractional shortening** $FS = \frac{LVEDD - LVESD}{LVEDD}$ **100%.** Percent change in Left Ventricular Cavity dimension at the base with systolic contraction. Limited by significant apical wall motion abnormalities

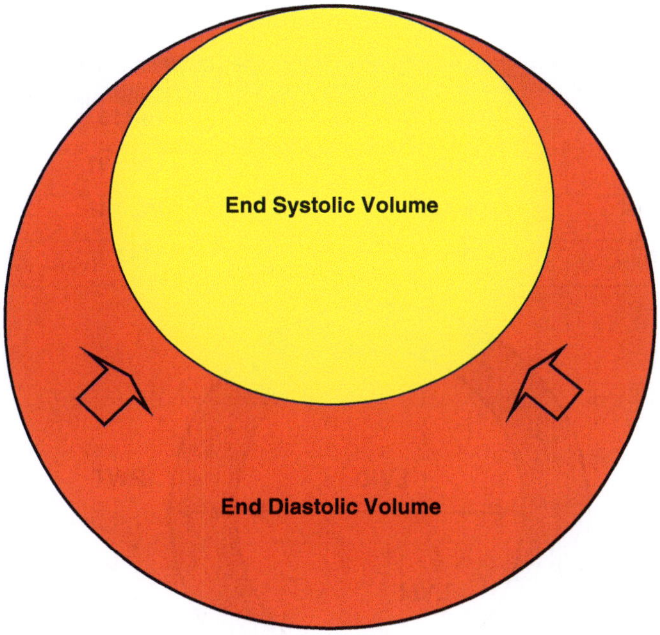

Fig. 46.2 Left ventricular ejection fraction. In normal subjects, the LV ejects more than half of its end-diastolic volume

$$LVEF = \frac{STROKE\ VOLUME = END\ DIASTOLIC\ VOLUME - END\ SYSTOLIC\ VOLUME}{END\ DIASTOLIC\ VOLUME}$$

Variable	Definition
Input	LV end-diastolic dimension (mm)
LVEDD	Correct for apical contraction
K	+10 % Normal apex 5 % Hypokinetic apex 0 % Akinetic apex -5 % Dyskinetic apex -10 % Apical aneurysm
Output	
LVEF	Ejection Fraction (%)
Normal	>55-60 %

Fig. 46.3 Left Ventricular Ejection Fraction (Simplified Quinones Equation). An even simpler adaptation uses the normally measured end-diastolic and end-systolic diameters of the Left Ventricular in the parasternal long axis view, with a correction of the apex as follows: (*LV* left ventricular)

$$LVEF = \frac{LVEDD^2 - LVESD^2}{LVEDD^2}\ 100\% + k$$

a

	Female	Male
Reference Range (g)	43-95	49-115
Mildly Abnormal	96-108	116-131
Moderately Abnormal	109-121	132-148
Severely Abnormal	≥122	≥149

b

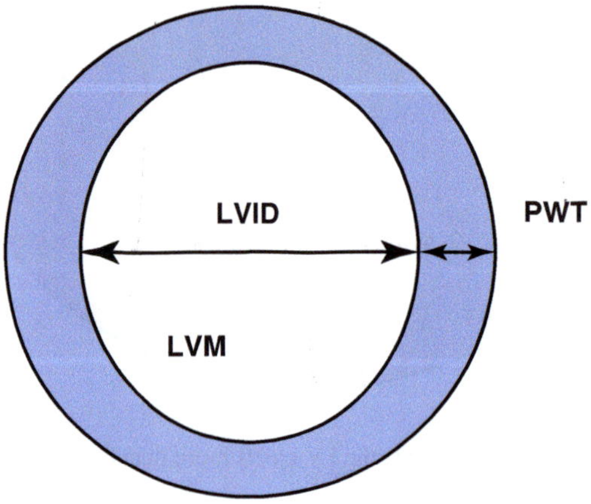

c

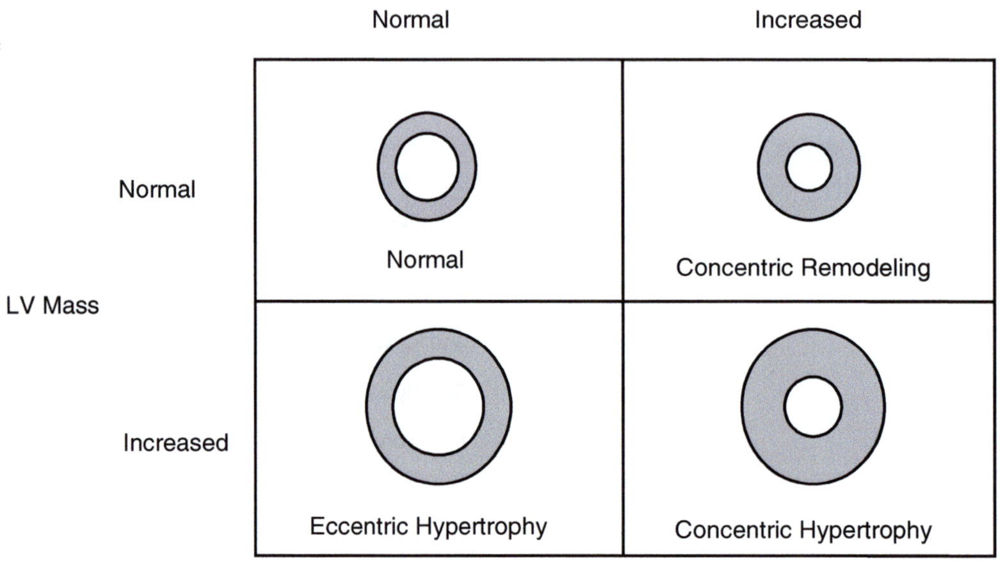

Fig. 46.4 (**a**) **Reference Ranges and Partition Values for Left Ventricular Mass Indexed To BSA (g/m²).** (**b**) **Left Ventricular Mass and Left Ventricular Mass Index:** Left ventricular mass and left ventricular mass indexed to body surface area estimated by Left Ventricular cavity dimension and wall thickness at end-diastole. Relative wall thickness (RWT) allows further classification of Left Ventricular mass increase as either concentric hypertrophy (RWT > 0.42) or eccentric hypertrophy (RWT ≤ 0.42). $\boldsymbol{LVMass\ (g)} = 0.8\ \{1.04[([LVEDD + IVSd + PWd]^3 - LVEDD^3)]\} + \mathbf{0.6}$. $\boldsymbol{RWT\left(Relative\ Wall\ Thickness\right) = \frac{2\ \ PWd}{LVEDD}}$. (**c**) Showing concentric and eccentric hypertrophy with normal and increased Left Ventricular Mass. Modified image from cardioserv.net; Inspiring excellence in imaging

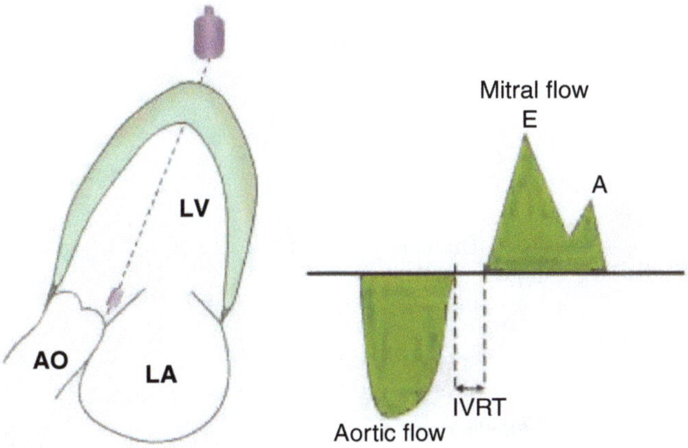

Fig. 46.5 Isovolumic relaxation time (IVRT): is an interval in the cardiac cycle, from the aortic component of the second heart sound, that is, closure of the aortic valve, to onset of filling by opening of the mitral valve. It can be used as indicator of diastolic dysfunction. It can be measured by simultaneous Doppler echocardiography, M-mode or tissue Doppler Imaging. Prolonged IVRT indicates poor and impaired myocardial relaxation. A normal IVRT is about 70 ± 12 ms, and approximately 10 ms longer in people over forty years. Modified image; Courtesy of Solomon SD. Echocardiographic instrumentation and principles of Doppler echocardiography. Essential echocardiography. Totowa, NJ: Humana Press; 2007 [13]

Variable	Definition
MR Vmax	Maximum mitral regurgitation velocity (m/sec)
SBP	Systolic Blood Pressure (mmHg)
LAP	Left Atrial Pressure (mmHg)

Fig. 46.6 **LAP estimation by mitral regurgitation jet and** Left atrial pressure (LPA) can be estimated by measuring the systolic blood pressure and the maximum mitral regurgitation velocity by spectral Doppler provided that there is no significant gradient across the aortic valve. $LAP = SBP - 4(MR\ Vmax)^2$ and $LVEDP = DBP - (AREDV)^2 \times 4$. *AREDV* Aortic Regurgitation End Diastolic Velocity

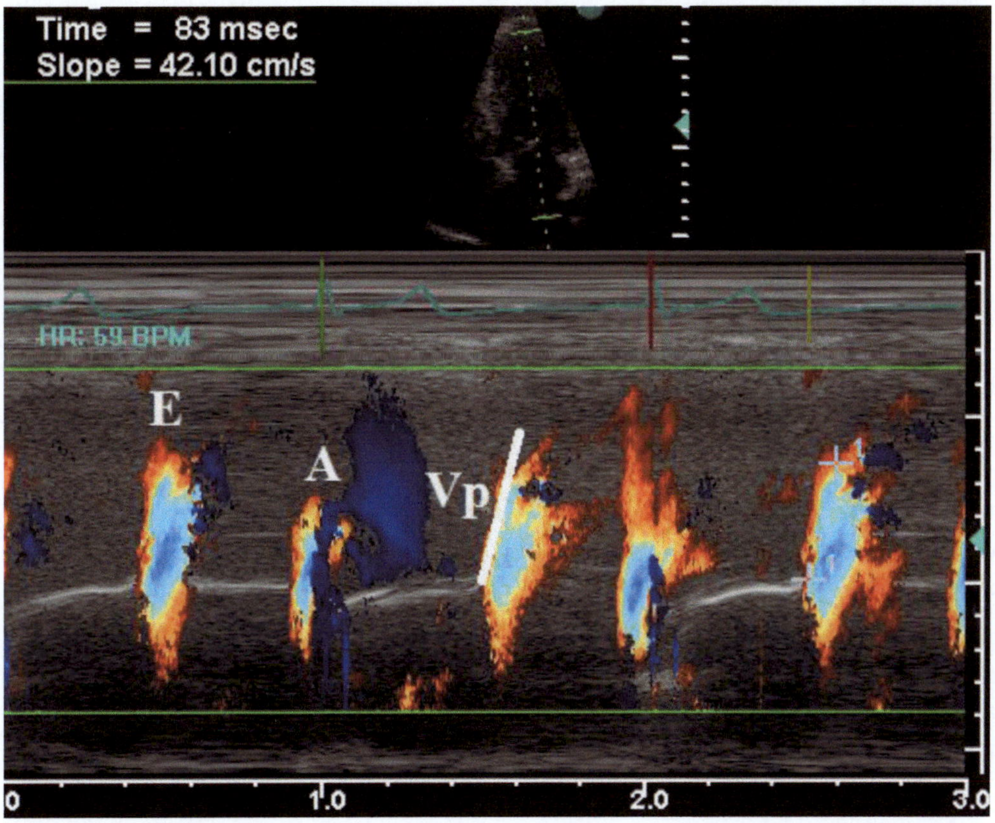

Fig. 46.7 Flow propagation velocity (Vp). Color M-mode Vp from a patient with depressed EF and impaired Left Ventricular relaxation. The slope was 42 cm/s. Value greater than 50 cm/s is considered normal

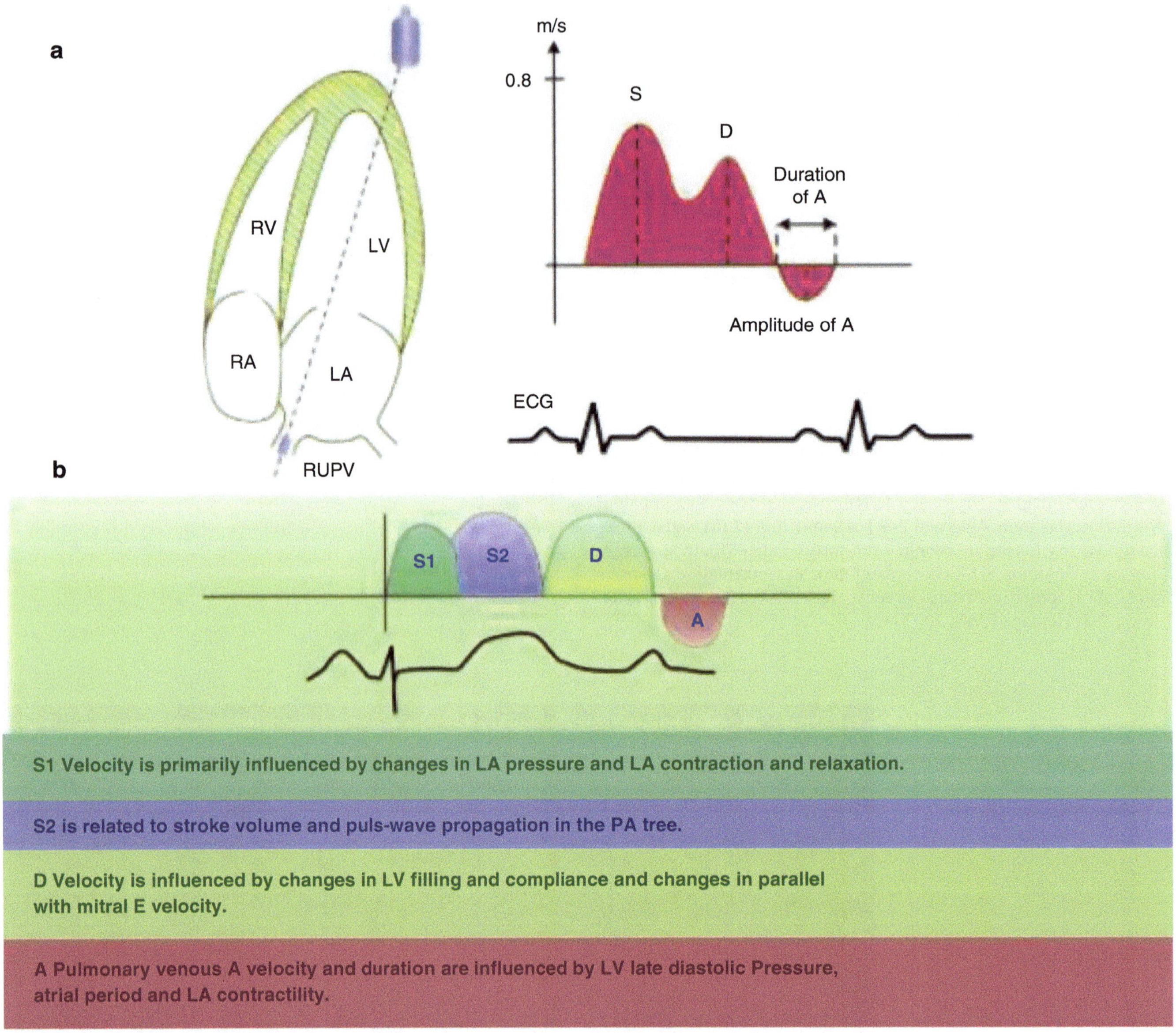

Fig. 46.8 (**a**, **b**) Echocardiography Doppler examination of the normal pulmonary venous flow. (**a**) The Doppler sample volume is inside the right upper pulmonary vein (RUPV); (**b**) schematic appearance of the pulmonary venous flow recorded using pulsed Doppler. *LA* left atrium, *LV* left ventricle, *RA* right atrium, *RV* right ventricle

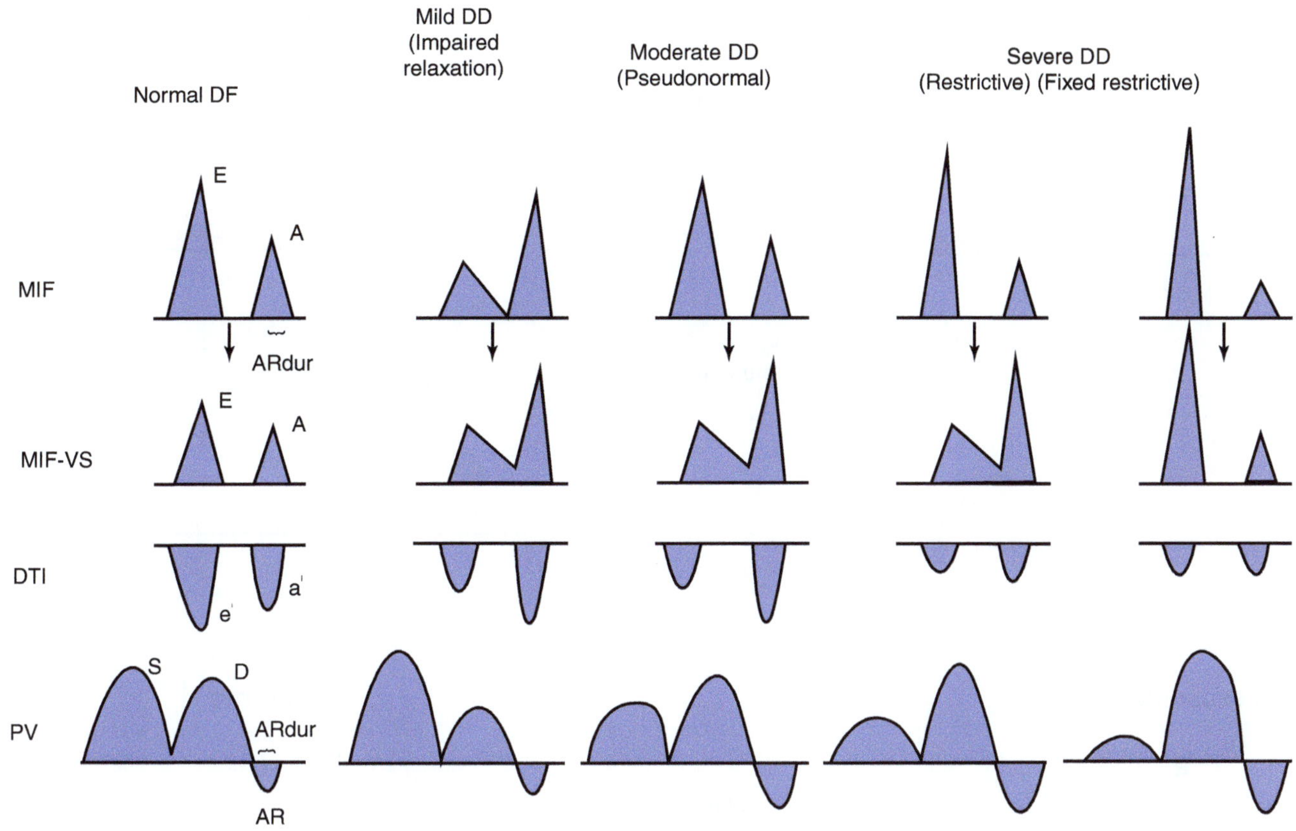

	Normal DF	Mild DD	Moderate DD	Severe DD (Restrictive)	Severe DD (Fixed restrictive)
Impaired LV relaxation		Yes	Yes	Yes	Yes
Reduced LV compliance		0-+	++	+++	++++
Elevated atrial pressure		0	++	+++	++++

Fig. 46.9 Diagram of various Doppler parameters for normal diastolic function (DF) and several stages of diastolic dysfunction (DD). *A* late diastolic mitral inflow velocity, *a′* late diastolic mitral annulus velocity, *AR* PV atrial reversal, *D* diastolic forward PV velocity, *DTI* Doppler tissue imaging, *E* early diastolic mitral inflow velocity, *e′* early diastolic mitral annulus velocity, *MIF* mitral inflow, *PV* pulmonary vein, *S* systolic forward PV velocity, *VS* Valsalva. (Modified from Redfield MM, Jacobsen SJ, Burnett JC Jr, et al. Burden of systolic and diastolic ventricular dysfunction in the community: appreciating the scope of the heart failure epidemic JAMA. 2003;289:194)

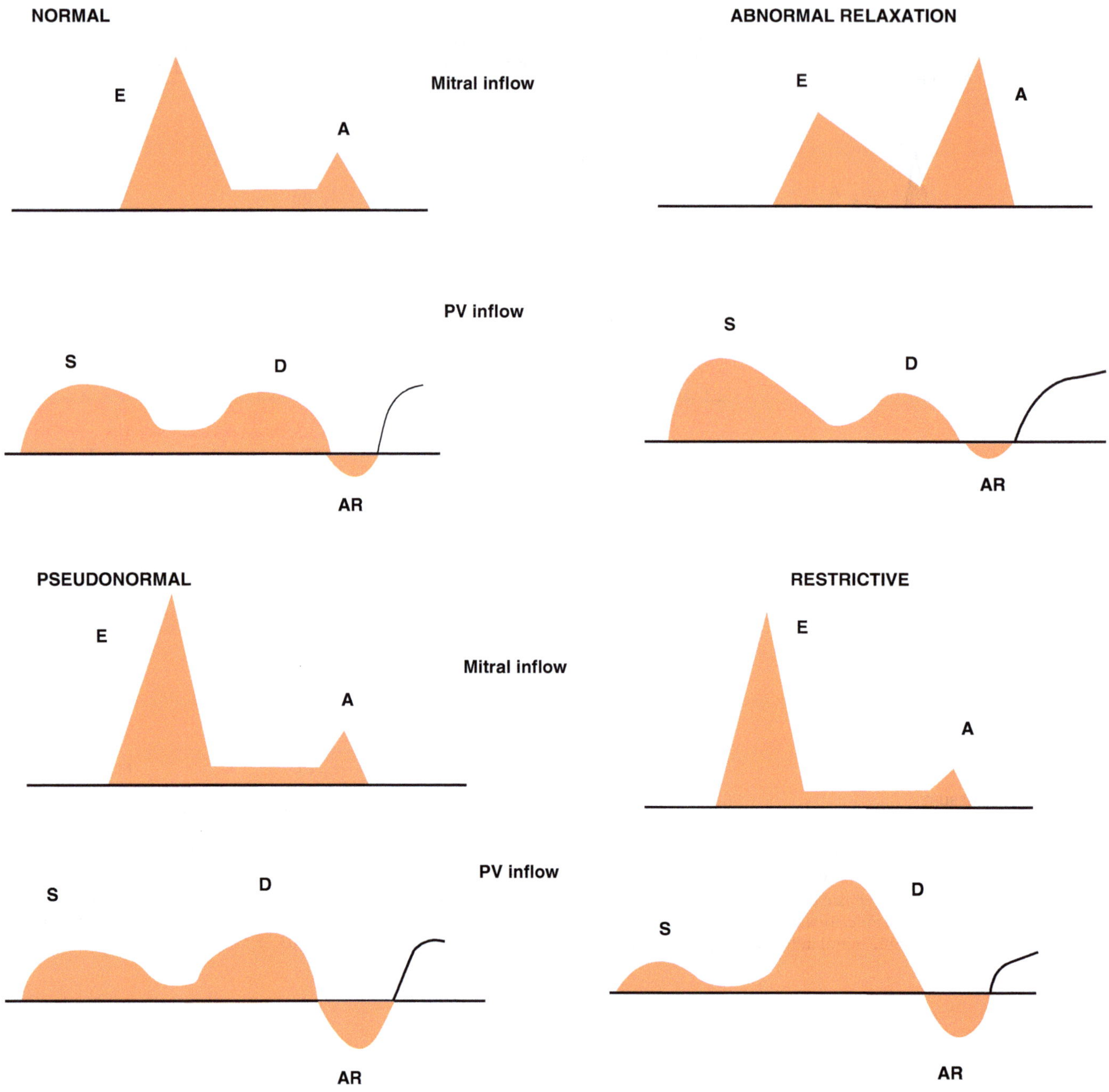

Fig. 46.10 Mitral inflow and Pulmonary vein inflow Doppler patterns in normal and abnormal diastolic functions. *S* systolic flow, *D* diastolic flow, *AR* atrial reversal flow. Modified image from: https://goo.gle/images/QTyhgZ

WALL MOTION	ENDOCARDIAL EXCURSION	ENDOCARDIAL THICKENING
Normal	Normal	30%
Hypokinesia	Decreased	10%-30%
Severe Hypokinesia	Minimal	<10%
Akinesia	None	None
Dyskinesia	Outward bulging in systole	Thinning during systole
Aneurysm	Outward bulging in systole and diastole	Scar-Thinning during systole and diastole

Fig. 46.11 Visual assessment of left ventricular wall motion by 2D echocardiography

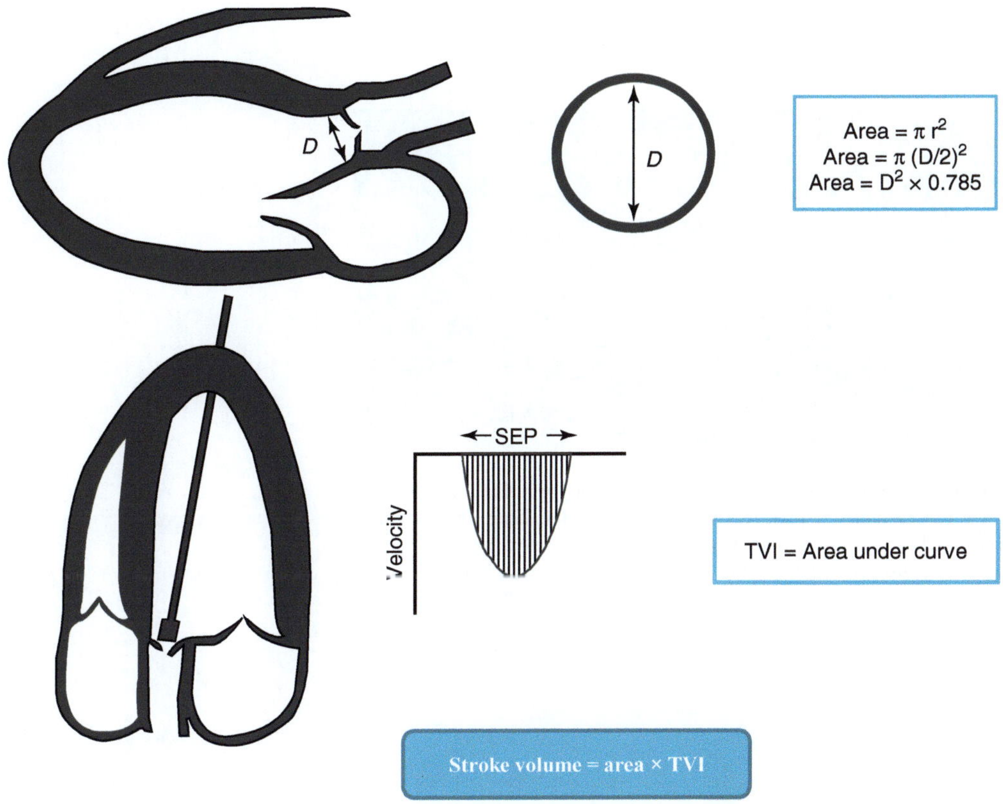

Fig. 46.12 The method for quantifying stroke volume. Two measurements are needed: area and time velocity integral. See text for details. *D* diameter; *SEP* systolic ejection period; *TVI* time velocity integral

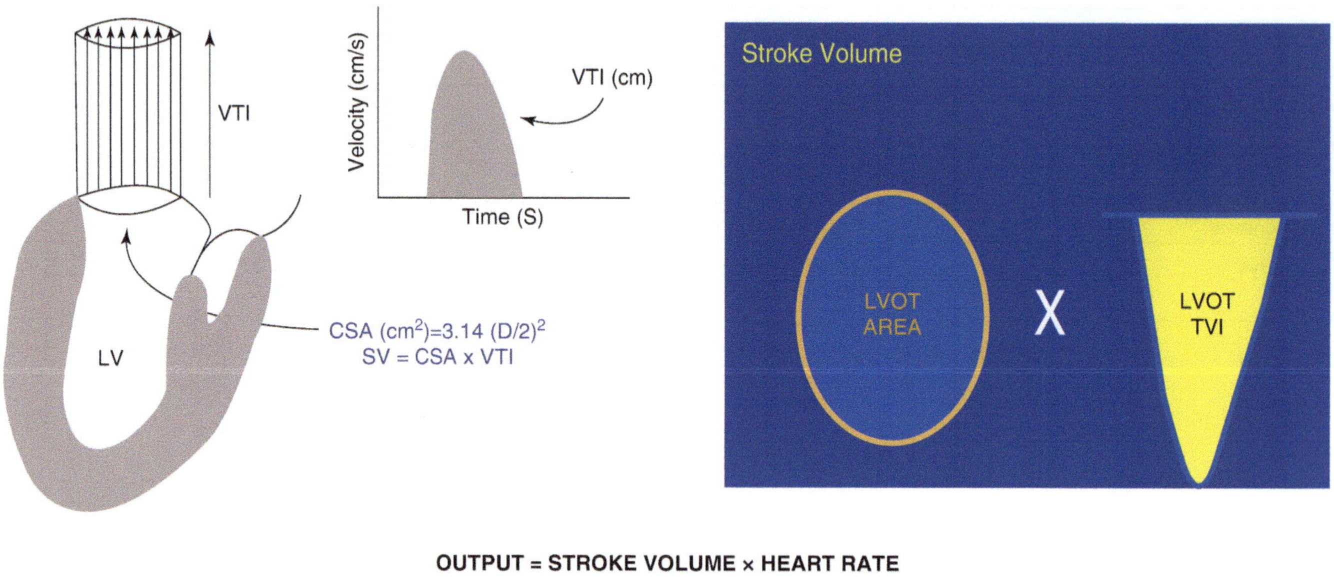

Fig. 46.13 Doppler stroke volume calculation

$$CSA = \left(\frac{D}{2}\right) \times \pi = D^2 \times 0.785$$

$$SV = D^2 \times 0.785$$

$$FLOW\ RATE = CSA \times FLOW\ VELOCITY$$

$$CO = SV\ HEART\ RATE$$

$$CI = \frac{CO}{BSA}$$

Fig. 46.14 Important basic Echocardiographic formula for assessment of SV, CO and CI. [The CSA of orifices in the heart is frequently assumed to be a circle, and it is determined from measurements of the orifice diameter; *CSA* circular cross-sectional area, *D* diameter, *SV* stroke volume, *CO* cardiac output, *CI* cardiac index, *BSA* body surface area]

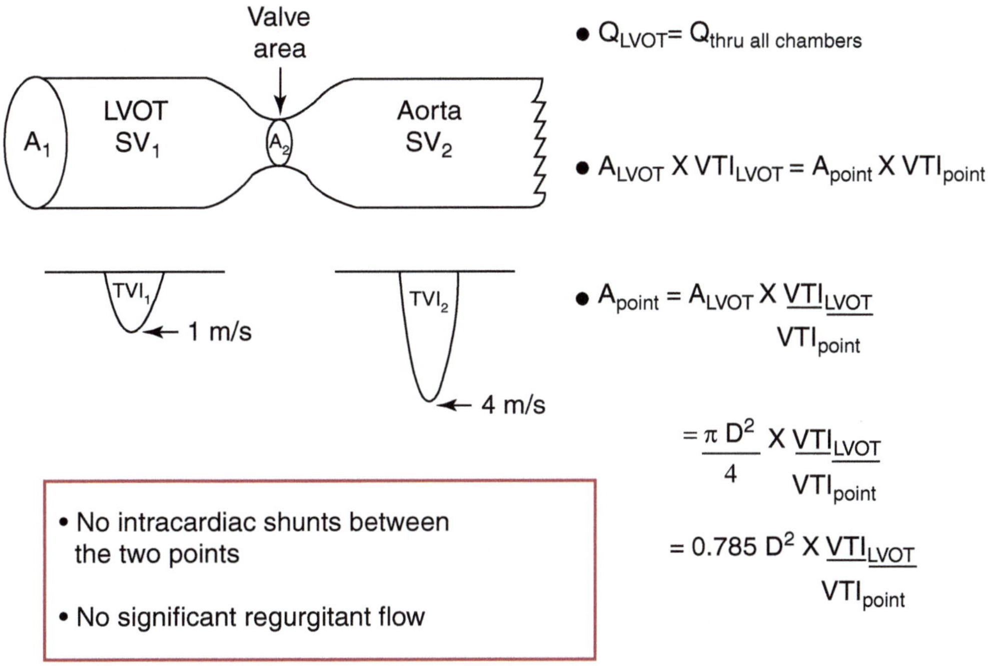

Fig. 46.15 Continuity equation

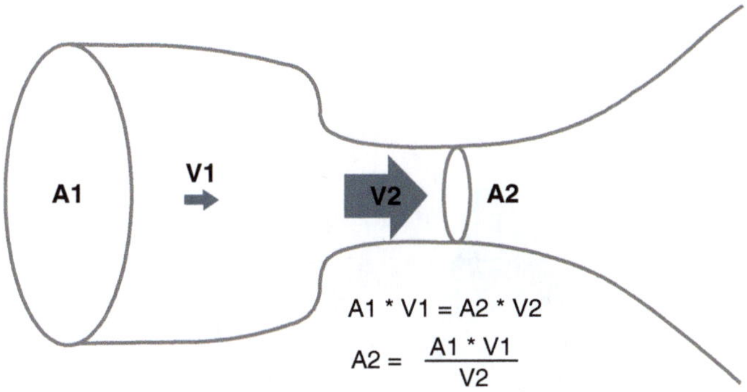

Fig. 46.16 Continuity equation showing by a simple schematic figure

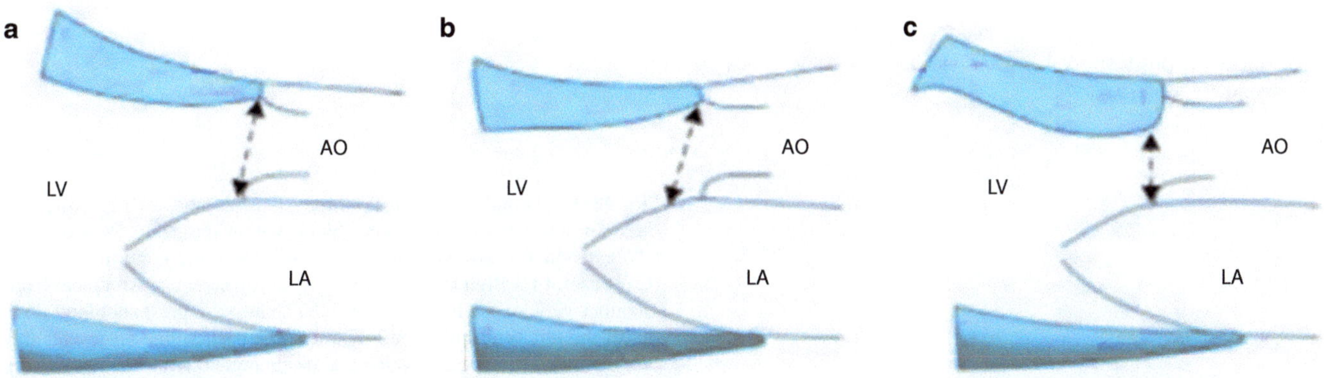

Fig. 46.17 (**a–c**) Measurement of aortic valve annulus and LVOT diameter by using 2D echocardiography; (**a**) Correct diameter; (**b**) Oblique angel over-estimating the size; (**c**) Sub-aortic septal hypertrophy that under-estimating the diameter. *AO* aorta, *LA* left atrium, *LV* left ventricle. Modified image; Courtesy to Solomon SD. Echocardiographic instrumentation and principles of Doppler echocardiography. Essential echocardiography. Totowa, NJ: Humana Press; 2007 [13]

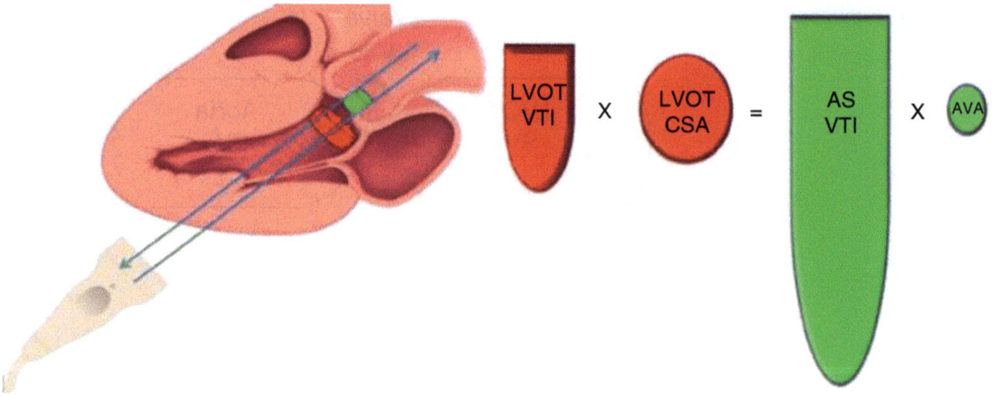

Fig. 46.18 Continuity equation for assessment of Aortic Valve area in Aortic Valve Stenosis

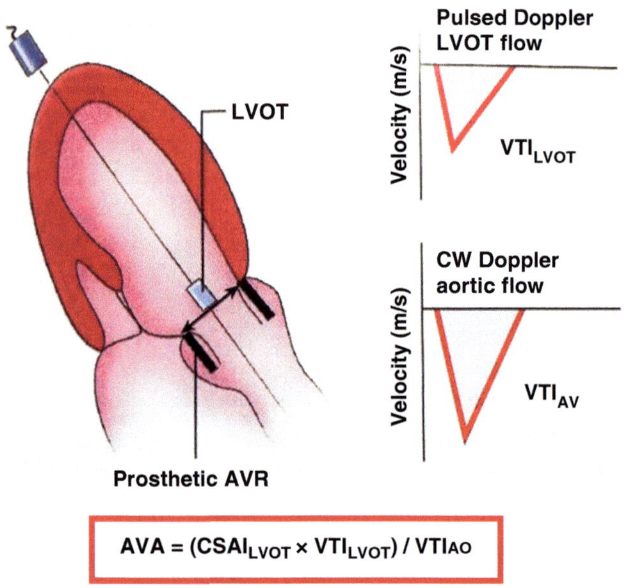

Fig. 46.19 The continuity equation can be used for calculation of aortic valve area (AVA) for an aortic valve replacement (AVR). Left Ventricularoutflow tract (LVOT) flow is recorded from an apical approach using pulsed Doppler with the sample volume positioned just proximal to the prosthetic valve. LVOT diameter is measured from a parasternal long-axis view for calculation of a circular cross-sectional area (CSA) of flow. Continuous-wave Doppler is used to record the flow signal across the prosthetic Valve from whichever window yields the highest velocity jet

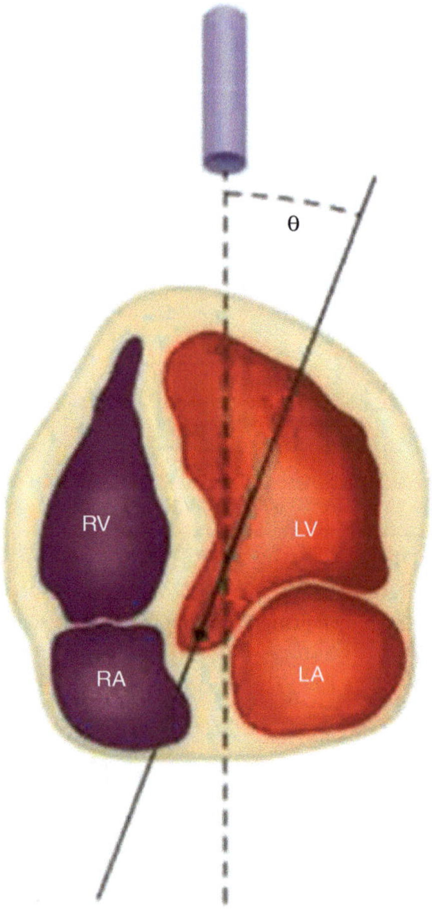

Fig. 46.20 Doppler echocardiography is a method for detecting the direction and velocity of moving blood within the heart. Pulsed wave (PW) useful for low velocity flow, e.g. MV flow; continuous Wave (CW) useful for high velocity flow, e.g. aortic stenosis; An apical five-chamber view of the heart is showed. The arrow represents blood flow out of the left ventricular outflow tract. The dashed line represents the Doppler ultrasoundbeam, which makes an angle θ with the blood flow. As long as the angle q remains < 20° there is insignificant effect on the accuracy of the velocity measurement

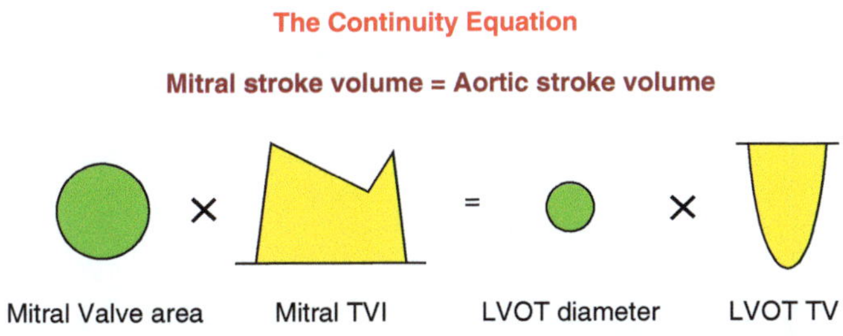

Fig. 46.21 Calculation of the Mitral Valve Area using the continuity equation

Simplified continuity equation

Based on the concept that in native aortic valve stenosis the shape of the velocity curve in the out flow tract and aorta is similar so that the ratio of LVOT to aortic jet VTI is nearly identical to the ratio of the LVOT to aortic jet maximum velocity.

$$AVA = CSA_{LVOT} \times V_{LVOT} / V_{AV}$$

This method is less well accepted be caused results are more variable than using VTIs in the equation.

Fig. 46.22 Simplified continuity equation according to LVOT and AV velocity

Dimension-less Ratio

- DVI is a dimension-less ratio of the proximal velocity in the LVOT to that of flow velocity through the prosthesis
- DVI = LVOT VTI / Prosthetic AV VTI
- DVI < 0.25 is highly suggestive of significant prosthetic valve obstruction

Fig. 46.23 DVI for assessment of AV prosthesis function and malfunction

Fig. 46.24 (**a**, **b**) Tei index or Myocardial performance index of left

a

Tei index or Myocardial performance index: It is an index that incorporates both systolic and diastolic time intervals in expressing global systolic and diastolic ventricular function. Systolic dysfunction prolongs prejection (isovolumic contraction time, IVCT) and a shortening of the ejection time (ET). Both systolic and diastolic dysfunction result in abnormality in myocardial relaxation which prolongs the relaxation period (isovolumic relaxation time, IVRT).

$$LV\ MPI = \frac{IVCT + IVRT}{LVET} = \frac{MCOT - LVET}{LVET}$$

Variable	Definition
Input	
MCOT	Mitral Valve Closure to Opening Time (ms)
LVET	LV Ejection time (ms)
Output	
LV MPI	LV Myocardial Performance Index
Normal	0.39 ± 0.05
Dilated Cardiomyopathy	0.59 ± 0.10

b

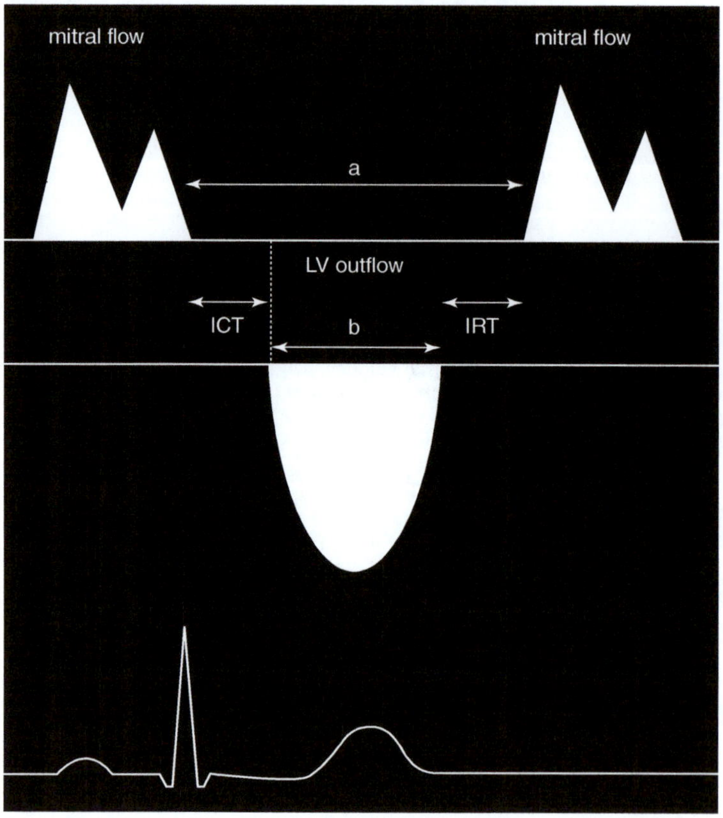

$$MPI = \frac{(a - b)}{b} = \frac{(ICT + IRT)}{ET}$$

Fig. 46.25 dP/dt Iso-volumic Phase Index of Left Ventricular Contractility

The Left Ventricular contractility dp/dt can be estimated by using time interval between 1 and 3 m/second MR velocity CW spectrum during isovolumetric i.e. before aortic valve opens when there is no significant change in LA pressure.

$$\frac{dp}{dt} = 32/T$$

Variable	Definition
T	Time (1 to 3 m/sec MR) (seconds. s)
dP/dt	dP/dt (mmHg/s)
Normal	≥ 1200 mmHg/s

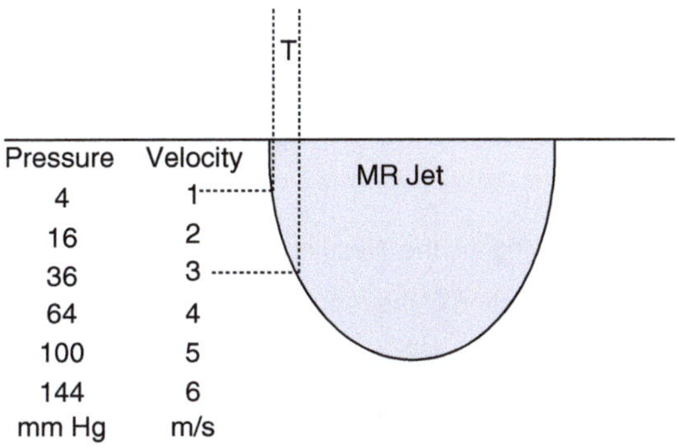

Variable	Definition
Input	
$2\pi r^2$	Proximal iso-velocity hemispheric Surface area at a radial distance (r) From the orifice
V_r	Aliasing velocity at the radial distance (r, cm/s)
V_{MR}	Peak velocity of the mitral regurgitant jet (m/s)
VTI	VTI of the mitral regurgitant jet (cm)
Output	
VFR	Volume Flow rate (mL/s)
ERO	Effective Regurgitant orifice (mm2)
R_{vol}	Regurgitant Volume (mL/beat)

$$VFR = 2\pi r^2 \times V_r$$

$$ERO = \frac{VFR}{V_{MR}}$$

$$R_{vol} = ERO \times VTI$$

Fig. 46.26 **PISA formula for (Mitral Regurgitation severity assessment)**: Quantification of mitral regurgitation using the value of conservation of mass by analyzing the proximal Isovelocity hemispheric Surface Area (PISA) of the flow convergeance of the ventricular side. This method is more precise for central regurgitant jets than eccentric jets, and for a circular orifice than a non-circular orifice

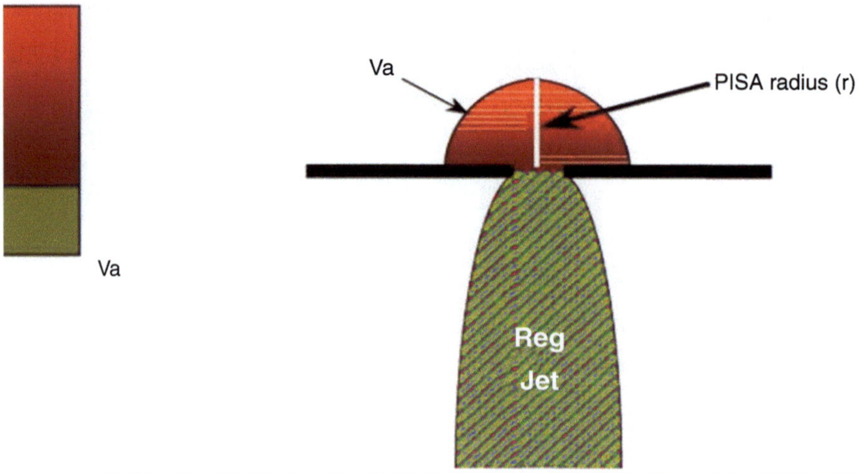

Regurgitant Flow = $2\pi r^2 \times V_{aliasing}$

EROA = Regurgitant Flow / Peak MR Velocity

Baseline shifting of the Nyquist limit toward the direction of the regurgitant flow results in a larger proximal iso-velocity surface area zone for optimal measurement of the proximal iso-velocity surface area region radius (right panel).

Fluid dynamic theory predicts that a flow approaches a circular finite orifice, it forms a series of concentric hemispheric shells with gradually decreasing area and increasing Velocity. Arrows refer to direction of flow as it approaches the proximal iso-velocity surface area region. R is the radius of a hemispherical shell. With principle of conservation of mass, flow through the regurgitant orifice = flow through the iso-velocity surface = $2\pi r^2 \times$ aliasing velocity

Fig. 46.27 Flow Convergence (PISA) Method for MR Severity with adjusting the Nyquist limit

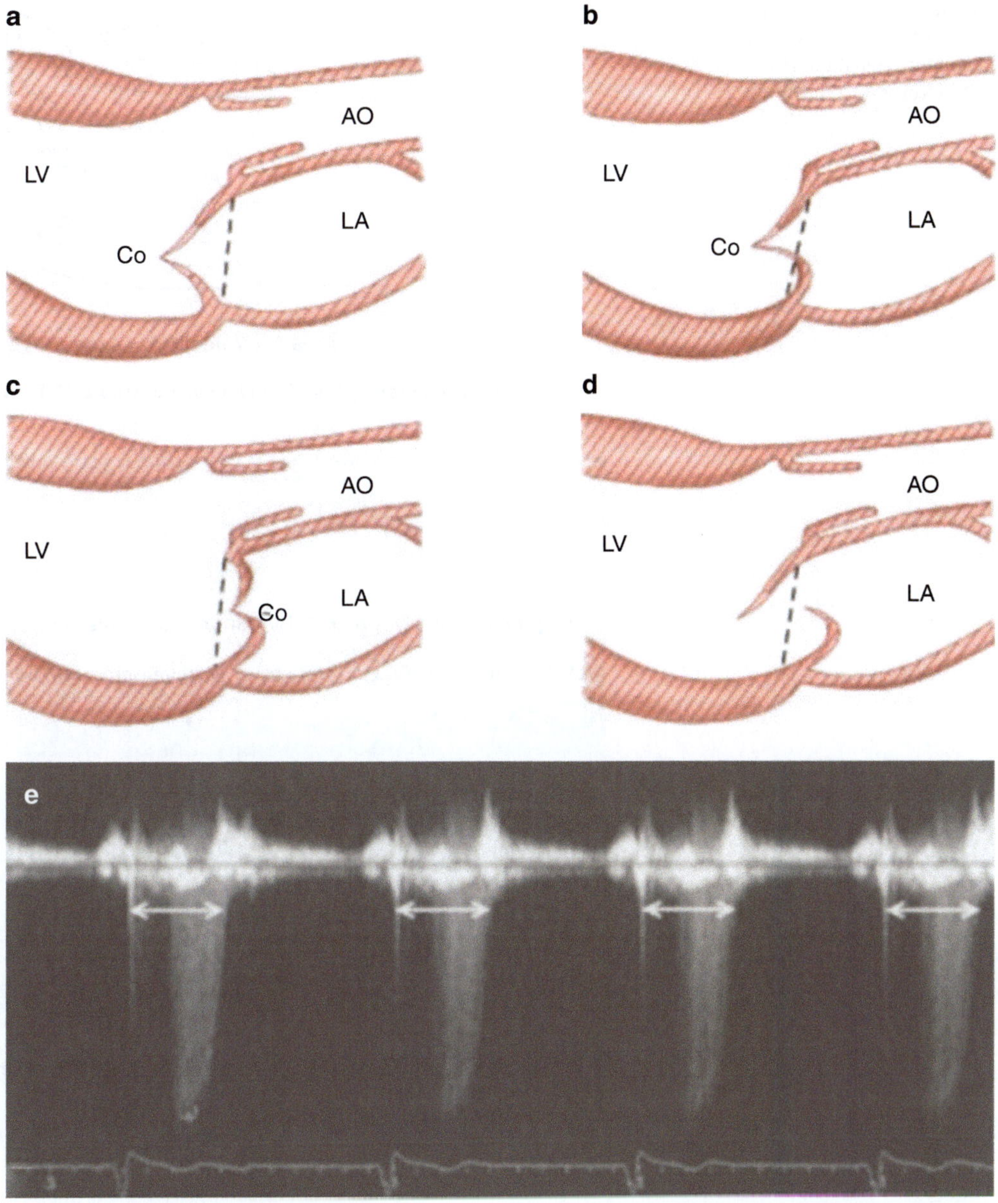

Fig. 46.28 (**a–e**) appearance of the mitral valve (MV) in longitudinal, parasternal long axis view cross-section (during systole); (**a**) Normal picture with the normal valvular coaptation (Co) that positioned in the foreground of the plane of the mitral valve annulus; (**b**) Ballooning of the small mitral valve leaflet; (**c**) prolapse of both mitral valve leaflets; (**d**) Ruptured chordae with eversion of the anterior mitral leaflet in the left atrium (LA); (**e**) interestingly, as Doppler flow pattern showing, frequently mitral valve prolapse resulting in mitral regurgitation in mid to late of systole with lower regurgitant volume *AO* aorta, *LMV* large mitral valve, *LV* left ventricle. Modified image; Courtesy of Solomon SD. Echocardiographic instrumentation and principles of Doppler echocardiography. Essential echocardiography. Totowa, NJ: Humana Press; 2007 [13]

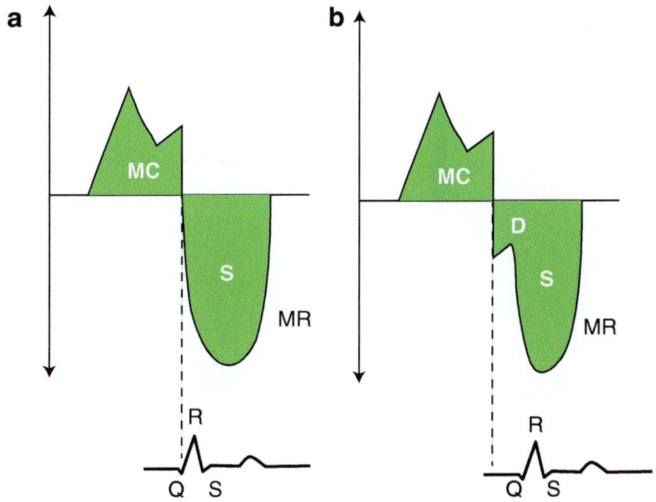

Fig. 46.29 (**a**, **b**) Mitral regurgitation (MR) recorded using continuous Doppler. (**a**) Systolic MR (S); (**b**) Diastolic MR (D) in concomitant with a systolic MR (S). The vertical line displays the beginning of the MR, which rises before the QRS wave. *MC* mitral closing. Modified image; Courtesy of Solomon SD. Echocardiographic instrumentation and principles of Doppler echocardiography. Essential echocardiography. Totowa, NJ: Humana Press; 2007 [13]

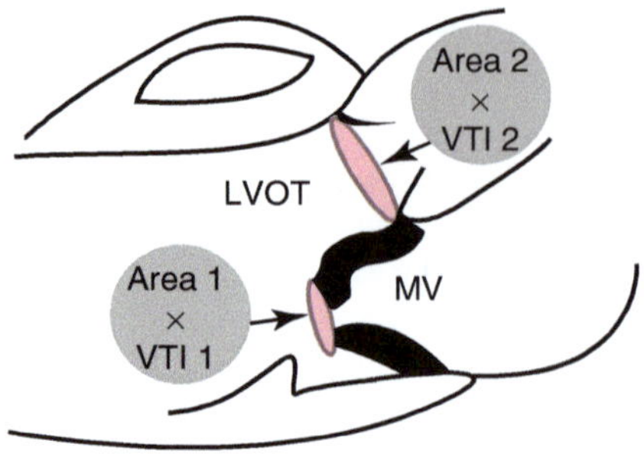

Area 1 × Velocity 1 = Area 2 × Velocity 2

Area MV × Velocity MV (CW Doppler) **= Area LVOT × Velocity LVOT** (PW Doppler)

a

$$MVA = \frac{\pi\,(radius\ LVOT)^2 \times Vmax_{LVOT^*}}{VTI_{MV^{**}}}$$

*** by pulsed wave Doppler, ** by continuous wave Doppler,**

LVOT, left ventricular outflow tract; VTI, velocity time integral; Π (pi) = 3.14

b

Proximal to a stenotic mitral orifice, PISA may not be a complete hemisphere but a portion of hemisphere because of mitral leaflets geometry on the atrial side.

$$MVA = 3.28 \times r^2 \times \frac{Aliasing\ velocity}{Peak\ MS\ velocity} \times \frac{alpha^\circ}{180^\circ}$$

Where alpha is the angle between two mitral leaflets on the atrial side

Fig. 46.30 (**a**) Mitral Valve Area in Mitral Stenosis: the Continuity Equation. (**b**) Mitral Valve area in Mitral Stenosis by PISA method

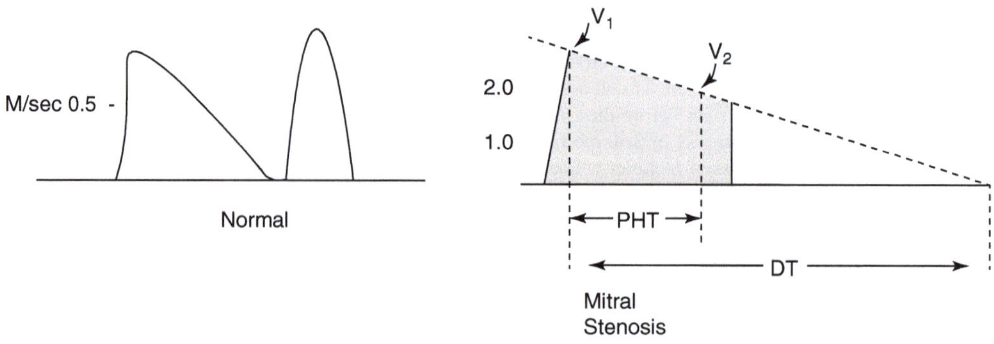

Fig. 46.31 Mitral Valve Area by (PHT)

Pressure half-time (PHT) is defined as the time interval in milliseconds between the maximum mitral gradient in early diastole and the time point where the gradient is half the maximum initial Value. The decline of the velocity of diastolic trans mitral blood flow is inversely proportional to valve area (cm^2), and mitral valve area (MVA) is derived using an empirical formula.

PHT is obtained by tracing the deceleration slope of the E-wave on Doppler spectral display of trans mitral flow. The deceleration slope is occasionally bimodal, the decline of the mitral flow velocity being more rapid in early diastole than during the following part of the E-wave. In these cases, it is recommended that the deceleration slope in mid-diastole rather than the early deceleration slope be traced.

Over-estimation of the MVA happens when PHT is shortened by concomitant important aortic insufficiency, decreased ventricular compliance, immediately after mitral balloon valvuloplasty and atrial septal defect.

$$MVA = \frac{220}{PHT}$$

$$RV\,MPI = \frac{IVCT + IVRT}{RVET} = \frac{TCOT - RVET}{RVET} \quad \text{(Fig. 46.32)}$$

Right ventricular fractional area change (RVFAC)

RVFAC expresses the percentage change in RV area between end-diastole and end-systole

It is obtained from a four-chamber view where the RV end-diastolic (RV-EDA) and end-systolic areas (RV-ESA) are measured (it is necessary to carefully delineate the free wall beneath the trabeculation), and the RV-FAC is calculated as follows (Fig. 46.33):

$$\mathbf{RV\,FAC(\%) = (RV\,EDA - RV\,ESA) / RV\,EDA \times 100}$$

The RV contractility dp/dt can be estimated by using time interval between 1 and 2 m/s on TR velocity CW spectrum during iso-volumetric contraction i.e. before pulmonic valve opens when there is no significant change in RA pressure.

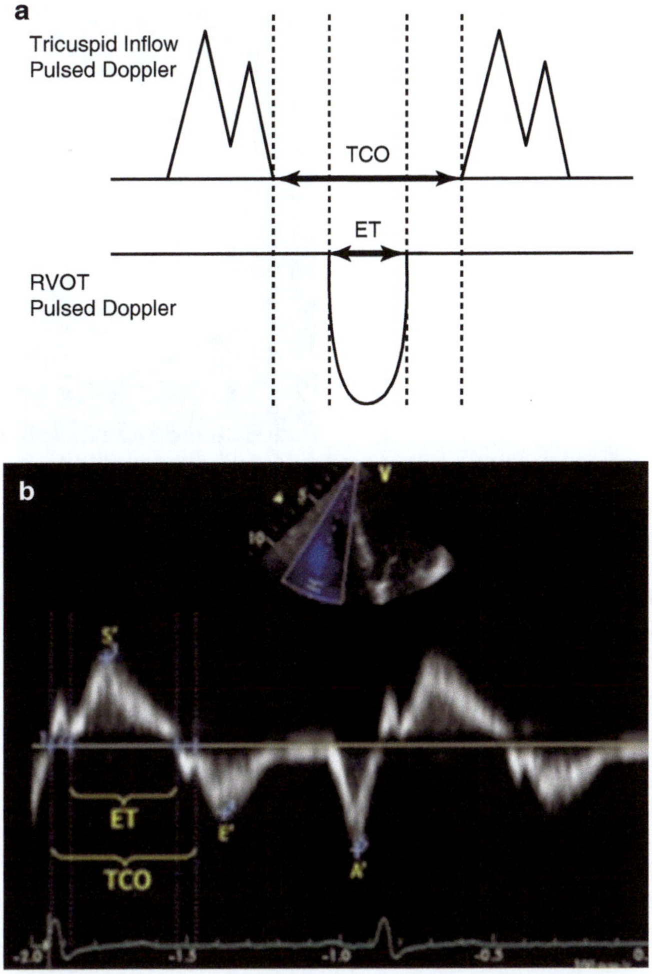

Fig. 46.32 (**a**, **b**) Calculation of the myocardial performance index (MPI) or tei index of RV by pulsed Doppler (**a**) and pulsed tissue Doppler (**b**). The tricuspid valve opening time (TCO) encompassed iso-volumic contraction time, ejection time (ET), and iso-volumic relaxation time. In the pulsed Doppler method, TCO can also be measured by the duration of the tricuspid regurgitation continuous-wave Doppler signal. MPI = (TCO−ET)/ET. Note that S′, E′, and A′ can also be measured from the same pulsed Doppler tissue image

Although the time from 1 to 2 m/s is most normally used, the best correlation between echocardiographic and invasive measures was found by using the time for the TR velocity to increase from 0.5 to 2 m/s (Fig. 46.34).

$$dp / dt = 12 / T$$

Fig. 46.33 Normal value for RV FAC: above 35%

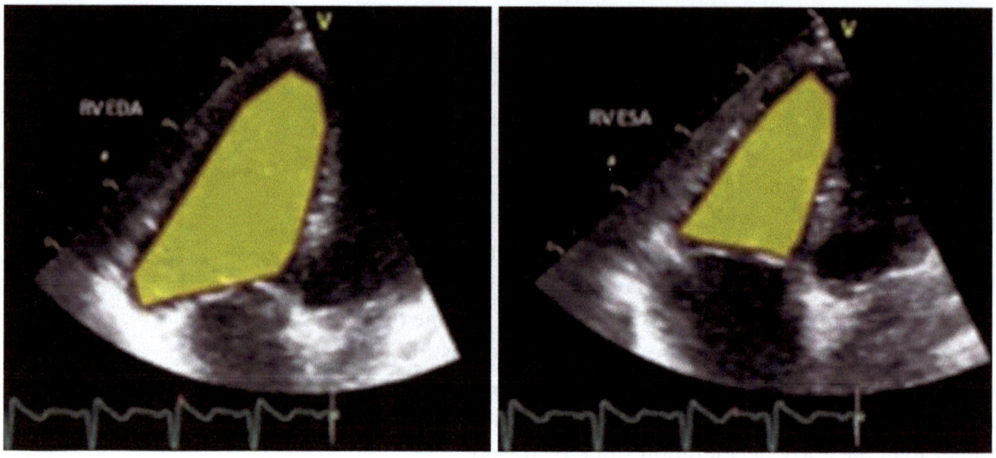

RV FAC (%) = (RV EDA-RV ESA) / RV EDA X 100

Fig. 46.34 dp/dt Iso-volumic phase index of RV contractility

Variable	Definition
T	Time (1 to 2 m/sec TR) (seconds, s)
dp/dt	dp/dt (mmHg/s)
Likely Abnormal	< 400 mmHg/s

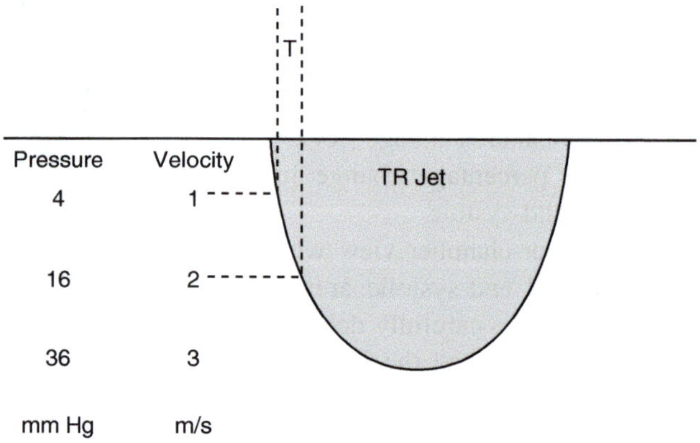

Fig. 46.35 (**a**, **b**) Calculation of "PA pressure or RVSP"

a

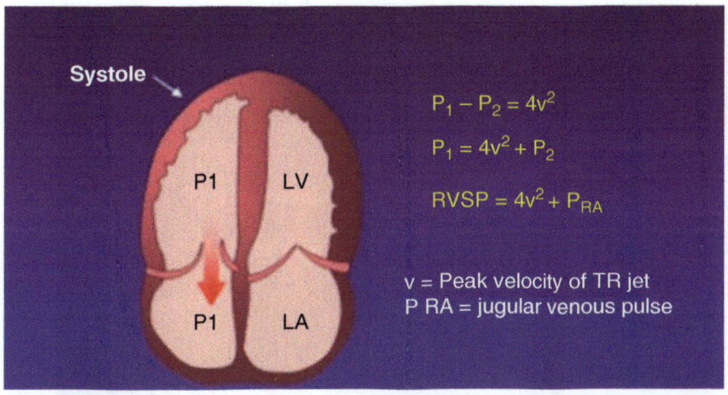

b

Input		
≤ 21mm	> 50%	Normal 3 (0-5)
Intermediate	Intermediate	Intermediate 8 (5-10)
> 21 mm	< 50%	High 15 (10-20)

Right ventricular systolic pressure (RVSP) can be estimated by measuring the TR jet maximum velocity by continuous wave (CW) spectral Doppler. If there is no significant stenosis at the right ventricular outflow tract, or the pulmonic valve, the RVSP is equivalent to the systolic pulmonary artery pressure (SPAP).

The RA pressure (RAP) can be estimated by the size and respiratory collapsibility of the inferior vena cava. For simplicity and uniformity of reporting, specific values of RAP, rather than ranges, should be used in the determination of RVSP.

Secondary indices of elevated RA pressure include:

1. **Restrictive filling**
2. **Tricuspid E/E' >6**
3. **Diastolic flow predominance in hepatic vein (HV) : HV systolic filling fraction Vs/(Vs+Vd) <55%**

In young athletes, IVC may be dilated in the presence of normal pressure. IVC is normally dilated and may not collapse in patients on ventilators, so it should not be used in such cases to estimate RA pressure.

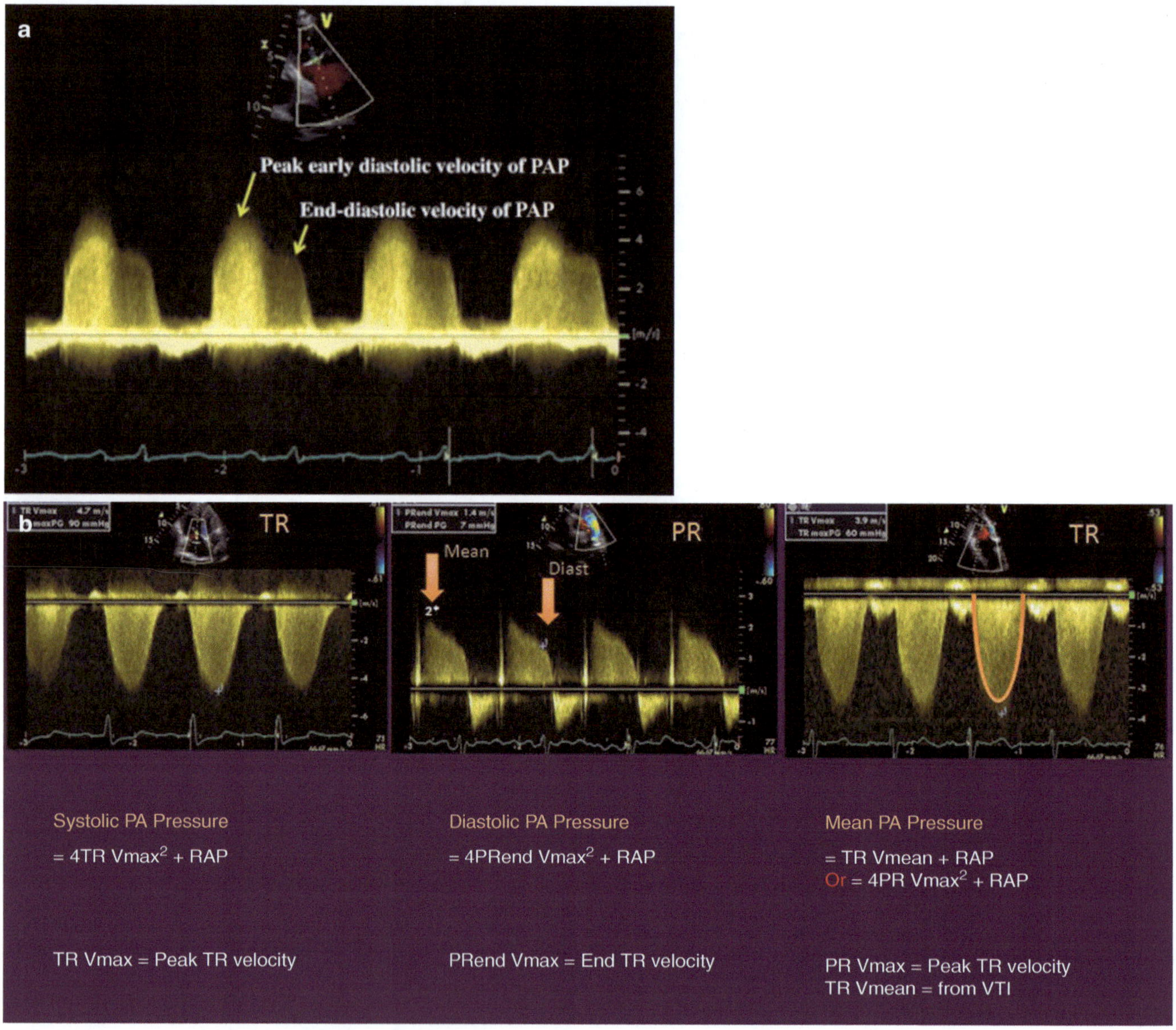

Fig. 46.36 (**a**–**c**) Calculation of PA systolic, mean and diastolic pressures

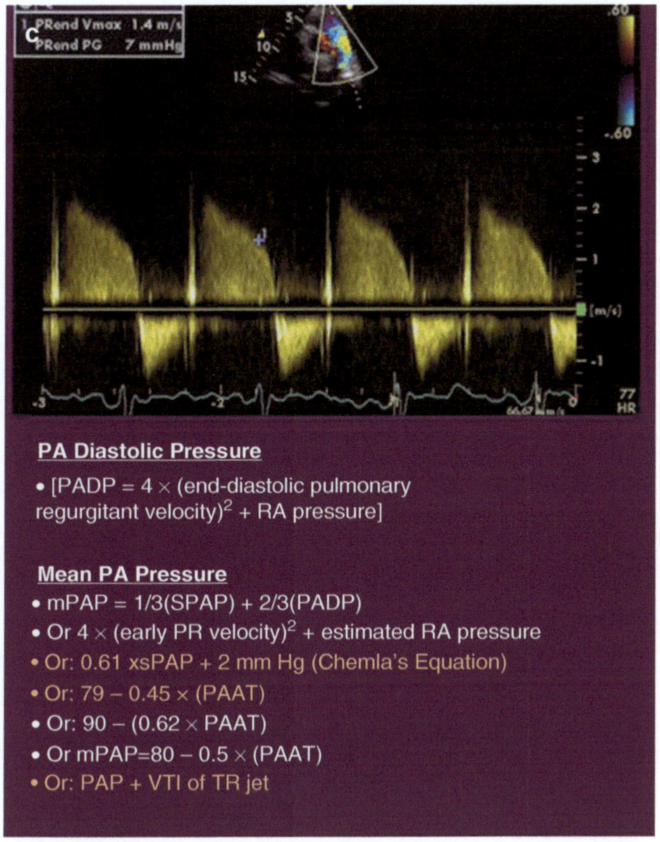

Fig. 46.36 (continued)

Fig. 46.37 Shunt study: Pulmonary-Systemic Flow Ratio (Qp/Qs)

QP/QS can be estimated by using 2-D echo and spectral Doppler measurements in patients who have intra-or extra-cardiac shunts e.g. atrial or ventricular Septal defects.

$$QP = RVOT\ VTI \times \pi \times \left(\frac{RVOT}{2}\right)^2$$

$$QS = LVOT\ VTI \times \pi \times \left(\frac{LVOT}{2}\right)^2$$

Qp/Qs Ratio = Qp/Qs

Variable	Definition
Input	
LVOT	Left ventricular outflow tract diameter (mm)
LVOT VTI	LVOT sub-valvular velocity time integral (cm)
RVOT	Right ventricular outflow tract diameter (mm)
RVOT VTI	RVOT sub-valvular velocity time integral (cm)
Output	
Qp/Qs	Pulmonary-Systemic Shunt Ratio

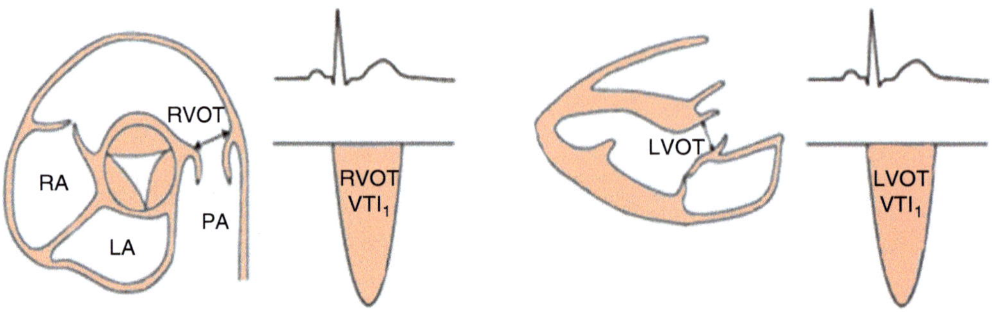

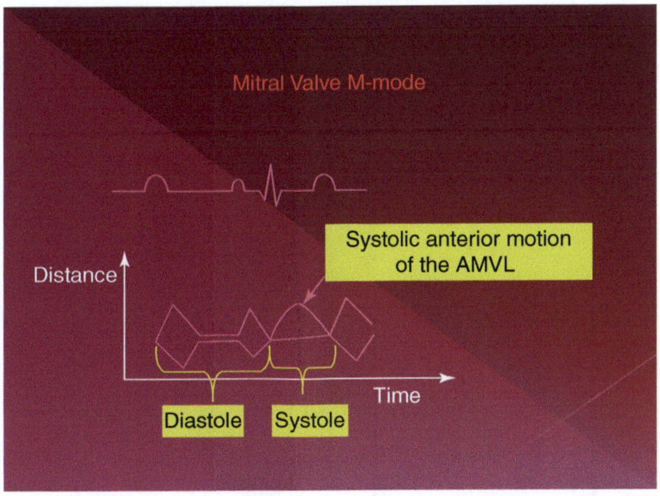

Fig. 46.38 Systolic anterior motion of the anterior mitral valve leaflet

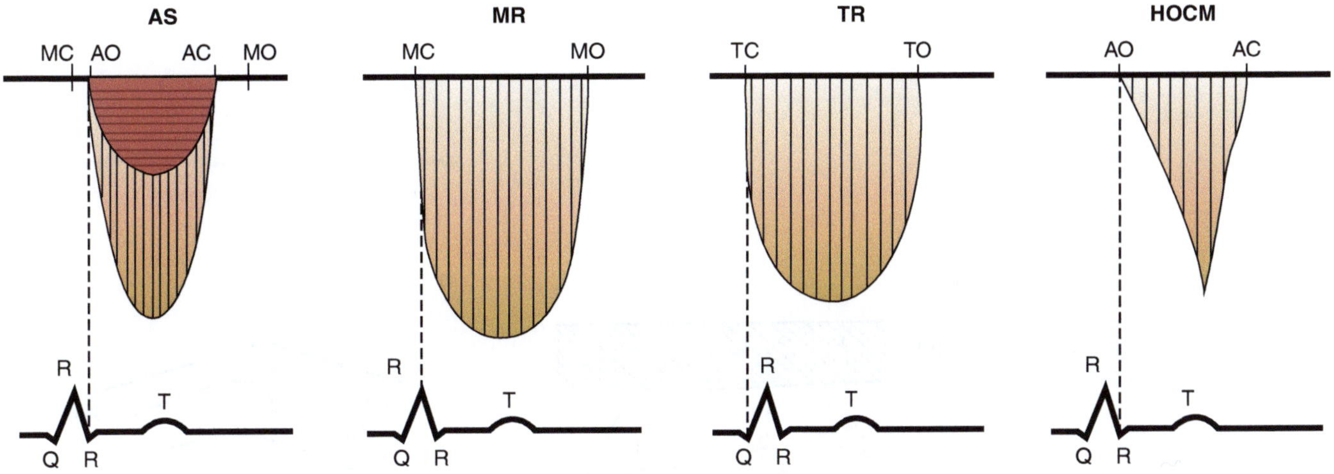

Fig. 46.39 Differential diagnosis between aortic valve stenosis (AS) and mitral valve regurgitation (MR), and also between the tricuspid valve regurgitation (TR) and hypertrophic obstructive cardiomyopathy (HOCM). Short ejection times for AS and HOCM and the extended ejection times for MR and TR. *MC* mitral closing, *AO* aortic opening, *AC* aortic closing, *MO* mitral opening, *TC* tricuspid closing, *TO* tricuspid opening. Modified image; Courtesy to Solomon SD. Echocardiographic instrumentation and principles of Doppler echocardiography. Essential echocardiography. Totowa, NJ: Humana Press; 2007 [13]

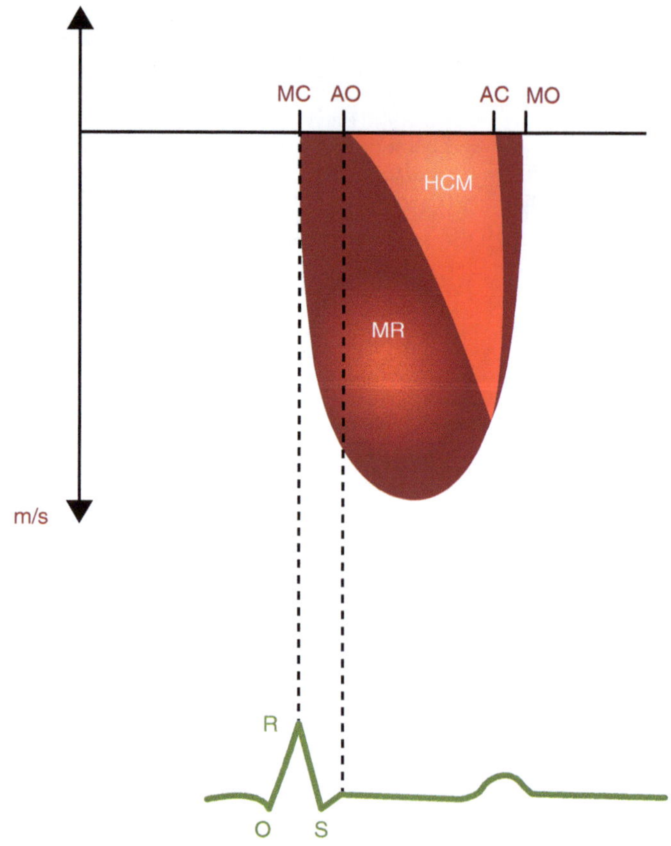

Fig. 46.40 Doppler flow shape in hypertrophic-obstructed cardiomyopathy (HOCM) from left ventricular outflow tract and the rounded flow of mitral regurgitation (MR) (superimposed two flows). Also the time between mitral closing (MC) and aortic valve opening (AO) is iso-volumic contraction time. *AC* aortic valve closing, *MO* mitral opening. Modified image; Courtesy of Solomon SD. Echocardiographic instrumentation and principles of Doppler echocardiography. Essential echocardiography. Totowa, NJ: Humana Press; 2007 [13]

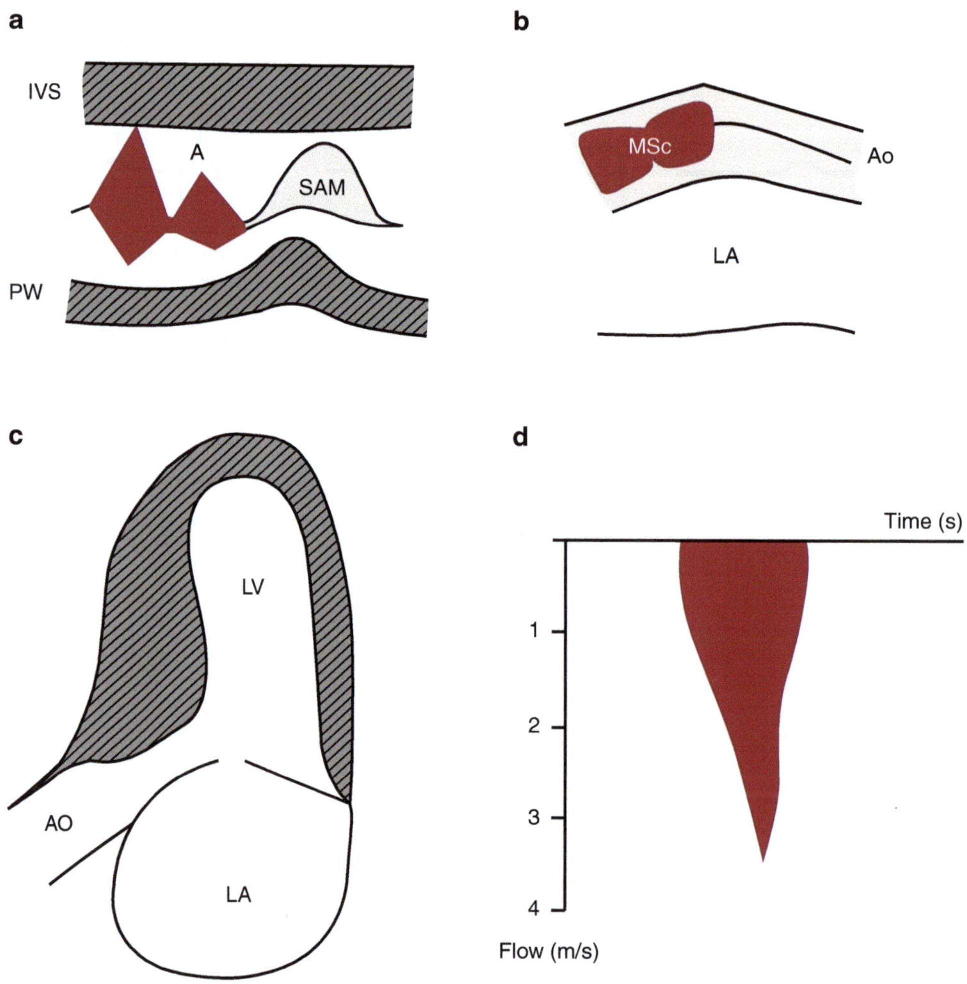

Fig. 46.41 (**a–d**) Echocardiography Doppler anomalies of hypertrophic obstructive cardiomyopathy (HOCM): (**a**) Abnormal systolic anterior motion (SAM) of the mitral valve in M-mode. (**b**) Partially mid-systolic closure (MSc) of the aortic valve in the M-mode. (**c**) Sub-aortic septal hypertrophy in 2D apical view. (**d**) Left ventricular outflow dynamic obstruction continuous Doppler flow. *AO* aorta, *IVS* inter-ventricular septum, *LA* left atrium, *LV* left ventricular, *PW* posterior wall

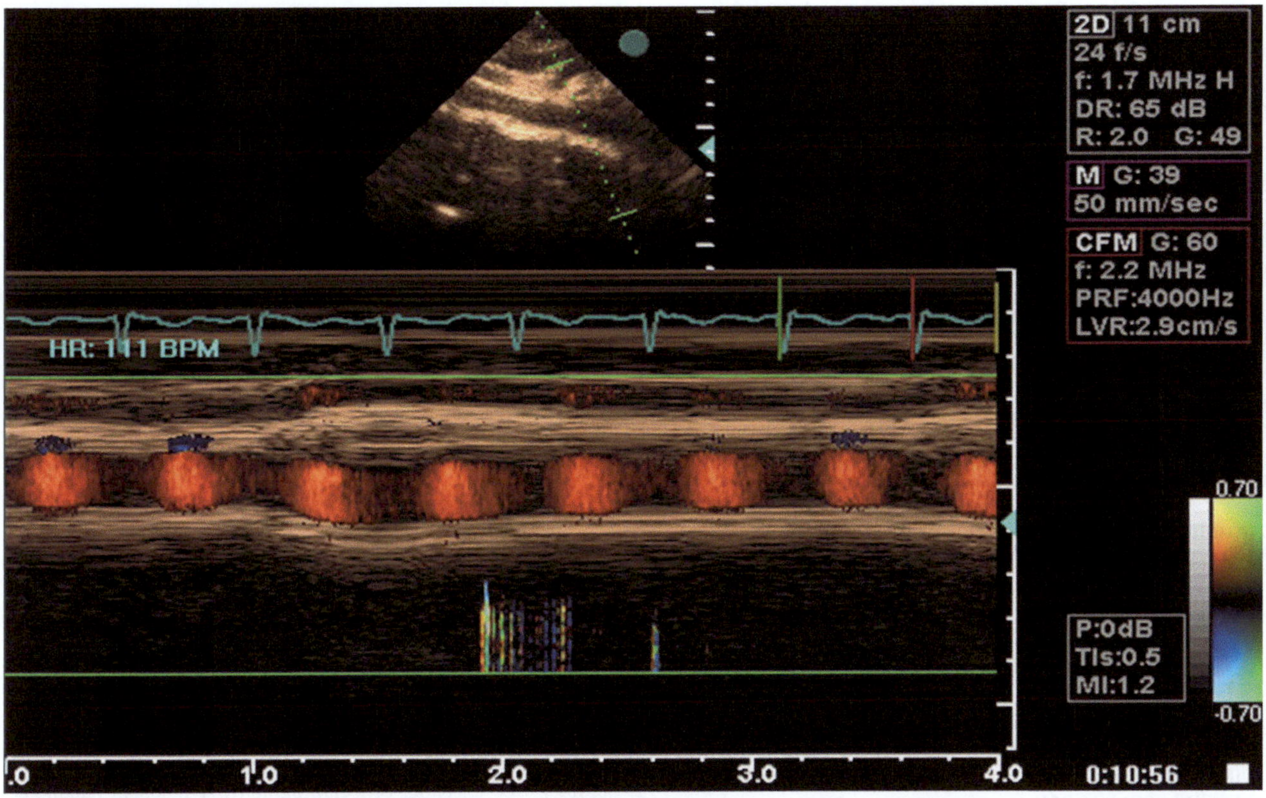

Fig. 46.42 Persistent ante grade flow in abdominal aorta in a patient with significant coarctation of Aorta

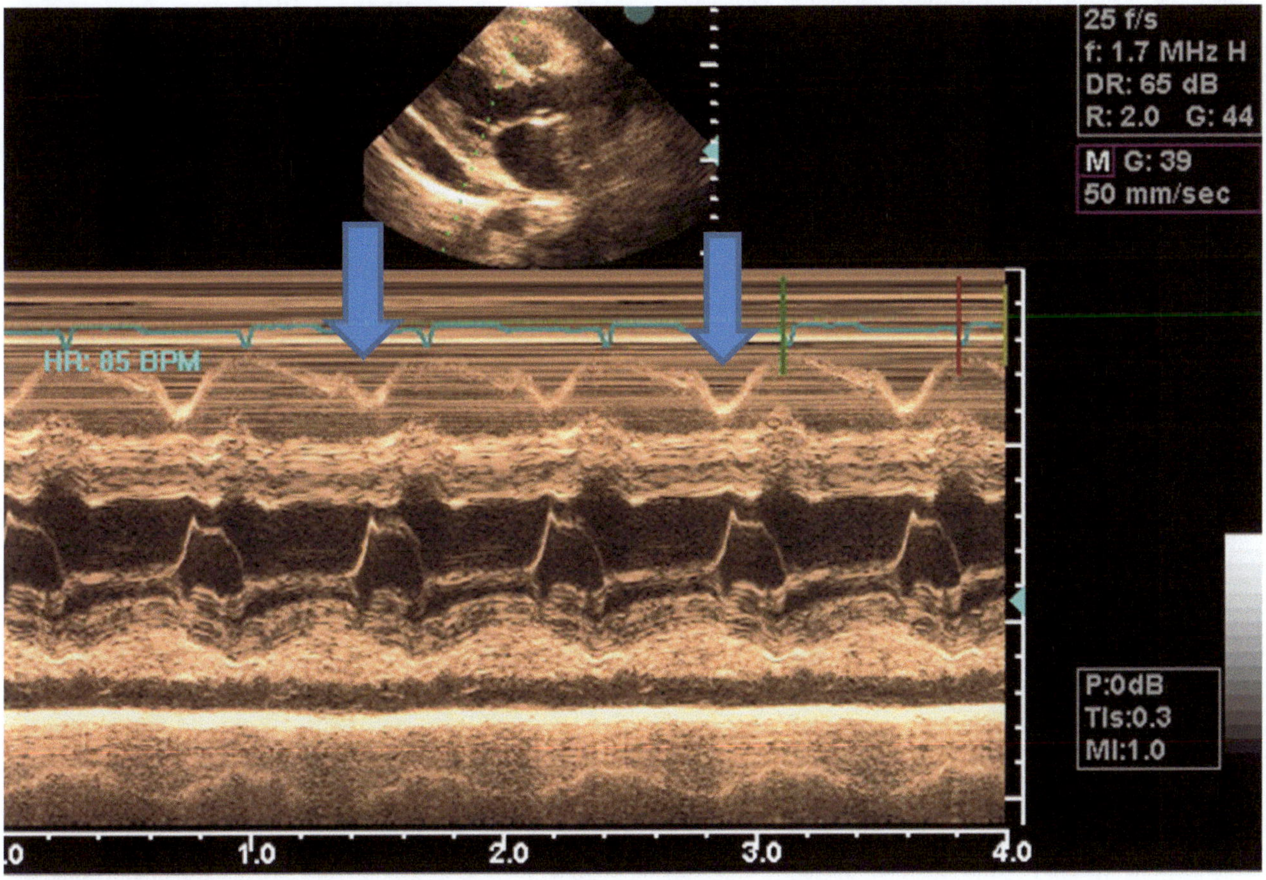

Fig. 46.43 Right ventricular outflow tract diastolic collapse in a patient with PE (arrows)

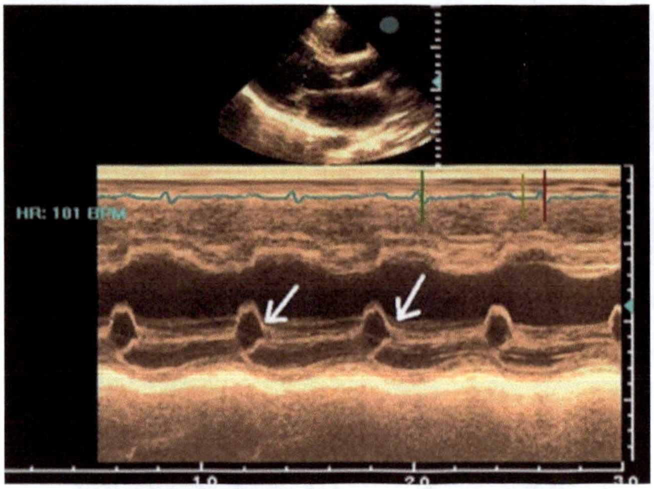

Fig. 46.44 M-mode study of the mitral valve shows early closure of mitral valve in the setting of acute aortic regurgitation (AR)

Bibliography

1. Ananthasubramaniam K, Dhar R, Cavalcante JL. Rule of multi-modality imaging in ischemic and non-ischemic cardiomyopathy. Heart Fail Rev. 2011;16:351.
2. Sadeghpour A, Alizadehasl A. Right ventricle: a comprehensive review from anatomy, physiology, and mechanics to hemodynamic, functional, and imaging evaluation. Arch Cardiovasc Imaging. 2015;3(4):e35717. https://doi.org/10.5812/acvi.35717.
3. Sadeghpour A, Kyavar M, Alizadehasl A. Comprehensive approach to adult congenital heart disease. 1st ed. London: Springer; 2014.
4. Banypersad SM, Pearce K. Successful accreditation in echocardiography, a self-assessment guide. Hoboken: Wiley; 2013.
5. Bossone E, D'Andrea A, D'Alto M, et al. Echocardiography in pulmonary arterial hypertension: From diagnosis to prognosis. J Am Soc Echocardiogr. 2013;26(1):1–14.
6. Vachiéry JL. Echocardiography in pulmonary arterial hypertension. Am J Cardiol. 2012;110(6 Suppl):16S.
7. Lancellotti P, Tribouilloy C, Hagendor A, et al. Recommendations for the echocardiographic assessment of native valvular regurgitation: an executive summary from the European Association of Cardiovascular Imaging. Eur Heart J Cardiovasc Imaging. 2013;14:611–44. https://doi.org/10.1093/ehjci/jet105.
8. Mann D, Zipes D, Libby P, Bonow R. Braunwald's heart disease. Textbook of cardiovascular medicine. 10th ed. Philadelphia: Elsevier Saunders; 2015.
9. Quiñones MA, Otto CM, Stoddard M, Waggoner A, Zoghbi WA. Recommendations for quantification of Doppler Echocardiography: a report from the Doppler Quantification Task Force of the Nomenclature and Standards Committee of the American Society of Echocardiography. American Society of Echocardiography Report. J Am Soc Echocardiogr. 2002;15:167–84.
10. Smiseth SF, Appleton CP, et al. Recommendations for the evaluation of left ventricular diastolic function by echocardiography: an update from the American Society of Echocardiography and the European Association of Cardiovascular Imaging. ASE/EACVI guidelines and standards. J Am Soc Echocardiogr. 2016;29:277–314.
11. Silbiger JJ. Mechanistic insights into ischemic mitral regurgitation: echocardiographic and surgical implications. J Am Soc Echocardiogr. 2011;24:707.
12. Solomon SD. Essential echocardiography. A practical handbook. New York City: Humana Press; 2007.
13. Solomon SD. Echocardiographic instrumentation and principles of Doppler echocardiography. In: Solomon SD, editor. Essential echocardiography. Totowa, NJ: Humana Press; 2007.
14. Williams LK, Frenneaux MP, Steeds RP. Echocardiography in hypertrophic cardiomyopathy diagnosis, prognosis, and role in management. Eur J Echocardiogr. 2009;10:iii9.

Index

A. Sadeghpour, A. Alizadehasl (eds.), *Case-Based Textbook of Echocardiography*,
https://doi.org/10.1007/978-3-319-67691-3

N

O

MIX
Papier aus verantwortungsvollen Quellen
Paper from responsible sources
FSC® C105338

If you have any concerns about our products,
you can contact us on
ProductSafety@springernature.com

In case Publisher is established outside the EU,
the EU authorized representative is:
Springer Nature Customer Service Center GmbH
Europaplatz 3, 69115 Heidelberg, Germany

Printed by Libri Plureos GmbH
in Hamburg, Germany